Pelvic Floor Disorders

Alain P. Bourcier, PT
*Specialist Continence Physiotherapist, Department of Urology, Tenon Hospital;
Director, Pelvic Floor Rehabilitation Services, Institut Français de Réadaptation Uro-Génitale;
Paris, France*

Edward J. McGuire, MD
*Professor of Surgery, University of Texas Medical School, Department of Urology,
Houston, Texas, United States*

Paul Abrams, MD, FRCS
*Professor of Urology, Bristol Urological Institute, Southmead Hospital,
Bristol, England*

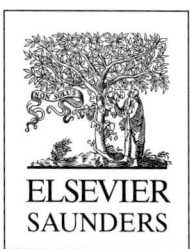

ELSEVIER
SAUNDERS

The Curtis Center
170 S Independence Mall W 300E
Philadelphia, Pennsylvania 19106

PELVIC FLOOR DISORDERS ISBN 0-7216-9194-3
Copyright © 2004, Elsevier Inc. All rights reserved.

No part of this publication may be reproduced or transmitted in any form or by any means, electronic or mechanical, including photocopying, recording, or any information storage and retrieval system, without permission in writing from the publisher. Permissions may be sought directly from Elsevier's Health Sciences Rights Department in Philadelphia, PA, USA: phone: (+1) 215 238 7869, fax: (+1) 215 238 2239, e-mail: healthpermissions@elsevier.com. You may also complete your request on-line via the Elsevier homepage (http://www.elsevier.com), by selecting 'Customer Support' and then 'Obtaining Permissions'.

NOTICE

Urology is an ever-changing field. Standard safety precautions must be followed, but as new research and clinical experience broaden our knowledge, changes in treatment and drug therapy may become necessary or appropriate. Readers are advised to check the most current product information provided by the manufacturer of each drug to be administered to verify the recommended dose, the method and duration of administration, and contraindications. It is the responsibility of the treating physician, relying on experience and knowledge of the patient, to determine dosages and the best treatment for each individual patient. Neither the publisher nor the editors assume any liability for any injury and/or damage to persons or property arising from this publication.

The Publisher

Library of Congress Cataloging-in-Publication Data
Pelvic floor disorders/[edited by] Alain Bourcier, Edward McGuire, Paul Abrams.
    p. ; cm.
ISBN 0-7216-9194-3
  1. Pelvic floor—Diseases. 2. Urinary incontinence. 3. Fecal incontinence. 4. Urogynecology.
I. Bourcier, A. II. McGuire, Edward J. III. Abrams, Paul.
  [DNLM: 1. Urologic Diseases—physiopathology. 2. Fecal Incontinence—physiopathology.
3. Pelvic Floor—physiopathology. 4. Sex Disorders—physiopathology. 5. Urinary
Incontinence—physiopathology. WJ 140 P393 2004]
RG482.P458 2004
617.5′5—dc22
                                                                                   2003066792

Acquisitions Editor: *Rebecca Schmidt Gaertner*
Developmental Editor: *Joanie Milnes*
Publishing Services Manager: *Joan Sinclair*
Project Manager: *Mary Stermel*

Printed in the United States of America

Last digit is the print number: 9 8 7 6 5 4 3 2 1

ACKNOWLEDGMENTS

I am grateful to my teachers, Shlomo Raz, Jerry Blaivas, Donald Ostergard, and Stuart Stanton, who have taught me so much. As leading investigators and clinicians in the field of pelvic floor disorders, they have helped to promote a worldwide interest in pelvic floor rehabilitation for many years.

It is also my pleasure to thank my friends, Paul Abrams and Edward McGuire, who assisted me in gathering many of the world's most prominent experts on various aspects of pelvic floor function to contribute to this book.

I'd also like to make a special dedication to my parents, to Sylvie, and to my children, Alexandre and Florent, for their encouragement and emotional support while I organized this edition.

I would like to thank Rebecca Schmidt Gaertner, Hilarie Surrena, and Joanie Milnes at Elsevier and Janine White at P.M. Gordon Associates, who helped to prepare the book and did excellent work. Without their assistance, this project would not exist.

—Alain P. Bourcier

CONTRIBUTORS

Paul Abrams, MD, FRCS
Professor of Urology, Bristol Urological Institute, Southmead Hospital, Bristol, England
Urodynamic Investigations
Urodynamic Evaluation

Karl-Erik Andersson, MD, PhD
Professor, Department of Clinical Pharmacology, Lund University Hospital, Lund, Sweden
Pharmacologic Treatment of Urinary Incontinence

Patrick Atienza
Chief, Department of Coloproctology, Diaconesses, Croix Saint Simon; Paris, France
Fecal Incontinence and Disorders of Defecation

Kazem M. Azadzoi, MD
Research Professor, Department of Medicine: Surgery/Urology, VAMC; Professor and Research Director, Urology Department, Boston University Medical School, Veterans Affairs Boston Healthcare System; Boston, Massachusetts, United States
Male and Female Sexual Dysfunction

Khawaja Azimuddin, MD, FRCS, MBBS
Assistant Clinical Professor of Surgery, University of New Mexico, Albuquerque, New Mexico; General and Colorectal Surgeon, Espanola Hospital, Espanola, New Mexico, United States
Rectal Prolapse

Kaven Baessler, MD
Urogynecology Subspecialty Trainee, Royal Women's and Mater Hospitals, Brisbane, Australia
Pregnancy, Childbirth, and Pelvic Floor Damage

Stuart B. Bauer, MD
Senior Associate, Department of Urology, Children's Hospital; Professor of Surgery, Harvard Medical School; Boston, Massachusetts, United States
Surgical Management of Children with Urinary and Fecal Incontinence

Jennifer R. Berman, MD
Assistant Professor of Urology, University of California, Los Angeles; Director, Female Sexual Medicine Center; Los Angeles, California, United States
Normal Sexual Function in Women
Sexual Dysfunction in the Female
Management of Male and Female Sexual Dysfunction

Laura Berman, PhD, LCSW
Assistant Clinical Professor of Urology, University of California, Los Angeles; Co-Director, Female Sexual Medicine Center; Los Angeles, California, United States
Management of Male and Female Sexual Dysfunction

Shalender Bhasin, MD
Division of Endocrinology, Metabolism, and Molecular Medicine, King-Drew Medical Center, Los Angeles, California, United States
Management of Male and Female Sexual Dysfunction

Jerry G. Blaivas, MD
Clinical Professor of Urology, Department of Urology, Weill Medical College of Cornell University, New York Weill Cornell Center, New York, New York, United States
Lower Urinary Tract Dysfunction in the Male

Alain P. Bourcier, PT
Specialist Continence Physiotherapist, Department of Urology, Tenon Hospital; Director, Pelvic Floor Rehabilitation Services, Institut Français de Réadaptation Uro-Génitale; Paris, France
Office Evaluation and Physical Examination
Colporectocystourethrography: The Dynamic Investigation
Electrical Stimulation
Biofeedback Therapy
Management of Incontinence in the Elderly

Kathryn L. Burgio, PhD
Professor of Medicine, University of Alabama at Birmingham; Associate Director for Research, Geriatric Research, Education, and Clinical Center; Birmingham VA Medical Center; Birmingham, Alabama, United States
Biofeedback Therapy

Guillaume Cargill, MD
Director, Institution Centre d'Explorations Fonctionnelles Digestives, Paris, France
Pelvic Floor Re-education in Bowel Diseases

Kevin V. Carlson, MD, FRCSC
Lecturer, Division of Urology, Department of Surgery, University of Calgary, Calgary, Alberta, Canada
Neurogenic Voiding Dysfunction
Management of Neurogenic Voiding Dysfunction

Contributors

Michael B. Chancellor, MD
Professor of Urology and OB/GYN, Department of Urology, University of Pittsburgh School of Medicine, Pittsburgh, Pennsylvania, United States
Lower Urinary Tract Dysfunction in the Male

Christopher R. Chapple, MD
Consultant Urological Surgeon, Department of Urology, The Royal Halamshire Hospital, Sheffield, United Kingdom
Pharmacologic Treatment of Urinary Incontinence

Emmanuel Chartier-Kastler, MD, PhD
Professor of Urology, Department of Urology, Pitié-Salpétrière Hospital; Neurourology, Department of Physical Medicine and Rehabilitation, Raymond Poincaré Hospital, Garches; Paris, France
Neuromodulation

Joanna K. Chon, MD
Assistant Professor, Thomas Jefferson University, Philadelphia, Pennsylvania, United States
Surgical Treatment in Men

Cyrus A. Chowdhury
Senior Research Associate, Female Sexual Medical Center, Department of Urology, University of California, Los Angeles, Los Angeles, CA, United States
Management of Male and Female Sexual Dysfunction

Calin Ciofu, MD
Urologiste, Department of Urologie, Hôpital Tenon, Paris, France
The Tension-Free Vaginal Tape Technique

Christos C. Constantinou, PhD
Associate Professor, Department of Urology, Stanford University School of Medicine VA Medical Center, Stanford, California, United States
Contribution of Magnetic Resonance Imaging in the Evaluation of Pelvic Floor Function

Henri Damon, MD
Exploration Fonctionnelle Digestive, Hopital E. Herriot; Gastroenterologist
Digestive Physiology Department, Hospices Civils de Lyon; Lyon, France
Investigation of Disorders of Anorectal Function

John O. L. De Lancey, MD
Professor of Gynecology, Department of Obstetrics and Gynecology, University of Michigan School of Medicine, Taubman Medical Center, Ann Arbor, Michigan, United States
Gross Anatomy and Functional Anatomy of the Pelvic Floor

Vincent Delmas, MD, PhD
Professor of Urology, Department of Urology, Bichat Hospital; Professor, Anatomy, Université René Descartes; Paris, France
Gross Anatomy and Functional Anatomy of the Pelvic Floor

Jean-Pierre Dentz, PT
Supervisor, Physical Therapy Division, Clinique de L'Estree, Stains, France
Incontinence Aids: Pads and Appliances

Pierre Desvaux, MD
Urology Department, Cochin Hospital, Paris, France
Normal Sexual Function in Men
Erectile Dysfunction

Ananias C. Diokno, MD
Professor of Urology, Department of Urology, William Beaumont Hospital, Royal Oak, Michigan, United States
Urinary Incontinence in the Elderly

Clare J. Fowler, FRCP
Department of Uro-Neurology, Institute of Neurology, University College London; Professor of Uro-Neurology, Institute of Neurology and Institute of Urology National Hospital for Neurology and Neurosurgery; London, United Kingdom
Electrodiagnosis

Niall T. M. Galloway, MB, FRCS(Ed)
Medical Director, Emory Continence Center, Emory University School of Medicine; Associate Professor of Urology, Emory Clinic; Atlanta, Georgia, United States
Extracorporeal Electromagnetic Stimulation Therapy

Stephen H. Garnett, BSc, MB, BS
Specialist Registrar, Department of Urology, Aberdeen Royal Infirmary, Aberdeen, Scotland
Urodynamic Investigations

Roger P. Goldberg, MD, MPH
Director of Urogynecology Research, Evanston Continence Center, Northwestern University Medical School, Evanston, Illinois, United States
Extracorporeal Electromagnetic Stimulation Therapy

François Haab, MD
Professor of Urology, Tenon Hospital, Paris, France
The Tension-Free Vaginal Tape Technique

H. Roger Hadley, MD
Dean and Professor of Surgery/Urology, School of Medicine, Loma Linda University, Loma Linda, California, United States
Artificial Sphincter: Transvaginal Approach

Wayne J. G. Hellstrom, MD
Professor of Urology, Tulane University Health Sciences Center; Tulane Cancer Center; New Orleans, Louisiana, United States
Management of Male and Female Sexual Dysfunction

Luc Henry, MD
Department of Radiology, Hopital E. Herriot; Hospices Civils de Lyon; Lyon, France
Investigation of Disorders of Anorectal Function

Julia H. Herbert, Grad Dip Phys, MCSP, SRP
Specialist Continence Physiotherapist, Bolton Primary Care Trust and Independent Practitioner; Ellesmere Physiotherapy Clinic; Manchester, United Kingdom
Pelvic Floor Muscle Exercises

Gerald J. Jarvis, MD
Gynecologist, Beechwood House, Wetherby, United Kingdom; Consultant Gynecologist, The BUPA Hospital, Leeds, United Kingdom
Bladder Retraining

Jean C. Juras, MD
Radiologist Specialist in Uro-Gynecology, Cardinet Radiologic Center, Paris, France
Office Evaluation and Physical Examination
Colporectocystourethrography: The Dynamic Investigation

Ditza Katz, PT, PhD
Co-Director, Women's Therapy Center, Plainview, New York, United States
Management of Vaginismus, Vulvodynia, and Childhood Sexual Abuse

Christopher E. Kelly, MD
Assistant Professor of Urology, NYU Medical Center; NYU Urology Associates; New York, New York, United States
Surgical Treatment of Stress Urinary Incontinence in Women

Indru T. Khubchandani, MD
Professor of Surgery, College of Medicine, Pennsylvania State University/Hershey Medical Center; Colon and Rectal Surgeon, Lehigh Valley Hospital; Allentown, Pennsylvania, United States
Rectal Prolapse

Carl G. Klutke, MD
Professor, Department of Surgery, Division of Urology, Washington University School of Medicine, St. Louis, Missouri, United States
Endoscopy in Benign Pelvic Floor Dysfunction

John J. Klutke, MD
Assistant Professor, USC Keck School of Medicine, Los Angeles, California, United States
Endoscopy in Benign Pelvic Floor Dysfunction

Jean François Lapray, MD
Radiologist, Radiology Center, Lyon, France
Standard Radiologic Studies in Women

Filippo La Torre
Professor of Surgery, Department of Surgical Services, University of Rome, La Sapienza, Rome, Italy
Fecal Incontinence and Disorders of Defecation

Gary E. Leach, MD
Director, Tower Urology Institute for Continence, Cedars-Sinai Medical Center, Los Angeles, California, United States
Surgical Treatment in Men

Albert C. Leung, MD
Resident, Department of Urology, Albert Einstein College of Medicine, Montefiore Medical Center, New York, New York, United States
Diagnostic Evaluation of Erectile Dysfunction

Oleg Loran, MD, PhD
Professor of Urology and Chairman, Department of Urology of Russian Medical Academy of Post Graduate Education, Moscow, Russia
Conventional and Minimized Pubovaginal Sling in Patients with Severe Stress Urinary Incontinence

Gunnar Lose, MD, DMSc
Professor and Chief Gynecologist, Department of Gynecology & Obstetrics, Glostrup County Hospital, University of Copenhagen, Copenhagen, Denmark
Pelvic Floor Re-education in Urogynecology

Anders Mattiasson, MD, PhD
Professor of Urology, Department of Urology, University Hospital, Lund, Sweden
Neurophysiology of the Lower Urinary Tract

Edward J. McGuire, MD
Professor of Surgery, University of Texas Medical School, Department of Urology, Houston, Texas, United States
Urodynamic Evaluation

Arnold Melman, MD
Professor and Chair, Department of Urology, Albert Einstein College of Medicine, Montefiore Medical Center, New York, New York, United States
Diagnostic Evaluation of Erectile Dysfunction

Sylvain Meyer, PT
Head, Urogynecology Unit, Department of Gynecology/Obstetrics, CHUV, Universite de Lausanne, Lausanne, Switzerland
Pelvic Floor Re-education in Urogynecology

François Mion, MD, PhD
Exploration Functionelle Digestive, Hopital E. Herriot; Professor of Physiology; Head of Digestive Physiology Department, Hospices Civils de Lyon; Lyon, France
Physiology of Anal Continence and Defecation
Investigation of Disorders of Anorectal Function

Diane Kaschak Newman, RNC, MSN, CRNP, FAAN
Co-Director, Penn Center for Continence and Pelvic Health, Division of Urology, University of Pennsylvania Medical Center, Philadelphia, Pennsylvania, United States
Lifestyle Interventions

Hiep T. Nguyen, MD, FAAP
Assistant Professor of Urology and Pediatrics, Department of Urology, University of California, San Francisco, San Francisco, California, United States
Surgical Management of Children with Urinary and Fecal Incontinence

Attilio Nicastro
Secretary of IPFDS, Chief IH, Department of General Surgery and Operative Unit of Colon Proctology, "Villa Pia" Hospital; Surgeon, Department of Coloproctology, European Hospital, Rome, Italy
Fecal Incontinence and Disorders of Defecation

Victor W. Nitti, MD
Associate Professor and Vice-Chairman, Department of Urology, New York University Medical Center, New York, New York, United States
Neurogenic Voiding Dysfunction
Management of Neurogenic Voiding Dysfunction

Pat D. O'Donnell, MD
Clinical Professor of Urology, Department of Surgery, Veterans' Administration Medical Center, Fayetteville, Arkansas, United States
Management of Incontinence in the Elderly

Kwang Tae Park, MD, PhD
Director HMT Incontinence & Medical Center; Chairman, Department of OB & GYN, Gaya Hospital; Seoul, Korea
Electrical Stimulation

Simon Podnar, MD, DSc
Assistant Professor of Neurology and Staff Neurologist and Clinical Neurophysiologist, Institute of Clinical Neurophysiology, Division of Neurology, University Medical Center, Ljubljana, Slovenia
Electrodiagnosis

Dmitry Pushkar, MD, PhD
Chairman, Department of Urology of Moscow State Medico-Stomatological University, Moscow, Russia
Conventional and Minimized Pubovaginal Sling in Patients with Severe Stress Urinary Incontinence

Shlomo Raz, MD
Professor, Department of Urology, University of California, Los Angeles School of Medicine; UCLA Female Urology, Pelvic Medicine Clinic; Los Angeles, California, United States
Dynamic Magnetic Resonance Imaging in the Evaluation of Pelvic Pathology

Larissa V. Rodriguez, MD
Assistant Professor, Department of Urology, University of California; UCLA Female Urology, Pelvic Medicine Clinic; Los Angeles, California, United States
Dynamic Magnetic Resonance Imaging in the Evaluation of Pelvic Pathology

Peter K. Sand, MD
Professor, Department of Obstetrics and Gynecology; Director, Division of Urogynecology; and Director, Evanston Continence Center; Evanston Northwestern Heathcare, Northwestern University, Feinberg School of Medicine, Evanston, Illinois, United States
Extracorporeal Electromagnetic Stimulation Therapy

Bernhard Schuessler, MD
Department of Obstetrics and Gynecology, Kantonssiptal Luzern Frauenklinik, Luzern, Switzerland
Pregnancy, Childbirth, and Pelvic Floor Damage

Farshad Shafizadeh, MD
Attending Physician, Department of Urology, Montefiore Medical Center, New York, New York, United States
Diagnostic Evaluation of Erectile Dysfunction

Michael B. Siroky, MD
Professor of Urology, Boston University; Associate Chief of Urology, Boston VA Healthcare System, Boston, Massachusetts, United States
Male and Female Sexual Dysfunction

Christopher P. Smith, MD, MBA
Assistant Professor and Co-Director, Neurourology Laboratory, Scott Department of Urology, Baylor College of Medicine, Houston, Texas, United States
Lower Urinary Tract Dysfunction in the Male

David Staskin, MD
Director, Sec. Voiding Dysfunction, New York Presbyterian Hospital; Associate Professor of Urology, Obstetrics and Gynecology, Weill-Cornell Medical College; New York, New York, United States
Lower Urinary Tract Dysfunction in the Female

Ross Lynn Tabisel, CSW, PhD
Co-Director, Women's Therapy Center, Plainview, New York, United States
Management of Vaginismus, Vulvodynia, and Childhood Sexual Abuse

Khai-Lee Toh, MBBS, FRCS(Ed), FRCSG
Associate Consultant, Section of Urology, Department of General Surgery, Tan Tock Seng Hospital, Singapore
Urinary Incontinence in the Elderly

Olivier Traxer
Urologist, Department of Urology, Urodynamics Unit, Tenon Hospital, Paris, France
The Tension-Free Vaginal Tape Technique

Guy Valancogne, PT
Centre Tête d'or, Lyon, France
Pelvic Floor Re-education in Bowel Diseases

Philip Edward Victor Van Kerrebroeck, MD, PhD, Fellow EBU
Chairman, Department of Urology, University Hospital Maastricht; Professor of Urology, University of Maastricht; Maastricht, The Netherlands
Neuromodulation

Richard M. Villet
Chief, Department of Gynecological Surgery, Dioconesses, Croix Saint Simon Hospital, Paris, France
Office Evaluation and Physical Examination
Colporectocystourethrography: The Dynamic Investigation

David B. Vodušek, MD
Professor of Neurology, University of Ljubljana; Professor of Neurology and Medical Director, Division of Neurology, University Medical Center; Ljubljana, Slovenia
Electrodiagnosis

Alain Watier, MD, LMCC, FRCP
Associate Professor of Gastroenterology, Centre Universitaire de Sante de l'Estrie Universite de Sherbrooke; Professor of Gastroenterology, CHUS Sherbrooke; Director, Pelviperinology Unit, CHUS-Hotel-Dieu; Quebec, Canada
Pelvic Floor Re-education in Bowel Diseases

Alan J. Wein, MD
Professor and Chairman, Division of Urology, University of Pennsylvania, Philadelphia, Pennsylvania, United States
Pharmacologic Treatment of Urinary Incontinence

Phillipe E. Zimmern, MD
Professor, Department of Urology, University of Texas, Southwestern Medical Center, Dallas, Texas, United States
Surgical Treatment of Stress Urinary Incontinence in Women

FOREWORD

Pelvic Floor Disorders is a unique work. It is not limited to one discipline but addresses all three major systems within the bony pelvis and its supporting structures, among the most important of which is the pelvic floor.

The pelvic floor not only contains the pelvic visceral organs within the pelvic cavity; it also controls individual and integrated functions, sustains proper anatomic relationships, and shares with the various visceral organs the basic mechanism that controls their function. The pelvic floor is the junction between these organs, with their autonomic innervation, and the pelvic floor musculature, with its somatic innervation; interaction between these two components can be facilitatory or inhibitory. Indeed, this is the only anatomic site where involuntary visceral organic function comes under voluntary control.

Although pelvic floor dysfunction has long been related to the lower urinary tract and, more recently, to lower gastrointestinal symptoms also, it is now considered an influential factor in the normal function and behavior of the genital system in both men and women. This volume addresses pathologic and clinical problems of the three pelvic visceral organs and relates them to the basic function and integrity of the pelvic floor.

The editors—three outstanding authorities—and the more than 30 contributors present an integrated multidisciplinary approach that adds to the book's originality. With extensive discussion of management by behavioral, pharmacologic, and surgical means, *Pelvic Floor Disorders* will be a much-used reference, not only for general urologists, gynecologists, and proctologists, but also for highly specialized practitioners within these disciplines. It is a pleasure to introduce this new text, and I enthusiastically endorse it as a valuable guide to an expanding field of interest.

Emil A. Tanagho, MD
San Francisco, California

PREFACE

Symptoms of urinary incontinence are common, and, at any age, incontinence can have a severe impact on the quality of life. Fecal incontinence is an under-reported, under-diagnosed condition. The symptoms can be of a multifaceted etiology and may include physiologic and psychological disability leading to a progressive feeling of isolation for patients. Sexual problems, which may be characterized as psychological, gynecologic, urologic, and neurologic, are common in both women and men and occur for several reasons.

This book is divided into five parts. Part I highlights basic sciences, including gross and functional anatomy, neurophysiology of the lower urinary tract, and normal sexual function in both men and women.

Part II relates to the pathophysiology of pelvic floor disorders and the conservative management of the lower urinary tract, disorders of anorectal function, and sexual function. This part contains information on the use of pelvic floor re-education in treating specific disease entities, such as childbirth damage, post-prostatectomy incontinence, and neuropathic voiding dysfunction.

Part III reviews the diagnosis and evaluation of pelvic floor disorders, including the office evaluation and physical examination and radiologic and MRI imaging.

Part IV explains rehabilitation techniques, such as lifestyle interventions, pelvic floor muscle training, electrical stimulation, bladder retraining, biofeedback, anti-incontinence devices, and incontinence aids.

Part V discusses pharmacologic and surgical techniques for managing pelvic floor disorders, including surgical treatments for men, women, and children.

As current constraints on the health care economy dictate that conservative treatment constitutes the principal form of management at a primary care level, we asked the contributors, who are leaders in the field of pelvic floor disorder, to make practical suggestions on pelvic floor rehabilitation techniques. One of the most important aspects of this book is the new concept of addressing all pelvic floor disorders in one work and allowing a multidisciplinary approach for diagnosis and conservative management. The book is recommended to physicians of all specialties and directed mainly to health care providers who treat patients with urinary or fecal incontinence or other manifestations of pelvic floor disorders.

CONTENTS

PART I
BASIC SCIENCES 1

1 Gross Anatomy and Functional Anatomy of the Pelvic Floor 3
JOHN O.L. DE LANCEY, MD, AND VINCENT DELMAS, MD, PHD

2 Neurophysiology of the Lower Urinary Tract 7
ANDERS MATTIASSON, MD, PHD

3 Physiology of Anal Continence and Defecation 14
FRANÇOIS MION, MD, PHD

4 Normal Sexual Function in Women 19
JENNIFER R. BERMAN, MD

5 Normal Sexual Function in Men 26
PIERRE DESVAUX, MD

PART II
PATHOPHYSIOLOGY OF PELVIC FLOOR DISORDERS 31

6 Pregnancy, Childbirth, and Pelvic Floor Damage 33
KAVEN BAESSLER, MD, AND BERNHARD SCHUESSLER, PROF. DR. MED.

7 Lower Urinary Tract Dysfunction in the Female 43
DAVID STASKIN, MD

8 Lower Urinary Tract Dysfunction in the Male 49
CHRISTOPHER P. SMITH, MD, MBA,
JERRY G. BLAIVAS, MD, AND MICHAEL B. CHANCELLOR, MD

9 Urinary Incontinence in the Elderly 57
ANANIAS C. DIOKNO, MD, AND KHAI-LEE TOH, MBBS, FRCS(ED), FRCSG

10 Neurogenic Voiding Dysfunction 66
KEVIN V. CARLSON, MD, FRCSC, AND VICTOR W. NITTI, MD

11 Fecal Incontinence and Disorders of Defecation 73
PATRICK ATIENZA, FILIPPO LA TORRE, AND ATTILIO NICASTRO

12 Rectal Prolapse 81
    INDRU T. KHUBCHANDANI, MD, AND KHAWAJA AZIMUDDIN, MD, FRCS, MBBS

13 Male and Female Sexual Dysfunction 89
    MICHAEL B. SIROKY, MD, AND KAZEM M. AZADZOI, MD

14 Sexual Dysfunction in the Female 121
    JENNIFER R. BERMAN, MD

15 Erectile Dysfunction 125
    PIERRE DESVAUX, MD

PART III
DIAGNOSIS AND EVALUATION OF PELVIC FLOOR DISORDERS 131

16 Office Evaluation and Physical Examination 133
    ALAIN P. BOURCIER, PT, JEAN C. JURAS, MD, AND RICHARD M. VILLET

17 Standard Radiologic Studies in Women 149
    JEAN FRANÇOIS LAPRAY, MD

18 Colporectocystourethrography: The Dynamic Investigation 164
    JEAN C. JURAS, MD, ALAIN P. BOURCIER, PT, AND RICHARD M. VILLET

19 Contribution of Magnetic Resonance Imaging in the Evaluation
    of Pelvic Floor Function 176
    CHRISTOS C. CONSTANTINOU, PHD

20 Dynamic Magnetic Resonance Imaging in the Evaluation
    of Pelvic Pathology 183
    LARISSA V. RODRIGUEZ, MD, AND SHLOMO RAZ, MD

21 Endoscopy in Benign Pelvic Floor Dysfunction 191
    JOHN J. KLUTKE, MD, AND CARL G. KLUTKE, MD

22 Urodynamic Investigations 198
    STEPHEN H. GARNETT, BSC, MB, BS, AND PAUL ABRAMS, MD, FRCS

23 Urodynamic Evaluation 208
    EDWARD J. MCGUIRE, MD, AND PAUL ABRAMS, MD, FRCS

24 Electrodiagnosis 216
    SIMON PODNAR, MD, DSC, DAVID B. VODUŠEK, MD, AND CLARE J. FOWLER, FRCP

25 Investigation of Disorders of Anorectal Function 235
    FRANÇOIS MION, MD, PHD, HENRI DAMON, MD, AND LUC HENRY, MD

26 Diagnostic Evaluation of Erectile Dysfunction 249
    FARSHAD SHAFIZADEH, MD, ALBERT C. LEUNG, MD, AND ARNOLD MELMAN, MD

PART IV
CONSERVATIVE TREATMENT: TECHNIQUES 267

27 Lifestyle Interventions 269
DIANE KASCHAK NEWMAN, RNC, MSN, CRNP, FAAN

28 Pelvic Floor Muscle Exercises 277
JULIA H. HERBERT, GRAD DIP PHYS, MCSP, SRP

29 Electrical Stimulation 281
ALAIN P. BOURCIER, PT, AND KWANG TAE PARK, MD, PHD

30 Extracorporeal Electromagnetic Stimulation Therapy 291
ROGER P. GOLDBERG, MD, MPH, NIALL T. M. GALLOWAY, MB, FRCS(ED), AND PETER K. SAND, MD

31 Biofeedback Therapy 297
ALAIN P. BOURCIER, PT, AND KATHRYN L. BURGIO, PHD

32 Bladder Retraining 311
GERALD J. JARVIS, MD

33 Incontinence Aids: Pads and Appliances 314
JEAN-PIERRE DENTZ, PT

34 Pelvic Floor Re-education in Bowel Diseases 320
GUY VALANCOGNE, PT, GUILLAUME CARGILL, MD, AND ALAIN WATIER, MD, LMCC, FRCP

35 Pelvic Floor Re-education in Urogynecology 331
SYLVAIN MEYER, PT, AND GUNNAR LOSE, MD, DMSc

36 Management of Incontinence in the Elderly 341
PAT D. O'DONNELL, MD, AND ALAIN P. BOURCIER, PT

37 Management of Male and Female Sexual Dysfunction 347
JENNIFER R. BERMAN, MD, SHALENDER BHASIN, MD, LAURA BERMAN, PHD, LCSW, CYRUS A. CHOWDHURY, AND WAYNE J. G. HELLSTROM, MD

38 Management of Vaginismus, Vulvodynia, and Childhood Sexual Abuse 360
DITZA KATZ, PT, PHD, AND ROSS LYNN TABISEL, CSW, PHD

PART V
PHARMACOLOGY AND SURGICAL TECHNIQUES 371

39 Pharmacologic Treatment of Urinary Incontinence 373
KARL-ERIK ANDERSSON, MD, PHD, CHRISTOPHER R. CHAPPLE, MD, AND ALAN J. WEIN, MD

40 Surgical Treatment of Stress Urinary Incontinence in Women 392
Christopher E. Kelly, MD, and Phillipe E. Zimmern, MD

41 The Tension-Free Vaginal Tape Technique 403
François Haab, MD, Olivier Traxer, and Calin Ciofu, MD

42 Artificial Sphincter: Transvaginal Approach 408
H. Roger Hadley, MD

43 Conventional and Minimized Pubovaginal Sling in Patients with
Severe Stress Urinary Incontinence 414
Dmitry Pushkar, MD, PhD, and Oleg Loran, MD, PhD

44 Surgical Treatment in Men 421
Joanna K. Chon, MD, and Gary E. Leach, MD

45 Surgical Management of Children with Urinary and
Fecal Incontinence 432
Stuart B. Bauer, MD, and Hiep T. Nguyen, MD, FAAP

46 Neuromodulation 450
Philip Edward Victor Van Kerrebroeck, MD, PhD, Fellow EBU,
and Emmanuel Chartier-Kastler, MD, PhD

47 Management of Neurogenic Voiding Dysfunction 454
Kevin V. Carlson, MD, FRCSC, and Victor W. Nitti, MD

Index 463

PART I

BASIC SCIENCES

CHAPTER 1

Gross Anatomy and Functional Anatomy of the Pelvic Floor

JOHN O.L. DE LANCEY ■ VINCENT DELMAS

What is the pelvic floor? The pelvic floor consists of all of the structures that close the bottom of the pelvis. Some of these structures are directly and totally involved in the static and the dynamic of the pelvis (e.g., the levator ani muscle and its fascia), and the others are indirectly and partially involved. All help to sustain the pelvic viscera and regulate their canals (anal canal, urethra, vagina), and all function interactively. A special focus is necessary on the musculofascial structures of the anterior perineal triangle, where the major consequences of defects are seen (e.g., incontinence, prolapse).

This chapter reviews the structures surrounding the urogenital hiatus of the female.

GROSS ANATOMY

The bony pelvic ring lies inferior to the abdominal cavity, and the levator ani muscles span this space. The borders of the opening spanned by the pelvic floor are the pubic bones anteriorly, the ischial spines laterally, and the sacrum posteriorly. Between the pubis and the spines lie the tendineus arches of the levator ani and the pelvic fascia. The sacrospinous ligament and its overlying coccygeus muscles lie between the spine and the sacrum. It is this polygonal opening that must be closed by the levator ani muscles.

From an organizational standpoint, the pelvic floor consists of two specific components, the levator ani and the coccygeus. The latter completes the pelvis floor posteriorly. The coccygeus forms a triangular structure whose apex attaches to the spine of the ischium. From the ischial spine the coccygeus forms a fibromuscular sheet that fans out medially and attaches to the lateral surface of the coccyx and S5. The coccygeus is nothing more than the musculotendinous internal surface of the sacrospinous ligament to which it is intimately attached. The coccygeus does not contribute to active movement of the pelvic floor.

Levator Ani

In practical terms, the pelvic floor is synonymous with the levator ani because this muscle forms the effective contractile support structure of the region. The muscle forms a broad, thin sheet that attaches anteriorly to the posterior surface of the body of the pubis and is suspended laterally from the pelvic wall as far posteriorly as the ischial spine. Between the pubis and the ischial spine the muscle is directly attached to (or sometimes slung from) the fascia covering the medial surface of the obturator internus. Anteriorly, the levator ani is absent in the midline. The part of the muscle that attaches to the pubis forms the medial portion of these fibers, and from the pubis this muscle attaches to the perineal body behind the prostate to form the levator prostate. In the female, these medial fibers attach to the lateral vaginal wall to form the pubovaginalis. Other fibers from the pubis pass behind the anorectal flexure, where they fuse with the deep part of the external anal sphincter to form the puborectalis. Other fibers run from the pubis and the fascia covering the obturator internus; these fibers are known as the pubococcygeus.

The part of the levator ani arising from the lateral wall of the pelvis posteriorly to the ischial spine is the iliococcygeus. The distinction between the end of the pubococcygeus and the start of the iliococcygeus is arbitrary because one merges imperceptibly with the other as a continuous sheet of muscle. Nevertheless, the fibers of the iliococcygeus run medially at different angles of obliquity to merge with the component parts of the pubococcygeus.

Parts of the levator collectively play an important role in maintaining the position of the pelvic viscera. In the female, contraction of the attachments of the levator ani to the vagina and external anal sphincter is responsible for the anterior movement of these viscera toward the pubic symphysis. On contraction of the pelvic floor, this anterior movement of the vagina produces occlusive forces on the urethra that cause its forward displacement.

Contraction of the levator ani is responsible for dynamic support of the urethra. Thus, the levator ani helps this sphincter to ensure continence and produce forceful support of the urethra (e.g., during coughing).

Innervation of the Levator Ani

The levator ani is innervated by somatic nerve fibers that emanate primarily from sacral root S3, to a lesser extent from S4, and minimally from S2, to form the nerve levator ani. The pudendal nerve is a mixed nerve that carries both motor and sensory fibers and is derived from the sacral plexus. Initially, the pudendal nerve lies superior to the sacrospinous ligament lateral to the coccyx. It runs on the cranial surface of the levator ani.

FUNCTIONAL ANATOMY

Support of the Pelvic Organs

The pelvic organs are supported by a combination of muscle and connective tissue. The levator ani muscles were discussed earlier, and the connective tissue attachments will now be considered. The pelvic organs are attached to the pelvic walls. The connecting tissue is known as the endopelvic fascia, a heterogeneous group of tissues including collagen, elastin, smooth muscle, blood vessels, and nerves. The fasciae and ligaments are often considered separately from the pelvic organs, as if they had a discrete identity, yet unless these fibrous structures have something to attach to (the pelvic organs), they can have no suspensory effect.

The overall geometry of this tissue determines its mechanical function. The endopelvic fascia attaches the uterus and vagina to the pelvic wall bilaterally. This fascia forms a continuous sheet-like mesentery that extends from the uterine artery at its cephalic margin to the point at which the vagina fuses with the levator ani muscles below. The part that attaches to the uterus is known as the parametrium, and the part that attaches to the vagina is the paracolpium.

The parametria are referred to clinically as the cardinal and uterosacral ligaments. These are two parts of the single mass of tissue. The uterosacral ligaments are the visible and palpable medial margin of the cardinal–uterosacral ligament complex, which has a considerable amount of smooth muscle. The paracolpium, as discussed later, attaches the vagina to the pelvic walls more directly.

Although these tissues are known as ligaments and fascia, they are not the same type of tissue seen in the fascia of the rectus abdominis muscle or the ligaments of the knee, both of which are composed of dense regular connective tissue. These supportive tissues consist of blood vessels, nerves, and fibrous connective tissue, and can be thought of as the mesenteries that supply the genital tract bilaterally. Their composition reflects their combined function as neurovascular conduits and supportive structures.

Regional variations in these tissues explain the differences between the types of pelvic support defects seen in women with pelvic organ prolapse (Fig. 1-1). The upper third of the vagina has the same suspensory tissues as the uterus. These long fibers elevate the upper portion of the vagina after the uterus is removed during hysterectomy. In the middle third of the vagina, the anterior and posterior vaginal walls are connected laterally to the pelvic walls. Continuous with the parametrium when the uterus remains in situ, this upper portion consists of the relatively long sheet of tissue that suspends the vagina by attaching to the pelvic wall. In the midportion of the vagina, the paracolpium attaches the vagina laterally and more directly to the pelvic walls. Ventrally, the vagina is attached to the arcus tendineus fascia pelvis. The combination of the vaginal wall and its attachments to the fascial arch comprise the structural layer that supports the bladder base and urethra. Dorsally, the vagina is attached to the inner surface of the levator ani muscles. This structure helps to restrain the rectum from being displaced forward.

These attachments, which stretch the vagina transversely between the bladder and the rectum, have functional significance. The structural layer that supports the bladder (pubocervical fascia) is composed of the anterior vaginal wall and its attachment through the endopelvic fascia to the pelvic wall. It is not a separate layer from the vagina, as sometimes inferred, but is a combination of the anterior vaginal wall and its attachments to the pelvic wall. Similarly, the posterior vaginal wall and the endopelvic fascia (rectovaginal fascia) form the restraining layer that prevents the rectum from protruding forward, blocking the formation of a rectocele, as discussed later.

In the distal vagina, the vaginal wall is directly attached to surrounding structures without intervening paracolpium. Anteriorly, the vaginal wall fuses with the

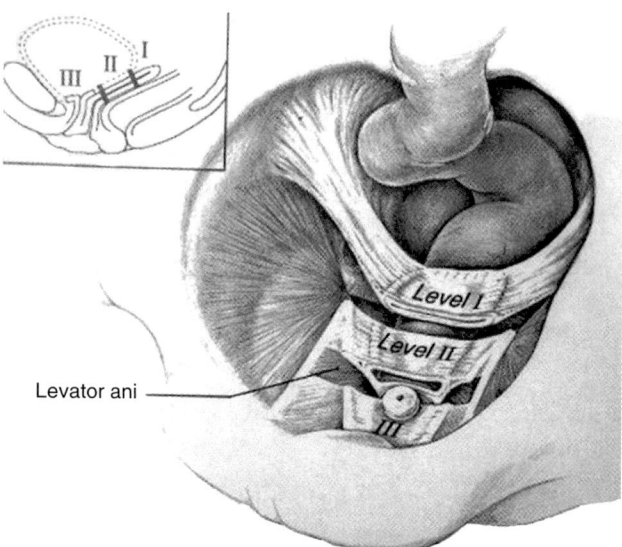

FIGURE 1-1 Different regions of vaginal support, showing anatomy after hysterectomy with hysterectomy scar shown at the vaginal apex. (From De Lancey, JOL: Anatomic aspects of vaginal eversion after hysterectomy. Am J Obstet Gynecol 166:1717, 1992.)

urethra and is attached to the arcus tendineus. Posteriorly, it fuses with the perineal body, whose position is maintained through connections to the ischiopubic rami by the perineal membrane. Laterally, it is attached directly to the levator ani muscles by the fibers of Luschka.

Damage to the upper suspensory fibers of the paracolpium causes a different type of prolapse than damage to the midlevel supports of the vagina. Defects in the support provided by the midlevel structures (pubocervical and rectovaginal fasciae) result in anterior and posterior vaginal wall defects (cystocele and rectocele); loss of the upper suspensory fibers of the paracolpium and parametrium causes vaginal and uterine prolapse. These defects occur in varying combinations, and this variation is responsible for the diversity of clinical problems encountered within the overall spectrum of pelvic organ prolapse.

Urethral and Anterior Vaginal Wall Support

Urethral support is an important factor in stress continence in women, because support in symptomatic women may be inadequate. This support is supplied by a combination of connective tissue and muscle arranged to resist the downward force created by increases in abdominal pressure. The urethra lies adjacent to, and is intimately connected with, the anterior vaginal wall. The connections of the vagina and urethra to the levator ani muscles and arcus tendineus fascia pelvis determine the structural stability of the urethra.

The arcus tendineus fascia pelvis is a fibrous band that is stretched between a fine tendon-like origin from the pubic bone anteriorly and an attachment to the ischial spine. The endopelvic fascia and the anterior vaginal wall form a layer that supports the urethra and vesical neck by connecting to the arcus tendineus. In this region, the medial portion of the levator ani muscles connects directly to the endopelvic fascia and vaginal wall. This muscular attachment permits contraction of the levator ani muscles to stabilize the urethra during a cough.

Urethral support depends on connective tissue and muscle action. If the connective tissue fails, then the urethral supports cannot stay in their normal alignment and stress incontinence often occurs. Conversely, if the muscles are damaged, as seen on magnetic resonance imaging, their action in supporting the urethra may be lost. Recent evidence shows that in primigravid women with stress incontinence, urethral support is preferentially lost during a cough, whereas mobility during the Valsalva maneuver is no different than in incontinent women.

Support of the Posterior Vaginal Wall and Rectum

The distal rectum is adjacent to the dense connective tissue of the perineal body. The perineal body is the central connection between the two halves of the perineal membrane (urogenital diaphragm). When the distal rectum is subjected to increased force directed caudally, the fibers of the perineal membrane become tight and resist further displacement. These fibers derive their lateral support from their attachment to the pelvic bones at the ischiopubic rami (Fig. 1-2). The ability of this layer to resist downward displacement depends on the structural continuity between the right and left sides of the perineal membrane.

The connection between the two halves of the perineal membrane extends cranially for a distance of approximately 2 to 3 cm above the hymenal ring. It is thickest and densest in the distal perineal body, and becomes progressively thinner toward its cranial margin. The lateral margin of the perineal body contains the termination of the bulbocavernosus muscle and terminations of the medial fibers of the levator ani muscle.

The midportion of the posterior vaginal wall is attached on either side of the rectum to the inner surface of the pelvic diaphragm by a sheet of endopelvic fascia. These fascial sheets attach to the posterior lateral vaginal wall, where the dorsally directed tension causes a posterior vaginal sulcus on each side of the rectum (Fig. 1-3). These endopelvic fascial sheets prevent ventral movement of the posterior vaginal wall. Most of the fibers of the endopelvic fascia attach to the vaginal wall, with only a few fibers passing from one side to the other.

The level II and level III supports are continuous with one another. Force applied to the anterior rectal wall in level II is resisted by the posterior vaginal wall and its attachments to the inner surface of the pelvic diaphragm. Pressure applied to the perineal body caudally in level III is resisted by the perineal membrane and the connection of the upper vaginal wall to the level II attachments that help to hold the cranial end of the perineal body in place.

Connective Tissue of the Pelvic Floor

Considerable confusion persists about the functional significance of the various fascial and ligamentous

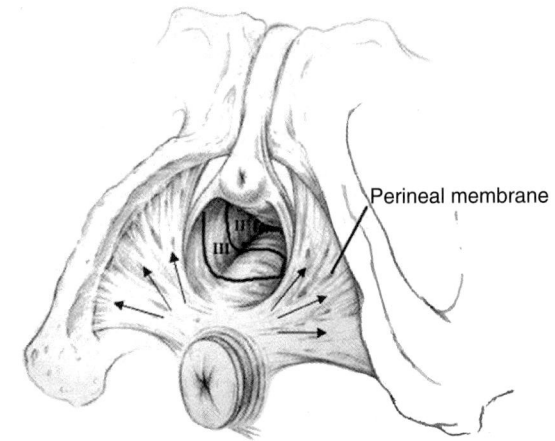

FIGURE 1-2 Support of the perineal body by the perineal membrane by its connection to the ischiopubic rami. (From De Lancey JOL: Structural anatomy of the posterior compartment as it relates to rectocile. Am J Obstet Gynecol 180:815, 1999.)

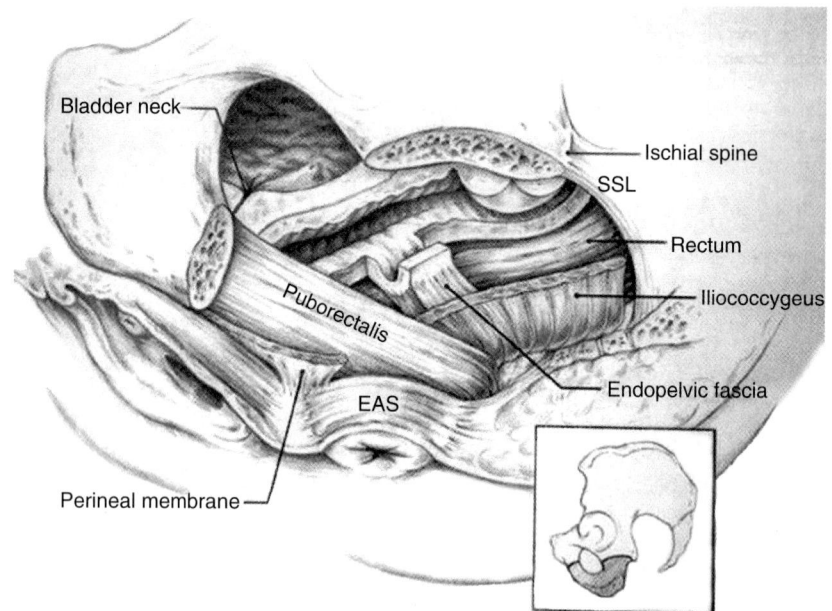

FIGURE 1-3 Lateral view of the pelvic floor structures. The ischium has been removed, as have portions of the iliococcygeus muscle and lateral vaginal wall. EAS, external anal sphincter; SSL, sacrospinous ligament. (From De Lancey JOL: Structural anatomy of the posterior compartment as it relates to rectocile. Am J Obstet Gynecol 180:815, 1999.)

structures that have been described and implicated in the support of pelvic organs. Some authors have noted the amount of connective tissue within quadripedal animals and have sought associations with the assumption of an upright posture. However, the connective tissue component of the levator ani has not received the same attention as the striated muscle component, although several investigators suggested that deficient or abnormal collagen may be the cause of pelvic floor dysfunction in humans. A histologic study of vaginal fascial connective tissue in women with and without uterine prolapse showed abnormal histologic changes in 7 of 10 patients with uterine descent. Other workers showed a significantly higher incidence of pelvic organ prolapse in women with hypermobile joints compared with a control group with clinical joint laxity, further implicating abnormalities of collagen in pelvic floor dysfunction. Clearly, further studies are needed to examine the role of contributing factors, such as age, estrogen activity, obesity, parity, delivery, sexual activity, and physical work, on the structure and function of the connective tissue component of the levator ani. These studies may further our understanding of the normal function of the pelvic floor.

CHAPTER 2

Neurophysiology of the Lower Urinary Tract

ANDERS MATTIASSON

All levels of the nervous system participate in a steady, ongoing interaction with the lower urinary tract, leading to a normal, harmonious micturition cycle. The different parts are in balance with each other and work together rhythmically, and this interaction can be seen as cooperation between two equal parts. Therefore, it is both appropriate and practical to consider the lower urinary tract and involved portions of the nervous system as a whole.[1] In this context, and from a functional–neurophysiologic point of view, the lower urinary tract should be seen in its broadest sense, including, in addition to the bladder and trigone or bladder neck, the urethra and vagina or prostate, pelvic floor, and adjacent structures as well as vessels and nerves. All parts of the system are highly dependent on volume (i.e., the functional status of the lower urinary tract and the nervous system are largely dependent on the degree of bladder filling).

Innervation of the lower urinary tract is both autonomous and somatic. Many neuron populations and signal substances or neuromodulators are involved at both central and peripheral levels.[2,3] At the central level, the pontine micturition center and the sacral segments of the spinal cord are of particular importance. The micturition reflex travels a long distance, from the lower urinary tract to the pons and back. The peripheral nervous projections in the target organs that mediate excitatory and inhibitory stimuli consist of excitatory pelvic cholinergic innervation to the bladder and smooth musculature of the urethra, adrenergic hypogastric innervation to the bladder and urethra (mediating both relaxation and contraction), and pudendal somatic innervation to the striated muscle of the external sphincter and pelvic floor.[4] Sensory afferent neurons run through all of these nerves. Nonadrenergic noncholinergic (NANC) nervous activity exerts its influence through a variety of transmitters and modulators on both the afferent and efferent sides. A higher degree of filling gives an increased afferent drive, which in varying ways is suppressed until bladder emptying is initiated.

The complexity of the system depends on the reciprocal functions being represented in all parts of the lower urinary tract. The variability in the requirements for functionality makes the apparently simple storing and emptying process of the micturition cycle more complex when described in neuromuscular terms.[5,6] The function and contractile ability of the bladder are central issues for studying the function of the lower urinary tract. The accessibility to this organ with urodynamic methods has probably contributed to this choice of focus. We now have an opportunity to expand our perspective, and by considering structure and function, we can view all parts of the lower urinary tract and all relevant levels of the nervous system simultaneously.

Communication between the nervous system and the lower urinary tract also appears to be of great importance, both functionally and structurally. For example, the target organ appears to produce substances with trophic effects on the nervous system, such as nerve growth factors. These substances appear to reflect the considerable adaptability that exists in relation to changes in functional requirements.[7,8]

Evolution has created the current nature of lower urinary tract innervation and receptor function. Thus, under the surface are more primitive cycles or programs that are not activated in the normal individual, but can be shown through disorders or injury. Much of our knowledge is based on observations in animal experiments, and extrapolations to humans can be tempting, if not always correct. In the gray area between what is normal and what represents pathophysiology, some things remain unclear. This chapter provides a brief systematic overview of how the lower urinary tract, in a broad sense (i.e., including the pelvic floor), depends on and works with the nervous system in normal physiologic conditions.

INNERVATION OF THE LOWER URINARY TRACT AND THE MICTURITION CYCLE

The fact that we can voluntarily control autonomously innervated organs is remarkable. Students treated with curare and receiving respiratory assistance could, on demand, both initiate and discontinue micturition.[9] The somatic innervation of striated muscles in the pelvic floor and the external sphincter is of great importance for closure as well as the entire micturition cycle. Autonomous peripheral innervation via the pelvic and hypogastric nerves flows laterally in the pelvis around the bladder, inner genitalia, and rectum in the plexus pelvicus. The part of this plexus that leads to the bladder is called the vesical plexus of autonomic nerves, and it contains both sympathetic and parasympathetic neurons.[3] Our traditional way of dividing nervous pathways in relation to immediate nervous centers, and then using terms such as afferent and efferent, and our method of naming nerves after the dominant signal substance, such as adrenergic and cholinergic, probably will need review, at least to some extent. Afferent nerves often have functions that are classically described as efferent, and many neurons contain more than one type of transmitter or neuromodulator. A double function (i.e., afferent and efferent) allows thresholds to be set for afferent signaling. In other words, the indirect tolerance of mechanical, chemical, or other effects is determined at the same time that signals are mediated in afferent direction toward the central nervous system.[10] Such dual functions seem to be represented by acetylcholine, purines such as adenosine triphosphate, calcitonin gene-related peptide (CGRP), and substance P.

Because the micturition reflex can be described as always ready to be triggered, adequate inhibition must be present during the filling phase of the bladder. Such inhibition, which also can be voluntarily inhibited, is important to the normal micturition cycle. Inhibition occurs at many levels, and not all have been identified. Cerebral influences inhibit the pontine micturition center[11]; inhibitory pathways (e.g., serotoninergic) descend from higher centers to the sacral spinal level[12]; inhibitory segmental interneurons are found in the sacral spinal cord[13]; a gating function (i.e., filtering of efferent nervous activity[14]) occurs at the pelvic ganglionic level; and finally, a dual inhibitory peripheral interaction occurs between peripheral adrenergic and cholinergic nerve endings.[15]

Nervous Control of the Lower Urinary Tract

Peripheral Nervous Control

As mentioned earlier, peripheral innervation of the lower urinary tract is often described as efferent pelvic cholinergic, hypogastric adrenergic, pudendal somatic, and sensory afferent. The efferent motor activity, especially cholinergic activation of the bladder, is usually emphasized, probably because we have more knowledge about the motor than about the sensory mechanisms in the lower urinary tract. Investigation of sensory mechanisms has been much more difficult than studies of motor activity, most of which have been performed in vitro on animal tissues.

Afferent Activity

Afferent nervous activity seems to be of paramount importance and could be described as the driving force for the micturition cycle. Unlike efferent activity, afferent nerves never seem to be completely inhibited (Fig. 2-1).

All types of peripheral nerves innervating the lower urinary tract mediate afferent activity. The activity is generated in both the bladder wall and the urethra. The bladder wall contains tension receptors, and superficially, in both the bladder and the urethral mucosa, there is a rich and complex innervation. Thin, myelinated A delta fibers relay information about the tension in the wall, whereas unmyelinated C fibers in the bladder wall, not at least in the mucosa, appear to mediate information about the degree of bladder filling. The afferent stream of impulses strengthens with increased bladder filling. At the same time, the resultant need for increased inhibition prevents the establishment of efferent excitatory activity to the detrusor musculature, inhibiting triggering of the micturition reflex, thus permitting continued undisturbed filling. Several substances affect the afferent nerve endings, such as neuropeptides, prostaglandins, acetylcholine, and nitric oxide (NO). Recently, purinergic activity mediated via the P2X receptor (and possibly also the P3X receptor) was found to be important for the sensory innervation of the bladder.[16,17] With larger volumes, it becomes increasingly difficult to suppress the reflex. In certain respects, increased bladder filling, even in normal individuals, brings about a more unstable situation in the system than occurs at lower degrees of filling. In other words, less disruption is needed to upset the balance at higher than at lower degrees of filling. The proximal urethra also contains many sensory nerves. These are probably important with regard to the ability to empty the bladder via positive feedback in the presence of urine. Therefore, the micturition reflex is triggered by sensory activity generated in the bladder and urethra. During voiding, intense bladder afferent discharge activates spinal bulbospinal reflex pathways that pass through the

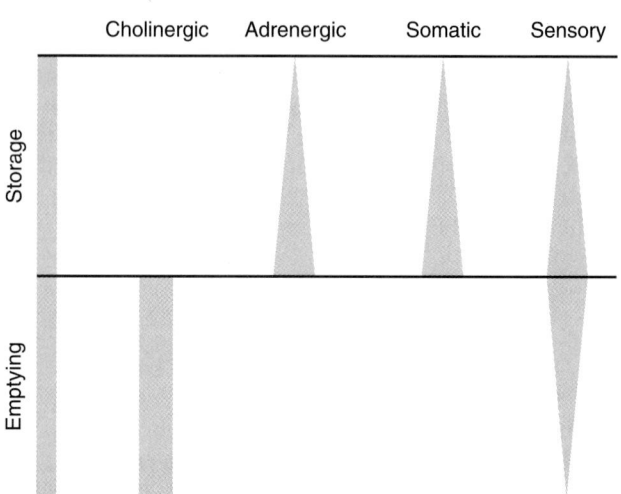

FIGURE 2-1 Lower urinary tract nervous activity "on-and-off" during the micturition cycle.

pontine micturition center. This stimulates the parasympathetic outflow to the bladder and internal sphincter smooth muscle and inhibits sympathetic and pudendal outflow to the bladder outlet.[11] Afferent discharges that occur during a bladder contraction have an important reflex function and appear to reinforce the central drive that maintains the detrusor contraction. Recently, we also learned that the reciprocal collaboration between the bladder and the urethra includes communication of afferent information from the urethra, which contributes to the positive feedback loop that guarantees complete emptying of the bladder via central and perhaps peripheral reflex arcs.

Several types of C fibers are found in the bladder wall, at least in certain species, but all fibers do not seem to be functional under normal circumstances (i.e., they are silent). They may be activated in various chemical and physical ways by injury or illness and therefore contribute to triggering activity in the bladder musculature. Perhaps the C fibers are protective. The role of the C fibers can be studied and used therapeutically by stimulation of vanilloid receptors on the C fibers with capsaicin or resiniferatoxin, substances that induce more or less complete transient emptying of the nerve terminal content of signal substances. The substances that are the actual messengers in these fibers have not been identified. Fine, unmyelinated fibers containing stimulating substances are located so superficially that they can be affected by the chemical composition of the bladder content. NO and adenosine triphosphate mediated via purinergic P2X receptors may play a part as messengers in this process.[16] The latter might be important for mediating filling sensation signals from the bladder.[17] Studies show that NO is released from the urothelium and nerves in the mucous membrane of the bladder, and noradrenaline may play a part in this release.[18] A release from the peripheral afferent nerves in a retrograde, antidromal direction takes place and helps to adjust the thresholds for excitation and contraction (i.e., the sensitivity of the system).

Efferent Activity

Cholinergic Activity. Cholinergic innervation of the lower urinary tract runs via S2–S4 in the pelvic nerves to the bladder and smooth musculature of the urethra. The bladder musculature has a dense innervation, and emptying of the bladder is effected via release of acetylcholine from cholinergic nerve endings, exciting the smooth muscle cells.[2] During emptying, the pressure on the outflow side is low while the bladder contracts, so that emptying can take place against the least possible resistance. Bladder contraction is caused by the release of acetylcholine from pelvic cholinergic neurons. Sliding of the contractile proteins under the influence of Ca^{2+} ions is induced intracellularly, via a chain of second messengers, by the stimulation of muscarinic receptors in the smooth bladder muscle cells, mainly of the M_3 type. The process that leads to activation of the contractile proteins is called the excitation–contraction coupling. There are two sources of Ca^{2+}, one extracellular that is made available for the cell via the Ca^{2+} channels in the cell membrane and one intracellular that is stored in the endoplasmic reticulum and released when needed, as part of the activation process.

Several subtypes of muscarinic receptors are found in the bladder. M_2 dominates quantitatively, whereas M_3 is the subtype that mediates the contractile response. The ratio between these is approximately 3:1. M_2 can also be of physiologic significance because it ensures the inhibition of other activity (e.g., adrenergic activity) as, for example, cyclic adenosine monophosphate activity, thereby helping to guarantee the vital emptying function. Receptors of the M_1 and M_4 subtypes are recovered prejunctionally. We do not know the roles of all of the subtypes.

The types of muscarinic receptors present in the lower urinary tract are not organ-specific, because drugs believed to affect them also affect other parts of the body. Many substances likely work together to ensure detrusor contraction and emptying of the bladder. In almost all types of animals, a contractile component is shown in tests with in vitro electrical field stimulation of detrusor preparations that are resistant to atropine, but sensitive to neurotoxins (atropine resistance). This type of response is also found in pathologic human bladder preparations, but is not seen in the normal human bladder. Many substances, such as peptides and purines, may still be involved in activating the bladder. The initial, phasic contractile response to bladder muscle stimulation is mediated via adenosine triphosphate acting on the P2X receptor, whereas the tonic contraction of long duration is a cholinergic response. It is logical to think of activation of the micturition reflex in several steps, as a cascade-like release of different substances. Bladder activation may be a condition for survival of all animal species and humans.

The emptying phase of the bladder is defined as the part of the emptying process in which the pressure in the bladder exceeds the pressure in the urethra, thus enabling urinary flow. However, the pressure in the urethra drops before flow is established. This drop in pressure precedes the initiation of bladder contraction, sometimes by several seconds. This is normally seen as a transition phase, but according to a new proposal, should be considered part of the emptying phase.[1] This small change in perspective probably means that neuromuscular activity other than cholinergic activity must be regarded as primary in the bladder-emptying phase. The mechanisms responsible for these functions are not fully known, but NO and various neuropeptides, such as CGRP, may be significant.[19-21] The abundant cholinergic innervation of the proximal urethra may contribute to funneling of the outflow from the bladder at emptying. This is the case in the urethra in rats,[22] but we do not know whether it is true for humans.

Adrenergic Outflow. Adrenergic innervation goes from Th10–L2 via the hypogastric nerves to the lower urinary tract and genitalia.[3] During filling, efferent adrenergic innervation activates the smooth muscle of the bladder outlet (i.e., the urethra) as well as the prostate in men. Noradrenaline is released from the adrenergic nerve terminals and especially stimulates alpha-1 receptors to activate the muscle cells of the bladder outlet or urethra, causing contraction. This contraction, especially of circular smooth muscle, contributes to the closing on the outflow side and thus to continence. Noradrenaline is released continually during the filling phase. Alpha-2 receptors are also present, but they are mainly localized prejunctionally and therefore participate in the automatic adjustment of transmitter release from the adrenergic nerve terminals.

To some extent, sparse adrenergic innervation of the bladder mediates relaxation of the detrusor musculature during filling by influencing beta receptors that mediate relaxation. Their physiologic role appears to be limited. In the human bladder, the dominating beta receptor seems to be beta-3.

The vesicosympathetic reflex is a negative feedback mechanism that allows inhibition of the bladder and thereby accommodates filling.[23] The adrenergic system does not appear to be vital to the function of the lower urinary tract, but an imbalance might occur if the adrenergic influence were manipulated. This system probably plays a role in various disorders. Adrenergic innervation, perhaps expressed as hyperinnervation, may have great significance for various disorders, such as obstruction and overactive bladder. This is seen in various animal models, and the situation might be similar in humans.

The stromal tissue component of the prostate also contains smooth muscle cells, and blockade of alpha-1 receptors is commonly used to relieve symptoms in patients with benign prostatic hyperplasia. Alpha receptors, especially alpha-1, are found in the spinal cord, and when these are influenced pharmacologically, the function of the lower urinary tract is affected.

NANC Nervous Influence. NANC mechanisms have significance for both efferent and afferent functions, peripheral as well as central. Besides purines, neuropeptides, such as substance P, CGRP, neurokinin A and B, neuropeptide Y, and vasoactive intestinal polypeptide (VIP), are present in the nerve fibers in the lower urinary tract. Their presence can be shown with immunohistochemical techniques, but the functional correlates are more difficult to study. Several neuropeptides probably have a neuromodulatory function, and some may be transmitters, together with classic substances, such as acetylcholine or noradrenaline. CGRP and the tachykinins substance P and neurokinin A and B are likely to be transmitters in sensory neurons. The release of neuropeptides is also believed to be significant for autofeedback at afferent nerve terminals (i.e., released peptides act at the threshold level at which the nerve terminal is discharging). Substance P and CGRP are abundant in submucosal sensory neurons, and substance P and VIP are present in the dorsal roots. Neurokinin A affects neurokinin receptors, NK2 in particular. Substance P, neurokinin A, and CGRP may also mediate neurogenic inflammation. Tachykinin receptor antagonists may affect bladder motility or reflexes that occur during different pathologic states, although they seem to have little influence on normal motor bladder function.[24]

Relaxation of the bladder neck and urethral smooth musculature appear to be mediated by NANC mechanisms. The first observations of NANC urethral relaxation were made almost 20 years ago.[25] A marked pressure drop in the urethra was induced preoperatively by stimulation at the sacral root level.[5] Relaxation on the outflow side occurs through several factors working together. Both somatic innervation and adrenergic nerve activity are inhibited. NANC mechanisms probably also play an important part in effective inhibition of neuromuscular activity that promotes filling. The fact that relaxation takes place on the outflow side and contraction makes funneling in the bladder neck area possible may be of significance.

NO appears to play a significant role,[19,26] and animal studies show that neuropeptides, such as CGRP, can induce considerable relaxation of the urethra in vitro and in vivo.[21,27] VIP seems to be important for other urogenital smooth muscle relaxation, as in erectile tissue, acting together with acetylcholine and NO. We do not know whether this constellation is also seen in the regulation of activity in the lower urinary tract, but VIP and Nitric Oxide Synthate (NOS) are colocalized in pelvic ganglionic cell bodies. We believe that NO plays an important role in both efferent and efferent nervous activity in the lower urinary tract.[19,26]

Somatic Nerve Function. Activation and inhibition of the striated musculature of the external sphincter and pelvic floor are vital for a smooth filling phase and effective emptying, respectively. The main efferent innervation of the rhabdosphincter originates in the motor neurons of Onuf's nucleus, located in the ventral horn of one or more segments of the sacral spinal cord.[3] With increased bladder filling, a reflexive increase occurs in the somatic pudendal flow to the striated musculature in the external sphincter and pelvic floor. An appropriate increase in pressure in the urethra occurs. Activation of the external sphincter musculature appears to be both phasic, or dynamic, and tonic, or static. Activation of the sphincter is inhibited at the same time that the emptying phase is initiated, and this continues throughout the emptying phase to ensure the least possible resistance against flow. A corresponding reduction in muscle activity is seen in the pelvic floor, again showing that all parts of the lower urinary tract are connected as one functioning unit.

The functional connection between the bladder and the pelvic floor or sphincter apparatus is reciprocal. The micturition reflex can be interrupted voluntarily, by contraction of the external sphincter or pelvic floor, or reflexively, for example, through dilation of the anal sphincter.[28,29] It is not known whether corresponding activation and inhibition occur in the external sphincter and affected parts of the pelvic floor. However, neuromuscular function in the areas of pudendal innervation is likely to be significant for the function of the lower urinary tract in health and disease.

Of considerable importance is the activation of the striated musculature in the external sphincter, mediated by the somatic nerve fibers in the pudendal nerve from S2–S4, the segments at which the cholinergic pelvic nerves originate. The degree of activity measured by electromyogram in the external sphincter and pelvic floor increases with the degree of bladder filling as more and more motor units are recruited. Increased tension in the external sphincter and pelvic floor activates tension receptors, producing afferent inhibitory feedback at the sacral level. This could explain why afferent activity from the bladder can be inhibited and helps to explain why voluntary control of the lower urinary tract is so effectively subordinate to the influence of the will. The existence of an inhibitory feedback function from the pelvic floor and urethral sphincter in humans has not been proved conclusively.

Central Nervous Influence on the Lower Urinary Tract

It is not likely that the pontine micturition center drives the micturition reflex by itself, like a pacemaker, although activation of the micturition reflex is often discussed in terms of a switch-like, on-and-off function.[23] However, as discussed earlier, this analogy may be too simple and does not include all of the different types of neuromuscular activity that affect the lower urinary tract. Figure 2-1 shows a possible pattern of nervous influence on the lower urinary tract during filling and emptying. For example, sensory activity is probably always "on" (i.e., during both filling and emptying). Facilitating and inhibiting stimuli of different origin balance each other during filling and emptying of the bladder.[30] The micturition reflex is discharged from the pons as a result of increasing afferent impulse traffic, which is a result of the filling of the bladder. In the pons, thresholds are set and coordination takes place.[31] The basal ganglia and the cerebellum also appear to be important to these objectives. This pontine and paraventricular gray area of the brain is inhibited by cerebral, conscious pathways developed early in life. Thus, on-and-off switching circuits in the brain and spinal cord are under voluntary control. Storage of urine is dependent in part on spinal reflex mechanisms that activate sympathetic and somatic pathways to the urethral outlet as well as on tonic inhibitory systems in the brain that suppress the parasympathetic outflow to the urinary bladder.[12,32,33] During storage, a low level of afferent discharge occurs as a result of bladder filling, which stimulates both adrenergic outflow to the bladder base and urethra and pudendal innervation of the external sphincter. A close relation between the nerve cells of Onuf's nucleus and the dendrites from autonomic nerve fibers suggests close connection and coordination at the spinal cord level.[34]

Functional imaging studies, such as cerebral positron emission tomography scans and magnetic resonance imaging scans, as well as experimental tracing techniques, have provided much new knowledge about the structure and organization of the central nervous system pathways and nuclei that control the lower urinary tract. Transneuronal virus tracing, injections of horseradish peroxidase into the end organ, and different coloring techniques have been used.[11,35] Glutamate, noradrenaline, acetylcholine, NO, and certain neuropeptides can be considered central nervous excitatory transmitters. Glutamic acid is the major excitatory transmitter in the central nervous system, and it appears to be important to the micturition reflex on several levels. Gamma-aminobutyric acid and enkephalin have an inhibiting tonic effect on the pontine micturition center. The monamines serotonin and noradrenaline promote filling.[36,37] Serotonin stimulates adrenergic nerve terminals and inhibits cholinergic nerve terminals. The serotoninergic pathways go from the paraventricular and pontine structures and the raphe nuclei to the sacral level.[11] Immunohistochemical studies show that many serotonin receptors are present in the dorsal horn, where they may influence incoming afferent stimuli, and in the ventral horn. In cats, serotonin appears to inhibit afferent sacral activity during the filling phase.[32,34] Adrenergic neurons exert an excitatory influence at the spinal cord level in a similar manner. This effect is probably mediated by alpha-1 receptors because it was inhibited by the selective alpha-1 blocker prazosin in animal studies.

Opioid receptors in the central nervous system also inhibit the micturition reflex. This inhibition is easily observed after spinal anesthesia with morphine derivatives, and can be used therapeutically.

The bladder musculature is inactive during filling, and excitatory stimuli are filtered or inhibited effectively so that the efferent cholinergic nerves of the bladder are not activated. At the same time, the afferent impulses from the bladder must be freely relayed to higher levels in the central nervous system so that the individual is conscious of the degree of bladder filling or, alternatively, warned of the need to empty the bladder.[38] As mentioned earlier, several central and peripheral mechanisms probably play a role in inhibiting activation of the micturition reflex.[40,41]

Sometimes it is appropriate to describe the collaboration between the nervous system and the lower urinary tract to evacuate the bladder in net terms, similar to vectors. A useful model with four different loops had been suggested.[39] This simplification is practical, because it does not require clinicians to describe individual pathway systems and signal substances, about which we have limited knowledge.

The four loops describe the following:

- **Cerebral inhibition of the pontine micturition center (loop I)**. Cerebral inhibition of the pontine micturition center is not yet developed in small children; it occurs during the first years of life. The neuronal correlation to this function is not known, but gamma-aminobutyric acid, enkephalins, and acetylcholine inhibit the pontine micturition center, and serotonin, for example, can inhibit descending motoric pathways starting at this level.[23] Dopamine has a stimulating affect.
- **Micturition reflex (loop II)**. The micturition reflex represents all levels from the pons to the lower urinary tract. In principle, it consists of an afferent limb and an efferent limb. The micturition reflex has a built-in drive that always discharges, but is stopped by inhibitory mechanisms at several levels. The afferent information from the lower urinary tract seems to be relayed continually, and the intensity of the signal traffic during the filling phase is proportional to the degree of bladder filling. The origin of efferent activity that leads to urethral relaxation and bladder contraction is inhibited at the pontine and spinal levels.
- **Coordination between the bladder and sphincter (loop III)**. Coordination between different parts of

the lower urinary tract is vital for maintenance of continence during the filling phase and for effective emptying, with the least possible resistance to flow, during the emptying phase. This coordination occurs in the pontine micturition center, under the influence of the basal ganglia and cerebellum.

- **Ability to deliberately interrupt micturition (loop IV).** The ability to voluntarily control the lower urinary tract, to release the inhibition of the micturition reflex or interrupt an ongoing micturition process, is of great importance. Normal individuals can interrupt the micturition reflex by squeezing.

CONCLUSION

Normal nervous control of the urinary tract is important for each individual as well as in an evolutionary perspective for the human race. It is a robust and normally effective system that has many components that perform reciprocal tasks. The communication pattern and trophic dependence among ingoing cellular elements, nerves, and muscle cells is not fully understood. We have probably just begun to understand the interdependency of the lower urinary tract and the central nervous system. For a long time, nervous activity in the lower urinary tract was labeled cholinergic, adrenergic, or somatic, but should also be seen as NANC. A greater understanding will be achieved when we learn more about afferent and efferent mechanisms, when the role of the urethra is included as frequently as the role of the bladder, and when the events in the central nervous system that are important for the action of the lower urinary tract are understood. The current goal-oriented, interdisciplinary clinical and research studies are likely to answer many of these questions.

REFERENCES

1. Mattiasson A: Characterisation of lower urinary tract disorders: A new view. Neurourol Urodyn 20:601–621, 2001.
2. Elbadawi A: Neuromorphologic basis of vesicourethral function: I. Histochemistry, ultrastructure and function of intrinsic nerves in the bladder and urethra. Neurourol Urodyn 1:3–50, 1982.
3. Gosling JA, Dixon JS, Jen PYP: The distribution of noradrenergic nerves in the human lower urinary tract. Eur Urol 36 (suppl 1):23–30, 1999.
4. Yoshimura N, De Groat WC: Neural control of the lower urinary tract. J Urol 4:111, 1997.
5. Torrens MJ, Morrison JFB (eds): The Physiology of the Lower Urinary Tract. New York, Springer-Verlag, 1987.
6. Mattiasson A: Physiology of continence. In O'Donnell (ed): Urinary Incontinence. St. Louis, Mosby, 1997, pp 25–33.
7. Steers WD, Kolbeck S, Creedon D, Tuttle JB: Nerve growth factor in the urinary bladder of the adult regulates neuronal form and function. J Clin Invest 88:1709–1715, 1991.
8. Persson K, Steers WD, Tuttle JB: Regulation of nerve growth factor secretion in smooth muscle cells cultured from rat bladder body, base and urethra. J Urol 157:2000–2006, 1997.
9. Lapides J, Sweet RB, Lewis LW: Role of striated muscle in urination. J Urol 77:247–250, 1957.
10. Maggi CA, Meli A: The sensory-efferent function of capsaicin-sensitive sensory neurons. Gen Pharmacol 19:1–43, 1988.
11. De Groat WC, Downie JW, Levin RM, et al: Basic neurophysiology and neuropharmacology. In Abrams P, Khoury S, Wein A (eds): Incontinence: First International Consultation on Incontinence, 1998, pp 105–154.
12. Morrison JFB, Spillane K: Neuropharmacological studies on descending inhibitory controls over the micturition reflex. J Auton Nerv Syst 16:393–397, 1986.
13. Wein AJ: Neuromuscular dysfunction of the lower urinary tract. In Walsh PC, Stamey TA, Vaughan ED (eds): Campbell's Urology, 6th ed. Philadelphia, Harcourt, 1992, pp 573–642.
14. De Groat WC, Saum WR: Synaptic transmission in parasympathetic ganglia in the urinary bladder of the cat. J Physiol 256(1):137–158, 1976.
15. Mattiasson A, Andersson KE, Elbadawi A, et al: Interaction between adrenergic and cholinergic nerve terminals in the urinary bladder of rabbit, cat and man. J Urol 137:1017–1019, 1987.
16. Burnstock G: Innervation of bladder and bowel. Ciba Found Symp 151:2–18; discussion 18–26, 1990.
17. Dunn PM, Zhong Y, Burnstock G: P2X receptors in peripheral neurons. Prog Neurobiol 65:107–134, 2001.
18. Birder LA, Apodaca G, de Groat WC, Kanai AJ: Adrenergic- and capsaicin-evoked nitric oxide release from urothelium and afferent nerves in urinary bladder. Am J Physiol 275:F226–F229, 1998.
19. Andersson KE, Persson K: Nitric oxide synthase and nitric oxide–mediated effects in lower urinary tract smooth muscles. World J Urol 12:274–280, 1994.
20. Bennett BC, Kruse MN, Roppolo JR, et al: Neural control of urethral outlet activity in vivo: Role of nitric oxide. J Urol 153:2004–2009, 1995.
21. Radzizewski P, Mattiasson A, Malmberg L, Soller W: CGRP and substance P induce pronounced motor effects in the female rat urethra in vivo. Scand J Urol Nephrol 37:275–280, 2003.
22. Masuda H, Tsujii T, Azuma H, Oshima H: Role of a central muscarinic cholinergic pathway for relaxation of the proximal urethra during the voiding phase in rats. J Urol 165:999–1003, 2001.
23. De Groat WC: Central nervous system control of micturition. In O'Donnell PD (ed): Urinary Incontinence. St. Louis, Mosby, 1997, pp 33–47.
24. Lecci A, Maggi CA: Tachykinins as modulators of the micturition reflex in the central and peripheral nervous system. Regul Pept 101:1–18, 2001.
25. Andersson KE, Mattiasson A, Sjogren C: Electrically induced relaxation of the noradrenaline contracted isolated urethra from rabbit and man. J Urol 129:210–214, 1983.
26. Brading AF: The physiology of the mammalian urinary outflow tract. Exp Physiol 84:215–221, 1999.
27. Parlani M, Conte B, Goso C, Szallasi A, Manzini S: Capsaicin–induced relaxation in the rat isolated external urethral sphincter: Characterization of the vanilloid receptor and mediation by CGRP. Br J Pharm 110:989, 1993.
28. Barrington F: The relation of the hindbrain to micturition. Brain 44:23, 1921.
29. Pompeius R: Detrusor inhibition induced from anal region in man. Acta Chir Scand Suppl 361:1–54, 1966.
30. Chai TC, Steers WD: Neurophysiology of micturition and continence in women. Int Urogynecol J Pelvic Floor Dysfunct 8:85–97, 1997.
31. Nishizawa O, Sugaya K, Shimoda N: Pontine and spinal modulation of the micturition reflex. Scand J Urol Nephrol Suppl 175:15–19, 1995.

32. McMahon SB, Spillane K: Brain stem influences on the parasympathetic supply to the urinary bladder of the cat. Brain Res 234:237–249, 1982.
33. De Groat WC: Anatomy of the central nervous pathways controlling the lower urinary tract. Eur Urol 34 (suppl 1): 2–5, 1998.
34. Thor KB, Morgan C, Nadelhaft I, et al: Organization of afferent and efferent pathways in the pudendal nerve of the female cat. J Comp Neurol 288:263–279, 1989.
35. Nadelhaft I, Vera PL, Card JP, et al: Central nervous system neurons labelled following injection of psudorabies virus into the rat urinary bladder. Neurosci Lett 143(1–2):271–274, 1992.
36. Danuser H, Bemis K, Thor KB: Pharmacological analysis of the noradrenergic control of central sympathetic and somatic reflexes controlling the lower urinary tract in the anesthetized cat. J Pharmacol Exp Ther 274:820–825, 1995.
37. Danuser H, Thor KB: Spinal 5–HT2 receptor–mediated facilitation of pudendal nerve reflexes in the anaesthetized cat. Br J Pharmacol 118:150–154, 1996.
38. Lumb BM: Brainstem control of visceral afferent pathways in the spinal cord. Prog Brain Res 67:279–293, 1986.
39. Bradley WE: Physiology of the urinary bladder. In Walsh PC, Gittes R, Perlmutter A, Stamey T (eds): Campbell's Urology, ed 5. Philadelphia, Saunders, 1986.
40. Levin RM: Overview of nerves and pharmacology in the bladder. Adv Exp Med Biol 462:237–240, 1999.
41. Thor KB, Muhlhauser MA, Sauerberg P, et al: Central muscarinic inhibition of lower urinary tract nociception. Brain Res 870:126–134, 2000.

CHAPTER 3

Physiology of Anal Continence and Defecation

FRANÇOIS MION

The physiology of anal continence and defecation is a complex process that involves both autonomous and voluntary reactions. The anus and rectum are essential in this physiologic act, but other factors also play a role, including stool consistency, motility and absorptive and secretive processes of the colon, and psychological and social factors. For example, the definition of normal bowel habits varies widely throughout the world, depending on factors such as diet, culture or religion, and individual psychosomatic feelings. This chapter discusses the rectoanal physiology associated with continence and defecation. Rectoanal physiology is very specialized and is closer to the physiology of the bladder than to that of the rest of the digestive tract.

CONTINENCE

Continence relies on a capacitive organ, the rectum, which acts as a reservoir, and a resistive component, the anal canal. It also requires a specific sensitivity that allows the individual to interpret rectal distension as a call to stool and to discriminate between flatus and liquid or solid stool.

Capacitive Compartment

The rectum is usually empty: stool is stored in the left and sigmoid colon. The rectosigmoid junction is a sharp angle that acts as an open sphincter. The motor activity of this area is significantly greater than that of the adjacent sigmoid and rectum, delineating a high-pressure zone. Stool fills the rectum only when propelled by peristaltic contractions of the colon.

The viscoelastic properties of the rectum allow this organ to accommodate large volumes of stool at low pressure. Intramural reflexes, mediated by nonadrenergic, noncholinergic neurons, also determine the receptive relaxation of the rectum. An electronic barostat, which maintains constant pressure in an intrarectal bag by inflating or releasing gas, allows rectal tone to be measured.

Although minor tone variations occur during fasting periods, the ingestion of a standard meal significantly and rapidly increases rectal tone.[1] This rectal response persists in patients with parasympathetic sacral nerve lesions.[2]

Distension of the rectal wall produces a conscious feeling of the need to defecate. Evoked potentials can be obtained in the cerebral cortex in response to rectal distension.[3] However, the capacitive characteristics of the rectum allow differing evacuation of stool; this phenomenon is associated with a disappearance of the conscious feeling of rectal fullness. This capacitive adaptation has its limits, however; for a certain degree of distension, an urgent need is felt, associated with a reflex relaxation of the internal and external anal sphincters.

The rectal sensation is dependent on the extrinsic parasympathetic nerve supply; in the absence of this innervation pathway, rectal distension is perceived only as vague abdominal discomfort. Integrity of the sensitive spinal cord pathways is mandatory for the sensation of rectal filling: lesions of the spinal cord above the lumbosacral level abolish rectal sensation.[4]

Resistive Compartment

The resistive compartment is represented by the anal sphincters.

The internal sphincter is composed of smooth muscle, and it corresponds to a thickening of the circular layer of the digestive muscle. This sphincter has permanent tonic contractile activity that is controlled in part by its extrinsic innervation. Destruction of the sacral nerves or a section of the hypogastric nerves significantly decreases anal pressure (Fig. 3-1). The nervous center is situated in the lumbosacral spinal cord, and anal pressure at rest is similar in normal subjects and patients with spinal cord lesions. Finally, internal sphincter activity is independent of rectal or anal afferent effects; anesthesia of the rectum or anus does not decrease anal pressure. The internal sphincter is mainly responsible for baseline continence; internal sphincter dysfunction causes passive soiling.

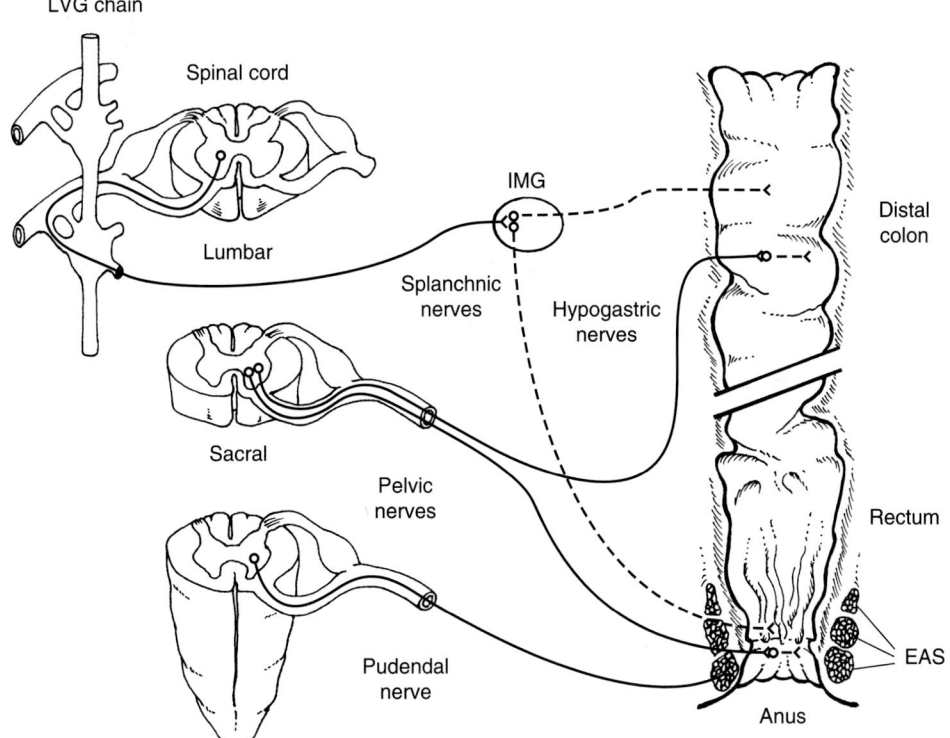

FIGURE 3-1 Motor innervations of smooth and striated muscles of the rectoanal region. EAS, external anal sphincter; IMG, inferior mesenteric sympathetic ganglia; LVG, laterovertebral ganglionic sympathetic chain.

The external sphincter is composed of striated muscle. This muscle is continuous with the puborectal part of the pelvic floor, the puborectalis muscle, which determines an 80-degree rectoanal angle. Two other muscular slings compose the external sphincter: the median sling is attached posteriorly to the coccyx, and the superficial sling is attached anteriorly to the anal skin (Fig. 3-2). This sphincter is characterized by tonic contractile activity and by bouts of reflex or voluntary phasic contractions.

The activity of these muscles creates a high-pressure zone (5–9 kPa) within the anal canal. At rest, this pressure is greater than the intra-abdominal or rectal pressure, thus guaranteeing anal continence. The rectoanal angle is also an important factor in continence. Certain actions, including speaking, singing, coughing, sneezing, lifting a load, and rising from a chair, increase intra-abdominal pressure to 20 kPa; this pressure is transmitted to the rectum. Continence is maintained by reflex contraction of the external sphincter and the puborectalis muscle. The origin of this reflex is spinal, and it is maintained in patients with suprasacral section of the spinal cord. Voluntary contraction of the external sphincter can significantly increase anal pressure for a limited time (1–2 minutes), when confronted with an urgent need to defecate.

Thus, reflex and voluntary contraction of the external sphincter acts fully as an emergency control of anal continence. Dysfunction of this sphincter is characterized by urgent stool and a short interval between the feeling of the need to defecate and defecation.

Passive mechanisms may help to maintain anal continence during increases of intra-abdominal pressure. Transmission of intra-abdominal pressure to the

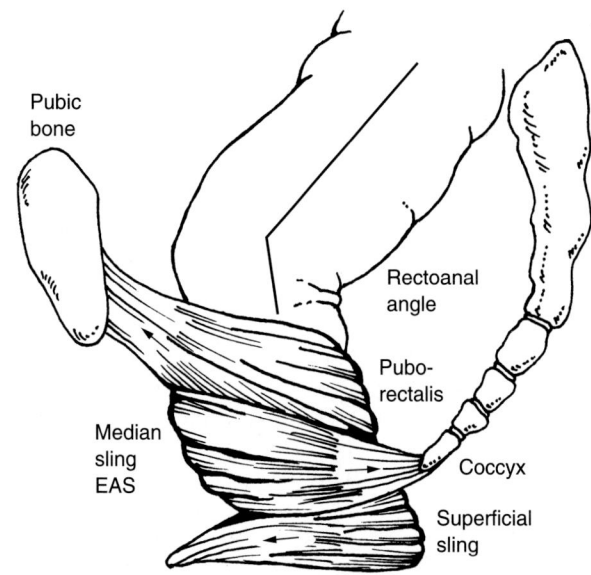

FIGURE 3-2 Triple-loop organization of the external anal sphincter (EAS). The upper sling is represented by the puborectalis muscle, attached anteriorly to the pubis; the median loop of the external sphincter is attached posteriorly to the coccyx; the third most superficial loop is attached to the perineal skin. (Adapted from Shafik A: A new concept of the anatomy of the anal sphincter mechanism and the physiology of defecation: The external anal sphincter. A triple-loop system. Invest Urol 12:412–419,1975).

side of the anal canal at the rectoanal junction may act as a flutter valve to maintain continence. Some described the existence of a flap valve in which the increase in intra-abdominal pressure flattens the anterior part of the rectum into the lumen at the level of the rectoanal angle.[5] Increases in intra-abdominal pressure are associated with proportional increases in anal pressure, although anal pressure always remains higher (Fig. 3-3). Thus, the conditions for a flutter or flap valve to act are not present physiologically. In anal incontinence, intra-abdominal pressure often exceeds anal pressure; the putative passive valves are insufficient to maintain continence.

Rectosphincteric Reflexes

Filling of the rectum with gas or stool distends the rectal wall and produces three different reflexes: propulsive rectal contraction (rectorectal reflex), relaxation of the internal sphincter (rectoanal inhibitory reflex), and contraction of the external sphincter (rectoanal excitatory reflex). In ambulatory persons, the sensation of flatus is associated with increased rectal pressure and decreased anal pressure.[6] This reflex activity persists after spinal cord lesions, but is suppressed by anesthesia of the rectal mucosa.

The efferent pathways responsible for relaxation of the internal sphincter involve nonadrenergic, noncholinergic neurotransmitters, such as nitric oxide[7] and vasoactive intestinal polypeptide.[8] The intramural nature of this inhibitory reflex is shown by its absence in Hirschsprung's disease, which is characterized by colorectal aganglionosis, and the reflex can be modulated by extrinsic nerves.

The rectoanal excitatory reflex protects continence and is acquired during toilet training in childhood. In newborns, rectal distension induces relaxation of both sphincters and stool passing. The afferent pathway involves the pelvic nerves, and the efferent limb involves the pudendal nerve. Puborectalis contraction persists after pudendal block, indicating that this muscle receives nerve endings from the pelvic plexus.

Sampling reflex is the rectosphincteric response to rectal distension.[9] Simultaneous contraction of the rectum and relaxation of the upper segment of the anal canal allows the rectal contents to enter the anal canal. The sensitive anal mucosa samples the physical nature of the contents (gas or liquid or solid stool) to determine the appropriate voluntary action (passing of flatus or voluntary contraction to maintain continence).

Integrative View of Anal Continence

Most of the time, stool is stored in the left and sigmoid colon. The rectum is usually empty, but its viscoelastic properties permit a relaxative adaptation to incoming stools and to differ evacuation. The primary role of the rectum is to create a delay between the rectal distension that elicits a conscious sensation of rectal feeling and the one that initiates reflex relaxation of both sphincters.

The resistive compartment is composed of the internal sphincter, which is responsible for baseline continence, and the external sphincter, which controls emergency continence. The puborectalis muscle also plays an important role by maintaining a permanent rectoanal angle. A more pronounced angle requires lower anal pressure to maintain continence. Finally, rectal and anal sensitivity plays a crucial role in continence: rectosphincteric reflexes constantly adapt pressures to the rectal contents and the social environment of the subject to determine the appropriateness of continence, passing flatus, or defecation.

DEFECATION

The controlling influence of the cerebral cortex makes defecation a complex process in humans. This process starts with a rectal sensation; often, the cortex inhibits this sensation and defecation is delayed. Conditioning is of great importance: acute lifestyle changes (e.g., traveling, hospitalization) can durably inhibit defecation.[10] Voluntary initiation of defecation is the rule in adults; however, perineal cutaneous stimulation causes reflex defecation in patients with spinal lesions.[4] Animal experiments confirmed the existence of a lumbosacral center that controls defecation.

Several motor actions are involved in defecation, and their timing differs from person to person. The squatting position, with the hips flexed more than 90 degrees, straightens the rectoanal angle.[11] X-ray defecography shows that the initiation of defecation is characterized by descent of the pelvic floor and relaxation of the

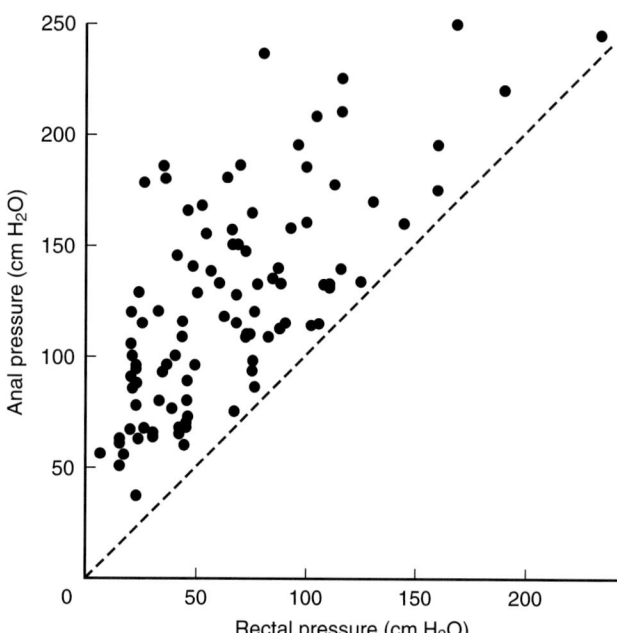

FIGURE 3-3 Variations in reflex anal pressure in relation to increasing intra-abdominal pressure. Measured anal pressures are always higher than rectal pressures in control subjects. (From Bannister JJ, Gibbons C, Read NW: Preservation of faecal continence during rises in intra-abdominal pressure: Is there a role for the flap valve? Gut 28:1242–1245, 1987. Reprinted with permission from BMJ Publishing Group.)

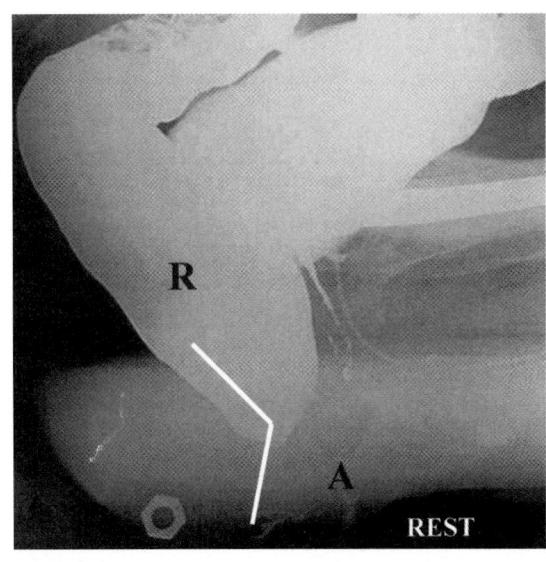

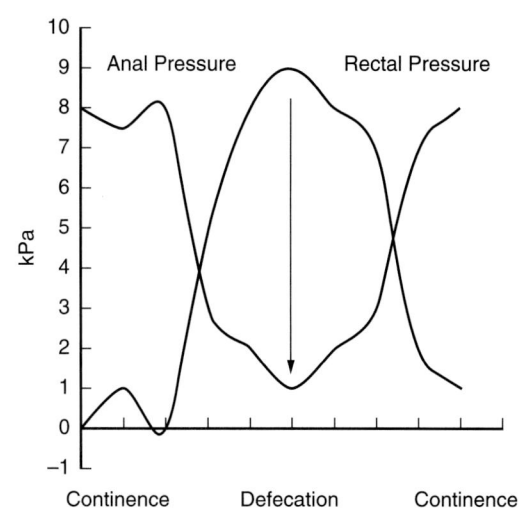

FIGURE 3-5 Variations in rectoanal pressure during defecation. The increased rectal pressure associated with relaxation of the anal sphincters allows evacuation of stool.

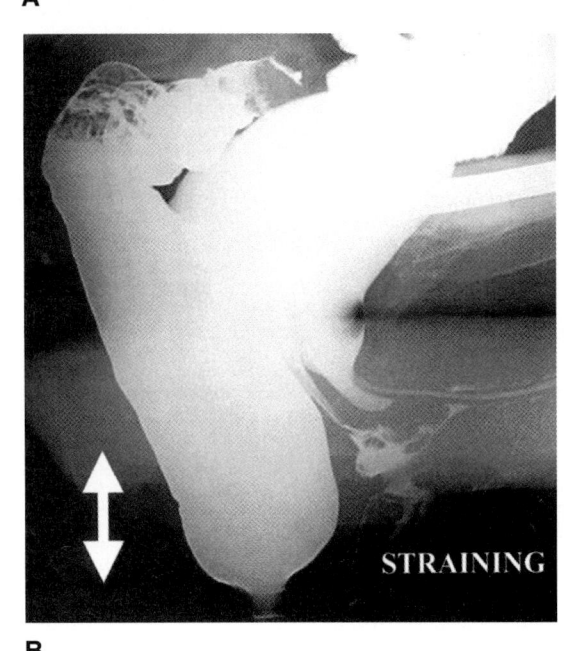

FIGURE 3-4 Pelvic viscerogram at rest (**A**) and during straining (**B**), showing lowering of the pelvic floor (*vertical arrow*) and disappearance of the rectoanal angle during straining. A, anus; R, rectum. (Courtesy of Dr. L. Henry.)

puborectalis muscle.[12] These two factors contribute to the disappearance of the rectoanal angle (Fig. 3-4). A voluntary straining effort (Valsalva maneuver) consists of a fixed lowered diaphragm, contraction of the abdominal muscles, and expiration with a closed glottis. This maneuver substantially increases intra-abdominal pressure.[10] Straining makes a fundamental difference compared with micturition, which is performed without abdominal contraction. Increasing intra-abdominal pressure overcomes anal pressure and leads to the passing of stool through the anal canal (Fig. 3-5). Unconscious mass peristalsis may occur simultaneously within the distal colon, clearing the bowel at once.[13] In other cases, stool is passed after several straining efforts. At the end of defecation, the puborectalis muscle and the external sphincter contract rapidly and complete the discharge of stool, and the rectoanal apparatus regains its baseline anatomic and functional characteristics.

REFERENCES

1. Bell AM, Pemberton JH, Hanson RB, et al: Variations in muscle tone of the human rectum: Recordings with an electromechanical barostat. Am J Physiol 260:G17–G25, 1991.
2. Leroi AM, Saiter C, Roussignol C, et al: Increased tone of the rectal wall in response to feeding persists in patients with cauda equina syndrome. Neurogastroenterol Motil 11:243–245, 1999.
3. Collet L, Meunier P, Duclaux R, et al: Cerebral evoked potentials after endorectal mechanical stimulation in humans. Am J Physiol 254:G477–G482, 1988.
4. MacDonagh R, Sun WM, Thomas DG, et al: Anorectal function in patients with complete supraconal spinal cord lesions. Gut 33:1532–1538, 1992.
5. Henry MM, Swash M: Faecal continence, defaecation and colorectal motility. In Henry MM, Swash M (eds): Coloproctology and the pelvic floor. London, Butterworths, 1985, pp 42–47.
6. Miller R, Lewis GT, Bartolo DC, et al: Sensory discrimination and dynamic activity in the anorectum: Evidence using a new ambulatory technique. Br J Surg 75:1003–1007, 1988.
7. O'Kelly T, Brading A, Mortensen N: Nerve mediated relaxation of the human internal anal sphincter: The role of nitric oxide. Gut 34:689–693, 1993.
8. Nurko S, Rattan S: Role of vasoactive intestinal polypeptide in the internal anal sphincter relaxation of the opossum. J Clin Invest 81:1146–1153, 1988.
9. Duthie HL, Bennett RC: The relation of sensation in the anal canal to the functional anal sphincter: A possible factor in anal continence. Gut 4:179–182, 1963.

10. Meunier P: Continence fécale et défécation. In Meunier P, Minaire Y, Lambert R (eds): La Digestion, 2nd ed. Paris, SIMEP, 1976, pp 176–182.
11. Tagart REB: The anal canal and the rectum: Their varying relationship and its effect on anal continence. Dis Colon Rectum 9:442–449, 1966.
12. Mahieu P, Pringot J, Bodart P: Defecography: I. Description of a new procedure and results in normal patients. Gastrointest Radiol 9:247–251, 1984.
13. Duthie HL: Physiology of the anus, rectum and colon. In Goligher J (ed): Surgery of the Anus, Rectum, and Colon, 5th ed. London, Baillière Tindall, 1984, pp 29–47.

CHAPTER 4

Normal Sexual Function in Women

JENNIFER R. BERMAN

Sexual function is a complex, multicomponent biologic process that comprises central mechanisms for regulation of libido and arousability and local mechanisms for arousal and orgasm in women. Both the central nervous system and peripheral nervous system are involved in normal sexual function in women.

Until recently, little basic science or clinical research has focused on female sexuality. One major barrier to research in this field is the absence of a well-defined diagnostic classification system. The 1998 American Foundation of Urologic Disease (AFUD) Consensus Conference updated the definitions and classifications based on current research and clinical practice. The definitions were broadened to include both psychogenic and organically based dysfunctions.

THE FEMALE SEXUAL RESPONSE CYCLE

Originally, Masters and Johnson outlined a progressive, three-phase sexual response cycle, consisting of arousal, orgasm, and resolution.[1] In 1974, Kaplan proposed another component, desire, and a new three-phase model, consisting of desire, arousal, and orgasm, with desire being the factor inciting the overall response cycle.[2] Subsequently, sexologists attempting to treat patients who chronically fail to initiate or respond to sexual stimuli added an initial phase of desire to the sexual response.[3] They characterized the female sexual response as consisting of four successive phases: excitement, plateau, orgasm, and resolution.[4,5] The American Psychiatric Association's *Diagnostic and Statistical Manual of Mental Disorders* (DSM-IV) describes the sexual response cycle as four related, but neurophysiologically discrete, phases: appetitive, desire, or libido; arousal or excitement; orgasm or climax; and refractory or resolution.[6] This phase model is the basis for the DSM-IV definition of female sexual dysfunction as well as the recent reclassification system proposed by the AFUD Consensus Panel in October 1998.[7] Others recently suggested that sexual function should be considered a circuit, with four main domains: libido, arousal, orgasm, and satisfaction. Each aspect may overlap or negatively or positively feed back on the other domains.[8]

During sexual arousal, the clitoris and labia minora become engorged with blood and increase in diameter. Masters and Johnson observed that, during sexual excitement, the labia minora increase in diameter by two to three times and consequently become everted, exposing their inner surface.[1]

FEMALE PELVIC ANATOMY

A formal understanding of female pelvic anatomy is fundamental to the evaluation and treatment of female sexual dysfunction. Although female pelvic anatomy comprises a continuum of organs interrelated in structure and function, it is helpful to group these organs into two categories: external and internal genitalia. The organs of the external genitalia are collectively known as the vulva, an area that is bound anteriorly by the symphsis pubis, posteriorly by the anal sphincter, and laterally by the ischial tuberosities. The vulva consists of the labia, interlabial space, clitoris, and vestibular bulbs. The organs of the internal genitalia include the vagina, uterus, fallopian tubes, and ovaries.

The Vagina

The vagina is a midline cylindric organ that connects the uterus with the external genitalia. It is usually 7 to 15 cm long, depending on the position of the uterus. It can easily dilate and expand for intercourse and childbirth. Anteriorly, two pleats of sensitive tissue, the labia minora (inner lips), surround the opening of the vagina and are further protected by the larger folds known as the labia majora (outer lips). The labia minora enclose an area called the vestibule, which contains the clitoris, urethral opening, and vaginal opening. The portion of the labia minora that covers the clitoris is known as the prepuce, or clitoral hood.

The wall of the vagina has three layers: an inner aglandular mucous membrane epithelium, an intermediary richly supplied vascular muscularis layer, and an outer adventitial supportive mesh. The middle muscularis portion is highly infiltrated with smooth muscle and an extensive tree of blood vessels that engorge during sexual arousal. The surrounding outer fibrosa layer provides structural support to the vagina. The vagina has many rugae that are necessary for distensibility of the organ; these are more prominent in the lower third. Smaller ridges increase frictional tension during intercourse.[9,10]

Blood Supply to the Vagina

The vagina has an extensive anastomotic network of blood vessels throughout its length. The main arterial supply arises from vaginal branches of the uterine arteries, pudendal arteries (vaginal branches), and ovarian arteries.

Innervation of the Vagina

Autonomic innervation of the vagina originates from two separate plexuses: the superior hypogastric and pelvic plexuses. Sympathetic fibers originate in the lateral gray column of T11–L2 and form the hypogastric plexuses. Parasympathetic fibers originate in the intermediolateral cell column of S2–S4 and synapse in the pelvic plexus. Sympathetic and parasympathetic nerve fibers leave the pelvic plexus and travel within the uterosacral and cardinal ligaments, along with the vessels, to supply the proximal two thirds of the vagina and the corporal bodies of the clitoris. Somatic motor fibers originate from the anterior horns of sacral cord levels S2–S4 and travel within the pudendal nerve to innervate the bulbocavernosus and ishiocavernosus muscles. Sensory fibers that innervate the introitus and perinuem travel within the perineal and posterior labial nerves to the pudendal nerve.[9,10]

Immunohistochemical studies show more nerve fibers in the distal vagina than in the more proximal part. When performing bladder suspension procedures and vaginal hysterectomies, it is important to be aware of this area of increased innervation because it plays an important role in sexual function.

Physiologic Changes in the Vagina during Sexual Arousal

During sexual arousal, genital vasocongestion occurs as a result of increased blood flow. The vaginal canal is lubricated by secretions from uterine glands and from a transudate that originates from the subepithelial vascular bed. These secretions are passively transported through the intraepithelial spaces, or intercellular channels. Engorgement of the vaginal wall raises pressure inside the capillaries and increases the transudation of plasma through the vaginal epithelium.[11] This vaginal lubricative plasma flows through the epithelium onto the surface of the vagina, initially forming sweat-like droplets that coalesce to form a lubricative film that covers the vaginal wall. Additional moistening during intercourse comes from secretions of the paired greater vestibular (Bartholin's) glands, although some believe that these glands have a more primal function of emitting an odiferous fluid to attract the male. In addition to lubricating, during sexual arousal, the vagina lengthens and dilates through relaxation of the vaginal wall smooth muscle. In human and animal models, sexual stimulation causes increased vaginal blood flow and decreased vaginal luminal pressure.[12] Despite many inaccurate accounts in physiology textbooks, vaginal lubrication during sexual arousal does not occur as a result of increased secretion from vaginal glands, cervical fluid, or Bartholin's glands.[13] On sexual arousal, the blood supply to the vaginal epithelium is rapidly increased by neural innervation via the sacral anterior nerves S2–S4.[14]

The vagina is the passageway between the vulva and the uterine cervix, and its function as the coital organ requires morphologic and physiologic versatility. The vagina undergoes marked physical changes in response to psychogenic and somatogenic erotic stimuli, and it can affect the perception of pleasurable sensation during coitus as a result of its pressure areas.

The Clitoris

In 1974, Kaplan described the clitoris as a "small knob" of tissue located below the symphysis pubis, a reflection of the shortcomings of anatomic literature at that time.[2] Current findings on dissection of adult female human cadavers have been interpreted to indicate that the organ is a triplanar complex of erectile tissue with a midline shaft lying in the medial sagittal plane. It is about 2 to 4 cm long and 1 to 2 cm wide, and bifurcates internally into paired curved crura that are 5 to 9 cm long. The external aspect of the clitoris includes the glans that is approximately 20 to 30 mm long, with a similar diameter.[13] The clitoris is not displayed as a three-dimensional structure, but rather as if it were flat against the pubic symphysis. In anatomy texts, the size of the clitoris is not depicted accurately, and its neurovascular supply is rarely described. The bulbs are often omitted, or if described, their relationship to other cavernous tissue is not described. Most of the female urogenital tissues are internal and relatively obscured, making investigations difficult.

The clitoris is an erectile organ similar to the penis, and it arises from the same embryologic structure, the genital tubercle. It is composed of three parts: the outermost glans, or head; the middle corpus, or body; and the innermost crura. The glans and body of the clitoris are 2 to 4 cm long, and the crura are 9 to 11 cm long.[9,10] The clitoris consists of fused midline erectile bodies (corpora cavernosa) that give rise to bilateral crura. The glans clitoris is visible as it emerges from the labia minora. The labia minora bifurcate to form the upper prepuce anteriorly and the lower frenulum posteriorly. Each corporus cavernosum is ensheathed by a thick, fibrous connective tissue structure, the tunica albuginea, which covers the lacunar sinusoids. These are surrounded by a trabecula of vascular smooth muscle and collagen fibers. The tunica albuginea in the clitoris is unilaminar, unlike the bilaminar structure found in the penis. Thus, no mechanism for venous trapping exists within the clitoris; consequently, sexual stimulation results in clitoral engorgement, but not erection. The two separate crura of the clitoris, formed from the separation of the most proximal parts of the corpora in the perineum, attach bilaterally to the undersurface of the pubis, along the ishiopubic rami. Studies show a strong link between increased age and decreased clitoral nerve cavernosal smooth muscle fibers, indicating that aging women undergo histologic changes in clitoral cavernosal erectile tissue.

Blood Supply to the Clitoris

The main arterial supply to the clitoris is via the iliohypogastric pudendal arterial bed. The internal pudendal artery is the last anterior branch of the internal iliac artery and traverses Alcock's canal to terminate as the inferior rectal, perineal, and common clitoral arteries. The common clitoral artery continues to the clitoris and bifurcates into a dorsal clitoral artery and two clitoral cavernosal arteries.

Physiologic Changes in the Clitoris during Sexual Arousal

With sexual stimulation, increased blood flow to the clitoral cavernosal arteries results in increased clitoral intracavernosus pressure and tumescence and protrusion of the glans. Studies show that, unlike the penis, the clitoris lacks a subalbuginealal layer between the erectile tissue and the tunica albuginea. In the male, this layer has a rich venous plexus that expands against the tunica albuginea during sexual excitement, reducing venous outflow and making the penis rigid. The absence of this venous plexus in the clitoris allows this organ to achieve tumescence, but not rigidity, during sexual arousal. Duplex ultrasonography of the clitoris shows that during sexual simulation, the clitoris increases in length and diameter and blood flow almost doubles.[12]

In conclusion, with effective sexual stimulation, the clitoris becomes tumescent, or swollen, but does not become erect or rigid.[15] As in the penis, nitric oxide (NO) may help to control clitoral flow; it also helps to regulate human clitoral corpus cavernosum smooth muscle tone.[16]

The Vestibular Bulbs

The vestibular bulbs, which are 3 cm long, are paired structures that lie along the sides of the vaginal orifice, directly beneath the skin of the labia minora. Although they are homologous to the corpus spongiosum of the penis and are composed of vascular smooth muscle, they are distinct in that they are separated from the clitoris, urethra, and vestibule of the vagina. Recent cadaver dissections showed that in young premenopausal women, the bulbs lie on the superficial aspect of the vaginal wall and do not form the core of the labia minora. Furthermore, considerable age-related variations in the dimensions of the erectile tissue are observed between young, premenopausal women and older, postmenopausal women.[17] The main arterial supply to the vestibular bulbs is via the bulbar, inferior perineal, and posterior labial branches of the internal pudendal artery.

The somatic sensory innervation of the labia minora travels via the perineal and posterior labial branches of the pudendal nerve. Autonomic innervation consists of sympathetic and parasympathetic fibers that travel with the vessels to reach the vestibular bulb.

In the labia minora, during sexual stimulation, blood flow increases, particularly to the vestibular bulbs. This increase in blood flow causes a twofold to threefold increase in the diameter of the labia, leading to eversion and exposure of its inner surface.

The Uterus

During sexual arousal, the uterine and cervical glands secrete mucus to lubricate the vagina. The cervix has the second highest concentration of vasoactive intestinal polypetide (VIP) of the female genitals, yet no function has been ascribed to the VIPergic innervation. The innervation of the uterus is closely proximate to the bladder and vagina, and pelvic dissection, as it is currently performed, can adversely affect a woman's sexual health by damaging uterine innervation. Uterine and other pelvic surgical procedures also can significantly affect female sexual response and function.

The cervix is a relatively insensitive structure, with no erotogenic capabilities per se.[13] However, some authors suggest that sexually pleasurable feelings can occur when it is jostled or buffeted by deep penile thrusting.[16]

Contact between the penis and the cervix was not observed in the missionary, or face-to-face, position, but Riley and colleagues[18] found that it could occur in the rear-entry sideways and rear positions. Even hysterectomy alone, without removal of the ovaries, can result in sexual dysfunction.[19] In some women who had the cervix or uterus removed, a significant loss in sexual arousal and orgasm by coitus was reported,[20] but others reported no differences.

After hysterectomy, women commonly experience decreased desire, decreased arousal, decreased genital sensation, and orgasmic dysfunction. The anatomic and physiologic basis for sexual dysfunction after hysterectomy is poorly understood. Our understanding of female neurovascular anatomy relative to normal sexual arousal and function is limited.

Other Anatomic Structures

Sevely[21] suggested that the female actually has two glans: that of the clitoris (clitoral glans) and that surrounding the urethra (female glans). The glans is mobile and is pushed into and pulled out of the vagina as a result of thrusting during coitus.[21] Given the complexity of the anatomy of the external female genitalia, the periurethral glans may be a further part of the corpus spongiosum.[22]

The female urethra is a short conduit. For nearly its entire length, it is surrounded by numerous venous or sinus channels that constitute the corpus spongiosum. It becomes further vasocongested during sexual arousal.[23]

Grafenberge[23] reported that digital stroking of the anterior vagina along the urethra, in the base of the bladder, sexually aroused female subjects. The area was rediscovered and renamed the G-spot. Investigators have described various locations, including the area along the entire length of the urethra and the anterior vaginal wall, which represents a part of the urethra that contains the periglandular or paraurethral tissue. Two other erotic pleasurable zones are also described: Halban's fascia[24,25] and the inner half of the anterior wall of the vagina.[26] It appeared that the digital technique would stimulate the urethra–G spot–Halban's fascia complex and need not imply a new, specialized area of the anterior vagina.[13]

The Pelvic Floor Muscles

The pelvic floor is a collection of tissues that span the opening within the bony pelvis. In addition to supporting the abdominal and pelvic organs and maintaining continence of urine and stool, the pelvic floor allows for intercourse and parturition. The pelvic floor musculature, in particular, the pelvic diaphragm that is formed by the levator ani muscles, urogenital diaphragm, and perineal membrane, is important for pelvic support. The perineal membrane that consists of the ischiocavernosus, bulbocavernosus, and superficial transverse perineal muscles is closely related to the vestibular bulbs and clitoris, and plays a role in sexual response. Voluntary contraction of these muscles can intensify orgasm of both the female and her male partner.

The levator ani muscle has two parts: the pubococcygeus and the iliococcygeus. During pelvic examination, these muscles can be palpated as a distinct ridge just above the hymenal ring along each lateral wall of the pelvis. This group of muscles pulls the rectum, vagina, and urethra anteriorly toward the pubic bones to compress the lumens closed. Kegel[27] and other authors claim that the pubococcygeal muscle contains sensory and motor elements of the orgasmic response and that its stimulation gives rise to sexual pleasure and can even induce orgasm.[13] Thus, the muscular contibution, particularly the medial puboccygeus muscles, functioning as lower vaginal constrictors, also facilitates clitoral vasocongestion by compressing venous drainage.

NEUROGENIC MEDIATORS OF THE FEMALE SEXUAL RESPONSE

Sexual responses (genital arousal, climax) are largely the product of spinal cord reflex mechanisms. These reflexes are mediated by genital afferents, primarily from the pudendal nerve. The efferent arm of the reflexes consists of complex, coordinated somatic, sympathetic, and parasympathetic activity.[13]

Within the central nervous system, the medial preoptic region, the anterior hypothalamic region, and related limbic hippocampal structures are activated during sexual arousal. On activation, these centers transmit electrical signals through the parasympathetic and sympathetic nervous systems. The neurogenic mechanisms that modulate vaginal and clitoral smooth muscle tone and vaginal and clitoral vascular smooth muscle relaxation are currently under investigation. The mechanisms underlying female sexual response remain to be elucidated; however, the following findings have been established:

- Female reflexes are similar to the cavernous nerve-mediated erectile response in males
- Sexual climax is also a spinal reflex
- Sensory information is relayed to supraspinal sites via the spinothalamic and spinoreticular pathways
- Neurons in the nucleus paragigantocellularis receive genital sensory information in males and females[28]

Nonadrenergic, Noncholinergic Mediated Responses

Immunohistochemical studies in human vaginal tissues show nerve fibers containing neuropeptide Y (NPY), vasoactive intestinal polypeptide (VIP), nitric oxide synthase (NOS), calcitonin gene-related peptide, and substance P.[29] Preliminary studies suggest that VIP and nitric oxide (NO) are involved in modulating vaginal relaxation and secretory processes. NO has been identified in human clitoral tissue and is hypothesized to be the primary mediator of clitoral and labial engorgement.[30] Organ bath analysis of rabbit clitoral cavernosal smooth muscle strips shows enhanced relaxation in response to sodium nitroprusside and L-arginine (both NO donors), supporting the above hypothesis.[25] Recently, phosphodiesterase type V, the enzyme responsible for degrading cyclic guanosine 3'5' monophosphate (cGMP), was isolated in human clitoral, vestibular bulb, and vaginal smooth muscle culture, and is inhibited by sildenafil citrate.[30]

Human and rabbit vaginal smooth muscle cells treated with the NO donor sodium nitroprusside, in the presence of sildenafil, have enhanced intracellular cGMP synthesis and accumulation. Prostaglandin E_1 and forskolin also produce a marked increase in intracellular cGMP.[31] In organ bath studies, sildenafil causes dose-dependent relaxation of female rabbit clitoral and vaginal smooth muscle strips, further suggesting a role for NO as a mediator of clitoral cavernosal and vaginal wall smooth muscle relaxation.[32] However, the exact identity of the relaxant nonadrenergic, noncholinergic neurotransmitter remains unclear. VIP is a nonadrenergic, noncholinergic neurotransmitter that, like NO, may play a role in enhancing vaginal blood flow, lubrication, and secretions. The vagina is heavily innervated with VIP-immunoreactive nerve fibers in close relation to the epithelium and blood vessels.[33] In organ bath studies, VIP also causes dose-dependent relaxation of rabbit clitoral cavernosal and vaginal smooth muscle tissue, suggesting a similar role for endogenous VIP as a nonadrenergic, noncholinergic neurotransmitter in clitoral and vaginal tissues (Min et al.).

Alpha-1 and Alpha-2 Adrenergic Responses

In men, adrenergic receptors in the brain centers are associated with penile erection, libido, and ejaculation. Agents that affect these receptors have been studied extensively and used to treat male erectile dysfunction. Alpha-adrenergic agonists, such as norepinephrine, activate sympathetic nerve terminals, resulting in contraction of penile trabecular smooth muscle and detumesence. Alpha-2 agonists cause similar responses. Activation of alpha-2 receptors results in a decrease in intracellular adenosine 3'5'monophosphate concentrations and potent contraction in blood vessels. Alpha-adrenergic mediators also appear to play a physiologic role in female sexual arousal.[34] Preliminary organ chamber experiments using rabbit vaginal tissue suggest that adrenergic mechanisms modulate smooth muscle tone. Exogenous norepinephrine (an alpha-1 and alpha-2 agonist) causes dose-dependent contraction of vaginal smooth muscle. Alpha-1 (prazosin and tamsulosin) and alpha-2 (delequamine) selective antagonists inhibit this contraction (Min et al.). These observations suggest that adrenergic nerves mediate contractile response. Furthermore, there appears to be a difference in the quality of the contractile responses in the upper and lower segments of the vagina. This observation is consistent with their different innervation and embryologic origin.

HORMONAL REGULATION OF FEMALE SEXUAL FUNCTION: THE ROLE OF ESTROGEN AND TESTOSTERONE

Estrogen

Estrogen plays a significant role in regulating female sexual function. Estradiol affects cells throughout the peripheral and central nervous systems and influences nerve transmission. A decline in serum estrogen levels causes thinning of the vaginal mucosal epithelium and atrophy of the vaginal wall smooth muscle. Decreased estrogen levels also result in a less acidic environment in the vaginal canal, which can lead to vaginal infections, urinary tract infections, incontinence, and sexual dysfunction.[35]

In animal models, estradiol administration results in expanded touch receptor zones along the distribution of the pudendal nerve, suggesting that estrogen affects sensory thresholds. In postmenopausal women, estrogen replacement restores clitoral and vaginal vibration and pressure thresholds to levels close to those of premenopausal women.[35] Estrogens also have vasoprotective and vasodilatory effects that cause increased vaginal, clitoral, and urethral arterial flow and maintenance of the female sexual response by preventing atherosclerotic compromise of the pelvic arteries and arterioles.[36]

With menopause and the associated decline in circulating estrogen levels, most women experience some degree of change in sexual function. Common sexual symptoms include loss of desire, decreased frequency of sexual activity, painful intercourse, diminished sexual responsiveness, difficulty achieving orgasm, and decreased genital sensation. In 1966, Masters and Johnson first published their findings of the physiologic changes in sexual function that occur in menopausal women.[1] We have since learned that symptoms related to alterations in genital sensation and blood flow are, in part, secondary to declining estrogen levels, and that there is a direct correlation between sexual symptoms and estradiol levels of less than 50 pg/mL.[35,36] Symptoms markedly decrease with estrogen replacement. To date, the only available treatments for menopause-associated sexual symptoms are hormone replacement therapy, commercial lubricants, psychotherapy, and antidepressant medication. Estrogen also plays a role in regulating vaginal and clitoral expression of NOS, the enzyme responsible for the production of NO. Aging and surgical castration cause decreased vaginal and clitoral expression of NOS and apoptosis of vaginal wall smooth muscle and mucosal epithelium. Estrogen replacement restores vaginal mucosal health, increases vaginal expression of NOS, and decreases vaginal mucosal cell death.[37] These findings suggest that medications, such as sildenafil, that mediate vascular and nonvascular smooth muscle via NO may have a potential role in the treatment of female sexual dysfunction, especially sexual arousal disorder.

Testosterone

The role of androgen deficiency in the pathophysiology of female sexual dysfunction is controversial. Most commercial assays for the measurement of total and free testosterone levels were developed to measure the much higher circulating concentrations in men. These assays lack the sensitivity and precision required to measure the low levels found in androgen-deficient women.[38] Because few normative data are available on serum total and free testosterone concentrations in healthy, menstruating women,[38] there is no consensus on the thresholds that can be used to define androgen deficiency in women. Until recently, the available testosterone formulations were designed to deliver the much higher dose required in hypogonadal men. However, two new formulations, the testosterone transdermal matrix patch for women and the testosterone gel, are now undergoing phase I and phase II studies.[39,40]

By acting within the brain, androgens influence sexual behavior, although a woman's libido is also determined by environmental, emotional, cultural, and hormonal factors.[41-43] The effects of androgens in the brain are mediated in part directly through the androgen receptor and through aromatization of testosterone to estradiol. Androgen receptors have been identified in the cortex, pituitary, hypothalamus, preoptic region, thalamus, amygdala, and brain stem. In addition, testosterone and estrogen exert nongenomic effects in the central nervous system.

Testosterone supplementation is associated with increased well-being, energy, and appetite, and improved somatic and psychological scores in surgically menopausal women.[41,44,45] Surgically menopausal women who were given suprapharmacologic doses of testosterone enanthate by intramuscular injection, alone or in combination with estrogen, reported increased sexual desire, fantasies, and arousal more than those given placebo or estrogen alone.[41] Testosterone and estradiol implants also increased sexual activity, satisfaction, pleasure, and frequency of orgasm more than estrogen alone.[44] In another recent study,[46] women who underwent hysterectomy and oophorectomy and received estrogen replacement (conjugated equine estrogen at least 0.625 mg/day orally) were randomized to receive placebo or transdermal testosterone 150 or 300 μg/day for 12 weeks each. The highest dose of testosterone resulted in a mean serum free testosterone level that was slightly above the physiologic range and significantly increased scores for frequency of sexual activity and orgasm. This treatment also increased sexual fantasies, masturbation, and positive well-being. Objectively, in a small number of women with hypothalamic amenorrhea, testosterone increased vaginal vasocongestion, as measured by vaginal photopletysmography during exposure to a potent visual stimulus.[46] Dehydroepiandrosterone (DHEA) replacement 50 mg/day for 4 months in women with adrenal insufficiency increased libido and well-being.[47] It is unclear whether these effects were secondary to the direct effect of DHEA on the brain or an indirect effect via an increase in androgen synthesis. In contrast, a cross-sectional study did not show correlation between sexual function and gonadal steroids. Although pharmacologic doses of testosterone undoubtedly improve overall sexual function, we do not know whether physiologic testosterone replacement can produce clinically meaningful changes in health-related outcomes.

All androgens carry the risk of inducing virilization in women. Early reversible manifestations include acne, oily skin, hirsutism, and menstrual irregularities. Long-term side effects, such as male pattern baldness, hirsutism, voice changes, and hypertrophy of the clitoris, are largely irreversible. Testosterone supplementation in supraphysiologic doses appears to decrease high-density lipoprotein cholesterol levels. Women with a history of breast cancer should not be prescribed testosterone because it is converted to estrogen by the aromatase enzyme.

CONCLUSION

Sexuality is not a singular phenomenon, but is composed of identifiably distinct, but interrelated processes. The components of sexual behavior associated with libido or sexual motivation (sexual desire, sexual fantasies, and satisfaction) and potency or sexual response (pelvic congestion and orgasmic contractions) are regulated by psychosocial and physiologic factors. During penile coitus, the internal and external anatomic structures, classified as erogenous friction and pressure sites, are stimulated by movements of the penile thrusting, which are transduced by specific nerve endings[48] and relayed via ascending sensory pathways to the brain. Stimuli that are psychologically acceptable and physiologically effective can create enough sexual excitement to activate an orgasmic response. Many anatomic structures play a role in sexual arousal up to orgasm. Sexual responses are largely the product of spinal cord reflex mechanisms that are mediated by genital afferents, primarily from the pudendal nerve. The spinal reflexes are under descending control, both inhibitory and excitatory, from a variety of supraspinal sites.[49]

Large gaps remain in our understanding of the central nervous control of female sexual function. It is likely that significant homology will be found between males and females in the control of sexual function, and there is need for more research in this area.[13]

REFERENCES

1. Masters WH, Johnson VE: Human Sexual Response. Boston, Little Brown, 1966.
2. Kaplan H: The New Sex Therapy. London, Baillière Tindall, 1974.
3. Kohn IJ, Kaplan SA: Female sexual dysfunction: What is known and what remains to be determined. Contemp Urol 54–72, 1999.
4. Kaplan HS: Hypoactive sexual desire. J Sex Marital Ther 3:3–9, 1977.
5. Leif HI: Inhibited sexual desire. Med Aspects Human Sex 7:94–95, 1977.
6. American Psychiatric Association: Diagnostic and Statistical Manual of Mental Disorders, 4th ed. Washington DC, American Psychiatric Association, 1994.
7. Berman JR, Berman L, Goldstein I: Female sexual dysfunction: Incidence, pathophysiology, evaluation, and treatment options. Urology 54:385–391, 1999.
8. Graziottin A: Libido. In: Yearbook of the Royal College of Obstetricians and Gynaecologists. London, Parthenon, 1996, pp 235–243.
9. Sjoberg I: The vagina: Morphological, functional and ecological aspects. Acta Obstet Gynecol Scand 71:84–85, 1992.
10. Weber AM, Walters MD, Schover LR, Mitchinson A: Vaginal anatomy and sexual function. Obstet Gynecol 86:946–949, 1995.
11. Levin RJ: The physiology of sexual function in women. Clin Obstet Gynaecol 7:213–252, 1980.
12. Park K, Goldstein I, Andry C, et al: Vasculogenic female sexual dysfunction: The hemodynamic basis for vaginal engorgement insufficiency and clitoral erectile insufficiency. Int J Impot Res 9:27–37, 1997.
13. Golstein I, Graziottin A, Heiman JR, et al: Female sexual dysfunction: In Jardin A, Wagner G, Khoury S, et al (eds): Erectile Dysfunction: 1st International Consultation on Erectile Dysfunction, July 1–3, 1999, pp 507–557.
14. Levin RJ, Mc Donagh RP: Increased vaginal blood flow induced by implant electrical stimulation of sacral anterior root in conscious woman: A case study. Sex Scand 22:471–475, 1993.
15. Toesca A, Stolfi VM, Cocchia D: Immunohistochemical study of the corpora cavernosa of the human clitoris. J Anat 188:513–520, 1996.
16. Park K, Moreland RB, Goldstein I, et al: Sildenafil inhibits phosphodiesterase type 5 in human clitoral corpus cavernosum smooth muscle. Biophys Res Commun 249:612–617, 1998.
17. O'Connell HE, Hutson JM, Anderson CR, Plenter RJ: Anatomical relationship between urethra and clitoris. J Urol 159:1892–1897, 1998.

18. Riley AI, Lees WR, Riley E: An ultrasound study of human coitus. In Benzener W, Cohen-Kettenis, Slob K, Van Son-Schoones N (eds): Sex Matters (Xth World Congress of Sexology). Amsterdam, Eccerpta Medica, 1992, pp 29–32.
19. Carlson KJ: Outcomes of hysterectomy. Clin Obstet Gynecol 40:939–946, 1997.
20. Kilkku P, Grinroos M, Hirvonen T, Raumano L: Supravaginal uterine amputation versus hysterectomy: Effects on libido and orgasm. Acta Obstet Gynecol Scand 62:147–152, 1983.
21. Sevely JL: Eve's secrets: A new perspective on human sexuality. London, Bloomsbury, 1987.
22. Van Turnhout AA, Hage WM, Van Diest PJ: The female corpus spongiosum revisited. Acta Obstet Gyn Scand 74:767–771, 1995.
23. Grafenberge E: The role of the urethra in the female orgasm. Int J Sex 3:135–148, 1950.
24. Singer I: The Goals of Human Sexuality. London, Wildwood House, 1973.
25. Minh HN, Smadia A, Herve de Sigalony JP: Le fascia de Halban: Son rôle dans ka phsysiologie sexuelle. Gynecologie 30:267–273, 1979.
26. Chua Chee A: A proposal for a radical new sex therapy technique for the management of vasocongestive and orgasmic dysfunction in women: The AFE zone stimulation technique. Sex Marital Ther 12:357–370, 1997.
27. Kegel A: Sexual function of the pubococcygeal muscle. West J Obstet Gynecol 60:521–524, 1950.
28. Hubscher CH, Johnson RD: Responses of medullary reticular formation neurons to input from the male gebitalia. J Neurophysiol 76:2474–2482, 1996.
29. Hoyle CH, Stones RW, Robson T, et al: Innervation of vasculature and microvasculature of the human vagina by NOS and neuropeptide containing nerves. J Anat 188:633–644, 1996.
30. Park K, Moreland RB, Goldstein I, et al: Sildenafil inhibits phosphodiesterase type 5 in human clitoral corpus cavernosum smooth muscle. Biochem Biophys Res Commun 249:612–617, 1998.
31. Traish A, Moreland RB, Huang YH, et al: Development of human and rabbit vaginal smooth muscle cell cultures: Effects of vasoactive agents on intracellular levels of cyclic nucleotides. Mol Cell Biol Res Commun 2:131–137, 1999.
32. Min K: Int J Impot Res 12 (suppl 3).
33. Helm G, Ottesen B, Fahrenkrug J, et al: Vasoactive intestinal polypeptide (VIP) in the human female reproductive tract: Distribution and motor effects. Biol Reprod 25:227–234, 1981.
34. Meston CM, Heiman JR: Ephedrine-activated physiological sexual arousal in women. Arch Gen Psychiatry 55:652–656, 1998.
35. Sarrell P: Sexuality and menopause. Obstet Gynecol 75:26, 1998.
36. Sarrel PM: Ovarian hormones and vaginal blood flow: Using laser Doppler velocimetry to measure effects in a clinical trial of post-menopausal women. Int J Impot Res 10 (suppl 2):S91–S93; discussion S98–S101, 1998.
37. Berman JR, McCarthy MM, Kyprianou N: Effect of estrogen withdrawal on nitric oxide synthase expression and apoptosis in the rat vagina. Urology 51:650–656, 1998.
38. Sinha-Hikim I, Arver S, Beall G, et al: The use of a sensitive equilibrium dialysis method for the measurement of free testosterone levels in healthy, cycling women and in human immunodeficiency virus-infected women. J Clin Endocrinol Metab 83:1312–1318, 1998. Published erratum appears in J Clin Endocrinol Metab 83:2959, 1998.
39. Javanbakht M, Singh AB, Mazer NA, et al: Pharmacokinetics of a novel testosterone matrix transdermal system in healthy, premenopausal women and women infected with the human immunodeficiency virus. J Clin Endocrinol Metab 85:2395–2401, 2000.
40. Mazer NA: New clinical applications of transdermal testosterone delivery in men and women. J Control Release 65:303–15, 2000.
41. Sherwin BB, Gelfand MM, Brender W: Androgen enhances sexual motivation in females: A prospective, crossover study of sex steroid administration in the surgical menopause. Psychosom Med 47:339–351, 1985.
42. Rako S: Testosterone supplemental therapy after hysterectomy with or without concomitant oophorectomy: Estrogen alone is not enough. J Womens Health 9:917–923, 2000.
43. Rako S: Testosterone deficiency: A key factor in the increased cardiovascular risk to women following hysterectomy or with natural aging? J Womens Health 7:825–829, 1998.
44. Davis SR, McCloud P, Strauss BJ, Burger H: Testosterone enhances estradiol's effects on postmenopausal bone density and sexuality. Maturitas 21:227–233, 1995.
45. Davis S: Androgen replacement in women: A commentary. J Clin Endocrinol Metab 84:1886–1891, 1999.
46. Shifren JL, Braunstein GD, Simon JA, et al: Transdermal testosterone treatment in women with impaired sexual function after oophorectomy. N Engl J Med 343:682–688, 2000.
47. Arlt W, Callies F, van Vlijmen JC, et al: Dehydroepiandrosterone replacement in women with adrenal insufficiency. N Engl J Med 341:1013–1020, 1999.
48. Krantz EK: Innervation of the human vulva and vagina. Obstet Gynecol 12:382–396, 1958.
49. Komisaruk BR, Gerdes CA, Whipple B: 'Complete' spinal cord injury does not block perceptual responses to genital self-stimulation in women. Arch Neurol 54:1513–1520, 1997.

CHAPTER 5

Normal Sexual Function in Men

PIERRE DESVAUX

FUNCTIONAL ANATOMY OF THE PENIS

The average length of the human penis is 8.8 cm when flaccid and 12.4 cm when stretched. Erect penile length varies from 12 to 20 cm, with an erect thickness of 3.5 cm. The penis is composed of three cylinders encased in a fascial sheath (Buck's fascia). The three cylinders are the corpus spongiosum and the two corpora cavernosa. The corpus cavernosum consists of a thick fibroelastic sheath (tunica albuginea) and spongy erectile tissue. The urethra-containing corpus spongiosum lies in the ventral groove formed by the paired corpora cavernosa. These structures form a unique vascular bed that consists of multiple blood-filled cavernous spaces (trabeculae) whose arterial blood supply arises from the resistance helicine arteries. The sinusoids are lined with endothelial cells that have a possible secretory function that may be important in the erectile process. The tunica albuginea is a multilayered structure of inner circular and outer longitudinal layers of connective tissue encompassing the paired corpora cavernosa. Three sets of peripheral nerves have a role in erectile function. At the T9 to L4 levels of the spinal cord, the intermediolateral column of gray matter gives rise to the sympathetic preganglionic fibers and the neurons interface with sympathetic chain neurons at the level of the spinal cord. Parasympathetic preganglionic fibers originate from the S2 to S4 and proceed to the pelvic or hypogastric plexus. Motor innervation of the penis derives from S2, S3, and S4 within the sacral nerves, which lead to the pudendal nerve. Neural innervation of the penis may be divided into autonomic (parasympathetic and sympathetic) and somatic (sensory and motor). The dorsal nerve of the penis may contain a parasympathetic component and play a direct role in erection. The sacral parasympathetic input is responsible for tumescence, and the thoracolumbar sympathetic pathway is responsible for detumescence. The arterial blood supply of the penis is primarily via the hypogastric artery. After giving off the perineal artery, the penile artery branches to form the bulbourethral, dorsal, and cavernous arteries. The bulbourethral artery supplies the urethra and glans, and the cavernosal arteries enter the corpora cavernosa at a point where the two crura converge. The venous drainage system of the penis occurs on three levels.[1] The superficial drainage system, which lies above Buck's fascia and primarily drains the penile skin, can also have connections with the deep dorsal vein. The intermediate drainage system consists of the deep dorsal vein and the circumflex veins. Along its course beneath Buck's fascia, the deep dorsal vein receives several circumflex and emissary veins that provide the main venous drainage of the glans penis. The deep drainage system consists of the cavernosal veins or crural veins that drain the deeper cavernous tissue. Emissary veins that drain the proximal corpora cavernosa join to form two to five cavernous veins that exit the dorsomedial aspect of the penile hilum. The veins of the three systems communicate variably with each other.

NEUROANATOMY AND PHYSIOLOGY OF SEXUAL FUNCTION

Sexual function is a complex, multicomponent biologic process that includes central mechanisms that regulate libido and arousability as well as local mechanisms that generate penile tumescence, rigidity, orgasm, and ejaculation. Both the central and the peripheral nervous systems are involved in normal sexual function in both men and women. Normal sexual activity as a whole depends on the integrity of the entire nervous system. The brain, spinal cord, sympathetic and parasympathetic systems, and motor and sensory elements of the peripheral nervous system participate in the initiation and coordination of sexual function.

Cerebral and Subcortical Centers

Sexual interest and initiative depend on cerebrocortical function, but the area (or areas) of the cerebral cortex that is most important in the experience of libido, sexual fantasy, and other more or less abstract elements of sexual activity is unknown.[2] The temporal and frontal lobes are believed to play vital roles in the elaboration of sexual interest and behavior, but this impression comes from observations of individuals who had injuries to these parts of the brain. Several regions of the brain modulate the psychogenic component of erection. These regions include the thalamic nuclei, rhinencephalon, and limbic structures. Integration of these areas occurs in the preoptic anterior hypothalamic area.[3]

Cerebrocortical areas are presumed to connect more or less indirectly to the genitalia through sympathetic pathways that exit the central nervous system at spinal cord levels T11–L2. As a result, psychic arousal through visual stimuli or fantasy evokes changes in the genitalia associated with arousal.[4,5] These centers are probably located in the brain, but their level of circumscription is controversial. The genital representations in the cerebrum that are the best documented probably play a relatively minor role in the initiation and organization of normal sexual function. Sensory information from the genitalia projects subcortically to the ventrolateral and intralaminar nuclei of the thalamus before being transmitted to the cerebral cortex.[4,6] The temporal lobe plays a role in a variety of sexual activities, although its precise function is uncertain.[7] Other cortical areas (e.g., cingulate gyrus, piriform cortex) also play a role in sexual function.[6] Several sites have been anatomically identified for their projection to the lumbosacral spinal cord, but their function in sexual response is unknown.[4]

The Limbic System

The limbic system includes cerebral and subcortical structures (amygdala, septal nuclei, hippocampus) that influence affect and emotional displays. The limbic system has inputs from centers in the cerebral cortex that connect through the limbic system to centers in the spinal cord that control penile erection and vaginal lubrication.[5] The posterior hypothalamus may play a more inhibitory role.[6] The hypothalamus is an essential site for reproduction and sexual behavior as well as for many homeostatic and motivated behaviors.[7] Because of the large number and complexity of these activities, it is difficult to precisely define the role of the hypothalamus in sexual arousal and performance; however, the paraventricular nucleus of the hypothalamus is probably responsible for control of genital responses.[4,8]

The Spinal Cord

Changes in the genitalia are mediated most directly by the spinal cord, paraspinal sympathetic ganglia, and parasympathetic nerves. In the spinal cord, the intermediolateral column of gray matter at the level of T11–L2 gives rise to sympathetic nerve fibers. The intermediolateral column at spinal levels S2–S4 gives rise to parasympathetic fibers. These fibers proceed to the pelvic and hypogastric plexus. In men, the cavernous nerve begins at the pelvic plexus and travels through the pelvic fascia to the prostatic capsule, where it crosses the posterolateral aspect of the prostate. The parasympathetic supply leaves the spinal cord through the ventral roots and forms the pelvic nerves. Sensory stimuli elicited in the glans, penis, and other perineal and inguinal areas originate in sensory receptors whose nerve fibers converge to form the dorsal nerve of the penis. This nerve joins other pelvic nerves to become the internal pudendal nerve, ascending to the dorsal root of the second, third, and fourth sacral vertebrae.[3,9,10] Motor innervation of the penis derives from the second, third, and fourth sacral vertebrae within the sacral nerves, which lead to the pudendal nerve that reaches the bulbocavernous and ischiocavernous muscles. Contraction of the ischiocavernous muscle plays an important role in the rigid erection phase by constricting and compressing the corpora cavernosa, whereas rhythmic contraction of the bulbocavernous muscle is important for the expulsion of semen during ejaculation.[3,4,9,10] These muscles are striated and innervated by somatic fibers carried in the pudendal nerve. During orgasm in men, sympathetic efferents induce the emission of semen. Impulses carried along the postganglionic sympathetic axons drive the rhythmic contraction of smooth muscle in the walls of the seminal vesicles, prostate, ductus deferens, and ampulla.[11] Reflex erection appears to depend predominantly on parasympathetic nerves, which inhibit the tonic contraction of smooth muscles of the penile arteries and cavernous muscles. The most vital penile arteries in erection are those that supply the corpora cavernosa.

The nucleus paragigantocellularis projects directly to pelvic efferent neurons and interneurons in the lumbosacral spinal cord.[12] Most of the neurons in the region stain positively for the neurotransmitter serotonin, and serotonin applied to the spinal cord inhibits spinal sexual reflexes.[12] Neurons in the nucleus paragigantocellularis receive genital sensory information.[7,13]

In men, parasympathetic fibers run in the pelvic nerves and synapse in terminal ganglia close to the target organs. The preganglionic fibers proceed to the pelvic or hypogastric plexus, which relays preganglionic and postganglionic fibers to the penis. Sensory stimuli elicited in the glans, penis, and other perineal and inguinal areas originate in sensory receptors whose nerve fibers converge to form the dorsal nerve of the penis. Parasympathetic efferents stimulate secretion from the bulbourethral glands, Littré's glands, seminal vesicles, and prostate.

Somatic Nerves

The somatic nerve that is most vital to reflex sexual activity in both men and women is the pudendal nerve. The levator ani is innervated by somatic nerve fibers that emanate primarily from sacral root S3, to a lessor extent from S4, and minimally from S2 to form the pudendal nerve. The pudendal nerve is a mixed nerve that carries both motor and sensory fibers and is derived from the sacral plexus. The nerve lies in the pelvis, crossing the ischial spine to the ischiorectal fossa via the lesser sciatic foramen. It extends forward in a fibrous tunnel (Alcock's canal) on the medial side of the obturator internus muscle. In both sexes, this nerve carries sensory information from the saddle area (i.e., perineal and perianal areas).

Stimulation of free nerve endings and pacinian corpuscles in the skin of the penis or clitoris and other erogenous zones around the perineum generates impulses that travel along the dorsal nerve of the penis and other branches of the pudendal nerve to the sacral spinal cord at S2–S4.[5,14] Motor innervation of the penis derives from S2–S4 within the sacral nerves, which lead to the pudendal nerve and reach the bulbocavernous and ischiocavernous muscles. In women, the pudendal nerve splits into two terminal branches after giving rise to the inferior hemorrhoidal nerve. One of these terminal branches is the perineal nerve, which carries sensory fibers from the vulva and carries motor fibers to muscles around the perineum. The pudendal nerves carry excitatory information from the perineum, parasympathetic stimuli to the penis, and somatic impulses to the bulbocavernous and ischiocavernous muscles.[2,15]

REGULATION AND HEMODYNAMICS OF MALE SEXUAL FUNCTION

The ability to achieve and maintain an erection is a fundamental part of male sexual function.[16] The hemodynamic events of penile erection can be divided into six phases.[17]

- Flaccid phase, or resting state. The minimal arterial blood flow that occurs is just enough to supply nutrients to the corpora.
- Latent phase, during which dominant arterial inflow occurs. On appropriate psychological or sexual stimulation, neurogenic impulses initiate erection. The corpora fill without pressure change for approximately 10 seconds.
- Tumescence phase, during which the penis expands and elongates. Intracavernous pressure begins to increase, and arterial inflow to the corpora gradually decreases.
- Full erection phase, during which complete penile expansion and elongation occurs. Arterial inflow decreases to near that of the flaccid phase and equals venous outflow.
- Rigid erection phase. Under stimulation of the pudendal nerve, the ischiocavernous muscles contract and further increase intracavernous pressure to several times the systolic blood pressure.
- Detumescence phase, which is the resolution phase. Venous flow increases and arterial flow decreases until the flaccid state is achieved. The opinion of the author is that latent phase could be combined with tumescence phase and full erection could be associated with rigid erection phase because of the chronology of the various sequences.

The penis is composed of three bodies of erectile tissue. The corpora cavernosa form a unique vascular bed consisting of sinuses (trabeculae) whose arterial blood supply arises from the resistance helicine arteries, which are fed from the deep penile cavernosal artery.[4,9,10] The cavernosal arteries and their branches, the helicine arteries, provide blood flow to the penis.[18] Helicine arteries deliver blood into the cavernosal sinuses.[9,19] Dilation of the helicine arteries increases blood flow and pressure in the cavernosal sinuses.[9,19] Blood pO_2 in the lacunae is 20 to 40 mm Hg when the penis is flaccid.[4,10] On erection, this venous-like flaccid blood pO_2 increases, with dilation of the heline arteries, to 90 to 100 mm Hg.[19] The tunica albuginea is a multilayered structure of inner circular and outer longitudinal layers of connective tissue that encompasses the paired corpora cavernosa.[18] The tunica albuginea varies in thickness from 1.5 to 3 mm, depending on the circular position.[20] The tunica albuginea is composed of fibrillar (mainly type I, but also type III) collagen arranged in organized arrays interlaced with elastin fibers.[20] The elastin content allows compliance of the tunica and helps to determine the length of the stretched penis. Histologically, like the corpus cavernosum, the corpus spongiosum is a spongy erectile tissue, but it does not provide structure to the erection. The intraspongiosal pressure is one third to one half of that in the corpora cavernosa. This lower pressure may prevent urethral blockage during ejaculation.[4,10]

The contraction of smooth muscle depends on the rapid rise of the intracellular free calcium concentration. Locally, detumescence of the erect penis is mediated by adrenergic nerve terminals whose neurotransmitter norepinephrine activates adrenergic receptors. Contraction of human penile arteries and trabecular smooth muscle is largely mediated by alpha-1 adrenergic receptors.[21] Adrenergic stimulation causes vasoconstriction of the penile arteries and contraction of the trabecular muscle. These changes result, respectively, in reduction of the arterial inflow and collapse of the lacunar spaces.[4] Contraction of the trabecular muscle causes decompression of the drainage venules from the cavernous bodies, allowing venous drainage of the lacunar spaces.[4,21] The peptide endothelin and some eicosanoids (prostaglandin F_2 alpha, thromboxane A2) may help to maintain penile flaccidity. Two endothelin receptors, ET A and ET B, mediate the biologic effects of endothelin in vascular tissue. ET A causes contraction in response to endothelin; ET B mediates an endothelium-dependent vasodilator response. The mechanism of intracellular transduction[4] for both receptors is activation of the metabolism of inositol phosphate, with release of intracellular calcium and activation of protein kinase C.

Dilation of the penile arteries is the first event in erection. It increases blood flow and pressure into the lacunar spaces. After arterial dilation, the trabecular muscle relaxes, increasing compliance of the lacunar spaces to its expansion and facilitating the accumulation of blood.[4] Many recent studies showed the role of the molecule nitric oxide (NO) in the urogenital tract and in sexual regulation. NO is produced by a family of isoenzymes known as NO synthases (NOS). The amino acid L-arginine and molecular oxygen is the substrate for NOS, forming NO and L-citrulline in equal amounts.[23] NO crosses the plasma membrane of the cells, targeting the enzyme guanylate cyclase and producing a conformational change in the molecule that increases its activity. The accumulation of 5′ cyclic guanosine monophosphate (cGMP) sets in motion a cascade of events at the intracellular level. These events induce a loss of contractile tone. Vasoactive intestinal peptide (VIP) in the autonomic nerves, prostaglandin E (PGE_1 and PGE_2, synthesized by smooth muscle), and neural or circulating catecholamines (norepinephrine and epinephrine) stimulate specific receptors coupled to Gs proteins that stimulate the adenylate cyclase that catalyzes the formation of cyclic adenosine monophosphate (cAMP).[2] Intracavernosal administration of VIP caused tumescence and rigid erection in some individuals.[23] The two molecules, VIP and NO, induce relaxation in the muscle by two different and potentially synergistic pathways: NO is released at low frequencies, and the largest release of VIP occurs at high frequencies. PGE_1 and PGE_2 are the most abundant prostanoids that are synthesized by penile smooth muscle. The stimulation by catecholamines of beta-adrenergic receptors causes relaxation of arterial and trabecular smooth muscle. The beta-2 subtype is probably the most important receptor mediating these effects.[24] In arteries, NO may directly stimulate the opening of potassium channels as well as the sodium-potassium adenosine triphosphatase. This last mechanism is seen in trabecular muscle.[25]

One mechanism by which cyclic nucleotides induce relaxation of smooth muscle is through the opening of potassium channels, hyperpolarizing the cell. This effect on K+ channels can be provoked by the cAMP-dependent protein kinase, the cGMP-dependent protein kinase, or cGMP itself.[1] Activation of the potassium channels (of the max-K+ type) by the action of PGE_1, an effect mediated by cAMP, has been shown.[26]

CONCLUSION

Normal penile erection requires coordinated involvement of the intact central and peripheral nervous systems, the corpora cavernosa and spongiosa, and a normal arterial blood supply and venous drainage.[4] The erectile state of the penis is determined by the tone of the corporal smooth muscle cells. When the cavernosal smooth muscle cells are relaxed, the tone is low and the penis is engorged with blood and erect. Conversely, when the cavernosal smooth muscle tone is high, the penis is flaccid.

Contraction of vascular smooth muscle in the corpora cavernosa is regulated by the noradrenergic pathway. Relaxation of the cavernosal smooth muscle trabeculae is regulated by the autonomic nervous system.[27-33] Although cholinergic, adrenergic, and nonadrenergic, noncholinergic mediators all play a role, an important biochemical regulator of cavernosal smooth muscle relaxation is NO derived from the nerve terminals that innervate the corpora cavernosa, the endothelial lining of the penile arteries, and the cavernosal sinuses.[27-33]

Erection is not necessarily a voluntary event, and psychogenic or visual stimuli can initiate a cortical erectile response. Through sensory tactile impulses, the somatic nervous system may also initiate and amplify the erectile response. The smooth muscles of the cavernous trabeculae and the arterioles constitute the central mechanism of erection by controlling tumescence and detumescence of the penis. Sexual drive is enhanced through the action of dopaminergic and adrenergic receptors and dopamine, apomorphine, alpha-2 blockers, yohimbine, substance P, gonadotropin-releasing hormone, alpha-melanocyte-stimulating hormone, and oxytocin are among the substances that positively influence sexual behavior.[17]

In summary, normal sexual function depends on autonomic reflexes in the pelvis and lumbosacral spine, hypothalamic–endocrine interactions, and cerebral activity.[2,8] Each element can operate somewhat independently, but sexual activity is truly normal only when all of the elements work in concert.

REFERENCES

1. Paick JS, Lue T: Anatomy of the penis. In Hashmat AI, Das S (eds): The Penis. Philadelphia, Lea & Febiger, 1993, pp 12–16.
2. Lechtenberg R, Ohl D: Normal sexual response. In Lechtenberg R, Ohl D (eds): Sexual Dysfunction: Neurologic, Urologic, and Gynecologic Aspects. Philadelphia, Lea & Febiger, 1994, pp 21–43.
3. Chuang AT, Steers WD: Neurophysiology of penile erection. In Carson CC, Kirby R, Goldstein I (eds): Textbook of Erectile Dysfunction. London, ISIS Medical Media, pp 59–72, 1999.
4. Saenz de Tejada I, Gonzalez Cadavid N, Heaton J, et al: Anatomy, physiology and pathophysiology of erectile function. In Jardin A, Wagner G, Khoury S, et al (eds): Erectile Dysfunction: WHO First International Consultation. Plymouth, Plybridge, 2000, pp 65–103.
5. Smith PJ, Talbert RL: Sexual dysfunction with antihypertensives and antipsychotic agents. Clin Pharm 5:373–384, 1986.
6. Horn LJ, Zasler ND: Neuroanatomy and neurophysiology of sexual function. J Head Trauma Rehabil 5:1–13, 1990.
7. Stasberg PD, Brady SM: Sexual functioning of persons with neurologic disorders. Semin Neurol 8:1–13, 1990.
8. Blumer D, Walker AE: The neural basis of sexual behavior. In Benson DF, Blumer D (eds): Psychiatric Aspects of Neurologic Disease. New York, Grune and Stratton, 1975, pp 199–217.
9. Andersson KE, Wagner G: Physiology of penile erection. Physiol Rev 75:191–236, 1995.
10. Nitahara KS, Lue TF: Microscopic anatomy of the penis. In Carson CC, Kirby R, Goldstein I (eds): Textbook of Erectile Dysfunction. London, ISIS Medical Media, 1999, pp 31–42.
11. De Groat WC, Booth AM: Autonomic systems to the urinary bladder and sexual organs In Dycj PJ, Thomas PK, Lambert EH, Bunge R (eds): Peripheral Neuropathy. New York, Saunders, 1989, pp 285–299.
12. Marson L, McKenna KE: A role for 5-hydrosytryptamine in descending inhibition of spinal sexual reflexes. Exp Brain Res 88:313–320, 1992.
13. Rose JD: Brainstem influences on sexual behavior. In Klemm WR, Verities RP (eds): Brainstem Influences on Sexual Behavior. New York, John Wiley & Sons, pp 407–463.
14. Deletis V: Intraoperative monitoring of the dorsal sacral roots: Minimizing the risk of iatrogenic micturition disorders. Neurosurgery 30:72–75, 1992.
15. Siroky MB: Neurophysiology of male sexual dysfunction in neurologic disorders. Semin Neurol 8:137–140, 1988.
16. Lue TF: Male sexual dysfunction. In Tanagho EA, Mc Aninch JW (eds): Smith's General Urology, 12th ed. Norwalk, CT, Appleton & Lange, 1998, pp 663–678.
17. Donatucci CF, Lue TF: Physiology of the penile tumescence. In Hashmat AI, Das S (eds): The Penis. Philadelphia, Lea & Febiger, 1993, pp 17–22.
18. Naylor AM: Endogenous neurotransmitters mediating penile erection. Br J Urol 81:424–431, 1998.

19. Christ GJ: The penis as a vascular organ: The importance of corporal smooth muscle tone in the control of erection. Urol Clin North Am 22:727–745, 1995.
20. Kim N, Vardi Y, Padma-Nathan H, et al: Oxygen tension regulates the nitrictic oxide pathway: Physiological role in penile erection. J Clin Invest 91:437–442, 1993.
21. Brock G, Hsu GL, Nunes L, et al: The anatomy of the tunica albuginea in the normal penis and in Peyronie's disease. J Urol 157:276–281, 1997.
22. Saenz de Tejada I, Kim N, Lagan I, et al: Modulation of adrenergic activity in penile corpus cavernosum. J Urol 142:1117, 1989.
23. Hatzichristou DG, Saenz de Tejada I, Kupferman S, et al: In vivo assessment of trabecular smooth muscle tone, its application in pharmacocavernosometry and analysis of intracavernous pressure determinants. J Urol 153:1126, 1995.
24. Knowles RG, Moncada S: Nitric oxide synthesis in mammals. Biochem J 298:249, 1994.
25. Ottesen B, Wagner G, Virag R, Fahrenkrug J: Penile erection: Possible role for vasoactive intestinal polypeptide as a neurotransmitter. Br Med J 288:9, 1984.
26. Christ H, Brink PR, Brooks S, Ney P: PGE1-induced alterations in maxi-K+ channel activity in cultured human corporal smooth muscle cells. J Urol 155:678A (abstract 1468), 1996.
27. Kwan M, Greenleaf WJ, Mann J, et al: The nature of androgen action on male sexuality: A combined laboratory-self-report study on hypogonadal men. J Clin Endocrinol Metab 57:557–562, 1983.
28. Salmimies P, Kockott G, Pirke KM, et al: Effects of testosterone replacement on sexual behavior in hypogonadal men. Arch Sex Behav 11:345–353, 1982.
29. Lugg JA, Rajfer J, Gonzalez-Cadavid NF: Dihydrotestosterone is the active androgen in the maintenance of nitric oxide-mediated penile erection in the rat. Endocrinology 136:1495–1501, 1995.
30. Andersson KE, Wagner G: Physiology of penile erection. Physiol Rev 75:191–236, 1995.
31. Christ GJ: The penis as a vascular organ: The importance of corporal smooth muscle tone in the control of erection. Urol Clin North Am 22:727–745, 1995.
32. Lue TF: Erectile dysfunction. N Engl J Med 342:1802–1813, 2000.
33. Lue TF, Tanagho EA: Hemodynamics of erection. In Tanagho EA, Lue TF, McClure RD (eds): Contemporary Management of Impotence and Infertility. Baltimore, Williams & Wilkins, 1998, pp 28–38.

PART II

Pathophysiology of Pelvic Floor Disorders

CHAPTER 6

Pregnancy, Childbirth, and Pelvic Floor Damage

KAVEN BAESSLER ■ BERNHARD SCHUESSLER

Vaginal delivery is an important cause of stress urinary and fecal incontinence and pelvic organ prolapse. Most epidemiologic studies link pelvic floor disorders and parity.[1-6] Until recently research had focused on fetal safety during labor; little research had been done on maternal morbidity. However, significant improvements have been achieved in fetal well-being and important information about latent and apparent maternal injuries during birth and its sequelae has emerged. There's a chance of nerve, muscle, and connective tissue damage after vaginal birth, which has been shown also in women with pelvic floor disorders.

As the population ages, apparent as well as latent injuries caused at birth may affect more women. More women will live to an older age and will be active enough to experience incontinence and pelvic organ prolapse. Although surgery for pelvic organ prolapse might be effective in restoring anatomy, functional outcomes have not been shown to be as satisfactory as anatomical results.[7-9]

This chapter summarizes the current research on childbirth and pelvic floor sequelae and provides an analysis of relevant knowledge to guide strategies for prevention. It discusses the effects of pregnancy and childbirth on the pelvic floor anatomy and function, the impact of intrapartum interventions, and the subsequent state-of-the-art management of childbirth.

PELVIC FLOOR TRAUMA DUE TO VAGINAL DELIVERY

The levator ani muscle supports the pelvic organs and helps to maintain continence. Vaginal delivery, especially during the second stage of labor when the baby's head emerges, distends the pelvic floor (Fig. 6-1). The status of the levator ani muscle can be assessed before and after childbirth by measuring the ability of this muscle to hold the perineal body in place both at rest and during training.[10] Vaginal delivery can lower the position of the perineum.[11-13]

Research shows, however, that 5 years after vaginal birth the perineum returns to its antepartum position.[14] Vaginal delivery also weakens pelvic floor muscles, a finding that is consistent regardless of the measurement technique used (e.g., vaginal cones,[15,16] standardized physical examination,[16-19] or intravaginal squeeze pressure[17,19,20-22]). Antepartum instruction on how to perform pelvic floor exercises seems important; in contrast with women who performed pelvic floor exercises, women who were not instructed did not regain antepartum pelvic floor contraction pressures 8 weeks after vaginal delivery.[21] One study found that 6 weeks postpartum 34% of women were not capable of an assessable voluntary pelvic floor contraction. This number decreased to 6% after 6 weeks of pelvic floor training with and without vaginal weights.[16]

Perineal ultrasound can be used to image the elevation of the bladder neck during a voluntary contraction of the levator ani muscle. A comparison of bladder neck elevation during pregnancy and 3 to 8 days postpartum revealed a significant decrease after vaginal delivery and a return to the antepartum position after 6 to 10 weeks.[23] In contrast, intravaginal contraction measurements remained significantly lower 6 to 10 weeks postpartum. This difference might be due a widened vagina, which reduces pressure transmission of the levator ani contraction to the intravaginal probe.[17]

Intact innervation of the levator ani muscle and anal and urethral sphincters is critical to normal pelvic floor function. In histologic and electrophysiologic studies that assessed neuromuscular pelvic floor damage, parous women, in contrast with nulliparous women, showed a decrease of type I muscle fibers (slow-twitch fibers) in the levator ani muscle and an increase of area and circumference of fibers.[24] Especially in the posterior part of the pubococcygeus muscle, pathologic changes were observed in incontinent women who gave birth vaginally.[25] These histologic characteristics are signs of reinnervation of striated muscle after partial denervation that may have occurred during vaginal delivery.

Single-fiber electromyogram and concentric-needle electromyogram can also identify partial denervation by

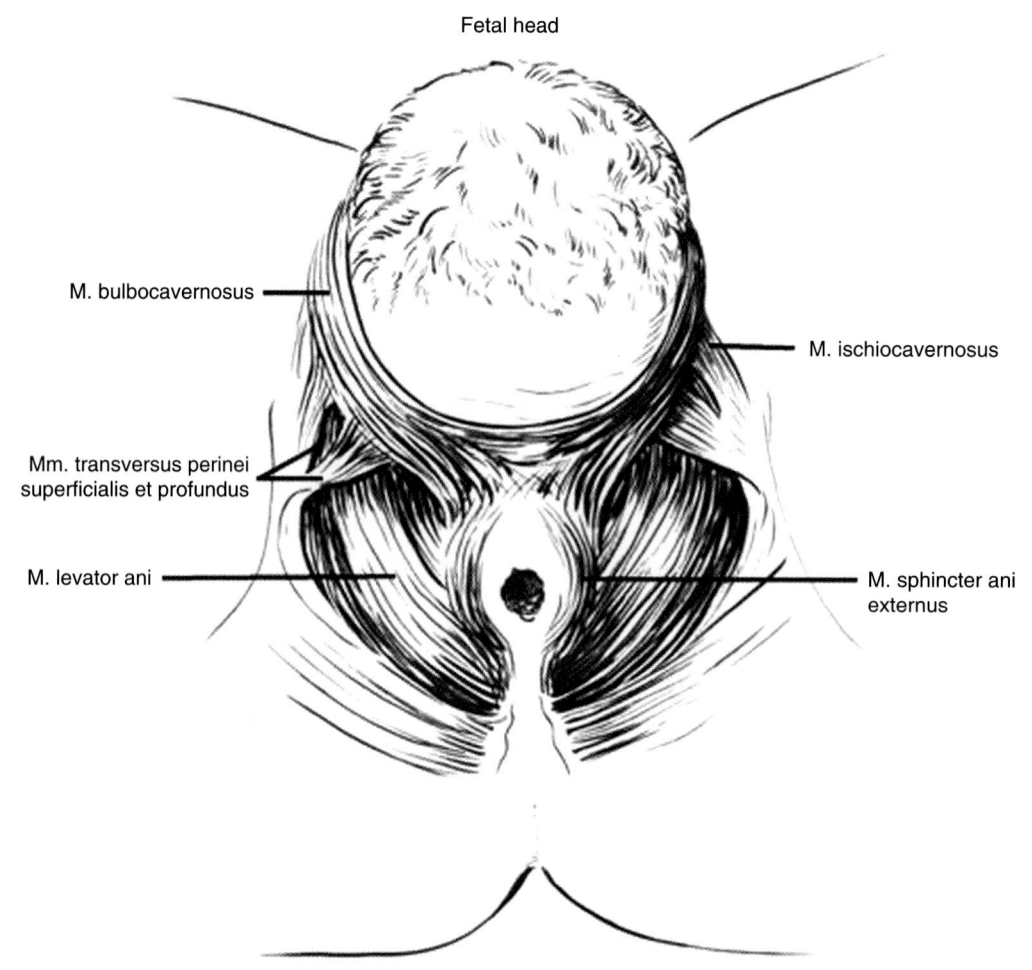

FIGURE 6-1 Pelvic floor distension during vaginal delivery. Note the stretching of the levator ani muscle and separation of the transverse perineal muscles.

signs of reinnervation. Vaginal delivery appears to result in pelvic floor denervation in up to 80% of women.[11,20,26] Pelvic floor denervation seems to progress with age.[14,24,27] Although no signs of reinnervation were found after elective cesarean section, changes were present after emergency cesarean sections when labor had already progressed.[20]

Prolongation of the pudendal nerve terminal motor latency (PNTML) is thought to be a result of pudendal nerve damage during vaginal delivery or excessive straining at defecation.[28] Although some question the value of the PNTML because only the fast conducting fibers are measured,[29] there is evidence of pudendal nerve damage caused by childbirth. Significantly prolonged PNTMLs have been found in women 2 to 3 days after vaginal delivery compared with a multiparous[11] and a nulliparous control group.[26] A 5-year follow-up found that prolongation of PNTML persisted.[14] In two prospective analyses,[13,30] PNTML was measured before and 6 to 8 weeks after vaginal delivery, demonstrating prolongation of latencies after vaginal delivery,[13,30] particularly after the first delivery.[13] Pregnancy itself caused no changes in PNTML.[30] Two-thirds of the women with an abnormally prolonged PNTML after delivery had normal measurements after 6 months.[13]

Case-control studies link pelvic floor disorders, nerve dysfunction, and childbirth. The studies indicate that fiber density is higher in parous than in nulliparous women and even higher in women with stress urinary incontinence or prolapse of pelvic organs.[26] An altered pelvic floor muscle activation pattern with absence and asymmetry of recruitment of motor units was described in stress incontinent parous women compared to nulliparous continent women.[31] Pudendal nerve terminal motor latency correlated with increasing parity in 126 perimenopausal women.[4]

The integrity of the urethral sphincter at rest as well as its performance under conditions of increased abdominal pressure ("pressure transmission") and during a voluntary pelvic floor contraction can be studied by urethral pressure profile measurements. Prospective urodynamic studies performed during pregnancy and 8 weeks postpartum revealed a notable decrease in urethral closure pressure,[32] functional urethral length,[19,32,33] and intraabdominal pressure transmission to the urethra during coughing after vaginal delivery.[34] The pressure transmission remained unchanged in women who underwent cesarean section.[34] One prospective study demonstrated no change of maximum urethral closure pressure and pressure transmission ratios 9 weeks postpartum, although there were no measurements immediately after childbirth.[19]

Compared with continent women and women who experienced urinary incontinence only during pregnancy, women with persistent urinary incontinence after childbirth were found to have a shorter functional urethral length, a lower urethral closure pressure, and a negative urethral closure pressure at coughing.[35,36] Bladder capacity was lower in pregnant than in nonpregnant women and increased 3 months postpartum,[37] although the capacity remained lower than normal.[37,38]

Reduced bladder neck support at rest and increased bladder neck mobility during straining after vaginal delivery compared to antepartum values have been demonstrated with perineal ultrasound.[19,23,39] The position of the bladder neck at rest and during straining was also lower postpartum compared with a control group of nulliparous women and with women who had elective cesarean sections.[23,39] Forceps assisted delivery resulted in an increased bladder neck excursion postpartum.[39]

It is still unclear how these described changes in the urethral sphincter unit contribute to the development or persistence of urinary incontinence after vaginal delivery. Up to 82% of women report symptoms of stress incontinence during pregnancy.[6,19,39–46] De novo postpartum stress urinary incontinence develops in 4% to 19% of women who give birth vaginally.[39,41-46] Compared with women who delivered by cesarean section, stress urinary incontinence is significantly more common after vaginal delivery.[19,43,44,47,48] Urodynamically investigated urinary symptoms show remarkably less urodynamic stress incontinence during pregnancy (9%) and postpartum (5%). Detrusor instability was demonstrated in 8% of women antepartum and in 7% postpartum.[37]

Long-term persistence of de novo postpartum stress incontinence has scarcely been assessed.[44,48,49] A 1-year postpartum study reported that 24% of primiparous women had persistent incontinence.[44] Another study found that stress incontinence persisted for at least one year postpartum in 75%.[48] One study followed 278 women for 5 years after their first delivery.[49] A validated questionnaire revealed significantly increased urinary incontinence during the 5 years of observation, being 19% for stress urinary incontinence and 11% for urge incontinence. Women with onset of urinary incontinence during the first pregnancy or puerperium had a significantly higher risk of incontinence 5 years postpartum than did women without urinary symptoms. Subsequent deliveries did not influence these incidences.[49]

The contribution of obstetrical factors to the development of stress incontinence is controversial. In some studies the duration of the second stage of labor[44,48,50] and birth weight[45,48] were associated with a higher incidence of stress incontinence. Other authors did not find significant correlations between stress incontinence and fetal head circumference,[43,52] second stage of labor,[44,47,48,51] or birth weight.[42,43,52,53] These studies are difficult to compare because their questioning techniques and definitions of incontinence vary widely. Also incontinence symptoms were more likely to be reported if they were more bothersome, and self-reporting was linked to a higher socioeconomic status.[54] A well-designed prospective study by Viktrup and colleagues showed that in a large sample size of 305 women, all obstetric risk factors that had shown a statistically significant correlation with the incontinence incidence immediately after delivery had vanished 3 months later.[44]

Great effort has been put into studies that assess predictive factors. Women with postpartum stress incontinence were found to have had greater bladder neck mobility during straining before delivery than continent women did.[39] Spontaneous perineal laceration >3 cm was not a risk factor for postpartum urinary incontinence.[45] One study found that, apart from vaginal delivery and multiparity, obesity was associated with the development of incontinence 3 months after childbirth[47]; Chaliha and colleagues did not observe the same association in a study of antenatal predictors of postpartum incontinence.[46] Markers of collagen weakness like striae, varicose veins, hemorrhoids, and joint hypermobility, were previously implicated in the pathogenesis of incontinence but failed to predict postpartum urinary and fecal incontinence.[46] Regular antepartum pelvic floor exercises significantly reduced the prevalence of postpartum incontinence,[39,47] whereas smoking was a possible risk factor for incontinence during pregnancy.[45]

For clinical consistency of the description of perineal trauma after childbirth, Abdul Sultan proposed the following classifications[55]:

First-degree tear: involving the vaginal epitheium only

Second-degree tear: involving the perineal muscles but not the anal sphincter

Third-degree tear: involving partial or complete disruption of the anal sphincter

(a) less than 50% of the external anal sphincter thickness torn
(b) 50% or more of the external anal sphincter thickness torn
(c) involving disruption of the internal anal sphincter.

Fourth-degree tear: involving torn anal epithelium

Clinically visible anal sphincter tears occur in up to 6.4% of vaginal deliveries.[45,56–66] With the advent of endoanal ultrasound it is possible to accurately, noninvasively, and painlessly image the anatomy of the anal sphincter without radiation. Occult, clinically not recognized, or not visible anal sphincter defects have been identified by endoanal ultrasound performed before and after delivery. Occult sphincter defects occur in up to 33% of primiparous and 4% of multiparous women after vaginal delivery.[46,63,67,68] In 16% of 79 primiparas only the internal anal sphincter was involved.[67] Unsuspected sphincter defects in women with fecal incontinence and in women attending a gynecology clinic for problems unrelated to the pelvic floor have also been described.[69,70] Figure 6-2 shows the normal anatomy of the female anal sphincter. In Figure 6-3 there is obstetric trauma with an external anal sphincter defect. An external and internal sphincter defect is seen in Figure 6-4.

An occult, sonographically identified anterior anal sphincter defect can be assumed if it does not extend for

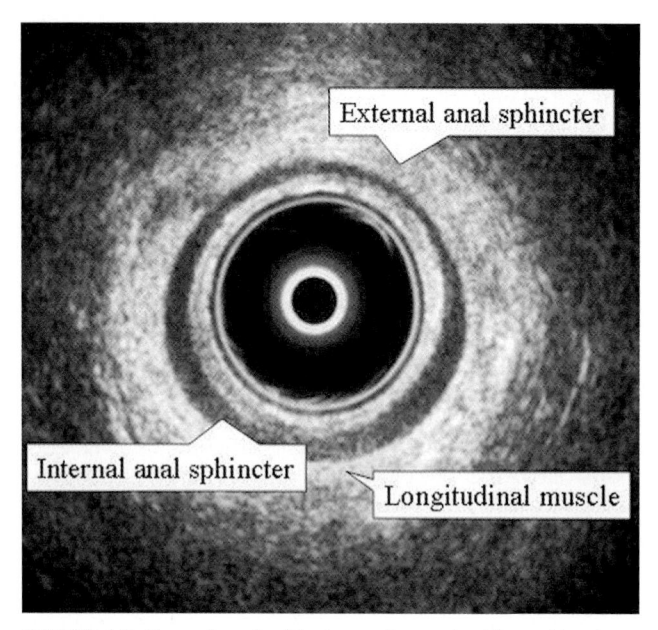

FIGURE 6-2 Normal anal sphincter anatomy at mid canal level.

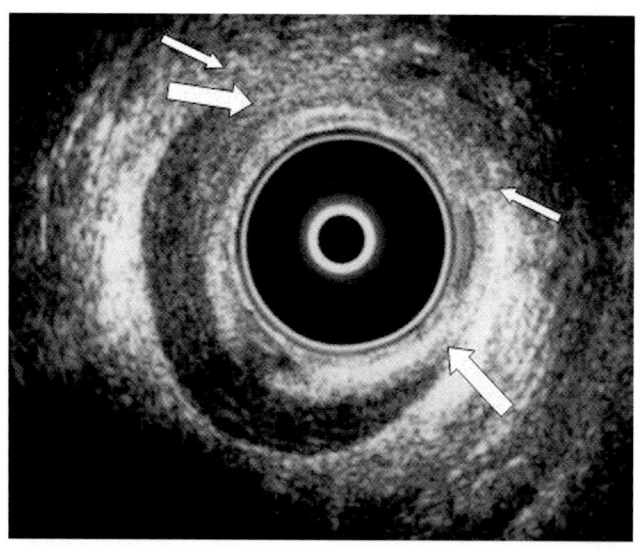

FIGURE 6-4 An external (*large arrows*) and internal anal sphincter defect (*small arrows*). Note the thickening of the remaining internal anal sphincter caused by retraction of the muscle ends.

more than a segment that corresponds to one hour on a clock face. Occult anterior sphincter defects that involve the full thickness of the external anal sphincter and extend for more than one segment on a clock face are significant defects, which were probably missed at delivery.[55]

Several obstetric risk factors for the development of sphincter lacerations have been identified. The use of midline episiotomy was associated with higher incidences of sphincter lacerations than in women who did not receive an episiotomy.[71-75] Use of fewer midline episiotomies resulted in an increase of intact perinea.[76] The first vaginal delivery was consistently found to result more frequently in anal sphincter tears.[64,66,72-80] The occipito-posterior presentation,[58,81] a higher birth weight,[58,64-66,73,78,80-82] prolonged second stage of labor,[63,64,83,84] and labor induction[80] were also associated with a higher sphincter laceration rate. Not all studies analyzed all obstetric factors, but no study revealed a negative correlation with these factors. Only one protective factor has been described: Klein and colleagues showed that a strong exercise profile (e.g., jogging, bicycling three or more times per week) is associated with fewer third- and fourth-degree tears.[73]

The contraction pressure of the anal sphincter decreases significantly after vaginal delivery.[14,19,58,63,85,86] Anal sphincter pressures at rest are also reduced after vaginal delivery but not after cesarean section.[12,63,67,87,88] Resting pressures tend to recover 1 to 6 months postpartum,[12,86,87] whereas squeeze pressures increase but do not reach antenatal values,[12,14,58,67,86,88] particularly if the anal sphincter was damaged.[87] The contraction pressure decreases more after anal sphincter ruptures than after spontaneous deliveries without perineal tears.[61,67,89] The decrement of resting pressure seems to be associated with a defect in the internal sphincter.[67]

Anal canal sensation has been assessed by mucosal electrosensitivity and was found to be impaired immediately after vaginal birth but not after cesarean section. Six months postpartum this difference disappeared.[87] Another study could not confirm these changes in anal sensation after vaginal delivery.[12] In 144 perimenopausal women, however, decreased anal sensibility correlated with increasing parity.[4]

After vaginal delivery, 0.04% to 6% of women develop new fecal incontinence.[2,19,46,52,61,63,90-92] This prevalence rises to levels of 17% to 50% after vaginal delivery complicated by anal sphincter rupture.[52,56,61,64,67,83,87,89,91,93,94] Most of these anal symptoms are transient, but 7% to 42% of women who were incontinent for feces immediately after childbirth with a sphincter tear, reported persisting symptoms 2 to 13 years after vaginal delivery.[89,93,95] In women without

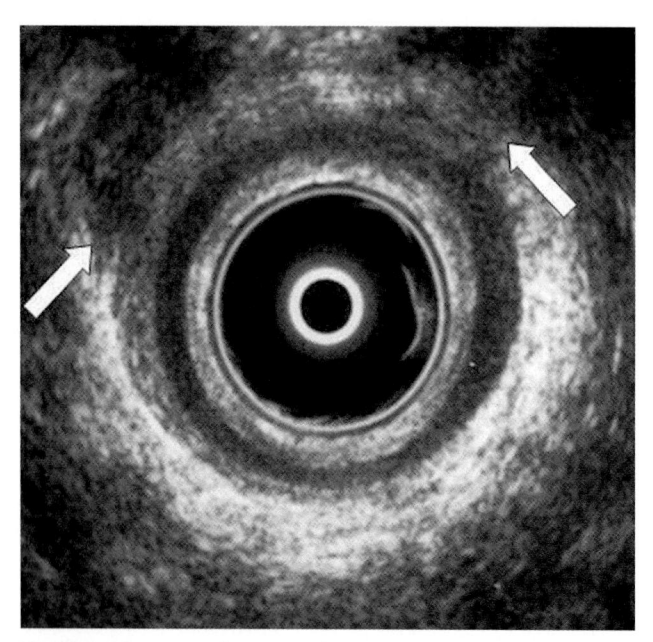

FIGURE 6-3 An anterior external anal sphincter defect (*arrows*).

sphincter lacerations, multiparity increased the incidence of permanent incontinence of flatus, being 8.3% after the third vaginal delivery.[2] Vaginal deliveries subsequent to a delivery with anal sphincter rupture and transient fecal incontinence resulted in recurrent transient anal incontinence in 39% and in permanent incontinence in 4%.[93] Maternal age was associated with the development of fecal incontinence and involuntary flatus 9 months postpartum.[92] Prolonged pudendal nerve terminal motor latency, instrumental delivery, and second stage of labor of more than 60 minutes were also associated with an increased risk of postpartum alteration of fecal continence.[63] Symptoms of fecal incontinence correlated with sphincter defects imaged by endoanal sonography[67,83,86] and with decreased anal pressures.[67,86] Emergency cesarean section performed at 4 to 7 cm of cervical dilatation did not necessarily prevent the development of anal incontinence.[90] Anal sexual intercourse was not a risk factor for postpartum anal incontinence.[83]

Only one long-term study contradicts the correlation between fecal incontinence and sphincter tears.[62] In a retrospective matched control study approximately 30 years postpartum, 29 women with anal sphincter disruption were compared with 89 women with episiotomy and 33 women who delivered by cesarean section. The prevalence of incontinence of flatus and feces did not differ significantly in the three groups (episiotomy group 31% and 18%, sphincter rupture group 43% and 7%, cesarean section group 36.4% and 0). No women who delivered by cesarean section developed fecal incontinence.[62] This study did not include clinical or sonographic examination, and thus it could not specify symptoms and clinical and latent sphincter defects.

In 40% to 85% of women who sustained a third-degree tear, endoanal sonography showed residual sphincter defects at ultrasound, indicating that the anal sphincter was inadequately repaired.[58,84] Primary sphincter repair usually employs the end-to-end technique. The overlap technique used by colorectal surgeons for secondary sphincter repairs appeared to be feasible for primary repair too.[96] The two techniques were compared in a randomized controlled trial.[7] The anatomic and functional outcomes of primary end-to-end repair and overlap repair were similar. Two thirds of women had persisting sphincter defects revealed by sonography, irrespective of the method of repair.[97]

INTRAPARTUM INTERVENTIONS: IMPACT ON PELVIC FLOOR ANATOMY AND FUNCTION

Episiotomy

Systematic reviews of episiotomy for vaginal birth concluded that the restrictive use of episiotomy is superior to routine episiotomy regarding perineal trauma, suturing, and healing. There are no differences regarding dyspareunia, urinary incontinence, and pain. Restrictive use of episiotomy increases anterior perineal trauma.[98,99]

Woolley[74] critically reviewed the professional literature on the benefits and risks of episiotomies from 1980 to 1994 after Thacker and Banta[75] had reviewed the literature from 1960 to 1980. Both reviews examined episiotomy benefit claims made in obstetrics textbooks: An episiotomy prevents perineal lacerations, is easier to repair, causes less pain, will heal better, is preferable to a spontaneous perineal tear, reduces the incidence of anterior perineal laceration, and relieves the baby's head of pressure that might lead to brain injuries. These claims have recently been questioned in controlled studies. Woolley[74] concluded in his systematic review that a mediolateral or midline episiotomy does not prevent damage to the anal sphincter and its sequelae. Episiotomy does not protect the newborn from intracranial hemorrhage or intrapartum asphyxia. Midline episiotomy carries a significantly higher risk of extension into the anal sphincter than no episiotomy. Episiotomy does prevent anterior lacerations, which are not considered severe complications. Episiotomy increases maternal blood loss. In the first week after vaginal delivery, perineal pain is more common after episiotomy than after a spontaneous perineal laceration. However, these differences disappear by 1 month postpartum.[74]

Studies that have been performed since this review confirm Woolley's[74] conclusions: Routine as well as selective midline episiotomies are associated with high incidences of sphincter lacerations.[65,72,73,100] A reduction in the use of midline episiotomies results in an increase of intact perinea. Mediolateral episiotomies do not prevent sphincter ruptures.[60,63,101,102] The second stage of labor is not related to the episiotomy rate. Most studies showed that reduced midline as well as mediolateral episiotomy rates result in an increase in anterior and vaginal lacerations,[73,101,103,104] which are considered minor injuries, and which do not increase postpartum pain.[103]

Only two retrospective case-control studies, from the Netherlands, report that mediolateral episiotomy protects against severe sphincter lacerations.[59,80] It was calculated that among primiparas 48 episiotomies would have to be performed to prevent one severe tear. This number rises to 106 episiotomies among multiparas. It was concluded that there is no justification for routine episiotomy.[59]

Perineal pain, disturbed wound healing, and dyspareunia are more common in women who delivered with a mediolateral episiotomy than with a midline episiotomy or with spontaneous perineal tears.[82,105-107] Vaginal tears, forceps extraction, and suture dehiscence were associated with perineal discomfort lasting longer than 1 month postpartum.[106] Women in the group with restricted use of episiotomy and women with an intact perineum started postpartum sexual intercourse earlier than women in a group with routine episiotomy.[82,108]

Prospective randomized controlled trials and retrospective studies have also failed to demonstrate a protective effect of the mediolateral or midline episiotomy on stress urinary incontinence after vaginal delivery.[44,52,108,109] In fact, two studies found a higher rate of stress incontinence when a mediolateral episiotomy was performed.[44,45] The incidence of stress urinary incontinence did not differ after episiotomies and spontaneous perineal tears.[52] An episiotomy neither increased nor decreased pudendal nerve terminal motor latency,[11,13,26] urethral closure pressure,[32] pelvic floor muscle strength,[22,110] or pelvic floor denervation.[20]

Vacuum and Forceps Extraction

Systematic reviews of vacuum extraction versus forceps for assisted vaginal delivery concluded that there is less maternal morbidity with the use of the vacuum extractor. Although serious neonatal injury is uncommon with either instrument, the vacuum is associated with an increase in neonatal cephalhematoma and retinal hemorrhage.[99,111]

There is a higher risk of sphincter laceration when the forceps are used than with vacuum extraction.[73,80,82–84,110–115] Occult sphincter defects that were visible only sonographically were also more common after delivery with forceps.[67] Symptoms of fecal incontinence correlate with sphincter defects and are seen in 38% of women who delivered with forceps, in 12% of women who delivered with vacuum extraction, and in 4% of spontaneous deliveries with a significant difference between forceps-assisted and spontaneous delivery.[67] In general, the risk of developing fecal incontinence is increased after operative vaginal delivery.[90] Women who delivered with forceps reported perineal pain more often than women who delivered with vacuum extraction.[112] With respect to neonatal morbidity, forceps delivery is associated with fewer cephalhematomata,[112,116] fewer sucking difficulties,[112] fewer retinal hemorrhages,[114] and fewer hyperbilirubinemia[114,117]; but the potential for facial injury[114] is higher with forceps-assisted delivery than with vacuum extraction. In a randomized controlled trial that compared vacuum and forceps extraction, hyperbilirubinemia rates did not differ.[116]

The higher risk of pelvic floor damage with forceps-assisted delivery than with vacuum extraction can be explained by the inability to flex or rotate the baby's head after the forceps are applied. Also, the additional volume occupied by the forceps passing the outlet may partly account for an increase in sphincter tears.[116]

Anesthesia for Vaginal Delivery

The role of epidural anesthesia or pudendal block in the occurrence of sphincter lacerations and postpartum incontinence is not clear. One study found epidural anesthesia during vaginal delivery lessened development of postpartum urinary stress incontinence in comparison to the pudendal block.[43] Another study found a higher incidence of stress incontinence in women who received epidural anesthesia than in women who had had no anesthesia.[51] A third study also observed an increase of stress incontinence in women who delivered with epidural anesthesia, especially if the second stage of labor was longer than 120 minutes.[50] Epidural anesthesia may be associated with a higher incidence of instrumental deliveries,[65,118] which may increase the rate of episiotomy and the occurrence of anal sphincter lacerations.

Position for Birth

The systematic Cochrane database review concluded that the adoption of any upright or lateral position for birth is associated with a shorter second stage of labor, fewer instrumental deliveries, and fewer episiotomies. However, there is an increased risk of blood loss of more than 500 mL.[119]

Several studies showed that the supine and lithotomy positions for childbirth had a negative effect on the perineum,[73,120,121] especially if stirrups were used.[122] The lateral position[121] and upright positions seem to protect the perineum[92,116] and tend to reduce forceps-assisted deliveries.[120]

CONCLUSION

It is evident that vaginal delivery can damage the pelvic floor. Some functional loss can be avoided by an elective cesarean section, but not necessarily by an emergency cesarean section.[20,90] Cesarean section carries other health risks, however, including a longer recovery. Elective cesarean section should be considered if the woman has an increased risk for functional loss of the pelvic floor. Elective cesarean section should be discussed with women who have had successful surgery for anal or urinary incontinence or pelvic organ prolapse or who have preexisting anal incontinence. To date the balance of hazards and benefits is unclear. As indicated by the strong desire of female London gynecologists to opt for an elective cesarean section,[123] it is likely that some women without obvious risk factors will ask for an elective cesarean section to protect the pelvic floor. The risks of cesarean section, such as an increase in postpartum hysterectomy, adhesions, ileus, placental implantation in subsequent pregnancies, and an increased risk of a respiratory distress syndrome in the newborn,[124] should be discussed carefully.

The impact of vaginal birth and intrapartum management on the connective tissue and on development or prevention of endopelvic fascia defects leading to cysto-, recto-, and enteroceles or loss of paravaginal support[125,126] has not been examined systematically and remains unclear.

The advantages of vaginal delivery without episiotomy are numerous. It is evident that it is possible to lower the mediolateral episiotomy rate in primiparas to 20% to 30% without increased risk of anal sphincter damage (Fig. 6-5).[108,109,127–129] Whether it is possible to further reduce this rate without an increase of third- or fourth-degree tears remains unclear. The general rate of episiotomy can be reduced only if midwives and doctors are sensitized and specially trained[102,109] and if continuity of midwifery care is provided.[130] Adoption of upright birth positions, perineal massage, warm compresses to the perineum, and flexion of and counterpressure to the baby's head may reduce both episiotomies and sphincter lacerations.[66,100,121,131–133]

Forceps-assisted delivery is associated with a higher risk of third- and fourth-degree tears than delivery with vacuum extraction. The increase of minor fetal risks

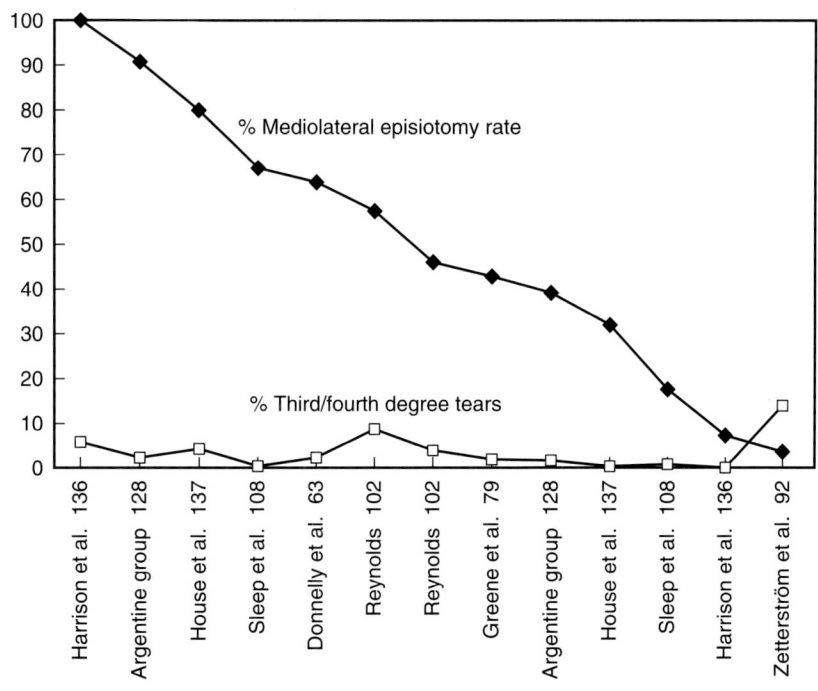

FIGURE 6-5 Rate of mediolateral episiotomy and corresponding rate of third- and fourth-degree perineal tears in nulliparous women.[63,79,92,102,108,128,136,137] Data include four randomized controlled trials comparing different episiotomy rates (routine and restricted use of episiotomy).[108,128,136,137]

following vacuum extraction are not strong arguments for routine use of forceps for delivery of mature fetuses when an instrumental delivery is required.

Prepartum pelvic floor exercises may lead to a decline of postpartum stress urinary incontinence[39,47] and an increase in postpartum pelvic floor contraction strength.[108,134] Obese women have a higher risk of urinary incontinence during pregnancy and postpartum.[45,47,135] Smoking is also a possible risk factor for urinary incontinence in pregnancy.[45] The odds for anal sphincter trauma are lower for women who regularly participate in sporting activities like jogging.[73] Pelvic floor exercises and a habit of regular exercise resulted in higher levator ani contraction pressures than did postpartal pelvic floor exercises alone. Research indicates that the woman herself can help prevent loss of pelvic floor function after childbirth. Regular athletic activities, pelvic floor exercises, and an upright birth position may reduce pelvic floor damage during childbirth.

REFERENCES

1. Foldspang A, Mommsen S, Lam GW, Elving L: Parity as a correlate of adult female urinary incontinence prevalence. J Epidemiol Community Health 46:595–600, 1992.
2. Ryhammer AM, Bek KM, Laurberg S: Multiple vaginal deliveries increase the risk of permanent incontinence of flatus and urine in normal premenopausal women. Dis Colon Rectum 38:1206–1209, 1995.
3. Mant J, Painter R, Vessey M: Epidemiology of genital prolapse: Observations from the Oxford Family Planning Association study. Br J Obstet Gynaecol 104:579–585, 1997.
4. Ryhammer AM, Laurberg S, Hermann AP: Long-term effect of vaginal deliveries on anorectal function in normal perimenopausal women. Dis Colon Rectum 39:852–859, 1996.
5. Gainey HL: Postpartum observation of pelvic tissue damage. Am J Obstet Gynecol 45:457–466, 1943.
6. Marshall K, Thompson KA, Walsh DM, Baxter GD: Incidence of urinary incontinence and constipation during pregnancy and postpartum: Survey of current findings at the Rotunda Lying-in Hospital. Br J Obstet Gynaecol 105:400–402, 1998.
7. Kahn MA, Stanton SL: Posterior colporrhaphy: Its effects on bowel and sexual function. Br J Obstet Gynaecol 104:82–86, 1997.
8. Baker KR, Beresford JM, Campbell C: Colposacropexy with Prolene mesh. Surg Gynecol Obstet 171:51–54, 1990.
9. Snyder TE, Krantz KE: Abdominal-retroperitoneal sacral colpopexy for the correction of vaginal prolapse. Obstet Gynecol 77:944–949, 1991.
10. Henry MM, Parks AG, Swash M: The pelvic floor musculature in the descending perineum syndrome. Br J Surg 69:470–472, 1982.
11. Snooks SJ, Setchell M, Swash M, Henry MM: Injury to innervation of pelvic floor sphincter musculature in childbirth. Lancet 8:546–550, 1984.
12. Small KA, Wynne JM. Evaluating the pelvic floor in obstetric patients. Aust NZ J Obstet Gynaecol 30:41–45, 1990.
13. Sultan AH, Kamm MA, Hudson CN: Pudendal nerve damage during labour: Prospective study before and after childbirth. Br J Obstet Gynaecol 101:22–28, 1994.
14. Snooks SJ, Swash M, Mathers SE, Henry MM: Effect of vaginal delivery on the pelvic floor: A 5-year follow-up. Br J Surg 77:1358–1360, 1990.

15. Röckner G, Jonasson A, Ölund A: The effect of mediolateral episiotomy at delivery on pelvic floor muscle strength evaluated with vaginal cones. Acta Obstet Gynecol Scand 70:51–54, 1991.
16. Fischer W, Baessler K: Postpartum pelvic floor conditioning using vaginal cones: Not only for prophylaxis against urinary incontinence and descensus. Int Urogynecol J 7:208–214, 1996.
17. Peschers U, Schaer G, Anthuber C, et al: Levator ani function before and after childbirth. Br J Obstet Gynaecol 104:1004–1008, 1997.
18. Sampselle CM: Changes in pelvic muscle strength and stress urinary incontinence associated with childbirth. J Obstet Gynecol Neonatal Nurs 19:371–377, 1990.
19. Meyer S, Schreyer A, De Grandi P, Hohlfeld P: The effects of birth on urinary continence mechanisms and other pelvic-floor characteristics. Obstet Gynecol 92:613–618, 1998.
20. Allen RE, Hosker GL, Smith ARB, Warrell DW: Pelvic floor damage and childbirth: A neurophysiological study. Br J Obstet Gynaecol 97:770–779, 1990.
21. Nielsen CA, Sigsgaard I, Olsen M, et al: Trainability of the pelvic floor. A prospective study during pregnancy and after delivery. Acta Obstet Gynecol Scand 67:437–440, 1988
22. Samples JT, Dougherty MC, Abrams RM, Batich CD: The dynamic characteristics of the circumvaginal muscles. J Obstet Gynecol Neonatal Nurs 17:194–201, 1998.
23. Peschers U, Schaer G, Anthuber C, et al: Changes in vesical neck mobility following vaginal delivery. Obstet Gynecol 88:1001–1006, 1996.
24. Dimpfl T, Müller-Felber W, Anthuber C, et al: Histomorphology of the pelvic floor muscles under specific consideration of age and parity. Neurourol Urodynam 15:333–334, 1996.
25. Gilpin SA, Gosling JA, Smith ARB, Warrell DW: The pathogenesis of genitourinary prolapse and stress incontinence of urine. A histological and histochemical study. Br J Obstet Gynaecol 96:15–23, 1989.
26. Snooks SJ, Swash M, Henry MM, Setchell M: Risk factors in childbirth causing damage to the pelvic floor innervation. Int J Colorect Dis 1:20–24, 1986.
27. Smith ARB, Hosker GL, Warrell DW: The role of partial denervation of the pelvic floor in the aetiology of genitourinary prolapse and stress incontinence of urine. A neurophysiological study. Br J Obstet Gynaecol 96:24–28, 1989.
28. Lubowski DZ, Swash M, Nicholls RJ, Henry MM: Increase in pudendal nerve terminal motor latency with defaecation straining. Br J Surg 75:1095–1097, 1988.
29. Fowler CJ: Prolongation of the pudendal terminal motor latency does equal denervation of the pelvic floor. Workshop: Prevention of incontinence. Annual Meeting ICS, Sept 23, 1997, Yokohama.
30. Tetzschner T, Sorensen M, Lose G, Christiansen J: Pudendal nerve function during pregnancy and after vaginal delivery. Int Urogynecol J 8:66–68, 1997.
31. Deindl FM, Vodusek DB, Hesse U, Schüssler B: Pelvic floor activity patterns: Comparison of nulliparous continent and parous urinary stress incontinent women. A kinesiological EMG study. Br J Urol 73:413–417, 1994.
32. Geelen JM van, Lemmens WAJG, Eskes TKAB, Martin CB: The urethral pressure profile in pregnancy and after delivery in healthy nulliparous women. Am J Obstet Gynecol 144:636–649, 1982.
33. Iosif S, Ingemarsson I, Ulmsten U: Urodynamic studies in normal pregnancy and in puerperium. Am J Obstet Gynecol 137:696–700, 1980.
34. Pigné A, Cotelle O, Kunst D, Barrat J: Consequences of pregnancy and delivery on the parameters of the urethral pressure profile. ICS Proceedings, p 119–120, 1985.
35. Iosif S, Henriksson L, Ulmsten U: Postpartum incontinence. Urol Int 36:53–58, 1981.
36. Iosif S, Ulmsten U: Comparative urodynamic studies of continent and stress incontinent women in pregnancy and in the puerperium. Am J Obstet Gynecol 140:645–650, 1981.
37. Chaliha C, Bland JM, Monga A, et al: Pregnancy and delivery: A urodynamic viewpoint. Br J Obstet Gynaecol 107:1354–1359, 2000.
38. Kerr-Wilson RHJ, Thompson SW, Orr JW, et al: Effect of labor on the post-partum bladder. Obstet Gynecol 64:115–117, 1984.
39. King JK, Freeman RM: Is antenatal bladder neck mobility a risk factor for postpartum stress incontinence? Br J Obstet Gynaecol 105:1300–1307, 1998.
40. Beck RP, Hsu N: Pregnancy, childbirth and the menopause related to the development of stress incontinence. Am J Obstet Gynecol 91:820–823, 1965.
41. Stanton SL, Kerr-Wilson R, Harris GV: The incidence of urological symptoms in normal pregnancy. Br J Obstet Gynaecol 87:879–900, 1980.
42. Iosif S: Stress incontinence during pregnancy and in puerperium. Int J Gynaecol Obstet 19:13–20, 1981.
43. Dimpfl T, Hesse U, Schüssler B: Incidence and cause of postpartum urinary stress incontinence. Eur J Obstet Gynecol Reprod Biol 43:29–33, 1992.
44. Viktrup L, Lose G, Rolff M, Barfoed K: The symptom of stress incontinence caused by pregnancy or delivery in primiparas. Obstet Gynecol 79:945–949, 1992.
45. Højberg K-E, Dalby Salvig J, Albertson Winsøw N, Lose G, Secher NJ: Urinary incontinence:prevalence and risk factors at 16 weeks of gestation. Br J Obstet Gynaecol 106:842–850, 1999.
46. Chaliha C, Kalia V, Stanton SL, Monga A, Sultan AH: Antenatal prediction of postpartum urinary and fecal incontinence. Obstet Gynecol 94:689–694, 1999.
47. Wilson PD, Herbison RM, Herbison GP: Obstetric practice and the prevalence of urinary incontinence three months after delivery. Br J Obstet Gynaecol 103:154–161, 1996.
48. MacArthur C, Lewis M, Bick D: Stress incontinence after childbirth. Br J Midwifery 1:207–215, 1993.
49. Viktrup L, Lose G: Lower urinary tract symptoms 5 years after the first delivery. Int Urogynecol J 11:336–340, 2000.
50. Jackson S, Barry C, Davies G, et al: Duration of second stage of labour and epidural anaesthesia: Effect on subsequent urinary symptoms in primiparous women. Neurourol Urodynam 14:498–499, 1995.
51. Viktrup L, Lose G: Epidural anesthesia during labour and stress incontinence after delivery. Obstet Gynecol 82:984–986, 1993.
52. Tetzschner T, Sorensen M, Lose G, Christiansen J: Anal and urinary incontinence in women with obstetric anal sphincter rupture. Br J Obstet Gynaecol 103:1034–1040, 1996.
53. Röckner G: Urinary incontinence after perineal trauma at childbirth. Scand J Caring Sci 4:169–172, 1990.
54. Burgio KL, Locher JL, Zyczynski H, et al: Urinary incontinence during pregnancy in a racially mixed sample: Characteristics and predisposing factors. Int J Urogynecol 7:69–73, 1996.
55. Sultan AH: Obstetrical perineal injury and anal incontinence. Clinical risk [editorial]. 5:193–196, 1999.

56. Go PMNYH, Dunselmann GAJ: Anatomic and functional results of surgical repair after total perineal rupture at delivery. Surg Gynecol Obstet 166:121–124, 1988.
57. Haadem K, Dahlström JA, Lingman G: Anal sphincter function after delivery: A prospective study in women with sphincter rupture and controls. Eur J Obstet Reprod Biol 35:7–13, 1990.
58. Sultan AH, Kamm MA, Hudson CN: Third-degree obstetric anal sphincter tears: Risk factors and outcome of primary repair. BMJ 308:887–891, 1994.
59. Anthony S, Buitendijk SE, Zondervan KT, et al: Episiotomies and the occurrence of severe perineal lacerations. Br J Obstet Gynaecol 101:1064–1067, 1994.
60. Fernando B, Leeves L, Greenacre J, Roberts G: Audit of the relationship between episiotomy and risk of major perineal laceration during childbirth. Br J Clin Pract 49:40–41, 1995.
61. Fornell EKU, Berg G, Hallböök O, et al: Clinical consequences of anal sphincter rupture during vaginal delivery. J Am Coll Surg 183:553–558, 1996.
62. Nygaard IE, Rao SSC, Dawson JD: Anal incontinence after anal sphincter disruption: A 30-year retrospective cohort study. Obstet Gynecol 89:896–901, 1997.
63. Donnelly V, Fynes M, Campbell D, et al: Obstetric events leading to anal sphincter damage. Obstet Gynecol 92:955–961, 1998.
64. Wood J, Amos L, Rieger N: Third-degree anal sphincter tears: Risk factors and outcome. Aust NZ J Obstet Gynaecol 38:414–417, 1998.
65. Röckner G, Fianu-Jonasson A: Changed pattern in the use of episiotomy in Sweden. Br J Obstet Gynaecol 106:95–101, 1999.
66. Samuelsson E, Ladfors L, Wennerholm UB, et al: Anal sphincter tears: Prospective study of obstetric risk factors. Br J Obstet Gynaecol 107:926–931, 2000.
67. Sultan AH, Kamm MA, Hudson CN, et al: Anal-sphincter disruption during vaginal delivery. N Engl J Med 329:1905–1911, 1993.
68. Varma A, Gunn J, Lindow SW, Duthie GS: Do routinely measured delivery variables predict anal sphincter outcome? Dis Colon Rectum 42:1261–1264, 1999.
69. Burnett SJD, Spence-Jones C, Speakman CTM, et al: Unsuspected sphincter damage following childbirth revealed by anal endosonography. Br J Radiol 64:225–227, 1991.
70. Frudinger A, Bartram CI, Spencer JAD, Kamm MA: Perineal examination as a predictor of underlying external anal sphincter damage. Br J Obstet Gynaecol 104:1009–1013, 1997.
71. Labrecque M, Baillargeon L, Dallaire M, et al: Association between median episiotomy and severe perineal lacerations in primiparous women. CMAJ 156:797–802, 1997.
72. Hueston WJ: Factors associated with the use of episiotomy during vaginal delivery. Obstet Gynecol 87:1001–1005, 1996.
73. Klein MC, Janssen PA, MacWilliam L, et al: Determinants of vaginal-perineal integrity and pelvic floor functioning in childbirth. Am J Obstet Gynecol 176:403–410, 1997.
74. Woolley RJ: Benefits and risks of episiotomy: A review of the English-language literature since 1980. Parts I and II. Obstet Gynecol Survey 50:806–835, 1995.
75. Thacker SB, Banta HD: Benefits and risks of episiotomy: An interpretive review of the English language literature, 1960–1980. Obstet Gynecol Surv 7:161–177, 1983.
76. Bansal RK, Tan WM, Ecker JL, et al: Is there a benefit to episiotomy at spontaneous vaginal delivery? A natural experiment. Am J Obstet Gynecol 175:897–901, 1996.
77. Green J, Soohoo SL: Factors associated with rectal injury in spontaneous deliveries. Obstet Gynecol 73:732–738, 1989.
78. Helwig JT, Thorp JM, Bowes WA: Does midline episiotomy increase the risk of third- and fourth-degree lacerations in operative vaginal deliveries? Obstet Gynecol 82:276–279, 1993.
79. Greene R, Gardeil F, Turner MJ: Data on episiotomy rates need analysis by parity. Am J Obstet Gynecol 176:498, 1997.
80. Poen AC, Felt-Bersma RJF, Dekker GA, et al: Third-degree obstetric perineal tears: Risk factors and preventive role of mediolateral episiotomy. Br J Obstet Gynaecol 104:563–566, 1997.
81. Combs CA, Robertson PA, Laros RK: Risk factors for third-degree and fourth-degree perineal lacerations in forceps and vacuum deliveries. Am J Obstet Gynecol 163:100–104, 1990.
82. Klein MC, Gauthier RJ, Robbins JM, et al: Relationship of episiotomy to perineal trauma and morbidity, sexual dysfunction, and pelvic floor relaxation. Am J Obstet Gynecol 171:591–598, 1994.
83. Abramovitz L, Sobhani I, Ganasia R, et al: Are sphincter defects the cause of anal incontinence after vaginal delivery? Dis Colon Rectum 43:590–598, 2000.
84. Kammerer-Doak DN, Wesol AB, Rogers RG, et al: A prospective cohort study of women after primary repair of obstetric anal sphincter laceration. Am J Obstet Gynecol 181:1317–1323, 1999.
85. Rieger N, Schloithe A, Saccone G, Wattchow D: The effect of a normal vaginal delivery on anal function. Acta Obstet Gynecol Scand 76:769–772, 1997.
86. Rieger N, Schloithe A, Saccone G, Wattchow D: A prospective study of anal sphincter injury due to childbirth. Scand J Gastroenterol 33:950–955, 1998.
87. Cornes H, Bartolo DCC, Stirrat GM: Changes in anal canal sensation after childbirth. Br J Surg 78:74–77, 1991.
88. Wynne JM, Myles JL, Jones L, et al: Disturbed anal sphincter function following vaginal delivery. Gut 39:120–124, 1996.
89. Sorensen M, Bondesen H, Istre O, Vilmann P: Perineal rupture following vaginal delivery: Long-term consequences. Acta Obstet Gynecol Scand 67:315–318, 1988.
90. MacArthur C, Bick DE, Keighley MRB: Faecal incontinence after childbirth. Br J Obstet Gynaecol 104:46–50, 1997.
91. Walsh CJ, Mooney EF, Upton GJ, Motson RW: Incidence of third-degree perineal tears in labour and outcome after primary repair. Br J Surg 83:218–221, 1996.
92. Zetterström JP, López A, Anzén B, et al: Anal incontinence after vaginal delivery: A prospective study in primiparous women. Br J Obstet Gynaecol 106:324–330, 1999.
93. Bek KM, Laurberg S: Risks of anal incontinence from subsequent vaginal delivery after a complete obstetric anal sphincter tear. Br J Obstet Gynaecol 99:724–726, 1992.
94. Crawford LA, Quint EH, Pearl ML, DeLancey JOL: Incontinence following rupture of the anal sphincter during delivery. Obstet Gynecol 82:527–531, 1993.
95. Haadem K, Dahlstrom JA, Ling L, Ohrlander S: Anal sphincter function after delivery rupture. Obstet Gynecol 70:53–56, 1987.
96. Sultan AH, Monga AK, Stanton SL: Primary repair of obstetric anal sphincter rupture using the overlap technique. Br J Obstet Gynaecol 106:318–323, 1999.
97. Fitzpatrick M, Behan M, O'Connell PR, O'Herlihy C: A randomized clinical trial comparing primary overlap with approximation of third-degree obstetric tears. Am J Obstet Gynecol 183:1220–1224, 2000.

98. Carroli G, Belizan J: Episiotomy for vaginal birth. Cochrane Database Syst Rev 2:CD000081, 2000.
99. Eason E, Labrecque M, Wells G, Feldman P: Preventing perineal trauma during childbirth: A systematic review. Obstet Gynecol 95:464–471, 2000.
100. Labrecque M, Baillargeon L, Dallaire M, et al: Association between median episiotomy and severe perineal lacerations in primiparous women. CMAJ 156:797–802, 1997.
101. Bansal RK, Tan WM, Ecker JL, et al: Is there a benefit to episiotomy at spontaneous vaginal delivery? A natural experiment. Am J Obstet Gynecol 175:897–901, 1996.
102. Reynolds LJ: Reducing the frequency of episiotomies through a continuous quality improvement program. Can Med Assoc J 153:275–282, 1995.
103. Thranov I, Kringelbach AM, Melchior E, et al: Postpartum symptoms. Episiotomy or tear at vaginal delivery. Acta Obstet Gynecol Scand 69:11–15, 1990.
104. Ecker JL, Tan WM, Bansal RK, et al: Is there a benefit to episiotomy at operative vaginal delivery? Observations over ten years in a stable population. Am J Obstet Gynecol 176:411–414, 1997.
105. Coats PM, Chan KK, Wilkins M, Beard RJ: A comparison between midline and mediolateral episiotomies. Br J Obstet Gynaecol 87:408–412, 1980.
106. Abraham S, Child A, Ferry J, et al: Recovery after childbirth: A preliminary prospective study. Med J Aust 52:9–12, 1990.
107. Larsson P-G, Platz-Christensen JJ, Bergman B, Wallstersson G: Advantage or disadvantage of episiotomy compared with spontaneous perineal laceration. Gynecol Obstet Invest 31:213–216, 1991.
108. Sleep J, Grant A: West Berkshire perineal management trial: Three year follow up. BMJ 295:749–751, 1987.
109. Sleep J, Grant A, Elbourne D, et al: West Berkshire perineal management trial. BMJ 289:587–590, 1984.
110. Gordon H, Logue M: Perineal muscle function after childbirth. Lancet 20:123–125, 1985.
111. Johanson RB, Menon BK: Vacuum extraction versus forceps for assisted vaginal delivery. Cochrane Database Syst Rev 2:CD000224, 2000.
112. Johansen RB, Rice C, Doyle M, et al: A randomised prospective study comparing the new vacuum extractor policy with forceps delivery. Br J Obstet Gynaecol 100:524–530, 1993.
113. Yancey MK, Herpolsheimer A, Jordan GD, et al:. Maternal and neonatal effects of outlet forceps delivery compared with spontaneous vaginal delivery in term pregnancies. Obstet Gynecol 78:646–650, 1991.
114. Williams MC, Knuppel RA, O'Brien WF, et al: A randomized comparison of assisted vaginal delivery by obstetric forceps and polyethylene vacuum cup. Obstet Gynecol 78:789–794, 1991.
115. Robinson JN, Norwitz ER, Cohen AP, et al: Episiotomy, operative vaginal delivery, and significant perineal trauma in nulliparous women. Am J Obstet Gynecol 181:1180–1184, 1999.
116. Bofill JA, Rust OA, Schorr SJ, et al: A randomized prospective trial of the obstetric forceps versus the M-cup vacuum extractor. Am J Obstet Gynecol 175:1325–1330, 1996.
117. Muise KL, Duchon MA, Brown RH: The effect of artificial caput on performance of vacuum extractors. Obstet Gynecol 81:170–173, 1993.
118. Echt M, Begneaud W, Montgomery D: Effect of epidural analgesia on the primary cesarean section and forceps delivery rates. J Reprod Med 45:557–561, 2000.
119. Gupta JK, Nikodem VC: Woman's position during second stage of labour. Cochrane Database Syst Rev 2:CD002006, 2000.
120. Gardosi J, Sylvester S, Lynch C: Alternative positions in the second stage of labour: A randomized controlled trial. Br J Obstet Gynaecol 96:1290–1296, 1989.
121. Albers LL, Anderson D, Cragin L, et al: Factors related to perineal trauma in childbirth. J Nurse Midwifery 41:269–276, 1996.
122. Borgotta L, Piening SL, Cohen WR: Association of episiotomy and delivery position with deep perineal laceration during spontaneous delivery in nulliparous women. Am J Obstet Gynecol 160:294–297, 1989.
123. Al-Mufti R, McCarthy A, Fisk NM: Obstetricians' personal choice and mode of delivery. Lancet 347:544, 1996.
124. Bowers SK, MacDonald HM, Shapiro ED: Prevention of iatrogenic neonatal respiratory distress syndrome: Elective repeat cesarean section and spontaneous labor. Am J Obstet Gynecol 143:186–189, 1982.
125. Richardson C, Lyon JB, Williams NL: A new look at pelvic relaxation. Am J Obstet Gynecol 126:568–574, 1976.
126. Youngblood JP: Paravaginal repair for cystourethrocele. Clin Obstet Gynecol 36:960–966, 1993.
127. Henriksen TB, Bek KM, Hedegaard M, Secher NJ: Episiotomy and perineal lesions in spontaneous vaginal deliveries. Br J Obstet Gynaecol 99:950–954, 1992.
128. Argentine Episiotomy Trial Collaborative Group. Routine vs selective episiotomy: A randomised controlled trial. Lancet 342:1517–1518, 1993.
129. Henriksen TB, Bek KM, Hedegaard M, Secher NJ: Methods and consequences of changes in use of episiotomy. BMJ 309:1255–1258, 1994.
130. Waldenström U, Turnbull D: A systematic review comparing continuity of midwifery care with standard maternity services. Br J Obstet Gynaecol 105:1160–1170, 1998.
131. Pirhonen JP, Grenman SE, Haadem K, et al: Frequency of anal sphincter rupture at delivery in Sweden and Finland: Result of difference in manual help to the baby's head. Acta Obstet Gynecol Scand 77:974–977, 1998.
132. Shipman MK, Boniface DR, Tefft ME, McCloghry R: Antenatal perineal massage and subsequent perineal outcomes: A randomised controlled trial. Br J Obstet Gynaecol 104:787–791, 1997.
133. Labreque M, Eason E, Marcoux S, et al: Randomized controlled trial of prevention of perineal trauma by perineal massage during pregnancy. Am J Obstet Gynecol 180:593–600, 1999.
134. Henderson JS: Effects of a prenatal teaching program on postpartum regeneration of the pubococcygeal muscle. J Obstet Gynecol Neonatal Nurs 12:403–408, 1983.
135. Rasmussen KL, Krue S, Johansson LE, et al: Obesity as a predictor of postpartum urinary symptoms. Acta Obstet Gynecol Scand 76:359–362, 1997.
136. Harrison RF, Brennan M, North PM, et al: Is routine episiotomy necessary? BMJ 288:1971–1975, 1984.
137. House MJ, Cario G, Jones MH: Episiotomy and the perineum: A randomized controlled trial. J Obstet Gynecol 7:107–110, 1986.

CHAPTER 7

Lower Urinary Tract Dysfunction in the Female

DAVID STASKIN

The purpose of a classification system is communication. The current understanding of the interrelationship between the bladder outlet and the pelvic floor requires modification of the current classification systems to acknowledge the effect of pelvic floor activity on lower urinary tract function. The value of grouping and interrelating these facts and concepts is measured by the ability of the modified classification system to provide a useful construct for organizing what is theorized and known as well as for introducing new information into the existing knowledge. The classification system should also act as a useful clinical tool for diagnosing and treating disease and facilitating communication among diverse practitioners and researchers. This chapter discusses the importance of pelvic floor activity in voiding abnormalities by integrating pelvic floor activity into commonly accepted classification systems of lower urinary tract function.

CLASSIFICATION: COMBINING SYMPTOMS AND FUNCTION

Several excellent methods for classifying voiding function and dysfunction currently exist. The classification of voiding dysfunction exclusively by symptoms is helpful, but lacks both sensitivity and specificity.[1,2] The classification of incontinence by symptoms is shown in Box 7-1. The symptoms of stress, urge, and overflow incontinence are not reliable indicators of the underlying pathophysiology, and a functional definition accompanies the symptoms. A more useful functional approach to voiding divides the lower urinary tract into the areas of the bladder and bladder outlet during storage and emptying, and classifies the activity as overactive, normoactive, or underactive.[3] The International Continence Society adopted this method. The "symptoms" are included to show the relationship between symptoms and underlying pathophysiology (Table 7-1).[4,5] An overactive bladder indicates an unwanted increase in detrusor pressure during urinary storage, and an underactive bladder indicates an unwanted failure to increase detrusor pressure during bladder emptying. An overactive outlet (obstruction during emptying) and an underactive outlet (decreased resistance during storage) are abnormalities in the function of the bladder neck and urethra. With this functional classification, the pathophysiology may be objectively confirmed with urodynamic findings. The neurogenic classification, based on the level of the neurologic lesion, can also be correlated with functional bladder activity and associated symptoms (Table 7-2).[6]

A FUNCTIONAL APPROACH: INCORPORATING PELVIC FLOOR ACTIVITY

The pelvic floor has two important functions in relation to lower urinary tract function:

1. The levator complex provides anatomic support to the bladder outlet.
2. The activity of the pelvic floor affects detrusor behavior.

The previous classification systems treat the bladder outlet as an isolated combination of smooth and skeletal sphincters, independent of pelvic floor activity, and they treat the bladder as an isolated smooth muscle organ under central and peripheral neurologic control. This concept does not account for the proposed interrelationships between the bladder, the bladder outlet, and the pelvic floor–levator complex.

For example, in classifying "genuine stress incontinence–underactive outlet," it is important to recognize that the anatomic support of the bladder outlet, which is critical to maintaining continence, is provided by constant levator tone in normal females.[7-9] After the pelvic floor undergoes anatomic or physiologic damage, the ability to identify, contract, or coordinate the external sphincter–levator complex may be critical to maintaining continence.

> **BOX 7-1 Symptomatic Classification Combined with Symptoms**
>
> **STRESS INCONTINENCE**
>
> **Symptom:** Involuntary loss of urine with activity (e.g., coughing, laughing, sneezing, lifting, straining).
>
> **Genuine stress incontinence:** Involuntary loss of urine caused by an increase in intra-abdominal pressure that overcomes the resistance of the bladder outlet in the absence of a true bladder contraction. The decrease in bladder outlet or urethral resistance may result from poor anatomic support of the bladder neck (urethral hypermobility), loss of urethral function (intrinsic sphincter deficiency), or low urethral closure pressure, alone or in combination.
>
> **Clinical confusion:** The patient describes the symptom of urine loss with activity, but the etiology of leakage is actually an uninhibited bladder contraction stimulated by a "stress maneuver." Similarly, many patients describe genuine stress incontinence accompanied by a sensation that is mistakenly identified as "urge." Finally, stress incontinence and urge incontinence may coexist.
>
> **URGE INCONTINENCE**
>
> **Symptom:** Loss of urine with the feeling of urgency, resulting in voiding before the ability to toilet.
>
> **Genuine urge incontinence:** Involuntary loss of urine caused by an increase in bladder pressure as a result of a true bladder contraction (detrusor motor overactivity). An involuntary contraction may occur as a result of a suprasacral (spinal or intracranial) neurologic lesion that causes uncontrolled reflex contractions (detrusor hyperreflexia). More commonly, it is idiopathic (detrusor instability). Patients may have other symptoms of "motor urgency" (frequency, urgency, nocturia) without urinary loss. "Sensory urgency" describes the sensation of urinary urgency without a true detrusor contraction (detrusor sensory overactivity).
>
> **Clinical confusion:** Because of an abnormality in sensation, the patient loses urine as a result of true motor activity of the bladder without the symptom of "urge." Conversely, frequency and urgency may be the result of phasic detrusor activity (low-level motor activity of the bladder consistent with an organ composed of smooth muscle) or a true contraction, but without actual urinary loss, suggesting sensory urgency. Finally, detrusor sensory activity and detrusor motor overactivity may coexist.
>
> **OVERFLOW INCONTINENCE**
>
> **Symptom:** Involuntary loss of urine caused by urinary retention as a result of inadequate bladder contractility or outlet obstruction. Urinary loss occurs when bladder pressure overcomes urethral resistance.
>
> **Clinical confusion:** Both stress and urge symptoms are associated with this condition. If the pathophysiology of overflow is outlet obstruction, the detrusor may be overactive or underactive. If the pathophysiology is an underactive detrusor, the outlet may be overactive, normoactive, or underactive.
>
> **FUNCTIONAL INCONTINENCE**
>
> **Symptom:** Involuntary loss of urine as a result of inability to perform toileting functions because of physical or mental limitations.
>
> **Clinical confusion:** The underlying pathophysiology of stress, urge, or overflow incontinence may coexist. In addition, it may be difficult to obtain an accurate history.

Although active contraction of the pelvic floor during increases in intra-abdominal pressure may not be a normal reflex, this learned behavior is critical to the understanding of pelvic floor therapy.

Inhibitory reflex arcs connecting the pelvic floor and bladder have been hypothesized in the human, but have not been defined. Clinically, an important relationship has been shown between resting and active contraction of the pelvic floor and "urge incontinence–overreactive bladder."[10] Pelvic floor activity may contribute significantly to both the reflex inhibition of the detrusor and the more practical ability to mechanically block bladder motor activity through sphincteric contraction until toileting is accomplished. The initiation of efficient voiding requires relaxation of the pelvic floor. The inhibition of detrusor initiation underactive bladder, or the inability to continue the detrusor contraction to achieve complete bladder emptying, may result from the failure to relax, or pseudodyssynergia, of the pelvic floor musculature.

A functional approach that incorporates pelvic floor activity is proposed; it should be refined as new scientific and clinical information is acquired (Box 7-2).

Underactive Outlet

The urethral sphincteric mechanism is responsible for "outlet resistance" during urinary storage. Resistance to urinary loss is supplied by the intrinsic closure pressure along the length of the urethra. The proximal sphincteric mechanism is a product of mucosa, submucosa, smooth muscle, and nonstriated skeletal muscle incorporating the bladder neck and proximal urethra. The distal mechanism, or "external" sphincteric mechanism, is located in the middle of the "anatomic urethra," and is intimately related anatomically and physiologically to the levator complex. During stress maneuvers, anatomic support facilitates the transmission of intra-abdominal pressure to both the proximal and distal areas. Anatomic support is provided by the anterior vaginal wall and its attachments to the pelvis as well as by the constant tone (slow-twitch fibers) of the anterior levator complex that surrounds this area.

TABLE 7-1 ■ Functional Approach To Voiding Dysfunctions

Bladder	Bladder Outlet
Overactive (urge)	Overactive (retention)
Normoactive	Normoactive
Underactive (retention)	Underactive (stress incontinence)

TABLE 7-2 ■ Neurogenic Classification

Bladder–Detrusor	Outlet–Sphincter
Hyper-reflexia (overactive: urge)	Uncoordinated (overactive: obstruction)
Normoreflexic	Coordinated
Areflexia (underactive: retention)	Denervated (underactive: stress)

Expected behavior of the bladder, internal sphincter, and external sphincter based on location of the lesion

Location of Lesion	Bladder	Internal Sphincter	External Sphincter
Infrasacral	Areflexic, Underactive	Innervated	Denervated, Underactive
Spinal	Hyper-reflexic, Overactive	Uncoordinated if located at T6 or above	Dyssynergic, Overactive
Suprapontine	Hyper-reflexic	Coordinated	Coordinated

Active contraction (fast-twitch fibers) of the levator complex can increase this support.

Active contraction is usually seen after pelvic muscle training, and may not be a "normal" reflex.[7-9,11,12]

Type I or II genuine stress incontinence indicates "poor anatomic support" associated with motion of the bladder neck and urethra. An understanding of the contribution of the pelvic floor shows that the pathophysiology of anatomic motion and the effects of hypermobility are multifactorial. Classically, an important event in maintaining continence is the preservation of intra-abdominal pressure transmission to the bladder neck and proximal urethra versus the bladder during stress maneuvers. The preservation or enhancement of the anatomic backboard beneath the bladder outlet facilitates the transmission of pressure to the proximal and distal sphincteric mechanism and preserves the anatomic relationships between the sphincteric components to maintain or increase closure pressure. The development of a "shearing force" as the posterior urethra wall rotates away from the anterior urethral wall can be prevented by satisfactory anatomic support. The external sphincter–levator complex in the midanatomic urethra is the most fixed point along the urethra and the area of maximal pressure transmission. Within this zone, transmission forces and active rhabdosphincter contraction augment closure pressure. Proper anatomic support provides an obvious mechanical advantage for pressure transmission, but just as importantly, allows efficient action of the individual structures by maintaining anatomic relationships.

Defects at many levels of the sphincteric mechanism may combine to decrease urethral resistance. Genuine stress incontinence type III (intrinsic sphincter deficiency), or low urethral closure pressure, is a deficiency in any of the intrinsic urethral functions discussed earlier, through atrophy, denervation, devascularization, or scarring. Pudendal nerve denervation during childbirth or aging may contribute to deficiencies in both anatomic support and intrinsic sphincter function by affecting the sphincter or levator support. In most patients, the complex etiology of genuine stress urinary incontinence is probably a mixture of anatomic support abnormalities and intrinsic sphincter abnormalities. Treatment may be directed at correcting the defect, compensating for the deficiency, or increasing the function of another component that contributes to urethral resistance.

Overactive Bladder

Bladder control is mediated by the central and peripheral nervous systems through complex voluntary pathways and reflex arcs. Central afferent control of the bladder smooth musculature may be in part mediated by reflex and voluntary contractions of the pelvic floor and sphincter musculature that suppress bladder contractility and prevent urge incontinence. Relaxation of the urethral sphincter during voiding and dyssynergic activity in patients with spinal cord injury has been documented. It is not known whether the specific anatomic areas of the urethra or pelvic floor (sphincter urethrae, compressor urethrae, urethrovaginal sphincter, bulbocavernosus, anal sphincter, levator complex) act in unison, individually, or at all in inhibition of the bladder in the neurologically intact person.

Underactive Bladder and Overactive Outlet

During the initial phase of bladder emptying, the pelvic floor and external sphincter relax to decrease urethral resistance and facilitate unobstructed urinary flow. This relaxation may also decrease the reflex inhibition of bladder contractility. Relaxation is followed by a detrusor contraction that continues until voiding is completed. Failure to empty the bladder may be caused by elevated outlet resistance or impaired contractility of the bladder. The most common clinical etiology of elevated outlet resistance in the female patient is obstruction after incontinence surgery. Neurogenic outlet obstruction is often seen after injury to the suprasacral spinal cord and is secondary to a loss of coordination between the bladder and sphincter

BOX 7-2   Expanded Functional Classification of Voiding Dysfunction, Including Pelvic Floor Activity

I. Outlet dysfunction: bladder outlet and pelvic floor
   A. Underactive outlet (decreased urethral resistance). Symptoms are those of genuine stress incontinence (GSI).
      1. Anatomic support defects (GSI-A; GSI types I and II). Pathophysiology: Anatomic motion results in decreased urethral resistance by two mechanisms:
         a. Unequal transmission of pressure to the bladder versus the outlet
         b. Shear forces that produce greater motion of the posterior versus the anterior wall of the urethra
            (1) Anatomic defects include the fascial, muscular, ligamentous, and bony pelvis.
            (2) Functional support: Constant levator tone or active contraction may involve denervation of the levators or loss of identification, strength, or coordination.
      2. Intrinsic sphincter dysfunction (ISD) [GSI-ISD; GSI type III; low urethral closure pressure]. Pathophysiology: Deficiency of the urethral closure mechanism as a result of decreased innervation or vascularization of the mucosa or trauma to the mucosa, submucosa, or smooth or skeletal musculature of the urethra
         a. Damage to the proximal urethral sphincter affects the bladder neck and proximal urethra (GSI-ISD-p)
         b. Damage to the external sphincter causes denervation or loss of voluntary or reflex control (GSI-ISD-d)
         c. Combined total proximal and external sphincter deficiency (GSI-ISD-t) also can occur
      3. Combined genuine stress incontinence (GSI-ISD). Pathophysiology: Both anatomic motion and sphincter dysfunction occur.
      4. Impaired inhibition of the detrusor causes decreased pelvic floor activity. Pathophysiology: Inability to contract the pelvic floor releases the detrusor reflex and decreases the ability to inhibit active contraction. Factors include:
         a. Neurologic (infrasacral) denervation (areflexia of the pelvic floor)
         b. Behavioral causes (inability to contract the pelvic floor because of the lack of identification, strength, or coordination)
         c. Mechanical causes (damage to pelvic floor structures with intact innervation)
   B. Overactive outlet (increased urethral resistance). Symptoms are those of overflow incontinence or retention and frequency or urgency.
      1. Anatomic obstruction (physical blockage). Pathophysiology: Increased outlet resistance as a result of compression or narrowing. Types include:
         a. Iatrogenic (e.g., caused by surgery for urinary incontinence)
         b. Other (congenital, inflammatory, neoplastic, or traumatic)
      2. Functional obstruction (inability to relax). Pathophysiology: Increased outlet resistance caused by failure of normal relaxation. Types include:
         a. Neurogenic: detrusor-sphincter dyssynergia (smooth or skeletal musculature)
         b. Behavioral: failure to relax the external sphincter or pelvic floor musculature
      3. Combined anatomic and functional obstruction
      4. Inhibition of detrusor activity as a result of increased pelvic floor activity. Pathophysiology: Inability to relax the pelvic floor inhibits the initiation of detrusor activity and the ability to initiate or continue a sustained detrusor contraction. Types include:
         a. Neurologic (suprasacral) overactivity or hyper-reflexia (dyssynergic pelvic floor activity)
         b. Behavioral (failure to relax the pelvic floor; may be learned, acquired, maladaptive, or psychogenic)
         c. Situational (voluntary inhibition as a result of environment or pain)
II. Bladder dysfunction
   A. Overactive bladder (increased intravesical pressure). Symptoms are those of urge incontinence, with or without sensation.
      1. Uninhibited detrusor contractions (motor urgency). Pathophysiology: Increased intravesical pressure overcomes urethral resistance or causes the sensation of urinary urgency.
         a. Bladder instability may be primary or secondary. Primary bladder instability may be idiopathic or may be caused by subclinical neurologic factors or by symptomatic phasic detrusor activity. Secondary bladder instability may be caused by obstruction or by reflex urethral relaxation.
         b. Detrusor hyper-reflexia may be suprapontine or suprasacral. The suprapontine (intracranial) type is caused by a neurologic lesion, and may occur with or without sphincter control. The suprasacral (spinal) type is also caused by a neurologic lesion, and may occur with or without sphincteric dyssynergia.
      2. Decreased compliance. Pathophysiology: Increased intravesical pressure occurs as a result of decreased accommodation. Types include:
         a. Fibrosis, caused by radiation, inflammation, or immune response.
         b. Neurologic, caused by loss or reversal of the accommodation reflex, which may be peripheral or may affect only the conus medullaris
      3. Combined detrusor contractions and decreased compliance
      4. Pelvic floor underactivity (see I A 4)
   B. Underactive bladder (decreased intravesical pressure). Symptoms are those of overflow incontinence or retention.
      1. Peripheral denervation or neuropathy. Pathophysiology: Decreased contractility occurs because neural input is absent. Causes include:
         a. Congenital, inflammatory, or neoplastic lesions, or trauma to the peripheral nerves
         b. Diabetes or another metabolic cause
      2. Detrusor myopathy. Pathophysiology: Contractility is decreased as a result of smooth muscle damage. Causes include:
         a. Fibrosis or collagen deposition
         b. Inflammation, obstruction, or overdistension
      3. Pharmacologic inhibition. Pathophysiology: Contractility is decreased as a result of receptor blockade. Causes include:
         a. Anticholinergics
         b. Smooth muscle relaxants, spasmolytics, or membrane stabilizers
      4. Pelvic floor overactvity (see I B 4)
III. Combined outlet and bladder dysfunction (I and II)
IV. Disorders of sensation
   A. Decreased sensation

> **BOX 7-2**   **Expanded Functional Classification of Voiding Dysfunction, Including Pelvic Floor Activity—cont'd**
>
> 1. Decreased bladder sensation. Pathophysiology: Causes include denervation and behavioral and pharmacologic factors. Patients may experience the following:
>   a. Decreased sense of fullness and normal urge response
>   b. Loss of sense of fullness or urge warning only with active contraction
>   c. Loss of sense of fullness or urge incontinence without appreciation of urge
>   d. Urinary retention without appreciation of distention
> 2. Decreased bladder outlet and pelvic floor sensation. Pathophysiology: Causes include denervation, myopathy, and behavioral and pharmacologic factors that impair the ability to identify, contract, and coordinate.
>   a. Bladder overactivity (see I A 4), with failure to inhibit
>   b. Bladder underactivity (see II B 4), with failure to initiate
>
>   c. Decreased bladder sensation (see IV A 1)
>   d. Sexual dysfunction or anorgasmia
> B. Increased sensation
>   1. Increased sensation of the bladder or bladder outlet. Pathophysiology: Causes include neuropathic, psychogenic, or inflammatory factors as well as mucosal permeability defects.
>   a. Frequency urgency symptoms
>   b. Suprapubic and pelvic pain syndromes
>   2. Increased sensation of the pelvic floor or bladder outlet. Pathophysiology: Causes include neuromuscular myalgia and neuropathic, inflammatory, or psychogenic factors.
>   a. Levator myalgia
>   b. Frequency, urgency, and pelvic pain syndromes
>   3. Combined deficit

(detrusor–sphincter dyssynergia). When emptying failure is caused by bladder dysfunction, it may caused by either detrusor smooth muscle pathology or insufficient neural stimulation of the detrusor. Insufficient neural stimulation may occur at the neuromuscular level (pharmacologic), as a result of nerve damage (neuropathy), or because of alterations in the central control of micturition (conus medullaris, spinal column, or brain). Impairment of detrusor contractility caused by the absence of pelvic floor relaxation is seen in spinal cord disease (failure to empty after adequate sphincterotomy as a result of incomplete detrusor contractions) and parkinsonism (failure to empty as a result of pelvic floor bradykinesia). Obstructive voiding symptoms in the neurologically intact female patient may be caused by insufficient relaxation of the pelvic floor–levator complex.

SENSORY DISORDERS

Traditional classification systems have focused on motor rather than sensory activity. Disorders of bladder and bladder outlet sensation may result from central or peripheral denervation, psychological disorders, or pharmacologic agents (e.g., pain medication). Further study is needed to determine the role of decreased sensation in pelvic floor function and the interaction between the pelvic floor and bladder in relation to the micturition reflexes. The pudendal nerve is responsible for innervation of the pelvic floor structures, genital skin, urethral mucosa, and anal canal. Proprioceptive information of the periurethral muscles and sensory innervation of the levator ani muscles are also mediated by the pudendal branches.

Bladder pain or increased sensation is a major clinical challenge. Urinary frequency, urgency, and suprapubic pressure often lead patients to seek diagnostic evaluation and result in therapy for bladder disorders, even in the absence of definitive findings of mucosal or smooth muscle abnormality. Pain that may originate from fascial, muscular, or neurologic etiologies within the pelvic floor should be included in the differential diagnosis of patients with urethral or bladder syndromes.

CONCLUSION

The effect of pelvic floor–levator complex dysfunction on presumed bladder symptoms and normal voiding behavior deserves increased attention. Effective therapy may be limited when the lower urinary tract is considered the sole source of the problem.[13,14]

REFERENCES

1. Versi E, Cardozo L, Anand D, Cooper D: Symptoms analysis for the diagnosis of genuine stress incontinence. Br J Obstet Gynaecol 98(8):815, 1991.
2. Bergman A, Bader K: Reliability of the patient's history in the diagnosis of urinary incontinence. Int J Gynaecol Obstet 32:255, 1990.
3. Wein AJ: Classification of neurogenic voiding dysfunction. J Urol 125:605, 1981.
4. Abrams P, Blaivas JG, Stanton SL, Andersen JT: The standardization of terminology of lower urinary tract function recommended by the International Continence Society. Int Urogynecol J 1:45, 1990.
5. Abrams P, Blaivas JG, Stanton SL, Andersen JT: The standardization of terminology of lower urinary tract function. Br J Obstet Gynaecol 97 (suppl 6):1, 1990.
6. Krane RJ, Siroky MB (eds): Classification of neuro-urologic disorders. In Clinical Neuro-Urology. Boston, Little, Brown, 1979.
7. Gilpin SA, Gosling JA, Smith ARB, Warrell DW: The pathogenesis of genitourinary prolapse and stress incontinence of urine: A histological and histochemical study. Br J Obstet Gynaecol 96:15, 1989.
8. Bo K, Stein R: Pelvic floor muscle function and urethral closure mechanism in young nullipara subjects with and without stress incontinence symptoms. Neurourol Urodynam 12(4):432, 1993.
9. Deindl F, Vodusek DB, Hesse U, Schussler B: Activity patterns of pubococcygeal muscles in nulliparous continent women: A kinesiologial EMG study. Brit J Urol 73:413, 1994.
10. Hald T, Bradley WE: The Urinary Bladder: Neurology and Dynamics. Baltimore, Williams & Wilkins, 1982.
11. Smith ARB, Hosker GL, Warrell DW: The role of pudendal nerve damage in the aetiology of genuine stress incontinence in women. Br J Obstet Gynaecol 96:29, 1989.

12. Snooks SJ, Badenoch D, Tiptaft R, Swash M: Perineal nerve damage in genuine stress incontinence: An electrophysiological study. Br J Urol 57:422, 1985.
13. Staskin D: Classification of voiding dysfunction. In Appell RA, Bourcier A, La Torre F (eds): Pelvic Floor Dysfunction: Investigations and Conservative Treatment Rome, Casa Editrice Scientifica Internazionale, 1999, p 1.
14. Staskin D: Classification of voiding dysfunction. In Cardozo L, Staskin D (eds): Textbook of Female Urology and Urogynecology. London, Isis Medical Media, 2001, p 83.

CHAPTER 8

Lower Urinary Tract Dysfunction in the Male

CHRISTOPHER P. SMITH ■ JERRY G. BLAIVAS ■ MICHAEL B. CHANCELLOR

In this chapter we will discuss four conditions of the bladder outlet that can cause significant lower urinary tract dysfunction in men. The four conditions occur at three locations: the bladder neck, the prostatic urethra, and the membranous urethra, or external urethral sphincter (Table 8-1).

Benign prostatic hyperplasia (BPH) is a common age-related pathological condition that affects men worldwide. Symptomatic BPH, currently referred to as lower urinary tract symptoms (LUTS), is a prevalent voiding disorder in aging men. Population-based studies show that the prevalence of LUTS increases with age and that moderate to severe LUTS occurs in nearly 25% of men older than 50 years.[1,2] The development of increased urinary symptoms is not sex-specific; women also develop urinary frequency, urgency, and urge incontinence with increasing age.[3] Scores on the American Urological Association Symptom Index are equivalent in men and women aged 55 to 79 years.[4] These observations suggest that LUTS in men and women may share some underlying etiologies.

There are two other relatively common but less well understood pathologies of the prostatic urethra. First, primary bladder neck obstruction is a condition in which the beginning or proximal part of the prostatic urethra is obstructed. Bladder neck obstruction is not caused by the gradual enlargement of the prostate gland with age but by hypertrophy of the bladder neck smooth muscle.[5] Clinical manifestations typically involve a man in his mid 40s and the etiology is usually unclear. The second pathology is prostatitis, inflammation of the prostate, which may be caused by infection or may be chronic.[6]

Neurogenic lower urinary tract dysfunction is a major problem in patients with a variety of neurological disorders. Neurogenic lower tract dysfunction can involve debilitating symptoms and lead to severe complications. Neurologic disease can also affect the bladder outlet, especially the innervation and coordination of the external sphincter. This condition is commonly called detrusor–sphincter dyssynergia (DSD).[7]

BENIGN PROSTATIC HYPERPLASIA

Benign prostatic hyperplasia (BPH), the most common benign tumor in men, is a benign enlargement of any or all cellular prostate components. The development of BPH generally begins in the fifth decade and may progress to the point where it results in voiding dysfunction. The specific biochemical factors that induce BPH development are unknown, although advancing age and testicular function are required.[8]

It has been estimated that a 60-year-old man has a 50% probability of developing histologic evidence of BPH; this probability rises to almost 100% in octogenarians.[1] Despite the almost universal development of histologic BPH with age, a significantly smaller proportion of men develop symptomatic BPH or require therapy for relief of obstruction.[9]

Almost all men, if they live long enough, will develop histologic evidence of BPH; however, not every man with histologic BPH will develop clinically significant symptoms of prostatic enlargement. Approximately 25% of all men who live to 80 years of age will eventually require treatment for symptomatic relief of prostatism (clinical BPH).[10] Prostate size is not the sole determinant of prostatism because other factors, such as the function of the detrusor muscle and the tone of the bladder neck and prostatic urethra mediated by the autonomic nervous system, also contribute.

Pathophysiology

Even though the etiology and pathogenesis of BPH are incompletely understood, BPH is clearly related to aging and active testicular endocrine function. Both prostatic growth and functional integrity depend on circulating androgen. Significant changes in secretory and proliferative capacity of the prostate occur with manipulation of the hormonal environment. The role of testicular androgens is underscored by the fact that BPH does not develop in men castrated before puberty or in those with

TABLE 8-1 ■ Anatomic Location with Associated Common Urologic Dysfunctions in Men

Location	Dysfunction
Bladder neck	Primary bladder neck obstruction
Prostatic urethra	Benign prostatic hyperplasia
	Prostatitis
Membranous urethra	Detrusor–sphincter dyssynergia

the genetic inability to produce either hormonally active androgens or androgen receptors.

The hypothalamic-pituitary-testes-prostate axis creates the hormonal milieu for the development of BPH. In response to decreased levels of circulating testosterone, the hypothalamus will release luteinizing hormone-releasing hormone (LHRH) in a pulsatile fashion into the hypothalamic-pituitary circulation. This results in the release of luteinizing hormone (LH) by the pituitary, which reaches the testes via the peripheral circulation. At the testis, luteinizing hormone binds to surface receptors on Leydig cells, which generate not only the extreme local levels of testosterone required for spermatogenesis but also circulating testosterone levels, which are modulated by this negative feedback loop. Testosterone reaches the prostate via general circulation, where it acts as a prehormone on the prostatic epithelial cell. At this site, it is converted by the enzyme 5-alpha-reductase to dihydrotestosterone (DHT), which binds to specific nuclear androgen receptors. Dihydrotestosterone promotes prostatic cell growth and proliferation. Despite decreases in plasma testosterone levels as men age, dihydrotestosterone levels in the prostate may remain stable.[10,11]

The role of estrogens in the pathogenesis of BPH is not clear. We do know that most serum estrogen in men is derived by aromatization from the conversion of circulating testosterone. Physiologic levels of estrogen might actually increase the nuclear androgen receptor content of the prostate cells, increasing androgen sensitivity and accelerating the development of BPH. As the process continues, enlargement of the prostate results. Microscopically, prostatic hyperplasia is characterized by nodules of benign adenoma. As the periurethral zone of the prostate enlarges, the outflow of bladder urine maybe obstructed. The physiologic dysfunction associated with BPH may therefore be related to the obstruction caused by the mass of tissue, a glandular static obstruction, a functional smooth muscular dynamic obstruction, or a combination of these factors.

Mechanical (Static) Obstruction

Mechanical or static obstruction is caused by the enlargement of the glands that surround the prostatic urethra, resulting in urethral compression. Pathologically, BPH develops as nodules that comprise both epithelial and stromal elements of the glands lining the proximal prostatic urethra. These nodules enlarge and coalesce within the anterior, posterior, and lateral walls of the prostate and form lobular masses of various shapes and sizes. Because the anterior lobe is usually only minimally involved, BPH is often designated as bilobar (lateral lobe enlargement only) or trilobar (both lateral and posterior lobe enlargement). Some patients have only posterior, median lobe hyperplasia, which may be obstructive. In these cases of BPH, the lateral lobes may be minimally enlarged while the median lobe grows infravesically to obstruct the bladder neck. This explains the variable correlation between rectally palpable prostatic size and the degree of obstruction. In the past treatment of the static component of BPH focused on surgical removal of the mass of hyperplastic prostatic tissue; more recent treatment uses anti-androgen agents to induce prostatic involution.

Smooth Muscle (Dynamic) Obstruction

The human prostate contains an abundance of alpha-1 adrenergic receptors, which modulate the contractility of prostatic smooth muscle. Stimulation of these receptors by norepinephrine and other alpha-active agents results in contraction of the smooth muscle and compression of the prostatic urethra, increasing the resistance to urinary flow.[3] Thus, the dynamic component of BPH may be a result of the increased smooth muscle tone of the bladder neck, prostatic adenoma, and prostatic capsule. Smooth muscle tone in these areas varies in response to local and systemic adrenergic stimulation. As such stimulation is mediated by variables such as emotion, temperature, and pain, the symptoms resulting from the consequent urethral compression may vary in severity and occurrence.

Clinical Manifestations

The symptoms of BPH are highly variable. They are generally related not only to the degree of urethral obstruction but also to the secondary alteration of bladder function. Some men are asymptomatic and others suffer from a plethora of symptoms.

Certain symptoms seem to be directly related to the degree of urethral obstruction. These obstructive symptoms include a decrease in the force and caliber of the urinary stream, hesitancy in voiding, inability to terminate micturition, a sensation of incomplete emptying, and occasionally urinary retention. Other symptoms reflect the changes of detrusor function caused by the obstruction. These irritative lower urinary tract symptoms include urgency, frequency, nocturia, and painful voiding.[7]

As the detrusor compensates, connective tissue deposition increases within the bladder wall. Up to 50% of men with BPH develop uninhibited detrusor contractions, which can be demonstrated during urodynamic testing. These contractions are directly related to obstruction at the bladder neck and prostatic urethra, resulting in symptoms of urgency, frequency, or incontinence. After relief of bladder outlet obstruction, uninhibited bladder contractions may persist, but they usually resolve spontaneously.

The American Urological Association (AUA) Symptom Index is a recently developed and validated questionnaire that quantifies the severity of voiding symptoms and can be used to determine treatment outcome.[9] Although the AUA Symptom Index may indicate the degree of lower urinary tract functional impairment, the symptoms and the index that quantify these symptoms are unfortunately not specific for BPH.[4] For example, the index has been used to monitor treatment effects in women with voiding symptoms. The AUA Symptom Index scores of a carefully monitored group of women with voiding dysfunction, verified by video-urodynamic evaluation, rivaled those of men with moderate and significant BPH. Furthermore, the AUA Symptom Index scores in this study decreased significantly after appropriate therapy was instituted. It is important for all physicians to be aware that voiding symptoms are not specific in patients with BPH. Treatment of patients with micturitional dysfunction should not be based on a specific set of symptoms.

Urinary Retention

Acute urinary retention can develop suddenly in asymptomatic patients or in those with only mild degrees of prostatism. This condition is painful because the inability to void creates a distended, palpable bladder. In this situation, catheter drainage of the bladder and subsequent prostatectomy are indicated to ensure enduring relief of obstruction. Acute urinary retention is the indication for prostatectomy in about 10% to 20% of patients who undergo this procedure. Some men develop acute urinary retention after ingestion of alpha-adrenergic agents, which are found in cough medicines and nasal decongestants. These drugs increase the smooth muscle tone in the prostatic urethra. This condition, combined with underlying prostatic enlargement, results in complete outflow obstruction and urinary retention. In addition, anticholinergic medications, such as antihistamines and antidepressants, may precipitate retention by a direct inhibitory effect on detrusor contractility, impairing the ability to generate adequate pressure to force urine through an obstructed prostatic urethra. Alternatively, acute urinary retention associated with BPH may be precipitated by conditions such as acute prostatitis, prostatic infarction, and acute bladder overdistension.

Chronic urinary retention develops infrequently in men with BPH. Many patients have minimal symptoms, although they may be afflicted with silent dilation of their upper tracts (hydronephrosis), or increased levels of serum urea nitrogen (uremia) and creatinine (azotemia), which indicates renal insufficiency. Unfortunately, the initial manifestation of chronic retention caused by BPH may be renal failure. This dreaded complication of BPH occurs in less than 1% of patients coming to prostatectomy.

Urinary Tract Infection

Urinary tract infection is not always a sequela of incomplete bladder emptying. However, once infection has occurred in those with significant residual urine, resolution is difficult to achieve without correction of the infravesical outlet obstruction. Outlet obstruction may lead to hyperplasia and hypertrophy of the detrusor musculature, resulting in bladder instability in 50% to 80% of patients. This condition may require 6 months of treatment to resolve. The expectant management of men with BPH requires careful attention to irritative symptoms. Urge incontinence is an indication of significant bladder decompensation, which can be resolved only with relief of the instigating obstruction. Left untreated, the irritative symptoms of detrusor instability can become irreversible.

Physical Findings

The most important physical sign of BPH is an enlarged, smooth, symmetrical prostate, as determined by digital rectal examination. The gland may be soft or somewhat firm, and diffuse nodularity may be present. The nodules, however, lack the hard consistency associated with carcinoma. The American Urological Association and the American Cancer Society recommend that all men older than 50 years have an annual digital rectal examination (DRE) and serum prostatic specific antigen (PSA) determination to rule out occult malignancy. Recent reports indicate such screening should begin at age 40 if a patient is symptomatic or has a family history of prostatic adenocarcinoma.[12]

Diagnostic Evaluation

A variety of additional diagnostic studies can be employed. Urinalysis may demonstrate white blood cells, bacteria, or microscopic hematuria. Urine culture will help determine whether the obstructed bladder harbors pathogenic bacteria. If obstruction has caused impairment of renal function, serum chemistry evaluation may detect abnormal electrolyte, urea nitrogen, and serum creatinine levels. An abdominal radiograph may reveal prostatic calculi, which often indicate chronic prostatitis.

The differential diagnosis of BPH involves several important conditions. The most important by far is prostate carcinoma. Most men with irritative or obstructive voiding symptoms have BPH. Such symptoms, however, can be caused by other conditions in 10% to 20% of male patients. Bacterial cystitis, nonspecific cystitis (e.g., radiation or interstitial cystitis), papillary transitional cell carcinoma, transitional cell carcinoma in situ, and bladder or ureteral calculi all can induce irritative symptoms that are suggestive of BPH. Obstructive symptoms can occur with a dyssynergic external sphincter mechanism, bladder calculi, bladder neck dysfunction, and urethral strictures. Strictures may develop not only after a nonspecific or gonococcal urethritis, but also after urethral trauma, catheterization, or a cystoscopic examination. As the stricture narrows the urethral lumen, urinary flow is obstructed. Symptoms such as decreased force of the urinary stream and intermittency then appear.

Ancillary diagnostic studies for these entities include intravenous urography, urethrography, urinary cytology, urine culture, urethral catheterization, cystometry, cystoscopy, and lumbar, suprapubic, and transrectal ultrasonography.

Urodynamic Evaluation

A carefully performed urodynamic evaluation is essential to an objective assessment of BPH and the response to therapy (Fig. 8-1). The urinary flow rate and cystometrogram are the cornerstones of urodynamics. Urinary flow rate determination is a helpful method for quantifying the efficiency of bladder emptying, measuring the rate of urine flow in mL/sec using a urinary flowmeter. A low rate of flow may be caused by the prostatic urethral obstruction of BPH, but one must remember that bladder outlet obstruction can also be caused by a dysfunctional bladder neck, a dyssynergic external sphincter, or a scarred and stenotic urethra. Furthermore, a diminished uroflow could be caused by impaired detrusor contractility (Fig. 8-2).[13]

A more advanced urodynamic evaluation of the patient with prostatic obstruction is obtained with the cystometrogram. In this study, as the bladder is slowly filled with fluid, the volumes are noted at which the patient reports the sensations of bladder filling, distension, and the urge to urinate. In addition, the occurrence and force of bladder contractions are monitored. The cystometrogram enables the diagnosis of uninhibited detrusor contractions, involuntary bladder contractions at low bladder volumes, and poor bladder contractions resulting from muscle decompensation or neuropathic detrusor dysfunction. Patients with outlet obstruction secondary to BPH and detrusor instability have symptoms of frequency, urgency, and often urge incontinence. Within 1 year of prostatectomy, these uninhibited contractions resolve in the majority (70% to 80%) of patients.

Neurogenic Bladder and BPH

Neurogenic vesical dysfunction is perhaps the most important entity that generates symptoms suggestive of BPH. Physicians should become familiar with the concept of neurologically mediated bladder disorders so that the voiding irregularity of an older male patient is not summarily attributed to an enlarged prostate gland. Cerebrovascular accidents can affect the central micturition control centers in the brain, impairing the ability to inhibit-

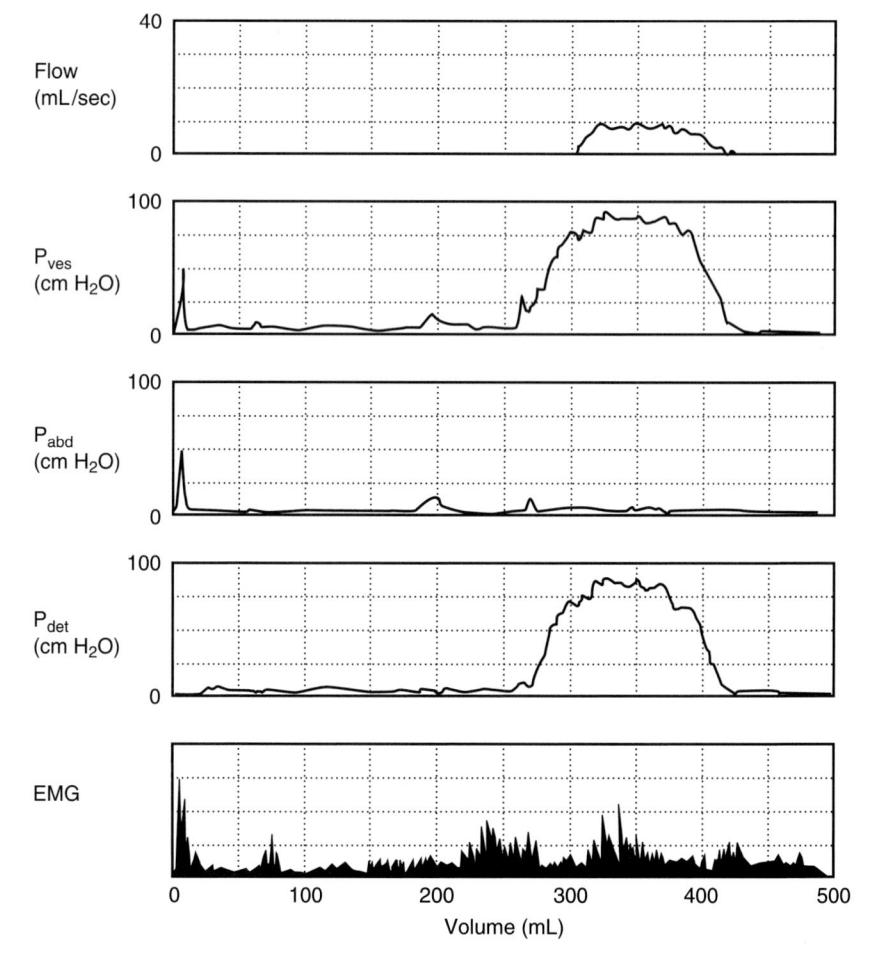

FIGURE 8-1 Pressure-flow study of a 66-year-old man without neurologic history and an American Urological Association (AUA) Symptom Index of 20. The maximum flow rate is 10 mL/sec at a volume of 325 mL. The patient developed a voluntary detrusor contraction without straining at 270 mL. Maximum voiding pressure was 92 cm H_2O. The diagnosis is bladder outlet obstruction based on high voiding pressure and low flow. P_{ves}, intravesical pressure; P_{abd}, intraabdominal pressure; P_{det}, subtracted detrusor pressure; EMG: pelvic electromyography.

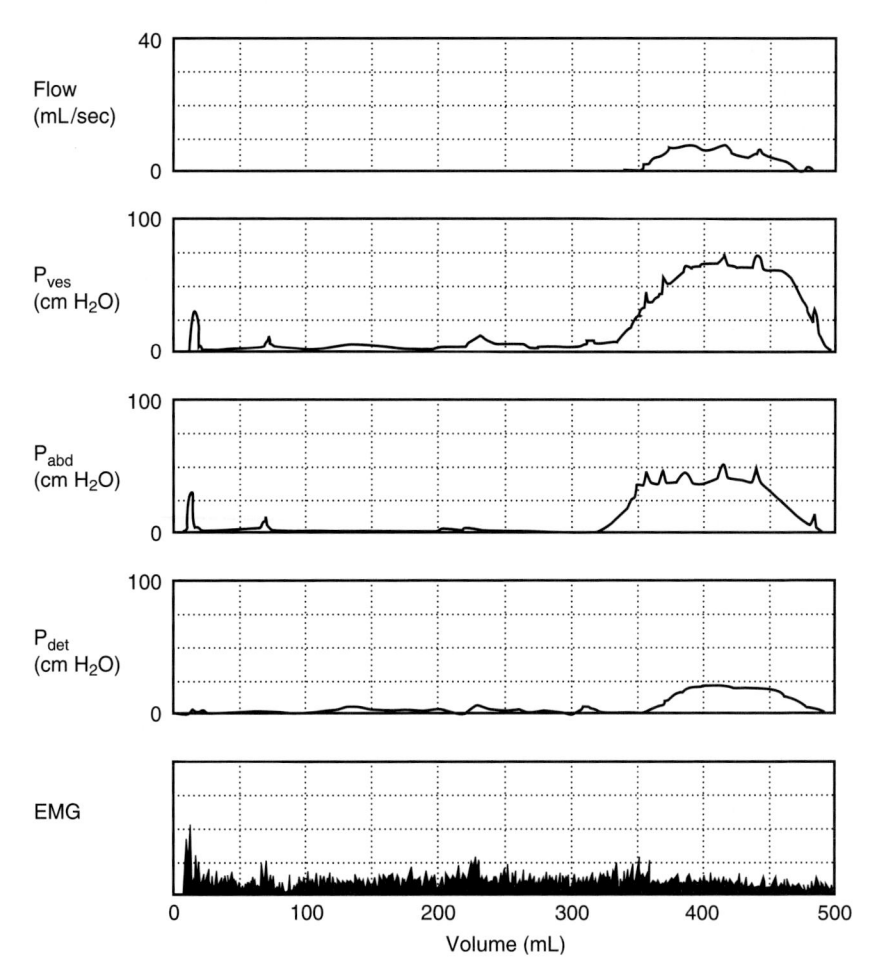

FIGURE 8-2 Pressure-flow study of a 58-year-old diabetic man with an American Urological Association (AUA) Symptom Index of 22. Although he voided with a low flow rate, a diagnosis of benign prostatic hyperplasia (BPH) would be incorrect. This patient has significant impaired bladder contractility and his elevated intravesical pressure is due to abdominal straining. The subtracted true detrusor pressure (P_{det}) only reached 25 cm H_2O. The diagnosis of bladder outlet obstruction involves high detrusor pressure and low flow. Diminished uroflow, by itself, is NOT diagnostic of BPH. Similarly, elevated intravesical pressure, by itself, is NOT diagnostic of BPH. P_{ves}, intravesical pressure; P_{abd}, intraabdominal pressure; EMG, pelvic electromyography.

spontaneous detrusor contractions.[6,14] This circumstance results in symptoms of frequency, urgency, and urge incontinence. Prostatectomy in these patients may indeed relieve obstructive symptoms, however, irritative symptoms can persist and develop into troublesome incontinence.

Functional bladder outlet obstruction can result from a number of neurologic lesions. Involvement of the central nervous system may affect voiding function, as in those patients with myelodysplasia or spinal cord injury.[15] Peripheral nervous injury, which can be caused by diseases such as diabetes mellitus and by trauma such as radical pelvic surgery (e.g., abdominoperineal resection), can also induce such changes. In these conditions the bladder muscle is hypotonic or even atonic and flaccid, unable to generate enough pressure to empty the bladder effectively.

In Parkinson's disease, the voluntary external sphincter may be the source of obstructive voiding symptoms. The bladder muscle and the urinary sphincters are controled by both the autonomic (parasympathetic: bladder muscle; sympathetic: bladder neck, prostatic urethra) and somatic (pudendal nerve: external striated sphincter) nervous systems. Neuropathic voiding dysfunction results from interference with bladder contraction or sphincter function.[16]

Men with neurologic impairment and symptoms of BPH require careful urodynamic assessment before decisions are made regarding prostatectomy and other treatments. This group of patients includes men with any disease process that affects nervous conduction, such as a herniated intervertebral disc, multiple sclerosis, cerebrovascular accident, diabetes mellitus, Lyme disease, spinal cord injury, neuromuscular disease, or with nervous injury caused by pelvic fracture or major abdominal and pelvic surgery. Prostatic resection in such patients without a thorough neurourologic evaluation can result in poor treatment outcome and exacerbated symptoms of frequency and incontinence. Irritative voiding symptoms, in the absence of obstructive symptoms, and any positive neurologic history should alert the clinician to the presence of a disease process other than, or in addition to, BPH.

Cystourethroscopy

Cystourethroscopic examination is effective in evaluating the patient with BPH. The use of a small rigid or flexible cystoscope enables the physician to perform this examination in the office with only local anesthesia. Cystoscopy helps to determine the size of the prostate, the degree of obstruction, the secondary changes of the bladder caused by the obstruction, and the presence of an enlarged median lobe, which may not be rectally palpable. Frequently, cystoscopy aides in the determination between the need for an open versus a transurethral approach to prostatectomy.

PRIMARY BLADDER NECK OBSTRUCTION

Primary bladder neck obstruction is an uncommon but not rare condition seen mostly in young and middle-aged men. Bladder neck obstruction is exceedingly rare in women. The etiology is unknown but it is most likely the result of neuromuscular overactivity and failure of the bladder neck to open wide during detrusor contraction. Many patients describe the inability to void in public, which can often be traced to childhood.[17] Surprisingly, the usual presenting symptoms are urinary frequency and urgency. Obstructive symptoms are usually not so prominent.[5] Many men are misdiagnosed with prostatitis or are labeled "problematic," especially after failing to improve with long courses of nonsteroidal antiinflammatory drugs (NSAIDs) or antibiotics.

A screening flow rate with postvoid residual (PVR) is a useful initial noninvasive test to identify patients at risk for this disorder.[17] However, the diagnosis of primary bladder neck obstruction is essentially a urodynamic one that includes high voiding pressure, low uroflow, narrowing at the bladder neck on fluoroscopic voiding cystourethrogram, and a relaxed external sphincter electromyogram (EMG) during micturition. Cystourethroscopy usually demonstrates an elevation or narrowing of the bladder neck and bladder trabeculation is often present.

The differential diagnosis includes bladder neck contracture, dysfunctional voiding (a learned behavior wherein the patient is unable to relax the external sphincter during attempts to void) urinary tract infection, prostatitis, and neurogenic bladder.

The treatment of choice is transurethral incision of the bladder neck, which is usually curative. The risk of retrograde ejaculation must be discussed with patients. This issue is important because many men with this disorder are young enough to desire fertility. A single incision at either the 5 o'clock or 7 o'clock position from proximal to the bladder neck on the trigone to the level of the verumontanum has yielded excellent results with a reduced risk of retrograde ejaculation.[18,19] Alpha-adrenergic blocking agents to relieve the obstruction or anticholinergics to treat the urinary frequency and urgency have not had much success. However, these drugs can be offered to patients who are unwilling to undergo surgery.

PROSTATITIS

Prostatitis is an enigmatic condition that is frustrating to many men and urologists. Some clinicians apply the diagnosis of prostatitis indiscriminately to men with any sort of voiding symptoms in whom there is no documented obstruction. Rarely does a man with the clinical diagnosis of "prostatitis" have a positive, documented bacterial infection of the prostate.

In our experience, urodynamic findings in prostatitis are similar to those of interstitial cystitis. Sensory urgency or a normal micturition are the two most common findings. Bladder compliance is normal and there is no obstruction. Often it is very difficult for middle-age men with prostatitis to void voluntarily during a urodynamic study. They are often nervous and cannot tolerate the gentle insertion of the small urodynamic catheter, even after application of copious urethral anesthetic jelly. Many cannot void with a urodynamic catheter in place in either the sitting or standing position. Urodynamic studies are not generally indicated for men with prostatitis unless there is a suspicion of urethral obstruction or bladder dysfunction.

DETRUSOR–SPHINCTER DYSSYNERGIA

Dyssynergia is a condition defined by the simultaneous contraction of two muscles whose actions oppose each other. When the external urethral sphincter contracts during a detrusor contraction, urinary flow is impeded by the resulting increased urethral resistance and, hence, the term detrusor-sphincter dyssynergia (DSD) (Fig. 8-3).[6] DSD can occur with any neurologic disease that affects the spinal cord between the pontine micturition center and the sacral 2–4 region, where the pelvic and pudendal nerves innervate the lower urinary tract.

More than 10,000 new traumatic spinal cord injuries occur every year in the United States. Eighty-five percent of these patients are men and 58% result in quadriplegia. Many of these patients have neurogenic vesical dysfunction associated with DSD.[20]

Complications of Sphincter Dyssynergia

Without appropriate treatment, up to 50% of patients with DSD develop serious urologic complications,[21] which include vesicoureteral reflux, ureterovesical obstruction, urolithiasis, and urosepsis. The primary risk factor is high intravesical pressure. It is essential to quantify intravesical pressures accurately during filling and at the point of urinary leakage. To avoid renal damage, voiding pressure should be less than 60 cm H_2O and the maximum filling pressure or leak point pressure should be less than 40 cm H_2O.

Therapy for Sphincter Dyssynergia

In patients with sufficient manual dexterity, the most reasonable treatment option is to abolish the involuntary detrusor contractions (to ensure continence) and then to institute intermittent self-catheterization (to empty the bladder).[21] Treatment options include either intermittent or continuous catheterization, external sphincterotomy, pharmacologic therapy, urinary diversion, biofeedback, and functional electrical stimulation. Several new minimally invasive alternatives to external sphincterotomy include UroLume stent placement across the external sphincter and injection of botulinum toxin into the external sphincter muscle.

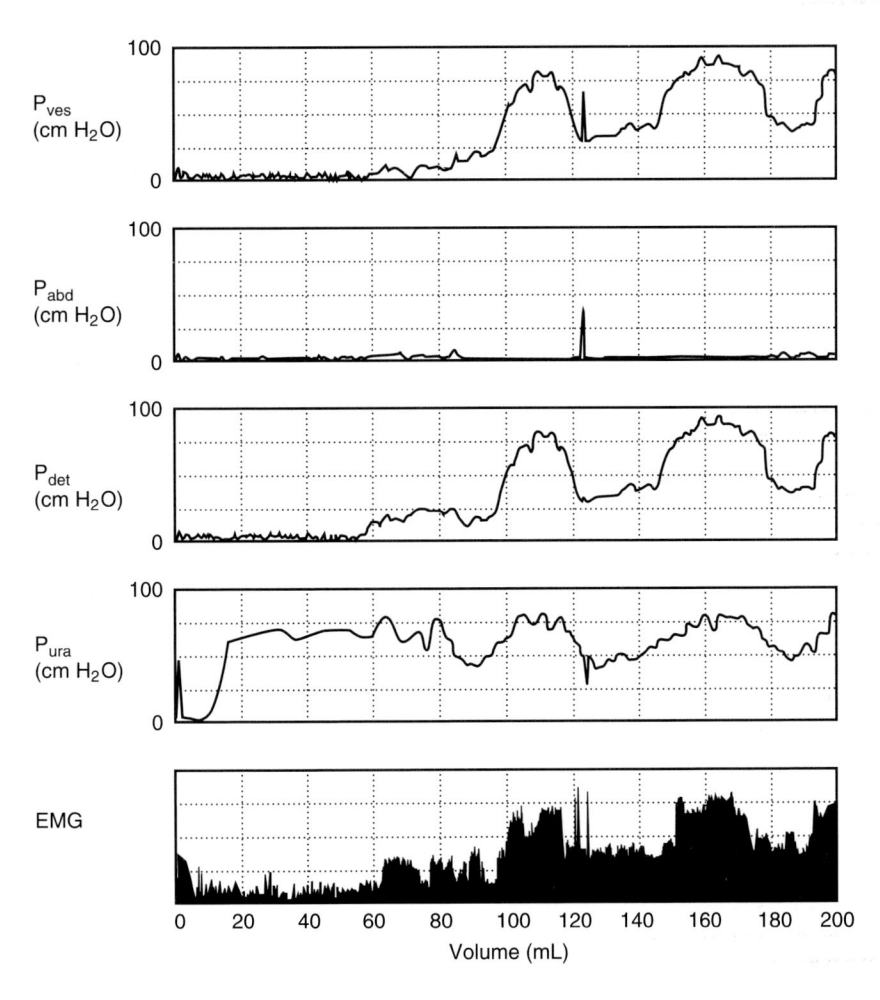

FIGURE 8-3 Pressure-flow study of a 34-year-old man with C5 spinal cord injury after an automobile accident 4 years ago. Although he is able to void and uses a condom catheter, this patient has had recurrent febrile urinary tract infections and autonomic dysreflexia. The urodynamic study demonstrates classic detrusor–sphincter dyssynergia. The patient develops involuntary detrusor contractions at 110 mL and 160 mL but the sphincter, instead of relaxing, develops increased spasticity. P_{ves}, intravesical pressure; P_{abd}, intraabdominal pressure; P_{det}, subtracted detrusor pressure; EMG, pelvic electromyography.

REFERENCES

1. Garraway WM, Collins GN, Lee RJ: High prevalence of benign prostatic hypertrophy in the community. Lancet 338:469–471, 1991.
2. Chute CG, Panser LA, Girman CJ, et al: The prevalence of prostatism: A population-based survey of urinary symptoms. J Urol 150:85–89, 1993.
3. Lepor H: The pathophysiology of lower urinary tract symptoms in the ageing male population. Br J Urol 81 (suppl 1):29–33, 1998.
4. Chancellor MB, Rivas DA: The American Urological Association symptom index for women with voiding symptoms: Lack of specificity for benign prostatic hyperplasia. J Urol 150:1706–1709, 1993.
5. Norlen LJ, Blaivas JG: Unsuspected proximal urethral obstruction in young and middle-aged men. J Urol 135:972–976, 1986.
6. Kakizaki H, Koyanagi T: Current view and status of the treatment of lower urinary tract symptoms and neurogenic lower urinary tract dysfunction. BJU Suppl 2 85:25–30, 2000.
7. Chancellor MB, Blaivas JG (eds): Practical neuro-urology: Genitourinary complications. In Neurologic Disease. Stoneham, Mass, Butterworth-Heinemann, 1995.
8. McConnell JD, Barry MJ, Bruskewitz RC, et al: Benign prostatic hyperplasia: Diagnosis and treatment. Quick Reference Guide for Clinicians. AHCPR Publication No. 94-0583. Rockville, MD, Agency for Health Care Policy and research, Public Health Service, U.S. Department of Health and Human Services, February 1994.
9. Barry MJ, Fowler FJ, Jr, O'Leary MP, et al: The American Urological Association symptom index for benign prostatic hyperplasia. J Urol 148:1549–1557, 1992.
10. Berry SJ, Coffey DS, Walsh PC, et al: The development of human benign prostatic hyperplasia with age. J Urol 132:474–479, 1984.
11. Walsh PG, Hutchins GM, Ewing IL: The tissue content of dihydrotestosterone in human prostatic hyperplasia is not supranormal. J Clin Invest 72:1772, 1983.
12. Walsh PC: Benign prostatic hyperplasia. In Walsh PC, Retick AB, Stamey TA, Vaughan ED (eds): Campbell's Urology, 6th ed. Philadelphia, WB Saunders, 1992, pp 1010–1024.
13. Chancellor MB, Blaivas JB, Kaplan SA, et al: Bladder outlet obstruction versus impaired detrusor contractility: Role of uroflow. J Urol 145:810–812, 1991.
14. Bruskewitz RC, Larsen EH, Madsen PO, et al: Three-year follow-up of urinary symptoms after transurethral resection of the prostate. J Urol 136:613–615, 1986.
15. Horton JA, Chancellor MB, Labatia I: Bladder management for the evolving spinal cord injury: Options and considerations. Top Spinal Cord Inj Rehabil 9:36–52, 2003.
16. Chancellor MB, Rivas DA, Manon-Espaillant R, et al: Evaluation of neurogenic bladder dysfunction and disability. Disability 6:1–17, 1997.
17. Kraus SR, Smith CP, Boone TB: Primary bladder neck obstruction in the male. AUA Update Series, vol. 19, no 8, 2000.

18. Kaplan SA, Te AE, Jacobs BZ: Urodynamic evidence of vesical neck obstruction in men with misdiagnosed chronic nonbacterial prostatitis and the therapeutic role of endoscopic incision of the bladder neck. J Urol 152:2063–2065, 1994.
19. Webster GD, Lockhart JL, Older RA: The evaluation of bladder neck dysfunction. J Urol 123:196–198, 1980.
20. Kaplan SA, Chancellor MB, Blaivas JG: Bladder and sphincter behavior in patients with spinal cord lesions. J Urol 146:113–117, 1991.
21. Chancellor MB, Bennett C, Simoneau A, et al: Sphincter stent versus external sphincterotomy in spinal cord injured men: Prospective randomized multicenter trial. J Urol 161:1893–1898, 1999.

CHAPTER 9

Urinary Incontinence in the Elderly

ANANIAS C. DIOKNO ■ KHAI-LEE TOH

Urinary incontinence (UI) poses a major problem for the elderly and has a profound effect on daily living.[1] Unfortunately, many accept it as part and parcel of aging and do not seek medical help.[2,3] This situation prevails in spite of evidence that up to 60% are concerned or worried about the incontinence.[1]

Much research has been devoted to UI, albeit in the younger sector of the community. Nevertheless, studies in the last 2 decades have greatly contributed to our understanding of the epidemiology of UI of the elderly. These studies have led to the realization that UI is highly prevalent in the elderly and its effects extend beyond the medical arena, negatively affecting the functional status and psychosocial well-being of the elderly.

FEMALE URINARY INCONTINENCE

Prevalence and Incidence

Prevalence of UI is defined as the probability incontinence within a defined population at a specified period of time. Incidence of UI is defined as the probability of becoming incontinent during a defined period of time. The incidence is helpful in determining the onset of UI as well as understanding the risk factors involved.

One of the earlier works, indeed a key publication, by Thomas and colleagues involved a postal survey of selected health districts in London and the surrounding area. The paper reported prevalence rates of 22.4% for those aged 65 through 74, 29.6% for those aged 75 through 84, and 32.4% for those aged 85 and older.[4]

The first definitive work on the epidemiology of urinary incontinence in the elderly in the United States, the MESA (Medical, Epidemiologic, and Social Aspects of Aging) study by Diokno and colleagues uncovered an equally high rate of 37.7% for those aged 60 and older who live in the community rather than in institutions.[5]

Since then many epidemiologic studies have been carried out, and recent reviews of the research cite prevalence rates ranging from 10% to 40%.[6–14] Chiarelli reports that the prevalence rate among elderly Australian females aged 70 through 75 years is 35.0%.[8] The EPICONT study in Norway, which involved more than 20,000 women, notes a gradual increase in prevalence until age 50 when it seems to plateau at about 30%. However, it begins to rise again at age 70.[8] Other researchers also observed this trend. In 1993 Molander reported that the prevalence rose from 13.9% in the birth cohort in 1920 to 24.6% in the birth cohort in 1900.[9] Likewise, Toba noted a trend rising from 59.3% among those aged 70 and younger, to 82.2% for those aged 90 and older.[15] Indeed, the prevalence of UI, as well as other lower urinary tract symptoms, increases with advancing age.[11]

Additionally, a significantly higher prevalence rate was noted among the institutionalized population. Rates ranging from 43% to 72% were repeatedly reported by various researchers on both sides of the Atlantic, as well as in the Far East.[6,15–19] Reasons to explain this phenomenon include admission criteria of the homes, which invariably would take in those in poorer health than the elderly living in the community, thus creating a selection bias.

There are unfortunately significant fewer reports comparing the incidence and prevalence of UI. Herzog reported a 1-year incidence of UI of 22.4% and Campbell and colleagues reported an incidence rate of UI among women in New Zealand to be about 10% in a 3-year period.[20,21]

The remission rate, that is, women who were incontinent at the baseline interview and had become continent by the time of the second interview 1 year later, was 11.2%. Similarly, 13.3% of the incontinent respondents at the second interview reported being continent in the third interview session. These data suggest that there is a significant portion of transient incontinence in the elderly.[21]

Types of UI

Several authors reported on the relative proportions of stress, urge, and mixed UI. However, findings differed as to the predominant type of UI among elderly females.

The MESA study found that mixed stress and urge UI was the most common in women, accounting for 55.5%, followed by stress at 26.7%, and urge UI at 9.0%.[5] Molander, on the other hand, found that urge UI was the most common at 49%.[22] Two earlier works noted stress UI to be the predominant type of UI among elderly females.[23,24]

Voiding Frequency

The MESA study established the pattern of voiding frequency among those aged 60 and older.[5] It appears that a normal frequency of urination is no more than eight times over a 24-hour period. Indeed, 88% of asymptomatic females—those not having UI, voiding difficulties, or irritative voiding symptoms—reported this frequency. Interestingly, the vast majority (93%) of these asymptomatic respondents also had nocturia, which was defined as the frequency of being awakened from sleep and getting up to void. In contrast, nocturia three times or more was experienced by 25% of women with irritative voiding and 24% of women with difficult bladder emptying.

MALE URINARY INCONTINENCE

Prevalence and Incidence

In stark contrast to female UI, there is significantly fewer data on male UI. Nevertheless, available data estimates that the male to female ratio of UI is in the order of 1 to 2 with figures ranging from 4% to 35% reported in the literature.[3,10] Earlier works by Yarnell and Thomas cited prevalence rates of 6.9% and 11%, respectively.[4,25] The study by Diokno and colleagues found a significantly higher rate of 18.9%.[5] More recent surveys quote rates ranging from 8.5% among those aged 65 and older to 28.2% for those aged 90 and older.[11,13]

These studies confirm that the problem of UI in the elderly has not abated despite tremendous advances in medical science. Furthermore, there appear to be no geographic or cultural boundaries; multiple studies conducted in different parts of the world consistently and uniformly point to a significantly high prevalence of UI among the elderly male.

Not only is the prevalence of UI high among the elderly male, but the rate increases as the population ages. Stratifying data obtained from the community, Schulman and colleagues noted a rise from 8.5% for males aged 65 through 69 to 13.8% for those older than 70 years.[13] Malmsten and coworkers observed a similar trend and noted the prevalence climbed from 6.1% for the 65-year-old males to 28.2% for men in their 90s.[11] As with UI in elderly women, the implications for aging men, particularly in developed countries, in terms of health care financing, nursing aid, and so on, are far reaching.

With regard to incidence, once again, there are significantly fewer reports about incidence than there are studies on prevalence. An early work found a 10% incidence over 3 years, although a higher rate of 10% over 1 year has been suggested.[21,26] Diokno and colleagues, in their study of community-dwelling elderly, noted an incidence of 9%.[20] On the other hand, as much as a third of incontinent elderly became continent later in life.[27] In the MESA study, the remission rate for older men with lower urinary tract symptoms over a 1-year period was 23%.[20]

Types of UI

Urge UI is consistently the predominant type among elderly males. This pattern is in contrast to female UI, as alluded to previously. In a literature review by Herzog, urge UI accounted for 40% to 80% of surveyed cases followed by mixed UI (10% to 30%) and then by stress UI (<10%).[27]

This situation has not changed since the time of Herzog's study in 1989. Recent reports found comparable data in their study populations. Damian and colleagues report that urge UI constituted 52.2% of male UI in their study of noninstitutionalized older people in Spain.[3] Both Schulman in Belgium and Ueda in Japan found that urge UI remains the primary type of UI in the elderly male.[2,13]

Voiding Frequency

The pattern of voiding frequency among elderly males was investigated as part of the MESA study. Among 500 asymptomatic men aged 60 and older, the vast majority (almost 80%) voided between four and eight times over a 24-hour period. Interestingly, 12% recorded frequency in excess of eight times a day and yet considered themselves asymptomatic. In addition, two thirds of these so-called asymptomatic elderly men had nocturia! In fact, 40% voided once, 17.8% twice, and 6.9% voided three or more times at night. Only one third did not have nocturia.[5]

PATIENT STRATEGIES TO CONTROL URINE LOSS

Patient strategies for coping with UI were investigated as well in the MESA study. The survey revealed that 55% of incontinent men used at least one method to control their urine loss; however, significantly more elderly females (69%) resorted to such strategies.[27] Use of absorbent products (e.g., sanitary napkins, toilet tissue, and absorbent garments) was the most popular method reported by 55% of female respondents. The second most common method used by 42% of the respondents was to locate a restroom immediately upon arrival at an unfamiliar destination. Voiding manipulations such as timed voiding or a conscious attempt to void before leaving home were practiced by 28% of incontinent women. Sixteen altered their diet and fluid intake and 12% did pelvic muscle exercises. Only 6% of women reported taking medications for their incontinence.[28]

MEDICAL CORRELATES, RISK FACTORS, AND ODDS RATIO

Multiple surveys have unearthed associations between many conditions and UI.[6,8,15,16,29] Key among these conditions is restricted mobility and indeed UI was found to be more prevalent among those with impaired mobility, those who require walking aids, those with a history of falling, and those with arthritis.

Additionally, those with concomitant lower urinary tract symptoms vis-à-vis poor stream, frequency, urgency, dysuria, and urinary tract infection were also more likely to have UI. Resnick described a specific physiologic condition, detrusor hyperactivity with impaired contractile function, that often renders the elderly incontinent.[30]

Other factors include functional impairment, for example, as a result of stroke.[2,16] Indeed, UI has been identified as an important prognostic factor for stroke but there remain gaps in our knowledge of the relationship between stroke and UI.[31]

Cognitive impairment secondary to dementia as well as use of antidepressants, antipsychotics, and antianxiety/hypnotic drugs were also identified as risk factors.[15,16] Many factors, particularly drug usage, are remediable, suggesting UI may respond to simple measures.

With regard to the observation that UI rises with age, Wetle noted that age itself does not contribute to UI. Rather, it is other effects of aging (e.g., diabetes mellitus, sleep disturbance, etc.) that lead to UI.[32]

Researchers have attempted to determine the odds ratio, which is defined as the odds of having a risk factor between persons having UI divided by the odds among those without. Using multivariate analysis, Brandeis arrived at odds of 4:2 for impairment in activities of daily living, 2:3 for dementia, 1:7 for trunk restraint, 1:4 for chair restraint, and 1:3 for confinement to bed.[16] Maggi and colleagues noted females with chronic obstructive pulmonary disease, parkinsonism, and a history of hip fracture were at higher risk of having UI with the odds ratios being 1:53, 2:27, and 1:38, respectively.[33]

Factors specific to female UI include a history of parent or sibling incontinence, vaginal infection, the use of female hormones, and menopause. Prior vaginal birth is a common cause of stress UI and nulliparous women have a lower prevalence.[4] Interestingly, the MESA study also found UI to be more prevalent among those who had incontinent episodes during pregnancy or in the postpartum period. Additionally, many nulliparous women were noted to be incontinent as well; however, the majority in this subgroup suffered from urge UI.[5] Vaginal surgery (e.g., hysterectomy and surgery for vaginal prolapse) were also identified as important medical correlates.[8]

Prostate surgery is a rising contributor to male UI. While the risk of developing UI following transurethral resection of the prostate is less than 1%, the complication rate for radical prostatectomy is much higher. Recent reports with at least a 12-month interval from the time of surgery revealed an incontinence rate of 8% to 10%.[34,35] The increasing number of radical prostatectomies performed may lead to an increase in male UI, but this may be tempered by improved surgical techniques and expertise.

VARIATION IN PREVALENCE RATES

The well-documented variation in prevalence rates is due to multiple factors, not least of which is the various methodologies adopted by different studies.[36] Some studies do not survey the general population but select their sample from health organizations, or sections of a city or community, and so on. Additionally, some population-based studies include patients from institutions located within their geographic boundary, thus confounding the prevalence rate because many people in institutions have different mechanisms of incontinence and different risk factors. Methods of data collection, such as postal survey or interviews either by phone or direct contact, undoubtedly contribute to the variation reported.

A major issue in epidemiologic research is the definition of UI. Unlike the traditional clinical or office setting where a diagnosis is made after a thorough history and clinical examination combined with appropriate investigations, most epidemiological studies rely on history as the sole diagnostic tool. Symptomatology invariably forms the basis of determining whether the respondents are continent or incontinent, as well as categorizing types of incontinence. For example, Diokno and colleagues invited respondents to a survey to have additional clinical examinations and found 83% agreement between self-reports and the clinical assessment.[37]

Furthermore, some studies regard UI as any episode of involuntary loss of urine, but others are more stringent and require regular urinary leakage. Holtedahl and Hunskaar calculated prevalence rates using different definitions of UI from the same sample population. The prevalence rate was 47% if the definition was any urinary leakage; it dropped to 31% if the definition required regular leakage.[38] These fundamental differences underscore the wide variation in reported rates.

PATHOPHYSIOLOGY OF URINARY INCONTINENCE IN THE ELDERLY

Although incontinence follows the same pattern in the elderly as in the general population, UI in the elderly is much more complex than in the younger population. The reason is the multifactorial nature of UI in the elderly. To compound the issue, many preexisting conditions could be considered possible causes of or contributors to UI. These conditions may or may not be contributing to the incontinence the patient is presently experiencing. UI in the elderly is, therefore, a challenge to the physician. So, it is the well-prepared clinician who can dissect through the multiplicity of etiologies, understand their relationships to the UI symptom, and, having considered all these factors, formulate a sound management strategy.

It is a well-known fact that patients may present with classic symptoms of either urge or stress UI. When one presents with involuntary urine loss that is preceded by an abrupt and strong desire to void and then loses urine, this is classically labeled as urge UI. However, when one presents with involuntary loss of urine in conjunction with increased abdominal pressure, as in coughing, sneezing, jumping, and so on, then this condition is labeled stress UI. In the elderly, it is not uncommon for the clinician to be confronted with a patient who complains of both urge and stress types of incontinence. We call this condition mixed UI. As discussed earlier, a major segment of the geriatric population suffers both types. Therefore, it is imperative for the clinician to sort out the type of UI that is afflicting the patient, determine which is the predominant complaint, and then seek to understand the mechanism and pursue possible causes of the UI. The authors use the MESA incontinence questionnaire not only to identify the type of incontinence but also the predominant type of incontinence afflicting the patient. (Fig. 9-1) This determination is made by tabulating the scores and identifying which type has the higher ratio.[39] Unfortunately, being able to identify the mixed nature of incontinence is not sufficient in the elderly. Not only do they present with mixed types but, in many instances, they present with confounding problems that one must also look into to completely understand the problem. In this regard, there are factors common to both male and female patients, but in other settings some factors are unique to gender. Resnick and Ouslander propose that transient or acute type of incontinence must be initially identified and, if present, treated.[40,41] One could then pursue the incontinence if it persists after eradicating or controlling the initial acute or transient factor.

Another problem in understanding the mechanism of UI in the elderly is that many patients present not only with mixed urge and stress UI but often also with unconventional incontinence symptoms such as massive loss of urine without urgency or warning, continuous small volume leaking day and night, or incontinence occurring only at night (enuresis). In these settings, the clinician must possess the necessary knowledge of the differential diagnoses of the mechanism of UI. With such knowledge, he or she can then proceed and determine the nature of the UI.

Likewise, the voiding symptoms associated with the urinary incontinence can provide a hint as to the mechanism of UI in the elderly. Incontinence may be associated with frequency of voiding day and night or night only, with urgency, or with voiding difficulty including hesitancy, straining to void, interrupted poor flow, and feeling of incomplete bladder emptying.

The mechanism of UI must be correlated not only with the current presenting symptoms but also with the patient's history. The presenting incontinence could have been modified by previous pelvic operations involving the gynecologic, urologic, or colorectal organs. The use of hormones by women, consumption of various medications, and the patient's habit of fluid intake and voiding frequencies could all influence the mechanism of incontinence.

Etiology and Mechanisms of Urge Incontinence

Urge UI, previously defined in this chapter as the involuntary loss of urine associated with an abrupt and strong desire to void (urgency), is a clinic or office diagnosis because this label is derived purely from history and not correlated with bladder function studies such as a cystometrogram (CMG). It implies that a patient with a clinical diagnosis of urge UI is also having uninhibited detrusor contraction (UDC) and this is the cause of the urge UI. However, such an assumption has never been confirmed. Indeed, UDC was not detected in spite of carefully conducted CMG studies.[37] These patients may be suffering from hypersensitive bladder as manifested by small capacity at first sensation or overall small capacity without involuntary detrusor contraction. This condition has been termed sensory urge bladder. Furthermore, some patients have small capacity at first sensation but have a normal overall bladder capacity. Others have normal capacity but constant sensation of urge throughout the CMG.

The discrepancy between the clinical diagnosis of urge incontinence and the CMG diagnosis of UDC can be attributed to many factors. One may surmise that the history taking is inaccurate. The elderly may be confused or misinformed or may misunderstand the physician conducting the interview. In most instances, however, the symptom is classic and the patient is extremely reliable, yet the CMG fails to demonstrate the presence of UDC.

One could also suggest that the CMG is inaccurate. It may not have the ability to trigger the UDC that occurs in real life but not during testing. We know some triggers, such as having the patient cough, stand, laugh, and so on, that provoke the occurrence of UDC during a CMG. Our experience with the MESA study in Ann Arbor, Michigan, showed that UDC may be observed not only in subjects with symptoms of urge UI but also in subjects who are continent and asymptomatic.[37] When CMG was performed in a group of 166 female volunteers, of which 53 had urge UI symptoms and 101 were either continent or had stress UI symptoms only, UDC was noted in both continent and urge incontinent subjects. The conclusion was that the accuracy of self-report in predicting the presence or absence of UDC on CMG was 72.1%. The sensitivity of self-report in predicting UDC on CMG was only 9.7%, whereas the specificity was 96.5%. These data suggest that most patients who have symptoms of urge will not manifest UDC on CMG, and if they do not have the symptom, they will probably not have UDC in CMG.

Indeed, urge UI has many causes and UDC is only one of them. The symptom of urge UI should not be considered synonymous with the presence of uninhibited detrusor contraction and, conversely, one should not assume that patients with UDC on CMG will have urge UI.

MESA URINARY INCONTINENCE QUESTIONNAIRE (UIQ)

Urge Incontinence Questions

1. Some people receive very little warning and suddenly find that they are losing, or about to lose, urine beyond their control. How often does this happen to you?
   _____Often (3)   _____Sometimes (2)   _____Rarely (1)   _____Never (0)

2. If you can't find a toilet or find a toilet that is occupied and you have an urge to urinate, how often do you end up losing urine and wetting yourself?
   _____Often (3)   _____Sometimes (2)   _____Rarely (1)   _____Never (0)

3. Do you lose urine when you suddenly have the feeling that your bladder is full?
   _____Often (3)   _____Sometimes (2)   _____Rarely (1)   _____Never (0)

4. Does washing your hands cause you to lose urine?
   _____Often (3)   _____Sometimes (2)   _____Rarely (1)   _____Never (0)

5. Does cold weather cause you to lose urine?
   _____Often (3)   _____Sometimes (2)   _____Rarely (1)   _____Never (0)

6. Does drinking cold beverages cause you to lose urine?
   _____Often (3)   _____Sometimes (2)   _____Rarely (1)   _____Never (0)

   TOTAL URGE SCORE_____
   URGE SCORE RATIO _____

Stress Incontinence Questions

1. Does coughing gently cause you to lose urine?
   _____Often (3)   _____Sometimes (2)   _____Rarely (1)   _____Never (0)

2. Does coughing hard cause you to lose urine?
   _____Often (3)   _____Sometimes (2)   _____Rarely (1)   _____Never (0)

3. Does sneezing cause you to lose urine?
   _____Often (3)   _____Sometimes (2)   _____Rarely (1)   _____Never (0)

4. Does lifting things cause you to lose urine?
   _____Often (3)   _____Sometimes (2)   _____Rarely (1)   _____Never (0)

5. Does bending over cause you to lose urine?
   _____Often (3)   _____Sometimes (2)   _____Rarely (1)   _____Never (0)

6. Does laughing cause you to lose urine?
   _____Often (3)   _____Sometimes (2)   _____Rarely (1)   _____Never (0)

7. Does walking briskly cause you to lose urine?
   _____Often (3)   _____Sometimes (2)   _____Rarely (1)   _____Never (0)

8. Does straining, if you are constipated, cause you to lose urine?
   _____Often (3)   _____Sometimes (2)   _____Rarely (1)   _____Never (0)

9. Does getting up from a sitting to a standing position cause you to lose urine?
   _____Often (3)   _____Sometimes (2)   _____Rarely (1)   _____Never (0)

   TOTAL STRESS SCORE_____
   STRESS SCORE RATIO _____

FIGURE 9-1 Instructions for scoring and obtaining ratio. Scoring of the Medical, Epidemiologic, and Social Aspects of Aging (MESA) questionnaire is done by adding the total score for each category, that is, urge category and stress category. For urge incontinence, the highest score is 18 based on six questions with a maximum score of 3 for each question. For stress incontinence, the highest score is 27 based on a question with a maximum score of 3 for each question. To determine predominance of either stress or urge incontinence, the percent score is obtained (by dividing the score by the maximum total possible score, for example, 9 urge score divided by 18 × 100 = 50% urge vs. 9 stress score divided by 27 × 100 = 33%). In this example, urge is considered predominant because the percent score of urge is greater than that of stress.

Other causes of urge UI could be categorized as local, regional, or central. Local causes include abnormalities in the bladder and urethra. The most common condition that must be excluded is an inflammatory condition that could trigger the symptom of urge and detrusor irritability leading to poor compliance and even spontaneous UDC. The inflammation may be related to infection or to noninfectious conditions such as the presence of a foreign body, new growth as in carcinoma in situ, residual effects of radiation to the bladder and urethra, and chemotherapy.

Another significant local factor is urethritis. Although bacterial urethritis is common in young women and usually manifests with frequency, dysuria, and at times urge UI, nonbacterial urethritis in elderly women is probably more often due to estrogen deficiency. Atrophic urethritis is associated with atrophic vaginitis and could be diagnosed easily. One could speculate that the thinning of the urethral and vaginal lining could expose the sensory nerve endings in this region, thus triggering a sensory hyperactivity that leads to symptoms of urgency and even urge UI. Several reports state that use of local estrogen to stimulate growth of the urethral and vaginal lining is effective in reducing the irritable bladder symptoms including urge UI.[42,43]

Regional pelvic organ factors that correlate with urge UI include gynecologic and colorectal problems. Severe constipation and diverticulitis at or near the wall of the bladder have been known to manifest as urge UI. Likewise, large ovarian and uterine tumors and pelvic masses in general may lead to increased detrusor irritability or trigger the development of UDC, resulting in urge UI.

A well-known mechanism of urge UI is the neurologic factor. Here, the classically described involuntary detrusor contraction that can overcome sphincteric resistance is considered the underlying cause. In this situation, during CMG testing, the patient can identify the impending UDC by a sudden urge to void and soon thereafter develop classic detrusor contraction, which the patient cannot consciously inhibit. However, at times, the patient can partially suppress the contraction only to have it recur soon after. When the patient feels a sudden strong urgency during bladder filling, suggestive of an impending UDC, there are two possible sphincteric reactions. This can be observed if sphincteric activity is being monitored simultaneously either with a pressure transducer at the mid-urethra or electromyogram. The sphincter may show transient relaxation and if allowed to continue, the patient may leak fluid around the urethral catheter at the height of the UDC. If, on the other hand, the patient is alert and tightens the sphincter voluntarily at the onset of urgency, no leakage will be observed.

Another urodynamic phenomenon that may be observed during CMG with urethral sphincter monitoring is involuntary urethral relaxation during bladder filling without associated UDC. If this occurs, leaking of fluid around the catheter may also be observed, especially if the bladder is at least half full. As mentioned earlier, uninhibited sphincter relaxation may also occur concomitantly with the UDC, and this urethral relaxation cannot be overcome voluntarily even when the patient is prompted to contract the sphincter.

Many neurologic conditions could lead to the development of urge UI. However, neurologic conditions do not necessarily lead to voiding dysfunction. The neurologic condition most frequently associated with urge UI is post-cerebrovascular accident (post stroke). This is believed to be caused by injury directly to the inhibitory areas in the brain center or due to partial interruption of cortical connections to the lower tracts.[44,45] Incontinence among stroke patients, as well as those with aphasia, is highly correlated with larger lesions.[46] Incontinence in stroke patients decreases over time, from a peak of 60% to as low as 20% at 6 months.[47]

Another common condition in the elderly that is highly correlated with urge UI is spinal stenosis. When the stenosis occurs at the cervical level, detrusor overactivity is generally the outcome. However, in lumbar stenosis, the outcome is uncertain and could lead to either an overactive or underactive detrusor. Recent reports suggest that laminectomy may improve voiding symptoms postoperatively.[48] However, the senior author has seen patients whose voiding symptoms remained despite relief of the stenosis.

Parkinson's disease is another neurologic condition frequently seen in the elderly that is associated with urge UI. In such cases, CMG invariably demonstrates UDC. Two exceptions are patients on anticholinergic therapy at the time of the test and patients in urinary retention, which is not an uncommon presentation for patients with Parkinson's disease. The bladder overactivity may be associated with sphincteric dysfunction, leading to some type of detrusor sphincter discoordination. Urinary retention in this group may be secondary to this phenomenon, to outlet obstruction, or to anticholinergic therapy. Because of the complexity of the mechanism of the voiding dysfunction among patients with Parkinson's disease, caution must be exercised before performing any surgical procedure that relieves the obstructive lesions but not the symptoms of the patient.

Although the prevalence of UI in patients with dementia is reported to be as high as 75%, incontinence in demented patients may not be attributable directly to the dementia itself but rather to all other factors that may be preexisting or coincident to dementia.[49] Therefore, it is necessary to be thorough in assessing the UI to be certain that the specific cause is identified. However, the presence of a factor that explains the incontinence must be balanced with the possible contribution of the cognitive impairment to the problem.

Urge UI associated with good bladder emptying, as manifested by absence of obstructive symptoms of hesitancy, straining to void, interrupted poor stream, and feeling of incomplete bladder emptying, is uncommon in elderly men but very common in elderly women. When such patients are confirmed to have good bladder emptying ability, evidenced by low postvoid residual urine volume, urge UI is then relatively simple to manage because therapy would then be directed primarily at detrusor overactivity. However, when the urge UI symptom is associated with symptoms of poor bladder emptying, it is necessary to rule out several conditions that could produce such a combination of symptoms. A common cause in men is outlet obstruction especially at the level of the prostate. In most cases, outlet obstruction should be managed first with a pharmacologic agent or surgical therapy followed by management of the urge component should it persist despite controlling or relieving the obstruction. If the voiding difficulty is discovered on urodynamic evaluation to be secondary to poor detrusor contractility, then the condition is called detrusor hyperactivity with impaired contractility (DHIC), as popularized by Resnick.[30] In this condition, unless there is obvious obstruction, the treatment is directed to emptying the bladder with intermittent catheterization and to controlling the urge component with pharmacologic agents.

Recently, Elbadawi, Yalla, and Resnick presented evidence that detrusor dysfunctions can be identified via electron microscopic studies.[50] They were able to characterize the ultrastructure of a normal aging detrusor that was defined as unobstructive, stable, and with normal contractility. They describe the normal aging detrusor as having preserved bundle and fascicle arrangement and structure, as well as virtually intact intrinsic axons. In contrast, they describe unobstructive overactive detrusor with normal contractility as having a distinctive disjunction ultrastructural pattern. The disjunction pattern is characterized by marked reduction or loss of intermediate cell junctions of normal detrusor and abundant, unique protrusion muscle cell junctions and ultra close simple abutments that are alien to the normal detrusor. Likewise, those with detrusor hyperactivity with impaired contractility manifest disjunction pattern but with interspersed distinctive degeneration patterns. Widespread marked degeneration of muscle cells and intrinsic nerves of detrusor characterize the degenerative pattern. The characteristic sarcolemmal features are often absent. In contrast, in detrusor overactivity associated with obstruction, they report myohypertrophy ultrastructural pattern superimposed on the disjunction pattern. Hypertrophic muscle cells, widely separated muscle cells, and abundant collagen between cell spaces and in the septa on interstitium characterize the myohypertropy pattern.

Etiology and Mechanism of Stress Urinary Incontinence

Stress UI is the involuntary loss of urine during coughing, laughing, or other physical activities that increase abdominal pressure. Like urge UI, stress UI is a clinical or office diagnosis based on history. In addition, stress UI may be confirmed by observing the patient leak fluid per urethra when asked to cough or strain with the bladder filled to near capacity. Furthermore, urodynamic studies may demonstrate leakage but uninhibited detrusor contraction during the moment of leakage must be excluded. Like urge UI, there are times that patients who present with classic UI yet do not manifest leakage at the time of urodynamic testing despite performing the provocative stress test, leak point pressure, or even under fluoroscopic observation. Such discrepancy has been attributed by some to poor patient reporting (i.e., mistaken history) but, in the senior author's view, it may be due to lack of sensitivity of the various tests to replicate the patients' real-life conditions. Another possible explanation is that the patient is very anxious during the test, causing her to tighten her pelvic floor muscles during the examination.

The MESA data suggest that the sensitivity of self-report that the provocative stress test will be positive is 39.5%. The specificity of self-report is 98.5%. This means the likelihood of a person who is not complaining of stress UI will have a negative stress test result is high. The study also found that the more severe the stress UI, the greater the likelihood that the provocative stress test will be positive. This observation suggests that there will be patients who present with stress UI but may not be confirmed with provocative stress test. There are many possible reasons for the discrepancy but it appears the mild nature of leakage could be one. Other possibilities include the status of pelvic organ prolapse. The presence of a severely prolapsing cystocele may mask an underlying stress leakage. In such cases, attempts should be made to reduce the cystocele with a pessary and the test repeated.

Simple genuine stress UI is uncommon in the elderly, especially among those who are frail. It is more common to encounter a mixed type of stress and urge UI with the urge component predominating. Nevertheless, should the stress component be dominant, it could very well be due to intrinsic sphincter deficiency (ISD). In this situation, the urethra and bladder neck is fixed or well supported as opposed to the mobile posteriorly rotating bladder neck seen in hypermobility. One explanation for the preponderance of intrinsic sphincter deficiency in this age group is the increased likelihood that these patients had previous bladder neck suspension or other pelvic organ and vaginal operations that distorted the anatomy of the bladder neck and urethra. Another reason is deterioration of nerves and muscles that innervate and support the bladder neck and urethra. Neuropathic disturbances may be a consequence of disorders that affect the spine, leading to lumbar stenosis or disk disease.

A problem frequently associated with UI in the elderly female is pelvic organ prolapse (POP). Pelvic organ prolapse may be a manifestation of weakness or herniation of the anterior, middle, posterior compartment or a combination of any or all of the compartments. A cystocele may be masking an underlying stress UI, which manifests paradoxically upon correction of the cystocele. If the cystocele is prolapsing beyond the introitus and is not reduced, incontinence is unlikely unless the bladder is chronically overdistended and overflow incontinence is the rule. However, if the cystocele is reducible and the patient discovers ways to reduce it, incontinence will be episodic depending on the location of the cystocele.

When there is persistent and severe prolapse of any compartment, patients invariably present with irritative voiding symptoms including urge and stress symptoms, as well as recurrent infections. It is not uncommon that elderly women are treated repeatedly for recurrent cystitis while the root problem is, in fact, pelvic organ prolapse. It is, therefore, imperative that a thorough pelvic examination be performed with an eye to quantifying the severity of the prolapse. The pelvic organ prolapse quantification technique (POPQ) adopted by the International Continence Society should be performed whenever pelvic examination is performed so as to communicate better the exact status of the prolapse.[51]

Stress UI in men is uncommon; however, it is common among men who have undergone radical prostatectomy for prostatic cancer. Even more rare is stress UI following a transurethral prostatectomy procedure for benign prostatic hyperplasia. However, stress UI is much more frequently encountered if transurethral resection of the prostate (TURP) is performed in patients who have undergone radiation therapy to the prostate. This is probably because radiation affected the membranous urethra and the surrounding striated muscle, which is the sole continence mechanism following a transurethral resection of the prostate.

Mechanism of Overflow Incontinence

Involuntary loss of urine associated with an overdistended bladder is termed overflow UI. This type of UI has a variety of presentations, including frequent or constant dribbling and irritative and stress symptoms. In general, it can be stated that overflow UI is really a variant of stress UI; the leakage occurs because the overdistended bladder has reached an intravesical pressure that periodically exceeds the urethral pressure. In contrast to stress UI, the patient with overflow UI is unable to empty the bladder effectively. Furthermore, the intravesical pressure necessary to cause leakage is higher in the overflow type. If the patient with an overdistended bladder has a urethral pressure that remains higher than the intravesical pressure, the patient will ultimately present with urinary retention instead. This group will present with symptoms of bladder pain or, if there is no pain or discomfort, possibly with azotemia, uremia, hydronephrosis, or possibly an accidentally discovered massively distended bladder. These patients feel they void "normally" or void small volumes without symptoms of incontinence.

Overflow UI may be due to an underactive or acontractile detrusor, which may be secondary to bladder outlet obstruction, drug usage, fecal impaction, neurologic conditions such as diabetic neuropathy and low spinal cord injury, or it may follow radical pelvic surgery. Vitamin B_{12} deficiency is also a possible cause of bladder weakness. The cause of many cases of detrusor weakness remains unknown.

In men, overflow UI associated with obstruction is commonly due to prostatic hyperplasia and less frequently to prostatic carcinoma and urethral strictures. Outlet obstruction is rare in women; however, it can occur as a complication of an anti-incontinence operation. Another cause of obstruction in women is severe pelvic prolapse, as described previously. Outlet obstruction can also occur in cases of detrusor sphincter dyssynergia in which the sphincter muscle inappropriately and involuntarily contracts rather than relaxes when the detrusor contracts.

Other Causes of Incontinence

Urine loss may be caused by factors outside the lower urinary tract, such as restricted mobility and impaired cognitive functioning. Many of these patients have multiple causes of incontinence and they may respond to specific therapies. UI can often be improved or even cured simply by improving the patient's functional status, treating other medical conditions, discontinuing certain types of medication, adjusting the hydration status, or reducing environmental barriers even if a lower urinary tract abnormality is present. It is, therefore, imperative that part of the evaluation of UI in the elderly be a thorough evaluation of physical status and cognitive function.

CONCLUSION

UI is a common problem faced by a significant portion of our geriatric community. Unfortunately, many accept it as part of the aging process without realizing that many contributory factors are pathologic and reversible. Recent research continues to add to our knowledge of the underlying mechanisms involved. The physician must sift through the multitude of pathologies because of the various types of UI, each with different mechanisms and etiologies, before formulating a management strategy. However, with proper understanding of the multifactorial nature of UI and improving methods for evaluating and managing UI, state-of-the-art approaches can certainly improve the quality of life of the elderly, enabling them to continue to live meaningful lives.

REFERENCES

1. Brocklehurst JC: Urinary incontinence in the community—analysis of a MORI poll. BMJ 27;306(6881):832–834, 1993.
2. Ueda T, Tamake M, Kageyama S, Yoshimura N, Yoshida O: Urinary incontinence among community-dwelling people aged 40 years or older in Japan: Prevalence, risk factors, knowledge and self-perception. Int J Urol 7:93–103, 2000.
3. Damian J, Martin-Moreno JM, Lobo F, et al: Prevalence of urinary incontinence among Spanish older people living at home. Eur Urol 34:333–338, 1998.
4. Thomas TM, Plymat KR, Blannin J, Meade TW: Pravelence of urinary incontinence. Br Med J 281:1243–1245, 1980.
5. Diokno AC, Brock BM, Brown MB, Herzog AR: Prevalence of urinary incontinence and other urological symptoms in the noninstitutionalized elderly. J Urol 136(5):1022–1025, 1986.
6. Aggazzotti G, Pesce F, Grassi D, et al: Prevalence of urinary incontinence among institutionalized patients: A cross-sectional epidemiologic study in a midsize city in northern Italy. Urology 56(2):245–249, 2000.
7. Bortolotti A, Bernardini B, Colli E, et al: Prevalence and risk factors for urinary incontinence in Italy. Eur Urol 37(1):30–35, 2000.
8. Chiarelli P, Brown W, McElduff P: Leaking urine: Prevalence and associated factors in Australian women. Neurourol Urodyn 18(6):567–577, 1999.
9. Hannestad YS, Rortveit G, Sandvik H, Hunskaar S: A community-based epidemiological survey of female urinary incontinence: The Norwegian EPICONT study. 53:1150–1157, 2000.
10. Ju CC, Swan LK, Merriman A, Choon TE, Viegas O: Urinary incontinence among the elderly people of Singapore. Age Ageing 20:262–266, 1991.
11. Malmsten UG, Milsom I, Molandr U, Norlen LJ: Urinary incontinence and lower urinary tract symptoms: An

epidemiological study of men aged 45 to 99 years. J Urol 158:1733–1737, 1997.
12. Molander U: Urinary incontinence and related urogenital symptoms in elderly women. Acta Obstet Gynecol Scand Suppl 158:1–22, 1993.
13. Schulman C, Claes H, Matthijs J: Urinary incontinence in Belgium: A population-based epidemiological survey. Eur Urol 32:315–320, 1997.
14. Fultz NH, Herzog AR: Prevalence of urinary incontinence in middle-aged and older women: A survey-based methodological experiment. J Ageing Health 12(4):459–469, 1986.
15. Toba K, Ouchi H, Iimura O, et al: Urinary incontinence in elderly inpatients in Japan: A comparison between general and geriatric hospitals. Ageing 8:47–54, 1996.
16. Brandeis GH, Baumann MM, Hossain M, et al: The prevalence of potentially remediable urinary incontinence in frail older people: A study using the Minimum Data Set. J Am Geriatr Soc 45(2):179–184, 1997.
17. Peet SM, Castleden CM, McGrother CW: Prevalene of urinary and faecal incontinence in hospitals and residential nursing homes for older people. BMJ 311(7012):1063–1064, 1995.
18. Sgadari A, Topinkova E, Bjornson J, Bernabei R: Urinary incontinence in nursing home residents: A cross-national comparison. Age Ageing 26 (suppl 2):49–54, 1997.
19. Ouslander JG, Palmer MH, Rovner BW, German PS: Urinary incontinence in nursing homes: Incidence, remission and associated factors. J Am Geriatr Soc 41(10):1083–1089, 1993.
20. Herzog AR, Diokno AC, Brown MB, et al: Two-year incidence, remission and change patterns of urinary incontinence in noninstitutionalized older adults. J Gerontol 45:M67–M74, 1990.
21. Campbell AJ, Reinken J, McCosk L: Incontinence in the elderly: Prevalence and prognosis. Age Ageing 14:65–70, 1985.
22. Molander U, Milsom I, Ekelund P, Mellstrom D: An epidemiological study of urinary incontinence and related urogenital symptoms in elderly women. Maturitas 12(1):51–60, 1990.
23. Iosif CS, Bekassy Z. Prevalence of genito–urinary symptoms in the late menopause. Acta Obstet Gynecol Scand 63(3):257–260, 1984.
24. Wells TJ, Brink CA, Diokno AC: Urinary incontinence in the elderly woman: Clinical findings. J Am Geriatr Soc 35:933–939, 1987.
25. Yarnell JW, St Leger AS: The prevalence, severity and factors associated with urinary incontinence in a random sample of the elderly. Age Ageing 8:81–85, 1979.
26. Campbell RT, Alwin DF: Quantitative approaches: Toward an integrated science of aging and human development. In Binstock R, George L (eds): Handbook of Aging and the Social Science, San Diego, Academic Press, 1995.
27. Herzog AR, Fultz NH, Normolle DP, et al: Methods used to manage UI by older adults in the community. J Am Geriatr Soc 37:339–347, 1989.
28. Herzog AR, Fultz NH: Prevalence and incidence of urinary incontinence in community-dwelling populations. J Am Geriatr Soc 38(3):273–281, 1990.
29. Diokno AC, Brock BM, Herzog AR, Bromberg J: Medical correlates of urinary incontinence in the elderly. Urology 36(2):129–138, 1990.
30. Resnick NM, Yalla SV: Detrusor hyperactivity with impaired contractile function: An unrecognized but common cause of incontinence in the elderly patients. JAMA 257:3076–3081, 1987.
31. Brittain KR, Peet SM, Casstleden CM: Stroke and incontinence. Stroke 29:524–528, 1998.
32. Wetle T, Scherr P, Branck LG, et al: Difficulty with holding urine among older persons in a geographically defined community: Prevalence and correlates. J Am Geriatr Soc 43:349–355, 1995.
33. Maggi S, Minicuci N, Langlois J, et al: Prevalence rate of urinary incontinence in community-dwelling elderly individuals: The Veneto study. J Gerontol A Biol Sci Med Sci 56(1):M14–M18, 2000.
34. Catalona WJ, Carvalhal GF, Mager DE, Smith DS: Potency, continence and complication rates in 1,870 consecutive radical retropubic prostatectomies. J Urol 162:433–438, 1999.
35. Benoit RM, Naslund MJ, Cohen JK: Complications after radical retropubic prostatectomy in the Medicare population. Urology 56:116–120, 2000.
36. Thom D: Variation in estimates of urinary incontinence prevalence I community: Effects of differences in definition, population characteristics and study type. J Am Geriatr Soc 46:473–480, 1998.
37. Diokno AC, Brown MB, Brock BM, et al: Clinical and cystometric characteristics of continent and incontinent noninstitutionalised elderly. J Urol 140:567–571, 1988.
38. Holtedahl K, Hunskaar S: Prevalence, 1-year incidence and factors associated with urinary incontinence: A population based study of women 50–74 years of age in primary care. Maturitas 28(3):205–211, 1998.
39. Diokno AC, Dimaculangan RR, Lim EU, et al: Office-based criteria for predicting type II stress incontinence without further evaluation studies. J Urol 161:1263–1267, 1999.
40. Resnick NM: Urinary incontinence in the elderly. Medical Grand Rounds 3:281–290, 1984.
41. Ouslander JG: Diagnostic evaluation of geriatric urinary incontinence. Clinics in Geriatric Medicine 2(4):715–730, 1986.
42. Semmens JP, Tsai CC, Semmens EC, Loadholt CB: Effects of estrogen therapy on vaginal physiology during menopause. Obstet Gynecol 66:15–18, 1985.
43. Raz R, Stamm WE: A controlled trial of intravaginal estriol in postmenopausal women with recurrent urinary tract infections. N Engl J Med 329:753–756, 1993.
44. Denays R, Tondeaur M, Noel P, Ham HR: Bilateral cerebral mediofrontal hypoactivity in Tc-99m HMPAO SPECT imaging. Clin Nucl Med 19:873–876, 1994.
45. Griffiths DJ, McCracken PN, Harrison GM, et al: Cerebral aetiology of urinary urge incontinence in elderly people. Age Ageing 23:246–250, 1994.
46. Gelber DA, Good DC, Laven LJ, Verhulst SJ: Causes of urinary incontinence after acute hemispheric stroke. Stroke 24:378–382, 1993.
47. DuBeau CE: Interpreting the effect of common medical conditions on voiding dysfunction in the elderly. Urol Clin North Am 23:11–18, 1996.
48. Deen HG Jr, Zimmerman RS, Swanson SK, Larson TR: Assessment of bladder function after lumbar decompressive laminectomy for spinal stenosis: A prospective study. J Neurosurg 80:971–974, 1994.
49. Skelly J, Flint AJ: Urinary incontinence associated with dementia. J Am Geriatr Soc 43:286–294, 1995.
50. Elbadawi A: Pathology and pathophysiology of detrusor in incontinence. Urol Clin North Am 22:499–512, 1995.
51. Bump RC, Mattiasson A, Bo K, et al: The standardization of terminology of female pelvic organ prolapse and pelvic floor dysfunction. Am J Obstet Gynecol 175:10–17, 1996.

CHAPTER 10

Neurogenic Voiding Dysfunction

KEVIN V. CARLSON ■ VICTOR W. NITTI

Neurogenic voiding dysfunction refers to a broad spectrum of functional abnormalities of the lower urinary tract, caused by a variety of neurologic diseases. These diseases can have a profound effect on the lower urinary tract, which may in turn compromise renal function. Normally, the lower urinary tract provides low-pressure storage of increasing volumes of urine and voluntary and complete evacuation of urine. This ensures protection of the kidneys and continence. Normal storage requires a compliant bladder (little change in pressure with large increases in volume) without involuntary contractions. It also requires a closed, competent outlet. A voluntary detrusor contraction of appropriate magnitude and duration with relaxation of the urinary sphincters and absence of significant obstruction is required for normal emptying. Neurologic disease can affect both storage and emptying functions of the lower urinary tract. In doing so it can cause symptoms such as incontinence and urinary retention or serious sequelae such as upper and lower urinary tract damage.

The principle objective in assessing patients with neurogenic voiding dysfunction is to determine the effects of the neurologic disease on the entire urinary tract so that treatment can be implemented to relieve symptoms and prevent damage to the upper and lower urinary tracts. The functional classification of voiding dysfunction proposed by Wein[1] provides a basis for the discussion of various diagnostic and treatment modalities (Box 10-1). In this system, all voiding disorders are related to the two phases of micturition, that is, storage and emptying. In each phase, the anatomic components of the lower urinary tract (i.e., the bladder and the bladder outlet) can be considered separately. Thus, one can have a storage disorder or an emptying disorder with each based on bladder or outlet dysfunction. A major advantage of this system is that it can be easily applied to urodynamic findings and treatment modalities, both of which are critical in the patient with neurologic dysfunction. Box 10-2 summarizes the effects of neurologic disease on storage and emptying functions.

It is important to keep in mind that symptoms of neurologic disease do not always indicate the magnitude of the disease's effect on the urinary tract. Serious sequelae can occur in the absence of symptoms. In addition, patients with neurologic disease are at risk for the same urologic and gynecologic problems as people of the same age without neurologic disease.[2] Having had a stroke does not prevent a woman from having stress incontinence. Finally, neurologic lesions can be "complete" or "incomplete." Therefore, the exact manifestations of a particular disease or lesion on a given patient are not absolutely predictable. A complete urologic evaluation of patients with neurogenic voiding dysfunction is therefore recommended.

This chapter begins with a brief review of the neuroanatomy and physiology of voiding. The neurourologic evaluation is then discussed, and a short overview of neurogenic voiding dysfunction (NVD) is given. This is followed by a section on management of neurogenic voiding dysfunction.

NEUROPHYSIOLOGY OF MICTURITION

Normal voiding is accomplished by activation of the micturition reflex. This reflex is a coordinated event characterized by relaxation of the striated urethral sphincter, contraction of the detrusor, opening of the vesical neck and urethra, and the onset of urine flow.[3] The micturition reflex is integrated in the pontine micturition center, which is located in the rostral brain stem. In addition, there is a sacral micturition center located at S2–S4 through which the bladder can contract independent of cortical and pontine input. The pontine micturition center through its neural pathways to the sacral micturition center is responsible for coordinated and voluntary voiding. Both the autonomic and somatic nervous systems play crucial roles in lower urinary tract function. Normal voiding occurs when the bladder responds to threshold tension via its mechanoreceptors. In order that this does not occur randomly, central nervous system inhibitory

> **BOX 10-1 Functional Classification of Voiding Disorders**
>
> **FUNCTIONAL CLASSIFICATION**
> - Emptying abnormality (failure to empty)
> - Storage abnormality (failure to store)
> - Emptying and storage abnormality
>
> **ANATOMIC CLASSIFICATION**
> - Bladder dysfunction
> - Bladder outlet dysfunction
> - Bladder and bladder outlet dysfunction

(cerebral cortex, basal ganglia, and cerebellum) and, to a lesser extent, facilitory (anterior pons and posterior hypothalamus) pathways coordinate urine storage and micturition.[4]

The pelvic, hypogastric, and pudendal nerves provide peripheral innervation to the bladder and internal and external sphincters. A detailed knowledge of the neuroanatomy of the pelvis is critical to anyone performing pelvic surgery because pelvic nerves are injured easily, and the consequences of such injury can be profound. A brief discussion follows; see Chapters 1 through 3 for a more formal discussion.

Parasympathetic efferent input to the bladder arises from the intermediolateral cell column of S2–S4 and travels as preganglionic fibers via the pelvic nerve (nervi erigentes) to the pelvic (inferior hypogastric) plexus located on both sides of the rectum from which postganglionic fibers innervate the bladder.[5] Efferent sympathetic nerves to the bladder and urethra arise from the intermediolateral cell column of T10–L2 as preganglionic fibers that travel to the pelvic plexus by two pathways. Short fibers travel to ganglia in the superior hypogastric plexus, from which arises the hypogastric nerve containing the postganglionic sympathetic efferents to the bladder and urethra.[4,6] The hypogastric nerves originate anterior to the bifurcation of the aorta and enter the pelvis below the endopelvic fascia, traveling medial to the iliac vessels and anterior to the sacrum. Longer fibers from the sympathetic trunks travel deep to the iliac vessels and fuse in front of the coccyx before sending branches to the pelvic plexus.

The pudendal nerve arises from the sacral plexus and carries somatic input from S2–S4 to the external sphincter. The sacral plexus lies on the pelvic surface of the piriformis, posterior to the iliac vessels and deep to the endopelvic fascia. The pudendal nerve follows the pudendal artery to the perineum, traveling dorsal to the ischial spine between the sacrotuberous and sacrospinous ligaments.

Storage and evacuation of urine depends on neural integration at the peripheral, spinal cord, and central levels. Normally, bladder distension causes low-level firing of afferent nerves, which causes reflex inhibitory response to the bladder via the hypogastric nerve and stimulatory response to the external sphincter from the pudendal nerve. With further distension, myelinated A delta fiber afferents are activated. Afferents travel up the spinal cord to the pontine micturition center. Here central input, mostly inhibitory, is received from suprapontine centers. If voiding is not desired, the voiding reflex can be interrupted. If voiding is desired, efferent output to the pelvic plexus at S2–S4 via the spinal cord is initiated. Ultimately, the stimulatory message is sent to the bladder via the pelvic nerve. At the same time inhibitory messages are sent to the hypogastric and pudendal pathways to allow relaxation of the sphincter mechanisms and coordinated voiding.

CLINICAL ASSESSMENT OF THE PATIENT WITH NEUROGENIC VOIDING DYSFUNCTION

Patients with neurogenic voiding dysfunction being evaluated for the first time should undergo a thorough history and physical examination, basic laboratory studies, upper tract imaging, and formal urodynamic studies. Patients should be reviewed at least annually, and the complete workup should be repeated if there are significant changes in the patient's neurologic status or in voiding symptoms, which can herald a change in the neurologic condition.

> **BOX 10-2 Effects of Neurologic Disease on Storage and Emptying Functions**
>
> **FAILURE TO STORE**
> **Bladder Dysfunction**
> - Detrusor hyper-reflexia (neurogenic detrusor overactivity)
> - Impaired contractility
>
> **Bladder Outlet Dysfunction**
> - Neurogenic intrinsic sphincter deficiency
>
> **FAILURE TO EMPTY**
> **Bladder Dysfunction**
> - Impaired contractility
> - Detrusor areflexia
>
> **Bladder Outlet Dysfunction**
> - Detrusor–external sphincter dyssynergia
> - Bladder neck dyssynergia

History

A complete neurologic, urologic, and gynecologic history and physical examination is essential for a thorough initial evaluation. A complete history of the patient's neurologic disease as well as how it affects daily activities is critical. It is important to understand how the neurologic disease affects the patient in general, specifically with respect to mobility and use of upper extremities.

Limitations of these functions can affect a patient's treatment options. Finally, it is important to know if the disease and its effects on urinary symptoms are stable or changing.

Noninvasive Testing

As part of the office evaluation, noninvasive studies such as uroflowmetry and measurement of postvoid residual urine can give an initial assessment of the patient's ability to empty the bladder. While nonspecific for underlying dysfunction, these provide an easy way to assess emptying and may prompt more comprehensive urodynamic testing. These simple tests are also useful for monitoring emptying in patients who have specific diagnoses and are being followed with observation or a specific treatment.

Basic laboratory investigations include renal function tests, electrolytes, urinalysis, and a urine culture. Patients with indwelling catheters, those on intermittent self-catheterization, and those who carry high residual urine volumes are at increased risk of urinary tract infections. Where secondary vesicoureteral reflux exists, the upper tracts are also at risk of infection and reflux nephropathy. For this reason, an upper tract study is indicated as a baseline. An ultrasound or intravenous urogram can be performed to assess for hydronephrosis and calculi. The ultrasound is also useful to evaluate for bladder calculi, which are reported in more than 30% of patients with indwelling catheters.[7] When videourodynamics are not available, a voiding cystourethrogram should be performed to assess for vesicoureteral reflux in high-risk patients. Where more detailed information on renal function is required, a nuclear renogram is obtained. Cystourethroscopy is indicated in select patients, particularly those with indwelling catheters. Besides evaluating for bladder calculi, it can detect epithelial changes. These patients carry a 5% lifetime risk of developing squamous cell carcinoma of the bladder.[8–10]

Urodynamics

The urodynamic study remains the mainstay of evaluating neurogenic voiding dysfunction. Urodynamics is covered in detail in Chapters 22 and 23. Here we will discuss the specific implications of urodynamic testing in the patient with neurologic disease. The purposes of the urodynamic evaluation in patients with neurologic disease are:

- To document the effect of neurologic disease on the lower urinary tract
- To assess for the presence of urologic risk factors
- To determine the etiology of symptoms

The urodynamic evaluation consists of several components including cystometrogram (CMG), abdominal pressure monitoring, electromyogram studies, and voiding pressure flow studies. Urodynamics can also be combined with simultaneous fluoroscopic imaging of the urinary tract (videourodynamics). Each component of the urodynamic test can be used to answer the preceding questions. It is often necessary to repeat a study several times to gain all the needed information.

The cystometrogram specifically determines the bladder's response to filling. Important parameters with respect to neurologic disease are bladder sensation, stability, storage pressures, and contractility. Involuntary detrusor contractions associated with neurologic disease are termed neurogenic detrusor overactivity by the International Continence Society.[11] During filling and storage, detrusor pressure is normally low (near zero). This low pressure is because the bladder is a highly compliant organ, which is able to store increasing volumes at low pressures. Pressures rising during storage, independent of a detrusor contraction, reflects impaired compliance (compliance = change in volume/change in pressure). Impaired compliance is not uncommon in neurogenic voiding dysfunction and can be dangerous (Fig. 10-1) . Impaired compliance is common with concomitant bladder outlet obstruction (e.g., detrusor–sphincter dyssynergia).

Storage can also be assessed during the filling phase of urodynamics. Incontinence is a common symptom in patients with neurogenic voiding dysfunction. Incontinence can be secondary to bladder dysfunction (neurogenic detrusor overactivity or impaired compliance) or sphincteric dysfunction (intrinsic sphincter deficiency). The detrusor or bladder leak point pressure (BLPP) can be used to assess incontinence secondary to bladder dysfunction.[12] The BLPP is the amount of detrusor pressure in the absence of an increase in abdominal pressure required to cause incontinence (see Fig. 10-1). The BLPP is a direct reflection of the amount of resistance provided by the external sphincter; that is, the higher the resistance (e.g., with detrusor–sphincter dyssynergia), the higher the BLPP. High storage pressures and high BLPPs can be dangerous to the upper urinary tract. McGuire and associates have shown that a BLPP of greater than 40 cm H_2O is associated with upper tract deterioration.[13] Incontinence secondary to sphincteric dysfunction can be measured by the valsalva or abdominal leak point pressure (ALPP).[14,15] The abdominal leak point pressure is the amount of abdominal pressure, in the absence of a rise in detrusor pressure, that is required to cause incontinence. Normally, there is no physiologic abdominal pressure that should cause incontinence and therefore there is no "normal ALPP." Unlike the BLPP, a high ALPP does not indicate danger to the upper tracts. ALPP is simply a measure of outlet resistance provided by the intrinsic urethral sphincter. If ALPP is demonstrated, sphincter dysfunction is implied.

Once filling and storage have been evaluated, attention can be turned to the voiding or emptying phase of micturition. If voiding is voluntary, the strength and duration of the detrusor contraction is assessed. Bladder contractility may be impaired in certain types of neurologic disease, particularly with lower motor neuron lesions. In addition, outlet resistance during voiding can be measured. The hallmark of bladder outlet obstruction is high pressure–low flow voiding. Several nomograms and formulas have been described to categorize obstruction, which can occur anywhere distal to the bladder.[16–19]

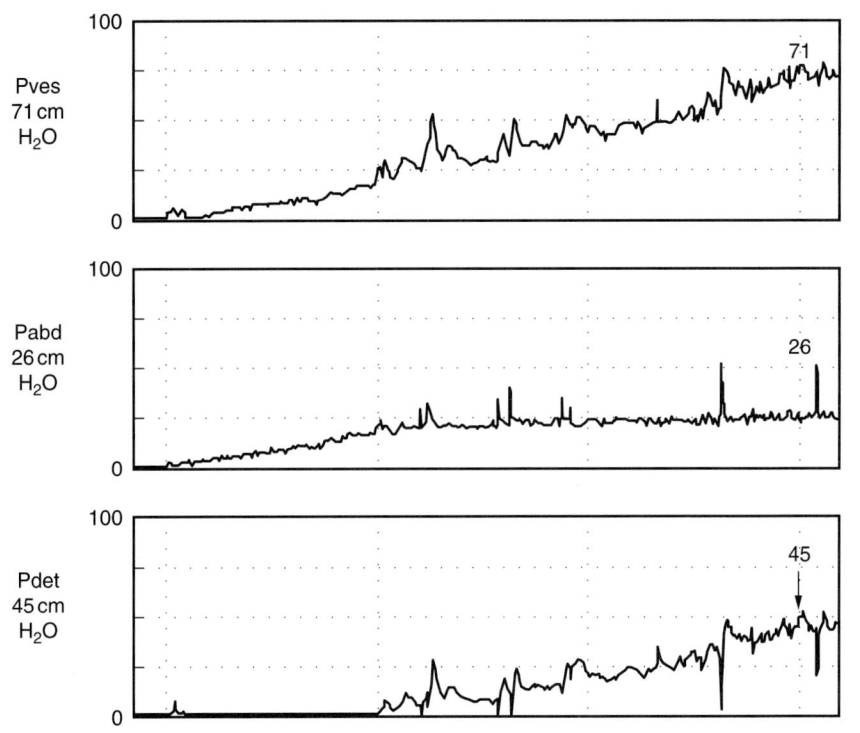

FIGURE 10-1 Impaired compliance. Note the rise in detrusor pressure as the bladder fills. The detrusor pressure is greater than 40 cm H_2O in the latter part of filling, indicating possible danger for the upper tracts. At the *arrow*, leakage was noted that corresponds to a bladder leak point pressure of 45 cm H_2O. P_{ves}, intravesical pressure; P_{abd}, abdominal pressure; P_{det}, detrusor pressure.

Normally, the external sphincter (and pelvic floor EMG) relaxes with a voluntary bladder contraction. Detrusor–external sphincter dyssynergia (DESD) occurs when the external sphincter contracts in response to a hyper-reflexic detrusor contraction (Fig. 10-2).[20] This contraction results in a functional obstruction, which can impair emptying and ultimately result in elevated storage pressures. True DESD occurs only with suprasacral spinal cord lesions.[3] Electromyographic (EMG) studies are used to evaluate external sphincter function. Electromyogram can be performed with surface or needle electrodes, the latter being more accurate and better qualifying sphincter dysfunction. Electromyographic studies are prone to various artifacts and must be interpreted with caution.

Videourodynamics (Fig. 10-3), or fluoroscopic evaluation of the urinary tract during urodynamics, is the most comprehensive and accurate way to assess neurogenic voiding dysfunction.[21] It allows determination of vesicoureteral reflux and the pressures at which it occurs, as well as detrusor and valsalva leak point pressure. Videourodynamics is also the best way to evaluate the bladder neck during storage and voiding (e.g., detrusor–internal sphincter dyssynergia). Internal sphincter dyssynergia can occur in high spinal cord injuries. Finally, confirmation of DESD and its effects on the lower urinary tract can be seen. In equivocal cases videourodynamics is an invaluable aid in the diagnosis of DESD. Urodynamic (and videourodynamic) findings that are associated with a high risk of urologic complications include:

- DESD
- Poor bladder compliance
- Sustained high-pressure detrusor contractions
- Vesicoureteral reflux

The integrity of the sacral reflex arc can be studied further with the evaluation of the latency time of the sacral-evoked potentials. This is done by stimulating the penile skin and recording the response with a needle electrode in the bulbocavernosus muscle. In patients with complete cauda equina lesions, the sacral-evoked response is either absent or significantly prolonged.[22] Evoked potentials provide a much more sensitive way of diagnosing neuropathy, especially occult, than classic EMG changes do.[23]

OVERVIEW OF NEUROGENIC VOIDING DYSFUNCTION

Neurologic diseases affect urinary tract function depending on which portions of the central and peripheral nervous systems are affected, therefore pathologic processes at each level of innervation must be considered in evaluations of neurogenic voiding dysfunction. In addition, the completeness of the lesion must be considered. The majority of neurologic diseases that affect urinary tract function can be divided into suprapontine lesions, suprasacral spinal cord lesions, sacral spinal cord lesions, and more peripheral lesions including cauda equina and pelvic plexus lesions. Some diseases, such as multiple sclerosis, can affect multiple areas of the nervous system. Thus the clinical effects can vary and be combined and unpredictable. Rather than discuss individual diseases, we will discuss the effects of specific lesions on voiding function.

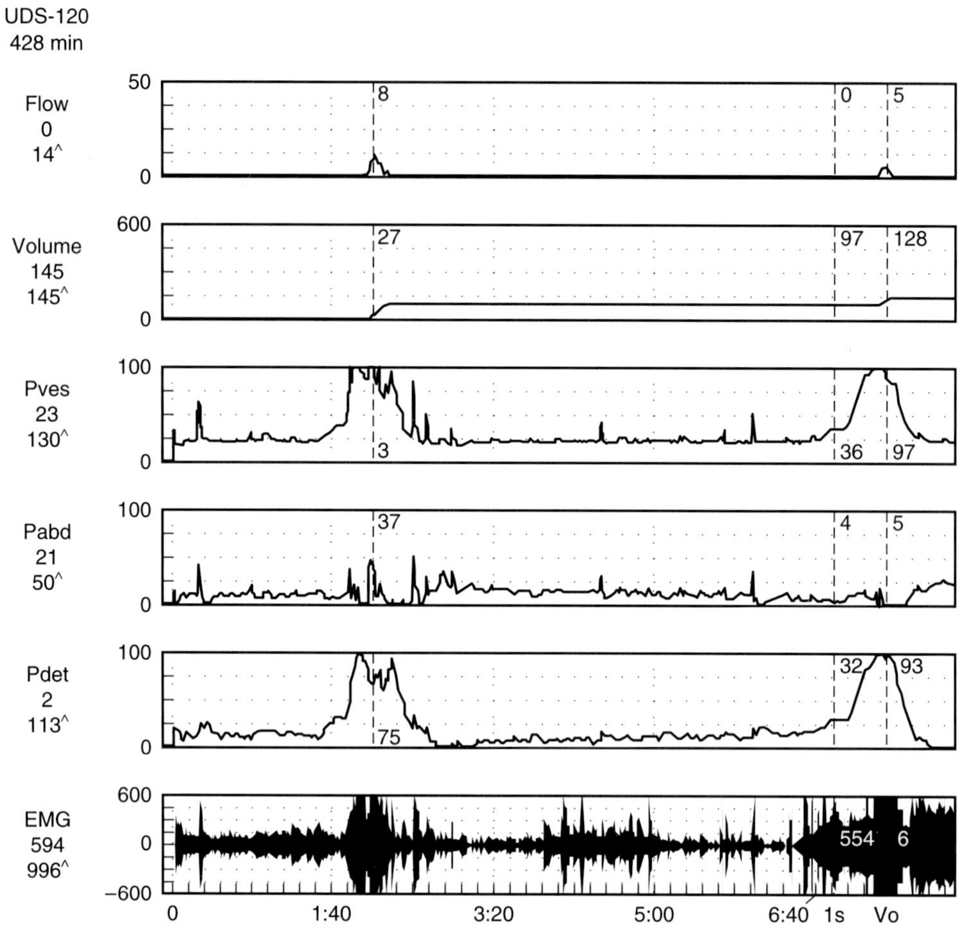

FIGURE 10-2 Detrusor–external sphincter dyssynergia in a female with a low spinal cord tumor. Note the two high-pressure involuntary contractions associated with increased external sphincter activity as measured by electromyogram (EMG). Incontinence is seen on the flowmeter. During the second involuntary contraction, the patient was asked to void and there was no relaxation of the external sphincter noted on the electromyogram tracing. P_{ves}, intravesical pressure; P_{abd}, abdominal pressure; P_{det}, detrusor pressure.

Suprapontine Lesions

Most of the suprapontine input to the pontine micturition center is inhibitory and therefore suprapontine lesions (e.g., cerebral atrophy, cerebrovascular accident, brain tumor) cause a loss of inhibitory input to the pontine micturition center. This loss results in uninhibited bladder contractions, but sphincter reflexes are not affected.[3,20] This condition can cause symptoms of urinary frequency, urgency, urge incontinence, and in severe cases, coordinated uninhibited voiding. Because sphincter activity is coordinated, there is little risk of upper tract damage because emptying is adequate and compliance changes generally do not occur. Although suprapontine lesions do not cause external sphincter dyssynergia, Parkinson's disease, which can cause generalized bradykinesia of skeletal muscles, can have a similar effect on the external striated sphincter (external sphincter bradykinesia).

Suprasacral Spinal Cord Lesions

Suprasacral spinal cord lesions also result in loss of supraspinal input. This loss usually results in uncontrolled activation of the micturition reflex with afferent stimulation from bladder distension, causing uninhibited detrusor contractions. Innervation to and from the sphincters can be interrupted, resulting in inappropriate contractions of the external (and in some cases internal) sphincter, causing DESD. In addition, afferent innervation is taken over by unmyelinated C fibers, instead of the myelinated delta fibers, which excite sacral neurons and trigger a bladder contraction.[24] With DESD the bladder contracts against a closed outlet with subsequent incontinence, retention, and eventual loss of bladder compliance. If the lesion is above the level of the sympathetic ganglia (T10–L1), detrusor–internal sphincter dyssynergia can also occur. The complexity of the voiding dysfunction and degree of detrusor overactivity, DESD, and internal sphincter dyssynergia depend on the level and completeness of the lesion. Theoretically, a complete spinal cord lesion will result in the development of a true spinal micturition reflex with DESD. Blaivas has shown that the incidence of neurogenic detrusor overactivity and DESD vary according to the level of the lesion.[3] Table 10-1 summarizes his findings.

In cases of acute spinal cord injury, there is usually a period of spinal shock, which can last from weeks to months. During this period the detrusor is usually areflexic, until the spinal micturition reflex is activated. In a small number of suprasacral cord lesions, the detrusor can remain areflexic.[3,25]

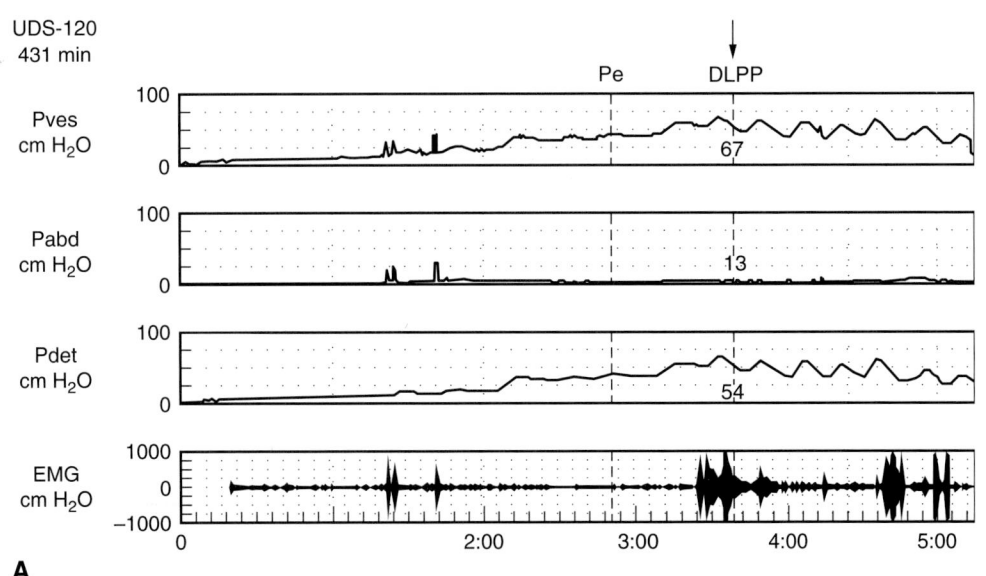

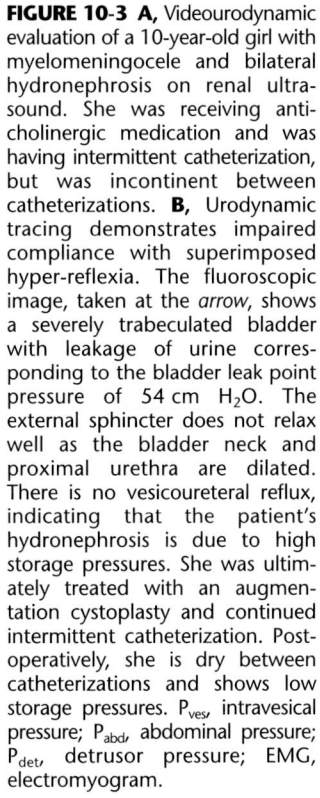

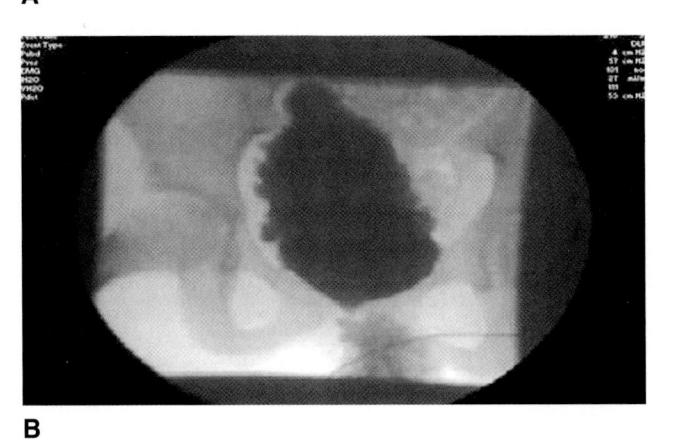

FIGURE 10-3 A, Videourodynamic evaluation of a 10-year-old girl with myelomeningocele and bilateral hydronephrosis on renal ultrasound. She was receiving anticholinergic medication and was having intermittent catheterization, but was incontinent between catheterizations. **B,** Urodynamic tracing demonstrates impaired compliance with superimposed hyper-reflexia. The fluoroscopic image, taken at the *arrow*, shows a severely trabeculated bladder with leakage of urine corresponding to the bladder leak point pressure of 54 cm H_2O. The external sphincter does not relax well as the bladder neck and proximal urethra are dilated. There is no vesicoureteral reflux, indicating that the patient's hydronephrosis is due to high storage pressures. She was ultimately treated with an augmentation cystoplasty and continued intermittent catheterization. Postoperatively, she is dry between catheterizations and shows low storage pressures. P_{ves}, intravesical pressure; P_{abd}, abdominal pressure; P_{det}, detrusor pressure; EMG, electromyogram.

TABLE 10-1 Urodynamic Findings in 550 Patients with Various Levels of Neurologic Lesions (including some with no lesion)

Neurologic Level	Number of Patients	Areflexia n (%)	Hyper-reflexia n (%)	DESD n (%)	Normal n (%)
Sacral	52	31 (60)	13 (25)	2 (4)	8 (15)
Lumbar	46	21 (46)	19 (41)	3 (7)	6 (13)
Thoracic	34	6 (18)	25 (73)	13 (38)	3 (9)
Cervical	39	3 (7)	34 (88)	21 (54)	2 (5)
Supraspinal	36	9 (25)	20 (55)	0	7 (20)
No neurologic Lesion	213	56 (26)	35 (16)	0	122 (57)

DESD, detrusor–external sphincter dyssynergia.
From Blaivas JG: The neurophysiology of normal micturition: A clinical study of 550 patients. J Urol 127:958–963, 1982.

Sacral Spinal Cord Lesions

As lesions approach the sacral cord, patients may present with various degrees of upper or lower motor neuron damage. This leads to a variety of clinical presentations, ranging from the hyper-reflexic suprasacral type bladder to the areflexic infrasacral. The external sphincter is similarly and variably affected, ranging from nonfunctional to DESD. Therefore, the typical combination of areflexic bladder and nonfunctioning sphincter is not always the case. Preservation of sphincter function with bladder denervation sometimes occurs. This observation can be attributed to the different locations of the detrusor and pudendal motor nuclei in the sacral cord.[26] A good example of the variability of sacral cord lesion is the patient with a low myelomeningocele, which can result in anything from a hyper-reflexic, poorly compliant bladder with DESD to a highly complaint, areflexic bladder with no sphincter function. Infrasacral cord and peripheral nerve lesions generally result in loss of sensation and contractility, leading to a large, highly compliant, areflexic bladder. The external sphincter may also be deficient of contractility and tone.

Cauda Equina and Pelvic Plexus Lesions

Bladder decentralization occurs in low myelodysplasia, in cauda equina injury, and following radical pelvic surgery and pelvic plexus injury. Classically, the behavior of a decentralized or lower motor neuron bladder has been described as areflexic, hypotonic, or flaccid and the sphincter as denervated.[23] Urodynamic abnormalities may be the only aberration documented in some patients with cauda equina injury and without other overt neurologic manifestations. Sphincter denervation—documented on electromyogram by a decreased interference pattern, fibrillation, positive sharp waves, and polyphasic potentials—has also been reported.[23] The bladder becomes areflexic but it is not always associated with low intravesical pressure. This paradoxical urodynamic reality after decentralization is difficult for many clinicians to recognize without formal urodynamic training.[27] After a lower motor neuron lesion, patients initially have a flaccid, areflexic, low-pressure bladder. However, the decentralized bladder is not denervated, and it may become poorly compliant and trabeculated over time.[24] Preservation of sphincter function with bladder denervation may occur not only because of the different location of the detrusor and pudendal motor nuclei in the sacral cord, but also because the dominant segment of the pelvic nerve usually arises one segment higher than that of the pudendal nerve.[28] Patients with intact sphincter function are much less likely to complain of incontinence (which is usually overflow incontinence) than are patients with sphincter denervation who may have significant stress incontinence. Thus, bladder and sphincter function must be evaluated independently. In these lower motor neuron lesions, bladder sensation is often preserved because numerous exteroceptive sensory nerves in the bladder trigone and vesical neck enter the thoracolumbar spinal segments, thus bypassing the sacral cord.[29] In patients with complete cauda equina lesions, the sacral-evoked response is either absent or significantly prolonged,[22] and this indicator is a more sensitive indicator of neuropathy than the classic electromyographic changes.[22]

REFERENCES

1. Wein AJ: Classification of neurogenic voiding dysfunction. J Urol 125:605–609, 1981.
2. Nitti, VW: Evaluation of the female with neurogenic voiding dysfunction. Int Urogynecol J 10:119–129, 1999.
3. Blaivas JG: The neurophysiology of normal micturition: A clinical study of 550 patients. J Urol 127:958–963, 1982.
4. Bhatia NN, Bradley WE: Neuroanatomy and physiology: Innervation of the urinary tract. In Raz S (ed): Female Urology. Philadelphia, WB Saunders, 1983, pp 12–32.
5. Wein AJ, Levin RM, Barnett DM: Voiding function and dysfunction. In Gillenwater JY, Grayhack JT, Howards SS, et al (eds): Adult and Pediatric Urology, 5th ed. Chicago, Yearbook Medical Publishers, 1991, pp 933–1100.
6. Norlen L: Influence of the sympathetic nervous system on the lower urinary tract and its clinical implications. Neurourol Urodynam 1:129–138, 1982.
7. Bunts RC: Management of urological complications in 100 paraplegics. J Urol 79:733–736, 1958.
8. Bejany BE, Lockhart JL, Rhamy RK: Malignant vesical tumors following spinal cord injury. J Urol 138:1390–1392, 1987.
9. Bickel A, Culkin J, Wheeler J: Bladder cancer in spinal cord injury patients. J Urol 146:1240–1241, 1991.
10. Broecker BH, Klein FA, Hackler RH: Cancer of the bladder in spinal cord injury patients. J Urol 125:196–197, 1981.
11. Abrams P, Cardozo L, Fall M, et al: The standardization of terminology of lower urinary tract function: Report from the Standardization Sub-Committee of the International Incontinence Society. Neurourol Urodynam 21:167–178, 2002.
12. Cespedes RD, McGuire EJ: Leak point pressures. In Nitti VW (ed): Practical Urodynamics. Philadelphia, WB Saunders, 1998, pp 94–107.
13. McGuire EJ, Woodside JR, Borden TA, et al: The prognostic significance of urodynamic testing in myelodysplastic patients. J Urol 126:205–209, 1981.
14. McGuire EJ, Fitzpatrick CC, Wan J, et al: Clinical assessment of urethral sphincter function. J Urol 150:1452–1455, 1993.
15. Wan J, McGuire EJ, Bloom DA, et al: Stress leak point pressure: A diagnostic tool for incontinent children. J Urol 150:700–702, 1993.
16. Abrams PH, Griffiths DJ: Assessment of prostate obstruction from urodynamic measurements and from residual urine. Br J Urol 51:129–134, 1979.
17. Schafer W: Principles and clinical application of advanced urodynamic analysis of voiding function. Urol Clin North Am 17:553–566, 1990.
18. Abrams P: Bladder outlet obstruction index, bladder contractility index and bladder voiding efficiency: Three simple indices to define bladder voiding function. BJU Int 84:14–15, 1999.
19. Blaivas JG, Groutz A: Bladder outlet obstruction nomogram for women with lower urinary tract symptomatology. Neurourol Urodynam 19:553–564, 2000.
20. Blaivas JG, Singa HP, Zayed AAH, Labib KB: Detrusor–external sphincter dyssynergia. J Urol 125:541–544, 1981.
21. Blaivas JG: Videourodynamic Studies. In Nitti VW (ed): Practical Urodynamics. Philadelphia, WB Saunders, 1998, pp 78–93.
22. Krane RJ, Siroky MB: Studies on sacral evoked potentials. J Urol 124:872–876, 1980.
23. Pavlakis AJ, Siroky MB, Goldstein I, Krane RJ: Neurourologic finding in Parkinson's disease. J Urol 129:80, 1983.
24. deGroat WC, Nadelhaft I, Milne RJ, et al: Organization of the sacral parasympathetic reflex pathways to the urinary bladder and large intestine. J Auton Nerv Syst 3:135–141, 1981.
25. Kaplan SA, Chancellor MB, Blaivas JG: Bladder and sphincter behavior in patients with spinal cord lesions. J Urol 146:113–117, 1991.
26. Kuru M: Nervous control of micturition. Physiol Rev 45:425, 1965.
27. Blaivas JG, Barbalias GA: Characteristics of neural injury after abdominal perineal resection. J Urol 129:84, 1983.
28. Bradley WE, Teague C: Spinal cord representation of the peripheral neural pathways of the micturition reflex. J Urol 101:220, 1969.
29. Bradley WE, Timm GM, Scott FB: Cystometry: V. Bladder sensation. Urology 6:654, 1975.

CHAPTER 11

Fecal Incontinence and Disorders of Defecation

PATRICK ATIENZA ■ FILIPPO LA TORRE ■ ATTILIO NICASTRO

FECAL INCONTINENCE

Definitions

Fecal incontinence has been defined in various ways, and no internationally accepted or accredited definition is currently available. The Royal College of Physicians proposed the definition, "the involuntary or inappropriate passage of feces."[1] Other experts define "functional fecal incontinence" as "recurrent uncontrolled passage of fecal material for at least one month, in an individual with a developmental age of at least four years."[2] It is important to distinguish between "anal incontinence," denoting loss of stool or flatus per anus, and "fecal incontinence," denoting any loss of solid or liquid stool.[3]

Idiopathic incontinence is often defined as incontinence that is not caused by trauma, congenital defects, or neurologic disease. Neurologic incontinence is often defined as fecal incontinence that is presumed to be caused by damage to the pudendal nerve during childbirth, rather than in association with neurologic disease. Neurogenic etiology of stress fecal incontinence was described in the 1980s, and the neurogenic hypothesis of stress incontinence arose from studies of idiopathic anorectal incontinence performed at St. Mark's Hospital and the London Hospital.[4,5] In this functional disorder of the anorectum, fecal incontinence occurs inadvertently, often without the patient's awareness until soiling of the underclothes is discovered. This form of fecal incontinence is predominantly a disorder of women, occurring especially after menopause. It is particularly associated with a history of difficult childbirth some years previously, but some cases occur in women who have never experienced childbirth. The latter women usually have a long history of constipation with prolonged straining at stool. A few patients have a history of previous persistent backache and sciatica or of laminectomy for lumbosacral disk prolapse.[6]

The anal canal is usually patent, and the patient may have a slight decrease in sensory acuity in the anal canal and at the anal margins.[7] Often the patient cannot distinguish between the presence of flatus and the presence of feces in the anorectum. The disorder progresses inexorably from minor dysfunction (e.g., incontinence of liquid stool) to frequent incontinence of formed stool.[4] During the last International Consultation on Incontinence, the committee proposed the following definition: "Anal incontinence is the involuntary loss of flatus, liquid or solid stool that is a crucial or hygienic problem."

Prevalence and Incidence of Anal Incontinence

It is difficult to establish the true prevalence of the problem in every country. Consequently, fecal incontinence is often underestimated because of the embarrassment and reluctance of patients to discuss this condition and the lack of attention by physicians when symptoms are detected.

The incidence of fecal incontinence common in institutionalized individuals varies between 0.5% and 5%, increasing to 18% in patients older than 18 years of age, 32% in the elderly, and 56% in patients with neuropsychiatric disorders.[8,9] The incidence of the disease in adults also varies according to sex; the occurrence of fecal incontinence in women who are 45 years of age is nine times higher than that in men of the same age. Women, particularly those younger than 65 years of age, are more at risk for anal incontinence than men. This increased risk is probably the result of obstetric injuries, as confirmed by the fact that many women are affected by temporary or permanent fecal incontinence after vaginal delivery. Enck and associates[10] reported that 30% of patients with gastroenteric disorders have fecal incontinence as a symptom, yet only 5% of the cases were entered in the patients' clinical records. The main risk factors observed are obstetric injury to the pudendal nerve, irritable bowel syndrome, diabetes, and anorectal surgery.[11,12] Underestimates of prevalence are common because many patients are reluctant to report symptoms of incontinence or to seek support services.[10,13] Prevalence also depends on the definition of incontinence used, and varies in different reports from 0.5% to 11%.[3] Fecal incontinence increases with age, disability that results in confinement to bed, dementia, and nursing home residence.[3,11,12,14]

Fecal incontinence has physically and psychologically disabling symptoms and is a significant social and public health issue. It has received medical attention only recently.[15]

Associations and Psychological Effect

Medical and Surgical Associations

Whereas the prevalence of fecal incontinence is probably approximately 2% to 3% and may increase with age to more than 10% in community-dwelling individuals, among nursing home residents, the prevalence approaches 50%.[3,16] Associations include diarrhea, dementia, impaired vision, fecal impaction, heart disease, arthritis, and loss of the ability to perform activities of daily living. Several specific diseases were associated with anal incontinence in case series, and mechanisms were investigated to explain the associations. Diseases include diabetes, multiple sclerosis, Parkinson's disease, spinal cord injury, and muscular dystrophy. Many of these conditions directly affect a patient's mobility, ability to perform activities of daily living, or cause of fecal impaction.[3] Additional etiologies include stroke and[17] hospitalization for acute illness.

Several operations could be associated with risk of anal incontinence including midline internal sphincterectomy, fistulotomy, ileoanal reservoir reconstruction, and total abdominal colectomy.[3] Anal and urinary incontinence commonly coexist, particularly in the elderly. Double incontinence is 12 times as likely as isolated fecal incontinence, and 10% to 25% of patients with urinary incontinence also have fecal incontinence.[18]

Psychological Effect

It is difficult to determine the full psychological effect of fecal incontinence. Little is known about the psychological aspects of fecal incontinence because no large-scale scientific studies have been conducted. Defecation is a profoundly private function,[15] and bowel dysfunction is the most fundamental of all personal problems, surpassing even sex in priority. Fecal incontinence is an embarrassing topic for the patient and for many caregivers. The sense of isolation and alienation that may accompany fecal incontinence can be reinforced by medical personnel who are unwilling or unable to discuss the topic openly. Because bladder and bowel control are learned in early childhood, loss of control often signifies a loss of adulthood and independence and causes an identification with the negative aspects of aging.[14] Various authors reported an association between fecal incontinence and anxiety, frustration, helplessness, depression, moodiness, sadness, pessimism, and decreased self-esteem. Continent women reported statistically greater emotional well-being and greater life satisfaction than did incontinent women in the same age category. Whatever the cause of fecal incontinence, loss of bowel control is one of the most devastating symptoms. Underestimation of prevalence is common due to the reluctance of patients to report or seek care.[19]

Incontinent women report more sexual dysfunction than continent control subjects. Depression and decreased libido, presumably arising from decreased feelings of self-worth, may be causes of sexual dysfunction. Embarrassment about odor or coital incontinence may be another reason for sexual difficulties. Finally, incontinence can be used as an excuse to avoid intercourse when more deep-rooted problems exist in a sexual relationship. It is unknown whether the relationship between sexual dysfunction and urinary incontinence would also be found in a group of women with isolated fecal incontinence or if double incontinence would exaggerate sexual dysfunction.[14,20]

Pathophysiology of Anal Incontinence

Introduction

Normal defecation and fecal continence require a complex interplay of several factors[21]:

- The continence mechanism works best when stool transit time is within the normal range. Even otherwise continent women may experience anal incontinence during an episode of severe diarrhea that overwhelms the continence system.
- The storage area in the rectum requires the rectal wall to be distensible, compliant, and capable of sending a sensory message.
- The voluntary muscles should be contracting during fecal storage and must be in the anatomically correct position to allow an acute anorectal angle, so that the fecal bolus is supported over the levator plate and not directly over the anal canal.
- The external anal sphincter should be circumferentially intact throughout its length.
- The neuromuscular integrity of the smooth and skeletal muscles is essential for optimal function.
- The integrity of the outflow system must be intact.

Thus, fecal continence is achieved by a combination of a competent, closed anal sphincter; normal anorectal sensation and sampling reflex; adequate rectal capacity and compliance; and conscious control.

Classification of Fecal Incontinence

Two types of history are typical in colorectal practice. Patients may have a history of prolonged or difficult childbirth with vaginal delivery, with occult sphincter damage,[22] or there may be a history of several years' duration of forceful straining at defecation. Incontinence may be passive, in which leakage of feces occurs without the patient being aware, or motor, in which the patient is aware of an urge to defecate, but cannot prevent the passage of feces.[3]

Incontinence is also divided into minor and major types.[23] Minor anal incontinence is occasional minor staining of the underwear or loss of control of flatus. At this level, the degree of social disability is likely to be minimal, and severe underlying disease or disorder is rare.

Simple anal pathology, such as third-degree hemorrhoids, a prolapsing anal polyp, or an anal fissure causing failure of normal local hygiene, may cause minor soiling. These conditions can be rapidly diagnosed on simple anal examination that includes proctoscopy. Persistent symptoms may indicate loss of internal anal sphincter control that may be the result of previous anal surgery (e.g., anal dilation, hemorrhoidectomy, sphincterotomy) or of complete rectal prolapse. In the latter case, the internal sphincter damage is probably the result of trauma caused by frequent prolapse of four layers of edematous rectal wall, giving rise to self-dilation. Less commonly, patients with damage to the striated component of the anal sphincter mechanism have major anal incontinence.

Major incontinence is frequent, uncontrollable passage of formed stool and represents significant disability. Severe gastrointestinal infection (e.g., cholera, shigella, amebiasis) and severe inflammatory bowel disease may lead to anal incontinence despite normal sphincter and pelvic floor function. In the presence of inflammatory bowel disease, the capacity of the rectum as a reservoir organ is reduced by fibrous tissue. Other patients considered to have major incontinence usually have a significant deficit of the external anal sphincter or pelvic floor muscles, sometimes in addition to a weak internal sphincter. Nerve conduction studies showed that in most cases denervation was secondary to damage to the pudendal nerves. This evidence strongly suggests that anal incontinence is usually neurogenic, arising from injury to the distal part of the innervation of the pelvic floor muscles.[23,24]

The cause of major incontinence, or total loss of control of solid stool, is poorly understood. Progressive loss of anal sphincter function occurs with no definite time of onset of symptoms. Initially, loss of control of flatus occurs, followed by seepage of fecal material onto the undergarments and incontinence to solid stool.[3]

The severity of fecal incontinence can be classified as minor (fecal seepage less than once a month), moderate (incontinence to solids more than once a month or to liquids more than once a week), or severe (loss of control of solids several times a week or loss of control of liquids daily).

Causes of Fecal Incontinence

Fecal incontinence is a complex physiologic function that depends on the interaction of multiple factors: stool consistency, enteral motility, rectal compliance and reservoir capacity, and functional integrity of the internal anal sphincter, external anal sphincter, and puborectalis muscle.

Stool Consistency

Insufficient stool consistency may lead to slight incontinence that usually disappears rapidly. Hyperinflux of liquid feces causes over-relaxation of the rectal reservoir that triggers the rectoanal inhibitory reflex. The internal anal sphincter relaxes, causing an immediate decrease in pressure in the anal canal and the urgent need to defecate. The urge to defecate is probably mediated by stretch receptors in the pelvic floor, and defecation is influenced by the size and consistency of the stool.[25]

Rectal Compliance

Repeated deferral of or ignoring the call to stool may lead to fecal impaction. Impaired anorectal sensation may be associated with an abnormal response of the external anal sphincter to rectal distension and, hence, incontinence.

A reduction in the reservoir capacity of the rectal ampulla may be caused by partial or total surgical exeresis of the bowels and by several specific diseases that may directly affect fecal impaction.[26] If it is damaged by radiation or Crohn's disease, the rectum becomes less compliant and increased rectal pressures may develop. In these cases, incontinence is caused by constant stimulation of the rectoanal inhibitory reflex, which is associated with reduced rectal sensation and misleading interpretation of the type of intraluminal content. As a result, feces pass repeatedly through the rectum (also as a result of the absence of Houston's valves, which may have been damaged or ablated), and come into direct contact with the anal canal that has been dilated by the inhibitory reflex, thus escaping control by the normal physiologic mechanism.[27]

Rectal Sensation

Diseases that alter mental condition (e.g., dementia, encephalopathy, stroke) and those that cause sensory neuropathy (e.g., diabetes) reduce conscious sensation and awareness of rectal saturation.[12] In these patients, once the fecal bolus reaches the rectum, it triggers the rectoanal inhibitory reflex. Because these patients do not perceive rectal distension, the internal sphincter relaxes, followed by fecal impaction and incontinence induced by hyper-reflux. Patients who have fecal incontinence usually have a high rectal sensation threshold; this high threshold is the cause of incontinence in 28% of the population. A high rectal sensation threshold was found in patients suffering from diabetes, peripheral neuropathy, descending perineal syndrome, fecal impaction, encopresis, spina bifida, and myelomeningocele.[28]

Anal Sensation and Rectoanal Inhibitory Reflex

The rectoanal inhibitory reflex allows rectal content to come into contact with the epithelium lining the anal canal. This area has a marked sensorial innervation that allows the distinction to be made between feces and flatus. The rectoanal inhibitory reflex deficit and the alteration in anal sensitivity may constitute an important factor in the pathogenesis of fecal incontinence. This condition is often associated with labor, descending perineal syndrome, or transanal mucosectomy.[29]

Internal Anal Sphincter

Relaxation of the internal anal sphincter during the rectoanal inhibitory reflex is followed by a gradual recovery of anal tone to allow the rectum to adjust to relaxation. In 25% of the population with fecal incontinence, a severe alteration in the internal anal sphincter has been found. Resting anal pressure is usually reduced in patients with fecal incontinence, often to a level similar to that recorded in the rectal lumen.[3] Marked descent of the pelvic floor may cause disruption of sympathetic innervation. The internal anal sphincter may relax inappropriately in response to relatively low amounts of rectal distension. Spontaneous relaxation of the internal anal sphincter without a compensating increase in contraction of the external anal sphincter may be an important pathogenic factor in fecal incontinence.[30]

External Anal Sphincter and Puborectalis Muscle

The external anal sphincter, the puborectalis muscle, and the levator ani muscle consist mainly of type I muscle fibers, which are typical of skeletal muscles with tonic contractile activity. The external anal sphincter is innervated by the inferior rectal and inferior hemorrhoidal branches of the pudendal nerves that reach this muscle by traversing Alcock's canal after passing out of the pelvis beneath the sacrospinous ligament. Although equally severely affected by the denervating process that damages the external anal sphincter, the puborectalis receives its innervation not from the pudendal nerves, but from direct motor branches derived from the same S2–S4 roots that project to its peritoneal surface from the lumbosacral plexus.[11] Repeated traction on the pudendal nerve leads to denervation and weakness of the external anal sphincter. Partial denervation injury may occur with repeated straining, with denervation occurring as a result of abnormal perineal descent. The pudendal nerve is stretched from its point in Alcock's canal, and there is a loss of myelinated and demyelinated nerves and fibrous replacement. In a study of these muscles, the histologic features of chronic partial denervation were recognized, especially in the puborectalis and external anal sphincter muscles.[31] Studies of small somatic afferent and efferent nerve fiber bundles innervating the external anal sphincter showed marked loss of myelinated and unmyelinated nerve fibers, with collagenous replacement. These features were consistent with denervation of the voluntary striated muscles that form the voluntary anal sphincter, as a result of damage to the innervation of these muscles at a distal site. The changes in the internal anal sphincter are believed to be caused by weakness of the striated muscle of the pelvic floor.[32]

Main Etiologies of Fecal Incontinence

The etiologic causes that lead to fecal incontinence may be classified as follows, and are listed in Boxes 11-1, 11-2, 11-3, and 11-4.[12]

Some of these causes were discussed earlier, and only causes that lead to alteration of the pelvic floor are discussed here. Fecal incontinence is often the result of obstetric damage or perineal descent and injury from stretching a nerve. Less frequently, it is associated with neurologic lesions or other medical conditions.

Effect of Childbirth

The effect of pregnancy and childbirth on innervation of the striated pelvic sphincter musculature was studied by Snooks and colleagues.[33] This study showed that the

---

BOX 11-1 Etiology of Fecal Incontinence: Altered Stool Consistency (Diarrheal States)

- Laxative abuse
- Infectious diarrhea
- Inflammatory bowel disease
- Irritable bowel syndrome
- Malabsorption syndrome
- Short-gut syndrome
- Radiation

BOX 11-2 Etiology of Fecal Incontinence: Reduced Rectal Reservoir Capacity or Compliance

- Inflammatory bowel disease
- Absent rectal reservoir
  - Low anterior resection
  - Coloanal anastomosis
  - Ileorectal anastomosis
  - Ileoanal reservoir
- Rectal ischemia
- Collagen vascular disease
  - Scleroderma
  - Dermatomyositis
  - Amyloidosis
- Rectal neoplasms
- Extrinsic rectal compression

BOX 11-3 Etiology of Fecal Incontinence: Reduced Rectal Sensation

- Upper motor neuron lesions: spinal cord lesions
  - Trauma
  - Cord compression
  - Ischemia
  - Multiple sclerosis
  - Syringomyelia
  - Tumor
- Upper motor neuron lesions: cerebral
  - Cerebrovascular disease
  - Dementia
  - Brain injuries
  - Stroke
  - Tumors (frontal lobe)
- Overflow incontinence
  - Fecal impaction
  - Psychotropic drugs
  - Encopresis
- Antimotility drugs

> **BOX 11-4 Etiology of Fecal Incontinence: Other**
>
> - Local sphincter pathology
>   - Congenital perineal anomalies (spina bifida, imperforate anus)
>   - Obstetric anal sphincter tears
>   - Trauma
>   - Perineal and pelvic neoplasms
> - Lower motor neuron pathway lesions
>   - Peripheral (intrapelvic) nerve lesions
>   - Pudendal, perineal, and intrapelvic nerve stretch lesions
>   - Obstetric nerve injuries
>   - Intrapelvic tumor and endometriosis
>   - Diabetic neuropathy
>   - Cauda equina lesions
>   - Lumbosacral spinal trauma
>   - Lumbosacral disk prolapse
>   - Lumbar canal stenosis
>   - Ankylosing spondylosis
>   - Idiopathic arachnoiditis of cauda equina
>   - Cauda equina tumors
> - Conus medullaris and sacral cord lesions
>   - Multiple sclerosis
>   - Multiple system atrophy
>   - Parkinson's disease
> - Enteric and bladder
>   - Sphincter overwhelmed by diarrhea
>   - Irritable bowel syndrome
>   - Procidentia
>   - Rectal prolapse

Pudendal Nerves Terminal Motor Latency (PNTML) was more increased in multiparas than in primiparas, and that prolonged labor, the use of forceps, and delivery of a large infant resulted in more pudendal nerve damage. Women who had cesarean deliveries show no evidence of damage to the innervation of the pelvic floor muscles. In multiparas, the PNTML was more likely still to be abnormal 2 months after delivery, indicating the development of cumulative and irreversible damage to the innervation of the pelvic floor muscles with increasing numbers of vaginal deliveries.

Stress urinary incontinence is closely related to idiopathic (stress) neurogenic fecal incontinence.[31] Approximately 15% of women with anorectal incontinence also have stress urinary incontinence (double incontinence), and in women in whom neurogenic fecal incontinence is the only symptom, the PNTML is abnormal, although it is not as increased as in those who also have stress urinary incontinence. The clinical features of the pelvic floor of women with stress urinary incontinence are similar to those of women with neurogenic (stress) fecal incontinence, especially in relation to perineal descent on straining.[11]

Direct measurement of the integrity of the motor innervation of the puborectalis muscle in these conditions shows that there is similar damage to the innervation of the pelvicaudal component of the pelvic floor musculature, in addition to that of the external anal sphincter and periurethral sphincter musculature.[5] When this damage is the direct result of childbirth, it is likely caused by stretching of the birth canal during delivery and by direct pressure or injury to the innervation of these muscles at the level of the lumbosacral plexus.

Approximately 40% to 60% of women with anal incontinence report a difficult childbirth. The hypothesis that childbirth might be a major factor in initiating denervation injury was investigated in the 1980s. The abnormalities found were most notable in multiparous women and correlated most strongly with a prolonged second stage of labor, the use of obstetric forceps, and delivery of a large infant. A difficult vaginal delivery may result in distal nerve damage from stretching of the pelvic floor (and its nerve supply) and probably also from direct compression by the fetal head of the nerves that lie in the sidewall of the pelvis. Sultan and associates[34] performed the only prospective study of 150 women (before and after childbirth) to show both occult anal sphincter trauma and pudendal nerve damage during childbirth in both primiparous and multiparous women. This study found a strong correlation between any defect and the development of symptoms. No relationship was seen between pudendal latency measurements and defecatory or urinary symptoms. In another study, Donnelly and colleagues[35] interviewed 210 nulliparas about bowel habits in the third trimester and performed anal vector manometry. At 6 weeks postpartum, the women returned and completed the same bowel symptom questionnaire and underwent anal vector manometry plus PNTML. Instrumental vaginal delivery and a passive second stage of labor prolonged by epidural analgesia were significantly associated with the greatest risk of anal sphincter trauma and impaired incontinence.

Constipation and Defecation Disorders

Denervation was also found in the pelvic floor muscles of patients with constipation and defecation disorders that cause excessive straining.[23,36] These patients often show the physical sign of perineal descent. In patients with abnormal descent, the perineum descends well below the bony outlet during a straining effort.[36] The terminal portion of the pudendal nerve in the adult is approximately 9 cm; in patients with abnormal descent of 2 to 3 cm, a stretching force to the distal portion of the pudendal nerve of 20% to 30% is exerted. Stretching of these nerves during straining may lead to secondary neuropathic damage.

A particular form of fecal incontinence occurs in descending perineum syndrome. In this case, incontinence has two causes, muscular and neurologic. Many patients with perineal descent have the same electrophysiologic abnormalities that are seen in patients with fecal incontinence. In the descending perineum, the perineal floor collapses more than 3 cm below the theoretical line linking the lower part of the pelvis to the coccyx in the anterior–posterior aspect and the two ischial tuberosities in the lateral aspect. This condition alters the stability of the muscles and the tendon ligaments from the anal canal to the pelvis, and leads to loss of muscular tone. Moreover, the pudendal nerve is strained in Alcock's canal and at its exit at the greater ischial tuberosity, with a consequent loss of postural and voluntary tone.

Other Important Etiologies

Traumatic damage to the pelvic floor that leads to disruption of the anorectal angle may cause significant incontinence. Impalement injuries to the perineum cause traumatic disruption of the rectum, anus, and surrounding musculature, and lead to varying degrees of fecal incontinence. This type of injury is occasionally seen after major pelvic injuries, when a fracture occurs across the bony ring of the pelvis. Damage to the external sphincter can occur with anal fistula surgery.

Anal sphincter injury may result from anorectal surgery, usually as a complication of treatment of a complex abscess or fistula. Prolapse of the rectum may also lead to fecal incontinence. Although this may reflect an associated traction injury to the pudendal nerves, recurring intrusion of the rectum through the anal canal may cause stretching of the anal levators and sphincters to the extent that normal muscle tone is lost.

Anal sexual activity may traumatize the sphincter mechanism to such a degree that the anus takes on the patent appearance seen in chronic rectal prolapse.

DISORDERS OF DEFECATION

Definition

Constipation is a misleading name because it does not necessarily mean the passage of hard or infrequent stools, as is commonly interpreted. It may also mean excessive straining at defecation or the passage of stools that are too small. All of these manifestations are interpreted by the patient as constipation, regardless of their possibly unrelated and different etiology, pathology, and treatment. At the same time, there is no agreement in the literature on the definition of constipation. Many definitions are used, describing the weight, frequency, and even consistency of stool. Devroede[37] defined constipation as fewer than three weekly stools in women or fewer than five weekly stools in men, despite a high-residue diet, or going longer than 3 days without a bowel movement. Moore-Gillon[38] defined constipation as defecation that is difficult, infrequent, or both. According to Drossmann and colleagues,[39] a patient who strains for more than 25% of the time at stool or passes two or fewer stools per week is constipated. Painter[40] classified as constipated any patient who strains to defecate and does not pass minimally one soft stool daily without effort. These discrepancies led to the challenge to study each manifestation of constipation separately. A useful guideline that is generally accepted as a normal range for bowel frequency is three times per day to three times per week. The most common symptoms associated with constipation are a feeling of having to strain at stool, abdominal pain or bloating, and dissatisfaction or a feeling of incomplete rectal emptying after passing stool.[41]

Pathogenesis

The causes of constipation can be varied and multifactorial. Constipation is a symptom of organic disease of the gastrointestinal tract and one of the most common chronic digestive disorders in the United States and in the developed Western countries. Concepts about defecation have been influenced by social and dietary customs.[42] It may be caused by endocrine factors, systemic diseases, psychologic factors, and neurologic diseases.[43] In some neurologic conditions, patients may suffer from constipation because of pelvic floor dyssynergia resulting in rectal outlet delay and prolonged straining.[44,45] Patients with chronic idiopathic constipation are divided into two main groups: those with colonic dysmotility and those with outlet obstruction. Three broad categories of disorders cause constipation: (1) systemic factors that affect normal colonic and rectal function, (2) primary colonic and anorectal factors, and (3) psychological factors.[41]

Anorectal abnormalities that interfere with normal defecation can be divided into three types: (1) dilation of the rectum or colon, such as megarectum or megacolon, (2) local anorectal abnormalities, and (3) chronic idiopathic constipation in which no structural abnormalities are present.

Colonic Abnormalities: Colonic Dysmotility

The myenteric plexus that regulates colonic motor function may be abnormal in some constipated patients. Some reports showed widespread abnormalities in the myenteric plexus of some constipated patients. Some of these patients had widespread gastrointestinal dysmotility with alterations in esophageal and gastric function as well.[46] The myenteric plexus that regulates colonic motor function may be abnormal in some constipated patients. Some of these patients have widespread gastrointestinal dysmotility.[47] Colonic dysmotility and slow transit may be generalized or localized to one segment.[48] The cause of this altered motility is unknown, and it has been related to neurogenic, myogenic, or psychogenic causes.[46] Krishnamurthy and associates[46] suggested that the detection of few or no argyrophilic, or silver-stained, neurons is an identifiable abnormality in patients with primary colonic dysmotility. Elderly people are at greater risk of dehydration, and low fluid intake in older adults has been related to slow colonic transit.[49] In addition, medications used to treat psychiatric disease may contribute to constipation.

Intestinal Transit and Motility: Rectal Inertia

As the fecal mass enters the rectum, the rectal detrusor contracts and the rectal neck relaxes in a reflex manner. Thus, anorectal dysmotility comprises rectal inertia and outlet obstruction. A subgroup of patients with constipation have delayed whole-gut transit, or slow-transit constipation.[43] Two types of delayed transit were identified: a delay in the entire colon, or colonic inertia, and a distal delay in the rectosigmoid colon.[47,50] This delay can be caused by neurologic, toxic, mechanical, or degenerative pathology, such as Hirschsprung's disease (congenital megacolon), Chagas' disease (trypanosomiasis), and volvulus (torsion of a loop of intestine), or by outlet obstruction. The delay allows large amounts of feces to accumulate in the rectum without initiating defecation. Manometric studies of the colon show decreased mass movements and a reduced urge to defecate with mass movements[51] in constipated patients. Concomitant studies with radiolabeled transit markers confirmed that some patients with constipation have impaired movement of colonic material after meals.

A common problem in these patients is difficulty delivering the hard, thick head of the stool column at the start of defecation. Excessive straining and great sphincter dilation are needed to allow stool to pass the rectal neck, which is commonly bruised.[52]

Pelvic Floor and Anorectal Abnormalities

Constipated patients who have no structural abnormality of the anorectum may have dysfunction of the pelvic floor musculature. In these patients, the anus does not open as a result of contraction rather than relaxation of the anal sphincter muscles on attempted defecation. This condition, known as anismus and pelvic floor dyssynergia, blocks normal rectal emptying by obstructing the outlet to the colon.[53]

Outlet obstruction is inability to completely expel stool that has reached the rectum because of failure of the rectal neck (anal canal) to open in front of the descending fecal mass.[52] Thus, rectal inertia may complicate chronic outlet obstruction and may affect treatment.

Normal defecation requires the coordination of pelvic floor muscles and anal sphincters with the rectal detrusor. Dysfunction of these muscles results in outlet obstruction. Defecation may be impaired by failure of the levator ani to open the anorectal angle. This abnormality is defined by anismus. A paradoxical increase in external and anal sphincter activity may be observed in patients with high spinal lesions. Some patients with anismus also have a selective disturbance in rectal sensation, suggesting that this combination is a disorder in the central nervous control of defecation. The true incidence of this paradoxical contraction of the puborectalis muscle on defecation is controversial, because some normal subjects also show this abnormality.[41,54]

Other Factors Involved in Constipation

Hypothyroidism, diabetes, and all causes of hypercalcemia, including hyperparathyroidism, can cause constipation. Diabetes warrants special mention because constipation is a very common symptom. In patients with long-standing diabetes, autonomic neuropathy may be a contributing factor to constipation.[41]

Diseases that cause structural changes include scleroderma and amyloidosis, which cause gradual destruction of intestinal muscle and nerves.

Neurologic abnormalities are often associated with constipation and can be divided into neurologic lesions that affect the central nervous system and lesions that affect the peripheral innervation of the colon. Any central neurologic disease may be associated with constipation. Drug therapy is probably the most common cause of constipation, after inadequate dietary intake of fiber. Many drugs cause constipation as a side effect, and most drugs aggravate constipation in some patients. Drugs commonly associated with constipation include anticholinergics, antidepressants, beta blockers, calcium channels blockers, diuretics, and phenothiazines.

CONCLUSION

Anal incontinence commonly coexists, particularly in the elderly. Anal incontinence occurs at all ages and in both sexes. The prevalence increases with age, and varies from 1.5% in children to 50% in nursing home residents. Fecal incontinence is a distressing symptom that is seen commonly in specialized anorectal practice. The most likely causes are obstetric trauma and chronic straining at stool.

Constipation, with its associated symptoms, is a common bowel problem. Women may be more susceptible to constipation because they normally have less frequent bowel actions. Many women have a normal bowel frequency of less than once a day and may normally pass stool only three times a week. Women are much more likely than men to have dysfunction of the pelvic floor muscles that may include anismus. Women with constipation may also have impaired awareness of rectal distension.

REFERENCES

1. Royal College of Physicians: Incontinence: Causes, management and provision of services. A Working Party of the Royal College of Physicians. J R Coll Physicians Lond 29:272–274, 1995.
2. Whitehead WE, Wald A, Diamant NE, et al: Functional disorders of the anus and rectum. Gut 45:1155–1159, 1999.
3. Norton C, Christiansen J, Butler U, et al: Anal incontinence. In Abrams P, Cardozo L, Khoury S, Wein A (eds): 2nd International Consultation on Incontinence. WHO. Plymouth, Plymbridge, 2001, pp 985–1043.
4. Parks AG: Anorectal incontinence. Proc R Soc Med 68:681–690, 1975.
5. Swash M, Snooks SJ, Henry MM: A unifying concept of pelvic floor disorders and incontinence. J R Soc Med 78:906–911, 1985.
6. Henry MM, Snooks SJ, Barnes PRJ, Swash M: Investigation of disorders of anorectum and colon. Ann Coll Surg Engl 67:335–360, 1985.
7. Roe AM, Bartolo DCC, Mortensen McNJ: A new method of assessment of anal sensation in various anorectal disorders. Br J Surg 73:310–313, 1986.
8. Johanson JF, Lafferty J: Epidemiology of fecal incontinence: The silent affliction. Am J Gastroenterol 91(1): 33–36, 1996.
9. Drossman DA, Sandler RS, Broom CM, McKee DC: Urgency and fecal soloing in people with bowel dysfunction. Dig Dis Sci 31:1221–1225, 1986
10. Enck P, Biefeld K, Rathman W, et al: Epidemiology of fecal incontinence in selected patient groups. Int J Colorectal Dis 6:143–146, 1991.
11. Swash M: The neurogenic hypothesis of stress incontinence. In Bock G, Wheland J, Mardsen CD (eds): Neurobiology of Incontinence. New York, John Wiley & Sons, Ciba Foundation Symposium, 1990, pp 151, 156–170.

12. La Torre F, Nicastro A: Faecal incontinence. In Appell RA, Bourcier A, La Torre F (eds): Pelvic Floor Dysfunction: Investigations and Conservative Treatment. Rome, Casa Editrice Scientifica Internazionale, 1999, pp 77–83.
13. Leigh RJ, Turberg LA: Faecal incontinence: The unvoiced symptom. Lancet 1:1349–1351, 1982.
14. McClellan E: Fecal incontinence: Social and economic factors. In Benson JT (ed): Female Pelvic Floor Disorders: Investigation and Management. New York, WW Norton, 1992, pp 326–332.
15. Mowlam V, North K, Myers C: Managing fecal incontinence. Nurs Times 82:55, 1986.
16. Tobin GW, Blocklehurst JC: Faecal incontinence in residents in homes for the elderly: Prevalence aetiology and management. Age and Ageing 15:41–46, 1986.
17. Nakayama H, Joergensen HS, Pedersen PM, et al: Prevalence and risk factors of incontinence after stroke: The Copenhagen stroke study. Stroke 28:58–62, 1997.
18. Nelson RL, Norton N, Cautley E, Furner S: Community based prevalence of anal incontinence. JAMA 274: 559–562, 1995.
19. Leigh RJ, Turnberg LA: Faecal incontinence: The unvoiced symptom. Lancet 1:1349–1351, 1982.
20. Bourcier A, Haab F, Ciofu C, et al: Sexual dysfunction in women attending an outpatient urodynamic clinic. No.133. Proceedings of the 28th Annual Meeting of the International Continence Society. Jerusalem, 1998.
21. Brubaker L: Anal Incontinence. In Cardozo L, Staskin D (eds): Textbook of Female Urology and Urogynecology. London, Isis Medical Media, 2001, pp 1007–1017.
22. Sultan AH, Kamm MA, Hudson CN: Anal sphincter disruption during vaginal delivery. N Engl J Med 329:1905–1911, 1993.
23. Henry MM: Fecal incontinence: Pathogenesis. In Benson JT (ed): Female Pelvic Floor Disorders: Investigation and Management. New York, WW Norton, 1992, pp 332–334.
24. Snooks SJ, Henry MM, Swash M: Abnormalities in central and peripheral nerve conduction in anorectal incontinence. J R Soc Med 78:294–300, 1985.
25. Ambioze WL, Pemberton JH, Bell AM: The effect of stool consistency on rectal and neorectal emptying. Dis Colon Rectum 34:1–7, 1991.
26. Wald A: Systemic diseases causing disorders of defecation and continence. Sem Gastrointest Dis 6:194–202, 1995.
27. Batignani G, Montaci I, Ficari F, Toreli F: What affects continence after anterior resection of the rectum? Dis Colon Rectum 34:329–331, 1991.
28. Read NW, Abouzekry I: Why do patients with fecal impaction have fecal incontinence? Gut 27:283–287, 1986.
29. Miller R, Batolo DCC, Cervero F, Mortensen NJ: Differences in anal sensation in continent and incontinent patients with perineal descent. Int J Colorectal Dis 4:45–49, 1989.
30. Sun WM, Read NW, Donnelly TC: Impaired internal anal sphincter in a subgroup of patients with idiopathic fecal incontinence. Gastroenterology 97:130, 1989.
31. Parks AG, Swash M, Urich H: Sphincter denervation in anorectal incontinence. Gut 18:656–657, 1977.
32. Swash M, Gray A, Lubowski DZ, Nicolls RJ: Ultrastructural changes in internal anal sphincter in neurogenic anorectal incontinence. Gut 29:1692–1698, 1988.
33. Snooks SJ, Swash M, Setchell M, Henry MM: Injury to innervation of pelvic sphincter musculature in childbirth. Lancet 2:546–550, 1984.
34. Sultan AH, Kamm MA, Hudson CN: Anal sphincter disruption during vaginal delivery. N Engl J Med 329:1905–1911, 1993.
35. Donnelly V, Fynes M, Campbell D, et al: Obstetric events leading to anal sphincter damage. Obstet Gynecol 92:955–961, 1998.
36. Snooks SJ, Barnes PRH, Swash M, Henry MM: Damage to the innervation of the pelvic floor musculature in chronic constipation. Gastroenterol 89:977–981, 1985.
37. Devroede G: Constipation: Mechanisms and management. In Sleisenger MH, Fordtran JS (eds): Gastrointestinal Disease, ed 2. Philadelphia, Saunders, 1978.
38. Moore-Gillon V: Constipation: What does the patient mean? J R Soc Med 77:108–110, 1984.
39. Drossmann DA, Sandler RS, McKee DC, Lovitz AJ: Bowel patterns among subjects not seeking health care. Gastroenterology 83:529–534, 1982.
40. Painter NS: Constipation. Practitioner 224:387, 1980.
41. Turnbull GK: Constipation. In Benson JT (ed): Female Pelvic Floor Disorders: Investigation and Management. New York, WW Norton, 1992, pp 407–424.
42. Johanson JF, Sonnenberg A, Koch TR: Clinical epidemiology of chronic constipation. J Clin Gastroenterol 11:525–536, 1989.
43. Whitehead WE, Taitelbaum G, Wiggley FM, Schuster MM: Rectosigmoid motility and myoelectric activity in progressive systemic sclerosis. Gastroenterology 96:428–432, 1989.
44. Bassotti G, Maggio D, Battaglia E: Manometric investigations of anorectal function in early stage and late stage of Parkinson's disease. J Neurol Neurosur Psychiatry 68:768–770, 2000.
45. Shafik A: A new concept of the anatomy of the anal sphincter mechanism and the physiology of defecation. Anorectal mobilization. A new surgical access to rectal lesions. Preliminary report. Am J Surg 142:629–635, 1981.
46. Krishnamurthy S, Schuffler MD, Rohrmann CA, Pope CE: Severe idiopathic constipation in associated with a distinctive abnormality of the colonic myenteric plexus. Gastroenterology 88:26–34, 1985.
47. Wald A: Colonic transit and anorectal manometry to chronic idiopathic constipation. Arch Intern Med 146:1713–1716, 1986.
48. Waldron D, Bowes KL, Kingma YJ, Cote KR: Colonic and anorectal motility in young women with severe idiopathic constipation. Gastroenterology 95:1388–1390, 1988.
49. Towers AL, Burgio KL, Locher JL, et al: Constipation in the elderly: Influence of dietary, psychological and physiological factors. J Am Geriatr Soc 42:701–706, 1994.
50. Chaussade S, Khyari A, Roche H: Determination of total and segmental colonic transit time in constipated patients. Dig Dis Sci 34:1168–1172, 1989.
51. Kumar D, Waldron D, Williams NS, et al: Prolonged anorectal manometry and external anal sphincter electromyography in ambulant human subjects. Dig Dis Sci 35:641–648, 1990.
52. Shafik A: Constipation. In Appell RA, Bourcier A, La Torre (eds): Pelvic Floor Dysfunction: Investigations and Conservative Treatment. Rome, Casa Editrice Scientifica Internazionale, 1999, pp 65–75.
53. Preston DM, Lennard-Jones JE: Anismus in chronic constipation. Dig Dis Sci 30:413–418, 1985.
54. Jones PN, Lubowski DZ, Swash M, Henry MM: Is paradoxical contraction of puborectalis muscle of functional importance? Dis Colon Rectum 30:667–670, 1987.

CHAPTER 12

Rectal Prolapse

INDRU T. KHUBCHANDANI ■ KHAWAJA AZIMUDDIN

The word *prolapse* is derived from the Latin term *prolapsus,* which means "falling down." *Prolapsus of rectum* was first described in 1500 BC in the Ebers Papyrus.[1] Frederick Salmon, the founder of St. Mark's Hospital, is credited with the first comprehensive description of rectal prolapse in 1831.[2]

The principal symptom in patients with rectal prolapse is the prolapse itself. In its early stages, the mass may extrude only on defecation, but in more advanced cases, extrusion occurs with slight exertion, such as coughing or sneezing. Initially, the patient may have rectal discomfort, a sense of incomplete evacuation, and tenesmus. As the condition progresses, the rectum may be completely extruded, excoriated, and ulcerated. As a result of mucosal congestion, irritation, and trauma, mucous discharge and bleeding occur, causing soiling of the underclothes and later resulting in perineal irritation and excoriation. Many patients have incontinence, with or without diarrhea and urgency. Others have constipation, with or without a history of straining.

PELVIC FLOOR ANATOMY

Any description of rectal prolapse is incomplete without a brief discussion of the anatomy of the pelvic floor. The bony pelvis surrounds and protects the pelvic organs, but provides little support. These organs are primarily supported by the tonic activity of the pelvic floor muscles. Instead of functioning as a rigid structure, the pelvic floor muscles provide a dynamic support to the pelvic contents by constantly adjusting their tension in response to momentary changes in intra-abdominal pressure.

The pelvic floor musculature consists of the bilaterally paired levator ani muscles. These muscles are attached to the bony pelvis anteriorly and posteriorly. Laterally, they are attached to the arcus tendineus, which overlies the muscles of the lateral pelvic wall. The puborectalis part of the muscle, after originating from the inner surface of the pubis, encircles the rectum and attaches to the perineal body posteriorly. There is extensive interweaving of the longitudinal fibers of the rectum, with the levator fibers creating a stable attachment between the rectum and this muscle (Fig. 12-1). This attachment provides the basis of firm fixation of the rectum to the pelvic floor, and is an important element in its stability. Without it, the rectum would slip down through the muscles during defecation.[3]

The pubococcygeus part of the muscle meets in the midline behind the rectum to form the levator plate. The levator plate consists of a thick band of connective tissue at the midline confluence of the two muscle complexes. It runs from the anorectal junction to the lowermost vertebral segments. In the erect posture, it normally lies almost horizontally as the fundamental pelvic support for the rectum and the vagina, both of which also rest horizontally and parallel to the levator plate (Fig. 12-2). Attenuation of the levator muscles results in downward tilting and sagging of the levator plate, which may lead to prolapse of the pelvic viscera.[4]

EPIDEMIOLOGY

Age

The peak incidence of rectal prolapse is in the sixth decade of life. Most female patients are elderly, whereas men have rectal prolapse at a younger age.[5–8] In men, the peak incidence of rectal prolapse declines after 40 years of age, whereas in women, it climbs steadily, reaching its maximum incidence in the seventh decade of life.[7]

Sex

Most patients with rectal prolapse are women. In a review of 536 patients treated at St. Mark's Hospital in London, Mann[7] reported that the female-to-male ratio was 6:1. Men are much less likely to have rectal prolapse,[3,5,9] and men who have rectal prolapse may have an associated neurologic or psychiatric abnormality.[5,8]

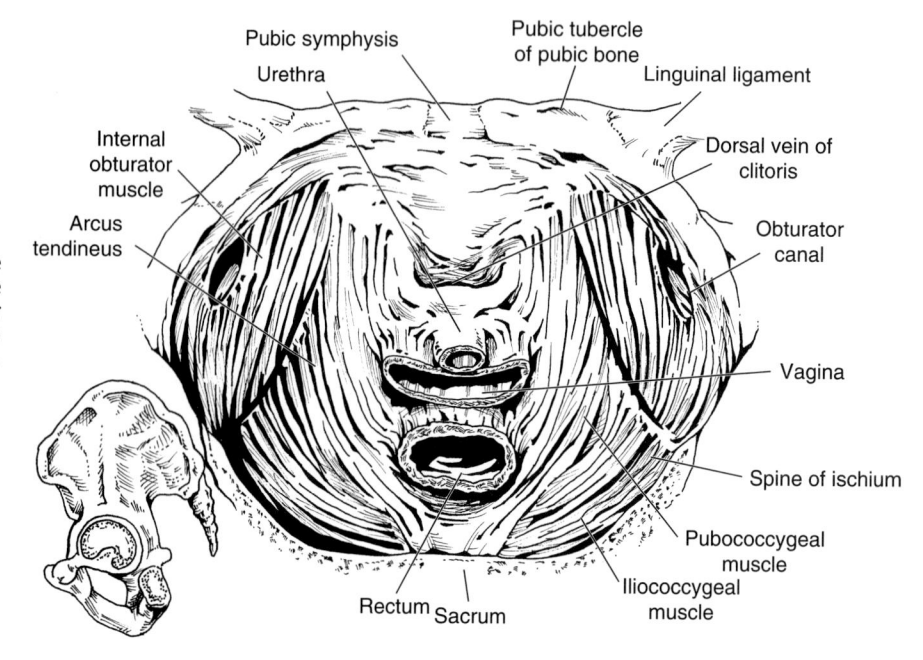

FIGURE 12-1 The longitudinal muscle fibers of the rectum blend with the external sphincter mechanism and levator ani. (From Anson BJ, McVay CG [eds]: Surgical Anatomy. Philadelphia, Saunders, 1971.)

Rectal prolapse is also seen in young men in Egypt and is associated with schistosomiasis.[10]

Parity

Although rectal prolapse is traditionally described in multiparous women with lax pelvic musculature, it also occurs in nulliparous women. In some series, one third to one half of the patients were unmarried and have had no children.[3,11,12] Unlike most multiparous women, nulliparous women with rectal prolapse have a normal pelvic floor and are more likely to be continent.[5,13] Most nulliparous women with prolapse are elderly.[5]

ETIOLOGY

The Sliding Hernia

In 1912, Moschowitz[14] proposed that rectal prolapse is a sliding hernia that extrudes through a defect in the pelvic floor. His theory was based on the observation that patients with rectal prolapse have an abnormally long and mobile pouch of Douglas. He theorized that the hernia sac slowly pushes through a weakened pelvic floor and ultimately presents through the anus as a complete prolapse (Fig. 12-3).

However, if the sliding anterior hernia theory were true, the anterior aspect of the prolapse would be longer or would precede the rest prolapse. In practice, prolapse is a circumferential event, with the apex presenting at the center of the prolapsed rectum. Therefore, a deep rectovaginal or rectovesical peritoneal pouch is likely the result, not the cause, of the prolapse.

Intussusception

In 1965, Devadhar[15] proposed that prolapse is a circumferential intussusception of the rectum. Later, Broden and Snellman[16] used cineradiography to show that rectal prolapse begins as an internal intussusception of the rectum. This view was confirmed by others who used radio-opaque markers applied to the rectal mucosa to show the intussusception.[13,17] They showed that prolapse starts as a circumferential intussusception of the rectum, approximately 6 to 8 cm above the anal verge, and that the anterior and posterior walls of the prolapse were of equal length. The lead point of the intussusception gradually proceeds through the levators and

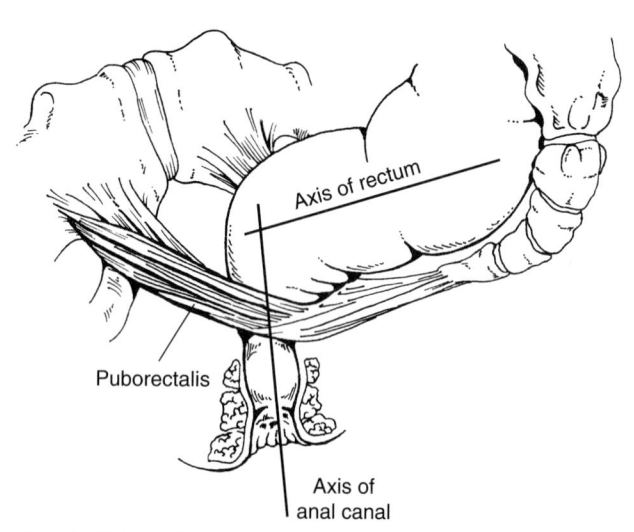

FIGURE 12-2 In the normal anatomic and erect position, the vagina and the lower part of the rectum lie in a horizontal plane. (From Nicholls RJ, Dozois RR (eds): Surgery of the Colon and Rectum. Edinburgh, Churchill Livingstone, 1997.)

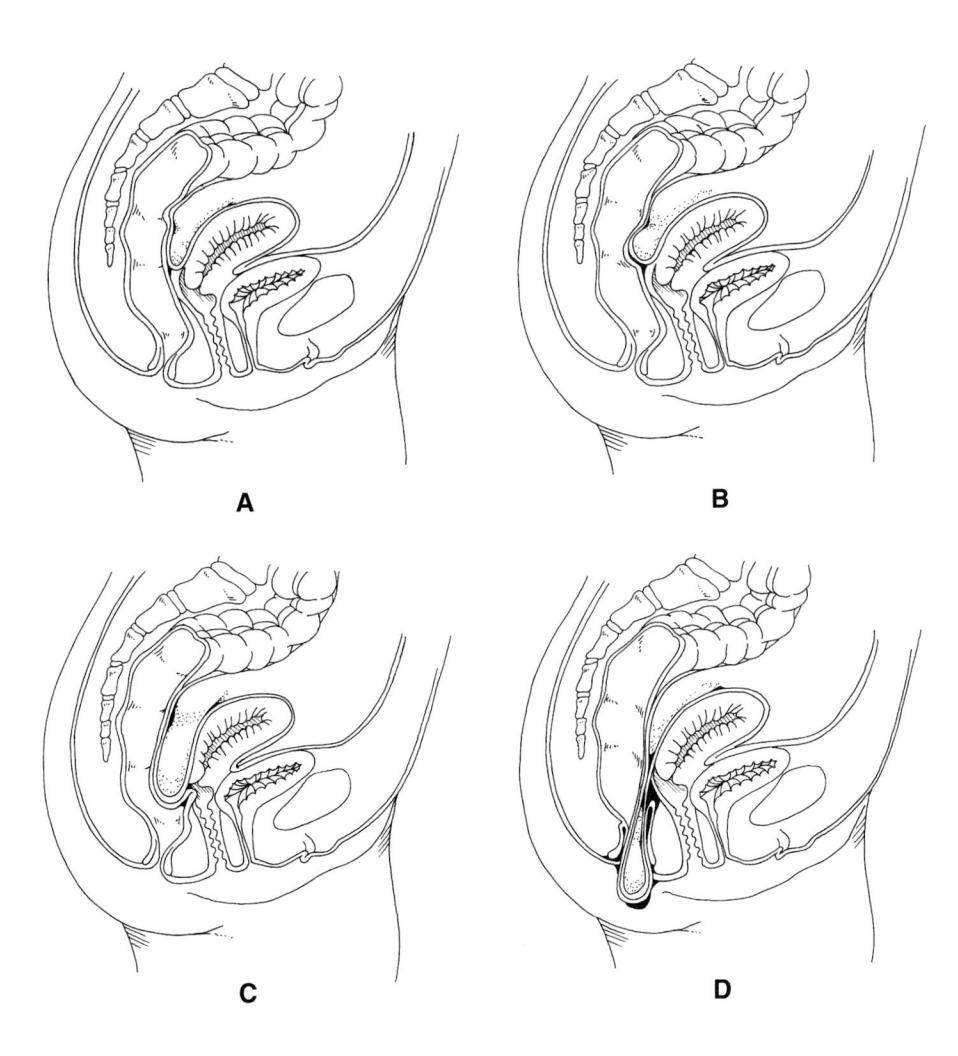

FIGURE 12-3 Rectal prolapse as conceived by Moschcowitz. **A**, Incipient prolapse. **B**, Partial prolapse. **C**, Incomplete prolapse. **D**, Complete prolapse. (From Gordon PH, Nivatvongs S [eds]: Principles and Practice of Surgery of the Colon, Rectum, and Anus, ed 2. St. Louis, Quality Medical Publishing. Reprinted from Ref. [03-182], p 504. Courtesy of Marcel Dekker Inc.)

sphincters, until the prolapse finally presents at the perineum (Fig. 12-4).

However, recently, the significance of intussusception has been challenged. The widespread use of videoproctography in recent years led to the discovery that many asymptomatic persons may also have an internal intussusception.[18–20] During defecography, the intussusception may appear as an unfolding of the upper rectum into the low rectal ampulla or anal canal. Mellgren[21] showed that rectal intussusception was not observed on the second examination in 38 of 41 patients and that only 1 of the 41 patients later had complete rectal prolapse. Thus, even though intussusception is the most likely theory for the pathogenesis of prolapse, internal intussusception is of uncertain significance.

Incomplete intussusception may be associated with inappropriate contraction of the pelvic floor during defecation, whereas complete prolapse is associated with a weak pelvic floor and eversion of the entire anorectal wall through the anal sphincters.[5]

Pelvic Floor Disorder

It is tempting to postulate that prolapse occurs because the rectum descends through a weak pelvic floor. Most patients with rectal prolapse are multiparous and have a weak and attenuated pelvic floor. However, in many patients with prolapse, the pelvic floor is normal. These include young men and women and as well as nulliparous women. Furthermore, cineradiography shows that the prolapse starts well above the pelvic floor, as in internal intussusception. Thus, laxity of the pelvic floor cannot be the only factor in the pathogenesis of this condition.

Electrophysiologic studies consistently show abnormalities in the pelvic floor muscles of patients with rectal prolapse. These abnormalities include dysfunction of the internal and external anal sphincters and the levator ani complex. The abnormalities in the external sphincter and puborectalis muscles may be related to the stretching of the pelvic floor and the consequent pudendal neuropathy that occur during periods of increased intra-abdominal pressure, pregnancy, and labor.[22–24] The stretched and lax pelvic floor results in sagging and downward tilting of the levator plate, thereby increasing the size of the hiatus through which the pelvic organs may prolapse downward (Fig. 12-5).

The theory that weakness of the pelvic floor muscles causes pelvic organ prolapse has been widely adopted by gynecologists, and may explain a spectrum of conditions that includes rectocele, cystocele, ureterovaginal prolapse, and rectal prolapse.

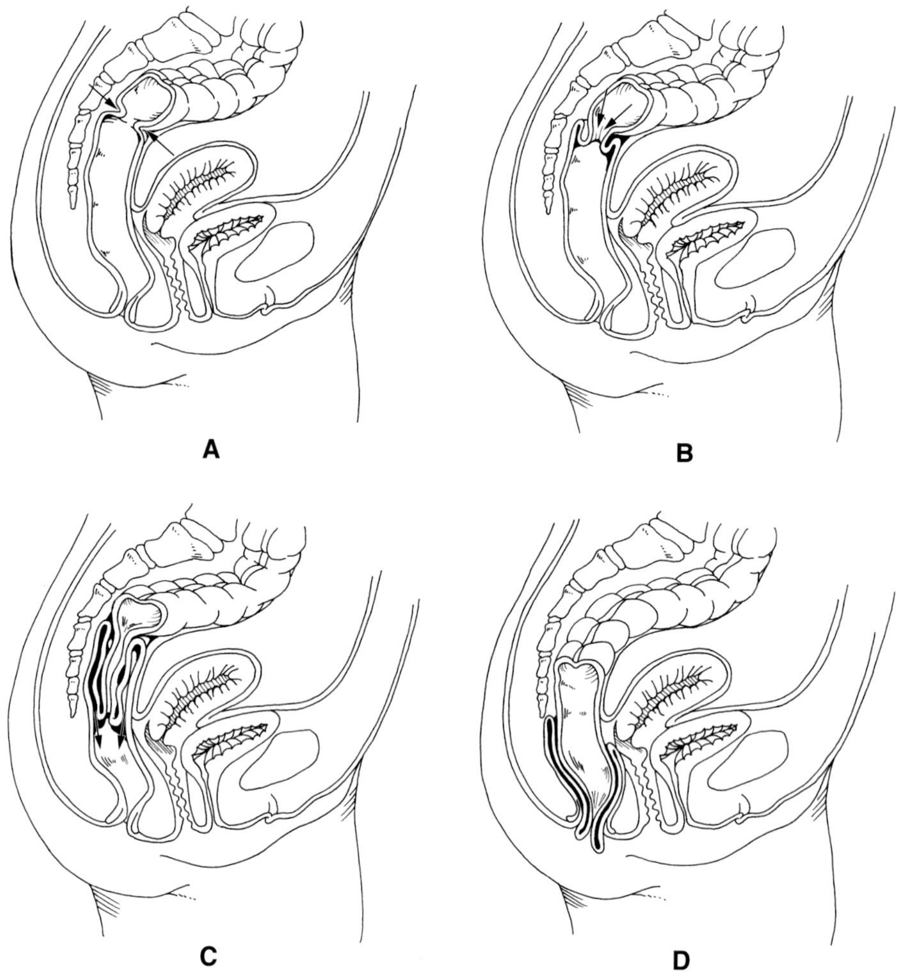

FIGURE 12-4 The intussusception theory of rectal prolapse. **A**, Starting point of intussusception. **B**, Early point of intussusception. **C**, Internal prolapse. **D**, Complete prolapse. (From Gordon PH, Nivatvongs S [eds]: Principles and Practice of Surgery of the Colon, Rectum, and Anus, ed 2. St. Louis, Quality Medical Publishing. Reprinted from Ref. [03-182], p 505. Courtesy of Marcel Dekker Inc.)

Electrophysiologic Basis of Prolapse

Sun and associates[23] reported the findings of electrophysiologic studies in 56 patients (21 with full-thickness rectal prolapse, 24 with anterior mucosal prolapse, and 11 with solitary rectal ulcer) and 30 normal individuals. During serial distension of the rectum, 76% of patients with rectal prolapse (but only 10% of normal volunteers) showed repetitive rectal contractions. The threshold rectal volume that is required to cause a desire to defecate and the maximum tolerable volume were significantly lower in the patients than in the normal subjects.

Similar findings were observed by Farouk and colleagues,[25] who performed ambulatory anorectal manometry in 35 patients with rectal prolapse, 32 patients with neurogenic fecal incontinence, and 33 normal subjects. High-pressure rectal "prolapse" waves with a median amplitude of 71 cm^2 and associated with inhibition of the internal anal sphincter were observed in patients with full-thickness rectal prolapse. These episodes lasted 30 to 150 sec and were not observed in the neurogenic group or in controls.

These findings suggest that in patients with prolapse, the rectum is hypersensitive and hyper-reactive. Because of this increased rectal sensitivity, patients may attempt to strain when very small volumes are present in the rectum, causing the rectum to prolapse into the weak anal canal. As the intussusception progresses, the sensitive rectum perceives this stimulus and the patient increases the straining efforts, leading to the vicious cycle of progressive prolapse, further straining, exacerbation of pelvic floor descent, and increasing neuropathic weakness of the levators. This cycle eventually leads to full-thickness rectal prolapse.[23]

Recently, Brown and associates[26] measured colonic intraluminal pressure by inserting a multilumen catheter in the colon. Compared with normal control subjects, patients with rectal prolapse did not increase the propulsive activity of the colon after ingestion of a meal. Furthermore, the patients had an uninhibited, overreactive, and nonpropulsive colon, similar to that seen in spinal cord injury.[27,28] The authors suggested that patients with rectal prolapse have a hindgut motility disorder that is undetected by standard colonic marker studies. The presence of such a disorder may explain the habitual straining that is commonly seen in patients with rectal prolapse.

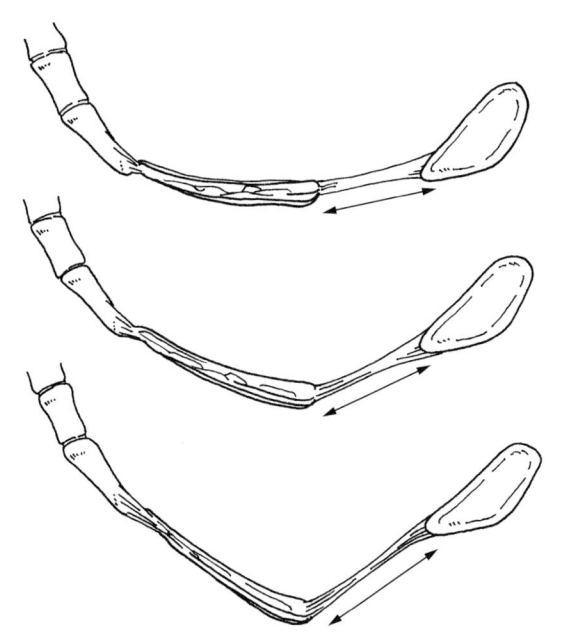

FIGURE 12-5 Widening and stretching of the levator hiatus, predisposing the patient to prolapse. (From Berek JS, Adashi EY, Hillard PA [eds]: Novak's Gynecology, ed 12. Baltimore, Williams & Wilkins, 1996.)

Summary

Despite the seemingly diverse opinions about the pathogenesis of rectal prolapse, clearly, these processes are not mutually exclusive. Invagination of the anterior rectal wall, clinically described as a sliding hernia, may not be different from an early intussusception that does not involve the entire circumference of the bowel. Once the intussusception begins, the hypersensitive rectum pushes the intussusceptum through the pelvic floor. Repetitive straining stretches and weakens the pelvic floor, damaging the pudendal nerves. The denervated anal sphincters are further relaxed, and the prolapse appears in the perineum.

PREDISPOSING FACTORS

Pregnancy and Labor

Pregnancy, labor, and vaginal delivery affect the pelvic floor in a variety of ways. Increased intra-abdominal pressure during pregnancy places a constant strain on the pelvic floor and predisposes it to weakness. During labor, the advancing fetal head may cause stretching, tearing, and separation of the pelvic floor muscles. The medial fibers of the pubococcygeal and puborectal muscles are especially likely to be affected.[4,29] The injury is worse when labor is prolonged, when the presenting part of the fetus is large, or when the bony pelvic outlet is narrow. Occasionally, the bony outlet is narrowed by an acute subpubic arch; in these cases, the presenting part of the fetus is likely to cause more stretching, tearing, and damage to the posterior vaginal and rectal support mechanisms.[4] The rectal attachments may be torn from the levator muscles and pelvic fascia. These changes weaken the pelvic floor and cause vertical tilting of the levator plate so that the rectum may prolapse through a widened levator hiatus.

In addition to the pelvic floor muscles, the pudendal nerve may be damaged during labor as a result of either longitudinal stretching with perineal descent or direct compression. Increases in pudendal nerve terminal motor latency and single-fiber density on electromyogram of the external anal sphincter are seen after normal vaginal delivery and are convincing evidence of nerve damage.[30-32] This injury leads to further atrophy and weakness of the pelvic floor musculature.

Conditions That Lead to Increased Intra-abdominal Pressure

In addition to pregnancy, increased intra-abdominal pressure is seen in a variety of conditions, including chronic cough, obesity, and chronic straining or constipation. This increased pressure may predispose patients to prolapse.

Conditions That Lead to Weakness of the Pelvic Floor Muscles

The changes associated with childbirth are further aggravated by aging, loss of estrogen stimulation, and obesity. Aging, in particular, leads to attenuation of connective tissue fascia and weakening of the pelvic floor muscles. Most multiparous women have prolapse late in life, when progressive weakening of the pelvic floor becomes apparent. Age-associated attenuation of the pelvic fascia and loss of estrogen after menopause are thought to play a role.

Connective Tissue Disorders

Connective tissue is the "glue" of the body. It holds the various tissues of the body together and maintains structural integrity. Understandably, disorders of connective tissue have been implicated in pelvic floor abnormalities. Marshman and associates[33] were the first to report an association between increased mobility of joints and rectal prolapse. Recently, Carley and Schaffer reported rectal prolapse in two patients with Ehler-Danlos syndrome.[34]

Neurologic Disorders

Neurologic disorders may predispose patients to rectal prolapse by compromising the pelvic floor musculature. Prolapse may develop in patients with progressive systemic sclerosis, spinal cord trauma, and tabes dorsalis, but this association is rare.[35,36] Prolpase is also reported in some patients with cauda equina lesions, particularly children with spina bifida.[37] Some paraplegic patients have solitary rectal ulcer syndrome, which may be a precursor to rectal prolapse.[38] These patients often have evidence of disordered colonic motility and rectal inertia.

More commonly, local nerve damage or degeneration may lead to weakness of the pelvic floor muscles. Although the most common cause of this injury is vaginal delivery, chronic straining and the prolapse itself may cause further stretch injury to the pudendal nerve fibers.[22,39] The damage may occur to the pudendal nerve directly, or small nerve endings may be pulled from individual muscle fibers.

Constipation

Many patients with rectal prolapse have a history of intractable constipation.[7,40] These patients have a delayed colonic transit time as well as disordered rectal emptying.[41] Chronic straining may predispose these patients to rectal prolapse. The role of colonic hypomotility was further confirmed by the observation that in laboratory animals, overexpression of hepatocyte growth factor in the digestive tract leads to intestinal pseudo-obstruction and anorectal prolapse.[42]

Psychiatric Illness

Many studies link rectal prolapse to psychiatric illnesses.[43,44] Although Goligher,[45] as a nonpsychiatrist, thought that one third of his patients were "rather odd," in recent years, the tendency to label patients with rectal prolapse as "psychotic" has decreased.[5] There does not appear to be any causal relationship between the two conditions, except that some patients may have a habitual tendency toward anal attentiveness and excessive straining. In this context, prolapse was described in some young female patients with anorexia nervosa and bulimia nervosa, perhaps as a result of chronic straining and purging.[8,46]

ASSOCIATED CHANGES IN PELVIC ANATOMY

A variety of associated anatomic abnormalities are commonly seen in patients with rectal prolapse. However, it is not clear whether these abnormalities are the cause or the effect of prolapse. The anatomic abnormalities include the following:

- An abnormally deep rectovesical or rectovaginal pouch
- Abnormally long mesentery of the small bowel in cases where small bowel is contained in the enterocele associated with the prolapse
- Redundant sigmoid colon that may contribute to a sigmoidocele
- Loss of sacral fixation of the rectum and elongation of the mesorectum; the rectum losses its normal horizontal position within the sacral hollow and assumes a near vertical position
- Obtuse anorectal angle; a straight anorectum on defecography is highly suggestive of prolapse
- Weak and patulous anal sphincter as a result of denervation and stretching

It is tempting to attribute an etiologic role to one or more of these factors. In the past, many operations were designed to correct these anatomic abnormalities. In recent years, the trend has shifted and most authorities now believe that these anatomic changes are caused by the recurring prolapse.

ASSOCIATED ABNORMALITIES

Incontinence

Incontinence occurs in 35% to 100% of patients with rectal prolapse.[11,12,41,47,48] It leads to perineal excoriation from fecal and mucous discharge and causes embarrassment and social isolation of the patient. Many theories have been proposed to explain the association of incontinence with prolapse.

The internal sphincter is abnormally relaxed in patients with rectal prolapse. This relaxation leads to low resting anal pressure and predisposes the patient to episodes of incontinence.[23,25,49-51] Neill and associates[24] reported that resting anal pressure is reduced in patients with rectal prolapse, with or without incontinence, whereas others believe that resting anal pressure is higher in continent patients with prolapse.[52,53] As the intussusception enters the rectum, it causes a rectoanal inhibitory reflex and relaxation of the internal sphincter. The resting anal pressure falls further, predisposing the patient to incontinence. The fact that this reflex is rarely elicited in patients with rectal prolapse indicates that the internal sphincter is already maximally inhibited in these patients.[25,49]

Others have focused on abnormalities of the external sphincter as the cause of incontinence in patients with rectal prolapse. The maximal squeeze pressure is reduced in patients with incontinence, but not in patients who are continent.[23,24,52] Many studies show evidence of denervation of the puborectalis and external sphincter muscles in incontinent patients with prolapse.[22,52] Parks and colleagues[22] showed denervation atrophy of external sphincter muscle fibers with consequent fibrosis on biopsy specimens. Others showed increased pudendal nerve terminal motor latency as evidence of injury to the pudendal nerves.[30,54] An increase in single-fiber nerve density is an indication of collateral sprouting and reinnervation of denervated muscle fibers as well as convincing evidence of previous nerve injury to the external sphincter.[24,30,55] Stretch injury to the pudendal nerves may occur as a result of perineal descent from repeated straining during defecation or labor.

Patients with rectal prolapse may have a hypersensitive and hyper-reactive rectum that reacts vigorously to rectal distension.[23] The less compliant rectum in these patients shows an impaired response to distension that predisposes them to incontinence.[56,57] An increase in colonic motility and a hyperactive sigmoid also may cause incontinence in patients with prolapse.[5,58]

It seems reasonable to conclude that the following three mechanisms act together to produce incontinence in patients with rectal prolapse: (1) the internal sphincter, which is inhibited as a result of the persistent rectoanal inhibitory reflex produced by the prolapsing intussusception; (2) the external sphincter, which is damaged by stretch injury to the pudendal nerve as the prolapsing rectum stretches the pelvic floor; (3) and the hypersensitive rectum produced by mechanical inflammation and ischemia of the prolapsing mucosa whose activity is exaggerated as it attempts to expel the prolapsing intussusception.

Constipation

Between 25% and 50% of patients with rectal prolapse also have constipation.[36,59,60] Symptoms range from infrequent defecation to the sensation of incomplete evacuation or obstructed labor. Some patients with rectal prolapse have slow colonic transit time.[24,36] Brown and colleagues[26] measured colonic intraluminal pressures with multilumen catheters in patients with prolapse. They showed that, even in patients with normal colonic motility on standard radiologic marker studies, there is evidence of poor colonic motility and a lack of propulsive activity.

On the other hand, Metcalf and Loening-Baucke[60] showed a paradoxical increase in external anal sphincter electromyographic activity during attempted defecation (when the external anal sphincter would be expected to relax) in patients with prolapse. This increased activity may lead to constipation and obstructed defecation.

Whatever the cause of constipation in patients with prolapse, it seems clear that the straining associated with constipation and obstructed defecation would lead to further exacerbation of the prolapse.

Pelvic Floor Abnormalities

Prolapse of the rectum is often associated with uterovaginal prolapse, cystocele, or rectocele. These patients have a weak and lax levator and attenuated endopelvic fascia. Therefore, generalized descent of the pelvic floor occurs, with prolapse of associated pelvic organs. Loygue and associates[6] reported that 54 of 200 women with rectal prolapse had an associated genital prolapse. Others reported a 16% to 50% incidence of pelvic organ prolapse in association with rectal prolapse.[5,8,44]

CONCLUSION

Rectal prolapse is a pelvic floor disorder with a multifaceted etiology. Factors that were previously believed to be causative may well be the effects of recurring prolapse and poor bowel habits. Further understanding of pelvic floor dysfunction will lead to better management options.

REFERENCES

1. Wassef R, Rothenberger DA, Goldberg SM: Rectal prolapse. Curr Probl Surg 23:297–451, 1986.
2. Salmon F: Practical Observations on the Prolapsus of the Rectum, ed 2. London, Whittaker, Treacher & Arnot, 1831.
3. Corman ML: Rectal prolapse, solitary rectal ulcer, syndrome of descending perineum and rectocele. In Corman ML (ed): Colon and Rectal Surgery, ed 4. Philadelphia, Lippincott-Raven, 1998, pp 401–448.
4. Thompson J: Surgical correction of defects in pelvic support. In Rock JA, Thompson JD (eds): Te Linde's operative gynecology, ed 8. Philadelphia, Lippincott-Raven, 1997, pp 951–1041.
5. Keighley MRB, Williams NS: Rectal prolpase. In Keighley MRB, Williams NS (eds): Surgery of the Anus, Rectum and Colon, ed 2. London, Saunders, 1999, pp 794–842.
6. Loygue J, Nordlinger B, Malafosse M, et al: Rectopexy to the promontory for the treatment of rectal prolapse: Report of 257 cases. Dis Colon Rectum 27:356–359, 1984.
7. Mann CV: Rectal prolapse. In Morson BC, Heinemann W (eds): Disease of Colon Rectum and Anus. London, Medical Books, 1969, pp 238–250.
8. Azimuddin K, Khubchandani IT, Rosen L, et al: Rectal prolapse: A search for the "best" operation. Am Surg 67(7): 622–627, 2001.
9. Huber FT, Stein H, Siewert JR: Functional results after treatment of rectal prolapse with rectopexy and sigmoid resection. World J Surg 19:138–143, 1995.
10. Abou-Enein A: Prolapse of the rectum in young men: Treatment with modified Roscoe Graham operation. Dis Colon Rectum 22:117–119, 1978.
11. Mortenson NJMcC, Vellacott KD, Wilson MG: Lahaut's operation for rectal prolapse. Ann R Coll Surg Engl 66:17–18, 1984.
12. Watts JD, Rothenberger DA, Buls JG, et al: The management of procidentia: 30 years experience. Dis Colon Rectum 28:96–102, 1985.
13. Thauerkauf FJ, Beahrs OH, Hill JR: Rectal prolapse: Causation and surgical treatment. Ann Surg 171:819–835, 1970.
14. Moschowitz AV: The pathogenesis, anatomy and cure of prolapse of the rectum. Surg Gynecol Obstet 15:7–21, 1912.
15. Devadhar DSC: A new concept of mechanism and treatment of rectal procidentia. Dis Colon Rectum 8:75–81, 1965.
16. Broden B, Snellman B: Procidentia of the rectum studied with cineradiography: A contribution to the discussion of causative mechanism. Dis Colon Rectum 11:330–347, 1968.
17. Pantanowitz D, Levine E: The mechanism of rectal prolapse. S Afr J Surg 13:53–56, 1975.
18. Hoffman MJ, Kodner JJ, Fry RD: Internal intussusception of the rectum: Diagnosis and surgical treatment. Dis Colon Rectum 27:435–441, 1984.
19. Berman IR, Harris MS, Leggett JT: Rectal reservoir reduction procedures for internal rectal prolapse. Dis Colon Rectum 30:765–771, 1987.
20. Choi JS, Hwang YH, Salum MR, et al: Outcome and management of patients with large rectoanal intussusception. Am J Gastroenterol 96:740–744, 2001.
21. Mellgren A, Schultz I, Johansson C, et al: Internal rectal intussusception seldom develops into total rectal prolapse. Dis Colon Rectum 40:817–820, 1997.
22. Parks AG, Swash M, Urich H: Sphincter denervation in anorectal incontinence and rectal prolapse. Gut 18:656–665, 1977.

23. Sun WM, Read NW, Carmel T, et al: A common pathophysiology for full-thickness rectal prolapse, anterior mucosal prolapse and solitary rectal ulcer. Br J Surg 76:290–295, 1989.
24. Neill ME, Parks AG, Swash M: Physiological studies of the anal sphincter musculature in fecal incontinence and rectal prolapse. Br J Surg 68:531–536, 1981.
25. Farouk R, Duthie GS, MacGregor AB, et al: Rectoanal inhibition and incontinence in patients with rectal prolapse. Br J Surg 81:743–746, 1994.
26. Brown AG, Horgan AF, Anderson JH, et al: Colonic motility is abnormal before surgery for rectal prolapse. Br J Surg 86:263–266, 1999.
27. Banwell JG, Creasey GH, Aggarwal AM, et al: Management of the neurogenic bowel in patients with spinal cord injury. Urol Clin North Am 20:517–526, 1993.
28. Longo WE, Ballantyne GH, Modlin IM: The colon, anorectum, and spinal cord patient: A review of functional alterations of the denervated hindgut. Dis Colon Rectum 32:261–267, 1989.
29. Ginsburg DA, Rovner ES, Raz S: Pelvic floor relaxation. In Graham SD Jr (ed): Glenn's Urologic Surgery, ed 5. Philadelphia, Lippincott-Raven, 1997, pp 135–144.
30. Snooks SJ, Swash M, Henry MM, et al: Risk factors in childbirth causing damage to pelvic floor innervation. Int J Colorect Dis 1:20–24, 1986.
31. Allen RE, Hosker GL, Smith AR, Warrell DW: Pelvic floor damage and childbirth: A neurophysiological study. Br J Obstet Gynaecol 97:770–779, 1990.
32. Smith AR, Hosker GL, Warrell DW: The role of partial denervation of pelvic floor in the etiology of genitourinary prolapse and stress incontinence of urine: A neurophysiological study. Br J Obstet Gynaecol 96:24–28, 1989.
33. Marshman D, Percy J, Fielding I, et al: Rectal prolapse: Relationship with joint mobility. Aust N Z J Surg 57:827–829, 1987.
34. Carley ME, Schaffer J: Urinary incontinence and pelvic organ prolapse in women with Marfan or Ehlers Danlos syndrome. Am J Obstet Gynecol 182:1021–1023, 2000.
35. Leighton JA, Valdovinos MA, Pemberton JH, et al: Anorectal dysfunction and rectal prolapse in progressive systemic sclerosis. Dis Colon Rectum 36:182–185, 1993.
36. Madoff RD: Rectal prolapse and intussusception. In Beck DE, Wexner SD (eds): Fundamentals of Anorectal Surgery. New York, McGraw-Hill, 1992, pp 89–103.
37. Nash DF: Bowel management in spina bifida patients. Proc R Soc Med 65:70–71, 1972.
38. Wang F, Frisbie JH, Klein MA: Solitary rectal ulcer syndrome (colitis cystica profunda) in spinal cord injury patients: 3 case reports. Arch Phys Med Rehabil 82:260–261, 2001.
39. Parks AG, Porter NH, Hardcastle JD: The syndrome of descending perineum. Proc R Soc Med 59:477–482, 1966.
40. Scaglia M, Fasth S, Hallgren T, et al: Abdominal rectopexy for rectal prolapse: Influence of surgical technique on functional outcome. Dis Colon Rectum 37:805–813, 1994.
41. Yoshioka K, Hyland G, Keighley MRB: Anorectal function after abdominal rectopexy: Parameters of predictive value in identifying return of continence. Br J Surg 76:64–68, 1989.
42. Takayama H, Takagi H, Larochelle WJ, et al: Ulcerative proctitis, rectal prolapse and intestinal pseudoobstruction in transgenic mice overexpressing hepatocyte growth factor/scatter factor. Lab Invest 81:297–305, 2001.
43. Altemeier WA, Culbertson WR, Schowengerdt C, et al: Nineteen years experience with the one-stage perineal repair of rectal prolapse. Ann Surg 6:993–1001, 1971.
44. Vongsangnak V, Varma JS, Watters D, et al: Clinical manometric and surgical aspects of complete prolapse of the rectum. J R Coll Surg Edinb 30:251–254, 1985.
45. Goligher JC: Prolapse of the rectum. In Goligher JC (ed): Surgery of the Anus, Rectum and Colon, ed 4. London: Ballière Tindall, 1980, pp 224–258.
46. Malik M, Stratton J, Sweeney WB: Rectal prolapse associated with bulimia nervosa. Dis Colon Rectum 40:1382–1385, 1997.
47. Andrews NJ, Jones DJ: Rectal prolapse and associated conditions. BMJ 305:243–245, 1992.
48. Stenchever MA: Management of genital prolapse in the geriatric patient. Geriatr Med Today 3:75–78, 1984.
49. Spencer RJ: Manometric studies in rectal prolapse. Dis Colon Rectum 27:523–525, 1984.
50. Williams JG, Wong WD, Jensen L, et al: Incontinence in rectal prolapse: A prospective manometric study. Dis Colon Rectum 34:209–216, 1991.
51. Farouk R, Duthie GS, Bartolo DCC, et al: Restoration of continence following rectopexy for rectal prolapse and recovery of the internal anal sphincter electromyogram. Br J Surg 79:439–440, 1992.
52. Matheson DM, Keighley MRB: Manometric evaluation of rectal prolapse and fecal incontinence. Gut 22:126–129, 1981.
53. Santini L, Pezzullo L, Caraco C, et al: Fecal incontinence and rectal prolapse, clinicofunctional assessment. Minerva Chir 50:741–745, 1995.
54. Percy JP, Swash M, Neill ME, et al: Electrophysiological study of motor nerve supply of pelvic floor. Lancet 1:16–17, 1980.
55. Jost WH, Ecker KW, Schimrigk K: Surface versus needle electrodes in determination of motor conduction time to the external anal sphincter. Int J Colorectal Dis 9:197–199, 1994.
56. Siproudhis L, Bellissant E, Jujuet F, et al: Rectal adaptation to distention in patients with overt rectal prolapse. Br J Surg 85:1527–1532, 1998.
57. Tsiaoussis J, Chrysos E, Glynos M, et al: Pathophysiology and treatment of anterior rectal mucosal prolapse syndrome. Br J Surg 85:1699–1702, 1998.
58. Keighley MRB, Shouler PJ: Abnormalities of colonic function in patients with rectal prolapse. Br J Surg 71:892–895, 1984.
59. Madoff RD, Williams JG, Wong WD, et al: Long-term functional results of colon resection and rectopexy for overt rectal prolapse. Am J Gastroenterol 87:101–104, 1992.
60. Metcalf AM, Loening-Baucke V: Anorectal function and defecation dynamics in patients with rectal prolapse. Am J Surg 155:206–210, 1988.

CHAPTER 13

Male and Female Sexual Dysfunction

MICHAEL B. SIROKY ■ KAZEM M. AZADZOI

The last quarter of the twentieth century has seen a complete revolution in our understanding of human sexual dysfunction. During most of the last century, male impotence was considered primarily a psychiatric illness or a manifestation of social maladjustment. For example, Young's 1926 textbook of urology does not mention or discuss erectile impotence or disorders of ejaculation. A 1935 marriage manual, although recognizing physical causes, ascribed most cases of impotence to "repressions and inhibitions."[1]

A new era began around 1970 as the organic nature of impotence, especially its relation to vascular insufficiency,[2] was increasingly recognized. This era was characterized by the application of objective diagnostic techniques and treatment aimed at the penis rather than the psyche. Surgical implants, penile revascularization, vacuum devices, and intracorporeal pharmacotherapy were developed during this period.

With the introduction of sildenafil citrate in 1998, we entered another new era, one of safe and effective oral pharmacotherapy for sexual dysfunction in both men and women. We are also witnessing increased interest in understanding and treating the sexual problems of women.

The subject of male and female sexual dysfunction is vast and cannot be adequately discussed in one chapter. We will concentrate our attention on the neurovascular mechanisms of male and female sexual dysfunction. Psychologic and endocrine mechanisms will not be discussed in depth.

DEFINITIONS

Organic sexual dysfunction in both sexes may encompass a wide variety of elements that include problems with libido, lubrication, erection, ejaculation, and orgasm. Because the various aspects of sexual function can be difficult to separate, the definition of sexual dysfunction can be problematic. The classification and definition of female sexual dysfunction is discussed later.[3]

Impotence means inability to perform sexually in the broadest sense. It is too broad a term to be useful in diagnosis. *Libido* is a term derived from psychoanalytic theory that describes sexual desire, drive, or interest in both sexes. Lack of libido in men may underlie many instances of impotence. *Erectile dysfunction* (ED) is the consistent inability to obtain or maintain an erection of sufficient rigidity to enable satisfactory sexual intercourse. Disorders of semen delivery include lack of *emission* (deposition of seminal fluid in the prostatic urethra), *anejaculation* (lack of ejaculation), and *retrograde ejaculation* (ejaculation through an incompetent bladder neck into the bladder). *Anorgasmia* is the persistent inability to achieve orgasm or delayed orgasm despite adequate sexual arousal.

FUNCTIONAL ANATOMY OF THE GENITAL ORGANS

The Male Genitals

The Penis

The penis is composed of paired corpora cavernosa and a corpus spongiosum that surrounds the urethra. The penis can be functionally divided into a pelvic and a pendulous part. The crurae (roots) of the corpora cavernosa are firmly attached to the under surface of the ischiopubic rami as two separate structures This is the main fixation point of the penis to the bony pelvis and this structure stabilizes the penis during sexual intercourse. The suspensory ligament is a fibrous fascial sheet that attaches and stabilizes the corpora cavernosa to the periosteum of the pubic bone. The suspensory ligament is a convenient dividing point between the pelvic and pendulous portions of the penis. In the pendulous portion of the penis, all three cylindrical structures are encased in a fascial sheath (Buck's fascia). The medial surfaces of the corpora cavernosa merge to become a common septum that extends all the way to the most distal aspect of the corpora cavernosa within the glans. The septum allows blood to pass from one corpus to the other corpus, thus equalizing intracavernosal pressure. This is not true in all species. In the dog, for example, the two corpora cavernosa do not communicate.[4]

The Corpora Cavernosa

The human tunica albuginea surrounds the cavernosal cylinders. It is a complex bilayered structure that has a thickness of 2 to 3 mm when flaccid.[5] The tunica must elongate, increase its girth, and withstand a large amount of axial loading when the penis is erect, yet it must be supple when the penis is flaccid. Approximately 5% of the tunica is elastin, which enables the penis to elongate and increase its girth. In the flaccid state, Loeb found the pendulous portion of the penis has an average length of 9.4 cm and circumference of 2.9 cm.[5] The average volume increase of the erect penis from the flaccid volume is about twofold.[6] The tensile strength of the tunica is approximately 1500 mm Hg, making this fascia one of the strongest in the body.[7]

Only recently has the complex arrangement of fibers in the tunica been recognized.[8,9] The fibers of the outer coat are oriented longitudinally while those of the inner coat are circular. The outer layer seems to be relatively deficient ventrally where the corpus spongiosum is in contact with the corpora cavernosa.[8] The multilayered arrangement of tunical fascia, in which one layer is able to slide up on the other, may occlude venous outflow through the emissary veins during tumescence. The emissary veins—small veins that pierce the tunica albuginea—transport blood from the lacunar spaces and subtunical venules to either the deep dorsal vein or the cavernosal and crural veins. Thus, the tunica may constitute one of the passive mechanisms of corporal veno-occlusive function.[10]

The erectile tissue of the corpora cavernosa consists of numerous sinusoids (lacunar spaces) among interwoven trabeculae of smooth muscles and supporting connective tissue.[11] The cavernosal sinusoids communicate widely, which enables blood entering the sinusoidal spaces to fill the corpora rapidly. This also enables the intracavernosal pressure to equalize rapidly. The peripheral sinusoids are smaller and have a greater individual surface area than central sinusoids. Since endothelial cells have an active role in relaxation of cavernosal smooth muscle, the greater surface area of peripheral sinusoids may be important in compression of subtunical veins and corporal veno-occlusion. Surrounding each endothelial-lined sinusoid is the trabecula, corresponding to the muscular wall of an artery surrounding the endothelial-lined arterial lumen. The trabeculae consist of approximately 45% smooth muscle and 55% connective tissue matrix.[12]

The Corpus Spongiosum

The corpus spongiosum, the third erectile structure of the penis, contains the urethra. The tunica albuginea of the corpus spongiosum is much thinner than that of corpora cavernosa. The pelvic portion of the corpus spongiosum, the urethral bulb, is attached to the inferior layer of urogenital diaphragm and receives blood from the bulbourethral artery. The pendulous portion lies in the ventral grove between the paired corpora cavernosa. Distally the corpus spongiosum expands to form a conical mass (glans penis) that sits over the distal tips of the corpora cavernosa. The internal structure is similar to that of corpora cavernosa except that the sinusoids are larger in diameter. At the glans penis the tunica albuginea is practically absent.

The major function of the glans penis is to act as a vascular cushion that facilitates vaginal intromission and not to provide penile rigidity. Although the glans penis is an erectile body, its mechanism of vascular trapping is fundamentally different from that of the corpora cavernosa. Essentially, the glans penis (and the corpus spongiosum) act as a large arteriovenous fistula during erection.[13] Especially during the initial phases of erection, a high arterial rate of flow is established through the glans penis with free egress of blood into the venous system. Contraction of the bulbocavernous and ischiocavernous muscles compresses the corpus spongiosum and also pulls Buck's fascia downward. This action compresses the dorsal veins as well as the corpus spongiosum, impeding the outflow of blood from the cavernosal sinuses as well as the corpus spongiosum.[14] In comparison to the efficient intrinsic veno-occlusive mechanism of the corpora cavernosa, the corpus spongiosum has an inefficient extrinsic mechanism that acts only for short periods of time. Because of these structural differences, intraspongiosal tissue pressure is limited to the arterial blood pressure, whereas intracavernosal tissue pressure may easily reach levels that are several times arterial pressure, especially during intercourse.

Arterial Inflow

The paired internal pudendal arteries, branches of the hypogastric artery, constitute the main arterial blood supply to the penis. The internal pudendal artery gives off the common penile artery, which itself divides into three branches: the bulbourethral, the dorsal, and the cavernosal arteries. The common penile artery courses next to the ischiopubic ramus and is therefore liable to injury during blunt perineal trauma. The bulbourethral branches supply the urethral bulb (and Cowper's gland), the corpus spongiosum, and the glans penis. The paired cavernosal arteries are primarily responsible for arterial inflow to the corpora cavernosa. The dorsal arteries provide arterial blood for the penile skin, subcutaneous tissues, and the glans penis. The dorsal arteries commonly provide numerous perforating branches, which pass through the tunica albuginea and anastomose directly with the cavernosal arteries.[15] These communicating branches make it possible to revascularize the cavernosal circulation by using an inferior epigastric to dorsal artery anastomosis.[16]

The cavernosal artery enters the corpora cavernosa at the point where the suspensory ligament attaches to the tunica as the two crura merge. Accessory arterial branches may also enter at the crus. Collateral circulation is common among the dorsal arteries, the cavernosal arteries, and the urethral branches. At the penile base, the cavernosal artery lies close to the septum between the corporal bodies. In the mid and distal penile shaft, it is more centrally located. Along its course, it gives off innumerable helicine arteries that supply the lacunar sinusoid spaces.

The helicine arteries constitute the primary resistance vessels controlling inflow to the sinusoidal spaces. In an important study in 1989, Banya and colleagues demonstrated that helicine arteries are but one of two circulatory pathways through the corpus cavernosum.[17] Using scanning electron microscopy of the human corpus cavernosum, they found that the cavernosal artery divides into two circulatory pathways: (1) arterioles leading into a capillary network that drain into a subtunical venous plexus and (2) helicine arteries that drain directly into the cavernous sinuses. The cavernous sinuses drain into that join venules at the periphery of the corpus cavernosum venules from the first pathway and leave the corpora as emissary veins. Thus, two circulatory routes are evident in the corpus cavernosum. These findings suggest that the penile erectile cycle is controlled by shunting of flow from the extrasinusoidal pathway to the intrasinusoidal pathway.

Venous Outflow

The *subtunical veins* are located intracavernosally immediately beneath the tunica albuginea.[10,17,18] Venules emanate from the peripheral sinusoidal spaces and travel beneath the tunica albuginea for some distance. These so-called subtunical venules coalesce to form the subtunical venular plexus before exiting through the tunica as the emissary veins. The primary site of corporal venoocclusion is passive compression or stretching of these subtunical venules.[10,17,18]

Outside the tunica albuginea, the venous outflow may again be divided into a pelvic and a pendulous portion. The *pelvic portions* of the corpora are proximal to the suspensory ligament. Emissary veins draining the proximal portion of the corpora cavernosa join to form two to five veins that exit the dorsomedial aspect of the penile hilum. These veins drain the bulbar, cavernous, and crural portions of the corpora and drain toward the preprostatic plexus and the internal pudendal veins.[19] The *pendulous portion* of the penis is drained by two separate systems that communicate variably with each other and vary widely in number and distribution. The *deep dorsal vein*, coursing beneath Buck's fascia, is usually a single vein between the right and left dorsal arteries and right and left dorsal nerves. On occasion, the vein bifurcates into several branches. Behind the symphysis pubis, the dorsal vein empties into the periprostatic venous plexus. Receiving blood from the circumflex and emissary veins, it provides the main venous drainage of the glans penis and distal two thirds of the corpus spongiosum, as well as the pendulous portion of the corpora cavernosa. The *superficial dorsal vein* runs subcutaneously between Colles' and Buck's fascia, often uniting near the root of the penis to form a single superficial dorsal vein, which in three quarters of cases drains into the left great saphenous vein.[19]

Innervation

The penis is innervated by autonomic (parasympathetic and sympathetic) and somatic (sensory and motor) nerves.[20]

The *parasympathetic nerves to the penis* arise from neurons in the intermediolateral cell columns of the second, third, and fourth sacral spinal cord segments (*pelvic nerves*). The preganglionic nerves enter the pelvic plexus, where they are joined by sympathetic nerves from the hypogastric plexus and nerves. Branches of this plexus innervate the rectum, bladder, prostate, and sphincters. Branches of the pelvic plexus that innervate the corpora cavernosa of the penis are called *cavernosal nerves*.[21] The cavernosal nerves are also preganglionic nerves that synapse with nitrergic nerves in or near the tunica albuginea. Stimulation of the pelvic or the cavernosal nerves causes penile erection in both animals[13,22,23] and humans.[24] However, it is still unclear whether the cavernous nerve is a purely parasympathetic nerve. Some sympathetic fibers emanating from the lumbosacral sympathetic chain exist in the pelvic nerve of the male rat.[25] The function of the sympathetic component of the cavernous nerve is unknown.

The cavernosal nerves pass posterolateral to the apex of the prostate and then proceed lateral to the membranous urethra and anterior to the bulbous urethra, where they enter the hilum of the penis.[21] This nerve is closely applied to the apex of the prostate and membranous urethra; it can be injured easily during radical pelvic surgery, transurethral prostatectomy, external sphincterotomy, or any procedure using electrocautery in that region.[15,21,26]

The *sympathetic nerves to the penis* originate from the 10th to 12th thoracic spinal segments and descend through the inferior mesenteric plexus, the hypogastric plexus, and the perivesical plexus. The *hypogastric nerve* is a discrete branch from these plexuses that enters the perivesical plexus, where it may communicate with parasympathetic nerve fibers. Stimulation of the hypogastric nerve or the sympathetic trunk causes no change in intracavernosal pressure, but stimulation during an established erection causes penile detumescence.[27] As mentioned, in the rat some sympathetic fibers travel to the penis via the cavernous nerves. Stimulation of the cut distal end of the pudendal nerve during erection also causes deturmescence.[27] Thus, it seems that some fibers also travel via the pudendal nerve, especially the sensory branch. At the same time, stimulation of the sympathetic nerves can also induce erection.[28] The mechanism of sympathetic proerectile activity is unclear. Sympathetic fibers may interact with nitrergic nerves in the corpus cavernosum to release nitric oxide (NO) or they may cause pelvic vasoconstriction and shunting of blood toward the penis. In patients with lesions of the parasympathetic pathway, this may be an alternative pathway that allows psychogenic erections.

Sensory nerves of the penis begin as free and specialized receptors primarily in the penile skin and glans. In the glans, the most numerous nerve terminals are free nerve endings (FNEs) present in almost every dermal papilla. Genital end bulbs are present throughout the glans, especially in the corona and near the frenulum. The ratio of free nerve endings to corpuscular receptors is approximately 10:1.[29] At an ultrastructural level, the genital end bulbs unique to the glans penis consist of axon terminals that resemble a tangled web of free nerve endings.[29] Simple, Pacinian, and Ruffini corpuscles are occasionally identified, predominantly in the corona of the glans. There are sensory nerves also in the urethra and corpora cavernosa, which relay pain and pressure sensation.

Temperature and nociceptive (pain) signals from free nerve endings travel via small-diameter, thinly myelinated, or unmyelinated nerve fibers; vibration, touch, and pressure use large-diameter, myelinated fibers.[29] All these nerve fibers converge to form the dorsal nerve of the penis,[30] which joins other perineal nerves to become the internal pudendal nerve and ascends to the dorsal roots of the second to fourth sacral nerves. The dorsal nerve appears to innervate the glans and the urethra separately, suggesting that it provides afferent impulses for sexual stimulation and for ejaculation.[30] Ascending pathways in the spinal cord include the spinothalamic tract to thalamus and to sensory cortex.

Somatic motor nerves to the penis originate from the ventral roots of sacral segments S2 through S4 and coalesce to form the pudendal nerves. These nerves pass into the perineum as the perineal nerve and innervate the bulbocavernous and ischiocavernous muscles. The major role of these muscles in penile erection is to provide temporary increases in intracavernosal pressure.[14] As mentioned, perineal muscle contraction can also cause increased intraspongiosal pressure. Voluntary perineal muscle contraction during erection can produce intracavernosal pressures of several hundred millimeters of mercury, albeit only for brief periods of time. These brief surges in intracavernosal pressure, with the resulting increased penile rigidity, aid in allowing successful vaginal penetration. However, perineal muscle contraction is not essential to penile erection; patients with paralysis of the pelvic floor can still be potent.[31]

Histochemistry

Human corpora cavernosum and spongiosum are richly innervated by cholinergic nerves.[32] These same nerves appear to contain neuronal nitric oxide synthase and vasoactive intestinal polypeptide.[32] Calcitonin gene–related peptide, a vasorelaxant, has also been localized in cavernosal nerves but its colocalization and role in penile erection are still unclear.[33] Adrenergic nerves are abundant in human cavernosal tissue, in particular around the helicine arteries.[34] Such nerves contain not only norepinephrine but also neuropeptide Y, another vasoconstrictor.[35–37]

Organs of Emission and Ejaculation

The organs of emission in the male consist of the tails of the epididymi, the vasa deferentia, the seminal vesicles, and the prostate. The vas deferens is a muscular propulsive tube that transports sperm from the epididymis to the ejaculatory duct. The seminal vesicle actually consists of a single tightly coiled tube that empties into the ejaculatory duct, mixing with the contents of the vas deferens. The glands of the prostate empty directly into the floor of the prostatic urethra. Accessory organs of emission include the bulbourethral glands (of Cowper) and periurethral glands (of Littre). Cowper's glands are two small pea-sized glands in the urogenital diaphragm. Each gland has a 2.5-cm excretory duct that opens in the floor of the bulbous urethra. The glands of Littre secrete mucus into the urethra. The organs of ejaculation consist of the urethra and the bulbospongiosus muscle that surrounds the bulb of the urethra. These muscles provide the contractile force that expels the semen out through the urethral meatus.

The Female Genitals

The female genital organs consist of the labia majora, labia minora, clitoris, bulbs (of the vestibule), and vagina. Although there are clearly many homologous structures in the male and female, female anatomy differs significantly enough to be described in its own right. Because the majority of female cadavers were postmenopausal women and significant changes follow menopause, many descriptions derived from cadaver dissection are inaccurate for younger and premenopausal women.

The *vulva* consists of the parts of the external visible female genitals—the labia majora, the labia minora, the glans of the clitoris, and the vestibule of the vagina. The *labia majora* represent the cleft female homologue to the male scrotum. They are two symmetrical folds of skin filled with fat connective tissue, nerves, and lymphatic vessels. The lateral surface is covered with variable amounts of coarse hair and the medial surface is hairless and contains a large number of sebaceous glands. The function of the labia majora is to protect and enclose the vaginal vestibule. The *labia minora* are thin, delicate folds of vascular, fat-free, hairless skin located on each side of the vaginal vestibule. The labia minora divide anteriorly to form the prepuce and frenulum of the clitoris. The glans of the clitoris is described in the next section. The *vestibule of the vagina* is the space enclosed by the labia minora and leads into the vagina itself. Anterior to the vestibule is the external urethral orifice and associated paraurethral (Skene's) glands. Posteriorly, the vestibule receives the orifices of the greater vestibular (Bartholin's) glands, which provide lubrication for the vestibule of the vagina and are homologues of the bulbourethral glands of the male.

The Clitoris

The *clitoris* is a small midline erectile body that is homologous to the male penis. It consists of a glans, a body, and crura. The glans is easily visible at the superior junction of the labia minora. The body, consisting of paired corpora with an incomplete septum between them, is 1 to 2 cm wide and 2 to 4 cm long.[38] The crura, 5 to 9 cm long, are attached to the ischial bone and covered by the ischiocavernosus muscle.[38]

Structural Support

Like the penis, the clitoris is attached to the pubis by specialized connective tissue supports. The so-called *suspensory ligament of the clitoris* has both superficial and deep components.[39] A superficial fibro-fatty ligament extends from within the fatty tissue of the mons pubis to the body of the clitoris and into the labia majora. In addition, a deep component originates on the symphysis pubis itself, extends to the body of the clitoris and then to the bulbs of the clitoris. The supporting structures of the clitoris thus appear to function less as suspensory ligaments and more as traction ligaments that transmit force from the labia majora, bulbs, and vaginal introitus to the clitoris. Some authors have suggested that the anterior vaginal wall acts to transmit forces generated during intercourse to the clitoris.[40]

Vascular Supply

Blood supply to the body of the clitoris is supplied by paired pudendal arteries that course lateral to the urethra along the pelvic aspect of the anterior vaginal wall.[38] These arteries give off the cavernous artery and the artery to the bulb. The body of the clitoris is composed of cavernous tissue surrounded by tough tunica albuginea. However, the clitoris seems to lack the subalbugineal plexus characteristic of the penis.[41] This finding suggests that, unlike the penis, the clitoris does not have a well-developed outflow occlusion mechanism and becomes erect mainly through increased blood flow.

Innervation and Histochemistry

The glans of the clitoris forms a cap that sits on the ends of the corporal bodies and is richly innervated by sensory nerve endings.[42] The deep dorsal nerves perforate the glans on the dorsal aspect of its junction with the corporal bodies. Recent studies have confirmed that the dorsal nerve of the clitoris is relatively large (more than 2 mm in diameter).[38] The cavernous nerve runs along with the cavernous artery as it enters the corporal bodies of the clitoris. Nerves containing neuronal nitric oxide synthase have been detected in both the body and the glans of the human clitoris,[43] suggesting that nitric oxide is involved in the control of clitoral smooth muscle tone. Nerve fibers containing vasoactive intestinal polypeptide (VIP), calcitonin gene–related peptide (CGRP), and substance P (SP) have also been described in human clitoral tissue.[37,44]

The Bulbs of the Vestibule

The female urethra, like the bulbous portion of the male urethra, is surrounded laterally by erectile tissue called the vestibular bulbs in most anatomy texts. Recent anatomic studies show that these erectile bodies are intimately related and lateral to the urethra rather than lateral to the vestibule of the vagina.[38] They are not, as often depicted in anatomic texts, located within the labia minora. Superiorly, the bulbs continue as the pars intermedia and terminate as the glans of the clitoris.[45] Thus, the bulbs represent the cleft female homologue to the bulb of the male urethra. The entire complex of spongy erectile tissue consisting of bulbs, pars intermedia, and clitoral glans corresponds to the corpus spongiosum of the male.[45]

The Vagina

Structure

The vagina is a muscular sheath that connects the uterus and the external genitalia. It has both sexual and reproductive functions and this dual function is reflected in various aspects of its structure, especially its vascular supply, its sensory and motor innervation, and its marked distensibility. The wall of the vagina consists of an inner lining of stratified squamous epithelium, an intermediate layer of smooth muscle, and an outer advential layer. The lining of the vagina is folded into numerous rugae, which are related to its extreme distensibility. The vaginal entrance is closed by the bulbocavernosus muscle, a striated muscle.

Vascular Supply

Corrosion studies of rat vagina have shown that the vaginal epithelium is intimately related to a dense capillary network in the subepithelial layer.[46] This vascular network may be related to the production of transudate during sexual arousal. Somewhat deeper, the loose submucosal layer contains a complex of numerous large veins and smooth muscle fibers that resemble cavernous tissue. The smooth muscle layer consists of an inner circular layer and a strong external longitudinal layer. The adventitial layer consists of connective tissue and a large plexus of blood vessels.

Innervation and Histochemistry

The vagina has a complex innervation that is not well understood. The pelvic nerves appear to subserve sensation from the vagina while the pudendal nerve subserves sensation from the labia and clitoris.[47] Afferent nerves in the vagina appear to contain substance P in both animal[47,48] and human[49] tissue samples, although SP-containing nerves appear to be sparse in the human vagina.[49] Nerves containing nitric oxide synthase (NOS) have been demonstrated in animal[50] and human vagina.[51] Nerves containing CGRP, neuropeptide Y, VIP, and peptide histidine-methionine (PHM) have also been found in human vaginae.[51,52]

PHYSIOLOGY OF MALE SEXUAL RESPONSE

Hemodynamics

The hemodynamic mechanisms of penile erection have been debated for some time.[13,18,27,53–56] Is erection primarily due to increased arterial inflow, decreased venous outflow, or a combination of the two? How is the inflow controlled? The presence of arterial polsters (von Ebner pads) was proposed by Conti as the major inflow controlling zone.[57] However, the work of Benson and others put much of this theory in doubt.[58] Is there a mechanism for corporal venous occlusion and is it necessary for penile erection? Some authors reported extensive flow in the dorsal veins during erection in dogs[53,54] as well as in humans.[59] However, we[13,18] and others[60,61] have demonstrated markedly decreased flow from the corpus cavernosum during erection. This discrepancy is probably accounted for by the fact that the glans and corpus spongiosum of the dog does not have a veno-occlusive mechanism and is drained primarily by the dorsal vein. What is the mechanism of corporal venous occlusion? Some authors have pointed to polsters and smooth muscle sphincters in the deep dorsal vein.[62] However, most studies indicate an intracavernosal point of occlusion due to compression of subtunical veins.[17,27,61]

Based on animal studies, the hemodynamic events of penile erection can be divided into several phases. In the *resting phase* the penis is flaccid; arterial inflow and venous outflow are minimal and approximately equal. The minimal arterial blood flow is just enough to provide nutrition to the penis. In studies of how blood flows through the corpora in the flaccid state,[27] we demonstrated that blood flow measured directly under the tunica albuginea was significantly higher than deep intracavernosal blood flow. Subtunical oxygen tension in the flaccid penis was consistent with a largely arterial circulation. These observations provide physiologic evidence of an important subtunical circulation that bypasses the sinusoidal spaces when the penis is flaccid. It is consistent with the anatomic findings of Banya describing two circulatory paths through the corpora[17] (Fig. 13-1).

With sexual stimulation, the second, or *arterial*, phase is initiated and is characterized by a marked increase in flow through the pelvic circulation and through the cavernosal arteries. In the canine model, we found that following pelvic nerve stimulation, arterial flow increases by a factor of 2.5 within 2 seconds of onset of stimulation.[18] The increase in arterial flow is followed 1 second later by a similar increase in venous outflow from the corpora cavernosa. Thus, we have physiologic evidence of an intracavernosal shunt that bypasses the sinusoids.[17] Spongiosal pressure begins to rise about 6 seconds after nerve stimulation and always remains below cavernosal pressure. During the second phase, intracavernosal pressure actually decreases as a result of active smooth muscle relaxation.

With the onset of the third, or *cavernosal*, phase, deep intracavernosal blood flow increases significantly followed by an increase in oxygen tension from a level consistent with venous blood to a level consistent with arterial blood. Cavernosal pressure begins to rise after a latency of about 11 seconds. There is also a significant decrease in subtunical blood flow. Eventually cavernosal pressure approaches arterial systolic pressure. This latency period is accounted for by relaxation of the smooth muscle of the cavernosal sinusoids and the time required for arterial blood to fill these spaces. Spongiosal pressure is maintained primarily by a high flow state through the glans penis and cavernosal pressure depends on a veno-occlusive mechanism. Contraction of the ischiocavernous muscles during this phase is similar to squeezing a closed space. This contraction may temporarily increase intracavernosal pressure to several times the systolic pressure (~300 mm Hg).

In the final, or *detumescence*, phase adrenergically mediated penile smooth muscle contraction occurs and blood flow through the subtunical space is reestablished.[27] Smooth muscle electromyography has shown that electrical activity of the corpus cavernosum is restored during detumescence.[62] The previously stretched and compressed subtunical venules open, venous outflow resistance falls, and venous outflow increases. Penile length and girth decrease until the penis is flaccid again.

Neurophysiology

Penile erection is a spinal reflex initiated by penile stimulation traveling through the dorsal penile nerve, as well as by visual, olfactory, and imaginary stimuli. The reflex involves both autonomic and somatic efferents. Especially in humans, it is heavily modulated by supraspinal influences.

Peripheral Control

Stimuli related to initiating and maintaining erection arise primarily in the glans and travel via the dorsal nerve of the penis.[30] Peripheral motor control of penile erection is established through control of smooth muscle tone in the sinusoidal trabeculae and arterioles in the corpora cavernosa. Smooth muscle tone in the corpora cavernosa is controlled through impulses from both the sympathetic and parasympathetic nervous systems as well as from endothelial-mediated mechanisms. The tone of the arterioles controls the amount of blood entering the cavernosal sinusoids and the tone of the trabeculae controls the amount of blood leaving the corpora.

Cholinergic Neurotransmission

Immunohistochemical studies have conclusively shown that the corpus cavernosum and the corpus spongiosum have rich cholinergic innervation.[32] These cholinergic nerves also stain positive for nitric oxide

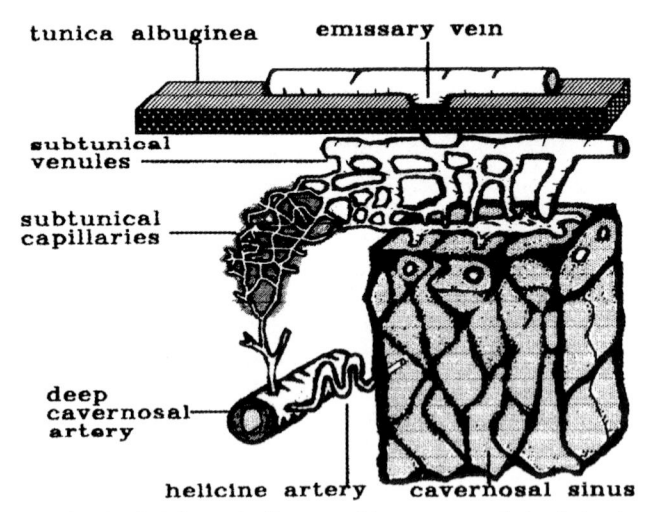

FIGURE 13-1 Schematic diagram of intracavernosal circulation in the dog showing deep cavernosal artery feeding both the sinusoidal space and the subtunical capillaries. (From Vardi Y, Siroky MB: A canine model for hemodynamic study of isolated corpus cavernosum. J Urol 138(3):663–666, 1987.)

synthase and VIP, suggesting that nitric oxide and VIP are released along with acetylcholine from cholinergic nerves.[32,63] All of these agents are, under most conditions, vasodilators and smooth muscle relaxants.

Acetylcholine, whether released from cholinergic nerves or applied directly to tissue, has a variety of effects. Intra-arterial[53,56] as well as intracavernosal[64] injection of acetylcholine can produce penile erection. These effects were only partially blocked by atropine but were abolished by removal of the endothelium.[65] While having no effect on flaccid cavernosal tissue, acetylcholine causes concentration-dependent relaxation of cavernosal tissue that was precontracted with norepinephrine.[66,67] The relaxant effect of acetylcholine is markedly attenuated by removal of the epithelium, indicating the release of an endothelial-derived relaxing factor from the epithelium under the influence of acetylcholine.[66] Acetylcholine may also act on adrenergic nerve terminals to suppress the release of norepinephrine.[65,66] Thus, there are at least three mechanisms by which acetylcholine may induce cavernosal smooth muscle relaxation: (1) corelease of nitric oxide and perhaps VIP from cholinergic nerve terminals, (2) release of nitric oxide from the vascular endothelium, and (3) suppression of norepinephrine release.

Nitric oxide plays a critical role in inducing smooth muscle relaxation and penile erection.[68,69] As mentioned, the sources of nitric oxide include autonomic nerves and vascular endothelium, including that of the lacunar spaces. Prior to its identification, nitric oxide was called endothelium-derived relaxing factor (EDRF). In the autonomic nerves, nitric oxide was previously identified as the nonadrenergic, noncholinergic (NANC) neurotransmitter. The enzyme nitric oxide synthase, existing as a constitutive as well as an inducible enzyme, produces nitric oxide from L-arginine. Nitric oxide induces reduction of cytosolic-free calcium as a result of activation of the soluble form of guanylate cyclase and increased cyclic guanosine monophosphate (cGMP) from guanosine triphosphate. Relaxation of the trabecular smooth muscle is blocked by methylene blue, which inhibits cGMP synthesis.[70]

Adrenergic Neurotransmission

Norepinephrine is the primary adrenergic transmitter in the penis and controls penile detumescence by inducing penile smooth muscle contraction. However, the regulation of adrenergic neurotransmission in the penis is complex and involves interaction with the cholinergic and nonadrenergic, noncholinergic neurons. For example, cholinergic nerves prejunctionally inhibit norepinephrine release from adrenergic nerves.[71] The presence of alpha- and beta-adrenergic receptors in penile blood vessels and cavernous smooth muscle has been demonstrated.[34,72] In the corporal smooth muscle, the primary adrenergic receptor is the alpha-1 receptor, and both alpha-1 and alpha-2 receptors are present in the cavernous artery.[73,74] Alpha-2 receptors are found both on prejunctional sites of the adrenergic nerves and on corporal smooth muscle cells.

On prejunctional sites, alpha-2 receptors mediate the feedback inhibition of norepinephrine neurotransmitter release from the adrenergic nerve.[71] Norepinephrine released from the adrenergic nerves binds to the prejunctional alpha-2 adrenoceptor on the adrenergic nerves and inhibits norepinephrine release. Thus, blockade of this reaction by selective alpha-2 receptor antagonists (e.g., yohimbine) enhances norepinephrine release and *inhibits* erection. At the same time, norepinephrine released from the adrenergic nerves binds to the prejunctional alpha-2 adrenoceptor on the nonadrenergic, noncholinergic nerves and inhibits nitric oxide synthesis and release. Blockade of this reaction by selective alpha-2 receptor antagonists (e.g., yohimbine) will enhance nitric oxide release and *facilitate* erection. The alpha-2 receptors on the smooth muscle cell also appear to be involved in the mediation of smooth muscle cell contraction. Specifically, alpha-2 agonists cause trabecular smooth muscle contraction. Blockade of these smooth muscle alpha-2 receptors by yohimbine or rauwolscine induces trabecular smooth muscle relaxation, facilitating erection.[75,76] The net effect of an agent such as yohimbine appears to be facilitation of erection, although most of its action may be on central rather than peripheral sites.

Peptidergic Neurotransmission

Neuropeptides have been identified in nerves that supply the penis, including vasoactive intestinal polypeptide, substance P, neuropeptide Y, somatostatin, peptide histidine-isoleucine, enkephalins, and calcitonin gene–related peptide.[32-37] The exact role of these substances is not well understood. Vasoactive intestinal polypeptide appears to serve as a cotransmitter with nitric oxide released from cholinergic nerves while neuropeptide Y, a vasoconstrictor, is released from adrenergic nerves.[77]

Paracrine Factors

Endothelin,[78] angiotensin,[79] prostaglandin $F_{2\alpha}$,[80] thromboxane,[80] and histamine[81] all have some vasoconstrictive actions. Whether these agents have a primary role or are modulators of vascular smooth muscle tone is unclear.

Endothelin is localized in the endothelial cell and to a lesser degree in the trabecular smooth muscle. Endothelins are potent constrictors that cause long-lasting contractions of corporal smooth muscle strips. Endothelin appears to have three isoforms called ET-1, ET-2, and ET-3 and two different receptors called ET A and ET B.[78] The ET A receptor is located on vascular smooth muscle and mediates contraction and proliferation while the ET B receptor is located on the endothelial cell and generally mediates vasodilation, perhaps through release of nitric oxide.

Angiotensin II is produced and secreted in physiologically relevant amounts in human cavernosal tissue.[82] Angiotensin II, a potent vasoconstrictor, is formed from angiotensin I by angiotensin-converting enzyme (ACE). Two subtypes of angiotensin II receptors (AT1 and AT2) have been characterized. It appears that male rabbit cavernosal tissue contains the AT1 receptor[83] and that angiotensin II causes a dose-dependent contraction of canine cavernosal smooth muscle, which is inhibited by giving angiotensin II receptor antagonist.[84]

Prostaglandins probably act as modulators of cavernosal smooth muscle tone by activating cyclic adenosine monophosphate (cAMP).[85,86] $PGF_{2\alpha}$, PGI_2, and especially thromboxane A_2 act as potent vasoconstrictors of cavernosal tissue while PGE_1 and PGE_2 have vasorelaxant effects.[87] In addition to direct vascular smooth muscle relaxation, PGE_1 may inhibit release of neuronal norepinephrine.[88] A variety of factors appear important in controlling the actions of prostaglandins. For example, the local production of prostanoids appears to be inhibited under hypoxic conditions.[89] Binding of PGE_1 to cavernosal tissue appears to vary widely among species and is suppressed by estrogens.[90] Furthermore, cavernosal relaxation in response to PGE_1 is markedly diminished after castration, indicating that androgens are a prerequisite for their action.[91]

Bradykinin has relaxant effects on human corpus cavernosum that are mediated through cAMP and cGMP.[79] Bradykinin appears to act on cavernosal BK2 receptors, leading to release of endothelial nitric oxide.[92] In contrast, histamine appears to induce an endothelium-independent relaxation of vascular tissue.[81,93]

The vasodilation induced by histamine seems to be mediated mainly by histamine H_2 receptors located on vascular smooth muscle, without the intervention of nitric oxide or relaxant prostanoids.[93]

Central Control

Compared with the peripheral nervous system, knowledge of central control mechanisms is much less complete. Much of it is derived from animal experiments and from observations in human patients with spinal cord injuries.

Spinal Mechanisms

Local segmental reflexes in the lumbosacral cord subserve penile erection in both normal and spinal cord–injured humans.[94–96] The dorsal nerve of the penis provides afferent input while the pelvic nerves provide the motor pathway. In the intact individual, these reflexes are under net tonic inhibitory control from higher centers.[97]

Supraspinal Mechanisms

In the male central nervous system, the erection centers include the septal portion of the hippocampus, the anterior cingulate gyrus, the anterior thalamic nuclei, the mammillothalamic tract, and the mammillary bodies. The medial dorsal nucleus of the thalamus and the medial preoptic area (MPOA) in particular appear to be important centers that control penile erection and sexual drive.[98,99] These centers send descending pathways via the medial forebrain bundle[98] and then into the dorsolateral columns of the spinal cord.

Central Neurotransmitters

Substances acting as neurotransmitters in the central nervous system and controlling penile erection include serotonin (5-hydroxytryptamine, 5-HT), dopamine, norepinephrine, nitric oxide, and many others.

Serotonin tends to inhibit penile erection at both spinal[100] and supraspinal sites.[101] Other known central inhibitors of sexual activity include gamma-aminobutyric acid,[102] prolactin,[103] and endogenous opioid peptides.[104] Serotoninergic nerves appear to be responsible for supraspinal inhibition of segmental penile erection reflexes.[99] Trazodone, a serotonin antagonist, has long been recognized as an agent that induces priapism, although the precise mechanism of action of trazodone in producing priapism is unclear.[105]

Dopamine and dopamine agonists such as apomorphine, when administered systemically, induce penile erection in experimental animals.[106] These effects are blocked by centrally acting dopamine receptor blockers (haloperidol) but not by peripherally acting dopamine blockers (domperidol), indicating that dopamine affects the central nervous system.[107] It is likely that dopamine induces penile erection by acting on oxytocin-containing neurons in the paraventricular nucleus of the hypothalamus.[107] Apomorphine has been reported to cause penile erection in humans, but these erections are usually only partial, not associated with sexual desire, and often accompanied by nausea.[108,109]

Norepinephrine has various effects on sexual function in the central nervous system. Central inhibition of alpha-2 adrenoceptors facilitates sexual function, whereas stimulation of these receptors inhibits sexual function.[110,111] Clonidine, a central alpha-2 receptor agonist used as an antihypertensive agent, is associated with impotence. Yohimbine, a central alpha-2 receptor blocker, can enhance sexual motivation.[112]

Oxytocin appears to facilitate erection at the spinal and supraspinal levels. Ascending sensory stimuli from the dorsal penile nerve appear to preferentially stimulate oxytocin-containing cells in the supraoptic nucleus. Electrical and tactile stimulation of the rat dorsal penile nerve stimulated 60% of the oxytocin cells in the contralateral supraoptic nucleus.[113] Oxytocin has been localized in descending pathways from hypothalamus to brain stem and autonomic centers in the spinal cord.[114] As mentioned, it is likely that dopamine's effects on penile erection are mediated by oxytocin-containing neurons in the hypothalamus.[107] In the rat, spinal autonomic neurons controlling penile erection appear to receive oxytocinergic innervation from the paraventricular nucleus of the hypothalamus, which facilitates erection.[115]

Nitric oxide (NO) was recently added to the list of compounds that act in the central nervous system to facilitate penile erection.[116] The paraventricular nucleus (PVN) of the hypothalamus is one of the richest areas of NO synthase in the brain and is also where dopamine and oxytocin act to induce penile erection. A role for nitric oxide is suggested by the ability of NO synthase inhibitors injected in the lateral ventricles or in the PVN of the hypothalamus to prevent penile erection induced by dopamine agonists and oxytocin. The inhibitory effect of NO synthase inhibitors was not observed when these compounds were injected concomitantly with L-arginine, the precursor of NO. It is likely that NO acts as an intracellular rather than an intercellular modulator.[117]

Opioids have long been recognized to interfere with erection. Recent work shows that morphine blocks erection by interfering with increased nitric oxide production.[118] It also blocks the actions of dopamine and oxytocin in producing erection.[119]

Adrenocorticotropin and related peptides (melanocortin) have been observed in many animal species to induce spontaneous penile erections and ejaculation.[120] Intracerebral injection of an NO synthase inhibitor appears to block erections caused by these peptides.[118] A synthetic analogue of alpha-melanocyte–stimulating hormone has been shown to be effective in treating impotence in man.[120]

Hormonal Factors

Androgens are essential in supporting male sexual development. However, the precise role of androgens in the postpubertal male is complex.[121] Castration may not always cause impotence in animals or in humans. Castration in rats prevents erections following injection of apomorphine[122] and oxytocin[123]; the efficacy of both agents is restored after exogenous testosterone is administered.[122,123] Testosterone[123] appears to be important in maintaining certain central dopaminergic pathways related to sexual arousal. In men, nocturnal erections appear to be androgen dependent, whereas visually stimulated erections appear not to be.[124] There may be a phylogenetically older system of sexual arousal that is androgen dependent and another androgen-independent system activated through the cerebral cortex.

Androgens appear to influence the peripheral nervous system, the reactivity of cavernosal smooth muscle, and the perineal striated muscles. Testosterone has been shown to affect peripheral parasympathetic ganglia,[125] dorsal penile nerve,[126] and NO synthase–containing nerves in the corpus cavernosum.[127] Castration of rabbits has reduced intracavernosal pressure and caused reduction of cavernosal smooth muscle content, effects that could be reversed by testosterone replacement.[128] Castration also produced failure of the veno-occlusive mechanism in rats by interfering with NO release in the corpora.[129] Finally, androgens appear to affect the function of the ischiocavernosus and bulbocavernosus muscles. Within 2 weeks of castration, there was a significant decrease in the weight of ischiocavernosus muscles and the size of their spinal motoneurons.[130] In humans, testosterone has been shown to increase the rigidity of nocturnal erections but not their frequency.[131]

PHYSIOLOGY OF FEMALE SEXUAL RESPONSE

Although we know less about female sexual physiology than male sexual function, our knowledge is increasing rapidly. The hemodynamic and neurogenic mechanisms of female sexual response are beginning to receive research attention both in animal models[132-136] and in human studies.[137-142]

Hemodynamics

As in the male, female sexual arousal involves several phases of hemodynamic components, which affect rather simultaneously the clitoris, vestibular bulbs, labia minora, and the vagina.

In the *resting phase*, the vagina is a sheath that contains a potential space with minimal blood flow and very low oxygen tension in the wall.[137,139] In the human vagina, blood flow at rest has been estimated at about 10 mL/min/100 gram tissue[141] and oxygen tension at between 4 mm Hg and 10 mm Hg.[137,142] In the rabbit clitoris, blood flow has been estimated at 2 mL/min/100 gram tissue.[133]

Corresponding to the *arterial phase* of penile erection, the earliest detectable sign of female sexual arousal based on animal studies is a significant increase in vaginal wall and clitoral blood flow.[133] There is a significant increase in clitoral cavernosal pressure as well. In the rabbit, clitoral cavernosal pressure increased from 6 mm Hg to about 10 mm Hg following pelvic nerve stimulation.[134] In the rat model,[135,136] there is a threefold increase in vaginal wall blood flow, which remains elevated as long as the nerve is stimulated. The possible relation of the dense capillary network just beneath the vaginal epithelium to the production of vaginal transudate was mentioned previously.[46] With the onset of increased vaginal blood flow, production of vaginal transudate ensues. A significant rise in tissue oxygen tension follows about 20 seconds later and indicates that the increased flow is due to increased inflow of arterial blood. In humans, vaginal oxygen tension increases from 4 to 8 times baseline during sexual stimulation[137,138] and vaginal wall blood flow increases about threefold[139-142] (Fig. 13-2). In humans, clitoral blood flow has been estimated to increase from 4 to 11 times baseline.[143]

The third or *plateau*, phase, which corresponds to the veno-occlusive phase of penile erection, is characterized by continued high blood flow and continued production of vaginal fluid transudate. The lack of veno-occlusion in the vaginal and clitoral circulation is a major factor that distinguishes the hemodynamic changes in the female from the male. Because of this, the circulatory changes in the female genitalia have been called vasocongestion.

The final or *resolution*, phase is characterized by slow return of blood flow to baseline values. In women, up to 20 to 30 minutes is required for vaginal oxygen tension to return to baseline.[137]

Changes in Vaginal Wall Tension

The smooth muscle of the vagina also responds to sexual arousal by relaxing and lengthening.[133] In rats, about 2 to 3 seconds after stimulation of the pelvic nerve, a biphasic response in vaginal wall tension begins. There is a rapid, short-lived increase in vaginal wall tension followed by a fall in tension to below baseline value, which indicates vaginal wall relaxation.[133,134]

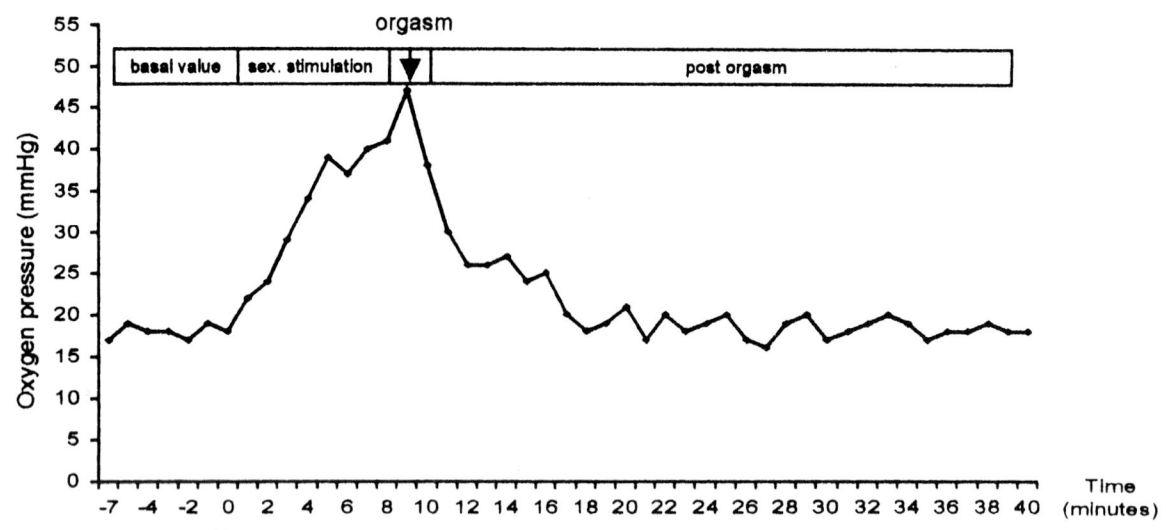

FIGURE 13-2 Normal female sexual function: labial surface oxygen tension showing increase during sexual stimulation, peak during orgasm and resolution. (From Sommer F, Caspers HP, Esders K, et al: Measurement of vaginal and minor labial oxygen tension for the evaluation of female sexual function. J Urol 165(4):1181–1184, 2001.)

Neurophysiology

Vaginal Blood Flow

The identity of the neurotransmitter(s) that control vaginal blood flow is currently unknown. Atropine does not affect the pelvic nerve–stimulated rise in vaginal blood flow in animals[133] or the rise in vaginal blood flow in human females.[144] This evidence suggest that muscarinic neurotransmission is probably not involved. The ability of sildenafil to enhance nerve-stimulated vaginal blood flow has been reported.[145]

This knowledge, of course, suggests the involvement of the NO-cGMP pathway.[145] At the same time, it has been reported that administration of VIP, either intravenously or by injection in the vaginal wall, increases vaginal blood flow and induces vaginal fluid production.[139,146] Peptide histidine-methionine (PHM) has effects similar to VIP but at lower potency.[147] Intravaginal prostaglandin E1 can also increase vaginal blood flow.[148] Although some authors have stated that VIP is the primary neurotransmitter in the vaginal circulation,[139] much more research in this area is required. Vaginal blood flow appears to undergo phasic shifts in conjunction with rapid eye movement (REM) sleep.[149]

Clitoral Smooth Muscle Tone

Angiotensin II is a potent constrictor of rabbit clitoral smooth muscle in muscle bath.[150] The clitoris has angiotensin II receptors of the AT1 variety.[150] Like the penis, electrical field stimulation induces nonadrenergic, noncholinergic (NANC) relaxation of clitoral smooth muscle.[151] The relaxation is inhibited by a NOS inhibitor and enhanced by sildenafil, suggesting involvement of the NO-cGMP system.[152]

Vaginal Muscle Tone

Pelvic nerve–stimulated increased vaginal tone is abolished by atropine and vercuronium bromide, a striated muscle relaxant, prevents the subsequent fall in vaginal tension.[134] These results suggest that vaginal contraction is due to smooth muscle under cholinergic control while vaginal lengthening or enlargement may be due to striated muscle contraction. How striated muscle contraction produces a decrease in vaginal pressure is unclear.

Central Control

Little is known about the central control of female sexual arousal. The medial amygdala appears to use vasopressin as a central neurotransmitter.[153] Oxytocin is also clearly involved; oxytocin serum levels measured before and after sexual stimulation in 12 healthy women were elevated significantly.[154] Although intravenous apomorphine, a centrally acting dopaminergic agent, has been shown to cause increased peak clitoral and vaginal wall blood flow,[155] the role of dopamine in female sexual behavior is not established.

Hormonal Factors

Ovarian hormones affect sensory nerves, central and peripheral neurons, and the vascular system.[156] In the central nervous system, estrogen induces sprouting of axons projecting to the lumbosacral spinal cord that control receptive behavior in female cats.[157]

Oophorectomy in rabbits diminishes vaginal and clitoral blood flow, effects which can be reversed with estrogen replacement.[158] Oophorectomy also causes thinning of vaginal epithelium and fibrosis of clitoral tissue.[158] In rat vagina, oophorectomy caused a decrease in expression of both nNOS and eNOS.[159] In contrast, it has been reported that oophorectomy in rabbits causes increased expression of nNOS and eNOS in clitoral and vaginal tissue[160] and that estradiol causes downregulation of NOS in rabbit vagina.[161] Thus, while it seems clear that oophorectomy reduces genital blood flow, the effects of estrogen on NOS are unclear at present.

In women, vaginal blood flow is under hormonal influence. Menopausal women are known to have significantly decreased vaginal blood flow[162]; intravenous administration of conjugated estrogen increases vaginal blood flow.[163] Menopause without hormone replacement also seems to reduce the vasodilating effect of VIP in the vagina.[164]

Androgens also appear to have a permissive role in female sexuality. Accumulating evidence indicates that many women with low circulating bioavailable testosterone report low libido, persistent fatigue, and diminished sense of well-being, for which testosterone therapy appears to be effective.[165] Whether the effects of testosterone are mediated via the androgen receptor or as a consequence of metabolism to estrogen is not known.

PATHOPHYSIOLOGY OF SEXUAL DYSFUNCTION

Erectile Dysfunction

Recent epidemiological studies have shown that erectile dysfunction (ED) affects an estimated 20 to 30 million American men with varying degrees of severity.[166-168] The Massachusetts Male Aging Study published in 1994 reviewed 1211 men between the ages of 40 and 70; 52% reported ED with 9.6% having mild, 22.2% moderate, and 17.2% complete or severe ED.[166] Approximately 2% of men are affected at 40 years of age and about 25% or more at 65 years of age. In men, erectile dysfunction is clearly related to various aspects of aging. Primary ED refers to the man who has never been able to achieve penile erection. Secondary ED refers to the man who once had normal penile erections and has subsequently lost erectile function completely or partially. The etiologies of ED are generally divided into psychogenic and organic categories. Approximately 80% of cases of ED are due solely or predominantly to organic causes.[169]

Psychogenic Erectile Dysfunction

Psychogenic ED is the persistent inability to achieve or maintain satisfactory erection due primarily to psychologic or interpersonal factors. The diagnosis is appropriate in cases where psychologic causes are predominant and not merely because no etiology is evident. It is imperative to appreciate that psychologic, interpersonal, situational, and organic etiologies of ED often coexist in the patient. An example of this is the *widower's syndrome* in which an elderly man with organic reasons for ED is also confronted with situational factors associated with depression related to the loss of his spouse and guilt over sexual activity with a new partner.

Pathophysiologic Mechanisms

The pathophysiology of psychogenic ED is only beginning to be investigated. Two pathophysiologic mechanisms have been proposed: direct motor inhibition by the cerebrum to the spinal centers[170] and excessive sympathetic tone or increased peripheral catecholamine levels that increase cavernous smooth muscle contraction.[171] Animal experiments show that stimulation of the sympathetic nerves can inhibit papaverine-induced erection.[172,173] Although there is some evidence of increased circulating norepinephrine in patients with psychogenic impotence,[174] some authors have failed to find such elevation.[175] Elevated sympathetic tone may explain why some patients respond poorly to injection therapy in an office setting but achieve prolonged erections when injecting at home.

Psychologic Mechanisms

Classically psychogenic ED has been attributed to proximate or remote psychologic causes.[176] Proximate causes include performance anxiety,[177] lack of adequate stimulation, and short-term conflicts in the relationship. Performance anxiety is a major cause of situational psychogenic impotence. As described originally by Masters and Johnson, it involves adopting a "spectator role" in which the male's focus is on his performance rather than on erotic stimulation. Some studies suggest that problems with attention and perception are found in males with psychogenic ED.[178] Anxiety itself is not the problem; rather it seems that cognitive distraction is inhibiting to men with psychogenic ED but not to normal men.[179]

This type of problem should be distinguished from psychogenic ED due to life stress, changes in mood, or depression.[180,181] The Massachusetts Male Aging Study found that certain conditions are predictors of erectile dysfunction, especially depression and a generally pessimistic attitude.[166] These are summarized in Table 13-1. Remote causes include childhood sexual trauma or abuse, sexual identity issues, unresolved parental issues, and religious or cultural inhibitions.[182,183]

Classification

An expanded classification of psychogenic impotence has been proposed by the International Society for Study of Impotence (Box 13-1). This classification takes into account some of the newer theories of centrally mediated inhibition.[170,171]

TABLE 13-1 ■ **Psychologic and Social Predictors of Erectile Dysfunction**

Variable	Odds Ratio
Marital change	1:41
Employment change	1:42
Unhappiness with life	2:30
Depressive symptoms	2:88
Pessimistic attitude	3:89

Data from Feldman HA, Goldstein I, Hatzichristou DG, et al: Impotence and its medical and psychological correlates: Results of the Massachusetts Male Aging Study. J Urol 151(1):54–61, 1994.

> **BOX 13-1 Classification of Psychogenic Erectile Dysfunction: From the International Society for Study of Impotence**
>
> I. Generalized Type
>   A. Unresponsiveness
>   1. Primary
>   2. Age related
>   B. Inhibition
> II. Situational Type
>   A. Partner related
>   1. Specific to relationship
>   2. Specific to sexual object preference
>   3. Inhibition due to partner conflict or threat
>   B. Performance related
>   1. Associated with other dysfunctions (rapid ejaculation)
>   2. Performance anxiety
>   C. Psychologic distress
>   1. Depression or major life stress

Organic Erectile Dysfunction

Organic ED is the persistent inability to achieve or maintain satisfactory erection due primarily to organic or physical factors. In contrast to psychogenic ED, organic ED is often a gradual deterioration of sexual function over months or years. Typically, the patient first notes a mild decrease in penile rigidity, then a decrease in the frequency of erections, followed by sporadic failure of erection with fatigue. Nocturnal erections gradually disappear, as do erections on awakening. In organic impotence, full erection may be achieved but frequently subsides quickly. Finally, many patients report a partial erection that is insufficient for vaginal penetration. Typically, libido is unaffected in organic ED, at least in the early stages, as is ejaculatory function.

A large number of diseases and conditions may lead to organic ED, including peripheral and central neurologic lesions, hypogonadism and other hormonal disturbances, pelvic atherosclerotic disease, microvascular disease, veno-occlusive dysfunction, Peyronie's disease, and drug therapies especially antihypertensive agents.[166,184–186] By far, the most frequent etiology of organic ED is vascular disease.

Vasculogenic Erectile Dysfunction

Vasculogenic erectile dysfunction consists of arteriogenic ED (cavernosal artery insufficiency) and veno-occlusive ED. Although frequently discussed separately, in reality these two mechanisms often coexist in the patient. In the process of penile erection, an adequate arterial inflow and pressure are critical. Arterial insufficiency may result from a variety of causes, but the majority of cases can be attributed to atherosclerosis, radiation,[187] and trauma,[188] including surgery. Risk factors for vasculogenic ED include increased age, diabetes mellitus, hypertension, uremia, heart disease, obesity, smoking, and use of various medications especially vasodilators, hypoglycemic agents, and antihypertensives.[189–191] Elevated serum cholesterol and decreased high-density lipoprotein are also associated with ED.[192] It is unclear whether cholesterol-lowering agents lead to reversal of ED. Current cigarette smoking magnifies the risk of ED significantly.[191,193] In the Massachusetts Male Aging Study, cigarette smoking at baseline almost doubled the likelihood of moderate or complete ED at follow-up. Cigar smoking and passive exposure to cigarette smoke also significantly predicted the presence of ED.[166]

Arterial Insufficiency. Atherosclerosis is the most prevalent disease of our time and its complications account for a high number of deaths and disabilities. It is characterized by the deposition of lipid in the vessel wall, leading to the formation of plaque. A thrombus is usually found secondary to atherosclerotic plaque disruption. Mural thrombosis, also at the site of plaque rupture, is an important mechanism in the progression of atherosclerosis. Animal models have shown that platelets, lipids, renin-angiotensin system, cytokines, and growth factors play roles in the evolution and progression of atherosclerosis.[194] Recently, elevated blood homocysteine has been identified as a risk factor for heart disease in the general population. The mechanism by which homocysteine induces atherosclerosis is unclear.[195]

Endothelial cell dysfunction is a central unifying mechanism in much of vasculogenic ED. This is due to the ubiquitous location of the endothelial cell in arteries and cavernous sinuses and the important role of the endothelial cell in controlling smooth muscle tone. Endothelial dysfunction is generally believed to be the inciting event in atherosclerosis, and it is probably important in ischemic manifestations as well.[196] The release of endothelium-derived vasoactive substances is not triggered only by acetylcholine, but also by shear forces exerted by the blood flowing through the blood vessel. Endothelial cell dysfunction is found in atherosclerosis, hypercholesterolemia, diabetes, uremia, coronary artery disease, and hypertension.

Endothelial cells, whether in the cavernosal artery or in the cavernosal sinuses, produce a variety of local paracrine factors that act to alter arterial vascular tone and growth.[196–198] These factors include angiotensin-converting enzyme, angiotensin, kinins, prostaglandins, endothelin, endothelium-derived relaxing factors (nitric oxide), prostaglandins, and histamine. Some of these substances (e.g., angiotensin, endothelin, and certain prostaglandins) are powerful vasoconstrictors while others (e.g., nitric oxide, certain prostaglandins, and histamine) are vasodilators. The endothelial cell is also the site of action of many factors and pharmaceutical agents.

The most important mechanism in endothelial cell dysfunction is imbalance between endothelium-dependent relaxation due primarily to nitric oxide and endothelium-dependent constriction due primarily to endothelin-1.[197] Numerous conditions characterized by an impaired availability of NO have been associated with enhanced synthesis of ET-1, and vice versa, suggesting that these two factors have a reciprocal regulation.[197] Experimental studies have provided evidence that endothelin-1 may influence NO production and that NO can inhibit endothelin synthesis. Of course, this does not rule out the likelihood that many other vasoactive agents play an important role.

Hypercholesterolemia, a common problem, interferes with penile erection.[199] It enhances the deposition of lipid in arterial vascular lesions, causing atherosclerosis and eventual luminal occlusion. The underlying mechanisms for these deleterious effects involve a local inflammatory response and release of cytokines and growth factors.[200] Experimentally, endothelium-dependent relaxation, but not relaxation induced by nitroprusside or electrical field stimulation, was impaired in the presence of hypercholesterolemia.[201] This suggests that hypercholesterolemia impairs NO production or release. In the presence of indomethacin, L-arginine improved endothelium-dependent relaxation of cavernosal tissue in hypercholesterolemic rabbits.[201] Reduction of elevated serum cholesterol has reversed impaired relaxation due to hypercholesterolemia.[202] Hypercholesterolemia also causes significant degeneration of smooth muscle cells with loss of intercellular contacts.[203]

Hypertension is highly associated with ED, which is significantly more common in hypertensive males than in the general population.[204–207] About 15% to 50% of hypertensive males report ED.[204–207] Hypertension affects arterial blood vessels by altering shear stress, which can lead to endothelial abnormalities such as altered production and activity of vasoactive substances, enhanced endothelial proliferation, and intimal permeability.[196] Animal work in the spontaneously hypertensive rat model has shown a direct correlation between systemic blood pressure and morphologic changes in vessels as well as in cavernous spaces of the erectile tissue.[208] Hypertension may also be associated with increased sympathetic activity,[209] which can also interfere with erection. However, the relation to hypertension may be overstated because many antihypertensive medications, especially beta blockers and thiazide diuretics, are associated with ED.[205]

Diabetes mellitus is highly associated with ED. About 50% of male diabetic patients complain of ED, which is correlated with diabetes duration and other diabetic complications.[210] Diabetes induces a wide variety of vasculopathic changes. Hyperglycemia itself may activate the intrarenal renin-angiotensin system, increase peripheral resistance, and cause hypertension.[211] Angiotensin-converting enzyme activity is elevated in diabetic patients.[212] Diabetic patients may also have a hypercoagulable state.

The plasma levels of many clotting factors, including fibrinogen, factor VII, factor VIII, factor XI, factor XII, kallikrein, and von Willebrand factor, are elevated in diabetes.[213] Conversely, the level of the anticoagulant proteins is decreased and platelets are activated.[213] These abnormalities have not yet been directly linked to ED experienced by diabetic men.

Diabetes is associated with penile arterial and sinusoidal endothelial cell dysfunction.[210,214] Diabetic men with impotence have impairment in both the autonomic and the endothelium-dependent mechanisms that mediate the relaxation of the smooth muscle of the corpora cavernosa.[214] Relaxation induced by acetylcholine was significantly less in tissue from diabetic men than in that from nondiabetic men, suggesting impairment of nitric oxide synthesis or release.[214] Similar findings were reported in an animal model of diabetic impotence.[215]

Endothelin levels are increased in diabetics[216] and endothelin may play a significant role in the vascular complications of diabetes.[217] Compared with age-matched healthy controls, in diabetic rabbits, a significant increase in ET B receptor binding sites was found in cavernosal tissue 6 months after induction of diabetes.[218] These receptor changes were accompanied by ultrastructural changes in the corpus cavernosum, which indicates an early, atherosclerosis-like process. Thus, endothelin-1, a powerful vasoconstrictor, may have a role in the pathophysiology of diabetic ED. This peptide may be released in an autocrine fashion, causing cavernosal smooth muscle cell contraction or proliferation.

Uremia is frequently associated with male erectile dysfunction, and the dysfunction usually is not corrected by hemodialysis. About 60% of male patients receiving hemodialysis complain of erectile insufficiency.[219] Although the pathophysiology of uremic ED is not well understood at present, accelerated atherosclerosis is certainly a major factor. In one study, cavernous artery occlusion was found in 80% and generalized corporal veno-occlusive failure in 90% of male uremic patients with ED.[220] Renal transplantation seemed effective in reversing or preventing these changes.[220] Experimentally, impairment of endothelial-dependent vasodilation has been demonstrated in vessels from uremic patients,[221] while others have found that response to acetylcholine is equivalent to that following nitroprusside in uremic patients.[222]

Trauma may cause vasculogenic ED in a variety of circumstances including pelvic trauma,[223] perineal trauma,[198,224] penile trauma,[225] and pelvic surgery.[226–228] The incidence of ED following pelvic fracture is about 40% when there is urethral injury and about 5% when there is no urethral injury.[223] Duplex ultrasound in patients with ED following pelvic fracture revealed a vasculogenic component in 80% of cases.[229] Other investigators, observing a high response rate to intracavernosal pharmacotherapy, have felt that ED following pelvic trauma was due to disruption of the cavernosal nerves.[230] Nevertheless, there is impressive evidence of penile vasculopathy in patients following pelvic trauma.[223]

Blunt trauma to the perineum may occur during sports or exercise, especially intensive bicycling.[231] In one sudy,[198] corporal veno-occlusive dysfunction was identified in 62% of the cases and cavernous artery insufficiency in 70%. Abnormal venous drainage was confined to the proximal corpora in 91% of cases. Thus, blunt perineal trauma may result in a crush injury to the arterial inflow bed and to the cavernosal smooth muscle. Traumatic veno-occlusive dysfunction is theorized to be the consequence of focal intracavernous wound repair and fibrosis. Localized lesions in the distal internal pudendal, common penile, or cavernosal arteries secondary to blunt trauma may also be seen.

Both radical cystectomy and radical prostatectomy can result in arterial insufficiency and ED. Penile blood pressure was found to be significantly lower in men with ED following radical cystoprostatectomy for cancer.[226] The addition of urethrectomy appears to considerably increase the risk of postoperative ED.[227] In a retrospective review of arterial inflow following standard nerve-sparing radical retropubic prostatectomy, 103 patients with ED who claimed normal erectile function prior to surgery underwent duplex color Doppler assessment following intracavernosal PGE$_1$.[228] Vascular insufficiency was found in 51% of these patients.[228] Although the literature is sparse, it seems clear that injury to the pudendal and cavernsosal vessels is common even when an attempt to spare the neurovascular bundle is made.

Radiation therapy for pelvic malignancy frequently leads to erectile dysfunction, although the effects may not be evident immediately after therapy. Following three-dimensional conformal radiotherapy, Kaplan-Meier estimates of the potency preservation rates at 1, 2, and 3 years after treatment are 100%, 83%, and 63%, respectively.[232] Total radiation dose did not affect potency rates. In patients who receive brachytherapy, potency is preserved in 50% at 2 years.[233]

The mechanism of radiation-induced impotence is clearly related to both vascular and neuronal injury, but their relative contributions remain unclear. One important factor appears to be the dose of radiation delivered to the bulb of the urethra. Patients who receive less than 4000 cGy to 70% of the bulb are much more likely to preserve their potency.[234] Excessive radiation to the bulb of the urethra is also a factor in brachytherapy-induced ED.[235] Interestingly, radiation dose to the neurovascular bundles does not seem to correlate with potency rates.[236] Postradiation ED appears to respond well to sildenafil, indicating that NO production is preserved.[235] Experimentally, it has been shown that radiation-induced ED in irradiated rats is associated with a decrease in nitric oxide synthase–containing nerves in the penis.[237] In rat penis, increased production of endothelin-1 has also been observed following pelvic radiation.[187] Maximal intracavernous pressure induced with electrostimulation decreased significantly with increasing radiation doses. Response to papaverine was significantly decreased in rats who received 2000 cGy or more, indicating smooth muscle replacement and fibrosis.

Corporal Veno-occlusive Dysfunction. Excessive venous outflow due to insufficiency of the corporal veno-occlusive mechanism constitutes an important pathophysiologic mechanism. Corporal veno-occlusive dysfunction, despite its name, is not due to abnormalities of the draining veins. The smooth muscle content of penile veins is no different in patients with veno-occlusive dysfunction and patients with normal erectile function.[238] Furthermore, only about 50% of men are successfully treated by penile vein ligation.[239] Thus, erection depends on the relaxing capabilities of the smooth muscle and the tensile strength of the tunica albuginea. Any impairment in cavernosal relaxation or in tunical strength can alter the ability to trap blood in the corporal spaces.

Veno-occlusive dysfunction may be primary or secondary, resulting from several possible pathophysiologic processes: (1) abnormalities of the tunica albuginea, (2) degeneration or dysfunction of the cavernosal smooth muscle, causing inadequate smooth muscle relaxation or excessive smooth muscle contraction, (3) abnormal venous drainage of the corpora cavernosa or iatrogenic venous shunts from operative correction of priapism. In patients with veno-occlusive dysfunction, cavernosography shows that 100% of patients leak into the deep dorsal vein, 70% via the crural veins, 40% via the glans, and 30% via the corpus spongiosum.[240] About 15% leak through the deep dorsal vein only, 35% leak through two sites, 30% through three sites, and 15% through four or more sites.[240]

TUNICA ALBUGINEA. As mentioned previously, the human tunica albuginea is a complex bilayered structure that must withstand a large amount of force when erect. Although the tensile strength of the tunica is one of the strongest in the body, it is subject to trauma and rupture. The multilayered arrangement of tunical fascia, in which one layer sliding on the other may occlude venous outflow during erection, may be disrupted by trauma and the subsequent healing process.

Penile fracture can occur when the penis is erect. This fracture is probably due to excessive intracavernosal pressure when the tunica albuginea is thinned out during erection. In the United States and Europe, the mechanism is most often due to excessive force during sexual intercourse.[241] In other parts of the world, self-manipulation in an attempt to induce detumescence is a common mechanism.[242] Most cases involve only one corpus; urethral injury occurs in up to 38% of cases.[241]

After primary surgical repair of the injury, most patients resume normal erectile function.[241,243] Studies of patients with ED after repair of penile fracture showed that corporal veno-occlusive dysfunction was the most common hemodynamic abnormality (84%).[244] In most cases (80%), leakage from a focal site on the penile shaft was demonstrated. Cavernous artery insufficiency was found less often (37%). The site-specific hemodynamic abnormalities were found not only in patients with a classical penile fracture with swelling and ecchymosis but also in patients with more minor injuries from masturbation or accidents. Thus, the cavernosal dysfunction does not seem to be due to bleeding but to the disruption of tunical integrity itself.

Peyronie's disease is an inflammatory lesion of the tunica albuginea and underlying cavernosal tissue that is probably secondary to repetitive penile trauma in most cases.[245] Aberrantly stained collagen, disrupted elastic fibers, and fibrin deposition have been detected histochemically in most Peyronie's plaque tissue.[246] Deposition of fibrin in plaque tissue is consistent with the hypothesis that repetitive microvascular injury occurs in Peyronie's patients. The injury causes inflammation in the tunica, which is followed by scarring and penile curvature. Beta blockers can sometimes result in Peyronie's disease for reasons that are unclear. The penile plaque or scar is inelastic, resulting in penile curvature that may interfere with intromission.

Slightly more than 20% of men with Peyronie's disease have ED.[247] Veno-occlusive failure appears more important than arterial insufficiency in the etiology of Peyronie's associated ED. In one study, 36% of the impotent men with Peyronie's disease had abnormal arterial blood flow and 59% had evidence of veno-occlusive dysfunction.[248] Upregulation of transforming growth factor beta 1 (TGF-B1) has been demonstrated in human plaque tissue.[249] In a rat model of Peyronie's disease,[250] erectile function measured by pressure response to cavernosal nerve stimulation and acetylcholine injection was significantly lower in rats with plaques than in control rats. Inducible NOS, generally found in macrophages, was significantly higher and constitutive NOS was downregulated in the corpus cavernosum of rats with Peyronie-like plaques. These results may provide a biochemical basis for the vascular abnormalities frequently found in patients with Peyronies's disease.

CAVERNOSAL SMOOTH MUSCLE. Dysfunction of the cavernosal smooth muscle may be due to degenerative changes, inadequate relaxation, or excess contraction. Corporal veno-occlusive dysfunction is correlated with loss of intracavernosal smooth muscle[251] and increased corporal collagen content.[252] In patients with veno-occlusive failure, a significant correlation was noted between flow to maintain erection and percentage of smooth muscle fibers, but there was no correlation with elastic fibers or endothelial cells.[251] The higher the smooth muscle content, the lower the flow required to maintain erection, and the higher the outflow resistance, the lower the pressure decay.[252] Smooth muscle content, normally 42% to 50% of cavernosal tissue, may decrease to as low as 13% in some cases.[252] Thus, degenerative changes in the cavernosal smooth muscle are associated with impaired veno-occlusive function.

Aging. Animals suffer deterioration in erectile function with aging just as humans do. Light microscopy showed degenerative signs of elastic fibers of aged rat specimens and the tissue demonstrated increased stiffness and abnormal compliance.[253] The percent of smooth muscle fell from 28% in young rats to 18% in aged rats.[254] Smooth muscle apoptosis and collagen deposition may be due to induction of inducible nitric oxide synthase (iNOS) expression and subsequent peroxynitrite formation in aging rat penis.[255] Erectile tissue from aged rats, when precontracted with norepinephrine, required a threefold increase in papaverine concentration to achieve full relaxation.[253] A decreased expression of caveolin-1, an NO transport protein, may explain some of the decreased relaxation in aged cavernosal tissue.[254]

Relatively few studies have examined aging per se as a factor in human erectile dysfunction. In an electron microscopic study of penile tissue obtained during penile prosthesis implantation, ultrastructural changes in the intracavernous smooth muscle endothelial cells and an increase in extracellular matrix were seen in aging patients.[256] Cavernosal tissue from older patients showed an increased reactivity to phenylephrine in vitro.[257]

Diabetes Mellitus. Aside from its effect on nerve conduction and atherosclerosis, diabetes has direct effects on cavernosal smooth muscle. In the streptozotocin diabetic rat model, the corpora demonstrate reduced smooth muscle.[258] In diabetic human cavernosal tissue, reduced ability to convert L-arginine to L-citrulline has been demonstrated, leading to reduced NO production.[259] In rat cavernosal cells grown in a high-glucose environment, protein kinace-C2 was upregulated and NO production was markedly reduced.[260] Advanced glycation products such as glycosylated hemoglobin are more prevalent in erectile tissue from diabetic than from control animals and cause impaired neuronal and endothelial NO-mediated relaxation.[261] Aminoguanidine, an agent that prevents formation of glycation products, reversed this impairment of diabetic penile tissue.[261] Superoxide dismutase, an enzyme that breaks down superoxide anions, also improves smooth muscle relaxation in diabetic tissue.[262] These findings indicate that generation of certain toxic molecules in diabetic tissue may impair relaxation responses. Also, ET-1 and ET A receptor binding has been reported increased in diabetic rat cavernosal tissue.[263] Increased numbers of endothelin receptors may contribute to increased contractility of cavernosal smooth muscle in diabetes.

Ischemia. Animals with atherosclerotic ischemia have been shown to have diminished intracavernosal equilibrium pressure and increased cavernosal pressure decay.[264,265] These findings suggest that cavernosal ischemia results in dysfunction of cavernosal smooth muscle and increased cavernosal leakage. Ischemia seems to result in impairment of endothelium-dependent relaxation of cavernosal tissue to acetylcholine.[266] Electrical field stimulation–induced neurogenic relaxation and cavernosal NOS activity were also significantly reduced by ischemia.[266] Finally, the basal release of cavernosal constrictor eicosanoids, prostaglandin $F_{2\alpha}$ and thromboxane A2 was significantly increased in ischemic cavernosal muscle.[267] These findings suggest that impairment of endothelium-dependent and neurogenic relaxation by ischemia occurs secondary to disruption of NO formation, as does increased output of constrictor eicosanoids in cavernosal tissue. Ischemia did not affect contraction to exogenous norepinephrine but did cause a significant increase in electrical field stimulation–induced neurogenic contraction.[267] This seems to suggest that ischemia enhances the release of neuronal norepinephrine. Dysfunction of ischemic cavernosal tissue thus seems to be characterized by impaired endothelium-dependent relaxation, increased output of constrictor eicosanoids, and enhanced release of norepinephrine.

Anoxia and Hypoxia. In the flaccid state, subtunical oxygen tension is consistent with arterial blood; deep intracavernosal oxygen tension is much lower.[27] With nerve or pharmacologic stimulation, sinusoidal blood oxygen begins to rise significantly. These observations indicate that the cavernosal smooth muscle is physiologically exposed to a wide range of oxygen tension. Oxygen tension in cavernosal blood has been reported as decreased in patients with both arteriogenic and veno-occlusive ED and it is quite likely that oxygen tension regulates cavernosal smooth muscle tone.[268] Under anoxic conditions, spontaneous contractile activity was eliminated in cavernosal muscle strips and basal tissue tension was reduced to a minimum.[269] Neither field stimulation nor pharmacologic agents (ATP, bethanechol, isoproterenol) could induce additional relaxation and alpha-adrenergic agonists produced little or no contraction. In an in vitro study[270] of rabbit corpus cavernosum tissue strips under hypoxic conditions (pO_2 = 10 mm Hg), contractions elicited by norepinephrine, endothelin-1, or potassium were attenuated. The hypoxia-induced relaxation was not affected by the removal of the endothelium. Reoxygenation resulted in an immediate recovery of tone.

Oxygen tension also regulates the ability of cavernosal smooth muscle to relax in response to various stimuli. When human and rabbit corpus cavernosum tissue strips were exposed to arterial-like pO_2 levels in organ baths, they relaxed in response to the endothelium-dependent dilator acetylcholine and to electrical stimulation of the autonomic dilator nerves.[271] These nitric oxide–mediated responses were progressively inhibited as a function of decreasing pO_2 levels. Relaxation in response to exogenous nitric oxide was not impaired in a low pO_2 environment. These results indicate that nitric oxide production is impaired under conditions of low pO_2, thus promoting vasoconstriction.

In organ culture, basal production of prostanoids, whether relaxant or vasconstrictive, was decreased under hypoxic conditions.[272] Although this inhibition was reversible on reoxygenation, the recovery was delayed, requiring at least 2 hours of exposure to 21% oxygen to reestablish prostanoid production.[273] When pO_2 was increased to 100 mm Hg, prostaglandin levels increased rapidly.[274] PGE_2 levels were higher than $PGF_{2\alpha}$, which were higher than PGD_2 levels. Thromboxane A_2 was undetectable. These data suggest that the amount and type of prostanoids produced by cavernosal smooth muscle is exquisitely sensitive to cavernosal oxygen tension in the penis.

Oxygen tension may also play a role in regulating structure by promoting synthesis of TGF-B1, a factor that promotes fibrosis.[275] It has been suggested that the function of nocturnal penile tumescence is the periodic exposure of cavernosal smooth muscle to arterial levels of oxygen, thus maintaining proper function of the cavernosal smooth muscle.[275] Many of the physiologic effects of aging on erectile function may be mediated by hypoxia. Whether prophylactic use of pharmacotherapy to induce erection can prevent many of the changes in penile structure associated with aging is at present unknown.

Acidosis. Contraction of corpus cavernosum smooth muscle following transmural electrical stimulation of constrictor nerves or exposure to norepinephrine was depressed under acidic (pH 6.9) conditions; control was (pH 7.4).[276] Relaxation responses to acetylcholine and electrical stimulation in phenylephrine-contracted tissues were unaffected by acidosis. Acidosis appears to impair trabecular smooth muscle contractility. Since acidosis is an early complication of ischemic priapism, it may be one of the factors that perpetuate priapism. The duration of priapism appears to correlate with the degree of intracavernosal acidosis.[277]

PRIMARY VENOUS LEAKAGE. Primary venous leakage from the cavernous bodies is rare and may be due to one or more fistulae from the cavernous bodies to the glans penis or to congenitally abnormal veins connecting the interior of the cavernous body to superficial veins.[278] Much more common is persistence of an iatrogenic fistula or a shunt created to treat low-flow priapism.[279]

Priapism is a prolonged, painful, penile erection that is unrelated to sexual stimulation. In general, an erection that lasts longer than 4 hours is considered priapistic. There are two pathophysiologic mechanisms in priapism, resulting in the names low-flow and high-flow priapism.[280]

Low-flow priapism, a failure of the detumescence mechanism, is much more common than high-flow priapism. It may be due to obstruction or thrombosis of draining venules, which leads to prolonged erection, ischemia, hypoxia, acidosis, and cavernosal smooth muscle dysfunction.[281] It is most often a complication of intracavernosal self-injection of pharmacologic agents. Low-flow priapism may be due to sickle cell disease,[282] heparin,[283] or psychotropic drugs.[284] This form of priapism is usually quite painful because of tissue ischemia. The glans is usually not involved in low-flow priapism. Penile blood aspirated from cavernous spaces has low pO_2 values consistent with venous blood or lower. Treatment must be given urgently to prevent penile fibrosis and erectile dysfunction.

High-flow priapism is usually due to trauma to the cavernosal artery,[285] although on rare occasions it has been due to sickle cell disease[286] or arteriovenous fistula.[287] The hallmark of this type of priapism is an increase in arterial inflow in the setting of normal venous outflow. High-flow priapism is thought to induce some cavernosal muscle relaxation due to high oxygen tension and shear stress associated with high flow.[288] Aspirated penile blood is bright red and has pO_2 values consistent with arterial blood. This form of priapism is not usually painful because it is nonischemic. Treatment is not urgent and may in some cases be nonsurgical.[289]

Neurogenic Erectile Dysfunction. This type of ED is the inability to obtain or maintain penile erection due to neurologic lesion or impairment. A vast number of neurologic diseases can affect erectile ability and in this chapter we attempt to discuss them only as examples of broad pathophysiologic mechanisms rather than as individual entities. An outline of well-known diseases that affect potency is presented in Box 13-2. Neurologic disorders may act through blocking or disorganizing central control, thus affecting penile sensation or interfering with the motor input to the penile vasculature.

SUPRASPINAL CENTRAL CONTROL. The crucial roles in sexual function of central dopamine, oxytocin, nitric oxide, norepinephrine, and serotonin have been reviewed.[100-119] Penile erection is completely dependent on central nervous system control. Clinical experience

---

BOX 13-2 Outline of Neurogenic Erectile Dysfunction

I. Central
   A. Parkinson's disease
   B. Epilepsy
   C. Dopamine blockade
II. Spinal Cord
   A. Trauma
   B. Multiple sclerosis
   C. Spina bifida
III. Peripheral Nerves
   A. Degenerative
   B. Trauma
   C. Toxins

with spinal cord injury clearly demonstrates that with appropriate afferent stimulation, the isolated spinal cord is fully capable of subserving penile erection. Inhibition of spinal sexual responses is mediated by the neurotransmitter serotonin. At the same time, the central dopaminergic system promotes penile erection. It is likely that dopamine can trigger penile erection by acting on oxytocinergic neurons in the paraventricular nucleus of the hypothalamus and perhaps on the sacral parasympathetic nucleus in the spinal cord.[107]

Parkinson's disease is a disorder of the basal ganglia characterized by tremor, akinesia, and rigidity. Although it is associated with degeneration of the dopamine-containing cells in the substantia nigra, the cause remains unknown.[290] The incidence of decreased erectile ability in Parkinson's disease has been reported at about 80%.[291] Dopaminergic agents, such as apomorphine, have been reported to produce penile erection in patients with Parkinson's disease.[292] Based on animal studies, this agent produces erection by stimulating central D_2 dopamine receptors, which leads to release of oxytocin from the paraventricular nucleus of the hypothalamus. This is one of clearest examples of ED due to a specific central neurotransmitter deficit and of its reversal by pharmacologic replacement.

Epilepsy, especially the temporal lobe variety, confers an approximately fivefold increase in risk of erectile dysfunction.[293] Loss of libido is also common in epileptic patients. These problems may be due to a combination of the epilepsy itself, antiepileptic drugs, and social constraints. The prevalence of ED among men with temporal lobe epilepsy is about 50%.[294] Abnormal nocturnal tumescence characterized primarily by decreased rigidity has been reported in most men with temporal lobe epilepsy and ED.[293]

A variety of endocrine abnormalities have also been found in epileptic patients with ED, most commonly hypogonadotropic hypogonadism.[294] Hyperprolactinemia and has also been described. Estradiol levels were significantly increased, resulting in decreased androgen/estrogen ratios and luteinizing hormone–releasing hormone (LHRH) infusion was less effective in releasing luteinizing hormone.[295] Interestingly, some antiepileptic agents such as valproate have been shown to increase androgen levels in men with epilepsy.[296] Lamotrigine, a newer anticonvulsant, has been reported to improve ED in men with epilepsy.[297] Temporal lobe epilepsy appears to be an interesting example of a neurologic condition that affects sexual function primarily through an endocrine mechanism.

Antipsychotic agents are commonly associated with erectile dysfunction[298] as well as parkinsonian-like side effects.[299] The dopamine hypothesis of schizophrenia implicates an enhanced dopaminergic function in the pathophysiology of the disorder.[300] Since dopamine acts as a prolactin release–inhibiting factor, any dopamine-blocking agent is likely to induce hyperprolactinemia. It is not surprising that many antipsychotic agents block or deplete dopamine and also cause hyperprolactinemia.[299] Dopamine and its effects on prolactin release thus serve as a fundamental connection among Parkinson's disease, antiparkinsonian drugs, schizophrenia, antipsychotic agents, epilepsy, and erectile dysfunction. The first generation of antipsychotic agents were typically associated with hyperprolactinemia. However, a newer class of antipsychotics (e.g., clozapine, olanzapine, quetiapine, sertindole, and ziprasidone) are not associated with significant prolactin increase[301]. The new antipsychotics appear to spare dopamine blockade and have a much lower incidence of sexual side effects.

SPINAL CONTROL. Spinal cord lesions may profoundly affect sexual function by interrupting or impairing neuronal traffic between the higher centers and the periphery. Lesions may be congenital such as those from spinal dysraphism[302] or acquired such as those from spinal cord trauma[303] and multiple sclerosis.[304]

Spinal Dysraphism. Spinal dysraphism is a developmental anomaly caused by impaired closure of the neural tube that includes spina bifida and myelomeningocele.[302] Occasionally, one finds tethered cord syndrome manifested by a thickened fiium terminale and a low positioned conus medullaris.[303] The patients generally present with sensory and/or motor deficits of the lower extremities combined with incontinence. The pathophysiology of this condition appears to be congenital deficits in spinal nerve roots combined with variable degrees of suprasacral dysfunction due to tethering of the spinal cord.[304] Spinal cord tethering appears to cause ischemia-hypoxia of the lower spinal cord, leading to a form of intermittent vascular myelopathy.[305]

Now that these patients have markedly increased life expectancy, erectile dysfunction has become a recognized problem. Estimation of the prevalence of ED in spinal dysraphism from the literature is difficult. In cases of tethered cord syndrome, surgical untethering seems to have little effect, either positive or negative, on sexual dysfunction.[305] Oral sildenafil in a dose of 50 mg appears to produce improvement in 80% of cases of spinal dysraphism with ED.[302] This suggests that cavernosal function is preserved in these patients. The efficacy of sildenafil in low doses suggests some element of lower motor neuron deficit in these patients.

Spinal Cord Trauma. The spinal cord injured (SCI) patient allows one to determine the role of various parts of the spinal cord in male sexual function. In general, penile erection is viewed as a segmental reflex located in the sacral spinal cord and is controlled by higher CNS centers. However, Chapelle and colleagues observed different types of reflex erection following complete spinal transsection at different levels.[306] In patients with lesions above the T10–T12 segments, reflex erection involves both corpus cavernosum and corpus spongiosum. If the lesion is below T12, the erection involves only the corpus cavernosum. This suggests that the thoracolumbar sympathetic outflow is essential for control of the corpus spongiosum and glans penis.

Patients with lesions below T12 may have psychogenic erections; they may respond to visual stimuli or sexual fantasy. In contrast, men with complete lesions above T12 require penile stimulation to achieve erection and do not respond to visual stimuli. This suggests two neural pathways innervating the genitals. The primary one is the sacral parasympathetic outflow and the second pathway exists through the thoracolumbar sympathetic outflow.

In theory, the second thoracic-lumbar pathway can compensate for the loss of the sacral pathway in cases of low spinal lesions. In an animal study, 85% of paraplegic rats with lesions below the thoracolumbar outflow had erection following hypothalamic stimulation.[307] In male paraplegics, preservation of the sympathetic skin response correlates with preservation of psychogenic erection.[308]

Sildenafil in doses of 50 mg improves erectile function in spinal cord injured patients.[309] However, the efficacy of sildenafil depends on sparing of either sacral (S2–S4) or thoracolumbar (T10–L2) spinal segments.[309] As mentioned, the thoracolumbar or sympathetic outflow is important in mediating psychogenic erections in male patients with spinal cord injuries and must be intact in order for sildenafil to be effective. The thoracolumbar outflow can be shown to be intact clinically by preservation of testicular sensation. The efficacy of sildenafil in the low paraplegic and its dependence on the thoracolumbar outflow suggest that some sympathetic fibers may stimulate NO production or release in the penis.

Multiple Sclerosis. Multiple sclerosis (MS) is a demyelinating disease of the central nervous system, often producing abnormalities in sexual function and urinary control.[310,311] Although autoimmunity is though to play a role, the cause of the demyelination is basically unknown. Cortical and subcortical gray-matter plaques are common in MS and have been related to disease duration, clinical course, and the level of neurologic disability.[312] These plaques occur primarily in the thalamus, basal ganglia, and rolandic cortex. Cortical atrophy is also a common finding. Spinal cord MS plaques are characteristically located in the periphery of the spinal cord, occupy less that two vertebral segments, and occupy less than half the cross-sectional area of the cord.[313] Approximately 75% of men with multiple sclerosis complain of erectile dysfunction.[310] Ejaculatory dysfunction and reduced libido are also more common among male MS patients.[311] In general, there seems to be an increase in symptoms of sexual disability over time and a strong correlation with bladder symptoms and bladder hyperreflexia.[310,314]

Penile arterial inflow and venous outflow were found to be normal in male MS patients with ED.[314] Abnormal pudendal evoked potentials were found in 90% of MS patients with ED but were normal in MS patients without ED.[315] Erectile failure was invariably associated with pyramidal signs in the lower limbs.[316] These findings suggest that erectile dysfunction in multiple sclerosis is due to spinal lesions situated in the suprasacral spinal cord. Additional sexual disability may be due to cortical atrophy and depression, both common in MS. As in other neurologic conditions, papaverine intracorporeal injections produced satisfactory erections in the majority of MS patients with ED.[316]

PERIPHERAL AUTONOMIC MOTOR DEFICITS. Peripheral autonomic motor deficits may result from lesions of the cauda equina,[317] the anterior nerve root,[318] or the peripheral nerves subserving erection.[319] It is important to remember, however, that no direct test of penile autonomic motor neuropathy exists.

Cauda equina syndrome is characterized by lower extremity paralysis and pain (sciatica); erectile failure may not be noticed. However, midline compression of the cauda may affect only the perineal innervation without lower extremity signs. The most common causes of such a condition are midline prolapse of a disk and tumor.[317] The sudden onset of bladder areflexia, sphincter incompetence, and erectile failure combined with saddle anesthesia should be viewed as highly suspicious for midline cauda equina compression. In 50% of cases the L5–S1 disk is prolapsed and recovery of sexual function after laminectomy may be slow.

Nerve root compression is most often due to a herniated intervertebral disk, but it can be secondary to other causes such as tumor. Chronic nerve compression is thought to result in local ischemia and inflammatory changes with resultant decreased nerve conduction velocity.[320] Impotence has been reported in association with herniated disk but the literature is sparse. Although reversal of impotence has been reported after surgery,[318] in many cases the impotence is psychogenic or related to chronic pain.

Polyneuropathy is often accompanied by autonomic dysfunction and can cause voiding abnormalities as well as ED.[321] In 341 patients who reported impotence, polyneuropathy was found in about 20%.[319] Some autonomic neuropathies are of acute onset, but most are chronic and of gradual onset. Conditions that primarily affect small nerve fibers or cause acute demyelination of small myelinated fibers are most likely to cause autonomic neuropathy. Examples include acute dysautonomia, familial and primary amyloidosis, Guillain-Barré syndrome, diabetes mellitus, porphyria, and Chagas' disease.

Aging. There is relatively little information on aging per se as a factor in neurogenic impotence. In a rat model the number of NOS-containing nerve fibers was significantly less in the old rats than in young and middle-aged rats.[322] The number of apomorphine-induced erections were significantly fewer and the response to intracavernous papaverine was significantly less in the old rats than in the young.[322] In contrast, vasoactive intestinal polypeptide (VIP) levels and distribution in the rat penis were not noted to deteriorate with aging.[323] Muscle weakness of the perineal floor may also be a factor in aging-associated ED.[324]

Diabetic Neuropathy. Diabetic neuropathy, although not the only cause of ED in diabetics, is clearly a major component.[325] Diabetic neuropathies include both focal neuropathies and diffuse polyneuropathy, which is the most common form. Despite intensive investigation, the pathophysiology of diabetic polyneuropathy is still unclear.[326] Microvascular disease appears to lead to autonomic fiber loss. There is impairment in the elaboration of trophic factors critical for peripheral nerves and their ganglia. In addition, diabetic nerves fail to regenerate as effectively as nondiabetic nerves.[326] As mentioned previously, glycosylated hemoglobin is more prevalent in erectile tissue from diabetic than in control animals and causes impaired neuronal NO-mediated relaxation.[263] Aminoguanidine, an agent that prevents formation of glycation products, reversed impaired cavernosal relaxation of diabetic penile tissue.[263]

Whatever the etiology, neuropathy reduces erectile response to visual stimulation in diabetics, whether they are insulin dependent or not.[325] Neurogenic relaxation of cavernosal smooth muscle in diabetic men is significantly reduced.[214] Acetylcholine synthesis and release were significantly reduced in the cavernosal tissue from diabetic patients compared to that from nondiabetic patients.[327] The impairment in acetylcholine synthesis worsened with the duration of diabetes. No differences in the parameters measured were found between insulin-dependent and noninsulin-dependent diabetic patients. A marked reduction was seen in VIP-like immunoreactivity in nerves associated with the cavernous smooth muscle, while acetylcholinesterase-positive stains were reduced in diabetic patients.[328] The noradrenaline content of the corpus cavernosum from diabetic patients was significantly lower than that of a non-neuropathic group.[328] These results indicate a marked effect on neuronal function in the penile tissues of diabetic patients.

Iatrogenic Nerve Trauma. Iatrogenic nerve trauma, generally due to surgery, constitutes an important cause of neurogenic ED. Trauma to the cavernous nerves may occur during radical prostatectomy,[329] radical cystoprostatectomy,[330] prectomy,[331] and transurethral prostatectomy (TURP).[332] The incidence of erectile dysfunction in men undergoing TURP has been estimated as 8%,[332] but incidence up to 50% has been reported.[333] The risk of ED following TURP is increased for prostate resection of less than 10 gm,[332] as is perforation of the capsule near the neurovascular bundle.[334] In one study the risk of ED was 28% if the capsule was perforated and 10% if it was not.[335] It seems likely that ED following TURP is related to heat transferred outside the prostatic capsule that can damage the neurovascular bundle.

In 1974, the nerve-sparing prostatectomy was developed in an attempt to preserve the neurovascular bundles near the prostate and thus preserve potency.[329] The technique has led to reduced urinary incontinence as well.[329] However, the assumption that postradical prostatectomy erectile dysfunction is due primarily to nerve trauma must be questioned. Most studies do not provide objective evidence of erectile function prior to surgery. In one recent study where preoperative studies were done,[331] only 17% of patients were found to have normal erectile function before surgery. After nerve-sparing radical retropubic prostatectomy, 63% of these patients had preserved erectile function. In those who became impotent, 60% were due to neurogenic factors and 40% were due to vascular factors. Cavernosal artery insufficiency after radical prostatectomy has been reported in approximately 40% of patients.[336] New onset of veno-occlusive dysfunction after radical prostatectomy has also been reported.[337] Thus, improved potency rates after "nerve-sparing" radical prostatectomy may be due to vascular sparing as well as to nerve sparing accomplished by the technique.

It is important to remember that the autonomic nerves lateral to the prostate are preganglionic nerves. They synapse with ganglia that lie close to the corpora cavernosa and these postganglionic nerves release NO and other neurotransmitters.[338] Thus, cutting the preganglionic fibers does not necessarily completely denervate the cavernosal smooth muscle. This may explain why bilateral cavernosal neurotomy in rats resulted in a moderate to severe deficit in erectile function but some animals were still able to obtain erection.[339] Bilateral cavernosal nerve section produced a marked decrease in electrical activity of cavernosal smooth muscle.[340] After bilateral cavernosal neurotomy in rats, NOS-positive nerve fibers were significantly decreased at 3 weeks and had not recovered at 6 months.[341] No erectile response could be elicited by pelvic nerve stimulation. After unilateral neurotomy, the NOS-positive nerve fibers were similarly decreased on the side of the neurotomy at 3 weeks, but by 6 months the number had increased significantly and approximated the level on the contralateral side.[341] Thus, unilateral nerve sparing appears to be sufficient to preserve erectile function.

Since several authors have found that stimulation of the hypogastric nerve can produce erection,[28,342,343] one might wonder what the effect of sympathectomy or cutting the hypogastric nerve might be on erection. Section of the hypogastric nerve in animals seems to have no effect on erection[339] and sympathectomy in humans seems to have no significant effect on potency.[344] However, when erection is induced by hypothalamic stimulation in animals, surgical or chemical sympathectomy seems to block these erections.[28] Thus, there is some experimental evidence that centrally mediated erections use sympathetic nerve pathways. However, because of alternative parasympathetic pathways, sympathectomy alone is insufficient to reduce potency.

SENSORY NERVE DEFICITS. The dorsal nerve of the penis is critical for sexual function.[30] It innervates the shaft of the penis and the glans penis, which provides most of the sensory input for reflex erection.[345] Decreased sensibility of the penis may be the primary etiology for erectile dysfunction.[346]

Somatic innervation of the penis may be tested by biothesiometry (vibration),[347] electrical stimulation,[348] sympathetic skin response,[349] and thermal sensitivity testing.[350] Electrical stimulation of the dorsal nerve can be used to determine nerve conduction velocity, bulbocavernosus reflex latency, or somatosensory latency. These various testing methods tend to correlate poorly because they stimulate different receptors and axonal populations.[351,352] In a direct comparison of thermal sensitivity and electrophysiologic testing, thermal sensitivity correlated much better with clinical assessment of erectile dysfunction.[353] This may be due to the fact that thermal testing stimulates the smaller unmyelinated sensory nerve fibers of the penis, whereas electrophysiologic testing stimulates the larger myelinated fibers.

Aging. Penile threshold to electrical and vibratory stimulation increases with age.[354–356] This phenomenon is seen in other parts of the sensory nervous system with aging.[357] In the penis there is a curvilinear rather than a linear relationship between penile threshold and aging. Sensory threshold rises with increasing slope as age increases.[354] Mean sensory thresholds occur at about 45 years of age and reach 2 standard deviations higher at about age 68.

Sexual Dysfunction. Sensory thresholds in men with ED are consistently higher than in age-matched controls.[358,359] Interestingly, men suffering from premature ejaculation as an isolated complaint were not found to have an abnormal penile sensory threshold.[359]

Effect of Erection. There is a significant elevation in threshold after intracavernous papaverine-induced erection and this elevation is particularly pronounced in men with ED.[358] There is thus a paradoxical decrease in penile sensitivity in all individuals during penile erection. Since elevation of skin temperature has been shown to decrease sensitivity to vibration,[360] this may be a possible mechanism for this phenomenon.

Testosterone Level. Untreated hypogonadal men were found to have a lower vibrotactile threshold and were slightly more sensitive to touch than were men with higher levels of androgen.[361] Testosterone replacement seemed to normalize the threshold values.

Diabetes Mellitus. Diabetes mellitus tends to affect small-diameter myelinated and unmyelinated sensory nerve fibers that are best assessed with thermal testing.[353,362] Sexually dysfunctional diabetic men have a higher threshold to vibration in the penis than potent diabetic men.[356,363] In a study comparing 35 diabetic patients with ED and 25 normal male subjects, cold threshold and warm threshold were much more sensitive parameters than vibration or standard electrophysiologic tests.[353]

Female Sexual Dysfunction

In contrast to the male, the pathophysiology of female sexual dysfunction is not easily categorized as vasculogenic, neurologic, or hormonal. Rather, it appears to involve multidimensional biologic, psychological, and interpersonal aspects. The prevalence of female sexual dysfunction is difficult to estimate because relatively few studies have been done in community settings. Female sexual dysfunction has been estimated to affect 20% to 50% of women and to increase in incidence with age.[364,365] In one study a standardized sexual function questionnaire was administered to 329 healthy women, aged 18 to 73 years. About 50% reported sexual intercourse at least weekly and about 28% reported no regular sexual activity.[365] Among these women, difficulty in achieving orgasm was reported by 15%, lack of lubrication by 14%, and dyspareunia by 11%. In a survey of about 3000 men and women, 43% of women and 31% of men complained of sexual dissatisfaction that lasted several months.[176] Sexual dysfunction in women correlated with age and with educational level.[176] The frequency of these sexual problems increases as menopause approaches and reaches a peak in the postmenopausal years.[176,365]

Classification and Definition of Female Sexual Dysfunction

Female sexual dysfunction has been classified into the four major categories of sexual desire disorders, sexual arousal disorders, orgasmic disorders, and sexual pain disorders.[366-369] Sexual desire disorders are subclassified into hypoactive sexual desire disorders and sexual aversion disorders. *Hypoactive sexual desire disorder* is the persistent or recurrent lack of sexual fantasies and thoughts or desire for sexual activity. *Sexual aversion disorder* is a persistent or recurrent fear of, aversion to, and avoidance of sexual contact with a partner. *Sexual arousal disorder* is defined as the persistent or recurrent inability to achieve or maintain sexual excitement. This may be expressed as lack of excitement, lack of lubrication, lack of vaginal and clitoral engorgement, or lack of expression of other somatic responses. *Orgasmic disorder* is the persistent or recurrent inability to achieve orgasm with sexual stimulation and arousal. *Sexual pain disorders* are subclassified into dyspareunia, vaginismus, and other sexual pain disorders. *Dyspareunia* is recurrent or persistent genital pain during sexual intercourse. *Vaginismus* is the recurrent or persistent involuntary spasm of outer vaginal musculature, which makes vaginal penetration difficult. Other sexual pain disorders include noncoital sexual pain, which is defined as recurrent or persistent genital pain caused by noncoital sexual stimulation. All types of sexual desire disorder are likely to lead to personal distress. Each category of female sexual dysfunction is divided to subtypes of chronic versus acquired, generalized versus situational, and organic versus psychogenic.

Pathophysiology

Role of Hormones

The role of hormones in female sexual function and dysfunction has long been discussed.[156,370,371] Sex hormones are produced primarily in the ovary; the exception is androgens, which are also made in the adrenal gland. Hormonally induced female sexual dysfunction may develop as a result of hypothalamic–pituitary axis dysfunction, surgical removal of the ovaries, natural menopause, premature ovarian failure, and long-term use of the birth control pill. Decline in circulating levels of estrogen is a major physiologic change during natural menopause.[370-372] The most common symptoms of hormonal dysfunction are decreased desire and libido, lack of vaginal lubrication, and inability to achieve sexual arousal.[372] Between 8% and 30% of menopausal women complain of dyspareunia. Many others experience marked decrease in vaginal sensation, reduced vaginal and clitoral engorgement, and decreased vaginal elongation during intercourse.

A regulatory role for estrogen in tissue structure has long been suspected. Estrogen may directly modulate physiologic smooth muscle cell growth,[373,374] inhibit mitogen-induced proliferation of vascular smooth muscle cells,[374] and inhibit the deposition of extracellular matrix proteins such as collagen.[374] These observations support the important role of estrogen in maintaining the normal physiology and structure of vascular structures such as the vagina and clitoris.

Effect of Estrogen Withdrawal. Although the precise mechanisms are unclear, estrogens appear to support the vasculature and epithelial lining of the female genital organs. Estrogen receptors have been identified in the vaginal walls of premenopausal but estrogen receptor beta was absent from the vaginal walls of postmenopausal women.[375] Studies in rats have shown that estrogen deprivation resulted in overall vaginal atrophy, diffuse intramural collagen accumulation, and thickening of the perivascular wall.[159] In rabbits oophorectomy caused significantly decreased vaginal and clitoral blood flow.[158] Impairment of vaginal and clitoral blood flow in the estrogen-deprived animals was associated with atrophic changes in the vaginal mucosal layer, decreased vaginal submucosal microvasculature, and loss of clitoral cavernosal smooth muscle. These effects could be reversed with estrogen replacement.[160] In women, vaginal blood flow appears to be strongly influenced by hormonal status. Estrogen appears to be capable of increasing vaginal blood flow in normal women.[376] Menopausal women have decreased vaginal blood flow[162] but intravenous administration of conjugated estrogen increases vaginal blood flow.[163]

Androgens also have an important role in female sexuality, especially in sexual desire and arousability.[377] The circulating level of androgens diminishes with menopause but to a much lesser extent than estrogen diminishes. Accumulating evidence indicates that many women with low circulating bioavailable testosterone complain of low libido, persistent fatigue, and a diminished sense of well-being.[165] Testosterone therapy appears to be effective in reversing these symptoms.[165] Whether the effects of testosterone are mediated via the androgen receptor or as a consequence of metabolism to estrogen is not known.

In a recent study comparing women with low sex drive and normal women, free testosterone was found to be significantly lower in the patients than in the control women.[378] In the control group, average daily sexual thoughts correlated positively with total testosterone, free testosterone, and free 5-dihydroxytestosterone. In both groups, average coital frequency correlated with free testosterone.[378] In contrast, some have reported no correlation between estrogen or androgen levels and sexual drive in women.[379] In a study of replacement therapy after oophorectomy, it was found that women who received both estrogen and androgen replacement reported higher rates of sexual desire, sexual arousal, and numbers of fantasies than those who were either given estrogen alone or who were untreated.[380] Androgens may be critical for the maintenance of libido in both premenopausal and postmenopausal women.

Psychological Factors

In women, psychological factors (e.g., history of sexual abuse, depression, anxiety, obsessive-compulsive disorders), sociocultural issues (e.g., beliefs regarding sexual activity), and interpersonal issues (e.g., partner availability, partner function, relationship with partner, communication with partner) affect sexual function in all age groups.[364,365] With aging may come additional psychological stresses, particularly loss of fertility, interruption of menstrual cycle, and the start of postmenstrual changes. Recently, however, there has been a large cultural shift with respect to negative implications of aging and menopause. The "baby-boom" generation, in contrast to its mothers and grandmothers, believe that aging need not necessarily cause asexuality, poor health, and loss of productivity.

Depression and Drugs. Female sexual dysfunction as a side of effect of psychiatric drugs is fairly common.[381,382] It is thought that heterocyclic antidepressants, monoamine oxidase inhibitors, benzodiazepines, and neuroleptics interfere with the adrenergic, cholinergic, and serotonergic pathways in women, which leads to sexual dysfunction. In particular, evidence seems to point to blockade or antagonism of adrenergic mechanisms that underlie normal orgasm.[383] Psychotropic drugs that have been reported to inhibit female orgasm include antipsychotic agents (e.g., thioridazine, trifluoperazine, and fluphenazine), the combination drug perphenazine-amitriptyline, antidepressants (e.g., phenelzine, isocarboxazid, tranylcypromine, amoxapine, clomipramine, imipramine, nortriptyline, and desipramine), and anxiolytic agents (e.g., diazepam, flurazepam, and alprazolam). Bupropion and nefazodone are exceptional in having a low rate of sexual side effects.[383]

Management of drug-induced female anorgasmia includes discontinuing the offending drug, reducing the dose, and substituting another class of agent. The use of bethanechol chloride and cyproheptadine has been reported as successful in resolving anorgasmia in female patients receiving antidepressants.[384] In recent years, however, it has been shown that sexual dysfunction in patients taking antidepressants may be, in large, related to the depression itself.[385] It is now believed that when a woman is experiencing intense conflict and depression, all phases of sexual response, in particular the ability to achieve orgasm, may be inhibited.

Neurologic Factors

Diseases of the central and peripheral nervous system can lead to female sexual dysfunction.

Spinal cord injury in women may be associated with orgasmic or lubrication failure.[386] Arousal may be secondary to audiovisual stimuli, fantasy, or genital stimulation. In women with complete suprasacral spinal cord injury above T6, audiovisual stimuli fail to cause a change in vaginal pulse amplitude.[387] However, in women with preservation of sensory function in T11–L2 dermatomes, psychogenically mediated genital vasocongestion is possible.[388] This suggests that, as in the male, the sympathetic outflow is an important pathway for psychogenic genital response in women.

Women with complete or incomplete suprasacral injury can achieve reflex genital response by manual stimulation but not when there is involvement of the sacral segments.[389] Orgasm is less likely in women with spinal cord injury and correlates poorly with the type of injury.[388]

Diabetes mellitus, which is known to cause erectile dysfunction in men, may interfere with female sexual function.[390–393] This issue, however, has been poorly investigated and it is unclear how diabetes affects female sexual function.[394] Jensen studied the sexual function of 80 diabetic women and 40 nondiabetic women.[393] A significantly larger number of diabetic women (11%) than nondiabetic women (7.5%) complained of lack of orgasm. A much greater number of diabetic women (24%) nondiabetic women (8%) reported difficulty in achieving vaginal lubrication. In the diabetic group, the incidence of sexual dysfunction was much greater in women with peripheral neuropathy (44%) than in diabetic women without neuropathy. The association of peripheral neuropathy and sexual dysfunciton in diabetic women has been noted by others.[395] Other studies have reported increased problems with vaginal lubrication in diabetic women.[392,396] Using vaginal photoplethysmographic measures of capillary engorgement, Wincze and colleagues showed that diabetic women demonstrated significantly less physiological arousal to erotic stimuli than controls, even though their subjective responses were comparable.[397]

Peripheral neuropathy is a common cause of erectile dysfunction but there is little literature about its effect on females. Clitoral neuropathy has been observed to cause sexual dysfunction.[398] In a test of female genital pressure and touch sensation, 32 neurologically intact women and 5 neurologically impaired women were tested.[399] A clear association was found between reduced vulvar sensitivity to pressure or touch and estrogen deficiency, sexual dysfunction, and neurologic impairment. Postmenopausal and hypoestrogenic women had significantly reduced sensitivity to pressure or touch compared with premenopausal and normoestrogenic women, respectively.

Vascular Factors

Vascular risk factors such as hypertension, diabetes, hypercholesterolemia, and smoking are associated with erectile dysfunction in men. The role of vasculopathy in female sexual dysfunction, however, has not been thoroughly investigated. The first phase of the female sexual response—vaginal lubrication, wall engorgement, and increased clitoral length and diameter—are all vascular responses. In the face of vascular insufficiency, symptoms such as delayed vaginal engorgement, diminished vaginal lubrication, and discomfort with intercourse may occur.[400] Diminished vaginal or clitoral arterial blood flow may result from atherosclerotic or nonatherosclerotic vascular disease due to pelvic or perineal trauma.[400]

Park and colleagues showed that vaginal and clitoral blood flow following electrical stimulation of the pelvic nerve were significantly less in rabbits with iliac atherosclerosis than in healthy animals.[133] In an animal model, pelvic atherosclerosis is associated with marked clitoral fibrosis and loss of cavernosal smooth muscle.[401] Histologic staining of ischemic vaginal and clitoral tissues from animals revealed diffuse fibrosis in both organs. Vascular supply to the vagina and clitoris appear to depend on estrogen support. In oophorectomized rabbits, nerve stimulation–induced peak vaginal and clitoral intracavernosal blood flow was significantly reduced.[158] Histologically, the percentage of clitoral cavernosal smooth muscle in the oophorectomized rabbits was significantly lower than in control animals. These observations support the existence of atherosclerosis-induced vasculogenic female sexual dysfunction, but the clinical significance remains to be determined.

In a study on the impact of arterial occlusive disease and chronic ischemia on vaginal and clitoral structure, human clitoral tissue from cadavers demonstrated that cardiovascular disease is associated with severe clitoral cavernosal fibrosis.[402] In this study, the percentage of clitoral cavernosal smooth muscle was significantly decreased in the presence of a cardiovascular disease–related mortality.

The use of vasodilating agents such as sildenafil[403,404] and alprostadil[405] appear to have significant effects in women. Alprostadil gel increases clitoral blood flow and reproduces many of the pleasurable sensations of sexual stimulation.[404]

In a pilot study of 48 women with arousal disorder, sildenafil induced significant improvement in poststimulation physiologic measurements including vaginal blood flow and lubrication.[403] Subjective complaints such as difficulty achieving orgasm and dyspareunia also improved significantly following 6 weeks home use of sildenafil. Similar results were obtained in a double-blind, placebo-controlled trial of sildenafil that examined women's subjective sexual responses.[404] Both arousal and orgasm improved with respect to placebo. The frequency of sexual fantasies and of sexual intercourse increased in the women treated with sildenafil. These observations suggest that, although women's sexual response is highly complex, intervention at only one level can affect many other aspects of sexual function.

REFERENCES

1. Stone HM, Stone A: A Marriage Manual: A Practical Guide-Book to Sex and Marriage. New York, Simon and Schuster, 1935, p 187.
2. Michal V, Kramar R, Bartak V: Femoro–pudendal bypass in the treatment of sexual impotence. J Cardiovasc Surg (Torino) 15(3):356–359, 1974.
3. Basson R, Berman J, Burnett A, et al: Report of the international consensus development conference on female sexual dysfunction: Definitions and classifications. J Urol 163(3):888–893, 2000.
4. Vardi Y, Siroky MB: A canine model for hemodynamic study of isolated corpus cavernosum. J Urol 138(3):663–666, 1987.
5. Loeb H: Harnrohrencapacitat und Tripperspritzen. Minch Med Wschr 46:1016–1019, 1899.
6. Knoll LD, Abrams JH: Application of nocturnal electrobioimpedance volumetric assessment: A feasibility study in men without erectile dysfunction. J Urol 161(4):1137–1140, 1999.
7. Bitsch M, Kromann-Andersen B, Schou J, Sjontoft E: The elasticity and the tensile strength of tunica albuginea of the corpora cavernosa. J Urol 143(3):642–645, 1990.
8. Hsu GL, Brock G, Martinez-Pineiro L, et al: Anatomy and strength of the tunica albuginea: Its relevance to penile prosthesis extrusion. J Urol 151(5):1205–1208, 1994.
9. Brock G, Hsu GL, Nunes L, et al: The anatomy of the tunica albuginea in the normal penis and Peyronie's disease. J Urol 157(1):276–281, 1997.
10. Fournier GR Jr, Juenemann KP, Lue TF, Tanagho EA: Mechanisms of venous occlusion during canine penile erection: An anatomic demonstration. J Urol 137(1):163–167, 1987.
11. Goldstein AM, Padma-Nathan H: The microarchitecture of the intracavernosal smooth muscle and the cavernosal fibrous skeleton. J Urol 144(5):1144–1146, 1990.
12. Nehra A, Azadzoi KM, Moreland RB, et al: Cavernosal expandability is an erectile tissue mechanical property which predicts trabecular histology in an animal model of vasculogenic erectile dysfunction. J Urol 159(6):2229–2236, 1998.
13. Vardi Y, Siroky MB: Hemodynamics of pelvic nerve induced erection in a canine model. I. Pressure and flow. J Urol 144(3):794–797, 1990.

14. Wespes E, Nogueira MC, Herbaut AG, et al: Role of the bulbocavernosus muscles on the mechanism of human erection. Eur Urol 18(1):45–48, 1990.
15. Breza J, Aboseif SR, Orvis BR, et al: Detailed anatomy of penile neurovascular structures: Surgical significance. J Urol 141(2):437–443, 1989.
16. Goldstein I: Overview of types and results of vascular surgical procedures for impotence. Cardiovasc Intervent Radiol 11(4):240–244, 1988.
17. Banya Y, Ushiki T, Takagane H, et al: Two circulatory routes within the human corpus cavernosum penis: A scanning electron microscopic study of corrosion casts. J Urol 142(3):879–883, 1989.
18. Vardi Y, Siroky MB: Hemodynamics of pelvic nerve induced erection in a canine model. II. Cavernosal inflow and occlusion. J Urol 149(4):910–914, 1993.
19. Moscovici J, Galinier P, Hammoudi S, et al: Contribution to the study of the venous vasculature of the penis. Surg Radiol Anat 21(3):193–199, 1999.
20. Rampin O, Bernabe J, Giuliano F: Spinal control of penile erection. World J Urol 15:2–13, 1997.
21. Paick JS, Donatucci CF, Lue TF: Anatomy of cavernous nerves distal to prostate: Microdissection study in adult male cadavers. Urology 42(2):145–149, 1993.
22. Lue TF, Takamura T, Schmidt RA, et al: Hemodynamics of erection in the monkey. J Urol 130(6):1237–1241, 1983.
23. Andersson PO, Bjornberg J, Bloom SR, Mellander S: Vasoactive intestinal polypeptide in relation to penile erection in the cat evoked by pelvic and hypogastric nerve stimulation. J Urol 138(2):419–422, 1987.
24. Brindley GS, Polkey CE, Rushton DN, Cardozo L: Sacral anterior root stimulators for bladder control in paraplegia: The first 50 cases. J Neurol Neurosurg Psychiatry 49(10):1104–1114, 1986.
25. Giuliano F, Facchinetti P, Bernabe J, et al: Evidence of sympathetic fibers in the male rat pelvic nerve by gross anatomy, retrograde labeling and high resolution autoradiographic study. Int J Impot Res 9(4):179–185, 1997.
26. Walsh PC, Donker PJ: Impotence following radical prostatectomy: Insight into etiology and prevention. J Urol 128(3):492–497, 1982.
27. Giuliano F, Rampin O, Bernabe J, Rousseau JP: Neural control of penile erection in the rat. J Auton Nerv Syst 55(1–2):36–44, 1995.
28. Giuliano F, Bernabe J, Brown K, et al: Erectile response to hypothalamic stimulation in rats: Role of peripheral nerves. Am J Physiol 273(6 pt 2):R1990–R1997, 1997.
29. Halata Z, Munger BL: The neuroanatomical basis for the protopathic sensibility of the human glans penis. Brain Res 371(2):205–230, 1986.
30. Yang CC, Bradley WE: Peripheral distribution of the human dorsal nerve of the penis. J Urol 159(6):1912–1916, 1998.
31. Kollberg S, Petersen I, Stener I: Preliminary results of an electromyographic study of ejaculation. Acta Chir Scand 123:478–483, 1962.
32. Hedlund P, Ny L, Alm P, Andesson KE: Cholinergic nerves in human corpus cavernosum and spongiosum contain nitric oxide synthase and heme oxygenase. J Urol 164(3 pt 1):868–875, 2000.
33. Stief CG, Benard F, Bosch R, et al: Calcitonin gene-related peptide: Possibly neurotransmitter contributes to penile erection in monkeys. Urology 41(4):397–401, 1993.
34. Andersson KE, Hedlund P, Alm P: Sympathetic pathways and adrenergic innervation of the penis. Int J Imp Res 12:S5–S12, 2000.
35. Mizusawa H, Hedlund P, Hakansson A, et al: Morphological and functional in vitro and in vivo characterization of the mouse corpus cavernosum. Br J Pharmacol 132(6):1333–1341, 2001.
36. Hauser-Kronberger C, Hacker GW, Graf AH, et al: Neuropeptides in the human penis: An immunohistochemical study. J Androl 15(6):510–520, 1994.
37. Cocchia D, Rende M, Toesca A, et al: Immunohistochemical study of neuropeptide Y-containing nerve fibers in the human clitoris and penis. Cell Biol Int Rep 14(10):865–875, 190.
38. O'Connell HE, Hutson JM, Anderson CR, Plenter RJ: Anatomical relationship between urethra and clitoris. J Urol 159(6):1892–1897, 1998.
39. Rees MA, O'Connell HE, Plenter RJ, Hutson JM: The suspensory ligament of the clitoris: Connective supports of the erectile tissues of the female urogenital region. Clin Anat 13(6):397–403, 2000.
40. Ingelman-Sundberg A: The anterior vaginal wall as an organ for the transmission of active forces to the urethra and the clitoris. Int Urogynecol J Pelvic Floor Dysfunct 8(1):50–51, 1997.
41. Toesca A, Stolfi VM, Cocchia D: Immunohistochemical study of the corpora cavernosa of the human clitoris. J Anat 188(pt 3):513–520, 1996.
42. Baskin LS, Erol A, Li YW, et al: Anatomical studies of the human clitoris. J Urol 162(3 pt 2):1015–1020, 1999.
43. Burnett AL, Calvin DC, Silver RI, et al: Immunohistochemical description of nitric oxide synthase isoforms in human clitoris. J Urol 158(1):75–78, 1997.
44. Hauser-Kronberger C, Cheung A, Hacker GW, et al: Peptidergic innervation of the human clitoris. Peptides 20(5):539–543, 1999.
45. van Turnhout AA, Hage JJ, van Diest PJ: The female corpus spongiosum revisited. Acta Obstet Gynecol Scand 74(10):767–771, 1995.
46. Shabsigh A, Buttyan R, Burchardt T, et al: The microvascular architecture of the rat vagina revealed by image analysis of vascular corrosion casts. Int J Impot Res 11 (suppl 1):S23–S30, 1999.
47. Peters LC, Kristal MB, Komisaruk BR: Sensory innervation of the external and internal genitalia of the female rat. Brain Res 408(1–2):199–204, 1987.
48. Traurig H, Saria A, Lambeck F: Substance P in primary afferent neurons of the female rat reproductive system. Naunyn Schmeidebergs Arch Pharmacol 326(4):343–346, 1984.
49. Lakomy M, Kaleczyc J, Majewski M, Sienkiewicz W: Peptidergic innervation of the bovine vagina and uterus. Acta Histochem 97(1):53–66, 1995.
50. Berman JR, McCarthy MM, Kyprianou N: Effect of estrogen withdrawal on nitric oxide synthase expression and apoptosis in the rat vagina. Urology 51(4):650–656, 1998.
51. Hoyle CH, Stones RW, Robson T, et al: Innervation of vasculature and microvasculature of the human vagina by NOS and neuropeptide-containing nerves. J Anat 188(pt 3):633–644, 1996.
52. Blank MA, Gu J, Allen JM, et al: The regional distribution of NPY-, PHM-, and VIP-containing nerves in the human female genital tract. Int J Fertil 31(3):218–222, 1986.
53. Dorr LD, Brody MJ: Hemodynamic mechanisms of erection in the canine penis. Am J Physiol 213(6):1526–1531, 1967.
54. Andersson PO, Bloom SR, Mellander S: Haemodynamics of pelvic nerve induced erection in the dog: Possible mediation by vasoactive intestinal polypeptide. J Physiol 350:209–224, 1984.

55. Vardi Y, Siroky MB: A canine model for hemodynamic study of isolated corpus cavernosum. J Urol 138(3):663–666, 1987.
56. Carati CJ, Creed KE, Keogh EJ: Vascular changes during penile erection in the dog. J Physiol 400:75–88, 1988.
57. Conti G: L'érection du pénis humaine et ses bases morphologico-vasculaires. Res Acta Anat 14:217–262, 1952.
58. Benson GS, McConnell J, Schmidt WA: Penile polsters: Functional structures or atherosclerotic changes? J Urol 125:800–803, 1981.
59. Shirai M, Ishii N: Hemodynamics of erection in man. Arch Androl 6:27–32, 1981.
60. Valji K, Bookstein JJ: The veno-occlusive mechanism of the canine corpus cavernosum: Angiographic and pharmacologic studies. J Urol 138:1467–1470, 1987.
61. Fournier GR, Junemann K-P, Lue TF, Tanagho EA: Mechanisms of venous occlusion during canine penile erection: An anatomic demonstration. J Urol 137:163–167, 1987.
62. Wagner G, Gerstenberg T, Levin RJ: Electrical activity of corpus cavernosum during flaccidity and erection of the human penis: A new diagnostic tool? J Urol 142:723–725, 1989.
63. Hedlund P, Alm P, Andersson KE: NO synthase in cholinergic nerves and NO-induced relaxation in the rat isolated corpus cavernosum. Br J Pharmacol 127(2):349–360, 1999.
64. Saenz de Tejada I, Blanco R, Goldstein I, et al: Cholinergic neurotransmission in human corpus cavernosum. I. Responses of isolated tissue. Am J Physiol 254(3 pt 2):H459–H467, 1988.
65. Aydin S, Ozbek H, Yilmaz Y, et al: Effects of sildenafil citrate, acetylcholine, and sodium nitroprusside on the relaxation of rabbit cavernosal tissue in vitro. Urology 58(1):119–124, 2001.
66. Stief CG, Bernard F, Bosch JLH, et al: Acetylcholine as a possible neurotransmitter in penile erection. J Urol 14:1444–1448, 1989.
67. Hedlund H, Andersson K-E, Mattiasson A: Pre- and post-junctional adreno and muscarinic receptor functions in the isolated human corpus spongiosum urethrae. J Auton Pharmacol 4:241–249, 1984.
68. Kim N, Azadzoi KM, Goldstein I, Saenz de Tejada I: A nitric oxide-like factor mediates nonadrenergic noncholinergic neurogenic relaxation of penile corpus cavernosum smooth muscle. J Clin Invest 88:112–118, 1991.
69. Rajfer J, Aronson WJ, Bush PA, et al: Nitric oxide as a mediator of relaxation of the corpus cavernosum in response to nonadrenergic, noncholinergic neurotransmission. N Engl J Med 326:90–94, 1992.
70. Waldman SA, Murad F: Cyclic GMP synthesis and function. Pharmacol Rev 39:163–196, 1987.
71. Saenz de Tejada I, Kim NN, Goldstein I, Traish AM: Regulation of pre-synaptic alpha adrenergic activity in the corpus cavernosum. Int J Impot Res 12 (suppl 1): S20–S25, 2000.
72. McConnell J, Benson GS: Innervation of human penile blood vessels. Neurourol Urodyn 1:199–210, 1982.
73. Costa PM, Soulie-Vassal L, Sarrazin B, et al: Adrenergic receptors on smooth muscle cells isolated from human penile corpus cavernosum. J Urol 150:859–863, 1993.
74. Levin RM, Wein AJ: Adrenergic alpha-receptors outnumber beta-receptors in human penile corpus cavernosum. Invest Urol 18:225–226, 1980.
75. Hedlund H, Andersson K-E: Comparison of the responses to drugs acting on adrenoceptors and muscarinic receptors in human isolated corpus cavernosum and cavernous artery. J Auton Pharmacol 5:81–88, 1985.
76. Klinge E, Sjostrand NO: Contraction and relaxation of the retractor penis muscle and the penile artery of the bull. Acta Physiol Scand 420 (suppl):1–88, 1974.
77. Kirkeby HJ, Jorgensen J, Ottesen B: Neuropeptide Y (NPY) in human penile corpus cavernosum and circumflex veins. J Urol 145:605–609, 1990.
78. Saenz de Tejada I, Carson MP, de las Morenas A, et al: Endothelin: Localization, synthesis, activity, and receptor types in human penile corpus cavernosum. Am J Physiol 261(4 pt 2):H1078–H1085, 1991.
79. Becker AJ, Uckert S, Stief CG, et al: Possible role of bradykinin and angiotensin II in the regulation of penile erection and detumescence. Urology 57(1):193–198, 2001.
80. Hedlund H, Andersson KE, Fovaeus M, et al: Characterization of contraction-mediating prostanoid receptors in human penile erectile tissues. J Urol 141(1):182–186, 1989.
81. Kim YC, Davies MG, Lee TH, et al: Characterization and function of histamine receptors in corpus cavernosum. J Urol 153(2):506–510, 1995.
82. Kifor I, Williams GH, Vickers MA, et al: Tissue angiotensin II as a modulator of erectile function. I. Angiotensin peptide content, secretion and effects in the corpus cavernosum. J Urol 157(5):1920–1925, 1997.
83. Park JK, Kim SZ, Kim SH, et al: Renin angiotensin system in rabbit corpus cavernosum: Functional characterization of angiotensin II receptors. J Urol 158(2):653–658, 1997.
84. Comiter CV, Sullivan MP, Yalla SV, Kifor I: Effect of angiotensin II on corpus cavernosum smooth muscle in relation to nitric oxide environment: In vitro studies in canines. Int J Impot Res 9(3):135–140, 1997.
85. Trigo-Rocha F, Hsu GL, Donatucci CF, et al: Intracellular mechanism of penile erection in monkeys. Neurourol Urodyn 13(1):71–80, 1994.
86. Minhas S, Cartledge J, Eardley I: The role of prostaglandins in penile erection. Prostaglandins Leukot Essent Fatty Acids 62(3):137–146, 2000.
87. Kirkeby HJ, Andersson KE, Forman A: Comparison of the effects of prostanoids on human penile circumflex veins and corpus cavernosum tissue. Br J Urol 72(2):220–225, 1993.
88. Italiano G, Calabro A, Aragona F, Pagano F: Effects of prostaglandin E1 and papaverine on non-neurogenic and neurogenic contraction of the isolated rabbit erectile tissue. Pharmacol Res 31(5):313–317, 1995.
89. Daley JT, Brown ML, Watkins T, et al: Prostanoid production in rabbit corpus cavernosum. I. Regulation by oxygen tension. J Urol 155(4):1482–1487, 1996.
90. Meghdadi S, Porst H, Stackl W, et al: Presence of PGE1 binding determines the erectile response to PGE1. Prostaglandins Leukot Essent Fatty Acids (2):111–113, 1999.
91. Bivalacqua TJ, Rajasekaran M, Champion HC, et al: The influence of castration on pharmacologically induced penile erection in the cat. J Androl 19(5):551–557, 1998.
92. Teixeira CE, Moreno RA, Ferreira U, et al: Pharmacological characterization of kinin-induced relaxation of human corpus cavernosum. Br J Urol 3:432–436, 1998.
93. Martinez AC, Prieto D, Raposo R, et al: Endothelium-independent relaxation induced by histamine in human dorsal penile artery. Clin Exp Pharmacol Physiol 27(7):500–507, 2000.
94. Chapelle PA, Durand J, Lacert P: Penile erection following complete spinal cord injury in man. Br J Urol 52:216–219, 1980.

95. Munro D, Horne HW, Paull DP: The effect of injury of the spinal cord and cauda equina on the sexual potency of men. N Eng J Med 239:903–911, 1948.
96. Talbot HS: A report on sexual function in paraplegics. J Urol 61:265–270, 1949.
97. Meisels RL, Sachs BD: Spinal transsection accelerates the developmental expression of penile reflexes in male rats. Physiol Behav 24:289–292, 1980.
98. MacLean PD, Ploog DW: Cerebral representation of penile erection. J Neurophysiol 25:29–55, 1962.
99. Slimp JC, Hart BL, Goy RW: Heterosexual, autosexual and social behavior of adult male rhesus monkeys with medial preoptic-anterior hypothalamic lesions. Brain Res 142(1):105–122, 1978.
100. Marson l, McKenna KE: A role for 5-hydroxytryptamine in descending inhibition of spinal sexual reflexes Exp Brain Res 88:313–320, 1992.
101. McIntosh TK, Barfield RJ: Brain monoaminergic control of male reproductive behavior. I. Serotonin and the post-ejaculatory period. Behav Brain Res 12:255–265, 1984.
102. Fernandez-Guasti A, Larsson K, Beyer G: GABAergic control of masculine sexual behavior. Pharmacol Biochem Behav 24:1065–1070, 1986.
103. Rehman J, Christ G, Alyskewycz M, Kerr E, Melman A: Experimental hyperprolactinemia in a rat model: Alteration in centrally mediated neuroerectile mechanisms. Int J Impot Res 12(1):23–32, 2000.
104. Pfaus JG, Gorzalka BB: Opiods and sexual behaviour. Neurosci Biobehav Rev 11:1–34, 1987.
105. Dornan WA, Malsbury CW: Neuropeptides and male sexual behavior. Neurosci Biobehav Rev 13:1–15, 1989.
106. Pehek EA, Thompson JT, Eaton RC, Hull EM: Apomorphine and haloperidol, but not domperidone, affect penile responses in rats. Pharmacol Biochem Behav 31:201–208, 1988.
107. Giuliano F, Allard J: Dopamine and sexual function. Int J Impot Res 13 (suppl 3):S18–S28, 2001.
108. Mulhall JP, Bukofzer S, Edmonds AL, George M: An open-label, uncontrolled dose-optimization study of sublingual apomorphine in erectile dysfunction. Clin Ther 23(8):1260–1271, 2001.
109. Heaton JP: Key issues from the clinical trials of apomorphine SL. World J Urol 19(1):25–31, 2001.
110. Giuliano F, Rampin O: Central noradrenergic control of penile erection [review]. Int J Impot Res 12 (suppl 1): S13–S19, 2000.
111. Bitran D, Hull EM: Pharmacological analysis of male rat sexual behavior. Neurosci BioBehav Rev 11:365–389, 1987.
112. Morales A: Yohimbine in erectile dysfunction: The facts. Int J Impot Res 12 (suppl 1):S70–S74, 2000.
113. Honda K, Yanagimoto M, Negoro H, et al: Excitation of oxytocin cells in the hypothalamic supraoptic nucleus by electrical stimulation of the dorsal penile nerve and tactile stimulation of the penis in the rat. Brain Res Bull 48(3):309–313, 1999.
114. Argiolas A, Melis MR, Stancampiano R: Role of central oxytocinergic pathways in the expression of penile erection. Regul Pept 45(1–2):139–142, 1993.
115. Chen K, Chang LS: Oxytocinergic neurotransmission at the hippocampus in the central neural regulation of penile erection in the rat. Urology 58(1):107–112, 2001.
116. Argiolas A: Nitric oxide is a central mediator of penile erection. Neuropharmacology 33(11):1339–1344, 1994.
117. Melis MR, Argiolas A: Role of central nitric oxide in the control of penile erection and yawning. Prog Neuropsychopharmacol Biol Psychiatry 21(6):899–922, 1997.
118. Melis MR, Succu S, Spano MS, Argiolas A: Morphine injected into the paraventricular nucleus of the hypothalamus prevents noncontact penile erections and impairs copulation: Involvement of nitric oxide. Eur J Neurosci 11(6):1857–1864, 1999.
119. Argiolas A, Melis MR, Murgia S, Schioth HB: ACTH- and alpha-MSH-induced grooming, stretching, yawning and penile erection in male rats: Site of action in the brain and role of melanocortin receptors. Brain Res Bull 51(5):425–431, 2000.
120. Wessells H, Fuciarelli K, Hansen J, et al: Synthetic melanotropic peptide initiates erections in men with psychogenic erectile dysfunction: Double-blind, placebo controlled crossover study. J Urol 160(2):389–393, 1998.
121. Mills TM, Lewis RW. The Role of androgens in the erectile response: A 1999 perspective. Mol Urol 3(2):75–86, 1999.
122. Heaton JP, Varrin SJ: Effects of castration and exogenous testosterone supplementation in an animal model of penile erection. J Urol 151(3):797–800, 1994.
123. Melis MR, Mauri A, Argiolas A: Apomorphine- and oxytocin-induced penile erection and yawning in intact and castrated male rats: Effect of sexual steroids. Neuroendocrinology 59(4):349–354, 1994.
124. Everitt BJ, Bancroft J: Of rats and men: The comparative approach to male sexuality. Annu Rev Sex Res 2:77–117, 1991.
125. Giuliano F, Rampin O, Schirar A, et al: Autonomic control of penile erection: Modulation by testosterone in the rat. J Neuroendocrinol 5(6):677–683, 1993.
126. Baba K, Yajima M, Carrier S, et al: Effect of testosterone on the number of NADPH diaphorase-stained nerve fibers in the rat corpus cavernosum and dorsal nerve. Urology 56(3):533–538, 2000.
127. Baba K, Yajima M, Carrier S, et al: Delayed testosterone replacement restores nitric oxide synthase-containing nerve fibres and the erectile response in rat penis. Brit J Urol 85(7):953–958, 2000.
128. Traish AM, Park K, Dhir V, et al: Effects of castration and androgen replacement on erectile function in a rabbit model. Endocrinology 140(4):1861–1868, 1999.
129. Dai YT, Stopper V, Lewis R, Mills T: Effects of castration and testosterone replacement on veno-occlusion during penile erection in the rat. Asian J Androl 1(1–2):53–59, 1999.
130. Nanasaki Y, Sakuma Y: Perineal musculature and its innervation by spinal motoneurons in the male rabbit: Effects of testosterone. J Nippon Med Sch 67(3):164–171, 2000.
131. Carani C, Scuteri A, Marrama P, Bancroft J: The effects of testosterone administration and visual erotic stimuli on nocturnal penile tumescence in normal men. Horm Behav 24(3):435–441, 1990.
132. McKenna KE, Chung SK, McVary KT: A model for the study of sexual function in anesthetized male and female rats. Am J Physiol 261(5 pt 2):R1276–R1285, 1991.
133. Park K, Goldstein I, Andry C, et al: Vasculogenic female sexual dysfunction: The hemodynamic basis for vaginal engorgement insufficiency and clitoral erectile insufficiency. Int J Impot Res 9(1):27–37, 1997.
134. Giuliano F, Allard J, Compagnie S, et al: Vaginal physiological changes in a model of sexual arousal in anesthetized rats. Am J Physiol Regul Integr Comp Physiol 281(1):R140–R149, 2001.
135. Vachon P, Simmerman N, Zahran AR, Carrier S: Increases in clitoral and vaginal blood flow following

clitoral and pelvic plexus nerve stimulations in the female rat. Int J Impot Res 12(1):53–57, 2000.
136. Min K, Munarriz R, Berman J, Kim N, et al: Hemodynamic evaluation of the female sexual arousal response in an animal model. J Sex Marital Ther 27(5):557–565, 2001.
137. Sommer F, Caspers HP, Esders K, et al: Measurement of vaginal and minor labial oxygen tension for the evaluation of female sexual function. J Urol 165(4):1181–1184, 2001.
138. Wagner G, Levin R: Oxygen tension of the vaginal surface during sexual stimulation in the human. Fertil Steril 30(1):50–53, 1978.
139. Henson DE, Rubin HB, Henson C: Labial and vaginal blood volume responses to visual and tactile stimuli. Arch Sex Behav 11(1):23–31, 1982.
140. Levin RJ: VIP, vagina, clitoral and periurethral glans—an update on human female genital arousal. Exp Clin Endocrinol 98(2):61–69, 1991.
141. Levin RJ, Wagner G: Orgasm in women in the laboratory—quantitative studies on duration, intensity, latency, and vaginal blood flow. Arch Sex Behav 14(5):439–449, 1985.
142. Wagner G, Ottesen B: Vaginal blood flow during sexual stimulation. Obstet Gynecol 56(5):621–641, 1980.
143. Lavoisier P, Aloui R, Schmidt MH, Watrelot A: Clitoral blood flow increases following vaginal pressure stimulation. Arch Sex Behav 24(1):37–45, 1995.
144. Wagner G, Levin RJ: Effect of atropine and methylatropine on human vaginal blood flow, sexual arousal and climax. Acta Pharmacol Toxicol (Copenh) 46(5):321–325, 1980.
145. Min K, Kim NN, McAuley I, et al: Sildenafil augments pelvic nerve-mediated female genital sexual arousal in the anesthetized rabbit. Int J Impot Res 12 (suppl 3):S32–S39, 2000.
146. Ottesen B, Pedersen B, Nielsen J, et al: Vasoactive intestinal polypeptide (VIP) provokes vaginal lubrication in normal women. Peptides 8(5):797–800, 1987.
147. Palle C, Bredkjaer HE, Ottesen B, Fahrenkrug J: Peptide histidine methionine (PHM) increases vaginal blood flow in normal women. Peptides 11(3):401–404, 1990.
148. Leffler CW, Amberson JI: Intravaginal prostaglandin E1 increases vaginal blood flow. Prostaglandins Leukot Med 9(6):587–589, 1982.
149. Abel GG, Murphy WD, Becker JV, Bitar A: Women's vaginal responses during REM Sleep. J Sex Marital Ther 5(1):5–14, 1979.
150. Park JK, Kim SZ, Kim SH, et al: Renin angiotensin system of rabbit clitoral cavernosum: Interaction with nitric oxide. J Urol 164(2):556–561, 2000.
151. Cellek S, Moncada S: Nitrergic neurotransmission mediates the non-adrenergic non-cholinergic responses in the clitoral corpus cavernosum of the rabbit. Br J Pharmacol 125(8):1627–1629, 1998.
152. Vemulapalli S, Kurowski S: Sildenafil relaxes rabbit clitoral corpus cavernosum. Life Sci 67(1):23–29, 2000.
153. Smock T, Albeck D, Stark P: A peptidergic basis for sexual behavior in mammals. Prog Brain Res 119:467–481, 1998.
154. Blaicher W, Gruber D, Bieglmayer C, et al: The role of oxytocin in relation to female sexual arousal. Gynecol Obstet Invest 47(2):125–126, 1999.
155. Tarcan T, Siroky MB, Park K, et al: Systemic administration of apomorphine improves the hemodynamic mechanism of clitoral and vaginal engorgement in the rabbit. Int J Impot Res 12(4):235–240, 2000.
156. Sarrel PM: Sexuality and menopause. Obstet Gynecol 75(suppl 4):26S–30S, 1990.
157. Van der Horst VG, Holstege G: Sensory and motor components of reproductive behavior: Pathways and plasticity. Behav Brain Res 92(2):157–167, 1998.
158. Park K, Ahn K, Lee S, et al: Decreased circulating levels of estrogen alter vaginal and clitoral blood flow and structure in the rabbit. Int J Impot Res 13(2):116–124, 2001.
159. Berman JR, McCarthy MM, Kyprianou N: Effect of estrogen withdrawal on nitric oxide synthase expression and apoptosis in the rat vagina. Urology 51(4):650–656, 1998.
160. Yoon HN, Chung WS, Park YY, et al: Effects of estrogen on nitric oxide synthase and histological composition in the rabbit clitoris and vagina. Int J Impot Res 13(4):205–211, 2001.
161. Al-Hijji J, Larsson B, Batra S: Nitric oxide synthase in the rabbit uterus and vagina: Hormonal regulation and functional significance. Biol Reprod 62(5):1387–1392, 2000.
162. Berman JR, Berman LA, Werbin TJ, et al: Clinical evaluation of female sexual function: Effects of age and estrogen status on subjective and physiologic sexual responses. Int J Impot Res 11 (suppl 1):S31–S38, 1999.
163. Abrams RM, Stanley H, Carter R, Notelovitz M: Effect of conjugated estrogens on vaginal blood flow in surgically menopausal women. Am J Obstet Gynecol 143(4):375–378, 1982.
164. Palle C, Bredkjaer HE, Fahrenkrug J, Ottesen B: Vasoactive intestinal polypeptide loses its ability to increase vaginal blood flow after menopause. Am J Obstet Gynecol 164(2):556–558, 1991.
165. Davis SR, Tran J: Testosterone influences libido and well being in women. Trends Endocrinol Metab 12(1):33–37, 2001.
166. Feldman HA, Goldstein I, Hatzichristou DG, et al: Impotence and its medical and psychosocial correlates: Results of the Massachusetts Male Aging Study. J Urol 151(1):54–61, 1994.
167. Lewis RW: Epidemiology of erectile dysfunction. Urol Clin North Am 28(2):209–216, 2001.
168. Laumann EO, Paik A, Rosen RC: Epidemiology of erectile dysfunction: Results from the National Health and Social Life Survey. Int J Impot Res 11 (suppl 1):S60–S64, 1999.
169. Levine LA: Erectile dysfunction: A review of a common problem in rapid evolution. Prim Care Update Obst Gyn 7(3):124–129, 2000.
170. Bancroft J: Central inhibition of sexual response in the male: A theoretical perspective. Neurosci Biobehav Rev 23(6):763–784, 1999.
171. Barlow DH: Causes of sexual dysfunction: The role of anxiety and cognitive interference. J Consult Clin Psychol 54(2):140–148, 1986.
172. Diederichs W, Stief CG, Lue TF, Tanagho EA: Sympathetic inhibition of papaverine induced erection. J Urol 146(1):195–198, 1991.
173. Diederichs W, Stief CG, Benard F, et al: The sympathetic role as an antagonist of erection. Urol Res 19(2):123–126, 1991.
174. Kim SC, Oh MM: Norepinephrine involvement in response to intracorporeal injection of papaverine in psychogenic impotence. J Urol 147(6):1530–1532, 1992.
175. Granata A, Bancroft J, Del Rio G: Stress and the erectile response to intracavernosal prostaglandin E1 in men with erectile dysfunction. Psychosom Med 57(4):336–344, 1995.

176. Laumann EO, Paik A, Rosen RC: Sexual dysfunction in the United States: Prevalence and predictors. JAMA 281(6):537–544, 1999.
177. Usta MF, Erdogru T, Tefekli A, et al: Honeymoon impotence: Psychogenic or organic in origin? Urology 57(4):758–762, 2001.
178. Cohen AS, Rosen RC, Goldstein L: EEG hemispheric asymmetry during sexual arousal: Psychophysiological patterns in responsive, unresponsive, and dysfunctional men. J Abnorm Psychol 94(4):580–590, 1985.
179. Cranston-Cuebas MA, Barlow DH: Cognitive and affective contributions to sexual functioning. Ann Rev Sex Res 1:119–161, 1990.
180. Lee IC, Surridge D, Morales A, Heaton JP: The prevalence and influence of significant psychiatric abnormalities in men undergoing comprehensive management of organic erectile dysfunction. Int J Impot Res 12(1):47–51, 2000.
181. Hartmann U: Psychological subtypes of erectile dysfunction: Results of statistical analyses and clinical practice. World J Urol 15(1):56–64, 1997.
182. Clarke M: Masturbatory guilt and sexual dysfunction. Aust Fam Physician 5(4):529–533, 1976.
183. Zargooshi J: Unconsummated marriage: Clarification of aetiology; treatment with intracorporeal injection. BJU Int 86(1):75–79, 2000.
184. Levine LA: Diagnosis and treatment of erectile dysfunction. Am J Med 109 (suppl 9A):3S–12S; discussion 29S–30S, 2000.
185. Morgentaler A: Male impotence. Lancet 354(9191):1713–1718, 1999.
186. Fabbri A, Aversa A, Isidori A: Erectile dysfunction: An overview. Hum Reprod Update 3(5):455–466, 1997.
187. Merlin SL, Brock GB, Begin LR, et al: New insights into the role of endothelin-1 in radiation-associated impotence. Int J Impot Res 13(2):104–109, 2001.
188. Munarriz RM, Yan QR, Nehra AJ, et al: Blunt trauma: The pathophysiology of hemodynamic injury leading to erectile dysfunction. J Urol 153(6):1831–1840, 1995.
189. Sullivan ME, Keoghane SR, Miller MA: Vascular risk factors and erectile dysfunction. BJU Int 87(9):838–845, 2001.
190. Ledda A: Diabetes, hypertension and erectile dysfunction. Curr Med Res Opin 16 (suppl 1):S17–S20, 2000.
191. Feldman HA, Johannes CB, Derby CA, et al: Erectile dysfunction and coronary risk factors: Prospective results from the Massachusetts Male Aging Study. Prev Med 30(4):328–338, 2000.
192. Schachter M: Erectile dysfunction and lipid disorders. Curr Med Res Opin 16 (suppl 1):S9–S12, 2000.
193. Tengs TO, Osgood ND: The link between smoking and impotence: Two decades of evidence. Prev Med 32(6):447–452, 2001.
194. Badimon L: Atherosclerosis and thrombosis: Lessons from animal models. Thromb Haemost 86(1):356–365, 2001.
195. Toohey JI: Possible involvement of sulfane sulfur in homocysteine-induced atherosclerosis. Med Hypotheses 56(2):259–261, 2001.
196. Bae JH: Noninvasive evaluation of endothelial function. J Cardiol 37 (suppl 1):89–92, 2001.
197. Rossi GP, Seccia TM, Nussdorfer GG: Reciprocal regulation of endothelin-1 and nitric oxide: Relevance in the physiology and pathology of the cardiovascular system. Int Rev Cytol 209:241–272, 2001.
198. Vapaatalo H, Mervaala E: Clinically important factors influencing endothelial function. Med Sci Monit 7(5):1075–1085, 2001.
199. Kim SC: Hyperlipidemia and erectile dysfunction. Asian J Androl 2(3):161–166, 2000.
200. Napoli C, Lerman LO: Involvement of oxidation-sensitive mechanisms in the cardiovascular effects of hypercholesterolemia. Mayo Clin Proc 76(6):619–631, 2001.
201. Azadzoi KM, Saenz de Tejada I: Hypercholesterolemia impairs endothelium-dependent relaxation of rabbit corpus cavernosum smooth muscle. J Urol 146(1):238–240, 1991.
202. Kim JH, Klyachkin ML, Svendsen E, et al: Experimental hypercholesterolemia in rabbits induces cavernosal atherosclerosis with endothelial and smooth muscle cell dysfunction. J Urol 151(1):198–205, 1994.
203. Junemann KP, Aufenanger J, Konrad T, et al: The effect of impaired lipid metabolism on the smooth muscle cells of rabbits. Urol Res 19(5):271–275, 1991.
204. Mikhailidis DP, Khan MA, Milionis HJ, Morgan RJ: The treatment of hypertension in patients with erectile dysfunction. Curr Med Res Opin 16 (suppl 1):S31–S36, 2000.
205. Burchardt M, Burchardt T, Baer L, et al: Hypertension is associated with severe erectile dysfunction. J Urol 164(4):1188–1191, 2000.
206. Muller SC, el-Damanhoury H, Ruth J, Lue TF: Hypertension and impotence. Eur Urol 19(1):29–34, 1991.
207. Toblli JE, Stella I, Inserra F, et al: Morphological changes in cavernous tissue in spontaneously hypertensive rats. Am J Hypertens 13(6 pt 1):686–692, 2000.
208. Palatini P: Sympathetic overactivity in hypertension: A risk factor for cardiovascular disease. Curr Hypertens Rep 3 (suppl 1):S3–S9, 2001.
209. Alexopoulou O, Jamart J, Maiter D, et al: Erectile dysfunction and lower androgenicity in type 1 diabetic patients. Diabetes Metab 27(3):329–336, 2001.
210. Ciarla MV, Bocciarelli A, Di Gregorio S, et al: Autoantibodies and endothelial dysfunction in well-controlled, uncomplicated insulin-dependent diabetes mellitus patients. Atherosclerosis 158(1):241–246, 2001.
211. Brands MW, Fitzgerald SM: Arterial pressure control at the onset of type I diabetes: The role of nitric oxide and the renin-angiotensin system. Am J Hypertens 14(6 pt 2):126S–131S, 2001.
212. Nicola W, Sidhom G, El Khyat Z, et al: Plasma angiotensin II, renin activity and serum angiotensin-converting enzyme activity in non-insulin dependent diabetes mellitus patients with diabetic nephropathy. Endocr J 48(1):25–31, 2001.
213. Carr ME: Diabetes mellitus: A hypercoagulable state. J Diabetes Complications 15(1):44–54, 2001.
214. Saenz de Tejada I, Goldstein I, Azadzoi K, et al: Impaired neurogenic and endothelium-mediated relaxation of penile smooth muscle from diabetic men with impotence. N Engl J Med 320(16):1025–1030, 1989.
215. Azadzoi KM, Saenz de Tejada I: Diabetes mellitus impairs neurogenic and endothelium-dependent relaxation of rabbit corpus cavernosum smooth muscle. J Urol 148(5):1587–1591, 1992.
216. Takahashi K, Ghatei MA, Lam HC, et al: Elevated plasma endothelin in patients with diabetes mellitus. Diabetologia 33(5):306–310, 1990.
217. Lam HC: Role of endothelin in diabetic vascular complications. Endocrine 14(3):277–284, 2001.
218. Sullivan ME, Dashwood MR, Thompson CS, et al: Alterations in endothelin B receptor sites in cavernosal tissue of diabetic rabbits: Potential relevance to the pathogenesis of erectile dysfunction. J Urol 158(5):1966–1972, 1997.

219. Rodger RS, Fletcher K, Dewar JH, et al: Prevalence and pathogenesis of impotence in one hundred uremic men. Uremia Invest 8(2):89–96, 1984–1985.
220. Kaufman JM, Hatzichristou DG, Mulhall JP, et al: Impotence and chronic renal failure: A study of the hemodynamic pathophysiology. J Urol 151(3):612–618, 1994.
221. Morris ST, McMurray JJ, Spiers A, Jardine AG: Impaired endothelial function in isolated human uremic resistance arteries. Kidney Int 60(3):1077–1082, 2001.
222. Cupisti A, Rossi M, Placidi S, et al: Responses of the skin microcirculation to acetylcholine and to sodium nitroprusside in chronic uremic patients. Int J Clin Lab Res 30(3):157–162, 2000.
223. Mundy AR: Pelvic fracture injuries of the posterior urethra. World J Urol 17(2):90–95, 1999.
224. Matthews LA, Herbener TE, Seftel AD: Impotence associated with blunt pelvic and perineal trauma: Penile revascularization as a treatment option. Semin Urol 13(1):66–72, 1995.
225. El-Bahnasawy MS, Gomha MA: Penile fractures: The successful outcome of immediate surgical intervention. Int J Impot Res 2000;12(5):273–277.
226. Bergman B, Sivertsson R, Suurkula M: Penile blood pressure in erectile impotence following cystectomy. Scand J Urol Nephrol 16(2):81–84, 1982.
227. Tomic R, Sjodin JG: Sexual function in men after radical cystectomy with or without urethrectomy. Scand J Urol Nephrol 26(2):127–129, 1992.
228. Blander DS, Broderick GA, Malkowicz SB, et al: Retrospective review of flow patterns following retropubic prostatectomy. Int J Impot Res 11(6):309–313, 1999.
229. Armenakas NA, McAninch JW, Lue TF, et al: Posttraumatic impotence: Magnetic resonance imaging and duplex ultrasound in diagnosis and management. J Urol 149(5 pt 2):1272–1275, 1993.
230. Mark SD, Keane TE, Vandemark RM, Webster GD: Impotence following pelvic fracture urethral injury: Incidence, aetiology and management. Br J Urol 75(1):62–64, 1995.
231. Sommer F, Konig D, Graft C, et al: Impotence and genital numbness in cyclists. Int J Sports Med 2001; 22(6):410–413, 2001.
232. Wilder RB, Chou RH, Ryu JK, et al: Potency preservation after three-dimensional conformal radiotherapy for prostate cancer: Preliminary results. Am J Clin Oncol 23(4):330–333, 2000.
233. Sanchez-Ortiz RF, Broderick GA, Rovner ES, et al: Erectile function and quality of life after interstitial radiation therapy for prostate cancer. Int J Impot Res 12 (suppl 3):S18–S24, 2000.
234. Fisch BM, Pickett B, Weinberg V, Roach M: Dose of radiation received by the bulb of the penis correlates with risk of impotence after three-dimensional conformal radiotherapy for prostate cancer. Urology 57(5):955–959, 2001.
235. Merrick GS, Wallner K, Butler WM, et al: A comparison of radiation dose to the bulb of the penis in men with and without prostate brachytherapy-induced erectile dysfunction. Int J Radiat Oncol Biol Phys 50(3):597–604, 2001.
236. Merrick GS, Butler WM, Dorsey AT, et al: A comparison of radiation dose to the neurovascular bundles in men with and without prostate brachytherapy-induced erectile dysfunction. Int J Radiat Oncol Biol Phys 48(4):1069–1074, 2001.
237. Carrier S, Hricak H, Lee SS, et al: Radiation-induced decrease in nitric oxide synthase-containing nerves in the rat penis. Radiology 195(1):95–99, 1995.
238. Claes H, Van de Voorde W, Vandeginste S, et al: A histopathological study of deep dorsal penile vein in venogenic impotence. Acta Urol Belg 62(4):61–67, 1994.
239. Wespes E, Delcour C, Preserowitz L, et al: Impotence due to corporeal veno-occlusive dysfunction: Long-term follow-up of venous surgery. Eur Urol 21(2):115–119, 1992.
240. Shabsigh R, Fishman IJ, Toombs BD, Skolkin M: Venous leaks: Anatomical and physiological observations. J Urol 146(5):1260–1265, 1991.
241. Mydlo JH: Surgeon experience with penile fracture. J Urol 166(2):526–528, 2001.
242. Zargooshi J: Penile fracture in Kermanshah, Iran: Report of 172 cases. J Urol 164(2):364–366, 2000.
243. Karadeniz T, Topsakal M, Ariman A, et al: Penile fracture: Differential diagnosis, management and outcome. Br J Urol 77(2):279–281, 1996.
244. Penson DF, Seftel AD, Krane RJ, et al: The hemodynamic pathophysiology of impotence following blunt trauma to the erect penis. J Urol 148(4):1171–1180, 1992.
245. Tunuguntla HS: Management of Peyronie's disease—a review. World J Urol 19(4):244–250, 2001.
246. Somers KD, Dawson DM: Fibrin deposition in Peyronie's disease plaque. J Urol 157(1):311–315, 1997.
247. Pryor J: Peyronie's disease and impotence. Acta Urol Belg 56:317–321, 1988.
248. Lopez JA, Jarow JP: Penile vascular evaluation of men with Peyronie's disease. J Urol 149(1):53–55, 1993.
249. El-Sakka AI, Hassoba HM, Pillarisetty RJ, et al: Peyronie's disease is associated with an increase in transforming growth factor-protein expression. J Urol 158:1391–1394, 1997.
250. Bivalacqua TJ, Diner EK, Novak TE, et al: A rat model of Peyronie's disease associated with a decrease in erectile activity and an increase in inducible nitric oxide synthase protein expression. J Urol 163(6):1992–1998, 2000.
251. Wespes E, Sattar AA, Golzarian J, et al: Corporeal veno-occlusive dysfunction: Predominantly intracavernous muscular pathology. J Urol 157(5):1678–1680, 1997.
252. Nehra A, Goldstein I, Pabby A, et al: Mechanisms of venous leakage: A prospective clinicopathological correlation of corporeal function and structure. J Urol 156(4):1320–1329, 1996.
253. Calabro A, Italiano G, Pescatori ES, et al: Physiological aging and penile erectile function: A study in the rat. Eur Urol 29(2):240–244, 1996.
254. Bakircioglu ME, Sievert KD, Nunes L, et al: Decreased trabecular smooth muscle and caveolin-1 expression in the penile tissue of aged rats. J Urol 166(2):734–738, 2001.
255. Ferrini M, Magee TR, Vernet D, et al: Aging-related expression of inducible nitric oxide synthase and markers of tissue damage in the rat penis. Biol Reprod 64(3):974–982, 2001.
256. Mersdorf A, Goldsmith PC, Diederichs W, et al: Ultrastructural changes in impotent penile tissue: A comparison of 65 patients. J Urol 145(4):749–758, 1991.
257. Christ GJ, Stone B, Melman A: Age-dependent alterations in the efficacy of phenylephrine-induced contractions in vascular smooth muscle isolated from the corpus cavernosum of impotent men. Can J Physiol Pharmacol 69(7):909–913, 1991.
258. Burchardt T, Burchardt M, Karden J, et al: Reduction of endothelial and smooth muscle density in the corpora cavernosa of the streptozotocin induced diabetic rat. J Urol 164(5):1807–1811, 2000.

259. Bivalacqua TJ, Hellstrom WJ, Kadowitz PJ, Champion HC: Increased expression of arginase II in human diabetic corpus cavernosum. In diabetic-associated erectile dysfunction. Biochem Biophys Res Commun 283(4):923–927, 2001.
260. Ganz MB, Seftel A: Glucose-induced changes in protein kinase C and nitric oxide are prevented by vitamin E. Am J Physiol Endocrinol Metab 278(1):E146–E152, 2000.
261. Cartledge JJ, Eardley I, Morrison JF: Advanced glycation end-products are responsible for the impairment of corpus cavernosal smooth muscle relaxation seen in diabetes. BJU Int 87(4):402–407, 2001.
262. Khan MA, Thompson CS, Jeremy JY, et al: The effect of superoxide dismutase on nitric oxide-mediated and electrical field-stimulated diabetic rabbit cavernosal smooth muscle relaxation. BJU Int 87(1):98–103, 2001.
263. Bell CR, Sullivan ME, Dashwood MR, et al: The density and distribution of endothelin 1 and endothelin receptor subtypes in normal and diabetic rat corpus cavernosum. Br J Urol 76(2):203–207, 1995.
264. Azadzoi KM, Siroky MB, Goldstein I: Study of etiologic relationship of arterial atherosclerosis to corporal veno-occlusive dysfunction in the rabbit. J Urol 155(5):1795–1800, 1996.
265. Azadzoi KM, Park K, Andry C, et al: Relationship between cavernosal ischemia and corporal veno-occlusive dysfunction in an animal model. J Urol 157(3):1011–1017, 1997.
266. Azadzoi KM, Goldstein I, Siroky MB, et al: Mechanisms of ischemia-induced cavernosal smooth muscle relaxation impairment in a rabbit model of vasculogenic erectile dysfunction. J Urol 160(6 pt 1):2216–2222, 1998.
267. Azadzoi KM, Krane RJ, Saenz de Tejada I, et al: Relative roles of cyclooxygenase and nitric oxide synthase pathways in ischemia-induced increased contraction of cavernosal smooth muscle. J Urol 161(4):1324–1328, 1999.
268. Tarhan F, Kuyumcuoglu U, Kolsuz A, et al: Cavernous oxygen tension in the patients with erectile dysfunction. Int J Impot Res 9(3):149–153, 1997.
269. Broderick GA, Gordon D, Hypolite J, Levin RM: Anoxia and corporal smooth muscle dysfunction: A model for ischemic priapism. J Urol 151(1):259–262, 1994.
270. Kim NN, Kim JJ, Hypolite J, et al: Altered contractility of rabbit penile corpus cavernosum smooth muscle by hypoxia. J Urol 155(2):772–778, 1996.
271. Kim N, Vardi Y, Padma-Nathan H, et al: Oxygen tension regulates the nitric oxide pathway. Physiological role in penile erection. J Clin Invest 91(2):437–442, 1993.
272. Daley JT, Brown ML, Watkins T, et al: Prostanoid production in rabbit corpus cavernosum. I. Regulation by oxygen tension. J Urol 155(4):1482–1487, 1996.
273. Daley JT, Watkins MT, Brown ML, et al: Prostanoid production in rabbit corpus cavernosum. II. Inhibition by oxidative stress. J Urol 156(3):1169–1173, 1996.
274. Moreland RB, Albadawi H, Bratton C, et al: O2-dependent prostanoid synthesis activates functional PGE receptors on corpus cavernosum smooth muscle. Am J Physiol Heart Circ Physiol 281(2):H552–H558, 2001.
275. Moreland RB: Is there a role of hypoxemia in penile fibrosis? A viewpoint presented to the Society for the Study of Impotence. Int J Impot Res 10(2):113–120, 1998.
276. Saenz de Tejada I, Kim NN, Daley JT, et al: Acidosis impairs rabbit trabecular smooth muscle contractility. J Urol 157(2):722–726, 1997.
277. Broderick GA, Harkaway R: Pharmacologic erection: Time-dependent changes in the corporal environment. Int J Impot Res 6(1):9–16, 1994.
278. Ebbehoj J, Wagner G: Insufficient penile erection due to abnormal drainage of cavernous bodies. Urology 13(5):507–510, 1979.
279. Kulmala RV, Lehtonen TA, Lindholm TS, Tammela TL: Permanent open shunt as a reason for impotence or reduced potency after surgical treatment of priapism in 26 patients. Int J Impot Res 7(3):175–180, 1995.
280. Melman A, Serels S: Priapism. Int J Impot Res 12 (suppl 4):S133–S139, 2000.
281. Moon DG, Lee DS, Kim JJ: Altered contractile response of penis under hypoxia with metabolic acidosis. Int J Impot Res 11(5):265–271, 1999.
282. Chakrabarty A, Upadhyay J, Dhabuwala CB, et al: Priapism associated with sickle cell hemoglobinopathy in children: Long-term effects on potency. J Urol 155(4):1419–1423, 1996.
283. Bick RL, Frenkel EP: Clinical aspects of heparin-induced thrombocytopenia and thrombosis and other side effects of heparin therapy. Clin Appl Thromb Hemost 5 (suppl 1):S7–S15, 1999.
284. Patel AG, Mukherji K, Lee A: Priapism associated with psychotropic drugs. Br J Hosp Med 55(6):315–319, 1996.
285. Touge H, Watanabe T, Fujinaga T, Kawabata M: Post-traumatic high flow priapism: A case report. Int J Urol 6(12):623–626, 1999.
286. Ramos CE, Park JS, Ritchey ML, Benson GS: High flow priapism associated with sickle cell disease. J Urol 153(5):1619–1621, 1995.
287. Harding JR, Hollander JB, Bendick PJ: Chronic priapism secondary to a traumatic arteriovenous fistula of the corpus cavernosum. J Urol 150(5 pt 1):1504–1506, 1993.
288. Bastuba MD, Saenz de Tejada I, Dinlenc CZ, et al: Arterial priapism: Diagnosis, treatment and long-term followup. J Urol 151(5):1231–1237, 1994.
289. Ilkay AK, Levine LA: Conservative management of high-flow priapism. Urology 46(3):419–424, 1995.
290. Sian J, Gerlach M, Youdim MB, Riederer P: Parkinson's disease: A major hypokinetic basal ganglia disorder. J Neural Transm 106(5–6):443–476, 1999.
291. Sakakibara R, Shinotoh H, Uchiyama T, et al: Questionnaire-based assessment of pelvic organ dysfunction in Parkinson's disease. Auton Neurosci 92(1–2):76–85, 2001.
292. O'Sullivan JD, Hughes AJ: Apomorphine-induced penile erections in Parkinson's disease. Mov Disord 13(3):536–539, 1998.
293. Guldner GT, Morrell MJ: Nocturnal penile tumescence and rigidity evaluation in men with epilepsy. Epilepsia 37(12):1211–1214, 1996.
294. Herzog AG, Seibel MM, Schomer DL, et al: Reproductive endocrine disorders in men with partial seizures of temporal lobe origin. Arch Neurol 43(4):347–350, 1986.
295. Murialdo G, Galimberti CA, Fonzi S, et al: Sex hormones and pituitary function in male epileptic patients with altered or normal sexuality. Epilepsia 36(4):360–365, 1995.
296. Rattya J, Turkka J, Pakarinen AJ, et al: Reproductive effects of valproate, carbamazepine, and oxcarbazepine in men with epilepsy. Neurology 56(1):31–36, 2001.
297. Husain AM, Carwile ST, Miller PP, Radtke RA: Improved sexual function in three men taking lamotrigine for epilepsy. South Med J 93(3):335–336, 2000.
298. Meinhardt W, Kropman RF, Vermeij P, et al: The influence of medication on erectile function. Int J Impot Res 9(1):17–26, 1997.

299. Montastruc JL, Llau ME, Rascol O, Senard JM: Drug-induced parkinsonism: A review. Fundam Clin Pharmacol 8(4):293–306, 1994.
300. Depatie L, Lal S: Apomorphine and the dopamine hypothesis of schizophrenia: A dilemma? J Psychiatry Neurosci 26(3):203–220, 2001.
301. Petty RG: Prolactin and antipsychotic medications: Mechanism of action. Schizophr Res 35 (suppl):S67–S73, 1999.
302. Palmer JS, Kaplan WE, Firlit CF: Erectile dysfunction in patients with spina bifida is a treatable condition. J Urol 164(3 pt 2):958–961, 2000.
303. Yamada S, Lonser RR: Adult tethered cord syndrome. J Spinal Disord 13(4):319–323, 2000.
304. Cornette L, Verpoorten C, Lagae L, et al: Closed spinal dysraphism: A review on diagnosis and treatment in infancy. EJPN 2(4):179–185, 1998.
305. Boemers TM, van Gool JD, de Jong TP: Tethered spinal cord: The effect of neurosurgery on the lower urinary tract and male sexual function. Br J Urol 76(6):747–751, 1995.
306. Chapelle PA, Durand J, Lacert P: Penile erection following complete spinal cord injury in man. Br J Urol 52(3):216–219, 1980.
307. Courtois FJ, Macdougall JC, Sachs BD: Erectile mechanism in paraplegia. Physiol Behav 53(4):721–726, 1993.
308. Courtois FJ, Gonnaud PM, Charvier KF, et al: Sympathetic skin responses and psychogenic erections in spinal cord injured men. Spinal Cord 36(2):125–131, 1998.
309. Schmid DM, Schurch B, Hauri D: Sildenafil in the treatment of sexual dysfunction in spinal cord-injured male patients. Eur Urol 38(2):184–193, 2000.
310. Goldstein I, Siroky MB, Sax DS, Krane RJ: Neurourologic abnormalities in multiple sclerosis. J Urol 128(3):541–545, 1982.
311. Zorzon M, Zivadi R, Bosco A, et al: Sexual dysfunction in multiple sclerosis: A case-control study. I. Frequency and comparison of groups. Mult Scler 5(6):418–427, 1999.
312. Bakshi R, Dmochowski J, Shaikh ZA, Jacobs L: Gray matter T2 hypointensity is related to plaques and atrophy in the brains of multiple sclerosis patients. J Neurol Sci 15;185(1):19–26, 2001.
313. Tartaglino LM, Friedman DP, Flanders AE, et al: Multiple sclerosis in the spinal cord: MR appearance and correlation with clinical parameters. Radiology 195(3):725–732, 1995.
314. Zorzon M, Zivadi R, Monti Bragadin L, et al: Sexual dysfunction in multiple sclerosis: A 2-year follow-up study. J Neurol Sci 15;187(1–2):1–5, 2001.
315. Kirkeby HJ, Poulsen EU, Petersen T, Dorup J: Erectile dysfunction in multiple sclerosis. Neurology 38(9):1366–1371, 1988.
316. Betts CD, Jones SJ, Fowler CG, Fowler CJ: Erectile dysfunction in multiple sclerosis: Associated neurological and neurophysiological deficits, and treatment of the condition. Brain 117(pt 6):1303–1310, 1994.
317. Tay EC, Chacha PB: Midline prolapse of a lumbar intervertebral disc with compression of the cauda equina. J Bone Joint Surg Br 61(1):43–46, 1979.
318. Choy DS: Early relief of erectile dysfunction after laser decompression of herniated lumbar disc. J Clin Laser Med Surg 17(1):25–27, 1999.
319. Vardi Y, Sprecher E, Kanter Y, et al: Polyneuropathy in impotence. Int J Impot Res 8(2):65–68, 1996.
320. Cornefjord M, Olmarker K, Otani K, Rydevik B: Effects of diclofenac and ketoprofen on nerve conduction velocity in experimental nerve root compression. Spine 26(20):2193–2197, 2001.
321. McDougall AJ, McLeod JG: Autonomic neuropathy. I. Clinical features, investigation, pathophysiology, and treatment. J Neurol Sci 137(2):79–88, 1996.
322. Carrier S, Nagaraju P, Morgan DM, et al: Age decreases nitric oxide synthase-containing nerve fibers in the rat penis. J Urol 157(3):1088–1092, 1997.
323. Amenta F, Cavallotti C, De Rossi M, et al: Vasoactive intestinal polypeptide levels and distribution in the penis of old rats. J Neural Transm 70(1–2):137–143, 1987.
324. Colpi GM, Negri L, Nappi RE, Chinea B: Perineal floor efficiency in sexually potent and impotent men. Int J Impot Res 11(3):153–157, 1999.
325. Ali ST, Shaikh RN, Siddiqi NA, Siddiqi PQ: Comparative studies of the induction of erectile response to film and fantasy in diabetic men with and without neuropathy. Arch Androl 30(3):137–145, 1993.
326. Zochodne DW: Diabetic neuropathies: Features and mechanisms. Brain Pathol 9(2):369–391, 1999.
327. Blanco R, Saenz de Tejada I, Goldstein I, et al: Dysfunctional penile cholinergic nerves in diabetic impotent men. J Urol 144(2 pt 1):278–280, 1990.
328. Lincoln J, Crowe R, Blacklay PF, et al: Changes in the VIPergic, cholinergic and adrenergic innervation of human penile tissue in diabetic and non-diabetic impotent males. J Urol 137(5):1053–1059, 1987.
329. Walsh PC: Anatomic radical prostatectomy: Evolution of the surgical technique. J Urol 160(6 pt 2):2418–2424, 1998.
330. Masui H, Ike H, Yamaguchi S, et al: Male sexual function after autonomic nerve-preserving operation for rectal cancer. Dis Colon Rectum 39(10):1140–1145, 1996.
331. Kawanishi Y, Lee KS, Kimura K, et al: Effect of radical retropubic prostatectomy on erectile function, evaluated before and after surgery using colour Doppler ultrasonography and nocturnal penile tumescence monitoring. BJU Int 88(3):244–247, 2001.
332. Tscholl R, Largo M, Poppinghaus H, et al: Incidence of erectile impotence secondary to transurethral resection of benign prostatic hyperplasia, assessed by preoperative and postoperative snap gauge tests. J Urol 153:1491–1493, 1995.
333. Bieri S, Miralbell R, Rohner S, Kurtz J: Influence of transurethral resection on sexual dysfunction in patients with prostate cancer. Br J Urol 78(4):537–541, 1996.
334. Bieri S, Iselin CE, Rohner S: Capsular perforation localization and adenoma size as prognostic indicators of erectile dysfunctional after transurethral prostatectomy. Scan J Urol Nephrol 31(6):545–548, 1997.
335. Hanbury DC, Sethia KK: Erectile function following transurethral prostatectomy. Br J Urol 75(1):12–13, 1995.
336. Aboseif S, Shinohara K, Breza J, et al: Role of penile vascular injury in erectile dysfunction after radical prostatectomy. Br J Urol 73(1):75–82, 1994.
337. Mulhall JP, Graydon RJ: The hemodynamics of erectile dysfunction following nerve-sparing radical retropubic prostatectomy. Int J Impot Res 8(2):91–94, 1996.
338. Ayajiki K, Hayashida H, Okamura T, Toda N: Influence of denervation on neurogenic inhibitory response of corpus cavernosum and nitric oxide synthase histochemistry. Brain Res 825(1–2):14–21, 1999.
339. Cruz MR, Liu YC, Manzo J, et al: Peripheral nerves mediating penile erection in the rat. J Auton Nerv Syst 76(1):15–2, 1997.
340. Basar MM, Yildiz M, Basar H, et al: Electrical activity of the corpus cavernosum in denervated rats. Int J Urol 6(5):251–256, 1999.

341. Carrier S, Zvara P, Nunes L, et al: Regeneration of nitric oxide synthase-containing nerves after cavernous nerve neurotomy in the rat. J Urol 153(5):1722–1727, 1995.
342. Andersson PO, Björnberg J, Bloom SR, Mellander S: Vasoactive intestinal polypeptide in relation to penile erection in the cat evoked by pelvic and by hypogastric nerve stimulation. J Urol 138:419–422, 1987.
343. Sjöstrand NO, Klinge EK: Principal mechanisms controlling penile retraction and protrusion in rabbits. Acta Physiol Scand 106:199–214, 1979.
344. Quayle JB: Sexual function after bilateral lumbar sympathectomy and aorto-iliac by-pass surgery. J Cardiovasc Surg (Torino) 21(2):215–218, 1980.
345. Yang CC, Bradley WE: Innervation of the human glans penis. J Urol 161(1):97–102, 1999.
346. Gerstenberg TC, Nordling J, Hald T, Wagner G: Standardized evaluation of erectile dysfunction in 95 consecutive patients. J Urol 141(4):857–862, 1989.
347. Breda G, Xausa D, Giunta A, et al: Nomogram for penile biothesiometry. Eur Urol 20(1):67–69, 1991.
348. Nogueira MC, Herbaut AG, Wespes E: Neurophysiological investigations of two hundred men with erectile dysfunction: Interest of bulbocavernosus reflex and pudendal evoked responses. Eur Urol 18(1):37–41, 1990.
349. Derouet H, Jost WH, Osterhage J, et al: Penile sympathetic skin response in erectile dysfunction. Eur Urol 28(4):314–319, 1995.
350. Yarnitsky D, Sprecher E, Vardi Y: Penile thermal sensation. J Urol 156(2 pt 1):391–393, 1996.
351. Bemelmans BL, Hendrikx LB, Koldewijn EL, et al: Comparison of biothesiometry and neuro-urophysiological investigations for the clinical evaluation of patients with erectile dysfunction. J Urol 153(5):1483–1486, 1995.
352. Dettmers C, van Ahlen H, Faust H, et al: Evaluation of erectile dysfunction with the sympathetic skin response in comparison to bulbocavernosus reflex and somato-sensory evoked potentials of the pudendal nerve. Electromyogr Clin Neurophysiol 34(7):437–444, 1994.
353. Lefaucheur JP, Yiou R, Colombel M, et al: Relationship between penile thermal sensory threshold measurement and electrophysiologic tests to assess neurogenic impotence. Urology 57(2):306–309, 2001.
354. Rowland DL: Penile sensitivity in men: A composite of recent findings. Urology 52(6):1101–1105, 1998.
355. Rowland DL, Greenleaf WJ, Dorfman LJ, Davidson JM: Aging and sexual function in men. Arch Sex Behav 22(6):545–557, 1993.
356. Rowland DL, Greenleaf W, Mas M, et al: Penile and finger sensory thresholds in young, aging, and diabetic males. Arch Sex Behav 18(1):1–12, 1989.
357. Era P, Jokela J, Suominen H, Heikkinen E: Correlates of vibrotactile thresholds in men of different ages. Acta Neurol Scand 74(3):210–217, 1986.
358. Rowland DL, Leentvaar EJ, Blom JH, Slob AK: Changes in penile sensitivity following papaverine-induced erection in sexually functional and dysfunctional men. J Urol 146(4):1018–1021, 1991.
359. Rowland DL, Haensel SM, Blom JH, Slob AK: Penile sensitivity in men with premature ejaculation and erectile dysfunction. J Sex Marital Ther 19(3):189–197, 1993.
360. Apkarian AV, Stea RA, Bolanowski SJ: Heat-induced pain diminishes vibrotactile perception: A touch gate. Somatosens Mot Res 11(3):259–267, 1994.
361. Burris AS, Gracely RH, Carter CS, et al: Testosterone therapy is associated with reduced tactile sensitivity in human males. Horm Behav 25(2):195–205, 1991.
362. Wellmer A, Sharief MK, Knowles CH, et al: Quantitative sensory and autonomic testing in male diabetic patients with erectile dysfunction. BJU Int 83(1):66–70, 1999.
363. Morrissette DL, Goldstein MK, Raskin DB, Rowland DL: Finger and penile tactile sensitivity in sexually functional and dysfunctional diabetic men. Diabetologia 42(3):336–342, 1999.
364. Spector I, Carey M: Incidence and prevalence of the sexual dysfunction: A critical review of the empirical literature. Arch Sexual Behav 19:389–408, 1990.
365. Rosen RC, Taylor JF, Leiblum SR, et al: Prevalence of sexual dysfunction in women: Results of a survey study of 392 women in an outpatient gynecological clinic. J Sex Marital Ther 19:171–188, 1993.
366. Vroege JA, Gijs L, Hengeveld MW: Classification of sexual dysfunctions: Towards DSM-V and ICD-11. Compr Psychiatry 39:333–337, 1998.
367. Leiblum SR: Definition and classification of female sexual disorders. Int J Impot Res Suppl 10:S104, 1998.
368. World Health Organization: ICD-10: International Statistical Classification of Diseases and Related Health Problems. Geneva: World Health Organization, 1992.
369. Basson R, Berman J, Burnett A, et al: Report of the international consensus development conference on female sexual dysfunction: Definitions and classifications. J Urol 163(3):888–893, 2000.
370. Berman JR, Goldstein I: Female sexual dysfunction. Urol Clin North Am 28(2):405–416, 2001.
371. Bachmann G: Physiologic aspects of natural and surgical menopause. J Reprod Med 46(suppl 3):307–315, 2001.
372. Sarrel PM: Effects of hormone replacement therapy on sexual psychophysiology and behavior in postmenopause. J Womens Health Gend Based Med 9 (suppl 1):S25–S32, 2000.
373. Krasinski K, Spyridopoulos I, Asahara T, et al. Estradiol accelerates functional endothelial recovery after arterial injury. Circulation 95:1768–1772, 1997.
374. Rosselli M, Keller PJ, Kern F, et al: Estradiol inhibits mitogen-induced proliferation and migration of human aortic smooth muscle cells. Circulation 90:I-87, 1994.
375. Chen GD, Oliver RH, Leung BS, et al: Estrogen receptor alpha and beta expression in the vaginal walls and uterosacral ligaments of premenopausal and postmenopausal women. Fertil Steril 71:1099–1102, 1998.
376. Sarrel PM. Ovarian hormones and vaginal blood flow: Using laser Doppler velocimetery to measure effects in a clinical trial of post-menopausal women. Int J Impot Res 10:S91–S93, 1998.
377. Beck JG: Hypoactive sexual desire disorder: An overview. J Consult Clin Psychol 63(6):919–927, 1995.
378. Riley A, Riley E: Controlled studies on women presenting with sexual drive disorder. I. Endocrine status. J Sex Marital Ther 26(3):269–283, 2000.
379. Schreiner-Engel P, Schiavi RC, White D, Ghizzani A: Low sexual desire in women: The role of reproductive hormones. Horm Behav 23(2):221–234, 1989.
380. Sherwin BB, Gelfand MM: The role of androgens in the maintenance of sexual functioning in oophorectomized women. Psychosom Med 49:397–409, 1987.
381. Segraves RT: Psychiatric drugs and inhibited female orgasm. J Sex Marital Ther 14(3):202–207, 1998.
382. Lesko LM, Stotland NL, Segraves RT: Three cases of female anorgasmia associated with MAOIs. Am J Psychiatry 139(10):1353–1354, 1982.

383. Segraves RT: Antidepressant-induced orgasm disorder. J Sex Marital Ther 21(3):192–201, 1995.
384. Shen WW, Sata LS: Inhibited female orgasm resulting from psychotropic drugs: A five-year, updated, clinical review. J Reprod Med 35(1):11–14, 1990.
385. Bartlik B, Kocsis JH, Legere R, et al: Sexual dysfunction secondary to depressive disorders. JGSM 2(2):52–60, 1999.
386. Sipski ML, Alexander CJ: Sexual activities, response and satisfaction in women pre- and post-spinal cord injury. Arch Phys Med Rehabil 74(10):1025–1029, 1993.
387. Sipski ML, Alexander CJ, Rosen RC: Physiological parameters associated with psychogenic sexual arousal in women with complete spinal cord injuries. Arch Phys Med Rehabil 76(9):811–818, 1995.
388. Sipski ML, Alexander CJ, Rosen R: Sexual arousal and orgasm in women: Effects of spinal cord injury. Ann Neurol 49(1):35–44, 2001.
389. Sipski ML, Alexander CJ, Rosen RC: Sexual response in women with spinal cord injuries: Implications for our understanding of the able bodied. J Sex Marital Ther 25(1):11–22, 1999.
390. Prather RC: Sexual dysfunction in the diabetes female: A review. Arch Sex Behav 17(3):277–284, 1988.
391. Schreiner-Engel P, Schiavi RC, Vietorisz D, et al: Diabetes and female sexuality: A comparative study of women in relationships. J Sex Marital Ther 11(3):165–175, 1985.
392. Tyrer G, Steel JM, Ewing DJ, et al: Sexual responsiveness in diabetic women. Diabetologia 24(3):166–171, 1983.
393. Jensen SB. Diabetic sexual dysfunction: A comparative study of 160 insulin treated diabetic men and women and an age-matched control group. Arch Sex Behav 10(6):493–504, 1981.
394. Enzlin P, Mathieu C, Vanderschueren D, Demyttenaere K: Diabetes mellitus and female sexuality: A review of 25 years' research. Diabet Med 15(10):809–815, 1998.
395. Leedom L, Feldman M, Procci W, Zeidler A: Symptoms of sexual dysfunction and depression in diabetic women. J Diabet Complications 5(1):38–41, 1991.
396. LeMone P: The physical effects of diabetes on sexuality in women. Diabetes Educ 22(4):361–366, 1996.
397. Wincze JP, Albert A, Bansal S: Sexual arousal in diabetic females: Physiological and self-report measures Arch Sex Behav 22(6):587–601, 1993.
398. Sax DS, Berman JR, Goldstein I: Female neurogenic sexual dysfunction secondary to clitoral neuropathy. J Sex Marital Ther 27(5):599–602, 2001.
399. Romanzi LJ, Groutz A, Feroz F, Blaivas JG: Evaluation of female external genitalia sensitivity to pressure/touch: A preliminary prospective study using Semmes-Weinstein monofilaments. Urology 57(6):1145–1150, 2001.
400. Goldstein I, Berman JR: Vasculogenic female sexual dysfunction: Vaginal engorgement and clitoral erectile insufficiency syndromes. Int J Impot Res 10 (suppl 2):S84–S90, 1998.
401. Park K, Tarcan T, Goldstein I, et al: Atherosclerosis-induced chronic ischemia causes clitoral cavernosal fibrosis in the rabbit. Int J Impot Res 12:111–116, 2000.
402. Tarcan T, Park K, Goldstein I, et al: Histomorphometric analysis of age-associated structural changes in human clitoral cavernosal tissue. J Urology 161:940–944, 1999.
403. Berman JR, Berman LA, Lin H, et al: Effect of sildenafil on subjective and physiologic parameters of the female sexual response in women with sexual arousal disorder. J Sex Marital Ther 27(5):411–420, 2001.
404. Caruso S, Intelisano G, Lupo L, Agnello C: Premenopausal women affected by sexual arousal disorder treated with sildenafil: A double-blind, cross-over, placebo-controlled study. BJOG 108(6):623–628, 2001.
405. Becher EF, Bechara A, Casabe A: Clitoral hemodynamic changes after a topical application of alprostadil. J Sex Marital Ther 27(5):405–410, 2001.

CHAPTER 14

Sexual Dysfunction in the Female

JENNIFER R. BERMAN

Female sexual dysfunction (FSD) is a multicausal, multidimensional medical problem that adversely affects physical health and emotional well-being. Because little basic science research has been done on female sexuality, our knowledge and understanding of the anatomy and physiology of normal female sexual response and the pathophysiology of FSD is limited. Based on our understanding of the physiology of the male erectile response, recent advances in technology, and heightened interest in women's health issues, the study of female sexual function and dysfunction is evolving. The epidemiology of FSD is not well understood, and several factors specific to the study of sexual function contribute to the current paucity of epidemiologic knowledge.

PREVALENCE AND INCIDENCE RATES

FSD is age-related, progressive, and highly prevalent, affecting 25% to 63% of American women.[1,2] In the National Health and Social Life Survey (NHSLS), which included 1749 women,[3,4] 43% of adult women reported sexual dysfunction. Although this study had a large sample size, included minorities, and used modern probability sampling, it was limited by its cross-sectional design. In addition, the NHSLS did not include women older than 60 years of age, nor did it adjust for menopausal status or medical risk factors. In another study of 448 women older than 60 years of age, two thirds of participants were sexually inactive, 12% of married women had difficulty with intercourse, and 14% experienced pain with intercourse. Sexual activity was strongly correlated with marital status.[3] Women older than 60 years of age were less likely to have sex if their partners were in poor health and if they had feelings of low self-worth.[4] Previous studies of older women did not include specific measures of female sexual arousal, orgasm, or satisfaction.

Incidence rates for FSD are unknown. The same disease processes and risk factors that are associated with erectile dysfunction in men, such as aging, hypertension, cigarette smoking, and hypercholesterolemia, are associated with sexual dysfunction in women.[5,6] However, in contrast to men, age is inversely associated with dysfunction in women. Younger age was a significant predictor for pain during sex, lack of pleasure, and anxiety about performance.[1] Women with a lower level of education were also more likely to experience pain during sex. Arousal disorder was higher and sexual pain was increased among women with urinary tract symptoms, emotional problems, or stress.[1]

Few epidemiologic data are available on the incidence of FSD because of small sample sizes, skewed sample populations, failure to sample nonresponders, and lack of uniform definitions of sexual dysfunction. The previous review of prevalence studies showed that the prevalence of most sexual dysfunctions is higher in clinical than in community samples. In recent studies,[1,7,8] the overall prevalence of dysfunction ranged from 19% to 42%; disorders of desire and arousal are the most common symptoms. Problems with dyspareunia ranged from 12% to 33%; problems with orgasm ranged from 5% to 23%. The NHSLS found a high overall prevalence of FSD (43%) in US women 18 to 59 years of age.

CLASSIFICATIONS AND DEFINITIONS OF FEMALE SEXUAL DYSFUNCTION

The first standardized method of classification of the various categories of FSD for use in research was published in 1980 as the *Diagnostic and Statistical Manual of the American Psychiatric Association* (DSM-III).[9] In the World Health Organization system, sexual dysfunction was defined as including "the various ways in which an individual is unable to participate in a sexual relationship as he or she would wish."[10]

The Sexual Function Health Council of the American Foundation of Urologic Disease established an interdisciplinary consensus conference panel consisting of a multinational group of experts in FSD. The panel included specialists from many relevant disciplines, including endocrinology, family medicine, gynecology, nursing, pharmacology, physiology, psychiatry, psychology, rehabilitation medicine, and urology. The objective of the panel was to evaluate and revise existing definitions and classifications of FSD. Specifically, medical risk factors and etiologies for FSD were incorporated into the existing psychologically based definitions. The definition of dysfunction was expanded to include both psychogenic and organic causes of desire, arousal, orgasm, and sexual pain disorders. FSD can stem from a variety of etiologies that are classified into three main categories[11]:

1. Organic causes include cardiovascular diseases (e.g., hypertension, coronary artery disease), endocrinopathies (e.g., diabetes, thyroid disorders), and neurologic diseases (e.g., multiple sclerosis, stroke).
2. Psychological factors include psychological problems (e.g., religious or social restrictions), traumatic experiences (e.g., sexual abuse), interpersonal problems (e.g., relationship difficulties, poor communication), and stressors (e.g., job loss, depression).
3. Drugs include those associated with disorders of desire (e.g., antipsychotics, antidepressants, barbiturates, beta blockers), those associated with arousal (e.g., anticholinergics, antihypertensives), and those associated with orgasmic dysfunction (e.g., antipsychotics, benzodiazepines, methyldopa).

The AFUD Consensus Panel classified FSD into several categories as described in the following discussion.

Hypoactive Sexual Desire Disorder

Hypoactive sexual desire disorder is persistent or recurring deficiency (or absence) of sexual fantasies or thoughts or lack of receptivity to sexual activity that causes personal distress. This disorder may result from psychological or emotional factors or from physiologic problems, such as hormone deficiencies and medical or surgical interventions. Further, sexual desire can be inhibited by any disruption of the female hormonal milieu caused by natural menopause, surgically or medically induced menopause, or endocrine disorders.

Sexual Aversion Disorder

Sexual aversion disorder is persistent or recurring deficiency (or absence) of sexual fantasies or thoughts or lack of receptivity to sexual activity that causes personal distress. This disorder is usually psychologically or emotionally based, and has a variety of causes, such as physical or sexual abuse or childhood trauma.

Sexual Arousal Disorder

Sexual arousal disorder is persistent or recurring inability to attain or maintain adequate sexual excitement that causes personal distress. Patients may experience a lack of subjective excitement or a lack of genital (lubrication or swelling) or other somatic response.

Disorders of arousal include, but are not limited to, lack of or diminished vaginal lubrication, decreased clitoral and labial sensation, decreased clitoral and labial engorgement, and lack of vaginal smooth muscle relaxation. These conditions may occur as a result of psychological factors; however, there is often a medical or physiologic basis, such as diminished vaginal or clitoral blood flow, previous pelvic trauma, pelvic surgery, or drugs.

Orgasmic Disorder

Orgasmic disorder is persistent or recurrent failure, difficulty, or delay in attaining orgasm after adequate sexual stimulation and arousal that causes personal distress. This may be a primary (never achieved orgasm) or secondary condition, and may be caused by surgery, trauma, or hormone deficiencies. Primary anorgasmia can be the result of emotional trauma or sexual abuse; however, other medical problems as well as drugs (e.g., serotonin reuptake inhibitors) can contribute to or exacerbate the problem.

Sexual Pain Disorders

Dyspareunia

Dyspareunia is recurrent or persistent genital pain associated with sexual intercourse. It can develop as a result of medical problems, such as vestibulitis, vaginal atrophy, or vaginal infection. The cause can be physiologic, psychological, or a combination of the two.

Vaginismus

Vaginismus is recurrent or persistent involuntary spasms of the musculature of the outer third of the vagina that interferes with vaginal penetration and causes personal distress. Vaginismus usually is a conditioned response to painful penetration or is caused by psychological and emotional factors.

Other Sexual Pain Disorders

Recurrent or persistent genital pain induced by noncoital sexual stimulation includes anatomic and inflammatory conditions, such as infections (e.g., herpes simplex virus), vestibulitis, previous genital mutilation, trauma, and endometriosis.

Each category of FSD can be subtyped depending on whether the disorder is lifelong or acquired, generalized or situational, and organic, psychogenic, or mixed in its pathophysiology. The etiology of any of these disorders may be multfactorial, and the disorders often overlap. Sexual arousal disorder is the focus of clinical and basic science research as well as treatment interventions. Human and animal models have been established to assess sexual arousal, and validated sexual arousal instruments are now available. An emerging hypothesis is that decreased sexual arousal as manifested by diminished genital engorgement may be related to inadequate pelvic arterial blood flow. Decreased genital blood flow ultimately leads to fibrosis of the vaginal wall and clitoral cavernosal smooth muscle.[12] Women with sexual arousal disorder report diminished vaginal lubrication, pain with intercourse, decreased vaginal and clitoral sensation, and difficulty achieving orgasm. Because different domains of sexual function in women are linked, enhancement of sexual arousal by improvements in vaginal lubrication, clitoral and labial engorgement, and genital sensation would be expected to improve both orgasmic ability and libido.[13] The potential role of pharmacotherapy in the treatment of female sexual arousal disorder is poorly understood.

ETIOLOGIES OF FEMALE SEXUAL DYSFUNCTION

Vasculogenic

High blood pressure, high cholesterol levels, smoking, and heart disease are associated with impotence in men and sexual dysfunction in women. The newly identified clitoral and vaginal vascular insufficiency syndromes are directly related to diminished genital blood flow as a result of atherosclerosis of the iliohypogastric–pudendal arterial bed.[14] Although many psychological and medical disorders may result in decreased vaginal and clitoral engorgement, arterial insufficiency is an important cause and should be considered in the evaluation of this disorder. Diminished pelvic blood flow as a result of aortoiliac disease leads to fibrosis of the vaginal wall and clitoral smooth muscle, resulting in vaginal dryness and dyspareunia.

Histomorphometric evaluation of clitoral erectile tissue from atherosclerotic animals shows clitoral cavernosal artery wall thickening, loss of corporal smooth muscle, and increased collagen deposition.[14] In human clitoral tissue, a similar loss of corporal smooth muscle occurs, with replacement by fibrous connective tissue in association with atherosclerosis of the clitoral cavernosal arteries.[12] Atherosclerotic changes that occur in clitoral vascular and trabecular smooth muscle may interfere with normal relaxation and dilation responses to sexual simulation.

Alterations in circulating estrogen levels associated with menopause contribute to age-associated changes in clitoral and vaginal smooth muscle. In addition, traumatic injury to the iliohypogastric-pudendal arterial bed as a result of pelvic fractures, blunt trauma, surgical disruption, or chronic perineal pressure from bicycle riding can decrease vaginal and clitoral blood flow and lead to sexual dysfunction.

Neurogenic

The same neurogenic disorders that cause erectile dysfunction in men can cause sexual dysfunction in women. These include spinal cord injury; diseases of the central or peripheral nervous system; diabetes; and complete upper motor neuron injuries that affect sacral spinal segments. Women with spinal cord injury have significantly more difficulty achieving orgasm than normal control subjects. Women with incomplete injuries retain the capacity for psychogenic arousal and vaginal lubrication.[15] The effects of specific spinal cord injuries on female sexual response and the role of vasoactive pharmacotherapy in this population are being investigated.

Hormonal

Dysfunction of the hypothalamic–pituitary axis, surgical or medical castration, premature ovarian failure, advanced age, and long-term birth control use are common causes of hormonally based FSD. The most common symptoms associated with decreased estrogen or testosterone levels are decreased desire and libido, vaginal dryness, and lack of sexual arousal. Estrogen improves the integrity of vaginal mucosal tissue and enhances arousal by improving vaginal sensation, vasocongestion, and secretions. Estrogen deprivation significantly decreases clitoral intracavernosal, vaginal, and urethral blood flow. Histologically, estrogen deprivation causes diffuse clitoral fibrosis, thinned vaginal epithelial layers, and decreased vaginal submucosal vasculature. Thus, a decline in circulating estrogen levels can adversely affect the structure and function of the vaginal and clitoral tissues, ultimately affecting sexual function. Serum testosterone concentrations in women decline with advancing age and are lower in older women than in younger women. However, unlike serum estradiol levels, serum testosterone levels do not decrease abruptly at menopause. A recent study of perimenopausal women showed conclusively that serum total and free testosterone concentrations change very little and might increase slightly in the perimenopausal transition.[16] Therefore, sexual dysfunction in healthy postmenopausal women cannot be attributed to androgen deficiency alone.[16,17]

Musculogenic

The pelvic floor muscles, particularly the levator ani and perineal membrane, participate in female sexual function and responsiveness. When voluntarily contracted, the perineal membrane, which consists of the bulbocavernosus and ischicavernosus muscles, contributes to and intensifies sexual arousal and orgasm. The bulbospongiosus and ischiocavernosus muscles are responsible for involuntary rhythmic contractions during orgasm. The levator ani also modulates vaginal receptivity and motor responses during orgasm. A hypertonic levator ani can contribute to the development of vaginismus, causing dyspareunia and other sexual pain disorders. A hypotonic levator ani can lead to vaginal hyoanesthesia, coital anorgasmia, and urinary incontinence during sexual intercourse or orgasm.

Psychogenic

In women, regardless of whether organic disease is present, emotional and relational issues significantly affect sexual arousal. Self-esteem, body image, and the quality of the relationship with her partner all affect a woman's ability to respond sexually. In addition, depression and other mood disorders are often associated with FSD. Furthermore, the drugs commonly used to treat depression can significantly affect the female sexual response. The most frequently used drugs for uncomplicated depression are the selective serotonin reuptake inhibitors. Women receiving these drugs often report decreases in desire, arousal, and genital sensation as well as difficulty achieving orgasm; however, several studies show improvements after the administration of sildenafil.

CONCLUSION

FSD is a common condition, with population estimates ranging from 22% to 43%. The epidemiology of FSD is not well understood, and it has been difficult to measure in nonclinical samples. Low physical and emotional satisfaction and low general happiness were significantly correlated with all three categories of sexual dysfunction (low desire, arousal disorder, and sexual pain). Both classification systems view sexual dysfunction as involving a combination of psychological and somatic components. Little is known about risk factors for FSD or changes over the natural history. More research is needed on the relationship between drugs and comorbidities and the occurrence of FSD.

REFERENCES

1. Laumann EO, Paik A, Rosen RC: Sexual dysfunction in the United States: Prevalence and predictors. JAMA 281:537–544, 1999.
2. Spector IP, Carey MP: Incidence and prevalence of the sexual dysfunctions: A critical review of the empirical literature. Arch Sex Behav 19:389–408, 1990.
3. Diokno AC, Brown MB, Herzog AR: Sexual function in the elderly. Arch Intern Med 150:197–200, 1990.
4. Mooradian AD, Greiff V: Sexuality in older women. Arch Intern Med 150:1033–1038, 1990.
5. Hsueh WA: Sexual dysfunction with aging and systemic hypertension. Am J Cardiol 61:18H–23H, 1988.
6. Scott RS, Hsueh GS: A clinical study of the effects of galvanic vaginal muscle stimulation in urinary stress incontinence and sexual dysfunction. Am J Obstet Gynecol 135:663–665, 1979.
7. Rosen RC, Taylor JF, Leiblum SR, Bachman GA: Prevalence of sexual dysfucntion in women: Results of a survey study of 329 women in an outpatient gynecological clinic. J Sex Marital Ther 19:171–188, 1993.
8. Read S, King M, Watson J: Sexual dysfucntion in primary medical care: Prevalence, characteristics and detection by the general practitioner. J Public Health Med 19(4):387–391, 1997.
9. Leiblum SR: Definition and classification of female sexual disorders. Int J Impot Res (suppl 2): S104, 1998.
10. World Health Organization: ICD-10: International Statistical Classification of Diseases and Related Health Problems. Geneva, World Health Organization, 1992.
11. Phillips NA: Female sexual dysfunction: Evaluation and treatment. Am Fam Physician 62:127–136, 141–142, 2000.
12. Tarcan T, Park K, Goldstein I, et al: Histomorphometric analysis of age-related structural changes in human clitoral cavernosal tissue. J Urol 161:940–944, 1999.
13. Berman JBL, Lin H, Cantey-Kiser J, et al: Effect of sildernafil on subjective and physiologic parameters of the female sexual response in women with sexual arousal disorder. J Sex Marital Ther 27(5):411–420, 2001.
14. Goldstein I, Berman JR: Vasculogenic female sexual dysfunction: Vaginal engorgement and clitoral erectile insufficiency syndromes. Int J Impot Res 10 (suppl 2):S84–S90; discussion S98–S101, 1998.
15. Sipski ML, Alexander CJ, Rosen RC: Orgasm in women with spinal cord injuries: A laboratory-based assessment. Arch Phys Med Rehabil 76:1097–1102, 1995.
16. Burger HG, Dudley EC, Hopper JL, et al: The endocrinology of the menopausal transition: A cross-sectional study of a population-based sample. J Clin Endocrinol Metab 80:3537–3545, 1995.
17. Davis S: Androgen replacement in women: A commentary. J Clin Endocrinol Metab 84:1886–1891, 1999.

CHAPTER 15

Erectile Dysfunction

PIERRE DESVAUX

Male sexual dysfunction can be classified as erectile dysfunction (ED), ejaculatory disorders, male orgasmic disorders, and poor desire. ED, previously referred to as impotence, is inability to attain or maintain an erection sufficient for satisfactory sexual intercourse. Sexual dysfunction is a more general term that includes libidinal, orgasmic, and ejaculatory dysfunction in addition to the inability to attain or maintain penile erection.[1]

PREVALENCE AND INCIDENCE RATES

The best data on the prevalence of ED emerged from two cross-sectional studies that used probability sampling techniques: the Massachusetts Male Aging Study (MMAS)[2,3] and the National Health and Social Life Survey (NHSLS).[4,5] The MMAS was a cross-sectional, community-based random sample epidemiologic survey of 1709 men, 40 to 70 years of age, in the greater Boston area. The men were surveyed first between 1987 and 1989.[2,3] Of these participants, 847 men were resurveyed between 1995 and 1997.[3] The survey showed that 52% of surveyed men were affected by ED to some degree; 17.2% reported minimal ED, 25.2% reported moderate ED, and 9.6% reported complete ED.

The NHSLS was a national probability survey of English-speaking Americans, 18 to 59 years of age, living in the United States in 1992.[4,5] In this survey, based on self-reports of difficulty in obtaining or maintaining erections, 7% of men between 18 and 29 years of age, 9% of men between 30 and 39 years of age, 11% of men between 40 and 45 years of age, and 18% of men between 50 and 59 years of age reported ED. These two landmark studies and data from several other studies are in agreement that ED is a common problem that affects 20 to 30 million men in the United States alone.[1] The prevalence of ED increases with age; it affects fewer than 10% of men younger than 45 years of age, but 75% of men older than 80 years of age.[2] Men with other medical problems, such as hypertension, diabetes, cardiovascular disease, and end-stage renal disease, have a significantly higher prevalence of ED than healthy men.[1,2]

Few longitudinal data are available on the annual incidence rates of ED. Most of the available information was derived from two studies. In the MMAS, of the 1290 men 40 to 70 years of age who were originally surveyed between 1987 and 1989, follow-up information was gathered from 847 men between 1995 and 1997. In this study, the crude incidence rate of ED in white men in the Boston area was 25.9 cases per thousand man-years. The incidence rate increased from 12.4 cases per thousand man-years for men 40 to 49 years of age to 29.8 cases per thousand man-years for men 50 to 59 years of age and 46.4 cases per thousand man-years for men 60 to 69 years of age. In another study, incidence rates were derived from a survey of 3250 men, 26 to 83 years of age, who were seen at a preventive medicine clinic between 1987 and 1991. In this study, the incidence rate of ED was less than 3 cases per thousand man-years among men younger than 45 years of age and 52 cases per thousand man-years among men 65 years of age or older. Based on these two studies, it was estimated that there are 600,000 to 700,000 new cases of ED each year in the United States alone.

The most scientific studies on prevalence of ED provide data for the United States, Europe, Asia, and Australia and show prevalance increases with age.[6] In 1993, a Danish study used a questionnaire to determine the prevalence of ED in 411 men who were 51 years of age. One hundred of these men were subsequently interviewed[7]: 4% of the 411 men reported having ED on more than a few occasions during the previous year, and 15% reported only occasional ED. However, only 7% considered the problem abnormal for their age, only 5% planned to consult a therapist, and only 2% considered their sexual problem to be part of a disease.[6] In other studies from Sweden and France, 5% of men reported sexual disability. Among these men, 69% reported that this disability was a problem for them, and of those with this perception, 75% were not sexually satisfied.[8] In the French study,[9] 7% of respondents reported having ED "often," and 47% reported having

ED "sometimes" or "quite seldom." In men 18 to 24 years of age, 11% reported ED alone and 22% reported ED and premature ejaculation. Shirai and associates[10] estimated that the prevalence rate of ED in Japan is 26%. In a large study conducted in Australia, 1409 men returned study questionnaires, for a participation rate of 88%.[11] Among the 707 who were 40 to 69 years of age, the prevalence of ED was 33.9% and 11.9% had complete impotence. Hypertension, ischemic heart disease, peripheral vascular disease, and diabetes mellitus were often associated with ED.[6]

Epidemiologic studies show that the best predictors of the risk of ED are age, history of diabetes mellitus, hypertension, drug use, and cardiovascular disease. Advancing age is an important risk factor. In both the MMAS and the NHSLS, the prevalence of ED increased with each decade of life.

In all studies, prevalence increased with age. Severity also increased with age: at 40 years of age, approximately 40% of men experienced ED, whereas nearly 70% of 70-year-old men had some degree of ED.[2] Although the incidence of ED increases with age, it is not an inevitable consequence of aging. After adjusting for age, the study determined that a higher probability of ED was directly associated with heart disease, diabetes, hypertension, drugs (antihypertensives, vasodilators), and depression. Among chronic diseases associated with ED, diabetes mellitus is the most important risk factor. In the MMAS, the age-adjusted risk of complete ED was three times higher in men with a history of treated diabetes mellitus than in those without a history of diabetes mellitus. Fifty percent of men with diabetes mellitus experience ED sometime during the course of their illness. In the MMAS, treated heart disease, treated hypertension, and hyperlipidemia were associated with a significantly increased risk of ED. Among men with treated heart disease and hypertension, the probability of ED was more than two times greater for smokers than for nonsmokers. Smoking also increases the risk of ED in men taking drugs for cardiovascular diseases. Cardiovascular disorders, including hypertension, stroke, coronary artery disease, and peripheral vascular disease, are associated with increased risk of ED. Approximately 80% of ED is primarily related to organic causes, and approximately 20% stems from psychological causes. Most cases have both organic and psychological components.[12]

RISK FACTORS

General Risk factors

General risk factors can be classified into three categories[4,6]:

1. **Health and lifestyle factors.** Men with emotional or stress-related problems are more likely to have sexual dysfunctions. Urinary tract symptoms appear to affect premature ejaculation and ED.
2. **Social status.** Men with poor health are at increased risk for all three categories of sexual dysfunction. Deterioration in economic position, indexed by falling household income, doubles the likelihood of ED, but has no association with the other two categories.
3. **Sexual experience.** Certain types of sexual experience increase the risk of sexual dysfunction. Men who were victims of adult–child contact or forced sexual contact are three times as likely to have ED and approximately twice as likely to have premature ejaculation as those who were not victims of adult–child contact.

Endocrine and Hormonal Factors[6,13,14]

The growth and development of the male reproductive tract is influenced by androgens, which are responsible for secondary sexual characteristics.[6,13] The effect on libido, sexual behavior, and the erectile mechanism remains unclear. In the MMAS, the largest male endocrine database, testosterone (free, albumin-bound, or total testosterone, or dihydrotestosterone), was not statistically significantly correlated with impotence. No correlation was found for any of the other 17 hormones measured, except for the adrenal androgen metabolite dehydroepiandrosterone sulfate.[2] Dihydrotestosterone and cortisol showed effects of small magnitude on minimal impotence only. Mulligan and Schmitt[15] concluded that testosterone enhances sexual interest. In their study, testosterone led to increased frequency of sexual acts and increased the frequency of sleep-related erections, but had little or no effect on fantasy or visually induced erections. ED has a clear association with the subject's aging but little correlation with testosterone serum levels.

Smoking

The use of tobacco is clearly a risk factor for ED. In the MMAS, cigarette smoking exacerbated the risks of impotence associated with cardiovascular disease and pharmacologic treatment[2,6]; however, an overall effect of current smoking was not determined, with complete impotence occurring in 11% of smokers and 9.3% of nonsmokers.[2]

Diabetes Mellitus

Diabetes mellitus is the most common disease to produce autonomic neuropathy as well as damage to the sensory and motor nerves. ED occurs in at least 50% of men with diabetes mellitus, with the onset of impotence occurring at an earlier age than in those without diabetes mellitus.[6,16] Diabetes mellitus may cause erectile difficulty because of its effects on tissue, including small arteries and arterioles; neurologic demyelinization; and sinusoid smooth muscle deterioration.[6] In a recent study[17] of the pathophysiology of ED and diabetes mellitus, 105 men (79 with non–insulin-dependent diabetes mellitus and 26 with insulin-dependent diabetes mellitus) underwent Doppler evaluation. The type of diabetes and a history of smoking or hypertension did not impact cavernosal artery peak systolic velocity between both groups.[6,17] Diabetes mellitus occasionally causes impotence as the initial symptom.

Drug-induced Dysfunction

Many prescription and illicit drugs substantially affect sexual interest, performance, and function. Of currently used prescription drugs, antihypertensive agents are most likely to interfere with sexual function; however, diuretics, neuroleptics, antiepileptics, and related drugs are also associated with ED. Major classes of prescription drugs associated with ED include vasodilators, antihypertensives, cardiac and hypoglycemic drugs, histamine-2 receptor antagonists, hormones, anticholinergics, and certain cytotoxic agents.[2] Antihypertensive drugs appear to be a major risk factor for ED. Impotence occurs in approximately 25% of men who take any type of antihypertensive drugs, and failed ejaculation is a problem for 26% of men who take these drugs.[18] The antihypertensive drugs that are most often implicated in impotence are thiazide diuretics, methyldopa, guanethidine, clonidine, and propanolol. Some drugs rarely produce sexual dysfunction; these include prazosin and calcium channel blockers. Diuretics are still widely used to manage hypertension, even though drugs with more limited side effects are available. Some investigators believe that thiazide diuretics lower serum zinc levels and that this interferes with testosterone secretion.[19,21] Regardless of whether they receive treatment, however, men with hypertension have a higher incidence of ED than the nonhypertensive population.[18]

Men with depression are at increased risk for impotence, possibly because of decreased testosterone levels.[2] Patients on psychotropic drugs such as antidepressants (monoamine oxidase inhibitors, tricyclic antidepressants, serotonin reuptake inhibitors) and antipsychotic drugs are definitely at greater risk of ED.[6,21] Antipsychotics with strong alpha-1 receptor affinity should be considered as substitutes for other prescription psychotropic drugs that are associated with ED. Histamine-2 receptor antagonists increase the risk of ED. Many anticholinergic drugs produce impotence, including anisotropine, dicyclomine, oxybutynin, and scopolamine. Alcohol abuse is a leading cause of ED and other disturbances of sexual dysfunction, and may cause either acute or chronic problems with male potency. Episodic erectile failure with acute intoxication is fairly routine.[20] This may be a direct chemical effect of alcohol on erectile mechanisms, but it also may be mediated by cerebrocortical disturbances induced by alcohol.[21] Amphetamines, marijuana, and methadone have the same effects on sexual function.

Neurologic Conditions

Although sexual problems commonly occur with diseases of the nervous system, they are usually overshadowed by the more disabling features of the neurologic damage. When the autonomic nervous system is affected preferentially, impaired sexual function is likely to be an early and significant symptom. In Parkinson's disease and Shy-Drager syndrome, sexual dysfunction may occur as a consequence of central and peripheral nervous system disease.[22,23] Chronic neurologic diseases that are correlated with increased risk of impotence include cerebrovascular accidents, temporal lobe epilepsy, multiple sclerosis, Chiari syndrome, Guillain-Barré syndrome, and encephalopathy. Sexual dysfunction is common with Parkinson's disease and multiple sclerosis. Patients with Parkinson's disease may have autonomic dysfunction, a complication that may cause impotence. The severity of the sexual dysfunction is likely to increase as Parkinson's disease progresses.[23] The prevalence of decreased erectile ability in patients with Parkinson's disease is high and had been reported at 80%.[24] Multiple sclerosis is a common neurologic condition that often causes sexual dysfunction as a result of spinal cord disease. Between 40% and 75% of patients with multiple sclerosis have altered sexual activity as an apparent consequence of the demyelinating disease; spinal cord demyelination causes impotence in 40% of patients.[23,25] ED is the most common type of sexual dysfunction observed in men with multiple sclerosis. Disturbed ejaculation, diminished libido, and problems with orgasm are also relatively common.

Peripheral nerve injury and neuropathy commonly causes sexual dysfunction, often in association with leg numbness, paresthesias, flaccid paraparesis, or areflexia in the legs, accompanied by constipation and urinary retention. Spinal cord disease may cause impotence, perineal dysesthesia, or other types of sexual problems, especially if the sacral segment of the cord is involved. Potency varies substantially with the level of spinal cord injury. Men with spinal cord injury have several associated sexual dysfunctions, including ED and alterations in ejaculation and orgasm.[23] Patients with lesions above the sacral parasympathetic center maintain reflexogenic erection. Patients with incomplete lesions can receive psychogenic input and maintain erectile function. Patients with significant lesions that affect the sacral parasympathetic center do not have reflex erections and have severe ED.[26,27] The incidence of ED after radical prostatectomy performed with the new nerve-sparing techniques varies from 35% to 68%, depending on surgical technique, clinical and pathologic tumor stage, and patient age. Both clinical cystectomy and clinical prostatectomy can affect arterial insufficiency and ED.[28]

Cardiovascular Disease

ED is associated with cardiovascular disease risk factors.[2] Many conditions that increase the risk of ED also increase the risk of cerebrovascular accident or myocardial infarction. Therefore, men who have cardiovascular risk factors should undergo a comprehensive medical evaluation and should be advised of the potential risks associated with sexual activity.[29] ED is highly correlated with many vascular factors, including cerebrovascular accidents, coronary bypass surgery, heart disease, hypertension, and arteriosclerosis.[6]

Other Chronic Diseases

Chronic renal failure is associated with impotence in up to 40% of patients, and patients with hepatic failure, particularly those with alcoholic cirrhosis, are also at increased risk for impotence.[16] Scleroderma is also a risk factor for ED. Impotence is reported in 12% to 60% of cases, and is the presenting symptom of systemic scleroderma in 12% to 21% of cases.[30]

CONCLUSION

As described in Chapter 5 (Normal Sexual Function in Men), normal sexual function requires the involvement and coordination of multiple regulatory systems. Alteration of psychological, hormonal, neurologic, or vascular factors may lead to ED; however, in many cases, a combination of factors is involved. In most cases, however, both organic and psychological components are involved. Normally, neurogenic dysfunction is differentiated from vasculogenic dysfunction. Events that interfere with the central nervous system and the peripheral nerves involved in sexual function can cause ED. In addition to the strictly neurologic bases for penile dysfunction, some diseases directly or indirectly cause vascular disturbances that impair erection or detumescence. Vasculogenic impotence can be caused by poor blood supply, excessive venous drainage, or a combination of the two. Vasculogenic impotence can be broken into two categories: poor blood supply and veno-occlusive dysfunction. Alterations in corpus cavernosal arterial inflow and corporal veno-occlusive dysfunction are thought to be the two most frequent causes of ED. Both conditions occur in patients with hypertension, myocardial infarction, and cerebrovascular diseases. A higher prevalence of ED is observed in patients with cardiovascular risk factors, hypertension, diabetes mellitus, peripheral vascular disease, a smoking habit, and depression with psychotropics.

Most cases of ED have both neurologic and vasculogenic causes, and the presence of a neurologic disorder or neuropathy does not exclude other causes.[12,31,32] The most common organic cause is vascular disease. Other organic causes include neurologic disorders and endocrine abnormalities. Psychological causes include performance anxiety, loss of self-confidence, and conflict or poor communication with the partner.

Boxes 15-1 and 15-2 summarize the medical conditions and risk factors that are commonly associated with sexual dysfunction.

BOX 15-1 Medical Conditions Associated with Sexual Dysfunction

- Cancer and its treatment (prostate, bladder, rectum)
- Coronary artery or peripheral vascular disease
- Depression
- Diabetes mellitus
- Endocrine disorders, hyperlipidemia
- Hypertension
- Peyronie's disease
- Trauma or surgery to the spine
- Vascular surgery

BOX 15-2 Risk Factors Associated with Male Sexual Dysfunction

- Diabetes mellitus
- Coronary artery or peripheral vascular disease
- Depression
- Smoking
- Hyperlipidemia
- High blood pressure

REFERENCES

1. Benet AE, Melman A: The epidemiology of erectile dysfunction. Urol Clin North Am 22:699–709, 1995.
2. Feldman HA, Goldstein I, Hatzichristou DG, et al: Impotence and its medical and psychosocial correlates: Results of the Massachusetts Male Aging Study. J Urol 151:54–61, 1994.
3. Johannes CB, Araujo AB, Feldman HA, et al: Incidence of erectile dysfunction in men 40 to 69 years old: Longitudinal results from the Massachusetts Male Aging Study. J Urol 163:460–463, 2000.
4. Laumann EO, Paik A, Rosen RC: The epidemiology of erectile dysfunction: Results from the National Health and Social Life Survey. Int J Impot Res 11 (suppl 1):S60–S64, 1999.
5. Laumann EO, Paik A, Rosen RC: Sexual dysfunction in the United States: Prevalence and predictors. JAMA 281:537–544, 1999.
6. Lewis R, Hatzichristou D, Laumann E, McKinlay J: Epidemiology and natural history of erectile dysfunction: Risk factors including iatrogenic and aging. Erectile function. In Jardin A, Wagner G, Khoury S, et al (eds): Erectile Dysfunction: WHO First International Consultation. Plymouth, Plymbridge, 2000, pp 21–51.
7. Solstad K, Hertoft P: Frequency of sexual problems and sexual dysfunction in middle aged Danish men. Arch Sex Behav 22(1):51–58, 1993.
8. Fugl-Meyer AR, Sjogren Fugl-Meyer K: Sexual disabilities: Problems and satisfaction in 18–74 year old Swedes. Scand J Sexol 2:79–105, 1999.
9. Bejin A: Epidemiologie de l'éjaculation prématurée et de son cumul avec la dysfonction érectile. Andrologie 9:211–225, 1999.
10. Shirai M, Takanama M, Tanaka T, et al: A stochastic survey of impotence population in Japan. Impotence 2:67, 1987.
11. Chew KK, Earle CM, Stuckey BGA, et al: Erectile dysfunction in general medical practice: Prevalence and clinical correlates. Int J Impot Res 12:41–45, 2000.
12. NIH Consensus Development Panel on Impotence: Impotence. JAMA 270:83–90, 1993.
13. Kwan M, Greenleaf WJ, Mann J, et al: The nature of androgen action on male sexuality: A combined laboratory–self-report study on hypogonadal men. J Clin Endocrinol Metab 57:557–562, 1983.

14. Gray A, Feldman HA, McKinley JB, Longcope C: Age, disease and changing sex hormone levels in middle aged men: Results of the MMAS. J Clin Endocrinol Metab 73:1016–1105, 1991.
15. Mulligan T, Schmitt B: Testosterone for erectile failure. J Intern Med 8:517–521, 1993.
16. Benet AE, Melman A: The epidemiology of erectile dysfunction. Urol Clin North Am 22:699–709, 1995.
17. Metro MJ, Broderick GA: Diabetes and vascular impotence: Does insulin dependence decrease the relative severity? Int J Impot Res 11:87–89, 1999.
18. Bulpitt CJ, Dollery CT, Carne S: Change in symptoms of hypertensive patients after referral to hospital clinic. Br Heart J 38:121–128, 1976.
19. Morley JE, Korenman SG, Mooredian AD, Kaiser FE: UCLA geriatric grand rounds: Sexual dysfunction in the elderly male. J Am Geriatr Soc 35:1014–1022, 1987.
20. Mendelson JH, Mello NK: Medical progress: Biologic concomitants of alcoholism. N Engl J Med 301:912–921, 1979.
21. Lechtenberg R, Ohl DA: Drug-induced dysfunction. In Lechtenberg R, Ohl DA (eds): Sexual Dysfunction. Philadelphia, Lea & Febiger, 1994, pp 55–70.
22. Siroky MB: Neurophysiology of male sexual dysfunction in neurologic disorders. Semin Neurol 8:137–140, 1988.
23. Lechtenberg R, Ohl DA: Sexual dysfunction with intracranial disesase. In Lechtenberg R, Ohl DA (eds): Sexual Dysfunction. Philadelphia, Lea & Febiger, 1994, pp 70–93.
24. Sakakibara R, Shinotoh H, Uchiyama A: Questionnaire-based assessment of pelvic organ dysfunction in Parkinson's disease. Auton Neurosci 92(1–2):76–85, 2001.
25. Litwiller SE, Frohman EM, Zimmern PE: Multiple sclerosis and the urologist. J Urol 161:743–757, 1999.
26. Saenz de Tejada I, Gonzalez Cadavid N, Heaton J, et al: Anatomy, physiology and pathophysiology of erectile function. In Jardin A, Wagner G, Khoury S, et al (eds): Erectile Dysfunction: WHO First International Consultation. Plymouth, Plymbridge, 2000, pp 65–103.
27. Brien SE, Heaton JPW, Adams MA: Interactions between apomorphine and sildenafil: Evidence for normalization of erections during hyperadrenergic stimulation (abstract). J Urol 161:219, 1999.
28. Blander DS, Broderick GA, Malkowicz SB: Retrospective review of low patterns following retropubic prostatectomy. Int J Impot Res 11(6):309–313, 1999.
29. Muller JE, Mittleman MA, Maclure M, et al: Triggering myocardial infarction by sexual activity. JAMA 275:1405–1409, 1996.
30. Nehra A, Hall SJ, Basile G, et al: Systemic sclerosis and impotence: A clinicopathological correlation. J Urol 153:1140–1146, 1995.
31. Miller TA: Diagnostic evaluation of erectile dysfunction. Am Fam Physician 61:109–110, 2000.
32. Montague DK, Reedy JL, Sadovsky R, Warnock JJ: Addressing the sexual health of our patients: Practical strategies and case studies. NFSHM. Cleveland, Cleveland Clinic Foundation Monographs, 2001, pp 1–56.

PART III

Diagnosis and Evaluation of Pelvic Floor Disorders

Office Evaluation and Physical Examination

ALAIN P. BOURCIER ■ JEAN C. JURAS ■ RICHARD M. VILLET

HISTORY

The general history should include questions about neurologic and congenital abnormalities as well as previous urinary infections and relevant surgery. Information must be obtained on medications with known or possible effects on the lower urinary tract. The general history should also include assessment of the patient's menstrual, sexual, bowel function, and obstetric history.

A questionnaire is useful in eliciting urinary and other symptoms associated with pelvic floor disorders. Many women are embarrassed to discuss these symptoms, and may need help to describe them. The questions can be grouped into four main areas:

1. Abnormal storage, including urinary stress incontinence, frequency and urgency, nocturia, and nocturnal enuresis
2. Abnormal voiding, including hesitancy, voiding difficulties, straining to void, incomplete emptying, poor stream, and postmicturition dribble
3. Abnormal sensation, including decreased sense of fullness and normal urge response, loss of sense of fullness, urinary retention, decreased pelvic floor activity, pelvic floor overactivity, and painful bladder
4. Anorectal diseases and sexual dysfunction, including incontinence to flatus, incontinence to liquid stool, incontinence to solid stool, straining to defecate, dyspareunia, and anorgasmia

The patient should be questioned about each symptom because she may not be able to describe these symptoms effectively or may be too embarrassed to mention them.[1,2] For many people, urinary symptoms are a taboo subject, and only 10% of spouses know about their partner's incontinence.[3] Different conditions can cause the same urinary symptoms. For example, overflow incontinence and detrusor instability can cause both urinary frequency and leakage. Overflow incontinence causes urinary frequency as a result of reduced functional bladder capacity because the bladder never empties completely. Detrusor instability causes urinary frequency because bladder capacity is reduced as a result of an overactive detrusor. Thus, the same symptom can be produced by two different mechanisms.[4] Symptoms of mixed incontinence occur in women in all diagnostic categories. Even when complex scoring systems are used, none of these methods discriminates between genuine stress incontinence and detrusor instability well enough to be of diagnostic value.[5]

The urinary history (Box 16-1) must include symptoms related to both the storage and the evacuation functions of the lower urinary tract. Many physicians ask the patient to complete a urologic questionnaire.

In the physician-patient interview one should obtain a description of main complaints and the assessment of severity of symptoms.

Urinary Symptoms

Frequency

Frequency is the number of times that a woman voids during her waking hours. Normal frequency is seven voids a day and once per night. Women who void infrequently can be at risk for difficulties.[6]

The frequency–volume chart is a specific urodynamic instrument that records fluid intake and urine output per 24-hour period. The chart gives objective information on the number of voidings, the distribution of voidings between day and night, and the volume of urine voided each time. The chart can also be used to record episodes of urgency and leakage and the number of incontinence pads used. The frequency–volume chart is very useful in the assessment of voiding disorders and in the follow-up treatment.[7] In patients with a high urine output per 24-hour period, it is also helpful to record fluid intake. Frequent voiding of small volumes during both day and night suggests a low-compliance bladder. Low volumes voided only during the daytime hours may be a sign of hypersensitivity (psychogenic) or hypermobility.

> **BOX 16-1   Urologic History**
>
> The urologic history should include the following:
> - Duration and characteristics of urinary incontinence
> - Times of voiding and episodes of incontinence
> - Precipitants and associated symptoms of incontinence
> - Number of episodes of incontinence and number of changes of incontinence pads, clothing, or protective devices
> - Degree of leakage (slight, moderate, or great) and descriptions of factors leading to symptoms
> - Other lower urinary tract symptoms
> - Fluid intake
> - Previous treatment and its effects on urinary incontinence
> - Alterations in bowel habits or sexual function

Nocturia

Nocturia is defined as rising from sleep to void more than once a night. This symptom should be differentiated from increased voiding by a woman because she is awake. Nocturia, or waking more than once a night to void, is a common and bothersome global symptom. It affects all ages, increasing significantly with age from 50 years onward. Up to the age of 70 years, more than a single void at night is considered abnormal.[4] After this age, every extra decade increases the normal upper limit of nocturnal voids by one. Thus, a normal 85-year-old woman may void three times at night. The main causes of nocturia are nocturnal frequency and nocturnal polyuria. Bladder problems that lead to nocturnal frequency include age, reduced bladder capacity, detrusor overactivity, and chronic retention. Nocturnal polyuria may be caused by increased urine production both day and night, as occurs with diabetes mellitus and cardiac failure. This change is probably related to an increased incidence of subclinical cardiac disease.

Urinary Incontinence

Questions about urinary incontinence should help to determine both the situation in which it occurs and the amount and types of sensation felt during the loss. This information helps to determine the cause of urinary leakage. The type of urinary incontinence is not a diagnosis, but is a symptom or sign. Severe urinary incontinence produces many symptoms that are common to different diagnostic categories.

Continuous urine loss is rare, occurring particularly at night, and is associated with fistulas or, occasionally, ectopic ureters. Fistulas are mainly caused by pelvic surgery, malignant disease, or radiation therapy. Obstetric fistulas are seen in women in developing countries. Women who report that they are never dry often have severe urinary incontinence. The severity of urinary incontinence can be quantified by the volume and frequency of episodes, the number of pads or changes of underwear required in a 24-hour period, and the magnitude of the provoking stimulus. Often, little relationship is found between the findings of urodynamic tests and the symptoms described by the patient.

Stress Incontinence

Stress incontinence is involuntary loss of urine with an increase in intra-abdominal pressure, such as coughing, sneezing, running, and lifting, that overcomes the resistance of the bladder outlet in the absence of a true bladder contraction. Urine is often lost in small, discrete amounts. The patient describes urine loss with activity, but the etiology of leakage may also be a "stress maneuver." For this reason, some patients have genuine stress incontinence accompanied by a sensation that is misinterpreted as urge. Stress incontinence is a symptom and a sign: the patient reports involuntary loss of urine during physical exertion and the examiner observes leakage from the urethra synchronous with physical exertion.

Urge Incontinence

Urge incontinence occurs with the symptom of urgency (a strong, sudden desire to void). Urge incontinence is a symptom: an involuntary loss of urine associated with a strong desire to void (urgency). Often, women describe an inability to get to the toilet in time. The patient may lose a few drops of urine before voiding or may lose the entire contents of the bladder. Some women describe at least one occasion where the urine has poured down the legs uncontrollably. Urge incontinence has many triggers, such as changes in temperature, physical exertion (e.g., opening a door), the sound of running water, and occasionally, orgasm.

Mixed Incontinence

Mixed urinary incontinence, which includes the symptoms of stress and urge incontinence, is very common. It is important to determine the balance between the two types of symptoms and to determine which symptoms cause the patient the most subjective discomfort. The duration of coexisting symptoms has prognostic value in determining the success of continence surgery.

Coital Incontinence

Urinary incontinence can occur during sexual intercourse, either on penetration or during orgasm. Urinary leakage on penetration is more likely to occur in women with urethral sphincter incompetence and an anterior vaginal wall prolapse. This type of urinary incontinence is not associated with urgency. Urinary incontinence can also occur with orgasm. The leakage is associated with urgency and is believed to be related to detrusor instability.[8,9]

Giggle Incontinence

Laughter can trigger partial or complete bladder emptying in some children well into the teenage years and intermittently in childhood. The condition occurs in both boys and girls, and is usually self-limiting. However, this problem often occurs in young women under the age of 20 as well. No anatomic dysfunction is noted, and the results of both urinalysis and upper tract visualization are normal. Two mechanisms have been postulated: (1) laughter induces a general hypotonic state that results in urethral relaxation or triggers the micturition reflex and (2) overriding central inhibitory mechanisms may occur.[10,11]

Nocturnal Enuresis

Nocturnal enuresis is urinary loss during sleep. This condition must be differentiated from waking with urgency and then leaking urine before arriving at the toilet, which is urge incontinence. Nocturnal enuresis can be primary or secondary. Primary nocturnal enuresis starts in childhood and can persist into adulthood, with the patient never having been consistently dry at night.[12] Secondary nocturnal enuresis is the recurrence of night-time incontinence in adulthood, after a period of night-time continence. The causes can be abnormal circadian secretion of antidiuretic hormone, detrusor instability, abnormal control of the micturition reflex, or an abnormal sleep pattern.[4]

Voiding Difficulties

Dysfunctional voiding usually causes urinary tract infections, urinary incontinence, and constipation. It is primarily considered a voiding disorder, but detrusor dysfunction is common.

Hesitancy

Occasional hesitancy is common in women, but only 7% of women who have persistent hesitancy have an obstruction.[13] Hesitancy is a delay in starting the urinary stream when the woman wishes to void. Hesitancy with a full bladder can indicate an obstruction when voiding, either because the urethral sphincter is not relaxing when the detrusor contracts (detrusor–sphincter dyssynergia), or because of stricture of the urethra. This symptom may also be caused by an acontractile detrusor muscle or by psychological inhibition of the voiding reflex. Women with detrusor instability may have hesitancy and poor stream as a result of the small volumes of urine that are passed frequently in response to urgency.

Poor Stream

Decreased urinary stream may be described as decreased force. To assess this symptom adequately, the volumes of urine voided should be recorded, assessed, and compared with the use of a frequency–volume chart. Reduced urine flow can be caused by reduced voided volume, bladder outflow obstruction (rare in women), or decreased bladder contractility.

Straining to Void

Intra-abdominal pressure is increased by a Valsalva maneuver, which increases intravesical pressure and can improve bladder emptying. If the urinary stream is impaired and intermittent, each transient increase in flow is associated with an increase in intra-abdominal pressure.

Incomplete Emptying

The sensation that urine is left in the bladder after micturition can be caused by fluid remaining in the bladder, abnormal bladder sensation, or aftercontractions of the bladder. These women do not always have increased postmicturition urinary residual volumes. Women with prolapse can have functional obstruction and may retain urine. Women with a pelvic organ prolapse (> stage 3) have incomplete emptying of the bladder. A severe cystocele can act as a sump, preventing complete emptying of the bladder.

Postmicturition Dribble

After voiding is completed, a woman may have intermittent urinary loss as a result of urethral diverticulum, cystourethrocele, or detrusor instability. The dribble may be associated with fluid left in the bladder after voiding or with a separate fluid collection.

Dysuria

Dysuria is often described as "burning on passing urine," and can be aggravated by sexual intercourse. As an isolated symptom, it is associated with urinary tract infection or urethritis. Pelvic inflammatory disease and endometriosis may also cause dysuria.

Bladder Pain

Suprapubic pain is associated with bladder inflammation, bladder stones, or tumor. The pain usually occurs after micturition, as the bladder mucosa closes down. Bladder pain is an indication for cystoscopy and bladder biopsy. Suprapubic pain can be associated with pathology outside the bladder, but within the pelvis.

Hematuria

Blood in the urine should always be investigated and should never be ignored. In women, it is often caused by urinary tract infections.

Neurologic History

Normal micturition is controlled by neural circuits in the brain and spinal cord that coordinate the activity of visceral smooth muscle in the urinary bladder and urethra with the activity of striated muscles. Injuries or diseases of the nervous system in adults are some of the causes of disruption of the voluntary control of micturition that lead to voiding dysfunction or incontinence. Because of the complexity of central nervous control of the lower urinary tract, incontinence can be caused by a variety of neurologic disorders as well as by changes in peripheral innervation and skeletal muscles. Bladder hyperactivity occurs after cortical inhibitory circuits are interrupted, basal ganglia function is disrupted, or the pathways from the brain to the spinal cord are damaged.[14]

Women should be questioned about any alteration in sensation and motor power in the legs or perineum. Fecal incontinence or sexual dysfunction associated with lower urinary tract symptoms may evoke a neurologic alteration. Among these neurological abnormalities, the most frequent are: Parkinson's disease, multiple sclerosis, and spinal cord lesions. Neurologic symptoms can also be caused by peripheral neuropathy associated with diabetes mellitus, cerebrovascular accidents, Parkinson's disease, or multiple sclerosis.

Gynecologic Symptoms and Previous Surgery

Clinically, urinary symptoms are an integral part of the transition from the premenopausal to the postmenopausal state. These atrophic changes increase susceptibility to urinary tract infections, and can cause storage symptoms (e.g., frequency, urgency), dysuria, vaginal dryness, and dyspareunia. Estrogen deprivation contributes to the problem. It is important to ask about changes in urinary symptoms during the menstrual cycle and to note whether menopause has occurred. Most women who have urologic symptoms have coexisting gynecologic pathology. Previous pelvic surgery and hysterectomy are often associated because these operations may interfere with innervation of the bladder, particularly after radical hysterectomy for carcinoma. Pelvic radiation therapy has profound effects on the bladder (e.g., fibrosis). It can also cause urgency and frequency. Spinal surgery and associated neurologic impairment must be recorded, particularly in relation to possible nerve damage. Operations on the large bowel, particularly those involving dissection at the side wall of the pelvis (e.g., abdominoperineal resection of the rectum) may cause denervation.

Potential Risk Factors and Drug History

Many variables affect urinary incontinence and pelvic floor dysfunction, and several possible risk factors or contributing variables may be identified.[15] These factors must be identified during the history to allow proper selection of conservative treatment techniques or surgical options.

Risk factors, such as smoking, menopause, vaginal childbirth, constipation, chronic cough, chronic straining for defecation, urogenital surgery, functional impairment, and occupational risks, must be investigated. Conditions that increase abdominal pressure can cause stress incontinence and worsen a minor problem. These conditions are also implicated in the development of vaginal prolapse. Cardiac and renal failure can cause frequency and nocturia as a result of polyuria. Endocrine disorders, such as diabetes mellitus or diabetes insipidus, may lead to polyuria and polydipsia. Other variables correlated with urinary incontinence include urinary tract infections, cystitis, fecal incontinence, the use of drugs (e.g., diuretics, benzodiazepines, anticholinergic drugs, opiates, antidepressants, antiparkinsonian agents, sympathetic). Caffeine, found in coffee and tea, is a diuretic and can lead to frequency and urgency. Other factors such as vaginal delivery, obesity, chronic straining, jobs with heavy lifting, and practice of sports may contribute to pelvic fecal dysfunction.

PHYSICAL EXAMINATION

Introduction

Universal agreement has not been reached on the components of the examination. It seems intuitive that the examination should include an assessment of the following features: bony architecture; tone and mass of the pelvic floor muscles; connective tissue support; epithelial lining of the vagina; size, location, and mobility of the uterus; adnexal structures; and innervation of the pelvic floor structures.[16] Increasing age, decreasing muscle strength, and parity are associated with prolapse. The anterior compartment is the most commonly affected vaginal segment. DeLancey and Hurd[17] reported that, when matched for age and parity, women with pelvic organ prolapse had a larger genital hiatus than women with no prolapse. In addition, women with recurrent prolapse after pelvic surgery had a larger genital hiatus than women cured by surgery. Few data link bladder, bowel, or sexual function to variations in the examination of women seeking routine gynecologic care. Data on women with urinary incontinence do not include detailed, specific information about pelvic examinations. Recognizing these shortcomings in our knowledge about what is normal and how findings change with age, we presume that function and physical examination findings are related in some patients.[17] Some women are cured of stress urinary incontinence, but acquire significant pelvic support defects, such as enterocele, cystocele, or vaginal vault prolapse, after surgery for stress urinary incontinence. In addition to postoperative support defects, these patients may acquire functional symptoms of urgency and emptying phase abnormalities.[18,19]

Before a patient undergoes conservative treatment or a surgical procedure, she should be evaluated for coexisting pelvic organ prolapse and dysfunctional defecation. Comprehensive treatment may include therapy for all of the anatomic and functional abnormalities that are identified.

In 1993, the International Continence Society (ICS) established an international multidisciplinary committee to standardize the terminology used to describe prolapse. The committee devised a site-specific quantitative description of support that describes the location of six defined points around the vagina (two anterior, two posterior, and two apical) with respect to their relationship to the hymen.

Once measurements are obtained, subjects are assigned to one of five ordinal stages:

- Stage 0   No prolapse is seen (i.e., all points are at their highest possible level above the hymen).
- Stage I   The criteria for stage 0 are not met, but the most distal portion of the prolapse is more than 1 cm above the level of the hymen.
- Stage II   The most distal portion of the prolapse is 1 cm or less proximal or distal to the plane of the hymen.
- Stage III The most distal portion of the prolapse is more than 1 cm below the plane of the hymen, but protrudes no further than 2 cm less than the total vaginal length.
- Stage IV   Complete eversion of the total length of the lower genital tract is seen.

In addition, the system calls for three other measurements: the anterior–posterior length of the genital hiatus, the length of the perineal body, and the total length of the vagina.

More recently, several authors compared the severity of pelvic organ prolapse noted on examination performed in the lithotomy position with the severity of prolapse noted on examination performed in other positions. Swift and Herring[20] directly compared measurements of pelvic organ prolapse obtained in the dorsal lithotomy position with measurements obtained in the same patients in the upright position. They found a high degree of correlation between values obtained in the two positions and no significant differences in the stage of prolapse. In another study, Barber and associates[21] reported a higher degree of prolapse in women who were examined at a 45-degree angle in a birthing chair. They also speculated that the 45-degree position predisposes patients to a greater degree of prolapse than does the standing position because sitting in the birthing chair opens the pelvic outlet and maximizes the effects of pushing. Consequently, when pelvic organ prolapse cannot be reproduced in the dorsal lithotomy position, the patient can be examined while she sits in the 45-degree position.[16]

The standardization document was formally adopted by the ICS in 1995 and by the American Urogynecologic Society and the Society of Gynecologic Surgeons in 1996. The ICS system used for staging of pelvic organ prolapse reliably describes the topographic position of six vaginal sites. It also describes perineal descent as well as the change in axis of the levator plate based on increases in measurements of the genital hiatus and perineal body. However, this system does not identify the specific defect in the pelvic support structures or the mechanisms responsible for the topographic changes, and cannot determine the surgical steps needed for successful repair.[16]

General Physical Examination

The patient's height and weight should be recorded so that the body mass index can be calculated. Abdominal examination should be performed to evaluate the condition of the skin and surgical incisions and to identify hernias or abnormal masses, including a full bladder.

Before the physical examination is undertaken, the patient should be informed that urinary leakage may occur and reassured that she should not be embarrassed if it occurs. The woman's mobility and mental state affect her ability to react to her incontinence problem, and may affect management.

Pelvic Examination

The external genitalia should be examined for dermatologic lesions and evidence of irritative or inflammatory conditions. The internal genitalia should be examined for estrogen deficiency, urine or abnormal vaginal secretions, pelvic organ prolapse, and abnormal pelvic masses. The well-estrogenized vagina has a thickened epithelium, with transverse rugae in its lower two thirds. The poorly estrogenized vagina has a thinned epithelium, with loss of transverse rugae.[22] Many authors showed that vaginal pH is usually 5 or lower in women with no infection and other definitive signs of good estrogen effect. The use of a pH indicator paper may help to evaluate estrogen status in women with no vaginal infection. The appearance of vaginal secretions may suggest a vaginal infection, and urine within the vagina suggests genitourinary fistula, hypospadias, or an ectopic ureter.

The urethra should be examined for discharge, inflammation, or fixation. If the patient reports a discharge or had recent onset of urgency and frequency, it may be useful to obtain swabs to culture for *Chlamydia* and gonococcus.

Vaginal dysfunction as a result of obstetric trauma or gynecologic causes should be assessed during a careful clinical examination. Because it is the weakest portion of the pelvic floor, the vagina is subjected to all vectors of gravity, and may be damaged by vaginal childbirth, estrogen deficiency, or pelvic surgery. Congenital shortening of the area between the fourchette and urethra is accompanied by a firm perineum, a thick hymen, and a small introitus. The normal length of the perineum is 3 cm between the inferior part of the introitus and the superior part of the anus (Fig. 16-1). A short distance (<2 cm) could be responsible for a gaping vagina, which is typically observed after vaginal childbirth. Introital laxity is usually obstetric in origin, and is accompanied by disturbed architecture of the musculature responsible for an enlarged vagina (Fig. 16-2). This defect is common after childbirth. The vagina may be torn away from its intrapelvic attachments, with subsequent loss of the superior vaginal sulcus. There may also be direct attenuation of the vaginal wall itself, manifested by loss of vaginal rugae and a thin appearance. Stretching and tearing of the levator ani muscles results in a longer, wider levator hiatus. In women with advanced pelvic relaxation, the perineum bulges downward (see Fig. 16-2); the vaginal introitus opens, exposing redundant mucosa; and the anus often appears everted. Vulvar episiotomy scars are commonly associated with dyspareunia. Mediolateral episiotomies tend to cause the problem more often than

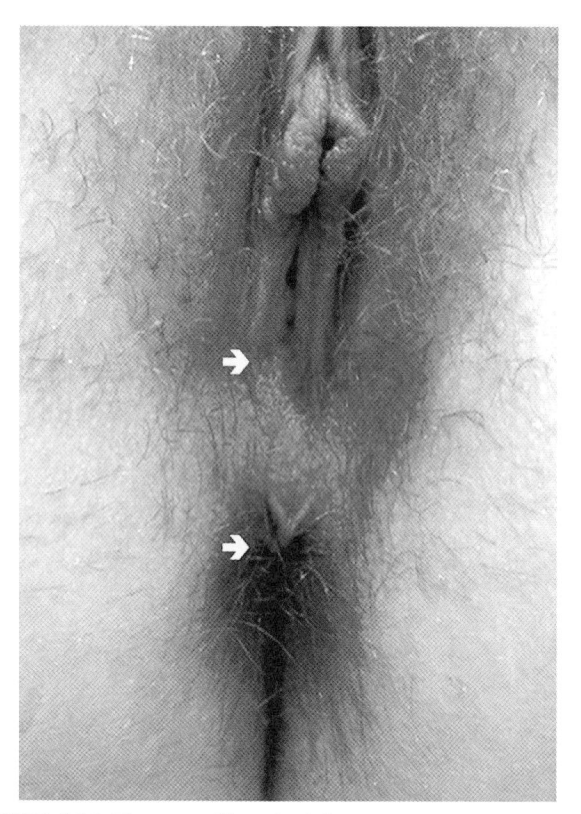

FIGURE 16-1 The normal length of the perineum is 3 cm from the inferior part of the introitus (top arrow) to the superior part of the anus (bottom arrow).

FIGURE 16-2 A short distance (<2 cm) can be responsible for a gaping vagina, which is usually observed after vaginal childbirth. Introital laxity is usually obstetric in origin, and the disturbed architecture of the musculature is responsible for the enlarged vagina.

midline episiotomies. Scars caused by perineoplasty or improperly performed posterior colporrhaphy are common, and vulvar diseases, including herpetic infection, radiation damage, and allergic reactions, must be noted. Iatrogenic shortening of the vaginal vault may also be observed in association with hysterectomy. Excessive removal of the apical vagina during hysterectomy results in shortened vaginal length. Organic features include excessive contraction of the vaginal orifice, vaginismus, and vulva vestibulitis syndrome. These conditions always cause introital dyspareunia and sometimes point tenderness and pain on vestibular touch, and must be evaluated carefully.

The anterior, superior, and posterior segments of the vagina should be examined for pelvic organ prolapse. Genital prolapse can be best assessed with the use of a Sims speculum while the patient is in the Sims (left lateral) position during coughing and straining (Fig. 16-3). When a patient states that she normally has a greater amount of prolapse than is detected on examination, she should be asked to stand erect and perform any provocative maneuvers that normally cause symptoms. In all women, a digital rectal examination is also performed to assess both resting and active sphincter tone and to detect fecal impaction or a rectal mass. Bimanual examination is performed to determine the size of the uterus and ovaries. Some women have coexisting pelvic disease that may require attention in addition to urinary incontinence. When hysterectomy or oophorectomy is indicated, there is no adverse effect on surgical success with

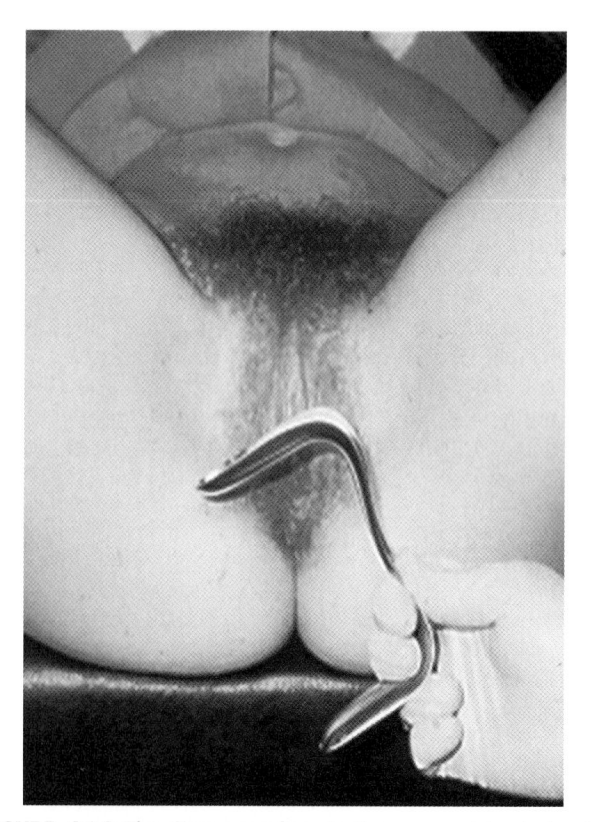

FIGURE 16-3 The Sims speculum is the appropriate device to identify vaginal compartment defects in patients with pelvic organ prolapse.

a colposuspension procedure. Pelvic masses are rarely the cause of urinary incontinence.

Urethral diverticula are occasionally congenital, but most are acquired. They may have simple or complex sacculation. Many patients with urethral diverticula are asymptomatic and need no treatment. Symptomatic patients have recurrent cystitis, frequency, dysuria, dyspareunia, urinary incontinence, and voiding difficulties. On clinical examination, a suburethral mass may be palpable, the urethra is usually tender, and if the sacculation communicates with the urethra, it may be possible to express a purulent exudate from the urethra.

Pelvic Relaxation and Pelvic Organ Prolapse

Symptoms of pelvic relaxation syndrome are varied because more than one vaginal compartment is often involved and more than one symptom is noted. Pelvic relaxation usually causes the following symptoms:

- Vaginal heaviness
- Pelvic pressure or irritation
- Protrusion through the introitus
- Vaginal wind
- Difficult defecation that requires digital maneuvers (The patient must insert her fingers into the vagina to reduce the posterior vaginal wall and make defecation possible.)
- Dyspareunia or lack of vaginal sensation during sexual intercourse

Stress urinary incontinence and pelvic organ prolapse are separate clinical entities that often coexist.[23] Significant protrusions of the vagina can obstruct voiding and defecation. Surgical repair of one pelvic support defect without repair of concurrent asymptomatic pelvic support defects appears to predispose the patient to accentuation of unrepaired defects and new symptoms.[24,25]

Anterior Vaginal Wall Descent

Hypermobility of the urethrovesical junction is demonstrated by having the patient perform a maximum Valsalva maneuver. In women with hypermobility, the increase in intra-abdominal pressure causes descent of the urethrovesical junction (bladder neck). Vaginal examination[16] may show loss of the transverse crease between the lower and middle thirds of the anterior vaginal wall and descent of the anterior vaginal wall.

Anterolateral protrusion into the vaginal canal may represent unilateral or bilateral detachment of the pubocervical fascia, along the anterolateral vagina sulcus, from its attachment to the arcus tendineus fascia pelvis (white line).[26] Central protrusions of the anterior vaginal wall may represent defects in the pubocervical fascia below the trigone and base of the bladder.

Apical Vaginal Wall Descent

After hysterectomy, descent of the cervix or vaginal apex below the level of the ischial spines suggests a defective vaginal suspension mechanism.[16] In some women, the intravaginal portion of the cervix becomes elongated, and as a result, the cervix extends into the lower vaginal canal, simulating prolapse; however, the fundus may have good support. In other women, the uterus may prolapse fully outside the hymen as uterine procidence.

Posterior Vaginal Wall Descent

The well-supported posterior vaginal wall should not cross the longitudinal axis of the vaginal canal. Posterior protrusions into the vaginal canal are most commonly caused by defects in the rectovaginal fascia that allow protrusions of the small bowel (enteroceles) or rectum (rectoceles). Distal loss of support in the posterior segment may cause a bulge that compresses the urethra and affects voiding.[16]

Neurologic Examination

All patients should undergo a simple neurologic examination that has three components: assessment of anal sphincter tone, evaluation of voluntary anal contraction, and evaluation for intact perineal sensation. When abnormalities are noted or neurologic disease or dysfunction is suspected, an extended neurologic examination should be performed.[16] This examination has four parts: mental status, sensory function, motor function, and deep tendon reflexes.[27]

Mental Status

Mental status is evaluated by observing the patient's level of consciousness, orientation, speech pattern, memory, and comprehension. Urinary dysfunction may be associated with changes in mental status caused by stroke, brain tumor, degenerative neurologic diseases, or acute or chronic infection of the central nervous system.

Sensory Function Evaluation

Lumbosacral dermatomes are tested for position, vibration, pinprick, light touch, and temperature.

Important sensory dermatomes are L1 (base of the penis, upper scrotum), L1–L2 (midscrotum, labia minora), L3 (front of the knee), S1 (sole and lateral area of the foot), S1–S3 (perineum and circumanal skin), and S2–S4 (sacral nerve roots innervating the external urethra and anal sphincter). The sensory examination includes cutaneous sacral reflexes.

The anal reflex (S2–S5) is stimulated by light stroking of the mucocutaneous junction of the circumanal skin, causing a visible contraction. Absence of this reflex suggests sacral nerve disease. In children, the disorder may be congenital. In women, the reflex may be lost as a result of trauma from vaginal childbirth.

Sphincter tone and volitional contraction must be assessed. Voluntary anal sphincter contraction indicates functioning pelvic floor innervation and sphincter muscle. Absent or decreased anal sphincter tone and voluntary anal contraction indicates a possible sacral or peripheral lesion. If the anal sphincter tone is present in the absence of voluntary anal contraction, a suprasacral lesion may be present.

The bulbocavernous reflex tests the innervation of all perineal striated muscles. It is a local sacral spinal cord reflex arc that reflects activity at S2–S4. The bulbocavernous reflex is elicited by squeezing the penis glans or the clitoris, causing a reflex contraction of the external anal sphincter. Absence of this reflex can indicate sacral nerve damage. It is absent in people with a complete lower motor neuron lesion.

Motor Function

To assess motor function, the following features are assessed: coordination, facial asymmetry, paresis, paralysis, tremor, mobility (e.g., cane, walker, wheelchair), and muscle atrophy. The tibialis anterior (L4–L5) and toe extensor (L1, S1) may be tested by dorsiflexion, plantar flexion, and toe extension.

Deep Tendon Reflexes

Deep tendon reflexes reflect the integrity of upper motor neuron and lower motor neuron function (Fig. 16-4). Upper motor neuron lesions are usually associated with detrusor overactivity (hyper-reflexia). Lower motor neuron damage causes an areflexic bladder. The evaluation includes lower deep tendon reflexes: quadriceps (L3–L4) and Achilles tendon (L5–S2). Children with complete spinal cord lesions above the conus medullaris may have hyperactive deep tendon reflexes, a hyper-reflexic bladder, skeletal spasticity, a pathologic toe sign (Babinski's sign), ankle clonus, and no skin sensation below the level of the lesion. Complete spinal cord lesions at or below the level of the conus medullaris may cause an areflexic bladder and skeletal flaccidity as well as absence of deep tendon reflexes, Babinski's sign, ankle clonus, and skin sensation below the level of the lesion.

Other Tests

Provocative Stress Testing

If stress urinary incontinence is suspected, provocative stress testing (direct visualization) can be performed by having the patient relax and then cough vigorously while the examiner observes for urine loss from the urethra. Optimally, these tests should be performed when the patient's bladder is full, but not when the patient has a precipitant urge to void. These tests can be performed with the patient in the standing or lithotomy position. If instantaneous leakage occurs with cough, then stress urinary incontinence is likely. If leakage is delayed or persists after the cough, then detrusor overactivity should be suspected. If the test is initially performed in the lithotomy position and no leakage is observed, then the test is repeated in the standing position. The patient is asked to cough and perform the Valsalva maneuver while the examiner observes for urinary leakage from the urethral meatus. Direct observation of urine leakage, with spurts at the same time as a cough or Valsalva maneuver, suggests urethral sphincteric incompetence. Bladder filling for stress testing may be performed conveniently in conjunction with catheterization for postvoid residual (PVR) measurement. Patients who have very little urine in their bladder and leak urine during a Valsalva maneuver may have intrinsic sphincter deficiency.[28]

Bonney's original stress test was performed to show urinary leakage during coughing.[29] Bonney described a test of bladder neck elevation to indicate the likelihood that stress incontinence can be cured with vaginal repair. The procedure is as follows:[4]

- The patient, whose bladder should not have been emptied recently, is told to cough violently, and the examiner notes the escape of urine.
- The examiner inserts the index and middle finger into the vagina and presses the anterior vaginal wall against the subpubic angle, without pressing on the urethra.
- The patient is told to cough again. If the pressure of the examiner's fingers prevents the leak, the result of the test is positive, indicating that any type of bladder neck suspension, if properly performed, will provide a cure. However, this test causes occlusion of the urethra that is not reproduced surgically. Thus, the result is positive, regardless of the urodynamic diagnosis or cause of urinary leakage; therefore, the test has no practical use.[30]

Subsequent modifications of the test require support of the urethrovesical junction during coughing in women who experience leakage during a stress test.

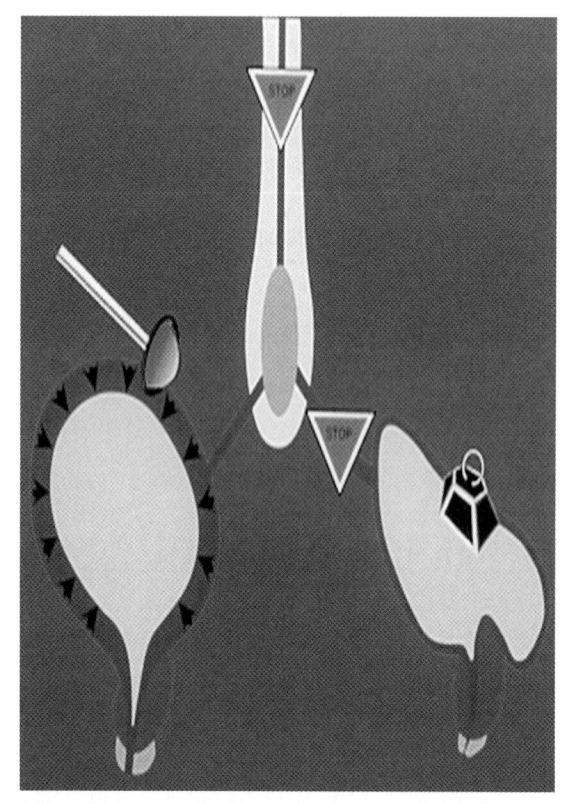

FIGURE 16-4 Neurologic evaluation includes a sensory examination of the cutaneous sacral reflexes, motor function, and the deep tendon reflexes.

These modifications are not reliable in selecting a surgical procedure or predicting cure.

Specific Test for Unmasked Incontinence

An important exception is the patient who has severe apical vaginal wall descent, or a "double bubble" prolapse (cystocele associated with rectocele). In this case, the patient with severe prolapse, which protrudes beyond the vaginal introitus during staining, remains paradoxically continent. This paradoxical continence is explained by kinking of the urethra as the prolapse is accentuated with stress. A stress test should be performed, with careful reduction of the prolapse with a pessary or with the lower half of a Sims or Collins speculum (Fig. 16-5). The device is positioned so that its leading edge is in the anterior fornix, or in the case of hysterectomy, at the vaginal apex. After the prolapse is reduced, a stress test is performed. The patient is asked to cough or strain again, and the examiner observes for urine loss from the urethra (Fig. 16-6).[31] This test may help to identify patients who have symptoms of incontinence after pelvic organ prolapse surgery.

Urethral Junction Mobility: Q-tip Test

Urethrovesical junction (bladder neck) mobility should be assessed in all women who have urinary incontinence.

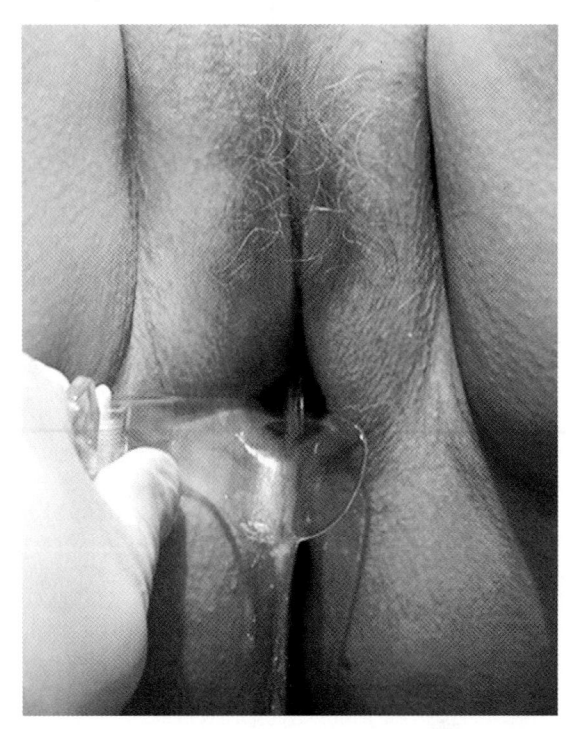

FIGURE 16-6 After the prolapse is reduced, urinary incontinence occurs. However, in this specific case, the large amount of leakage is the result of both sphincter incompetence and bladder instability.

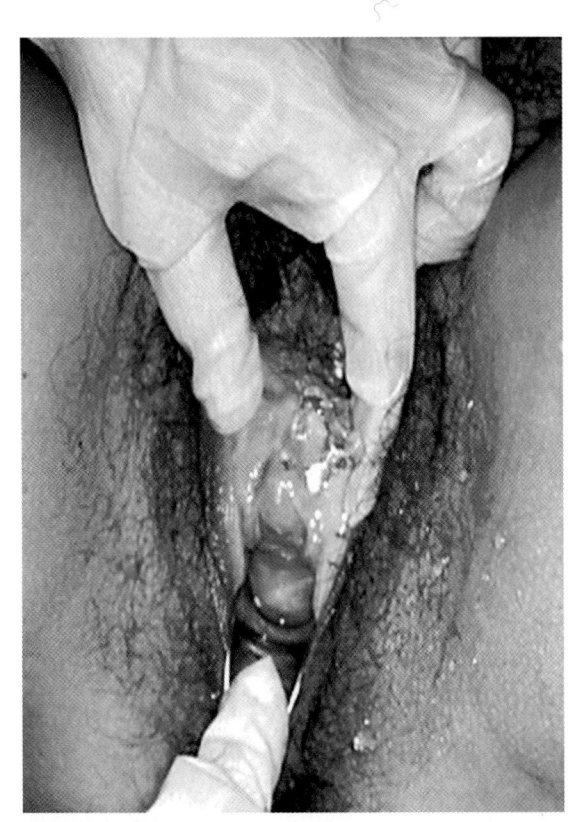

FIGURE 16-5 Specific test for unmasked incontinence. The patient who has severe prolapse that protrudes beyond the vaginal introitus during straining remains paradoxically continent. A stress test is performed, with careful reduction of the prolapse with the lower half of a Sims or Collins speculum.

Those with genuine incontinence are classified into several categories based on an assessment of urethral support and function. The choice of therapy may be affected by the assessment of bladder neck mobility. One method used to assess bladder neck mobility is visual inspection. When a woman with good bladder neck support is in the lithotomy position, the urethral meatus is horizontal to the floor. When she increases intra-abdominal pressure, the examiner can observe for posterior rotation of the anterior vagina and deflection of the meatus toward the ceiling, both signs of some loss of support. The patient may be asked to contract the pelvic muscles to determine whether urethral support improves with muscle contraction, a sign that pelvic floor training may be therapeutic.

The mobility of the urethra and bladder neck can be evaluated by inserting a sterile, lubricated Q-tip cotton bud into the urethra to the level of the bladder neck. The patient is then asked to strain. The rotation of the bladder neck around the symphysis pubis causes the Q-tip bud to move cranially. The angle of the Q-tip bud is measured relative to the horizon, using an orthopedic goniometer. The resting and straining angles are measured, and the difference between the two is calculated. A change of more than 30 degrees shows a hypermobile urethra.

This test does not establish the diagnosis of stress incontinence and does not add information to the history and examination.[32] However, some clinicians consider it the most appropriate continence procedure in patients with genuine stress incontinence, and it may predict failure of incontinence surgery.

Q-tip testing does not diagnose any form of incontinence, although it may be useful in differentiating stress urinary incontinence caused by hypermobility from that caused by intrinsic sphincter deficiency. Other tests to document bladder neck mobility include cystourethrography, ultrasonography, and videocystourethrography.

Postvoid Residual Measurement

PVR measurement is recommended for patients with urinary incontinence. Specific PVR measurement can be accomplished within a few minutes of voiding, either by catheterization or by ultrasound.

Review of the literature does not show a specific maximum PVR that is considered normal, nor is there documentation of the minimal PVR that is considered abnormal. The Agency for Health Care Policy and Research (AHCPR) guidelines state that, in general, a PVR of less than 50 mL is considered adequate bladder emptying and a PVR of greater than 200 mL is considered inadequate emptying. Because PVR may vary, one measurement may not be sufficient.[33] Women with pelvic organ prolapse may need to reduce their prolapse to void. Women with pelvic organ prolapse and a large PVR should be evaluated for voiding phase dysfunction (e.g., outlet obstruction, detrusor hypofunction).

FUNCTIONAL ASSESSMENT OF THE PELVIC FLOOR MUSCLES

Introduction

The use of pelvic floor physical therapy for muscle training is an important initial approach for patients with pelvic floor dysfunction. The pelvic floor muscles include the levator ani complex as well as the more distal muscles of the urogenital diaphragm. These muscles act as a distinct physiologic unit to assist with the proper support and function of the pelvic organs. Because different names are used for the same group of muscles, descriptions can be confusing. The terms pelvic floor and pelvic diaphragm refer to all of the muscular components that close the pelvic cavity and their respective parietal fascial coverings.

The levator ani muscles include the pubococcygeus (puborectalis), iliococcygeus, and ischiococcygeus muscles. The levator ani muscles exhibit constant resting tone, as does the external anal sphincter. A properly maintained pelvic floor performs four functions:

1. Supports the pelvic viscera
2. Helps to maintain urinary continence
3. Helps to constrict the vaginal hiatus
4. Controls flatus and fecal continence

The pelvic floor complex consists of the visceral pelvic fascia, the pelvic diaphragm, and the urogenital anal triangles, with superficial and deep genital muscles. The levator muscles are innervated by motor efferents from S2–S4 on their pelvic surface and by branches of the pudendal nerve on their perineal surface.[34–37]

The levator ani muscle is a heterogeneous mixture of type I (aerobic–oxidative) and type II (anaerobic-glycolytic) fibers of large diameter. Seventy percent of fibers within the periurethral levator ani are slow-twitch (type I) fibers, and 30 % are fast-twitch (type II) fibers. The slow-twitch fibers of the levator ani maintain the tonus of the pelvic floor, thereby providing support for the pelvic viscera. The fast-twitch fibers are activated mainly during events that increase intra-abdominal pressure.[38,39] Both resting tone and voluntary contractions are important. Because of the histomorphologic differences in pelvic floor muscles, both types of contractions must be evaluated and considered in any program of pelvic floor re-education.

Basic evaluation of the pelvic floor muscles can help physicians and caregivers to evaluate the patient's ability to produce voluntary contractions and maintain a contraction during stressful situations. Careful investigation of pelvic floor function is mandatory. Two basic techniques are used to evaluate the pelvic floor muscles:

1. Digital palpation or manual muscle testing of pelvic floor function[40,41]
2. The functional stop test[42,43]

These tests do not provide a complete evaluation of the strength and function of the pelvic floor. A thorough clinical examination of an incontinent patient or a patient with pelvic floor dysfunction includes functional testing, which consists of digital and apparatus-based tests. Valid clinical parameters are required to assess pelvic floor muscle strength.

To provide effective treatment, therapists need the following information:

- Symmetry of the levator ani bundles
- Scarring and changes in the connective tissue
- Volume of the muscles
- Importance of the defects in the pelvic floor muscles
- Resting tone of the muscles
- Voluntary perineal command
- Strength of contractions
- Endurance of contractions
- Results of sacral reflex tests
- Fast-twitch fiber capability and assessment of coordination (the patient should be instructed to contract the pelvic floor muscle by coughing)

Although digital palpation and manual testing (Fig. 16-7) are sufficient for clinical purposes, reproducible quantification before and during treatment requires the use of other scientific tests (Box 16-2). Vaginal palpation is performed with the index finger. A well-developed pubococcygeus muscle is manifested by firm tone throughout the length of the vagina. In case of pelvic relaxation with a wide open hiatus (see Fig. 16-3), the vaginal walls offer little resistance and feel thin and loose, as if detached from the surrounding structures. The pubococcygeus muscle, which lies in the middle third of the vagina, can be palpated on the lateral wall when the index finger is introduced to a depth of 3 to 5 cm beyond the vaginal introitus (see Fig. 16-7). The areas in which contractions can be palpated vary with the position of the pubococcygeus. Normally, the contraction can be felt throughout the length of the muscle. During pelvic relaxation, the pubococcygeus muscle sags and tension is slight near the vaginal outlet.

The integrity and volume of the pelvic floor muscles are best assessed with ultrasonography and magnetic

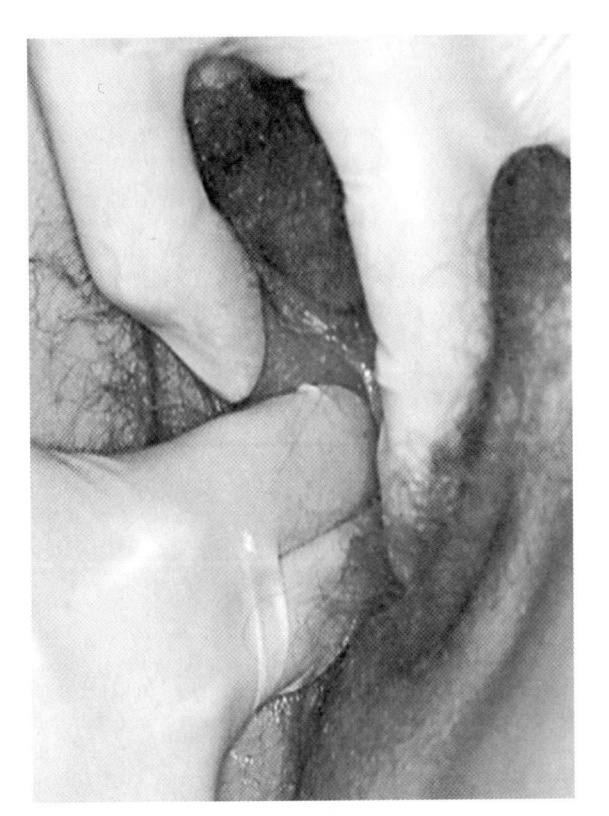

FIGURE 16-7 Manual muscle testing of the pelvic floor muscles. Digital evaluation provides information about the patient's ability to relax as well as on the duration and symmetry of the contraction.

| BOX 16-2 | Pelvic Floor Re-education Related to Assessment |

Techniques used by urotherapists and nurse practitioners:

- Inspection and observation of the perineum
- Vaginal and rectal palpation
- Manual muscle testing of pelvic floor muscles
- Functional stop test
- Perineometry
- Vaginal cones
- Pelvic floor evaluation with electromyography and biofeedback
- Q-tip testing

Techniques used by physicians:

- Sonography
- Urodynamics with urethral pressure measurement
- Colporectocystourethrography
- Electrodiagnosis
- Magnetic resonance imaging of the pelvic floor
- Biopsy

resonance imaging. Contractility is quantified with ultrasonography and colporectocystourethrography. Physiologic behavior and kinesiologic conditions can be assessed with electrodiagnosis.

No technique is available to allow the therapist to differentiate definitively between patients who will benefit from training and those who will not. Classification is possible only according to the complexity of the cases and the scientific value of the investigational techniques (Box 16-3).

Techniques of Functional Assessment

Manual Muscle Testing

Testing incorporates standard muscle assessment scales and differentiates between fast-twitch and slow-twitch muscle components. Proficiency in manual testing requires comprehensive and detailed knowledge of muscle function, including the origin and insertion of muscles. The examiner must understand synergic and antagonist muscle actions as well as the importance of the substitution of suboptimal muscle groups. The initial evaluation begins by identifying the muscles that will be graded. Assessment of strength and isolation is of critical importance. Digital assessment of pelvic muscle strength is likely to be clinically useful.

Manual evaluation provides information about the patient's ability to relax and the duration and symmetry of contractions. Grades of 0 and 1 mean that the patient cannot generate a pelvic floor contraction and usually compensates by recruiting large muscle groups (e.g., gluteals, adductors, abdominals). Grades 2 and 3 indicate a weak squeeze and a poor lift. Grade 4 indicates a good squeeze and a good hold with lift. Grade 5 describes a strong squeeze with a good lift, and implies a very strong grip of the examiner's fingers as well as repeatable contractions.

A patient with a grade of 3 or less should seek further medical testing and undergo pelvic floor exercise training. A patient who has a grade of 4 or 5 at the first visit should maintain this condition and use her muscles functionally.

| BOX 16-3 | Practical and Scientific Value of Investigational Techniques |

Important practical value, less scientific value:

- Manual muscle testing of pelvic floor function[40,41]
- Functional stop test[42,43]
- Perineometry[44–46]
- Vaginal cones[47,48]
- Pelvic floor evaluation with electromyography and biofeedback[49–51]

Moderate practical value, good scientific value:

- Q-tip testing[52,53]
- Sonography[54–57]

No practical value, important scientific value:

- Urodynamics with urethral pressure measurement[58–61]
- Colporectocystourethrography[62–64]
- Electrodiagnosis[65–67]
- Magnetic resonance imaging of the pelvic floor[68–72]

Functional Stop Test

The functional stop test is a self-administered test of the pelvic floor complex. This technique is used for evaluation only, and should never be performed as a pelvic exercise program because it can disrupt the normal voiding reflexes. Patients must be advised that this testing procedure should not be repeated as an exercise.

The functional stop test is performed once daily at the beginning of the pelvic training program. Later, it is performed a maximum of twice monthly to assess changes in muscle function. The test is performed while the patient sits on a toilet in a relaxed position to avoid abdominal participation. After urinating for 5 seconds, the patient attempts to stop the urine flow for a maximum of one or two trials. Patients who cannot interrupt the urine flow or slow the stream are graded 0. Partial deflection of the urine stream that cannot be maintained is graded 1 (trace). Maintenance of deflection in the urine flow is graded 2 (poor). The ability to stop the urine flow completely is graded 3 (fair). Grades 4 (good) and 5 (normal) are difficult to assess with the functional stop test.

We have noted[41] no relationship between pelvic floor power (grades 0–5) and the results of the functional stop test (grades 0–3). Patients can have good results on tests of the pelvic floor muscles (grade 4) and have a partial deflection finding (grade 1) on the functional stop test. Both evaluations are necessary to obtain information about the power of the levator ani muscles (grade 0–5) and the activity of the urethral sphincter by assessing interruption or deflection of urine flow (grade 0–3).

Perineometry

Digital assessment of pelvic muscle strength is likely to be used clinically, buy it is not helpful for the patient who is exercising without receiving timely feedback on performance and progress. Many devices have been designed to measure the dynamic characteristics of the circumvaginal muscles. Arnold Kegel was the first to describe and promote pelvic muscle exercises (Kegel exercises), and began his work in the late 1940s and early 1950s.[44] He combined visual observation with the use of the pressure perineometer to assess pelvic floor contraction. Traditionally, the device consists of an air-filled vaginal probe connected to a manometer that registers pressure changes caused by contraction of the perivaginal muscles. He postulated that the pressure generated in the vagina reflects the contraction of pelvic floor muscles, and that it can be used as a biofeedback signal for self-teaching and objective self-evaluation of progress. The Kegel perineometer is a pressure-sensing device that is inserted into the vagina and provides numeric values and visual feedback on muscle contractions.

Other instruments are available for assessment and feedback. A perineometer provides feedback on the strength and duration of pelvic contractions. Different devices use the same method of assessment, with a pressure balloon covered with a disposable condom. Many devices are available in different countries, allowing both assessment and biofeedback training.

The use of these devices has disadvantages. Care must be taken to ensure that the pressure increase is the result of contraction of the pelvic floor muscles and is not transmitted abdominal pressure. This is most easily carried out by observing the drawing in of the perineometer during a voluntary contraction and by palpating the abdominal muscles. The practical use of a perineometer in the supine position does not reflect the function of the pelvic muscle or allow for evaluation in the positions that often lead to leakage.[44,45]

Another type of perineometer that was described by Samples and associates[46] provides an accurate measurement of pressure. This method uses a balloon that is individually fitted into the intravaginal space. Each balloon is filled with sterile water. Intraballoon pressures are measured with a transducer that is inserted into a strip chart recorder during contractions of the circumvaginal muscles. The intravaginal pressure exerted by these muscles is measured by the intravaginal balloon device. The technique used to assess and control abdominal pressure is original. A small (1×2 cm), flat, pressure-sensitive intravaginal balloon device is placed in the posterior vagina. Posterior vaginal pressure is highly correlated with rectal measurement of intra-abdominal pressure, as in urodynamic studies. Increases in abdominal pressure are recorded when circumvaginal muscle contractions occur. Other instruments are available for evaluation with feedback of abdominal activity. Another channel provides information obtained from surface electrodes about muscle events. More sophisticated software-driven equipment is available from several manufacturers. These devices provide health care providers with objective data on muscle events and are necessary for a thorough functional assessment of the pelvic floor muscles. This method is described later.

Vaginal Cones

Vaginal cones were designed as a biofeedback method for testing and exercising the pelvic floor muscles. They were constructed as a series of tampon-like cones of equal shape and volume, but different weight. These cones may be used as an evaluation method that measures how long a patient can hold a cone of a given weight inside the vagina while exercising. As it is generally accepted that as muscle strength increases heavier cones can be retained, various protocols were proposed. One disadvantage of this method is the variation that occurs in vaginal diameters and pelvic organ defects (e.g., cystocele, rectocele). Therefore, comparing the weight of the cone and the time that the patient can hold it in the vagina provides a rapid method of assessment that has no side effects. A disparity between the size of the cone and the size of the vagina or the finding of different intrasubject pelvic floor muscle tonus during testing decreases the reliability of this test. Some women can retain heavy cones, despite a weak pelvic floor. In the case of an enlarged introitus, the mismatch may be caused by a transverse position of the cone in the vagina.

Electronic Perineometry and Computerized Electromyographic Monitoring

A common error in contracting the pelvic floor muscles is to recruit other muscles, such as the gluteal, adductor, and abdominal muscles, which may mask the strength of the contraction of the pelvic floor muscles. Even in patients with good results on manual muscle testing, electromyographic activity of the lower rectus abdominis muscle increases during a maximum contraction. To ensure valid measurement of pelvic floor muscle strength, perineometry must first register the inward lift and squeeze of the muscle by digital palpation and then observe the inward movement of the probe as a sign of a proper contraction.

The electromyographic response to pelvic floor contraction is an alternative method of monitoring baseline or resting tone, strength, endurance, and other activity patterns. Surface electromyography provides information about muscle events and assesses the magnitude and timing of overall muscle contraction and relaxation, with the objective of obtaining data on normal and abnormal function of the pelvic floor muscle.

Different techniques are used to ensure accuracy in recording the details of pelvic floor muscle function. These data are used to select a specific pelvic muscle training program. Biofeedback is more effective than verbal feedback based on vaginal palpation for teaching patients to improve selective voluntary pelvic floor muscle contraction. In patients with a weak pelvic floor (grade 1 or 2), this information is helpful in the selection of a program of re-education.

Q-tip Test

This test was described earlier. As part of a pelvic floor training program, this test allows the therapist to determine whether the patient can contract the pelvic muscles correctly. A grade of less than 3 indicates poor displacement. When a patient recruits the abdominal muscles, no displacement occurs and the Q-tip can usually be expulsed or directed cephalad. This test improves and quantifies voluntary perineal command by measuring changes in angle displacement. During voluntary contraction, the mobile urethra moves towards the symphysis causing the Q-tip stem to move gradually downward. Modification of the angle is dependent on the extent of the pelvic floor contraction.

Ultrasonography

The use of visualizing techniques to show the urethrovesical junction is one of the most important aims of pelvic floor rehabilitation. This method efficiently shows elevation of the urethrovesical junction by voluntary or reflex contraction of the pelvic floor muscles. Because disturbed or normal contraction of the pelvic floor muscles causes displacement of the bladder base and urethrovesical junction, ultrasonography can be used to provide functional assessment. Easy visualization of bladder neck movement during pelvic floor muscle contractions allows demonstration of the relevant structures for the patient.

Ultrasonography shows the correct contraction and activation of the pelvic floor muscles in demonstrating and recording movement of the bladder neck toward the symphysis. Thus, additional information can be obtained about the mobility of the urethrovesical junction, particularly in patients with pelvic relaxation. A video recorder can be used to produce a permanent record of scans obtained under different stressful conditions. This record provides accurate and reproducible data that can be used to measure perineal activity and the position and displacement of the bladder neck.

Urethral Pressure Profile

A variety of voluntary activities on the urethral closure pressure profile can be used to assess the dynamics of the sphincteric unit. For example, this method can be used to evaluate the effectiveness of the contraction of the voluntary urethral sphincter and the paraurethral muscles. Urethral pressure profile testing can be performed during a "hold maneuver" (Kegel's urethral pressure profile). Kegel's urethral pressure profile can also be used to assess how effectively an individual patient can contract the pelvic floor muscles. A normal reaction indicates an increase in closure pressure; the patient substantially increases the strength of urethral closure with no abdominal straining. In some cases, the Kegel effort is accompanied by a significant Valsalva effort, with a resultant increase in abdominal and vesical pressure. The net effect is a decrease in the total profile area. In cases of incorrect contraction, an increase in intra-abdominal pressure is seen with a decrease in closure pressure. In some cases, when the pressure becomes negative during this maneuver, leakage occurs.

Using the method of Brown and Wickham, measurements are taken with the patient at rest and during pelvic floor contraction.[41] The bladder is filled with 150 mL of water or 0.9% (normal) saline, and the mean value of two consecutive profiles is recorded. A microtransducer can also be used to record urethral pressure profiles at rest and under stress, and before and after a course of pelvic exercises. In case of the paradoxical perineal command ("pusher group") with the recruitment of abdominal muscles, intravesical pressure increases. Patients with good (grade 4) and normal (grade 5) results during digital testing show higher resting functional urethral length and maximal urethral closure pressure, both at rest and under stress. In patients with normal (grade 5) results on pelvic floor testing, an increase of 20 to 30 cm H_2O is observed during voluntary contraction.

A catheter is used simultaneously with electromyography to record the urethral pressure profile and the activity of the skeletal muscle component of the urethral sphincteric mechanism. This method is used to identify dysfunction of periurethral striated muscle.

Colporectocystourethrography

Colporectocystourethrography allows visualization of the dynamic changes in the pelvic organs that are caused by contraction of the pelvic floor muscles. This test allows objective measurement of changes in bladder neck position, anorectal angle, and displacement of the upper vagina and uterus. In order to clearly understand the functional anatomy of the female, levator ani muscle testing is performed with a radiopaque substance. Vaginal colpography, in which the vaginal walls are coated with a thin layer of barium cream, provides radiographic information about the normal configuration of the muscles. The levator ani plate tenses and rises as a consequence of a reflex muscular contraction, causing a greater horizontal inclination that provides additional functional support. During contraction, simultaneously, the muscle sling shortens in a dorsoventral and cranial direction, with narrowing of the vaginal hiatus and upward displacement of the anterior pelvic organs. Colporectocystourethrography can be used to show the decrease in the anorectal angle, the urethrovesical junction, and a lift of the bladder base that occur after successful physiotherapy.

The disadvantages of this radiologic evaluation are the radiation dose needed and the time required to prepare the patient. For these reasons, this method cannot be used in routine practice.

Electrodiagnosis

Electrophysiologic methods are used to evaluate the function of the striated muscles and nervous system. The muscles used for recording depend on the aims of investigation. Routine electromyography of the pelvic floor muscles in urodynamic laboratories is a single-channel recording that shows activity in the urethral or anal sphincter. The sphincters always react in the same way. However, this is not the case in the presence of pathology. Selective recordings from the sphincter muscles can be obtained only by needle-type electrodes. To make electromyographic recordings less invasive, various surface electrodes are used. These are divided into the following types:

- Small skin surface electrodes applied to the perineal skin
- An anal plug used to record the activity of the anal sphincter
- A catheter mounted with ring electrodes used to record urethral sphincter activity

It is generally assumed that the pelvic floor muscles act in a coordinated fashion, but differences are noted in normal women. Peripheral neuropathic disorders may cause important changes in the pattern of muscle activity. At most detection sites, in normal women, the pubococcygeus shows activity patterns similar to those of the urethral and anal sphincters. Coordinated behavior is observed in normal conditions, with an increase in activity seen during bladder filling and periods of increased intra-abdominal pressure. In patients with pelvic floor dysfunction, the patterns of activation and the coordination between the two sides of the vagina may be lost. In patients with possible neurogenic involvement (pelvic floor neuropathy), neurophysiologic studies are of considerable importance. Applied tests, such as motor unit electromyography, bulbocavernosus reflex, motor-evoked potentials, and somatosensory-evoked potentials, are tailored to the neurologic condition affecting the pelvic floor muscles. In cases of pelvic floor denervation, when conservative treatment is recommended, electrodiagnosis is suggested before undergoing therapy.[65-67]

Magnetic Resonance Imaging of the Pelvic Floor

The use of magnetic resonance imaging to analyze the musculature of the pelvic floor has contributed greatly to the current understanding of pelvic floor dysfunction. In the supine position, the female pelvic floor is dome-shaped at rest.[71] During voluntary contraction, the levator musculature straightens and becomes more horizontal. With bearing down, the muscles descend and become basin-shaped, and the width of the genital hiatus widens. Bo and colleagues[72] used magnetic resonance imaging to evaluate the changes seen with pelvic floor contraction in continent and incontinent women in an upright sitting position. They showed inward movement with pelvic floor contraction (average, 10.8 mm) and outward movement with straining (average, 19.1 mm). The levator ani muscle is not easy to visualize with magnetic resonance imaging. Only the pubococcygeus can be visualized with unisectional imaging. The advantages of this method include:

- Recognition of asymmetry between the two sides of the levator ani
- Demonstration of the relationship with the obturator internus muscle
- Visualization of defects within the pelvic floor muscles
- Determination of muscle volume[68-70]

CONCLUSION

History and examination alone cannot diagnose female urinary disorders, but can be used to guide future investigations and management. In some cases, an obvious cause can be found, avoiding the need for further investigations. Pelvic floor muscle training may last for 3 to 6 months, depending on whether it is combined with additional techniques (e.g., biofeedback). Therefore, the effect of therapy must be monitored through reevaluation. The pelvic floor muscles should be assessed regularly, according to the number of sessions prescribed and the grade of the pelvic muscles at the first interview. All of the previously described evaluation techniques allow comparison of clinical data before and after treatment.

With this assessment, it is possible to select patients according to pathology and thus to determine the most suitable treatment.[73-75]

REFERENCES

1. Khullar V, Damiano R, Tooz-Hobson P, Cardozo LD: Prevalence of faecal incontinence among women with urinary incontinence. Br J Obstet Gynecol 105:1211–1213, 1998.
2. Bourcier A, Haab F, Ciofu C, et al: Sexual dysfunction in women attending an outpatient urodynamic clinic. No. 133. Proceedings of the 28th Annual Meerting of the International Continence Society. Jerusalem, 1998.
3. Brocklehurst JC: Urinary incontinence in the community: Analysis of a MORI poll. BMJ 306:832–834, 1993.
4. Khullar V, Cardozo L: History and examination. In Carozo L, Staskin D (eds): Textbook of Female Urology

and Urogynaecology. London, Isis Medical Media, 2001, pp 154–163.
5. Wise BG, Cutner A, Cardozo L: Do detailed symptoms questionnaires negate the need for urodynamic investigations? Neurourol Urodynam 11:353–355, 1992.
6. Swinn MJ, Lowe E, Fowler CJ: The clinical features of nonpsychogenic urinary retention. Neurourol Urodynam 17:383–384, 1998.
7. Abrams P, Blaivas JG, Anderssen JT: The standardization of terminology of lower urinary function recommended by the International Continence Society. Int Gynecol J 1:45–58, 1990.
8. Sutherst JR: Sexual dysfunction and urinary incontinence. Br J Obstet Gynecol 86:387–388, 1979.
9. Bourcier A, Juras J: Prevalence and incidence of urinary incontinence and relaxation in young female patients. In La Torre F, Nicastro A (eds): Abstracts of Proctological and Perineal Diseases. Rome, 1997, pp 93–100.
10. Glahn BE: Giggle incontinence (enuresis rissoria): A study and an aetiological hypothesis. Br J Urol 51:363–366, 1979.
11. Arena MG, Leggiadro N: Enuresis rissoria: Evaluation and management. Funct Neurol 2:579–582, 1987.
12. Foldspang A, Mommsen S: Adult female urinary incontinence and childhood bedwetting. J Urol 152:85–88, 1994.
13. Abrams P: The clinical contribution of urodynamics. In Abrams P, Feneley R, Torrens M (eds): Urodynamics. Berlin, Springer-Verlag, 1983, pp 118–174.
14. Morrson J, Steers WD, Brading A, et al: Neurophysiology and neuropharmacology. In Abrams P, Cardozo L, Khoury S, Wein A (eds): 2nd International Consultation on Incontinence: WHO. Plymouth, Plymbridge, 2001, pp 83–163.
15. Hunskaar S, Burgio K, Diokno AC, et al: Epidemiology and natural history of urinary incontinence (UI). In Abrams P, Cardozo L, Khoury S, Wein A (eds): 2nd International Consultation on Incontinence: WHO. Plymouth, Plymbridge, 2001, pp 167–201.
16. Shull BL, Hurt G, Laycock J, et al: Physical examination. In Abrams P, Cardozo L, Khoury S, Wein A (eds): 2nd International Consultation on Incontinence: WHO. Plymouth, Plymbridge, 2001, pp 375–388.
17. DeLancey JOL, Hurd WW: Size of the urogenital hiatus in the levator ani muscles in normal women and women with pelvic organ prolapse. Obstet Gynecol 91:364–368, 1988.
18. Shull BL, Baden WF: A six year experience with paravaginal defect for stress urinary incontinence. Am J Obstet Gynecol 160:1432–1440, 1989.
19. Stanton SL, Cardozo LD: Results of colposuspension operation for incontinence and prolapse. Br J Obstet Gynecol 86:693–697, 1979.
20. Swift SE, Herring M: Comparison of pelvic organ prolapse in the dorsal lithoytomy compared with the standing position. Obstet Gynecol 91:961–964, 1998.
21. Barber MD, Lambers AR, Visco AG, Bump RC: Effect of patient position on clinical evaluation of pelvic organ prolapse. Obstet Gynecol 96:18–22, 2000.
22. Fantl J, Cardozo L, McClish V: The Hormones and Urogenital Therapy Commitee: Estrogen therapy in the management of urinary incontinence in postmenopausal women: A meta analysis. Obstet Gynecol 83:12–18, 1994.
23. Jackson SL, Weber AM, Hull TL, et al: Fecal incontinence in women with urinary incontinence and pelvic organ prolapse. Obstet Gynecol 89:423–427, 1997.
24. Shull BL, Baden WF: A six year experience with paravaginal defect repair for stress urinary incontinenec. Am J Obstet Gynecol 160(6):1432–1440, 1989.
25. Stanton SL, Cardozo LD: Results of colposuspension operation for incontinence and prolapse. Br J Obstet Gynecol 86:693–697, 1979.
26. Richardson AC, Lyon JB, Williams NL: A new look at pelvic relaxation. Am J Obstet Gynecol 126:568–674, 1976.
27. Abrams P, Blaivas JG, Stanton SL, Andersen JT: The standardization and terminlogy of lower urinary tract function recommended by the International Continence Society. Int Urogynecol J 1:45–58, 1990.
28. McLenman MT, Bent AE: Supine empty stress test as a predictor of low Valsalva leak point pressure. Neurourol Urodynam 17:121–127, 1998.
29. Berkely C, Bonney V: Textbook of Gynecological Surgery, 3rd ed. London, Cassell, 1935.
30. Bhatia NN, Bergman A: Urodynamic appraisal of the Bonney test in women with stress urinary incontinence. Obstet Gynecol 62:696–699, 1983.
31. Bump RC, Fantl JA, Hurt WG: The mechanism of urinary continence in women with severe uretrovaginal prolapse: Results of barrier studies. Obstet Gynecol 72:291–295, 1988.
32. Karram MM, Bhatia NN: The Q-tip test: Standardization of the technique and its interpretation in women with urinary incontinence. Obstet Gynecol 71:807–811, 1988.
33. Hall AF, Theofradtous JP, Cundiff GC, et al: Inter and intra-observer reliability of the proposed International Continence Society, Society of Gynecology Surgeons and American Urogynecologic Society pelvic organ prolapse classification system. Am J Obstet Gynecol 175:1467–1471, 1996.
34. Raz S: The anatomy of pelvic support and stress incontinence. In Raz S (ed): Atlas of Transvaginal Surgery. Philadelphia, Saunders, 1992, p 1.
35. DeLancey JOL, Richardson AC: Anatomy of genital support. In Benson JT (ed): Female Pelvic Floor Disorders: Investigations and Management. New York, WW Norton, 1992.
36. DeLancey JOL: Functional anatomy of the female lower urinary tract and pelvic floor. In Bock G, Whelan J (eds): Neurobiology of Incontinence. New York, John Wiley & Sons, Ciba Foundation Symposium, 1990, pp 57–76.
37. Staskin DR, Zimmern PE, Hadley HR, Raz S: The pathophysiology of stress incontinence. Urol Clin North Am 12:271, 1985.
38. Gosling JA, Dixon JS: Histomorphology of pelvic floor muscle. In Schüssler B, Laycock J, Norton P, Stanton S (eds): Pelvic Floor Re-Education. Berlin, Springler-Verlag, 1994, p 28.
39. Gosling JA, Dixon JS: Structural aspects of pelvic floor. In Bourcier A (ed): Pelvic Floor Rehabilitation Monograph Series. Libertyville, Hollister, 1994, p 1.
40. Laycock J: Clinical evaluation of the pelvic floor. In Schüssler B, Laycock J, Norton P, Stanton S (eds): Pelvic Floor Re-Education. Berlin, Springler-Verlag, 1994, pp 42–48.
41. Bourcier AP, Bonde B, Haab F: Functional assessment of pelvic floor muscles. In Appell RA, Bourier A, La Torre F (eds): Pelvic Floor Dysfunction: Investigations and Conservative Treatment. Rome, Casa Editrice Scientifica Internazionale, 1999, pp 97–107.
42. Brubaker L, Kotarinos R: Pelvic floor rehabilitation: The role of muscle training. American Urogynecologic Society quarterly report 11:1–3, 1993.
43. Wallace K: Female pelvic floor functions, dyfunctions, and behavior approaches to treatment. Clin Sports Med 13:457–459, 1994.
44. Kegel AH: Physiologic therapy for urinary stress incontinence. JAMA 146:915–917, 1951.
45. Shepherd AM, Montgomery E, Anderson RS: Treatment of genuine stress incontinence with a new perineometer. Physiotherapy 69(4):113–116, 1983.

46. Samples JT, Dougherty MC, Abrams RM, Batch CD: The dynamic characteristics of the circumvaginal muscles. J Obstet Gynecol Nurs 194,1988.
47. Plevnik S: New method for testing and strenthening of pelvic floor muscles. Proceedings of the 15th Annual Meeting of the International Continence Society, London, Sept 3–6, 1985.
48. Peattie AB, Plevnilz S, Stanton SL: Vaginal cones: A conservative method of treatment of genuine stress incontinence. Br J Obst Gynecol 95:1049–1053, 1988.
49. Kasman G: Use of integrated electromyography for the assessment and treatment of musculoskeletal pain: Guidelines for physical medicine practitioners. In Cram JR (ed): Surface EMG for Clinical Recordings. Nevada City, Clinical Resources, 1990, p 255.
50. Schartz MS: Single-site versus multisite and single-site versus multomodality monitoring and biofeedback and the issue of microcomputer-based-systems. In Scharwtz MS (ed): Biofeedback: A practioner's Guide. New York, Guilford Press, 1987, p 219.
51. Deindl FM, Vodusek DB, Hesse U, et al: Pelvic floor activity patterns in nulliparous women. Neurol Urodynam 10:385–387, 1991.
52. Crystle D, Charme L, Copeland W: Q-tip test in stress urinary incontinence. Obstet Gynecol 38:313–315, 1971.
53. Schüssler B, Hesse V: Q-tip testing. In Schüssler B, Laycock J, Norton P, Stanton SL (eds): Pelvic Floor Re-education. Principles and Practice. London, Springer-Verlag, 1994, pp 49–50.
54. Bahtia NN: Ultrasound in gynecologic urology. In Ostergard DR (ed): Gynecologic Urology and Urodynamics. Baltimore, Williams & Wilkins, 1985, p 219.
55. Kolb H, Hanzal E, Bernaschek G: Sonographic urethrocystography: Methods and application in patients with genuine stress incontinence. Int Urogynecol J 2:25, 1991.
56. Mostwin JL, Yang A, Sanders R, Genadry R: Radiography, sonography and magnetic resonance imaging for stress incontinence: Contributions, uses and limitations. Urol Clin North Am 22:539, 1995.
57. Beco J: Echographie endovaginale en urologie: L'urèthre. In Perrot N, Boudhene F (eds): Echographie Endovaginale. Paris, Masson, 1991, p 107.
58. Constantinou CE: Resting and stress urethral pressures as a clinical guide to the mechanism of continence in the female patient. Urol Clin North Am 12:247, 1985.
59. Meyer S, DeGrandi P, Schmidt N, et al: Urodynamic parameters in patients with slight and severe genuine stress incontinence: Is the stress profile useful? Neurol Urodynamics 13:21, 1994.
60. Haab F, Zimmern PE, Leach GE: Female stress urinary incontinence due to intrinsic sphincteric deficiency: Recognition and management. J Urol 156:3, 1996.
61. Hilton P: The role of urodynamics in pelvic floor re-education. In Schüssler B, Laycock J, Norton P, Stanton S (eds): Pelvic Floor Re-Education. Berlin, Springler-Verlag, 1994, p 51.
62. Bethoux A, Bory S, Huguier M, Lan LS: Une technique radiologique d'exploration des prolapsus génitaux et des incontinences d'urine: Le colpocystogramme. Ann Radiol 8:809, 1965.
63. Schüssler B, von Obernitz N, Frimberger J, et al: Analysis of successful treatment of SUI by pelvic floor re-education: A urodynamic and radiological study. Neurourol Urodynam 9:433, 1990.
64. Brubaker L, Retzky S, Smith C, Saclarides T: The role of dynamic proctograms in the evaluation of women with genital prolapse. Presented at the 12th Annual Meeting of the AUGS. Port Beach, CA, Oct 1991.
65. Burgio KL, Engel BT, Quilter RE, Arena VC: The relationship between external anal and external urethral sphincter activity in continent women. Neurol Urodynam 10:555, 1991.
66. Dmochowski RR, Ganabathi K, Zimmern PE, Leach GE: Coaxial needle electromyography (EMG) as an adjunct to clinical neurologic testing (abstract 428). J Urol 153(2):335A, 1995.
67. Swash M: The neurogenic hypothesis of stress incontinence. In Bock G, Whelan J (eds): Neurobiology of Incontinence. New York, John Wiley & Sons, Ciba Foundation Symposium, 1990, pp 151, 156.
68. Yang A, Mostwin JL, Saunders RC, Genadry RR: Reassessment of conventional concepts of pelvic floor and urethral weakness using dynamic fastscan MRI and high resolution endocavitary surface coil imaging of the urethra (abstract 771). J Urol 151(2):420A, 1994.
69. Christensen LL, Constantinou CE: Resonance magentic image in female incontinence. In Appell RA, Bourcier A, La Torre F (eds): Pelvic Floor Dysfunction: Investigations and Conservative Treatment. Rome, Casa Editrice Scientifica Internazionale, 1999, pp 173–181.
70. Butler PF: Physical principles of magnetic resonance imaging. In Fishman Javitt MC, Stein HL, Lovecchio JL (eds): Imaging of the Pelvis. Boston, Little Brown, 1990, pp 1–10.
71. Hjartardottir S, Nilsson J, Petersen C, Lingman G: The female pelvic floor: A Dome, not a Basin. Acta Obstet Gynecol Scand 76:567–571, 1997.
72. Bo K, Lilleas F, Talseth T, Hedland H: Dynamic MRI of the pelvic floor muscles in an upright sitting position. Neurourol Urodynam 20:167–174, 2001.
73. Blaivas JG, Olsson CA: Stress incontinence: Classification and surgical approach. J Urol 139:727, 1988.
74. Bourcier AP: Pelvic floor rehabilitation. Int Gynecol J 1:31, 1990.
75. Tapp A, Cardozo L, Hills B, Barnick C: Who benefits from physiotherapy? Neurol Urodynam 7:259, 1988.

CHAPTER 17

Standard Radiologic Studies in Women

JEAN FRANÇOIS LAPRAY

Although it is not a new technique, retrograde dynamic and voiding cystography (RDVC), which shows the two essential functions of the bladder, continence and micturition, still remains the most common urologic examination for the study of urinary incontinence. However, the use of ultrasound to show the morphologic and dynamic features of the urethra is increasing.

For the evaluation of genital prolapse, the idea of a unified pelviperineal disease contradicts the previous idea of segmentation of the three compartments (anterior–urologic, middle–genital, and posterior–anorectal) and attempts to analyze the inter-relationships of the different types of prolapse.[1] This new concept also leads to the consideration of cystography as the first step in colpocystodefecography, which eventually may be replaced by dynamic magnetic resonance imaging (MRI) after this technique is fully developed (open MRI) and becomes widely available.

RETROGRADE DYNAMIC AND VOIDING CYSTOGRAPHY

Standard Retrograde Dynamic and Voiding Cystography[2]: Method

Standard RDVC is the first step in colpocystodefecography. It is a tailor-made examination that begins with questioning of the patient by the radiologist, who must obtain the patient's cooperation and verify that the patient fully understands the procedure. The examination should be performed in the first part of the menstrual cycle, and any pad or vaginal tampon must be removed. The examiner must ensure that no urinary infection is present.

Plain x-ray is obtained, and includes the entire urinary tract, from the upper pole of the kidney to the urethral meatus. During the examination, both functional signs (e.g., painful filling of the bladder, urgency) and physical signs (e.g., urethral stenosis at the urethral catheterization site, explosive micturition) are observed.

Retrograde filling of the bladder (sodium and meglumine amidotrizoate, iode: 146 mg/mL) is interrupted at 150 mL, the opacified catheter (8 Fr) is taped onto the thigh, and the dynamic phase is performed. The patient stands upright, with the legs slightly apart. Lateral views are obtained at rest and during a Valsalva maneuver. An opaque metric ruler is placed on the table to allow measurements on the x-ray films. Sometimes an important prolapse must be pushed backward with a forceps and a cotton pad to permit free mobilization of the organs before the lateral view is taken.

The table is then lowered to allow the bladder to fill (≥ 500 mL) until the patient feels a strong desire to void. The voiding lateral views are obtained during maximum flow, with the patient sitting on a special commode. These views include at least two exposures that focus on the bladder neck and the entire urethra.

After the patient empties the bladder in the toilet, the postvoiding view is obtained. Like the plain x-ray, this view includes the entire urinary tract.

Descending Cystography

This second part of the intravenous pyelogram follows the same protocol as RDVC, except that voiding views are taken before the dynamic views, after the study of the upper tract. The density of the bladder can be enhanced by the use of isosmolar contrast media at intravenous injection.

Colpocystodefecography

This examination has two phases. The first is RDVC, and the second is defecography, which is performed after vaginal, rectal, and small bowel opacification, and is adapted from the technique described by Kelvin and associates[3] and Maglinte and associates.[4]

First Phase

The examination begins with a large anteroposterior radiograph to ensure that the small bowel opacification resulting from the absorption of 500 mL barium sulfate suspension, administered 90 minutes before the procedure, is correct.

The examination starts with a bladder study, as described earlier, unless complete filling of the bladder occurs and the voiding views are obtained first. Less than 100 mL contrast material is left in the bladder for defecography. Sometimes it is necessary to empty the bladder partially through catheterization, until 100 mL remains, because a volume of more than 200 mL may mask another prolapse.

Second Phase

Vaginal opacification and rectal repletion with barium paste are performed to permit defecography to be performed with the patient sitting on a special commode. Lateral views that include the entire pelvis and perineum are obtained during rectal evacuation and total emptying of the bladder, which may occur simultaneously. The patient can be asked to repeat the vaginal or para-anal maneuver that she uses to empty the rectocele. After the patient empties the bladder and rectum, a final lateral view is taken during maximum straining. This view usually shows peritoneocele most effectively.

Dosimetry

Radiation is not negligible; it ranges from 10 mGy for cystography to 20 to 25 mGy for colpocystodefecography. The dose is decreased by numerization. Therefore, unnecessary exposure must be avoided.[2]

Standard Retrograde Dynamic and Voiding Cystography: Analysis and Results

Retrograde Dynamic and Voiding Cystography[2]

This analysis includes morphologic and dynamic studies. The elements of the analysis are summarized in Table 17-1.

Morphologic Study

The plain x-ray shows lithiasis, spinal alterations or lesions that could suggest a neurologic bladder, or signs of constipation.

Bladder capacity and detrusor aspect can be seen during bladder filling, with progressive unfolding of the bladder wall. The full bladder appears rounded, with a regular wall. The normal capacity is approximately 400 to 500 mL.

Dynamic Study

For isolated cystography, the pubococcygeal or pubosacrococcygeal line used with MRI or colpocysto-

TABLE 17-1 ■ Bladder and Urethra Analysis

Type of Test	Important Area	Conditions Detected
Plain x-ray		Lithiasis, spine Constipation
Repletion	Detrusor	Capacity Functional aspect, reflux
Straining views	Bladder neck Trigone	Mobility Type and grade of the ptosis
Voiding views	Urethra	Bladder neck funneling Mobility Stenosis, bending Periurethral abnormalities
Postvoiding view		Postvoiding residual urine, vesico-ureteric reflux

defecography is often difficult to draw because a better image is obtained when the posterior part of the pelvis is left unseen. In this case, the main criterion for bladder base descent is the horizontal line through the inferior margin of the pubic symphysis. Normally, with straining, the bladder moves slightly downward and backward and its inferior and posterior aspects become slightly convex.

Normally, regardless of the patient's position during straining or at rest, no part of the bladder is located under the horizontal line at the inferior margin of the pubic symphysis (Fig. 17-1). This is even more evident for the pubosacral line, which is higher than the pubic symphysis line. The bladder neck or urethrovesical junction (UVJ) moves downward 1 cm from the decubitus to the standing position. From rest to strain, it always remains closed.

Voiding Study

Voiding views show the urethral morphology. During micturition, the bladder becomes spherical because of detrusor contraction and the two margins of the bladder neck open symmetrically. The caliber must be harmonious, without sudden rupture between the bladder neck and the small retromeatal dilation (Fig. 17-2). The axis of the proximal urethra is 35 degrees on the vertical axis (urethral inclination), and the bladder base has an angle of 100 degrees with the posterior urethra (posterior urethrovesical angle). The symphysis orifice distance, measured at rest as the distance on a horizontal line from the symphysis to the internal urethral orifice, is normally 31 ± 6 mm.[5]

The situation of the bladder base and bladder neck must also be appraised on the voiding views. As a result of voiding difficulties or insufficient straining in the upright position, the bladder base or bladder neck may appear lower than on the straining views. No residual urine is seen on the postvoiding view.

Colpocystodefecography

The bladder position is analyzed in the same way as during RDVC. The analysis focuses on the interdependence of the different prolapses in accordance with filling and emptying of the organs. An opaque and graduated rule taped to the table can be used to measure the radiologic enlargement.

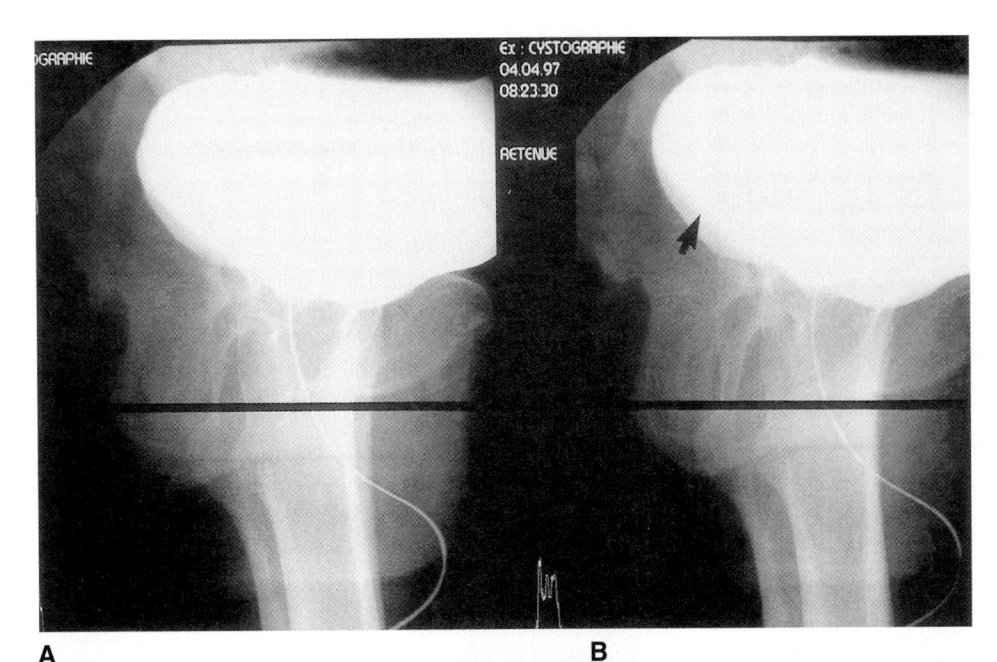

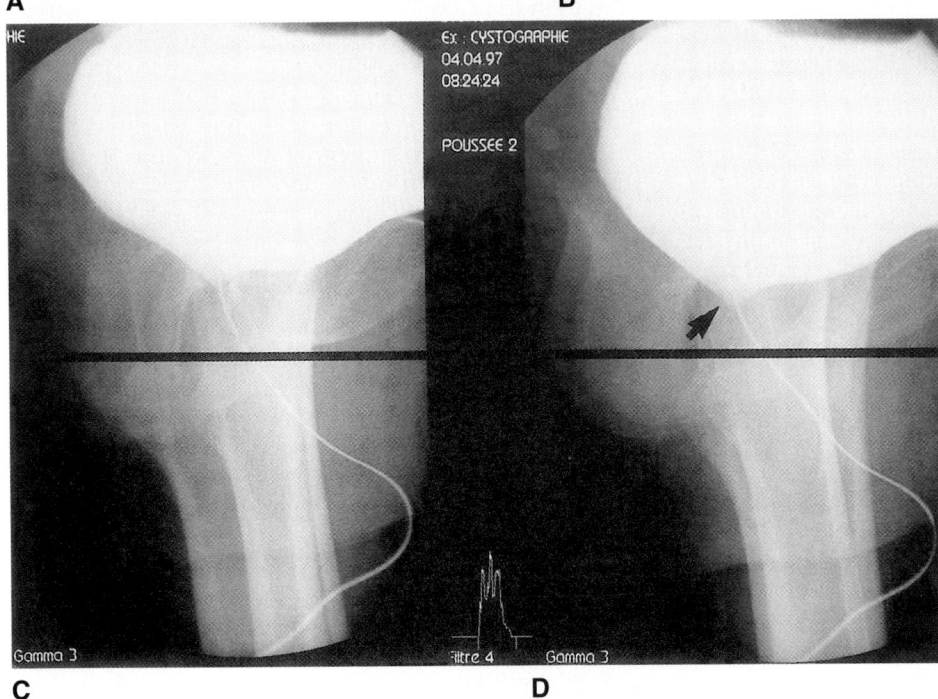

FIGURE 17-1 Retrograde dynamic and voiding cystography: dynamic views. Normally, there is no part of the bladder under the horizontal line at the inferior margin of the pubis at rest (**A**) or at strain (**B**). While retaining, the posterior part of the bladder base is more flattened and vertical (*arrow*). Note that the second effort of strain (**D**) is stronger (bladder neck: *arrow*) than the first one (**C**). (From Lapray JF: Imagerie de la vessie et de la dynamique pelvienne de la femme. Masson, Paris, 1999, p 237.)

The normal and pathologic features of these compartments are described in other chapters. Nevertheless, it is important to discuss the advantages of colpocystodefecography for a study of vesicourethral disorders because it shows associated static abnormalities and, most importantly, competition between prolapses. Box 17-1 shows the criteria for the middle and posterior compartment analysis.

URINARY INCONTINENCE

Urinary incontinence is involuntary loss of urine through the urethra as a result of sphincter or bladder dysfunction. This definition excludes urinary leakage as a result of ectopic ureteral insertion in the urethra or vagina, urogenital fistulas, and dribbling from urethral diverticula.

Dynamic study of the UVJ was initiated by bead chain cystography.[6] The goal was to differentiate urinary stress incontinence with hypermobility of the UVJ that can be surgically cured by restoring it to its normal position from urinary stress incontinence caused by intrinsic

---

BOX 17-1 | **Analysis of the Middle and Posterior Compartments**

Vaginal and uterine descent (grade)
Rectovaginal wall rectocele, enterocele, and contents
Tonus of the pelvic floor (descending perineum)
Anorectal dynamics (rectal prolapse, quality of evacuation)

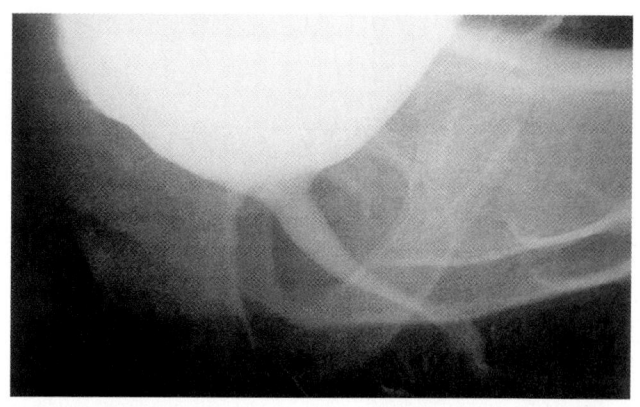

FIGURE 17-2 Retrograde dynamic and voiding cystography: normal urethra. On this lateral voiding view, the two margins of the bladder neck are symmetrical. The posterior urethra and the retromeatal segment are larger than the middle part. (From Lapray JF: Imagerie de la vessie et de la dynamique pelvienne de la femme. Masson, Paris, 1999, p 237.)

sphincteric deficiency. Treatment of intrinsic sphincteric deficiency is more complex than hypermobility of the UVJ, and includes slings, periurethral injections, and the use of an artificial urinary sphincter.[7] However, the recent introduction of tension-free vaginal tape will modify the classic surgical indications.

The diagnosis of urinary incontinence is made through questioning and physical examination. The role of imaging and urodynamics is to analyze and quantify the mechanisms of incontinence in light of the findings on physical examination, which remains the initial and essential step.

Urinary Stress Incontinence

Genuine urinary stress incontinence (GSI) has two mechanisms that may be associated: UVJ hypermobility and bladder neck incompetence. Many patients have a combination of both factors.[8]

Urethrovesical Junction Hypermobility

Straining lateral views and voiding views obtained during cystography or colpocystodefecography show a low situation of the UVJ (below the pubic symphysis or the pubococcygeal line) or an abnormal mobility greater than 2 cm between rest and straining (or voiding) views (Fig. 17-3). Besides voiding, urethral marking is necessary to identify the bladder neck. However, UVJ hypermobility does not mean urinary incontinence. Anatomic changes in the posterior urethrovesical angle of less than 100 to 115 degrees, in the angle of inclination of less than 30 to 45 degrees, and in the symphysis orifice distance of less than 20 mm denote urethroceles, but do not correlate with urinary stress incontinence.[9]

Measurement of the bladder neck descent and these angles allows geometric characterization of the situation and motion of the bladder neck, but there is no correlation between these angles and urinary stress incontinence.[2] Urinary incontinence is a syndrome, not a radiologic diagnosis (Fig. 17-4). Most authors agree that cystourethrography cannot discriminate between stress incontinence and continence. Likewise, the degree of urinary stress incontinence does not correlate with the type or degree of suspension defect.[5]

Bladder Neck Incompetence

Bladder neck incompetence is the radiologic equivalent of intrinsic sphincter deficiency. Whereas intrinsic deficiency corresponds to a cause of urinary stress incontinence, intrinsic deficiency of the closure system defined by urodynamic criteria (closure pressure or Valsalva leak-point

FIGURE 17-3 Urethrovesical junction hypermobility (**A**) at rest and (**B**) at strain. PU line (*dotted line*). (From Lapray JF: Imagerie de la vessie et de la dynamique pelvienne de la femme. Masson, Paris, 1999, p 237.)

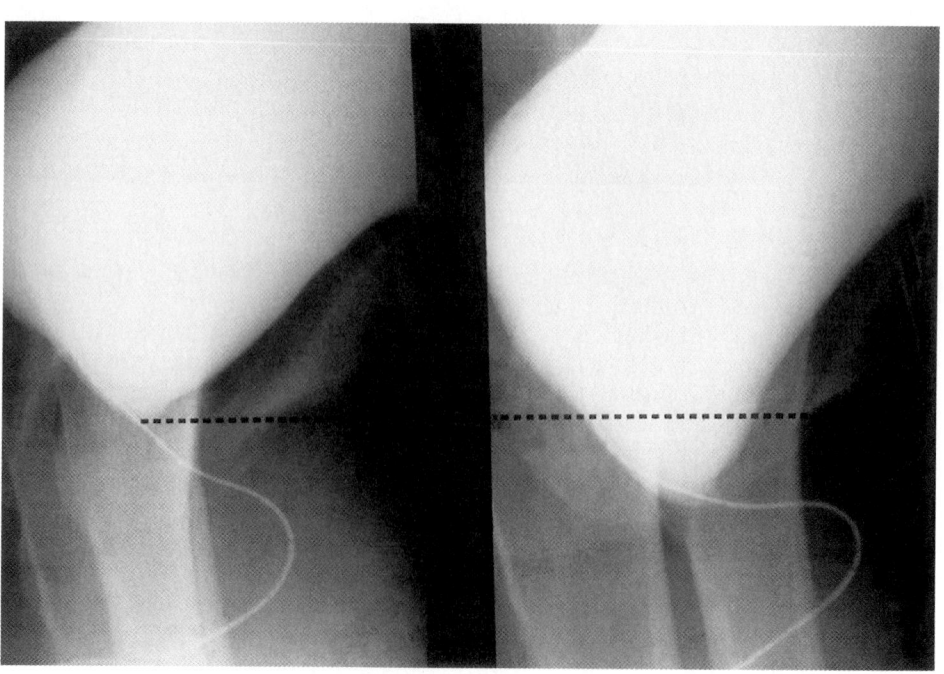

A   **B**

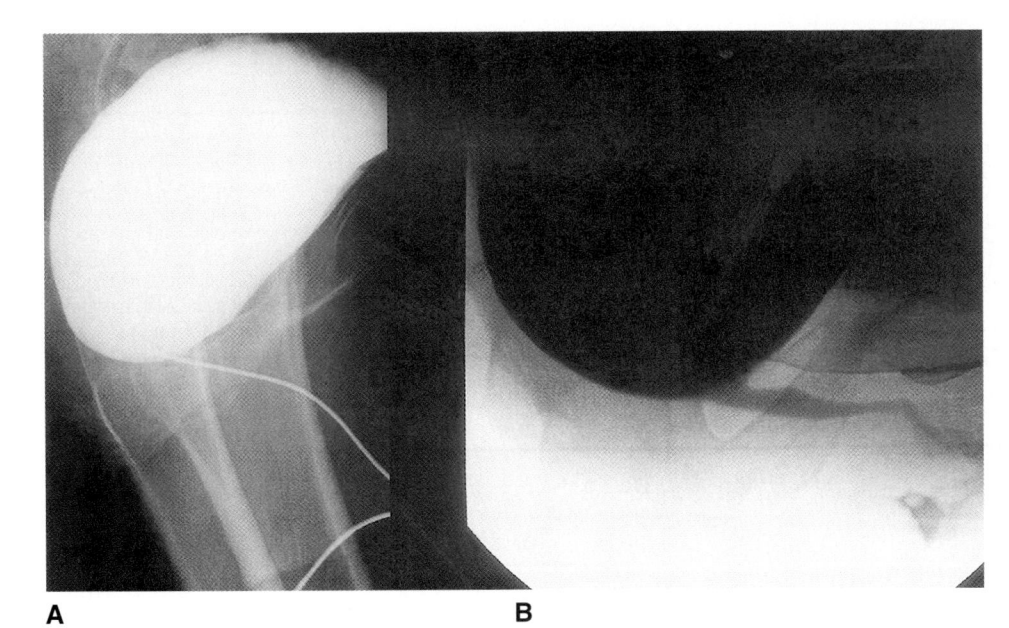

FIGURE 17-4 20-year-old woman without urinary incontinence (repeated urinary infections). The urethral angles are abnormal. (**A**) straining, (**B**) voiding. (From Lapray JF: Imagerie de la vessie et de la dynamique pelvienne de la femme. Masson, Paris, 1999, p 237.)

pressure), bladder neck insufficiency is the iconographic display of a result: easy opening of the UVJ, which may or may not be linked to intrinsic sphincter deficiency (Fig. 17-5). Thus, the UVJ can open too easily for reasons other than intrinsic sphincter deficiency, especially urge incontinence as a result of detrusor instability.[9] Therefore, images that are compatible with the diagnosis of intrinsic sphincter deficiency, or even suggestive of intrinsic sphincter deficiency, must be correlated with urodynamic criteria. This is the advantage of videourodynamics, which shows fluoroscopic images and manometric readings simultaneously. If simultaneous manometric data are not available, the images must be interpreted in conjunction with urodynamic results or at least with questioning of the patient.

In the typical, pure form of bladder neck incompetence, for example, persistent urinary stress incontinence after colposuspension, bladder neck incompetence can be suspected based on a cystographic straining lateral view showing opening of the bladder neck without mobility. Opening of the bladder neck in association with bladder neck hypermobility can correspond to other mechanisms. Other than an important intrinsic sphincter deficiency with a very large opening of the UVJ and leakage at rest, the finding of mild bladder neck opening at rest is not a good criterion for bladder neck incompetence.[2,10]

Cystographic voiding lateral views can provide other evidence of bladder neck incompetence: vesicalization of the urethra with a large UVJ (Fig. 17-6). Funneling of the bladder neck makes it impossible to determine with precision the borders of the bladder and urethra.

In major intrinsic sphincter deficiency, the bladder neck and urethra are permanently open, making correct filling of the bladder and upright views impossible. To obtain a minimal appraisal of the cervicourethral morphology, with the table in the horizontal position, it is often necessary to obtain oblique views of the bladder neck during filling and spontaneous evacuation of the bladder. In this case, the morphologic findings correspond to type III of the Blaivas and McGuire classifications.[11]

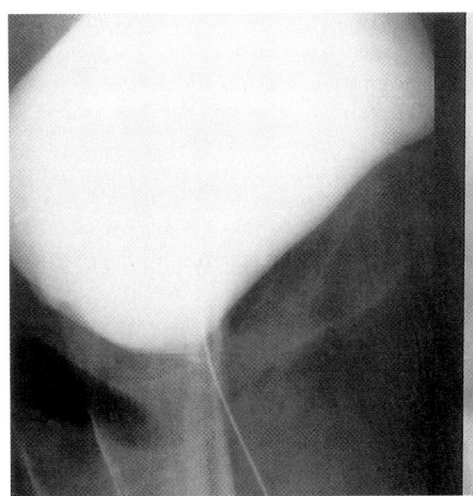

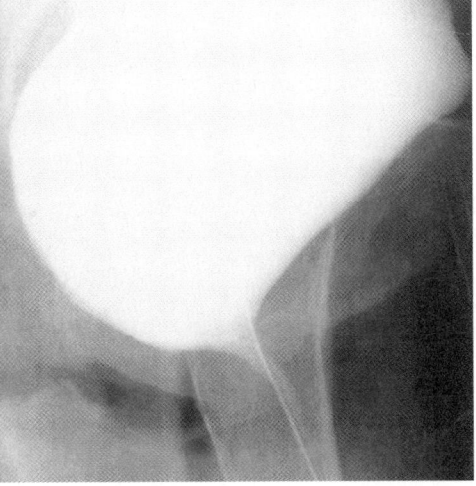

FIGURE 17-5 Bladder neck incompetence. At rest (**A**) or at strain (**B**), there is no mobility of the bladder neck. The bladder neck opening is evident with urinary leakage (without visible contraction of the detrusor). (From Lapray JF: Imagerie de la vessie et de la dynamique pelvienne de la femme. Masson, Paris, 1999, p 237.)

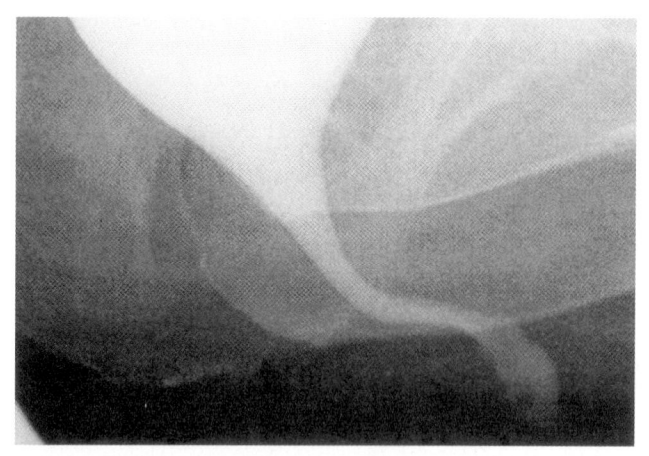

FIGURE 17-6 Open bladder neck. Lateral voiding view: Bladder neck funneling. Slight retromeatal dilation.

Detrusor Instability and Other Types of Incontinence

Imaging is of less interest in this disorder than in urethral causes of incontinence.

Detrusor Instability

The role of imaging is modest in detrusor instability, which is suggested by clinical investigation and confirmed by urodynamics. Nevertheless, symptoms such as urgency during retrograde bladder filling, which limits bladder filling, and explosive micturition, are observed on cystography. However, the role of imaging and urethrocystoscopy is important in the search for etiologies that include lower urinary tract dysfunction, prolapses, and neurologic disease. The two other causes of vesical incontinence are rare. Urinary incontinence related to overflow is rare in the female compared with the male. Urinary incontinence with poor bladder compliance does not show radiologic signs, except indirect signs, such as a small, painful bladder during retrograde filling, sometimes with a high-pressure vesicoureteric reflux.

Mixed Incontinence: Classifications

Mixed incontinence includes both urinary stress incontinence and bladder instability. All degrees and all associations of causes are seen.

Several radiologic classifications have been proposed (Tables 17-2 and 17-3).[11,12] There is agreement in these classifications that type III urinary stress incontinence corresponds to true intrinsic sphincter deficiency. These classifications do not include the role of the following associated abnormalities that can interfere with treatment:

- Bladder capacity, either very small (<200 cm³), which can explain frequency and urgency by itself, or enlarged (>600 to 700 cm³, even 1 L), or hypoactive, leading to overflow leakage and the risk of postoperative retention
- Detrusor aspect that is smooth or shows spots of rectilign margins, sometimes with diverticula

TABLE 17-2 ■ Radiologic Classification of Blaivas and Olsson[11]

Type	Description
0	Absence of GSI, BN hypermobility <2 cm
I	At rest, BN closed At strain, BN open, hypermobility <2 cm
IIa	At rest, BN closed > inferior margin of the pubis At strain, BN open + hypermobility ≥2 cm
IIb	At rest, BN closed < inferior margin of the pubis
III	At rest, BN and proximal utrethra open

GSI, genuine urinary stress incontinence; BN, bladder neck.

TABLE 17-3 ■ Classification of McGuire[12]

Type	Description
0	Absence of GSI
I	UVJ hypermobility <3 cm (with or without cystocele) C_p >20 cm H_2O
II	UVJ hypermobility ≥3 cm C_p >20 cm H_2O
III	Failure of previous surgery or C_p <20 cm H_2O

GSI, genuine urinary stress incontinence; C_p, closing proximal urethral pressure; UVJ, urethrovesical junction.

- Associated urologic abnormalities, including vesicoureteric reflux and urethral diverticula
- Caliber of the urethra, which is determined through calibration, although voiding views show bending related to cervicocystoptosis
- Residual urine volume

PELVIC ORGAN PROLAPSE

Imaging plays a major role in the evaluation of cystocele. In the analysis of anterior compartment descent, the role of imaging is:

- To eliminate another cause of anterior vaginal wall descent and confirm cystocele
- To identify defects and the type and grade of bladder descent
- To visualize factors associated with continence, including mobility and competence of the bladder neck, bladder capacity, detrusor aspect, urethral morphology, and residual urine
- To detect (during colpocystodefecography or dynamic MRI) other possible associated defects that can mask or be masked during the physical examination
- To show the fascia and ligamentous muscular structures (ultrasound and MRI)

Cystocele

Cystoptosis is the descent of any part of the bladder below the horizontal line through the inferior margin of the pubis (pubic symphysis line). The pubosacrococcygeal line that runs from the inferior border of the pubis to the sacrococcygeal joint can be used, especially in MRI, although it appears slightly higher.[13,14] However, in the anterior compartment, the pubic symphysis line and the pubosacral line are not far apart (Fig. 17-7).

Types of Cystocele[2]

Cervicocystoptosis is the descent of both the UVJ and the bladder base (Fig. 17-8). Cervicoptosis is the descent of the UVJ. It is rarely seen as an isolated descent and is often associated with bladder neck incompetence. It suggests bladder neck descent, with compression of the posterior bladder base. When detected, colpocystodefecography or dynamic MRI should be performed to show prolapse of the middle or posterior compartment of the pelvis.

Cystoptosis without cervicoptosis (isolated descent of the bladder base with the bladder neck fixed in a high, retropubic position) is usually seen after surgical colposuspension.

Grades of Cystocele

RDVC allows cystocele to be classified according to the same criteria used for physical examination (Table 17-4).

According to Zimmern,[15] descent of the bladder less than 2 cm below the inferior margin of the pubic symphysis corresponds to prolapse above the introitus, cystoptosis of between 2 and 5 cm corresponds to prolapse extending to the introitus, and ptosis greater than 5 cm corresponds to external prolapse.[2] The size of the cystocele is often reduced on voiding views because of detrusor contraction.

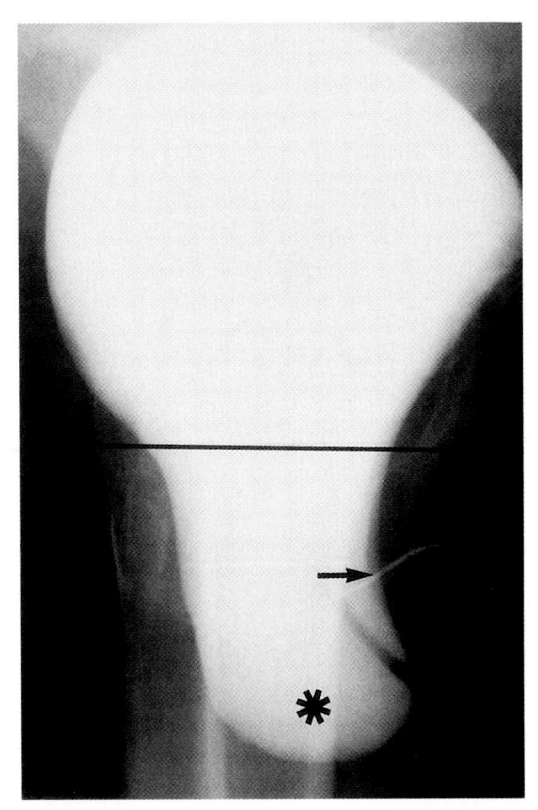

FIGURE 17-8 Cervicocystoptosis. Descent of both the bladder neck (*arrow*) and the bladder base (*asterisk*) under the pubic symphysis line. Note the urethral notch under the bladder neck. (From Lapray JF: Imagerie de la vessie et de la dynamique pelvienne de la femme. Masson, Paris, 1999, p 237.)

On physical examination or with cystography or sonography, it is also possible to classify the situation of the UVJ on a constructed orthogonal graph at the inferior edge of the pubic symphysis, where one axis corresponds to the long axis of the pubic symphysis (Fig. 17-9).[16] This construction has been used during sonography to measure UVJ mobility.[17,18]

In a large cystocele, the ureteral notch is often visible on the lateral aspect of the bladder (see Fig. 17-8). Rarely, ureterohydronephrosis as a result of plicature of the distal ureter is observed.[19] In a large cystocele, sonography is performed to visualize dilation of the upper urinary tract, particularly if uterine prolapse is present. Residual urine is common in a large cystocele, and lithiasis can occur.

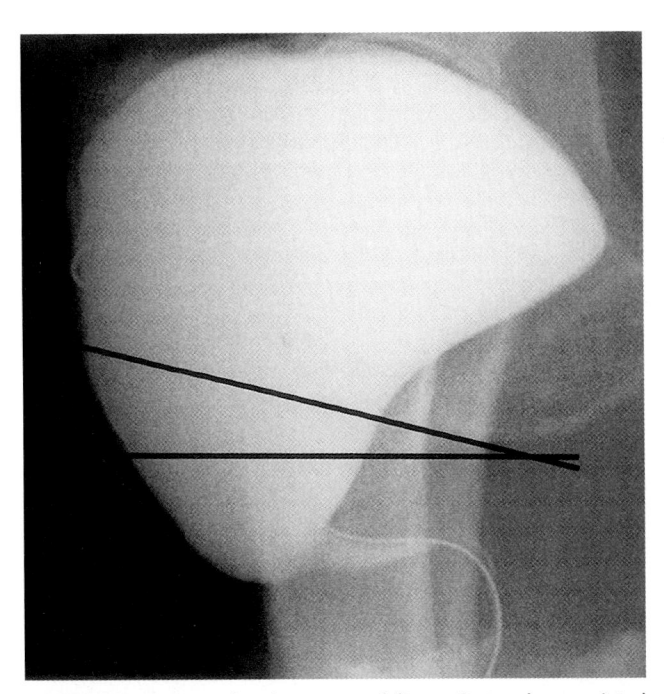

FIGURE 17-7 PU and pubococcygeal lines. Cystocele associated with urinary leakage. Pubic symphysis line (bottom line) and Pubosacro coccygeal line (top line) are not distant for the anterior compartment. (From Lapray JF: Imagerie de la vessie et de la dynamique pelvienne de la femme. Masson, Paris, 1999, p 237.)

TABLE 17-4 ■ Radiologic Classification of Cystocele at Rest and During Straining

Grade	0	1	2	3
Prolapse at physical examination	0	Above the introitus	Extending to the introitus	Below the introitus
Bladder base descending below the pubic symphysis	0	<2 cm	>2 cm <5 cm	>5 cm

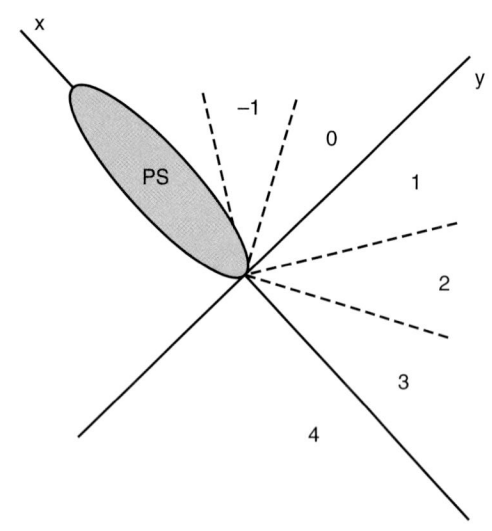

FIGURE 17-9 Bladder neck mobility measurement. The abscissa axis (x) is the grand axis of the PS. A line (y) is drawn orthogonally at the inferior edge of the PS, allowing the construction of various quadrants. The normal bladder neck position is 0. The −1 position is generally observed after surgical colposuspension. Positions 1,2,3,4 represent increasing degrees of bladder neck descent permitting a classification. (Adapted from Haab F, Cortesse A, Jacquetin B, et al: Classification des cystocèles: CUROPF (work in progress). Presented at the 94ème Congrès de l'Association Française d'Urologie, Paris, Nov 2000. Unpublished.)

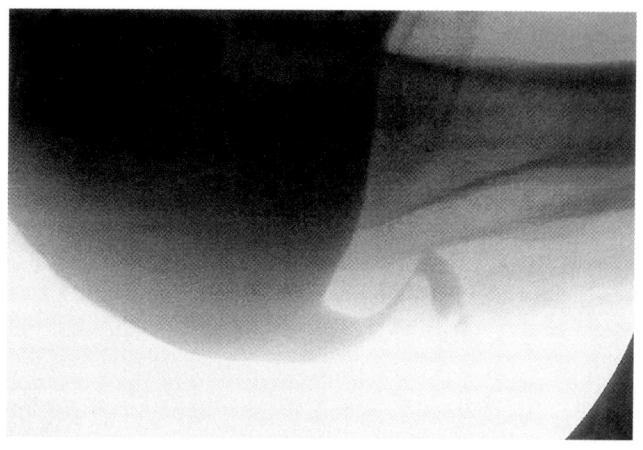

FIGURE 17-10 Cystocele: lateral voiding view. In this case the bladder neck is large, but it is difficult to differentiate an associated BNI from a bladder neck dilation due to the bending of the urethra.

Urinary Incontinence

Cystocele may be associated with urinary stress incontinence as a result of surgical treatment. In some cases, preexisting urinary stress incontinence can be cured by isolated cystocele repair. In other cases, urinary stress incontinence initially appears after cystocele repair. Women with prolapse and coexisting incontinence should be offered a continence procedure rather than simple vaginal repair.[20] Some studies suggest that one fourth of women with anterior wall relaxation, with or without incontinence symptoms, have occult genuine urinary stress incontinence.[8,20] Different mechanisms that may be associated could explain the continence in patients with large cystocele: pressure dissipation, urethral kinking, and urethral compression.[21]

When cystoptosis is associated with bladder neck descent, the diagnosis of simultaneous bladder neck incompetence is difficult,[22] although an opened bladder neck or bladder neck funneling in the voiding views is an important sign that suggests associated bladder neck incompetence (Fig. 17-10).

The insertion of a vaginal pack or a ring pessary during videourodynamic studies enhances the detection of urinary stress incontinence.[8,20,21,23] However, in RDVC without simultaneous urodynamic recording, on the straining views, while the cystocele is pushed backward, it is impossible to assert that the bladder neck is not compressed during the maneuver or, if leakage occurs, to eliminate a detrusor contraction that is possibly initiated by the maneuver.

Other Pelvic Floor Defects

Competition among different prolapses may occur. The role of colpocystodefecography is to unmask all of the prolapses and show them at their maximum degree. The procedure is started with exploration of the bladder, because in the prolapse competition, cystocele and uterine prolapse often dominate.[2,7,24] At the end of the urinary phase, it is sometimes necessary to push an external prolapse backward or to drain the bladder with a catheter, leaving no more than 50 to 100 mL iodine contrast material in the bladder for the second part of the examination (defecography). The analysis of the first part (urinary phase) is identical to the analysis described earlier for RDVC.

The second part of the examination shows posterior pelvic floor disorders with different abnormalities that are often associated, such as vaginal dome descent anterior rectocele, rectal intussusception, descending perineum, or enterocele (Fig. 17-11). Peritoneocele without small bowel content (e.g., fat, sigmoid colon) appears as an

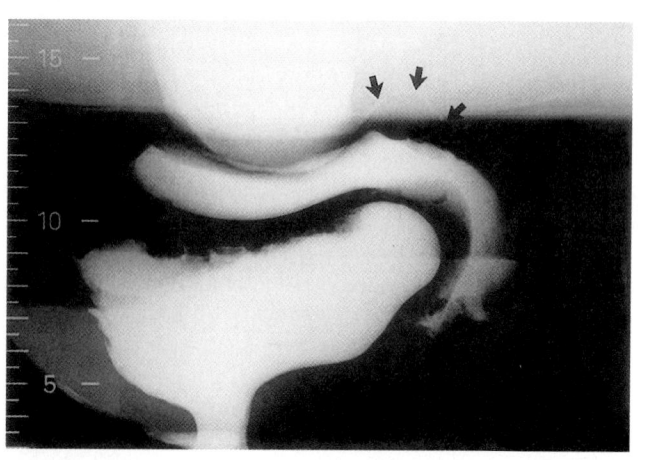

FIGURE 17-11 Colpocystodefecography: competition between a cystoptosis and an anterior rectocele. The enterocele can only appear after emptying of these two prolapses. Urethra (*arrows*). (From Lapray JF: Imagerie de l'insuffisance sphinctérienne. In Amarenco G, Serment G [eds]: L'insuffisance sphinctérienne de la femme, Paris, Elsevier, 2000, pp 87–108.)

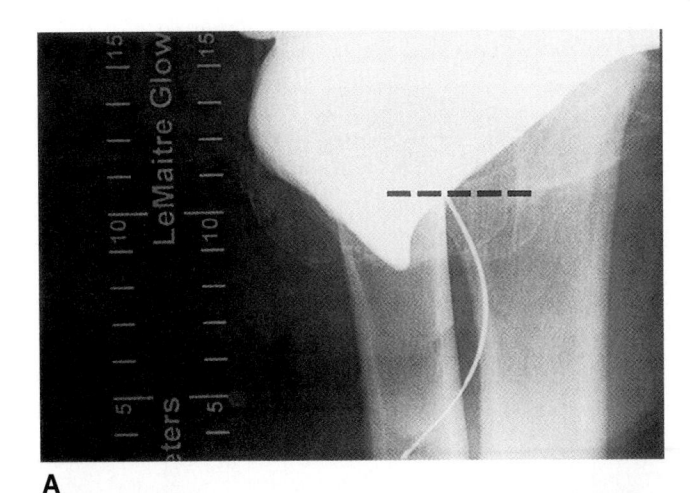

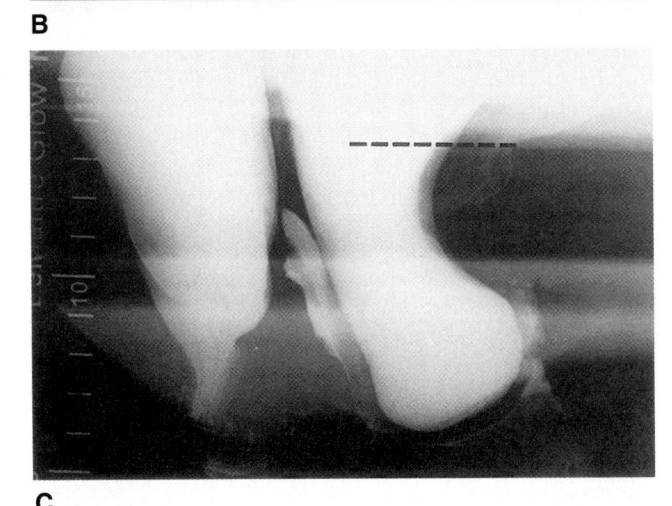

FIGURE 17-12 Importance of cystoptosis: variations according to the straining intensity in the same patient. Dotted line indicates pubic symphysis line. **A,** At rest, grade 1 cystoptosis. **B,** At strain, grade 2 cystoptosis with grade 1 cervicoptosis. **C,** At defecography, grade 3 cystoptosis. This tends to prove that defecation corresponds to the maximum strain. (From Lapray JF: Imagerie de la vessie et de la dynamique pelvienne de la femme. Masson, Paris, 1999, p 237.)

of dynamic MRI over colpocystodefecography. In our opinion, "peritoneography" has no more indication.

Maximum vaginal wall descent is usually observed during defecography, when abdominal pressure is greatest (Fig. 17-12).

ULTRASOUND OF THE LOWER URINARY TRACT

Technical Aspects

The perineal, introital (i.e., sectorial probe placed behind the external urethral meatus), endovaginal, and transrectal views have replaced the suprapubic view.[7,17,25,26] All of these methods can be used to study the morphology and mobility of the UVJ.[26] The endocavitary views and particularly the endovaginal view are not adapted when vaginal prolapse is present because the prolapse can be pushed back by the probe.[27]

Ultrasonography is performed with the patient in the dorsal lithotomy or standing position.[26] The left lateral decubitus position is used for the transrectal view. Some studies have been performed with a special chair that allows prolapse to occur naturally in an upright seated position.[7] To allow a reliable comparison of the different measurements, for the same patient, all examinations should be performed in the same position.

The bladder is usually half-filled (≤250 mL) during this part of the procedure. However, the bladder neck and proximal urethra are more mobile when the bladder is nearly empty. Funneling of the proximal urethra is more easily observed when the bladder is full.[28]

In some studies, the UVJ is marked, often with a urodynamic catheter during simultaneous urodynamic testing, although high-frequency transducers allow excellent delineation of the UVJ.[26] To better detect bladder neck funneling in the perineal view, Schaer and associates[29] proposed transurethral injection of ultrasound contrast medium.

Urinary Incontinence

Assessment of Urethrovesical Junction Mobility and Bladder Neck Funneling

Most authors report that the normal UVJ mobility between rest and straining is 1 cm or less (Fig. 17-13).[26,30] UVJ mobility is measured unidirectionally, between the middle of the inferior margin of the pubic symphysis and the internal urethral orifice (the upper and ventral point of the bladder neck, between the urethral and bladder walls),[27] either with an orthogonal construction with the grand axis of the pubis at the inferior margin of the pubic symphysis,[17] or sometimes with the rotation angle of the bladder neck (Fig 17-14).[31]

Although not essential for a positive diagnosis of UVJ hypermobility, two-directional measurements more nearly reflect reality. In urinary stress incontinence, the bladder neck does not fall vertically, but rotates gradually to a point at which funneling of the urethra occurs or worsens. This funneling occurs because the anterior wall of the urethra is

enlargement of the rectovaginal space. Peritoneocele is often seen only on the last straining view, obtained after complete emptying of the bladder and rectum (see Fig. 17-11). However, in contrast to MRI, a posterior peritoneocele above an anterior rectocele will not appear so clearly on colpocystodefecography. This is one advantage

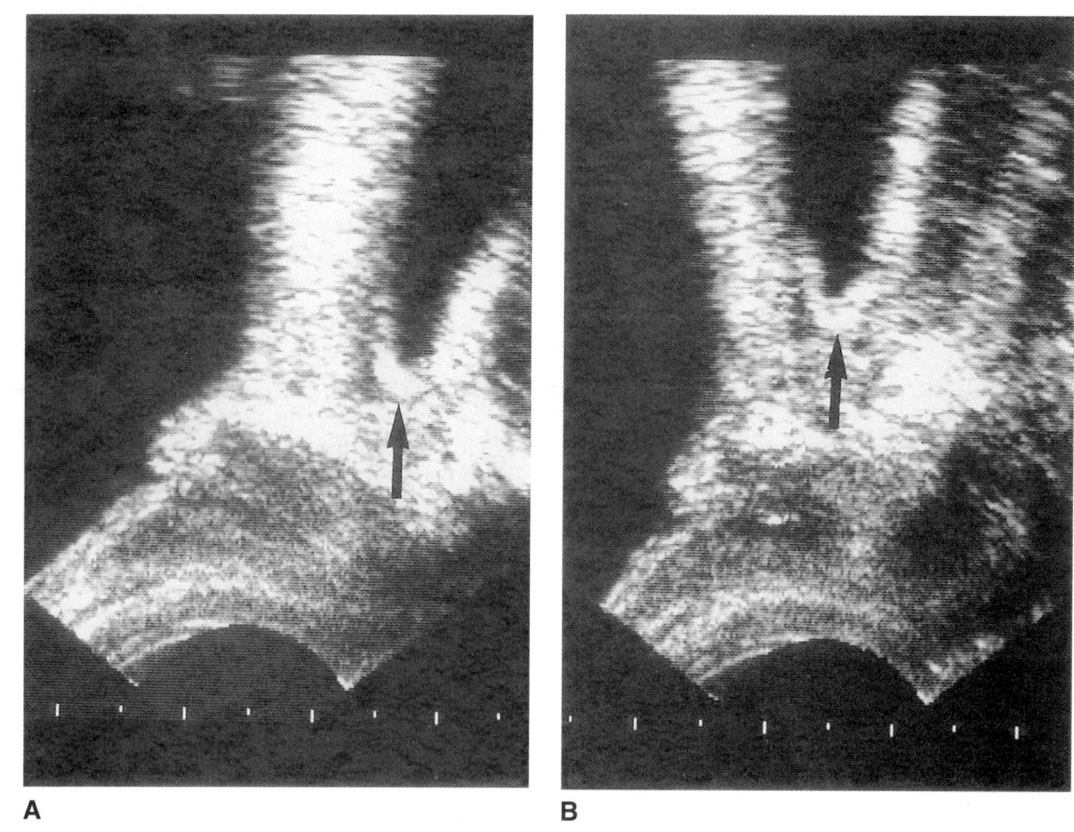

FIGURE 17-13 Normal mobility of the bladder neck. The distance between the internal orifice of the bladder neck between rest (**A**) and strain (**B**) is <10 mm from the pubic symphysis (PS) on a horizontal line. Endovaginal view with sectorial probe. Arrows indicate the inferior margin of the pubic symphysis.

stopped by its attachments, while the posterior wall follows the movement of the vagina.[7] In urinary stress incontinence, UVJ hypermobility is defined by most authors as mobility of 1 cm or more between rest and strain.

Ultrasonography showing real-time UVJ mobility on a thin, precise slice offers an advantage over an x-ray that shows a summation of all layers on a static view.

Funneling is diagnosed when a slight separation of the internal urethral orifice is seen at strain (or when ultrasound contrast agent enters the bladder neck),[31] and is graded more severely when it appears extensive or occurs at rest[7] (Fig. 17-15). A method has been proposed to allow quantification of the depth and diameter of bladder neck dilation.[17]

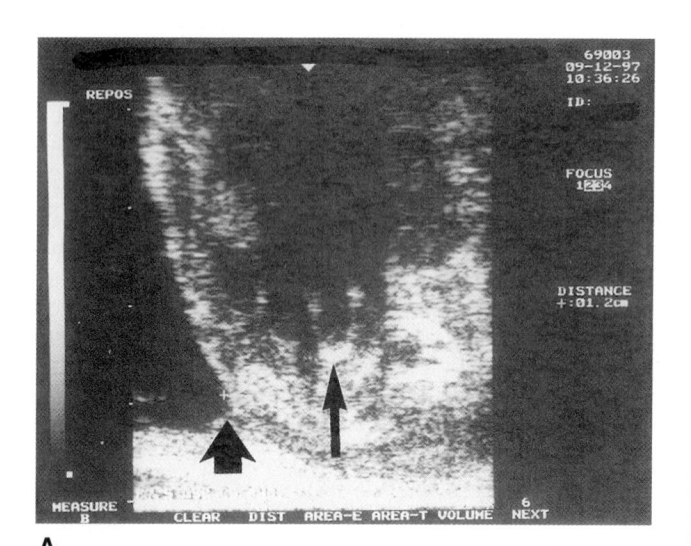

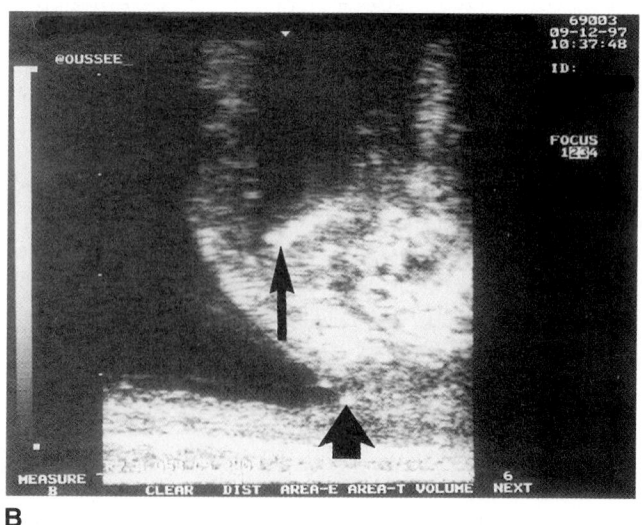

FIGURE 17-14 Urethrovesical junction hypermobility. Bladder neck mobility (*thick arrow*) of 2 cm from the PS (*thin arrow*) on a horizontal line between rest (**A**) and strain (**B**). Endovaginal view with linear probe. (From Lapray JF: Imagerie de la vessie et de la dynamique pelvienne de la femme. Masson, Paris, 1999, p 237.)

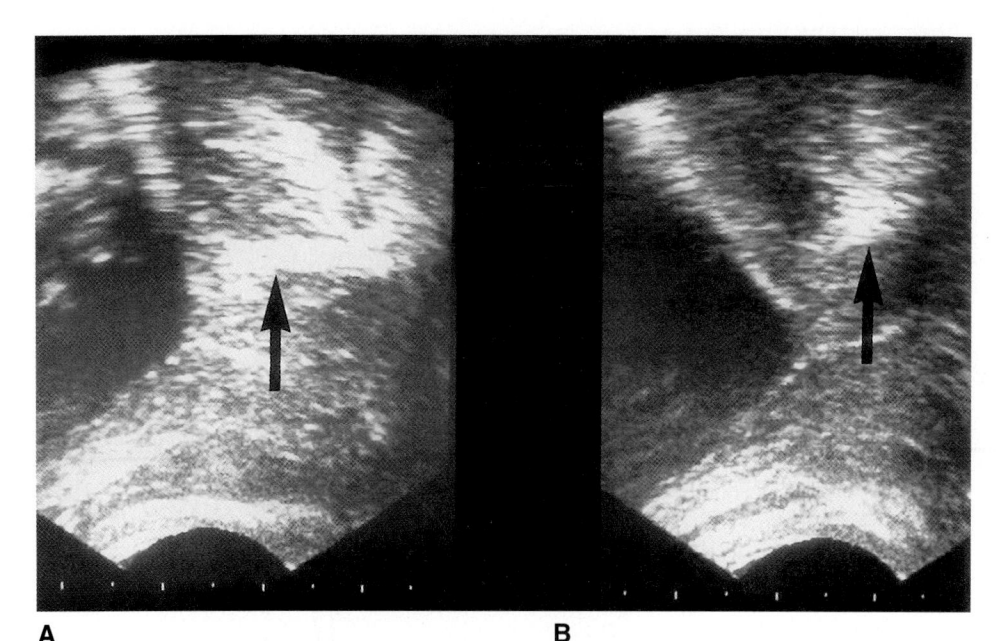

FIGURE 17-15 Bladder neck incompetence. Funneling of the bladder neck without mobility at rest (**A**) and with strain (**B**) Transrectal view with sectorial probe. The arrows indicate pubic symphysis. (From Lapray JF: Imagerie de l'insuffisance sphinctérienne. In Amarenco G, Serment G [eds]: L'insuffisance sphinctérienne de la femme, Paris, Elsevier, 2000, pp 87-108.)

All ultrasonography methods have advantages and limitations (Table 17-5). The quality of imaging is better with endocavitary views. However, endocavitary views, especially the endovaginal method, may cause distortion of the UVJ anatomy as a result of compression from the probe. The mobility and opening of the UVJ must not be manipulated during straining, and measurements should be obtained in a perfect horizontal and sagittal plane. The endovaginal linear probe should not be pushed in the cul-de-sac, and the pressure exerted on the urethra with a sectorial probe should remain low. Because of these requirements, the examination is very operator-dependent.

The artifacts have been studied (Table 17-6),[26,27] and the transrectal method, although sometimes difficult for the patient, seems to be a good compromise.[7] Detrusor contraction is even more difficult to detect with ultrasonography (unless simultaneous urodynamic monitoring is performed) than with x-ray.

Bladder neck incompetence is as difficult to detect with ultrasonography as with cystography, especially in the case of cystocele with bladder neck descent. Therefore, some ultrasonography studies are directed toward the assessment of morphologic abnormalities of the urethral sphincter.

Morphologic Studies of the Urethral Sphincter

The width of the urethra (Fig. 17-16), measured 1 cm below the UVJ, appears reduced in postmenopausal women,[32] and sphincter volume is increased in women with electromyographic signs of outlet obstruction.[33] On transrectal sonography of the urethra, Kuo[34] noticed that the urethral peripheral striated muscular area was significantly smaller in subjects with type III urinary stress incontinence shown by videourodynamic study than in subjects with type 0 incontinence and in continent subjects. Other intraurethral and Doppler color ultrasonography studies show similar findings.[33,35-37]

Classification of Cystocele

Using a perineal view, Schaer and associates[38] proposed the following classification of cystoceles in four grades, identical to clinical or radiologic assessment:

TABLE 17-5 ■ Comparison of Ultrasonography Methods

Method	Perineal	Introital	Endovaginal	Transrectal
Probe (MHz)	5	5	7.5	7.5
Quality of imaging	+	+	++	++
Direct measurement of bladder neck mobility	+	±	++	++
Simultaneous UD	0	0	++	++
Voiding views	0	0	+	+

UD, urodynamics.

TABLE 17-6 ■ Importance of Ultrasonography and Urodynamic Artifacts Between Ultrasonography Methods

Method	Perineal	Introital	Endovaginal	Transrectal
Bladder neck mobility	0	±	+	0
Posterior urethrovesical angle	0	0	++	−
Closure pressure	0	+	+	0
Functional length of urethra	0	++	±	0
Transmission	0	+	±	0

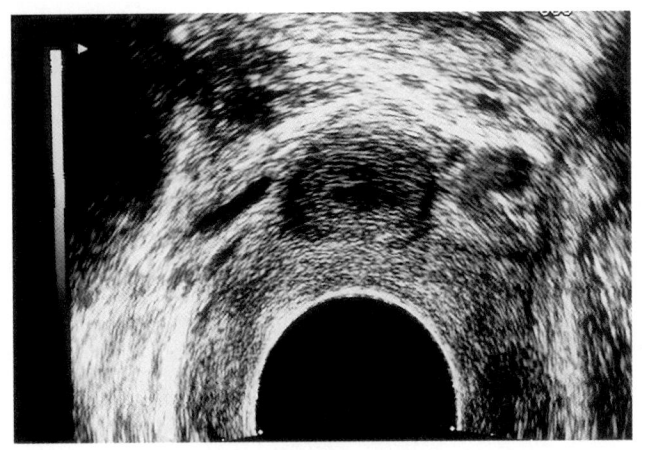

FIGURE 17-16 Endovaginal axial view of the upper third of the urethra. Note the hypoechoic external ring that corresponds to the peripheral striated muscular area.

- Grade 0 = No visible descent of the bladder base
- Grade 1 = Descent of the bladder base that does not reach the introitus
- Grade 2 = Descent of the bladder base that reaches the introitus
- Grade 3 = Descent of the bladder base below the introitus, pushing the ultrasonography probe away (Fig. 17-17)

Other Contributions of Ultrasound

Ultrasonography is the preferred method for the assessment of postvoiding residual urine and the detection of upper-tract dilation or pelvic masses and gynecologic diseases. It is also the most common imaging method used to study periurethral structures and abnormalities and to detect urethral diverticula.

Through the perineal and introital views, ultrasonography also allows rough assessment of prolapses of the other compartments. Recent studies reported the use of ultrasonography to evaluate the supporting structures (decreased thickness of the levator ani with aging and in incontinent women).[39] Sonography remains the first imaging tool in endocavitary evaluation of the anal sphincter, although the role of MRI is increasing.

THE ROLE OF IMAGING

Comparison of Physical Examination and Imaging

Physical examination remains the initial and essential step for patients with urinary incontinence or prolapse. However, this examination has limitations; moreover, when examined with colpocystodefecography, most patients (95%) with a clinical symptom specific to a single pelvic compartment had multiple coexisting compartment defects.[1]

In pelvic organ prolapse, physical examination is often less accurate than imaging, especially colpocystodefecography.

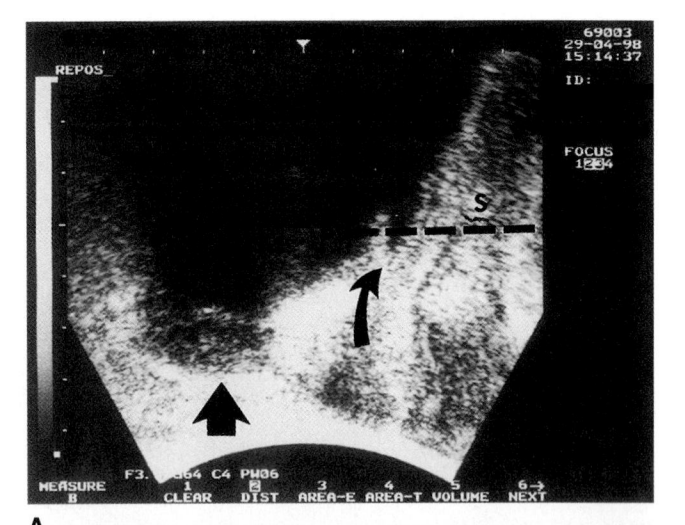

FIGURE 17-17 Cystocele: perineal view. At rest (**A**), grade 2 cystocele (*arrow*). Bladder neck (*curved arrow*). At strain (**B**), grade 3 cystocele (*arrow*): the probe is pushed out and the pubic symphysis (*dotted line*) is no longer visible. (From Lapray JF: Imagerie de la vessie et de la dynamique pelvienne de la femme. Masson, Paris, 1999, p 237.)

raphy. Altringer and colleagues reported correlation of only 74% for important anterior vaginal wall descent and 61% for posterior prolapse.[40] Hock[41] and Kelvin and associates[14] reported the same conclusions.[1,14,41]

These discrepancies can probably be explained by the conditions under which the clinical examination is performed.[41] On physical examination, the patient is lying or standing compared with the sitting position used in defecography. Furthermore, physical examination is performed with vaginal touch or the use of a speculum, with the risk of pushing the prolapse backward. Finally, physical examination uses palpation rather than observation with imaging. In urinary stress incontinence, the Q-tip test gives only an idea of the anatomic defect, and therefore has a lower specificity than imaging.[26]

All of the imaging methods can differentiate UVJ mobility from bladder neck incompetence when they are not associated, and each method has advantages and limitations.[7]

Urinary stress incontinence is a clinical diagnosis and does not necessarily imply the visualization of the leakage through the urethra.

Hypermobility and Bladder Neck Incompetence

The finding of bladder neck mobility between rest and strain of 2 cm or greater on x-ray or 1 cm or greater on ultrasonography or spontaneous situation of the bladder neck below the pubic symphysis corresponds to bladder neck hypermobility. Studies comparing the assessment of bladder neck position and mobility with cystography and ultrasonography show a good correlation.[42] However, these examinations cannot discriminate between stress incontinence and continence.[5]

Opening of the bladder neck during straining (without hypermobility or detrusor contraction) and micturition suggests bladder neck incompetence. However, the usefulness of RDVC and ultrasonography is limited because of detrusor instability, which is not detectable unless a manometric reading is obtained simultaneously.[9]

Retrograde Dynamic and Voiding Cystography and Colpocystodefecography

This radiologic technique provides dynamic views in the upright position and voiding views in the sitting position. Voiding views in the sitting position can be obtained with ultrasonography, but are rarely used, and, at the moment, cannot be obtained with MRI, although defecography can be performed with this technique.[43] Advantages of RDVC include objective images that are of better quality than videourodynamic images; images that are easy to read if the radiologist is familiar with the technique and range of findings; and low cost.[7] This technique allows precise quantification of UVJ mobility and bladder base descent, and permits a global approach to the lower urinary tract, with emphasis on voiding views to identify the morphology of the bladder neck.

Disadvantages of this technique are the need to expose the patient to radiation; the static images that provide very little information about periurethral structures and the pelvic floor muscles; and the focus on the anterior compartment of the pelvic floor. This last deficiency is eliminated by colpocystodefecography, which shows with precision vaginal descent, rectocele, perineal descent, and peritoneocele. The inclusion of defecation in the procedure ensures that the study provides maximum strain, which is difficult to determine with RDVC or ultrasonography unless abdominal pressure is monitored simultaneously. The most significant inconveniences are increased radiation and the need for a more complex examination. However, a skilled team can shorten the examination and maximize patient comfort.

Ultrasonography

Ultrasonography allows an analysis of UVJ mobility and morphology, even with coughing. Beaking and funneling of the bladder neck suggest bladder neck incompetence. Sonography is useful in assessing the position of the surgical slings, particularly of the probes during urodynamic studies, where it represents a good morphologic complement. It is still the simplest method for periurethral soft tissue analysis (urethral diverticula). Advantages include avoiding exposure to radiation, giving continuous real-time imaging, low cost, and current availability. The technique has been promoted mainly by gynecologists.

On the other hand, there is no standardization of the techniques and measurements used.[26] Increasing pressure of the probe can affect the bladder neck position, and when an associated prolapse is present, the endovaginal view becomes inaccurate. Furthermore, this technique requires considerable experience and some knowledge of urodynamics.[7]

New technical developments (three-dimensional, color Doppler, and intraurethral techniques) to permit assessment of the sphincter and pelvic floor muscles remain in the investigational phase.

CONCLUSION

The role of imaging is to allow matching of the treatment to the patient's condition. As noted by Brubaker and associates,[44] the goal of imaging is to prevent "the persistence of an uncorrected defect, recurrence in an adequately corrected defect, or complications from an unnecessary operation performed for a defect that was not present."

Although pelvic floor diseases require a global approach, the indications are different for isolated urinary incontinence and for prolapse. The recent availability of the new surgical technique of tension-free vaginal tape could change the treatment of urinary stress incontinence (Fig. 17-18).

If surgical treatment is planned after a failure of pelvic floor rehabilitation, imaging will provide a good morphologic complement to urodynamics to attempt to distinguish UVJ hypermobility from bladder neck incompetence. The indication for imaging appears uncontested after failed operations, when there is an associated prolapse, or when the clinical diagnosis is in doubt. In the same context, colpocystodefecography should be performed on patients with prolapse. Retrograde dynamic and voiding cystography can be used to complement MRI as long as dynamic MRI does not provide voiding views. The use of imaging will probably increase with the development and availability of dynamic MRI.

Too often considered an accessory procedure compared with urodynamic techniques that provide more data on detrusor and sphincter function, imaging should find a deserved place alongside urodynamics, with its numerous indications in the assessment of urinary incontinence and pelvic floor disorders. Cystourethrography is not indicated in primary uncomplicated urinary stress incontinence or

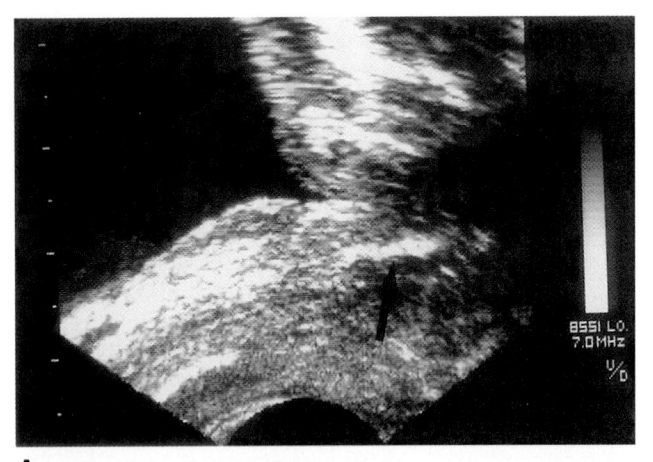

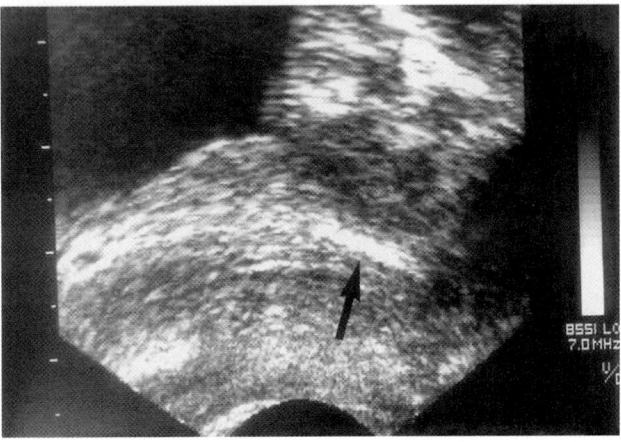

FIGURE 17-18 Tension-free vaginal tape (sagittal transrectal view). Note the difference between the situation of the vaginal tape (*arrows*) at rest (**A**) and during straining (**B**). The vaginal tape becomes horizontal. (From Lapray JF: Imagerie de l'insuffisance sphinctérienne. In Amarenco G, Serment G (eds): L'insuffisance sphinctérienne de la femme, Paris, Elsevier, 2000, pp 87–108.)

urge incontinence. Although dynamic MRI is the imaging method of the future, RDVC has an important place among the imaging techniques in the preoperative evaluation of complicated or recurrent female pelvic floor organ prolapse or urinary incontinence.

REFERENCES

1. Maglinte DT, Kelvin FM, Fitzgerald K, et al: Association of compartment defects in pelvic floor dysfunction. AJR 172:439–444, 1999.
2. Lapray JF: Imagerie de la vessie et de la dynamique pelvienne de la femme. Masson, Paris, 1999, p 237.
3. Kelvin FM, Maglinte DT, Benson JT, et al: Dynamic cystoproctography: A technique for assessing disorders of the pelvic floor in women. AJR 163:368–370, 1994.
4. Maglinte DT, Kelvin FM, Hale DS, et al: Dynamic cystoproctography of female pelvic floor defects and their interrelationships. AJR 169:769–774, 1997.
5. Artibani W, Andersen JT, Ostergard DR, et al: Imaging and other investigations. In Abrams P, Khoury S, Wein A (eds): First International Consultation on Incontinence, June 28–July 1, 1998, Monaco. Choisy le Roy, Graph'Imprim, pp 401–445.
6. Hodgkinson CP: Relationships of the female urethra and bladder in urinary stress incontinence. Am J Obstet Gynecol 65:560–573, 1953.
7. Mostwin JL, Yang A, Sanders R, et al: Radiography, sonography, and magnetic resonance imaging for stress incontinence. Urol Clin North Am 22:539–549, 1995.
8. Versi E, Deirdre JL, Griffiths DJ: Videourodynamic diagnosis of occult genuine stress incontinence in patients with anterior vaginal wall relaxation. J Soc Gynecol Invest 5:327–330, 1998.
9. Pelsang RE, Bonney WW: Voiding cystourethrography in female stress incontinence. AJR 166:561–565, 1996.
10. Kelvin FM, Maglinte DDT, Hale D, et al: Voiding cystourethrography in female stress incontinence (letter to the editor). AJR 167:1065–1066, 1996.
11. Blaivas JG, Olsson CA: Stress incontinence: Classification and surgical approach. J Urol 139:727–731, 1988.
12. McGuire EJ: Urodynamic findings in patients after failure of stress incontinence operations. Prog Clin Biol Res 78:351–360, 1981.
13. Healy JC, Halligan S, Reznek RH: Patterns of prolapse in women with symptoms of pelvic floor weakness: Assessment with MR imaging. Radiology 203:77–81, 1997.
14. Kelvin FM, Maglinte DT, Hale DS, et al: Female pelvic organ prolapse: A comparison of triphasic dynamic MR imaging and triphasic fluoroscopic cystocolpoproctography. AJR 174:81–88, 2000.
15. Zimmern PE: The role of voiding cystourethrography in the evaluation of the female lower urinary tract. Probl Urol 23–41, 1991.
16. Haab F, Cortesse A, Jacquetin B, et al: Classification des cystocèles: CUROPF (work in progress). Presented at the 94ème Congrès de l'Association Française d'Urologie, Paris, Nov 2000. Unpublished.
17. Schaer GN, Perucchini D, Munz E, et al: Sonographic evaluation of the bladder neck in continent and stress-incontinent women. Obstet Gynecol 93:412–416, 1999.
18. Kuo HC: Transrectal sonography of the female urethra in incontinence and frequency-urgency syndrome. J Ultrasound Med 15:363–370, 1996.
19. Delaere K, Moone W, Debruyne F, et al: Hydronephrosis caused by cystocele. Urology 24:364–365, 1984.
20. Hextall A, Boos K, Cardozo L, et al: Videocystourethrography with a ring pessary in situ: A clinically useful preoperative investigation for continent women with urogenital prolapse? Int Urogynecol J 9:205–209, 1998.
21. Ghoniem GM, Walters F, Lewis V: The value of the vaginal pack test in large cystoceles. J Urol 152:931–934, 1994.
22. Lapray JF: Imagerie de l'insuffisance sphinctérienne. In Amarenco G, Serment G (eds): L'insuffisance Sphinctérienne de la Femme. Paris, Elsevier, 2000, pp 87–108.
23. Gardy M, Kozminski M, DeLancey J, et al: Stress incontinence and cystoceles. J Urol 145:1211–1213, 1991.
24. Kelvin FM, Maglinte DT: Dynamic cystoproctography of female pelvic floor defects and their interrelationships. AJR 169:769–774, 1997.
25. Johnson JD, Lamensdorf H, Hollander IN, et al: Use of transvaginal endosonography in the evaluation of women with stress urinary incontinence. J Urol 147:421–425, 1992.
26. Demirci F, Fine PM: Ultrasonography in stress urinary incontinence. Int Urogynecol J 7:125–132, 1996.
27. Beco J: Reducing uncertainty for vesico-urethral sonography in women. Acta Urol Belg 63:13–29, 1995.
28. Dietz HP, Wilson PD: The influence of bladder volume on the position and mobility of the urethrovesical junction. Int Urogynecol J 10:3–6, 1999.

29. Schaer GN, Koechli OR, Schuessler B, et al: Usefulness of ultrasound contrast medium in perineal sonography for vizualization of bladder neck funneling: First observations. Urology 47:452–453, 1996.
30. Brandt FT, Albuquerque DC, Lorenzato FR, et al: Perineal assessment of urethrovesical junction mobility in young continent females. Int Urogynecol J 11:18–22, 2000.
31. Kuo HC: Transrectal sonographic investigation of urethral and paraurethral structures in women with stress urinary incontinence. J Ultrasound Med 17:311–320, 1998.
32. Yang JM: Factors affecting urethrocystographic parameters in urinary continent women. J Clin Ultrasound 24:249–255, 1996.
33. Noble JG, Dixon PJ, Rickards D, et al: Urethral sphincter volumes in women with obstructed voiding and abnormal sphincter electromyographic activity. Br J Urol 76:741–746, 1995.
34. Kuo HC: The relationships of urethral and pelvic floor muscles and the urethral pressure measurements in women with stress urinary incontinence. Eur Urol 37:149–155, 2000.
35. Heit M: Intraurethral ultrasonography: Correlation of urethral anatomy with functional urodynamic parameters in stress incontinent women. Int Urogynecol J 11:204–211, 2000.
36. Beco J, Léonard D, Léonard F: Study of the female urethra's submucous vascular plexus by color Doppler. World J Urol 16:224–228, 1998.
37. Frauscher F, Helweg G, Strasser H, et al: Intraurethral ultrasound: Diagnostic evaluation of the striated urethral sphincter in incontinent females. Eur Radiol 8:50–53, 1998.
38. Schaer GN, Koechli OR, Schuessler B, et al: Perineal ultrasound for evaluating the bladder neck in urinary stress incontinence. Obstet Gynecol 85:220–224, 1995.
39. Bernstein I, Juul N, Gronvall S, et al: Pelvic floor muscle thickness measured by perineal ultrasonography. Scand J Urol Nephrol Suppl 137:131–135, 1991.
40. Altringer WE, Saclarides TJ, Dominguez JM, et al: Four-contrast defecography: Pelvic "flooroscopy." Dis Colon Rectum 38:695–699, 1995.
41. Hock D: La colpocystodéfécographie: Étude morphodynamique du pelvis féminin. Lyon Chir 92:243–250, 1996.
42. Kolbl H, Bernaschek G, Wolf G: A comparative study of perineal ultrasound scanning and urethrocystography in patients with genuine stress incontinence. Arch Gynecol Obstet 244:39–45, 1988.
43. Schoenenberger AW, Debatin JF, Guldenschuh I, et al: Dynamic MR defecography with a superconducting, open-configuration MR system. Radiology 206:641–646, 1998.
44. Brubaker L, Retsky S, Smith C, et al: Pelvic floor evaluation with dynamic fluoroscopy. Am J Obstet Gynecol 82:863–868, 1993.

CHAPTER 18

Colporectocystourethrography: The Dynamic Investigation

JEAN C. JURAS ■ ALAIN P. BOURCIER ■ RICHARD M. VILLET

DIAGNOSTIC METHODS OF EVALUATION

Most women with pelvic floor dysfunction have multiple defects that affect various functions. Pelvic prolapse is a common problem that affects women of all ages and is much more widespread than previously thought. Pelvic prolapse leads to surgical intervention in an estimated 11% of all women by 80 years of age,[1] especially after hysterectomy, with a reported prevalence of up to 16%.[2,3] In 1996, in the United States, an estimated 600,000 hysterectomies were performed, and 90,000 were performed for pelvic prolapse. Patients often see urologists or gynecologists because of urinary incontinence or voiding difficulties. To prevent or treat urinary stress incontinence or repair prolapse, surgeons must become familiar with the evaluation and treatment techniques for pelvic prolapse. The most common problem after surgery is the need to repair defects of the posterior or middle compartment in patients who undergo uretropexy for urinary stress incontinence. Wiskind and colleagues[4] reported 24% of cases of vaginal prolapse after surgery for urinary stress incontinence. Often, in a patient with prolapse, surgical relief leads to unmasked, or hidden, incontinence. The preoperative rates are high when a single defect is repaired, and the surgeon must tailor the technical procedure to the patient. Careful evaluation is needed. It is helpful to make the differentiation preoperatively to ensure proper repair and avoid relapse or treatment failure.

Pelvic examination for pelvic prolapse is always performed with the patient resting and straining while supine to define and grade the different compartments involved. When a patient complains of heaviness or bulging and pelvic organ prolapse is not observed, have patient assume an erect posture. Provocative maneuvers may confirm symptoms and allow grading of different compartments. Physical examination also must evaluate other concomitant types of prolapse. Unfortunately, the clinical evaluation is difficult to complete. Electrophysiologic and urodynamic techniques are specific evaluations of the lower urinary tract, but do not yield valuable information about gross anatomic alterations. A variety of static and dynamic imaging techniques are used in the investigation of pelvic floor relaxation and anorectal disorders. Therefore, studies that provide only static anatomic information are of limited value. One area of anatomic investigation that recently made progress is cross-sectional imaging of the pelvic floor with magnetic resonance imaging (MRI). This technique shows the specific anatomy of women with pelvic organ prolapse. Others advocate dynamic MRI as an excellent imaging technique for evaluating pelvic prolapse.[5,6] There are some contradictions between authors who recommend MRI as a noninvasive alternative to colpocystorectography for diagnosing enterocele and vaginal vault prolapse[7] and those who report that MRI is inferior to this radiologic study for detecting cystocele and enterocele.[8] In that case, the authors reported that MRI has less sensitivity than colpocystodecography for detecting prolapse involving the anterior and middle compartments.

Another radiologic technique used with a different approach can be applied to record events with the patient in the upright position. With this technique, the patient performs all of the normal or exaggerated maneuvers (e.g., resting, holding, straining). This combined radiologic study is known as dynamic cystocolpography. The radiologic investigation is known as colporectocystourethrography (CRCU). It was introduced in France by Bethoux and colleagues[9,10] as colpocystogram, and later developed by Richter and associates[11] in Europe and Brubaker and associates[12] in North America.

This radiologic investigation allows indirect visualization of the pelvic floor muscles and accurate assessment of the entire pelvic floor, including changes in the topography of the pelvic viscera. The most profound changes in the pelvic floor occur in the standing position, usually when the patient is straining or lifting. Although a thorough clinical examination is possible in the office setting, the examination can be easier to perform during radiologic evaluation and can be reproduced radiologically with dynamic colporectocystography. When physical examination does not definitively differentiate a large defect from a minimal pelvic floor defect with concomitant pelvic prolapse (enterocele), this radiographic study may be useful.

PATHOPHYSIOLOGY

With the increasing number of patients referred to gynecologists and urologists for the treatment of pelvic prolapse, familiarity with pelvic anatomy and evaluation is essential. Urinary incontinence and pelvic organ prolapse are separate entities that often coexist, and protrusions of the vagina can alter either voiding or defecation. Surgical repair of one pelvic organ without repair of concurrent asymptomatic pelvic support defects may lead to new symptoms that affect bowel function, sexual function, and other pelvic organ prolapse.[13,14]

A review of the pathophysiology[15-20] is needed to provide a better understanding of this specific evaluation. The vagina may be divided into three anatomic sections.[15,19] The upper third of the vagina, called the vaginal vault apex, is supported by the cardinal and uterosacral ligaments. These structures also help to support the cervix and uterus. The broad ligaments play a role in attaching the lateral uterine walls to the lateral pelvic side walls. The middle third of the vagina is supported by lateral attachments to the pubococcygeal muscles. The distal third of the vagina, which is in close proximity to the urethra, is the least mobile portion. It has multiple periurethral attachments and connections to the surrounding urogenital diaphragm structures.

Posterior connections of the vagina include attachments to the central tendon of the perineum and to the transverse perineal muscles. The levator hiatus is a space bordered by the levator ani muscles through which the upper vagina, bladder, pouch of Douglas, and rectum pass.

Anterior Vaginal Wall Prolapse: Cystocele

Anterior prolapse is responsible for cystocele that involves herniation of the bladder base into the vagina (Fig. 18-1). In the case of urethral hypermobility, vaginal wall prolapse may be referred to as cytourethrocele. There are two main types of cystoceles. Between 70% and 80% of cystoceles are caused by lateral defects, in which the anterior cardinal ligaments to the pelvic side walls are disrupted, and 5% to 15% of central defects result from the connective tissue of the visceral fascia. In severe prolapse, it is possible to have both defects. Several classifications of cystoceles are proposed. We commonly use the Baden and Walker classification.[21]

Grade I (bladder descent toward the introitus with straining) and grade II (bladder descent to the introitus with straining) cystoceles may cause urinary stress incontinence, but usually are asymptomatic. Patients with cystocele accompanied by urethral hypermobility may have urinary stress incontinence. Patients with grade III cystocele (bladder outside of the introitus with straining) may have vaginal bulging, vaginal mass or fullness, and sometimes voiding symptoms. Grade IV cystocele (bladder outside of the introitus at rest) may cause obstructive or irritative voiding symptoms and the need to lean forward or reduce the prolapse manually to void (Fig. 18-2). At this high grade of cystocele, ureteral obstruction and recurrent urinary tract infection may occur.[19] In patients with high-grade cystocele, hydronephrosis may result from ureteral kinking. When a cystocele is present after anti-incontinence surgery, patients with a well-supported bladder neck may have obstructive voiding symptoms as a result of urethral kinking.[15,19,22]

Apical and Posterior Vaginal Wall Prolapse

Vaginal Apical Prolapse: Enterocele

Enterocele involves peritoneal herniation between the uterosacral ligaments at the vaginal apex (Fig. 18-3). This condition causes a bulge at the top of the vagina, and identification of the viscera occupying the enterocele location (e.g., small bowel, sigmoid colon) in combination with other findings is difficult. It is also difficult to differentiate this type of enterocele from a coexisting

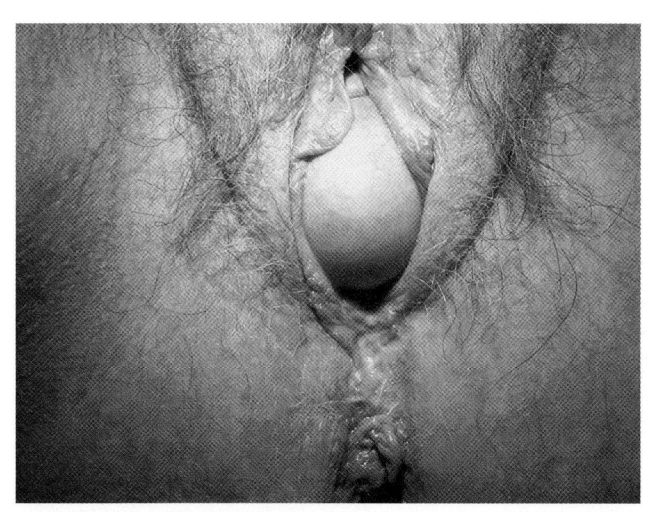

FIGURE 18-1 Grade II (moderate) cystocele in a parous woman with a pelvic organ prolapse. As she strains, the urogenital hiatus opens to allow prolapse of the anterior vaginal segment.

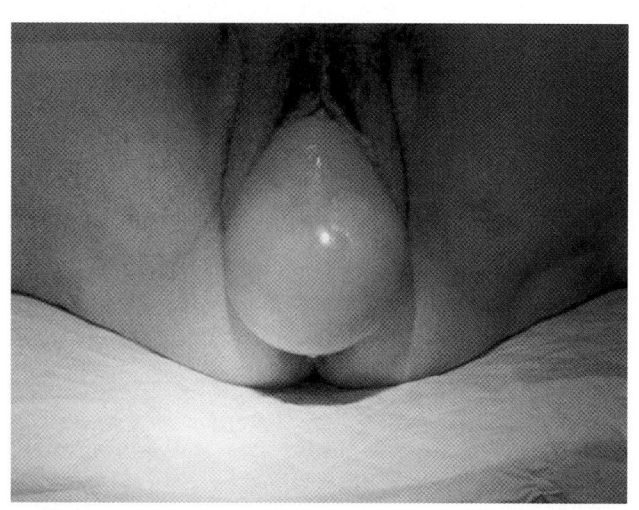

FIGURE 18-2 Grade IV (severe) cystocele. At rest, the patient does not strain, and the advanced prolapse may obstruct a well-supported bladder neck.

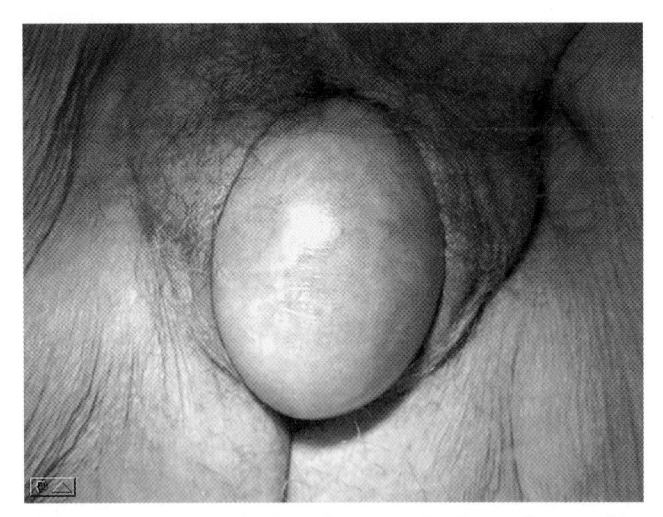

FIGURE 18-3 Enterocele. Posterior protrusion is usually caused by defects in the rectovaginal fascia, allowing protrusion of the small bowel.

large rectocele or enterocele (Fig. 18-4). Different types of enterocele are described. Traction enterocele, the most common type, occurs when the pouch of Douglas is pulled down by a prolapsing uterus.[22] Acquired enterocele accounts for 5% to 27% of cases. It usually develops after abdominal bladder neck suspension, which causes a widely open and unprotected cul-de-sac.[23] Women with enterocele are often asymptomatic, but they may have a mass at or beyond the introitus as well as perineal pressure. A bulge higher in the posterior vagina may represent enterocele or high rectocele. Enterocele is differentiated from vault prolapse by posterior vaginal wall shortening, which is indicative of vault prolapse.

Vaginal Apical Prolapse: Vaginal Vault Prolapse

Upper vaginal eversion is a result of weakening of the vaginal apex, usually after previous surgery, such as hysterectomy or enterocele repair.[22,24] Women describe perineal pressure, dyspareunia, or the sensation of a mass protruding from the vagina. They also have difficulty voiding and must reduce the prolapse manually to facilitate bladder emptying. Posterior vaginal wall foreshortening indicates vault prolapse, whereas an apical bulge without posterior wall shortening is consistent with enterocele.

Vaginal Apical Prolapse: Uterine Prolapse

Women with uterine prolapse (Fig. 18-5) often have perineal pressure, dyspareunia, or a mass at the introitus.[25] They may describe urinary incontinence or difficult urination, consistent with obstruction. Examination with the patient standing is important to determine the degree of prolapse (i.e., the level to which the cervix falls).

Posterior Vaginal Wall Prolapse: Rectocele

Rectocele (Fig. 18-6) is a protrusion of the rectum into the posterior vagina caused by a weakened rectovaginal septum and perineal body.[20,22,23] Patients are often asymptomatic, but they may also notice a sensation of the stool becoming stuck as it moves through the rectum. They often must insert a finger into the vagina to reduce herniation and facilitate stool evacuation. Symptoms that are not attributable to rectocele are chronic constipation, perineal pressure, dyspareunia, and fecal incontinence. A similar classification is used to determine the grade of the rectocele: grade I rectocele is protrusion with straining, grade II is protrusion to the introitus, and grade III is protrusion outside of the introitus. During physical examination, the physician's finger is directed anterior to detect rectal herniation into the vagina or through the introitus.

Urinary Stress Incontinence

The mechanisms of urinary stress incontinence depend on two factors that may be isolated or combined: urethral junction hypermobility and urethral sphincter deficiency.

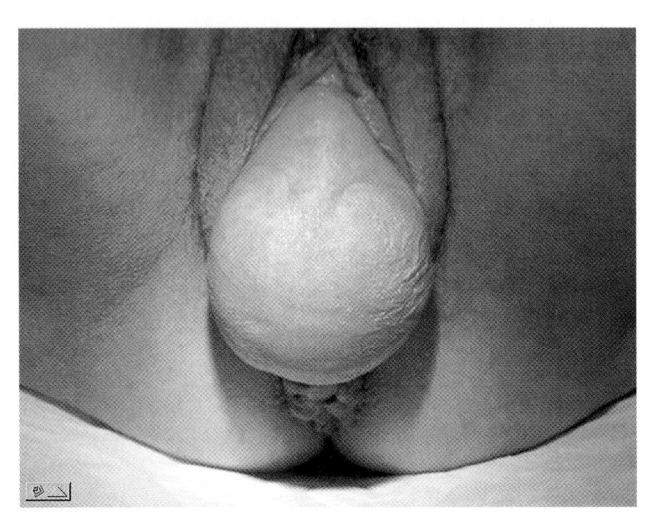

FIGURE 18-4 Posterior vaginal wall descent with difficulty differentiating between rectocele and enterocele.

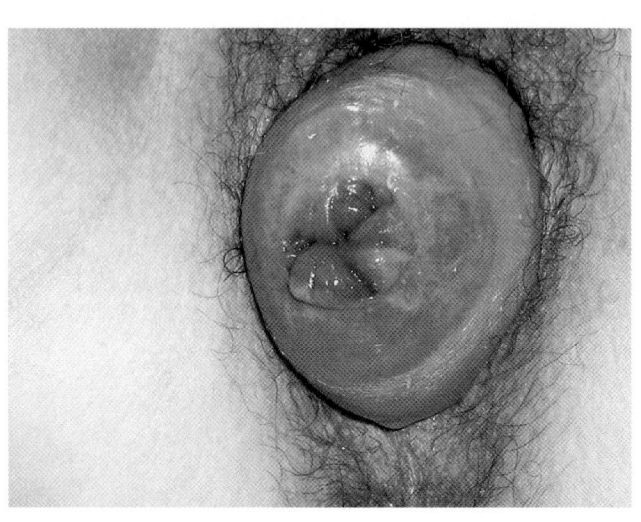

FIGURE 18-5 Uterine prolapse. The uterus prolapses fully outside the hymen as uterine procidentia.

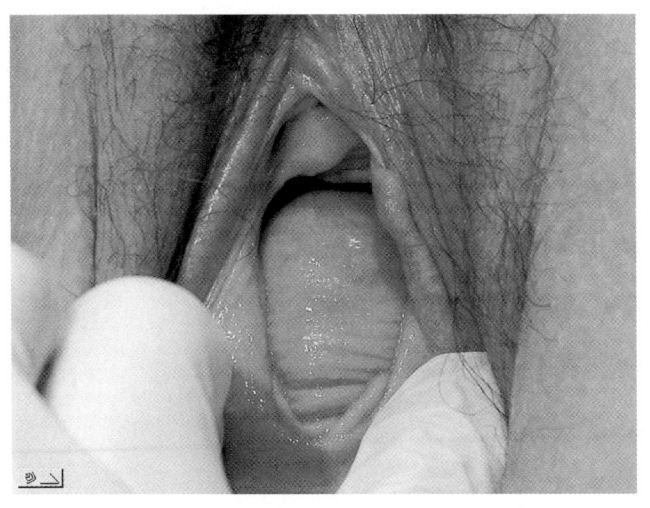

FIGURE 18-6 Rectocele. Distal loss of support in the posterior segment may result in a bulge that compresses the urethra and affects voiding.

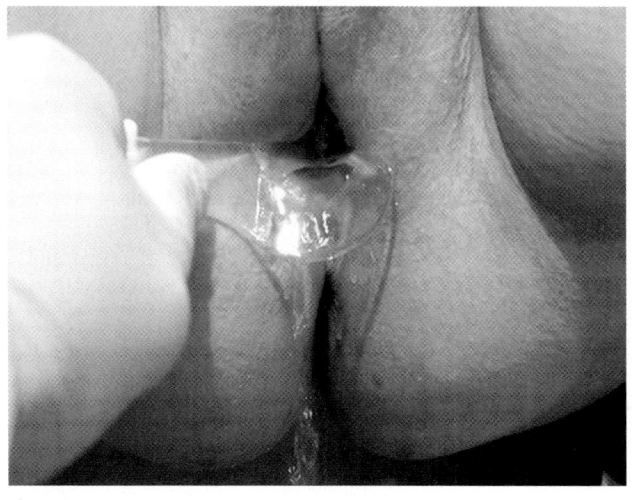

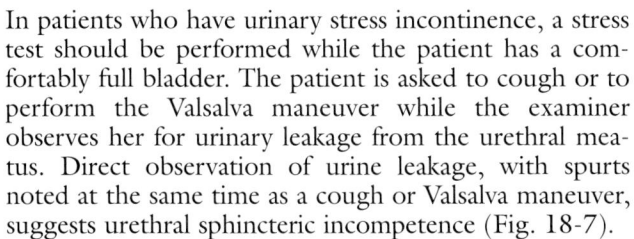

FIGURE 18-8 Unmasked incontinence as a result of severe uterovaginal prolapse. The stress test is performed with the posterior blade of a speculum to reduce the prolapse.

In patients who have urinary stress incontinence, a stress test should be performed while the patient has a comfortably full bladder. The patient is asked to cough or to perform the Valsalva maneuver while the examiner observes her for urinary leakage from the urethral meatus. Direct observation of urine leakage, with spurts noted at the same time as a cough or Valsalva maneuver, suggests urethral sphincteric incompetence (Fig. 18-7).

In patients with severe uterovaginal prolapse or a posterior vaginal wall defect, such relaxation causes coexisting loss of urethrovesical junction support, but the patient remains paradoxically continent. These patients should undergo a stress test, regardless of whether they have urinary leakage (Fig. 18-8). This test may help to identify patients with urinary stress incontinence who will have symptoms only after prolapse reduction surgery. The basis of this paradoxical continence is mechanical urethral obstruction that may be caused by physical kinking of the urethra because the prolapse is accentuated by stress.[24]

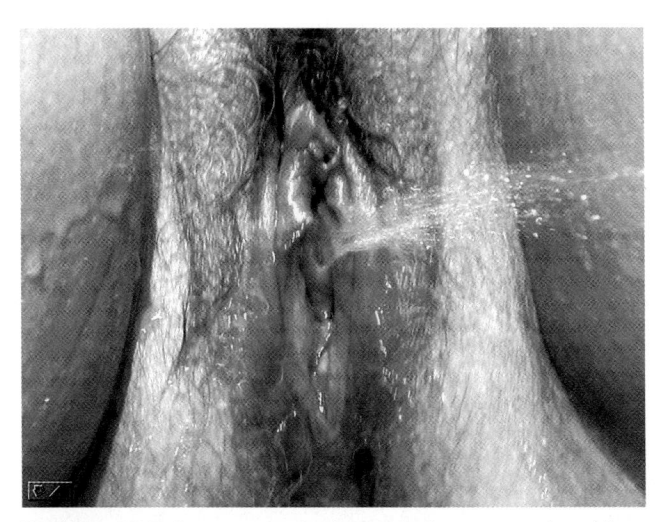

Anterior compartment visualization allows the bladder and urethra to be seen. Cystocele may be defined by a straining view of standing CRCU that shows descent of the bladder base below the inferior aspect of the symphysis pubis. Lateral views are essential for evaluating urethral and bladder base descent. The mobility of the urethra, its location relative to the bony pelvis, and its degree of competency, as shown by funneling, can be determined. Others advocate CRCU in all women with anterior pelvic prolapse to unmask occult urinary stress incontinence. Evaluation of the middle compartment is important when the prolapsing structure is difficult to evaluate, particularly when the patient also has a prolapsing central mass. Identification of the viscera occupying this location is essential, and can affect surgical management.

Evaluation of the posterior compartment provides useful information about the differentiation between a rectocele and an enterocele, puborectalis contractility, anal closing forces, and relaxation of the pelvic floor muscles. Enteroceles are often identified after repeated straining, and for this reason, they may not found be on clinical examination.

TECHNIQUE

To evaluate pelvic floor disorders,[9,10,26] barium is placed into the urethra, bladder, vagina, and rectum to opacify fully the pelvic organs. The patient is placed in the supine position on a mobile x-ray table. The bladder is then catheterized (Fig. 18-9A) with a small-caliber 8 Fr, and 50 to 60 mL fluid contrast medium (Fig. 18-9B) is instilled (Telebrix 35, Labo Guerbet, Roissy, France). This amount is sufficient to allow visualization of the bladder base and bladder neck. A syringe of 3 mL barium sulfate sterile cream is instilled into the urethra (Fig. 18-9C). Two speculum blades are introduced simultaneously and

FIGURE 18-7 Stress test. Leakage during a cough with a comfortably full bladder. The patient is asked to cough or perform the Valsalva maneuver while the examiner observes for urinary leakage from the urethral meatus.

FIGURE 18-9 Techniques used for the different sequences of dynamic fluoroscopy. **A**, Bladder catheterization done in a sterile manner with a small-caliber (8 Fr) catheter. **B**, The bladder is filled with 50 to 60 mL fluid contrast material (Telebrix 35, Labo Guerbet, Roissy, France). **C**, Barium sulfate cream (3 mL) is instilled into the urethra. **D**, Two speculum blades are introduced simultaneously and remain separated. A paste of thickened barium powder and water is placed into the vagina with a lubricated syringe. **E**, A tube with 50 mL barium paste (Micropaque, Labo Guerbet, Roissy, France) is introduced into the rectum.

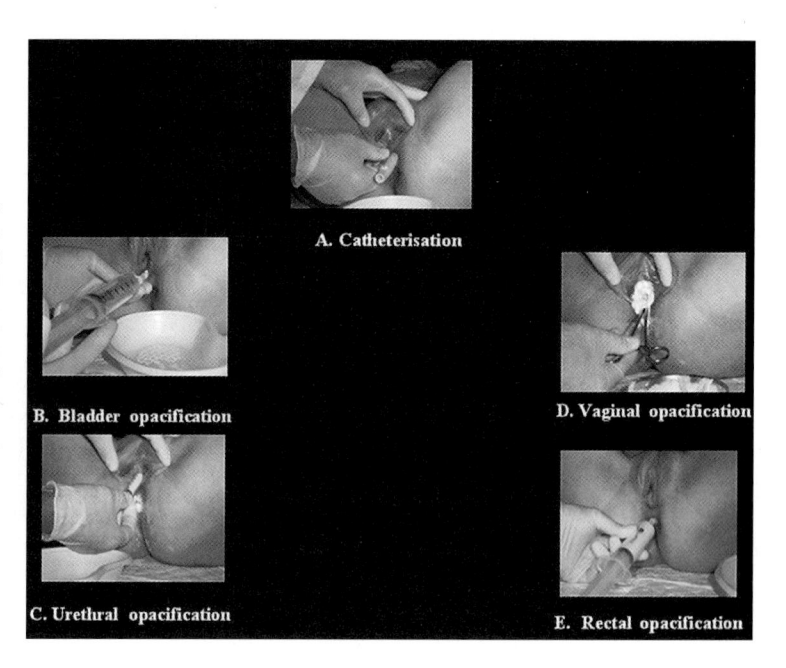

remain separated. A paste of thickened barium powder and water is placed into the vagina (Fig. 18-9D) with a lubricated syringe. Later, 50 mL commercially available paste (Micropaque, Labo Guerbet, Roissy, France) is inserted into the rectum (Fig. 18-9E). The uterus is no longer systematically identified.

Other authors use a similar technique, but use[27,28] a radiolucent commode. Between 1 and 2 hours before entering the fluoroscopic suite, the patient ingests 2 cups low-density barium sulfate suspension and drinks 8 oz cold water. The patient then sits on a specific commode that is attached to the fluoroscopic table for radiographic examination of the pelvis (E-Z EM, Westbury, NY). Two lateral films are obtained, one with the patient at rest and one with the patient straining hard. After the vagina and rectum are opacified, two other films are obtained during evacuation. A seated position seems to be more physiologic because patients normally sit for voiding and bowel evacuation. In the study of pelvic floor defects, the standing position most nearly replicates the real-life situation.

Other authors[12,29] finalize this preparation with two radiopaque markers placed on the surface of the perineum. One marker is placed as close as possible to the anus, and the other is placed on the perineal body, between the vagina and the rectum, allowing adequate assessment of the structures in relationship to the perineal body.

When all contrast agents have been administered,[26,30,31] the patient is placed in the upright position. The correct lateral view (Fig. 18-10) is confirmed by the finding of hip joints overlying each other. A view of the pelvis is obtained, and x-rays are taken with the patient at rest (first position), with the patient squeezing the pelvic floor muscles "as if trying to stop her urine flow" (second position), and finally with the patient straining in attempted defecation (third position). The dynamic portion of this examination is performed as the patient evacuates the contrast material from the rectum. Dynamic images are recorded under video control or with rapid filming sequences to highlight structural alterations and show the relationships between pelvic organs. Maximum straining to show defects may be difficult to obtain because of emotional factors, particularly embarrassment or humiliation.

NORMAL PELVIC FLOOR

As experience with CRCU has accumulated, it has become clear that the normal range of appearances is wider than initially appreciated. Many radiologic reports of normal findings are based on studies of asymptomatic persons who are presumed to be normal. Different parameters can be measured, such as the anorectal angle, the position of the anorectal junction, the urethrovesical junction, anterior and posterior vaginal defects, and the efficacy of pelvic floor contraction.

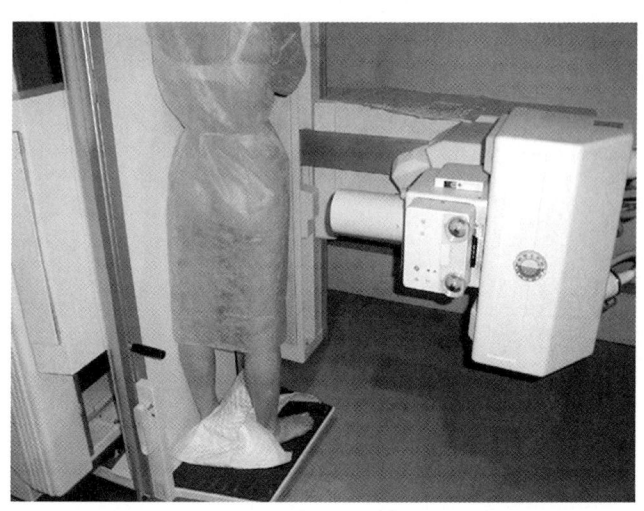

FIGURE 18-10 Pelvic views are obtained with the patient in a standing position. The correct lateral view is confirmed by the observation that the hip joints are overlying each other.

1. At rest (Fig. 18-11), the dorsal wall of the rectum lies on the posterior levator plate, forming the upper side of the anorectal angle. The urethra and the bladder base are attached to the medial border of the levator ani. Normally, the bladder base is horizontal and does not descend below the inferior border of the symphysis. In the absence of bladder contraction, funneling of the bladder base usually does not occur at rest. During the first position (CRCU at rest), the inferior margins of the bladder and urethra are affected by muscle activity: the levator ani muscles maintain constant neural stimulation of fatigue-resistant striated muscle.[32] This constant constriction of the vagina by the levator ani muscles eliminates any opening within the pelvic floor, through which prolapse could occur.[32,33]
2. In the second position (Fig. 18-12), active contraction of the pelvic floor muscle has influenced the attached organs with a compression, caused by narrowing of the urogenital hiatus. During voluntary pelvic floor contraction, the levator ani musculature straightens and the muscle sling shortens in a dorsoventral direction.[34]
3. In the third position, during straining (Fig. 18-13), the patient is asked to push hard, straining as if attempting to defecate. Straining allows visualization of the effects of relaxation on the pelvic viscera. The levator plate moves downward, causing a descent of the anorectal junction and an opening of the genital hiatus. As the puborectalis muscle relaxes, the vagina and bladder base descend and the urethral axis is modified. The urethrovesical junction moves less than 10 mm on maximal strain. Small rectoceles (<2 cm deep) that empty completely are common in asymptomatic subjects. The normal cul-de-sac may extend 1 to 2 cm below the vaginal apex; therefore, an enterocele should be diagnosed only when small bowel herniation extends deeper into the rectovaginal space.
4. The fourth position is an additional position that is not necessary for each evaluation (Fig. 18-14). Because some prolapse elements compete, one prolapse may hide another. Therefore, in some cases, a technical variation is used. Vaginal examination can be performed with the posterior blade of a Graves or monovalve speculum in the vagina to retract the posterior vaginal wall.[26,31] The posterior wall of the vagina is depressed while the patient strains, allowing the examiner to observe the vaginal wall for descent and assess the position of the bladder and urethra. Others suggested reducing prolapse with a Pozzi clamp, a vaginal pessary, or vaginal packing to show urinary stress incontinence.

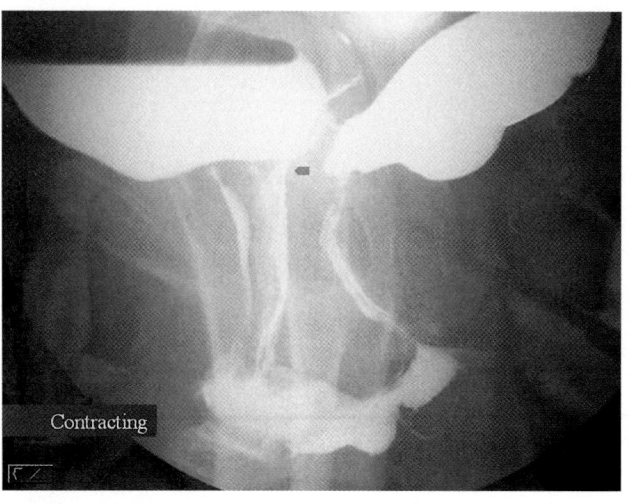

FIGURE 18-12 Colporectocystourethrography during contraction. On active contraction, the anterior movement of the vagina produces occlusive forces on the urethra and anterior movement of the viscera toward the pubic symphysis. Arrow shows an upward displacement of the proximal vagina.

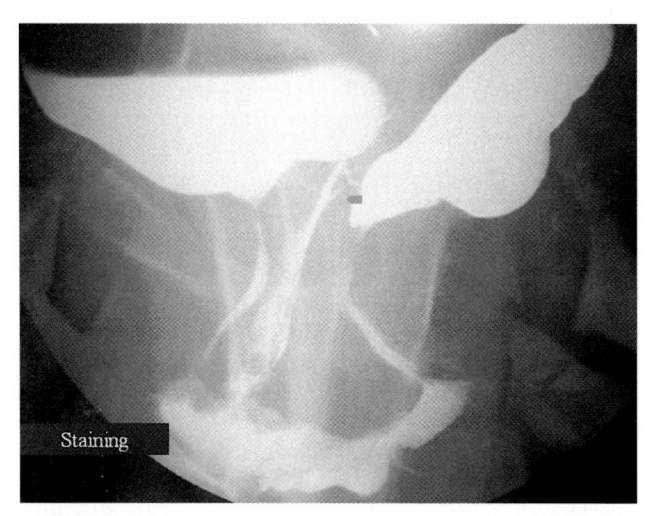

FIGURE 18-13 Colporectocystourethrography during straining. The levator plate moves downward, causing descent of the anorectal junction and opening of the genital hiatus, with widening of the anorectal angles. Arrow indicates the modification of the axis of the proximal vagina with a loss of the midurethral angulation. The levator plate relaxes and becomes less horizontal.

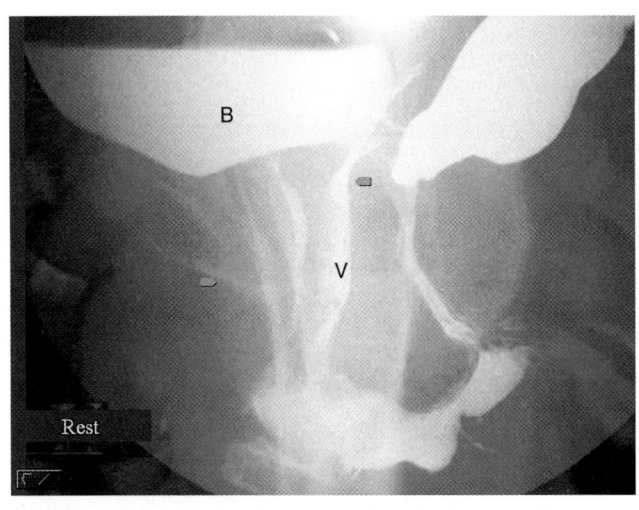

FIGURE 18-11 Lateral radiograph of the pelvis. At rest, the patient has contrast material in the bladder (B), vagina (V), and rectum. The bladder base should be horizontal and should not descend below the inferior border of the symphysis. Top arrow shows normal vaginal support. The proximal vagina rests horizontally on the levator plate forming an angle of approximately 110 degrees with the axis of the distal vagina. Bottom arrow represents the inferior border of the symphysis pubis.

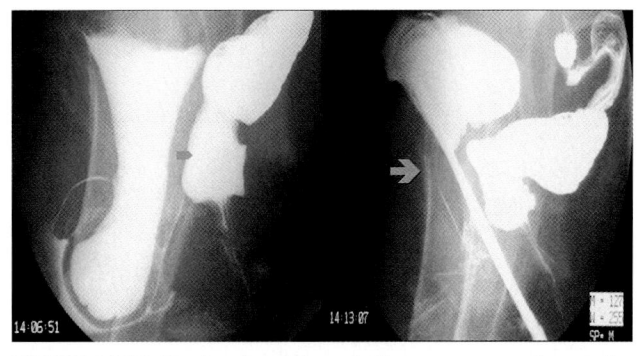

FIGURE 18-14 The fourth position of colporectocystourethrography, with reduction of the prolapse with a monovalve speculum. Left arrow indicates the rectum. Right arrow indicates the depression of the anterior wall of the vagina (reduction of the cystocele with a monovalve speculum).

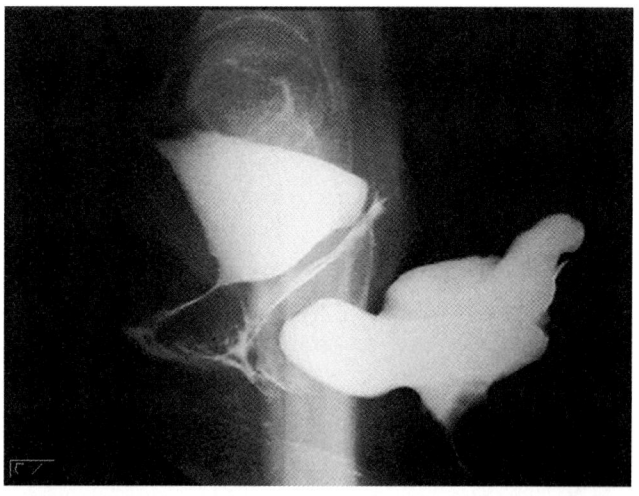

FIGURE 18-15 Lateral upright colporectocystourethography during straining shows loss of pelvic support and moderate cystocele.

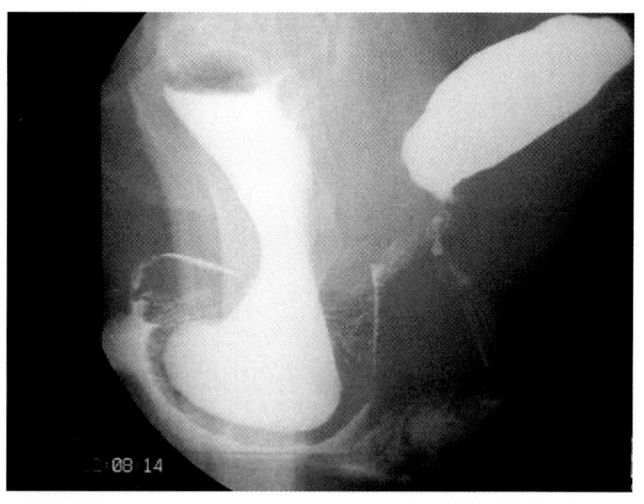

FIGURE 18-16 Voiding dysfunction with obstruction caused by a large prolapsing cystocele (grade IV cystocele with lateral and central defects). The cystocele causes functional obstruction of the bladder neck during voiding as a result of urethral kinking.

When performed by a skillful and experienced team, this radiologic examination is well accepted and well tolerated by most patients. However, it is important both to explain the procedure and to reassure the patient before the evaluation is performed.

ABNORMALITIES OF THE PELVIC FLOOR: FLUOROSCOPIC FINDINGS

Anterior Vaginal Defects

Site-specific analysis of pelvic organ support begins with evaluation of the anterior segment: the urethra, urethrovesical junction, and bladder. As the patient strains maximally in a standing position, mobility and descent of the distal anterior vaginal wall can be seen. As noted earlier, we classify cystoceles according to the Baden and Walker classification.[21]

When the patient voids, the urethrovesical junction normally opens with a funnel-shaped configuration. Movement of the urethrovesical junction on straining can be measured accurately by exactly superimposing the rest and strain films,[8,26,30,31] thereby determining the distance that the junction moved on straining. Most patients with urinary stress incontinence show hypermobility of the urethrovesical junction, with anteroinferior movement occurring on straining. A funnel-shaped junction at rest is an abnormal finding consistent with an intrinsic sphincter deficiency. Although the splinting effect of a catheter can cause funneling, its small size (5 Fr) makes this finding unlikely.

Disruptions in endopelvic fascial support produce cystoceles. Cystocele causes prolapse of the urinary bladder below the pubic symphysis and intrinsic pressure on the anterior and superior aspects of the vagina. The spectrum of appearances is wide, ranging from minimal bulging of the bladder base (Fig. 18-15) to classic grade IV cystocele (Fig. 18-16). In such cases, the top half of the urethra is kinked and departs from the urethral segment of the vagina. Of course, the funnel-shaped configuration, cystocele, and urethral hypermobility can happen together to various degrees. Kelvin and associates[35] assume that the size of a cystocele varies with patient position and degree of straining. They also emphasize that reflex contraction of the levator ani may provide better support to the bladder in the standing position used for CRCU than during sitting. They also state that the size of the cystocele is underestimated compared with the appearance seen on straining during or after evacuation with dynamic cystoproctography.[28,35]

Pelvic Relaxation of the Middle Compartment

When support of the cardinal uterosacral ligament is poor, the cervix descends from its normal position at or above the level of the ischial spines. The severity of middle compartment relaxation ranges from mild uterine descent to total uterovaginal prolapse when the uterus is present. Middle compartment support may exist in association with defects of the anterior compartment, the posterior compartment, or both. After hysterectomy, relaxation of the middle compartment may range from mild vaginal vault descent, through vaginal vault prolapse, to complete vaginal eversion. Vaginal vault prolapse or uterine descent can be observed. Descent of the cervix or vaginal apex can be observed as well as the vaginal cuff after hysterectomy and demonstrated with CRCU. Because contrast material is placed in the vagina during fluoroscopic evacuation, vaginal vault prolapse or uterine descent can be visualized easily.[9,31] Radiologic investigation can confirm the findings of physical examination and can be used to grade the degree of uterine prolapse. With minimal prolapse, the uterus reaches the midvaginal area; with moderate prolapse, the uterus reaches from midvagina to the introitus; and with severe prolapse, the uterus is always outside the introitus (Fig. 18-17). If the support structures are weakened, the cervix can invaginate and migrate downward on a vertical axis into the vagina.

Posterior Vaginal Defects

Posterior Vaginal Wall Prolapse: Rectocele

Relaxation of the posterior compartment may involve the upper, middle, or lower portion of the posterior vaginal wall and result in a variety of disorders, such as rectocele, enterocele, and perineal defects.[13]

Rectocele is protrusion of the rectum into the posterior vagina, and is caused by a weakened rectovaginal septum and perineal body.[18,22,23] Defects of the posterior vaginal wall or supporting attachments result in rectoceles that can cause a spectrum of symptoms. Many patients are asymptomatic, but others notice a sensation of the stool becoming stuck as it moves through the rectum. They have a distressing sensation of obstructed defecation and incomplete evacuation. The straining efforts that accompany these feelings may aggravate minor degrees of damage and can result in progressive injury. Some patients describe posterior vaginal splinting or the need to insert a finger into the vagina to reduce herniation and facilitate stool evacuation. Most rectoceles are located anteriorly and become evident in the early or middle stages of the examination. The contour of the rectoceles varies, as does their location with respect to the perineal body.[36,37] Rectoceles are easily observed during CRCU and may have a heterogenous appearance (Fig. 18-18). Rectoceles that retain contrast material after the rectum is emptied are considered abnormal.[38,39]

Vaginal Apical Prolapse: Enterocele

The cul-de-sac is normally located at or above the level of the ischial spines, and contains no small bowel. If support is lost, the epithelium overlying the cul-de-sac may become thin and shiny and the peritoneal lining may be distended by the intestines.

Enterocele involves peritoneal herniation between the uterosacral ligaments at the vaginal apex. Palpation of small bowel or visualization of peristalsis in the cul-de-sac confirms enterocele. Diagnosic testing for such defects was performed as early as 1962.[37] The normal depth of the cul-de-sac and the perineal descent required for classification are still being investigated. With CRCU, the presence of enterocele can be assumed using the standard finding of "widening of the rectovaginal septum."[14] Some authors[12] found that instead of assuming the presence of an enterocele using this standard finding, direct opacification of the small bowel and evaluation by dynamic rectocolpocystography provided a more reliable study of this type of herniation. Enteroceles are clinically divided into four types (congenital, pulsion, traction, and iatrogenic) on the basis of anatomy and etiology. When enteroceles are large and prolapsing, visualization is not difficult. Radiologically, the typical appearance is detachment between the posterior vaginal wall and the anterior rectal wall (Fig. 18-19).

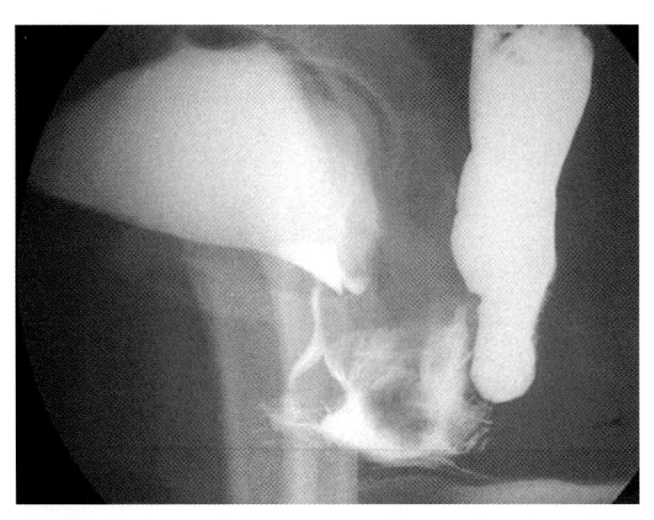

FIGURE 18-17 Grade IV uterine and vaginal vault prolapse (procidentia), with descent of the uterus through the introitus.

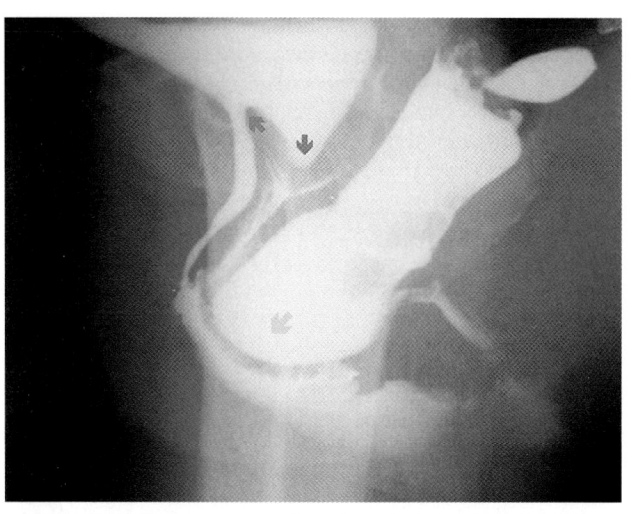

FIGURE 18-18 A large rectocele with slight bulging of the bladder base, consistent with a small cystocele that was not detected clinically. Top arrow indicates a hyper correction of the bladder neck after colposuspension procedure. Middle arrow indicates a grade I cystocele. Bottom arrow indicates a grade III rectocele.

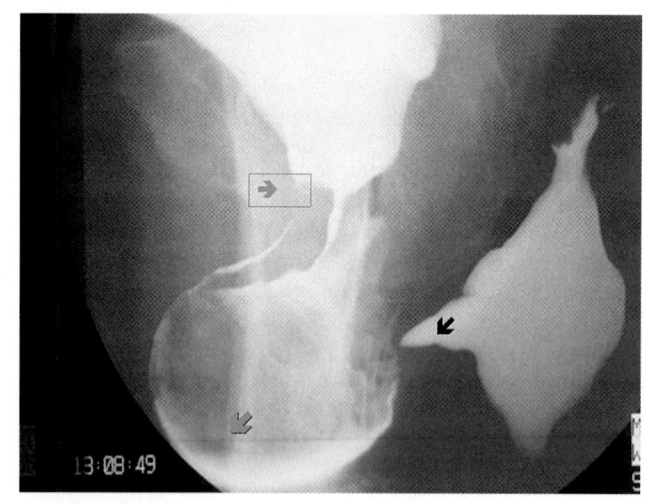

FIGURE 18-19 Enterocele. Multiple small bowel loops have herniated into the pelvis, causing vaginal deformity and an associated posterior compartment defect. Top arrow indicates a normal position of the bladder neck. Middle arrow indicates a posterior compartment defect. Bottom arrow indicates a large enterocele.

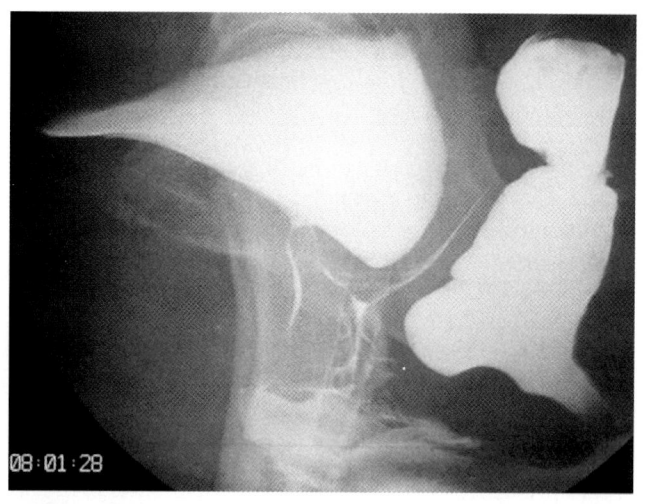

FIGURE 18-20 Low position of the sling after anti-incontinence surgery.

Discrimination between an enterocele and a rectocele can be clinically difficult. A "double bubble," the discrete appearance of a hernia sac anterior to the surface of the rectum, is a helpful clinical sign of enterocele, but is not common. The patient may need to strain to force the intestine into the elongated cul-de-sac.

Puborectalis Muscle Dysfunction

When a patient has a severe pelvic muscle defect or very weak contraction of the pelvic floor muscles, she cannot contract the puborectalis muscle. As a result, neither compression nor narrowing of the genital hiatus occurs. On the other hand, with attempts at defecation, the anorectal angle should become more obtuse.[38,39] When the puborectalis relaxes, the angle between the anus and the rectum remains acute. Another important abnormality is the descending perineum, which may be initiated by abnormal bowel habits with straining. It is defined radiologically by measuring the descent of the anorectal junction on straining.

OTHER ABNORMAL FINDINGS

In addition to the abnormalities of the pelvic floor described earlier, the most common causes of abnormalities after surgery that are detected by CRCU[26,29,31,40] are the following:

- **Improper position of the sling.** If the sling is too low and is situated below the bladder neck (Fig. 18-20), a urethral kink causes dysuria or urinary retention. Alternatively, if the sling is situated above the bladder neck (Fig. 18-21), urinary incontinence may occur as a result of urethral sphincter deficiency.
- **Distortion of the urethra by a sling that is too tight** (Fig. 18-22). This distortion usually occurs after suburethral sling procedures. CRCU shows urethral stenosis.
- **Distortion of the trigone.** The bladder neck remains fixed, and marked descent is observed around the fixed point (Fig. 18-23).
- **Postoperative complications.** After vaginal surgery, patients may have urge incontinence during stressful situations because of vault or middle compartment prolapse. The uterus prolapses, pulling the bladder neck with it. The mechanism is probably related to the somatic afferent pathways that have receptors in the bladder neck that can induce voiding reflexes (Fig. 18-24).

Another interesting finding is the abnormality of the lower urinary tract that occurs with urethral pathology. If the bladder neck abnormality cannot be seen on standard radiography (i.e., intravenous pyelogram), the urethral

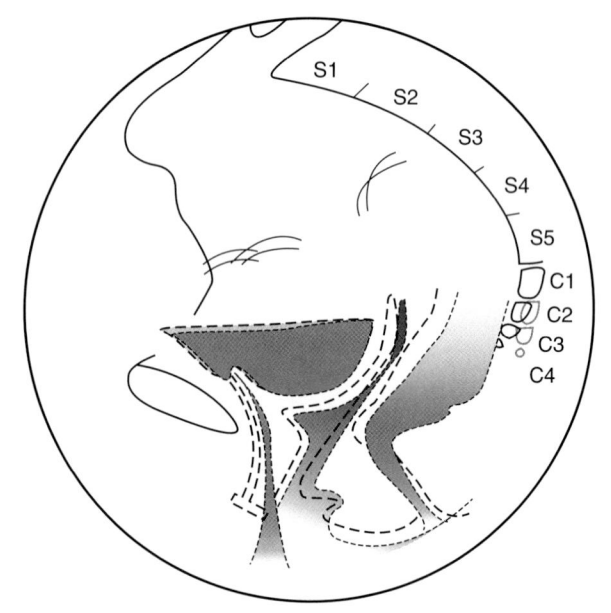

FIGURE 18-21 Improper position of the sling after anti-incontinence surgery (above the bladder neck).

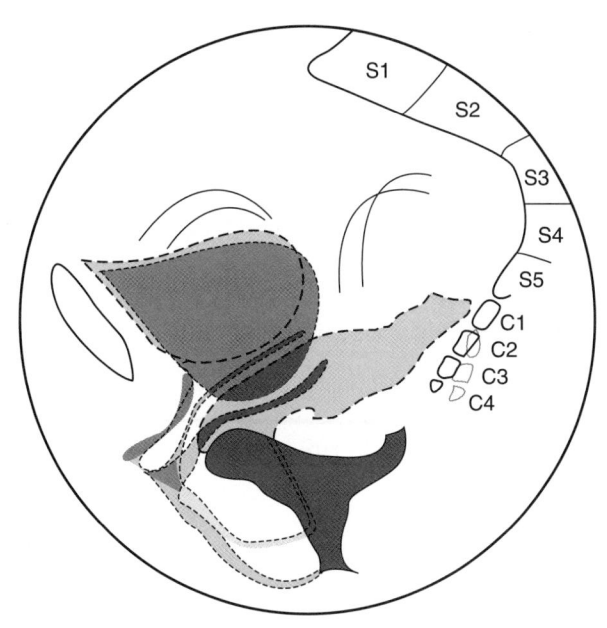

FIGURE 18-22 Urethral distortion because of the improper position of a sling that is too tight and causes stenosis.

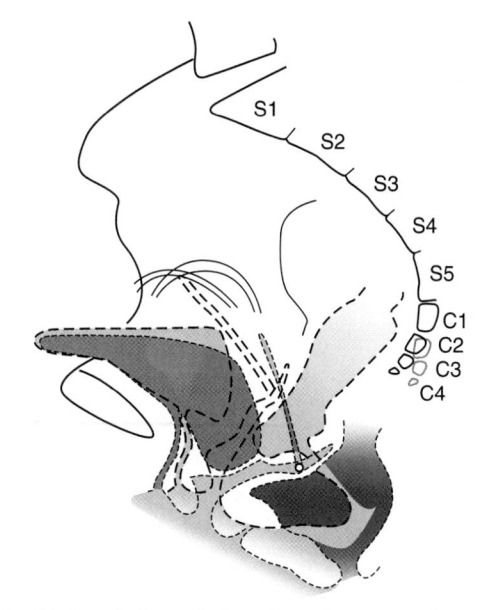

FIGURE 18-24 Bladder dysfunction after vaginal surgery for cystocele repair, with remaining uterus prolapse leading to urge incontinence.

pathology can be seen clearly on CRCU. With this technique, it is possible to show the following:

- **Urethral diverticula.** Women with this disorder have chronic dysuria, dyspareunia, recurrent urinary tract infection, and sometimes postvoid dribbling (Fig. 18-25).
- **Postsurgical stricture and stenosis.** Narrowing of the meatus is common, and the threshold between normal and pathologic findings may be difficult to determine.
- **Fistulas** (Fig. 18-26). Vesicovaginal fistula is an abnormal communication between the bladder and vagina. The most important cause is poor obstetric care, and obstetric fistulas are rare in developed countries. Surgical trauma after gynecologic procedures causes approximately 90% of vesicovaginal fistulas,[41] with the number of cases increasing as pelvic laparoscopic surgery becomes more common.[42] Although urethrovaginal and vesicorectal fistulas are less common and more difficult to diagnose, good films can be obtained in an upright position. If retrograde dynamic voiding cystography and urethrocystoscopy show evidence of a vesicovaginal fistula, CRCU is one of the best methods for radiologic evaluation of such ureterovaginal fistulas.

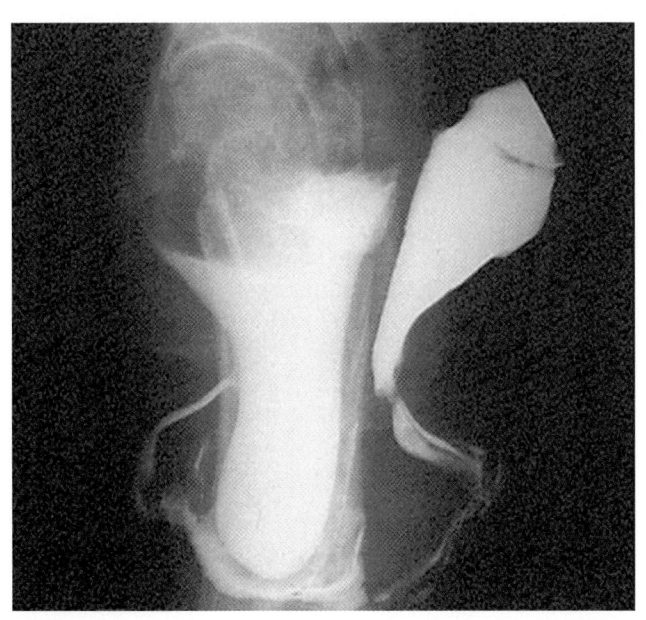

FIGURE 18-23 Distortion of the trigone. Fixed bladder neck and bladder prolapse.

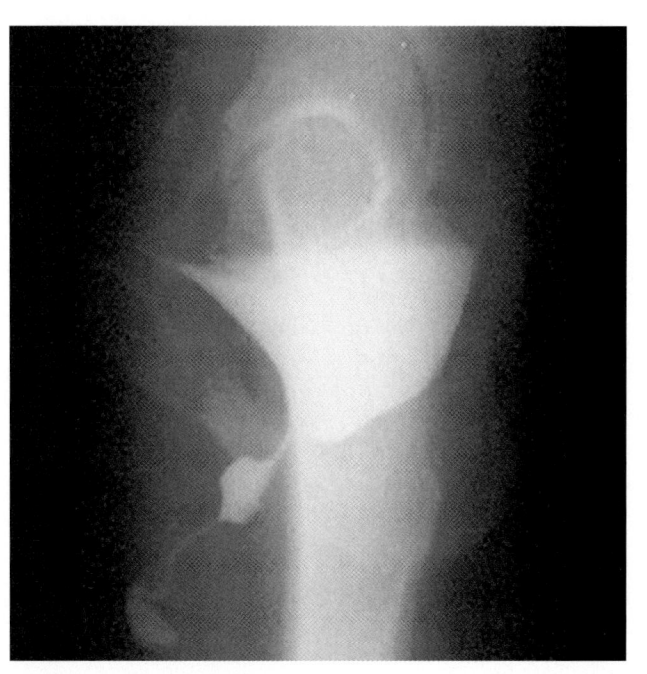

FIGURE 18-25 Urethral diverticulum.

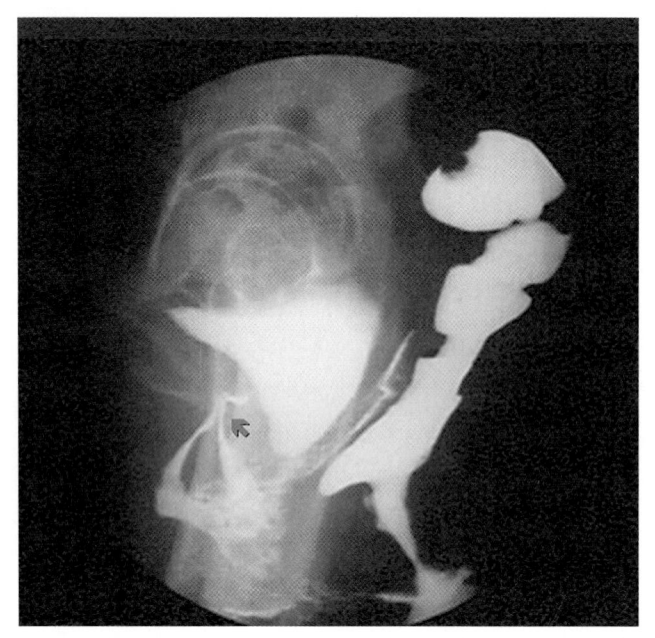

FIGURE 18-26 Uretrovaginal fistula after surgical procedure. The arrow indicates the localization of the vesicovaginal fistula.

CONCLUSION

For patients who have not undergone surgery, CRCU usually is not indicated as long as physical examination allows adequate assessment of pelvic relaxation of the different compartments.

However, it is important to avoid concluding prematurely that a posterior colpocele responds to a rectocele, because it could be an enterocele. Nevertheless, this type of radiologic investigation is imperative in women with unsuccessful surgery, relapse, or postsurgical incontinence. In elderly women in whom physical examination is difficult, this type of examination may be helpful, especially if vaginal stenosis is present. The effectiveness of pelvic floor training programs could include using radiologic investigation as evidence. Schüssler and associates[43] conducted a study in which this method was used before and after pelvic floor re-education for urinary stress incontinence. Compared with patients whose treatment was unsuccessful, patients who achieved cure had a greater decrease in anorectal and urethrovesical inclination and a greater lift of the bladder base and posterior rectal wall.

The relationship of the bladder and urethra to the pubosacral line determines whether urethral prolapse exists. Radiographically, this relationship is determined during upright voiding cystourethrography, often in conjunction with videourodynamic evaluation. Relaxed and strained images taken in a true lateral projection show urethral hypermobility, the degree of prolapse, and the presence of cystocele, rectocele, and enterocele. Radiologic visualization of the pelvic floor may also be helpful, especially after surgery.

CRCU permits visual assessment of the interrelationship of the urethra, bladder, vagina, rectum, and pelvic floor muscle activity. If urodynamic studies are necessary in patients with lower urinary tract symptoms, fluoroscopic studies are gaining in importance in the evaluation of pelvic floor dysfunction.

REFERENCES

1. Olsen AL, Smith VJ, Bergstrom JO: Epidemiology of surgically managed pelvic floor organ prolapse and urinary incontinence. Obstet Gynecol 89:501, 1997.
2. Hagstad A, Janson PO, Lindsedt G: Gynaecological history, complaints, and examinations in a middle-aged population. Maturitas 7(2):115, 1985.
3. Graves EJ, Kozak LJ: Detailed diagnoses and procedures: National Hospital Discharge Survey, 1996. Vital Health Stat 13:1, 1998.
4. Wiskind AK, Creighton SM, Stanton SL: The incidence of genital prolapse after the Burch colposuspension. Am J Obstet Gynecol 167:395, 1992.
5. Comiter CV, Vasavada SP, Barbaric ZL, Raz S: Grading pelvic prolapse and pelvic floor relaxation using dynamic magnetic resonance imaging. Urology 54:454, 1999.
6. Lienemann A, Anthuber C, Baron A: Dynamic MR colpocystorectography assessing pelvic floor descent. Eur Radiol 7:1309, 1999.
7. Yang A, Mostwin JL, Rosnehein NB, Zerhouni EA: Pelvic floor descent in women: Dynamic evaluation with fast MR Imaging and cinematic display. Radiology 179:25, 1991.
8. Vanbeckevoort D, Van Hoe L, Oyen R: Pelvic floor descent in females: Comparative study of colpocystodefecography and dynamic MR imaging. J Magn Reson Imaging 9:373, 1999.
9. Bethoux A, Bory S, Huguier M, Lan CS: Une technique radiologique d'exploration des prolapsus génitaux et des incontinences d'urine: Le colpocystogramme. Ann Radiol 8:809–819, 1965.
10. Bethoux A, Bory S, Huguier M: Radio-cinétique viscérale pelvienne: Le colpocystogramme. EMC Radiodiagnostic. Paris, Masson, A10, 34:630, 1967.
11. Richter K, Hausegger K, Lissner J, et al: Die Dochtmethode: Eine vervollkommnete Art der Kolpozystorectographie. Geburtshilfe Frauenheilkd 34:711, 1974.
12. Brubaker LP, Retsky S, Smith C, Saclarides T: Pelvic floor evaluation with dynamic fluroscopy. Obstet Gynecol 82:1, 1993.
13. Smith C, Brubaker LP, Saclarides TJ: Fluoroscopic evaluation of pelvic floor support. In Brubaker LP, Saclarides T (eds): The Female Pelvic Floor: Disorders of Function and Support. Philadelphia, FA Davis, 1996, pp 81.
14. Shull BL, Baden WF: A six-year experience with paravaginal defect repair for stress urinary incontinence. Am J Obstet Gynecol 160(6):1432, 1989.
15. Raz S, Slothers L, Chopra A: Vaginal reconstructive surgery for incontinence and prolapse. In Walsh PC, Retik AB, Vaughan ED (eds): Campbell's Urology, ed 7. Philadelphia, JB Lippincott, 1992.
16. Zimmern PE, Leach GE, Ganabathi K: The urological aspects of vaginal wall prolapse: Part 1. Diagnosis and surgical indications. AUA Update Series, vol XII, lesson 25, 1992, p 193.
17. DeLancey JO: Anatomy and biomechanics of genital prolapse. Clin Obstet Gynecol 36:897, 1993.
18. Jackson SL, Weber AM, Hull TL, et al: Fecal incontinence in women with urinary incontinence and pelvic organ prolapse. Obstet Gynecol 89:423, 1997.
19. Bump RC, Mattiasson A, Bo K, et al: The standardization of terminology of female pelvic organ prolapse and pelvic floor dysfunction. Am J Obstet Gynecol 175:10, 1996.

20. Kobashi K, Leach GE: Pelvic prolapse. J Urol 164:1879, 2000.
21. Baden WF, Walker TA: Physical diagnosis in the evaluation of vaginal relaxation. Clin Obstet Gynecol 15:1055, 1972.
22. Stanton SL, Cardozo LD: Results of the colposuspension operation for incontinence and prolapse. Br J Obstet Gynaecol 86:693, 1979.
23. Foote JE, Zimmzern PE, Leach GE: Vaginal reconstruction for pelvic floor laxity. In Webster G, Kirby R, King L (eds): Reconstructive Urology. Boston, Blackwell Scientific, 1993, p 819.
24. Zimmern PE, Leach GE: Repair of enterocele and rectocele, perineal repair, and vault suspension. Urol Clin North Am 2:47, 1993.
25. Richardson DA, Bent AE, Ostergard DR: The effect of uterovaginal prolapse on urethrovesical pressure dynamics. Am J Obstet Gynecol 146:901, 1983.
26. Zafiropulo M: Le colpocystogramme. In Kujas A, Coussement A, Villet R (eds): Imagerie dynamique des troubles pelvi-périnéaux de la femme. Paris, Vigot, 1998, p 19.
27. Benson JT, Kelvin FM: Dynamic cystoproctology. In Blaivas J (ed): Atlas of Urodynamics. Baltimore, Williams and Wilkins, 1996, p 126.
28. Kelvin FM, Maglinte D, Hornback JA, Benson JT: Pelvic prolapse: Assessment with evacuation proctography (defecography). Radiology 184:547, 1992.
29. Brubaker L, Heit MH: Radiology of the pelvic floor. Clin Obstet Gynecol 36:1, 1993.
30. Lapray JF, Grandjean JP, Leriche B: Radiologie. In Lafray JP (ed): Imagerie de la Vessie et de la Dynamique Pelvienne de la Femme. Paris, Masson, 1999, p 165.
31. Zafiropulo M, Bourcier A, Juras J: Colporectocystourethrography. In Appell RA, Bourcier AP, La Torre F (eds): Pelvic Floor Dysfunction: Inversigations and Conservative Treatment. Rome, Casa Editrice Scientifica Internationale, 1999.
32. Parks AG, Porter NH, Melzak J: Experimental study of the reflex mechanism controlling muscles of the pelvic floor. Dis Colon Rectum 5:407, 1962.
33. DeLancey JOL: The anatomy of the pelvic floor. Curent Opin Obstet Gynecol 6:313, 1994.
34. Klarskov P, Jepsen PV, Dorhp S: Reliability of voiding colpo-cysto urethrography in female urinary incontinence before and after treatment. Acta Radiol 26:685, 1988.
35. Kelvin FM, Maglinte DDT, Benson JT: Dynamic cystoproctography: A technique for assessing disorders of the pelvic floor in women. Am J Roentgenol 163:368, 1993.
36. Oettle GJ, Roe AM, Bartolo DCC, McMortensen MJ: What is the best way of measuring perineal descent? A comparison of radiographic and clinical descent methods. Br J Surg 72:999, 1985.
37. Lash AF, Levin B: Roentgenographic diagnosis of vagina vault hernia. J Obstet Gynecol 20:427, 1962.
38. Shorvon PJ, McHugh S, Diamante NE: Defecography in normal volunteers: Results and implications. Gut 30:1737, 1989.
39. Karasick S, Karasick D, Karasick SR: Functional disorders of the anus and rectum: Findings on defecography. AJR 160:777, 1993.
40. Zafiropulo M: Les prolapsus génitaux. In Villet RM, Buzelin JM, Lazorthes F (eds): Les Troubles de la Statique Pelvi Périnéale de la Femme. Paris, Vigot, 1995, p 71.
41. Stothers L, Chopra A, Raz S: Vesicovaginal fistula. In Raz S (ed): Female Urology, ed 2. Philadelphia, Saunders, 1996, p 490.
42. Kadar N, Lemmerling L: Urinary tract injuries during laparoscopically assisted hysterectomy: Causes and prevention. Am J Obstet Gynecol 170(1):47, 1994.
43. Schüssler B, Von Obernitz N, Frimberger J, et al: Analysis of successful treatment of SUI by pelvic floor re-education: A urodynamic and radiological study. Neurourol Urodynam 9:433, 1990.

CHAPTER 19

Contribution of Magnetic Resonance Imaging in the Evaluation of Pelvic Floor Function

CHRISTOS C. CONSTANTINOU

In recent years, the use of magnetic resonance imaging (MRI) of pelvic floor structures has contributed to our understanding of the mechanism of urinary continence as well as to our understanding of the way that some surgical procedures are likely to work. MRI of the pelvic floor documents the static anatomic position of the various muscle groups, their attachments, and their juxtaposition with respect to the bladder and urethra. However, stress incontinence is a dynamic physiologic event, and with current technology, it cannot be captured by MRI in real time. Because efforts to strengthen the pelvic floor can cure or at least minimize stress urinary incontinence, it is useful to examine the anatomy of the pelvic floor under both relaxed and contracted states and to extrapolate from these two images the net effect of a contraction. This approach can be used to identify the relevant muscle groups that contribute to continence. Before the anatomic components of the pelvic floor are examined, it is appropriate to consider some physiologic events involved in maintaining closure of the urethra during stress. To maintain urinary continence, patients rely on reflex and voluntary mechanisms of bladder and urethral function. The guarding reflex is an important involuntary control mechanism associated with the recruitment of fast neuromuscular contraction of periurethral skeletal muscles and the pelvic floor. Similarly, the voluntarily controlled mechanisms initiated by willful contraction of periurethral skeletal muscles involve the urethra and its attachments to the pelvis. Both voluntary and reflex control mechanisms activate neuromuscular recruitment of skeletal muscles that compress or displace the urethra. MRI findings are compared with the resting and dynamic urethral pressures obtained in a matched population of subjects to show the effects of voluntary and reflex pressures along the urethra. This comparison was done to show the extent to which intrinsic and extrinsic urethral closure mechanisms are responsible for maintaining closure. These findings are discussed in terms of the effect of pelvic floor exercises and electrical or magnetic stimulation on strengthening the skeletal muscles that are responsible for responding to incontinence-producing forces. In this context, the effect of endoscopic surgery on the mechanisms of urethral closure is used to show the importance of individual pelvic floor muscle groups and the significance of their attachment and mechanical properties.

ANATOMIC CONSIDERATIONS

Recently, Hjartardottir and associates[1] raised the issue of whether the female pelvic floor is a dome or a basin. These authors noted that classically and based on necropsy observations, the muscles of the pelvic floor (levator ani and coccygeus muscles) have been described as having the shape of a basin. In a previous study by Hugosson and colleagues,[2] MRI showed a dome-shaped pelvic floor in live subjects when muscular tonus was present. Conventional and fast-sequence MRI was used to examine the normal anatomy and dynamic movements of the female pelvis. Nulliparous and parous healthy women without signs or symptoms of pelvic relaxation were studied in the supine position at rest, during voluntary pelvic contractions, and while bearing down. The results showed a dome-shaped levator ani muscle at rest. During voluntary pelvic contractions, the muscle straightened, becoming more horizontal, and during bearing down, it descended, becoming basin-shaped. The width of the genital hiatus was the same in both groups at rest, and widened during bearing down. The bladder base was lifted upward and forward during voluntary pelvic contractions, but during bearing down, it descended. At rest, the rectum had a posterior angle that decreased during voluntary pelvic contractions and increased during bearing down. The authors interpret these findings to show that the female pelvic floor is shaped like a dome, not a basin. Clearly, this type of MRI can prove valuable in the anatomic and dynamic analysis of healthy women, and offers new information about the female pelvic floor. However, it is important to remember that these studies were performed in the supine position. As the new generation of MRI machines is introduced that allows the subject to remain in the upright position, these studies must be performed again to determine the role of gravity on pelvic floor configuration.

Mouritsen[3] compared the use of MRI with ultrasonography in the study of bladder support to determine their relative diagnostic value in different types of urinary incontinence. They studied patients with congenital incontinence, hypermobility of the bladder neck, and urethral wall abnormalities. The authors concluded that dynamic ultrasonography should be used as the initial imaging technique to study bladder support. Bladder neck hypermobility, which indicates a defect in adjunctive closure forces, is better correlated to stress incontinence than bladder morphology diagnosed during static cystography. Voiding cystography has a role in the diagnosis of dysfunction of the lower urinary tract. Clinical use of MRI is just beginning, and this technique seems relevant for studies of urethral pathology.

EFFECT OF PARITY

Recently, Handa and associates[4] provided an important contribution to our knowledge about the applications of MRI. These authors reviewed the literature on the effects of childbirth on the muscles, nerves, and connective tissues of the pelvic floor,[4] and developed an overview of the structure and function of the pelvic floor to provide a context for subsequent data. This review identified original sources from a computerized search of English language articles published during the last decade. Additional sources were identified from references cited in relevant research articles. This search was performed to obtain evidence to support an association between childbirth and anal incontinence, urinary incontinence, and pelvic organ prolapse. In addition, the authors provided recommendations to prevent these sequelae. Articles were accumulated on the anatomy of the pelvic floor, the association of childbirth and neuromuscular injury, and biomechanical and morphologic alterations in muscle function and connective tissue structure. The authors provided functional data on the long-term effects of childbirth on continence and pelvic organ support, and summarized the effects of obstetric interventions on the pelvic floor. The authors concluded that childbirth was associated with a variety of muscular and neuromuscular injuries of the pelvic floor that are linked to the development of anal and urinary incontinence and pelvic organ prolapse. Risk factors for pelvic floor injury include forceps delivery, episiotomy, a prolonged second stage of labor, and increased fetal size. Cesarean delivery appears to be protective, especially if the patient does not experience labor before delivery. The consensus of this study is that the pelvic floor plays an important role in continence and pelvic organ support. The study also suggests that obstetricians may be able to reduce pelvic floor injuries by minimizing forceps deliveries and episiotomies, allowing passive descent in the second stage of labor, and selectively recommending elective cesarean delivery. Hayat and colleagues[5] used serial MRI examinations to study changes in the pelvic floor in the postpartum patient. Assessment of the urethrovesical angle, the length of the urethra, the distance from the symphysis to the proximal and distal vagina, the length of the vagina, the width and length of the sphincters, and the presence of sphincter defects was done in the sagittal plane. The sphincter, abnormal distance between the symphysis and the midurethra, and the vagina and rectum were assessed in the axial plane. Only the distance between the symphysis and distal vagina changed significantly over time, and no significant correlations were noted between birth weight and MRI parameters.

DYNAMICS OF PELVIC FLOOR CONTRACTION

To obtain dynamic data on the anatomic changes produced during voluntary pelvic floor contraction, Christensen and associates[6] used image processing to highlight the anatomic changes between the relaxed and the contracted pelvic floor. In these studies, MRI was used to visualize the effect of voluntary pelvic floor contractions on the abdominal structures, with particular emphasis on determining the dynamic relationship between the bladder and surrounding organs. The pelvic floor was imaged in asymptomatic female volunteers using MRI views obtained in seven coronal and seven sagittal planes. Relative displacement of the bladder as a result of voluntary pelvic floor contraction was measured, and the changes between the relaxed and the contracted stage were identified. Measurements obtained from sagittal images show superior bladder wall, posterior, and gluteal movement. These observations show that voluntary contractions of the pelvic floor produce anatomic displacement of the bladder in the superior direction, indicating that pelvic floor contraction provides increased levator muscle support. There is no significant displacement of the anterior aspect of the bladder, whereas the posterior wall shows maximum movement. Subsequent MRI evaluation by the same authors was carried out with a larger number of healthy volunteers.[6] One way to visualize the changes occurring in the pelvic floor as a result of voluntary contraction is to image the pelvic floor structures with MRI at rest and during willful contraction. Analysis of subsequent image processing can identify the magnitude of displacement produced by specific pelvic floor muscles during contraction. Figure 19-1A shows an axial view of an MRI obtained in the resting state. Figure 19-1B

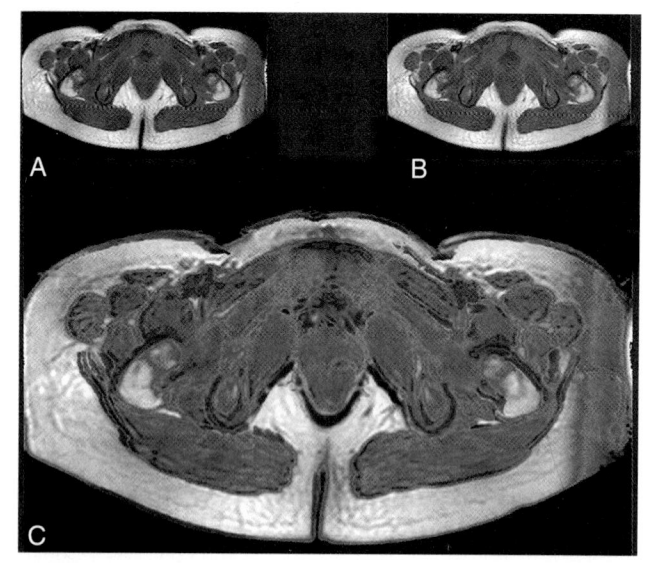

FIGURE 19-1 Axial magnetic resonance images obtained (**A**) at rest and (**B**) during voluntary pelvic floor contraction. **C**, Composite image showing the differences to identify the effect of contraction. As indicated, the major compressive effect is seen around the vagina.

shows the same axial view, with the subject voluntarily contracting the pelvic floor, as would occur during physiotherapy. Figure 19-1C shows a composite image of Figure 19-1A and B, with the differences associated with pelvic floor contraction highlighted. As shown, in this plane, pelvic floor contraction typically compresses the vagina toward the symphysis pubis. Clearly, pelvic floor contractions recruit a large number of muscles. For this reason, different viewing planes and orientations should be used. One viewing plane that provides a more generalized perspective of voluntary pelvic floor contraction is the midline sagittal (Fig. 19-2). Using the same schema as Figure 19-1, this section shows displacement of the rectum and abdomen. The rest of the pelvic floor can best be viewed at the coronal plane shown in Figure 19-3. In this plane, the support of the bladder by the pelvic floor can be clearly identified. The MRI scan used to generate these data is shown in the inset showing the location of the pelvic floor with respect to the surrounding structures. Finally, in Figure 19-3, the thickness of the boundary of the pelvic floor denotes the range of movement from the resting state to the contractile state.

These studies quantify the magnitude and direction of pelvic floor displacement using MRI scans obtained in the axial, sagittal, and coronal planes in asymptomatic young women. Comparison of these images with information obtained on postmenopausal women shows that the range of displacement of the urethra and vagina in older women is significantly lower. In addition, compared with control subjects, women with parity 2 to 3 showed left–right asymmetry of pelvic floor contractions. Imaging was performed in consecutive coronal, sagittal, and transverse planes, with the pelvic floor relaxed and contracted. These studies showed significantly larger displacement produced by contracting the pelvis in younger subjects. Thus, aging reduces the amount by which

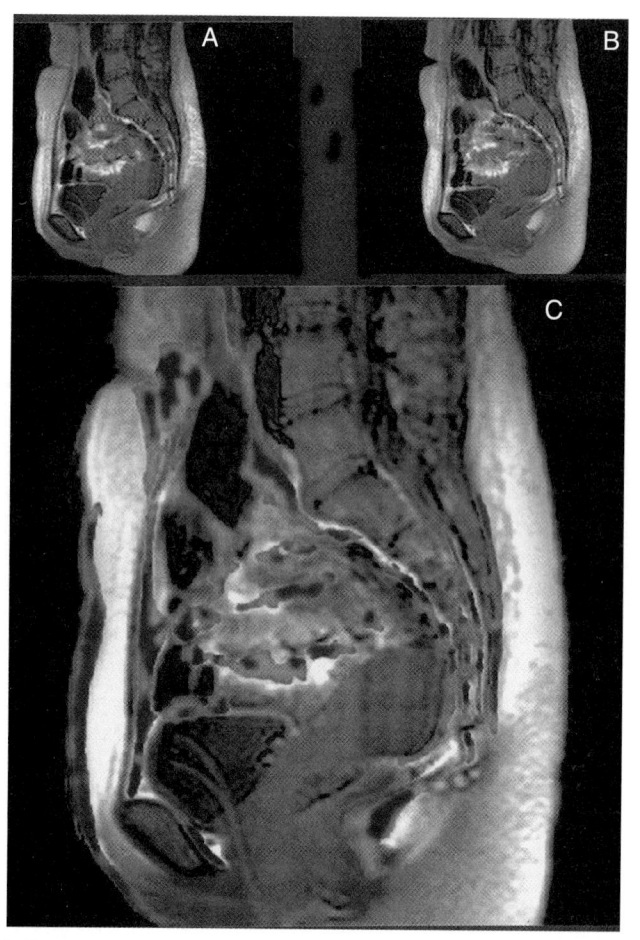

FIGURE 19-2 Saggital magnetic resonance image constructed in the same way as Figure 19-1. **A**, At rest. **B**, During voluntary pelvic floor contraction. **C**, Composite image. In this plane, the bladder is clearly identified with a catheter in place, and the path of the urethra can be traced. As shown, the effect of contraction in this plane is best visualized at the anal sphincter.

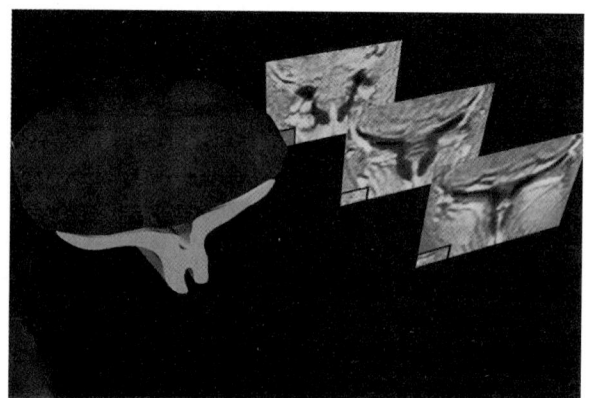

FIGURE 19-3 Composite image reconstructed from three coronal magnetic resonance imaging planes (*insert*), showing displacement of the pelvic floor and bladder.

abdominal structures can be moved by the pelvic floor. Although the authors did not perform analogous investigations in incontinent women, Mostwin and colleagues[7] showed that in symptomatic women, straining produces significant displacement from the reference line (sagittal pubococcygeal line), whereas normal women show minimal displacement.[7] Using MRI, these authors noted that stress incontinence is only one symptom of local pelvic prolapse that may be part of a more global pelvic prolapse that involves the levator musculature, pudendal innervation, connective tissue deterioration, and prolapse of other components. These observations are consistent with those of DeLancey, and underscore the importance of using MRI to identify the component suitable for treatment.

Techniques of Data Acquisition and Resolution

There are conflicting reports about the techniques used in image acquisition, particularly the use of a body coil versus an endovaginal coil. This question was examined by Tan and associates,[8] who visualized the anatomy of the female pelvic floor and urethra from images obtained with an endovaginal coil and compared them with those obtained with a quadrature body coil. These authors suggest that compared with the body coil, endovaginal MRI provides excellent visualization of the pelvic floor and the zonal anatomy of the urethra. Pelvic floor structures as well as the levator ani muscles and urogenital diaphragm are clearly shown with the endovaginal coil. In volunteers, the endovaginal coil was used to show a new ligamentous structure, the urethropelvic sling, which connects the urethra to the levator ani muscle and contributes to the supporting mechanism of the urethra.

MRI provides a detailed view of the anatomy of the pelvic floor structures that are critical to the maintenance of urinary continence and of the anal sphincters that are responsible for fecal continence. It is important to examine the information obtained from that perspective. An important contribution was made by Schafer and colleagues,[9] who compared anal endosonography with MRI in healthy volunteers. MRI was performed to obtain consecutive slices in the sagittal and angled axial (perpendicular to the anal canal) planes. Although the thickness of the sphincter muscles in the dorsal projection could be measured with ultrasound, when both measures were compared, differentiation among the mucosa, submucosa, and internal anal sphincters was not possible with MRI.

In an earlier study of the pelvic floor, Goodrich and colleagues[10] used MRI to provide a dynamic analysis and evaluation of patients before and after surgical repair to evaluate the structures involved in pelvic support. This study is particularly important because the authors calibrated their system by evaluating control subjects and incontinent women. In this way, they clearly showed the value of analyzing and assessing pelvic floor relaxation and understanding the anatomic changes that occur before and after surgical repair. Clinically, the increased sensitivity of MRI in grading prolapse makes this type of examination useful in evaluating women who have symptoms of pelvic floor relaxation, but who have negative findings on clinical examination. These workers used conventional spin-echo MRI and dynamic snapshot GRASS MRI at various levels of the Valsalva maneuver to describe and quantitate the anatomy of pelvic floor relaxation in female volunteers. These studies were done to characterize the normal anatomy and obtain reference measurements for comparison with changes caused by surgical repair. On clinical pelvic examination, these authors showed that static and dynamic MRI scans were more sensitive in assessing and grading pelvic floor relaxation. Their quantitative analysis suggested a widening of the levator hiatus and a more vertical lie of the levator plate postoperatively. In contrast, postoperatively, the descent of the pelvic organs on maximal straining was the same as that in normal volunteers. The posterior urethrovesical angle was more than 110 degrees in almost all of the continent women who were examined.

Kirschner-Hermanns and colleagues[11] evaluated the contribution of MRI of the pelvic floor to the examination to understand the effect of anatomy and underlying pathology on urinary incontinence. These authors examined patients with stress incontinence and healthy volunteers. These MRI studies showed that the urethra is not connected to the levator ani or fixed to the deep perineal muscle layers. The sharp angulation of the levator ani that is seen in healthy volunteers is lost in most subjects with stress incontinence (65%). In addition, these observations showed degeneration of the levator ani muscle in approximately 45% of patients with stress incontinence. These authors concluded that the extent of damage to the levator can be clearly identified with the aid of MRI.

Understanding the physiologic mechanisms involved in the maintenance of urinary continence requires an understanding of the causes of urine loss. Except for incontinence originating from the detrusor, invariably, urine loss occurs after a stress-related event, such as coughing, sneezing, or changing position, when the distribution of pressure within the pelvic floor changes transiently. Transient pressure changes within the pelvic floor stimulate a proportional increase in closure of the urethral lumen. Such closure of the urethra increases urethral pressure, possibly as a result of the combination of active and passive compression of the lumen. The magnitude of stress pressures within the pelvic cavity and outside the urethra relative to pressures within the lumen can be conveniently viewed as a transmission ratio. Practically, the pressure transmission ratio incorporates a dimensionless fraction of urethra pressure divided by pelvic cavity pressure. This measurement can be made by determining urethral and bladder pressure while the patient coughs. The intuitive advantage of the transmission ratio is that its value is independent of the strength of the cough. A transmission ratio of greater than 1.0 indicates that the totality of urethral is greater within the urethra than within the pelvic cavity, and suggests active closure of the urethra. A maximun transmission value of less than 1.0 indicates that pelvic pressure is higher than urethral pressure; therefore, the possibility of stress-initiated leakage is high. Furthermore, the region of maximum transmission of pressure is at the distal end of the urethra. Basic investigations performed in normal, healthy female subjects show that a transmission ratio of greater than 1.0 can be consistently measured.

In women with stress incontinence, the maximum transmission ratio is less than 1.0, as shown in Figure 19-4. The configuration of pressure transmission values with respect to urethral length (see Fig. 19-4) shows that the outline of the curve of the women with stress incontinence is similar to that of control subjects, except that it does not reach values of greater than 1.0. The similarity of the outline of the transmission curve in control subjects and women with stress incontinence is an important indication that the mechanism for producing transmission pressures of more than 1.0 is in place, but is quantitatively of insufficient magnitude.

The mechanism responsible for the success of surgery for stress incontinence becomes evident when its effect on pressure transmission is considered (see Fig. 19-4). As seen in Figure 19-4, the postoperative response of the urethra to incontinence-inducing stress, such as coughing, is restoration of the transmission ratio to greater than 1.0. Immediate postsurgical restoration of the maximum transmission ratio to greater than 1.0 has been interpreted anatomically. Petros and Ulmsten[12] expanded on the observations of Einhorning[13] and Constantinou[14] to explain the effect of surgery on alterations in mechanical support of the urethra.

Drawing from existing information on muscle damage as the principal, collateral, or connective tissue cause, Petros and Ulmsten introduced the integral theory of continence in 1990.[15-18] The premise of this theory is the prediction that defects of the vagina or its supporting ligaments adversely affect the dynamics of the pelvic floor and the ability of interacting forces to coordinate opening and closing of the urethra.[19] Furthermore, regardless of the surgical approach used, whether highly invasive, such as endoscopic bladder neck suspension, or minimally invasive, such as slings to repair these defects, the ultimate end point is directly based on this theory. Although this concept has verified experimentally by showing the role of vaginal tissue in the transmission of muscle forces, laxity of the vagina can produce urinary dysfunction.[20]

The surgical success reported by Petros and Ulmsten[12] points the way to the diagnosis of defects associated with female urinary incontinence on the basis of the mechanical properties of the surrounding muscles. Although this assertion requires a leap of faith, nonetheless, these authors make a significant contribution to the current knowledge by focusing on the importance of the various muscular elements that contribute to or are involved in opening and closing the urethra. Petros[20] went further in his analysis, identifying the four directional forces generated by the anterior portion of the pubococcygeus, the longitudinal muscles of the anus, the levator plate, and the bulbocavernosus. He emphasized the importance of the ligaments in anchoring soft tissue and, in some cases, serving as a fulcrum for organ movement. These considerations have been important in identifying the anatomically significant structures to be imaged by MRI or other emerging functional techniques. Furthermore, from such imaging it may be possible to identify the zones of elastic vaginal tissue, located anteriorly, centrally, and posteriorly, that assist other connective tissues in transmitting muscle forces to other anatomic structures.

Although these structures can be visualized with imaging techniques, a method is needed to measure the parameters associated with each factor through routine clinical examination. Although many approaches and devices are used to measure the strength of pelvic floor contractions, they are susceptible to artifact and cannot accurately discriminate the symmetry, magnitude, and direction of closure forces. This information can be best obtained by adding detail to techniques such as finite element models, similar to those used by other studies to model the deformation of soft tissue, given interaction with exerted forces. Similar modes include those investigating the deformation of skeletal muscle during contraction and skin after plastic surgery.

Using fast MRI techniques, Gousse and associates[21] evaluated pelvic organ prolapse as well as other female pelvic pathology by prospectively correlating clinical findings with imaging findings from 100 consecutive cases. With the patient supine, relaxed, and straining, midsagittal and parasagittal views were obtained. The anterior vaginal wall, bladder, urethra, posterior vaginal wall, rectum, pelvic floor musculature, perineum, uterus, vaginal cuff, ovaries, ureters, and interaperitoneal organs were evaluated to identify pathologic conditions, including pelvic prolapse. Comparison of MRI findings with the findings on physical examination shows that this type of MRI appears to be an important addition to the comprehensive evaluation of the female pelvis. These authors suggest that, in addition to the superb anatomic detail obtained, and except for rectocele, this technique provides accurate staging of pelvic floor prolapse and reliable detection of pelvic organ

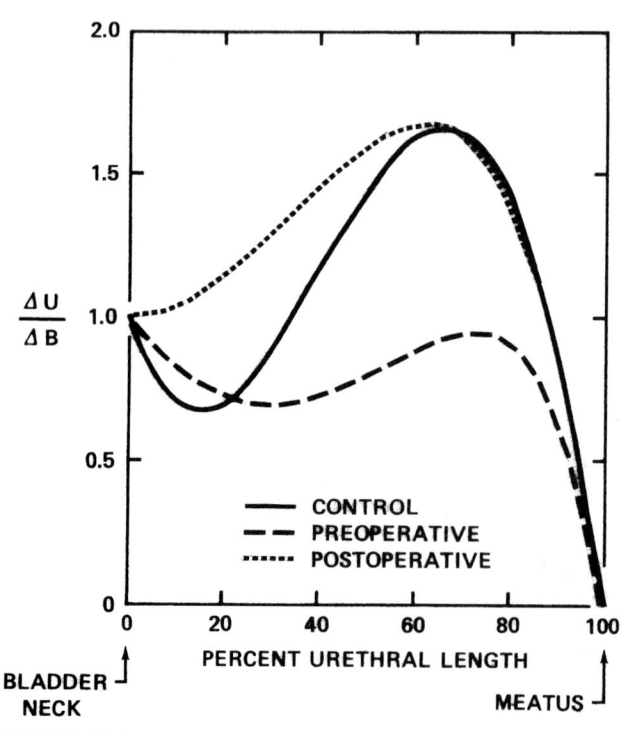

FIGURE 19-4 Transmission of bladder (B) pressure to the urethra (U) during coughing. The values in normal control subjects, incontinent preoperative patients, and postoperative patients are shown.

pathology. When urinary continence is being assessed, it would be useful to include images of the pelvic floor that show voluntary contraction because these muscles would best show the integrity of the pelvic floor musculature.

UTILITY OF MAGNETIC RESONANCE IMAGING IN URINARY CONTINENCE

In evaluating the significance of pelvic floor function in urinary continence, it is useful to identify the specific anatomic components that help to support the pelvic contents. To accomplish this goal, it is useful to examine the considerations proposed in a recent critical report by DeLancey,[22] where the influence of pelvic floor anatomy was directly linked to stress urinary incontinence. This report appropriately frames our current state of knowledge and also addresses the issue of where we should go. DeLancey[22] considers the importance of imaging in localizing the specific muscle structures and nerves of the pelvic floor that produce urinary incontinence when damaged. The nature of the injury defines the damage to each element of the continence mechanism. Consequently, it is appropriate to select the treatment plan based on the abnormality found in any given subject. This concept is best illustrated when considering a woman who has lost all neural control of the pelvic muscles. Under such circumstances, physical therapy to strengthen the pelvic floor would be futile and would simply lead to frustration. Conversely, the patient with neurologically intact, but otherwise weak muscles can achieve continence with exercise. On the basis of these considerations, an appropriate therapeutic approach should be chosen, taking into consideration the neuronal integrity of the system, not simply the diagnosis of stress urinary incontinence. The issue may be approached more systematically by asking questions about the status of each part of the continence mechanism. Kinder and associates[23] reported an indirect approach that considered the neuronal circuitry of the lower urinary tract, with particular focus on the influence of central and peripheral neuronal control of the micturition cycle.[23] This study introduced a new technique to describe the neuronal circuitry involved in the regulation and control of the lower urinary system and its control mechanisms, based on flowcharts and verified with four qualitative models. Because the mechanisms of the reflex arcs and supraspinal connections are not well defined, currently, we cannot characterize systematically the components involved in micturition and continence, as suggested by DeLancey.[22] Because of these limitations, little is known about supraspinal interconnections and their function in micturition control. Considerations include the role of the pelvic floor musculature in the control of the lower urinary tract, in particular, compression of the urethra. Nonetheless, the flowcharts presented by Kinder and associates[23] provide the foundation for the future design of a single, complete, qualitative model of the central and peripheral nervous connections and control mechanisms. Input data for the model promoted by Kinder and associates[23] could be obtained by studying the neuronal activity of the pelvic floor. Toward this end, in a kinesiologic electromyographic study, Deindl and associates[24] evaluated pelvic floor activity patterns in continent nulliparous women and parous women with stress urinary incontinence. Using these neurophysiologic methods, they searched for damage to neuromuscular structures that may be injured during pregnancy or after delivery. Simultaneous electromyographic recordings of the left and right pubococcygeus muscles were obtained with wire electrodes and compared with the findings in continent women. The authors found that activation patterns in the parous women with stress urinary incontinence were similar to those observed in the continent nulliparous women. However, two significant exceptions were noted: (1) On voluntary squeezing, significant differences were noted in the holding time between the parous patients with stress urinary incontinence and the nulliparous continent control subjects. (2) Approximately half of the parous women with stress urinary incontinence had an empty bladder and asymmetrical and uncoordinated levator activation patterns. These observations suggest that childbirth appeared to induce both quantitative and qualitative changes in the pelvic floor that jeopardized the continence mechanism. Furthermore, sphincter weakness appeared to result not only from the loss of motor units but also from altered activation patterns in the remaining units. These observations support DeLancey's suggestions about the importance of identifying neuronal abnormalities before relevant treatment planning can occur.[22]

CONCLUSION

MRI of the pelvic floor has provided the answers to many questions about the mechanisms of action of constituent muscles as they relate to urinary continence. As with any new imaging modality, important questions often arise, and perhaps more significantly, weaknesses and limitations that were not recognized earlier can emerge. Many of the considerations discussed in this chapter were described by Artibani and colleagues.[25] At the current state of technologic development, MRI is performed with the patient in the supine position, which is not the anatomically correct posture to simulate the action of skeletal musculature. Upright MRI systems are now becoming more commonplace, and are likely to provide important new information about the effects of abdominal content weight bearing on the pelvic floor. Perhaps more important is the limited resolution of MRI scans of pubourethral structures that are potentially critical in the supporting the urethra. In this context, it remains to be shown functionally to what extent these structures contribute evidence to substantiate the hammock hypothesis.

REFERENCES

1. Hjartardottir S, Nilsson J, Petersen C, Lingman G: The female pelvic floor: A dome—not a basin. Acta Obstet Gynecol Scand 76(6):567–571, 1997.
2. Hugosson C, Jorulf H, Lingman G, Jacobson B: Morphology of the pelvic floor. Lancet 337(8737):367, 1991.

3. Mouritsen L: Techniques for imaging bladder support. Acta Obstet Gynecol Scand Suppl 166:48–49, 1997.
4. Handa VL, Harris TA, Ostergard DR: Protecting the pelvic floor: Obstetric management to prevent incontinence and pelvic organ prolapse. Obstet Gynecol 88(3):470–478, 1996.
5. Hayat SK, Thorp JM Jr, Kuller JA, et al: Magnetic resonance imaging of the pelvic floor in the postpartum patient. Int Urogynecol J Pelvic Floor Dysfunction 7(6):321–324, 1996.
6. Christensen LL, Djurhuus JC, Lewis MT, et al: MRI of voluntary pelvic floor contractions in healthy female volunteers. Int Urogynecol J 6:138–152, 1995.
7. Mostwin JL, Genadry R, Sanders R, Yang A: Anatomic goals in the correction of female stress urinary incontinence. J Endourol 10(3):207–212, 1996.
8. Tan IL, Stoker J, Lameris JS: Magnetic resonance imaging of the female pelvic floor and urethra: Body coil versus endovaginal coil. Magma 5(1):59–63, 1997.
9. Schafer A, Enck P, Furst G, et al: Anatomy of the anal sphincters: Comparison of anal endosonography to magnetic resonance imaging. Dis Colon Rectum 37(8): 777–781, 1994.
10. Goodrich MA, Webb MJ, King BF, et al: Magnetic resonance imaging of pelvic floor relaxation: Dynamic analysis and evaluation of patients before and after surgical repair. Obstet Gynecol 82(6):883–891, 1993.
11. Kirschner-Hermanns R, Wein B, Niehaus S, et al: The contribution of magnetic resonance imaging of the pelvic floor to the understanding of urinary incontinence. Br J Urol 72(5):715–718, 1993.
12. Petros PE, Ulmsten U: An integral theory and its method for the diagnosis and management of female urinary incontinence. Scand J Urol Nephrol Suppl 153:1–93, 1993.
13. Enhorning G: Simultaneous recordings of intravesical and intraurethral pressure. Acta Chir Scand 20:309:317, 1967.
14. Constantinou CE: Resting and stress urethral pressures as a clinical guide to the mechanism of continence in the female patient. Urol Clin North Am 12:247–258, 1985.
15. Swash M, Henry MM, Snooks SJ: Unifying concept of pelvic floor disorders and incontinence. J R Soc Med 78:906–911, 1985.
16. DeLancey J: Structural support of the urethra as it relates to stress incontinence: The hammock hypothesis. Am J Obstet Gynecol 170(6):1713–1723, 1994.
17. Jeffcoate TNA: Anatomy in Principles of Gynaecology, ed 4. London, Butterworths, 1975, pp 17–52.
18. Petros PE, Ulmsten U: An integral theory of female urinary incontinence. Acta Obstet Gynecol Scand 69 (suppl 153):1–79, 1990.
19. Petros PE, Ulmsten U: Bladder instability in women: A premature activation of the micturition reflex. Neurourol Urodynam 12:235–239, 1993.
20. Petros PE, Ulmsten U: Urethral pressure increase on effort originates from within the urethra, and continence from musculovaginal closure. Neurourol Urodynam 14:337–350, 1995.
21. Gousse AE, Barbaric ZL, Safir MH, et al: Dynamic half Fourier acquisition, single shot turbo spin-echo magnetic resonance imaging for evaluating the female pelvis. J Urol 164(5):1606–1613, 2000.
22. DeLancey JO: Stress urinary incontinence: Where are we now, where should we go? Am J Obstet Gynecol 175(2):311–319, 1996.
23. Kinder MV, Bastiaanssen EH, Janknegt RA, Marani E: Neuronal circuitry of the lower urinary tract: Central and peripheral neuronal control of the micturition cycle. Anat Embryol 192(3):195–209, 1995.
24. Deindl FM, Vodusek DB, Hesse U, Schussler B: Pelvic floor activity patterns: Comparison of nulliparous continent and parous urinary stress incontinent women. A kinesiological EMG study. Br J Urol 73(4):413–417, 1994.
25. Artibani W, Andersen J, Ostergaard DR, et al: Imaging and other investigations. In Abrahms P (ed): Incontinence. WHO/UICC, Plymbridge Ltd., Plymouth, UK 1999, pp 401–445.

Dynamic Magnetic Resonance Imaging in the Evaluation of Pelvic Pathology

Larissa V. Rodriguez ■ Shlomo Raz

Pelvic floor dysfunction encompasses a variety of fascial and anatomic defects that can affect the anterior wall, posterior wall, and apex of the vagina. Because cystocele, rectocele, uterine prolapse, enterocele, and vault prolapse often coexist, all of the components of the pelvic floor must be evaluated thoroughly. Although patients may have symptoms isolated to one compartment of the pelvic floor, most patients have concomitant defects in other compartments.[1] Because surgical failures have been attributed to a lack of thorough preoperative evaluation of the female pelvis as well as to inadequate diagnosis and staging of pelvic floor dysfunction,[2] accurate diagnosis of coexisting abnormalities is essential in planning reconstructive procedures. Although most diagnoses of pelvic floor prolapse are made based on the findings of a detailed physical examination, various studies show that pelvic examination has poor sensitivity and specificity in the diagnosis of various forms of pelvic floor prolapse.[3-5]

Previously, pelvic ultrasonography was the study of choice for evaluation of the female pelvis.[6] Subsequently, fluoroscopy has been used to evaluate the bladder and rectum and to aid in the diagnosis of cystocele and rectocele.[3-4,7] Recently, magnetic resonance imaging (MRI) has been used in the diagnostic evaluation of pelvic floor dysfunction. MRI provides outstanding anatomic detail of the pelvic floor, including rectocele, cystocele, enterocele, and uterine prolapse, in a single, noninvasive study that does not expose the patient to ionizing radiation.[8-17] MRI also provides a thorough multiplanar evaluation of the pelvic contents, including the uterus, ovaries, ureters, kidneys, and levator muscles, as well as the urethra. This type of evaluation is unavailable with any other imaging modality.[10,12-16,18,19] Therefore, dynamic MRI appears to be the ideal modality to evaluate the female pelvis and identify the components of pelvic floor dysfunction.

Besides its utility in the diagnosis of organ prolapse, MRI provides useful information about ureteral obstruction, hydronephrosis, and uterine and ovarian pathology. This information is essential in the management of women with pelvic floor disorders. In addition, MRI is the study of choice for the evaluation of urethral pathology. One disadvantage of MRI is that it is not a functional study. The ureters and renal pelvis can be evaluated only if the collecting system is filled with fluid. Administration of gadolinium (magnetic resonance urogram) is necessary for more effective evaluation of the collecting system. In addition, MRI is not adequate for use in evaluating renal or ureteral calculi. Computed tomographic urogram continues to be the study of choice in the evaluation of the upper tracts.

MAGNETIC RESONANCE IMAGING

Technique

Very fast single-shot MRI sequences for the evaluation of pelvic prolapse were recently developed, and allow excellent visualization of the pelvic floor in women.[14,15,20] The patient is placed in the supine position, with the legs slightly spread apart and the knees bent and supported by a pillow. There is no need for bowel preparation, premedication, instrumentation, or organ opacification with contrast medium. The MRI torso coil is centered at the symphysis pubis. Images are acquired in the sagittal plane with single-shot fast spin echo (SSFSE) or half-Fourier acquisition, single-shot turbo spin echo (HASTE) sequences. Single midsagittal views are obtained during 3 seconds of suspended respiration, with the patient relaxed and during various degrees of progressive abdominal straining. The total MRI room time is approximately 10 to 15 minutes, and the cost is comparable to that of radiographic or fluoroscopic methods.

Two sets of images are obtained. The first set consists of static sagittal and parasagittal images that show the pelvis from the left to the right side wall. These images provide information on pelvic anatomy and pathologic abnormalities, and are used to select the midsagittal plane for the dynamic second set of images. This static sequence also allows anatomic delineation of the pelvic side walls and the muscular and fascial components of the pelvic floor.[14,15,20] The static set consists of 17 to 20 sequential images that are acquired independently in approximately 18 seconds. Static images are typically acquired with an SSFSE pulse sequence using a 128 × 256 matrix with a repetition time of 4000 msec, an echo time of 22.5 msec, slice thickness of 5 mm, and a field of view of 28 cm.

The second set of images consists of relaxed and straining midsagittal views that are used to assess the degree of pelvic floor relaxation and organ prolapse. A 128 × 256 matrix is used, with a repetition time of 4000 msec, an echo time of 90 msec, a field of view of 28 cm, and slice thickness of 5 mm. Images can be looped for viewing on a digital station as a cine stack.

Grading of Pelvic Floor Relaxation

To evaluate descensus, certain anatomic landmarks are used, as shown in Figures 20-1 and 20-2. The pubococcygeal line marks the distance from the pubis to the coccyx, and serves as a fixed anatomic reference. The width of the levator hiatus is measured as the distance from the pubis to the pubococcygeus muscle (H-line). The hiatus is formed by the puborectalis muscle, and encompasses the urethra, vagina, and rectum. The M-line shows the relaxation of the muscular pelvic floor by measuring the descent of the levator plate from the pubococcygeal line. Using these three simple measurements, an MRI classification of the degree of organ prolapse has been described.[14] In the normal population, during straining, the hiatus (H-line) is less than 6 cm long and does not descend (M-line) more than 2 cm below the pubococcygeal line. The upper urethra, urethrovesical junction, bladder, upper vagina, uterus, small bowel, sigmoid colon, mesenteric fat, and rectum are all located above the H-line. A combination of hiatal enlargement and pelvic floor descent constitutes relaxation. As the pelvic floor descends, so do the organs above it. The grading system for prolapse of any pelvic organ is based on 2-cm increments below the H-line. By determining the degree of visceral prolapse beyond the H-line, the degree of rectocele, enterocele, cystocele, and uterine descent can be graded on a scale of 0 to 3, as follows (Table 20-1).

- 0 = No descent
- 1 = Minimal descent
- 2 = Moderate descent
- 3 = Severe descent

PELVIC PROLAPSE

Enterocele

Enteroceles may be simple or complex. Simple enteroceles exist when there is no associated vault prolapse and the cuff of the vagina is well supported. Complex enteroceles are associated with vault prolapse and tend to coexist with other forms of prolapse of the anterior or posterior vaginal wall. As a result of vaginal crowding, an enterocele is often missed on physical examination when it is accompanied by other significant prolapse.[6] In addition,

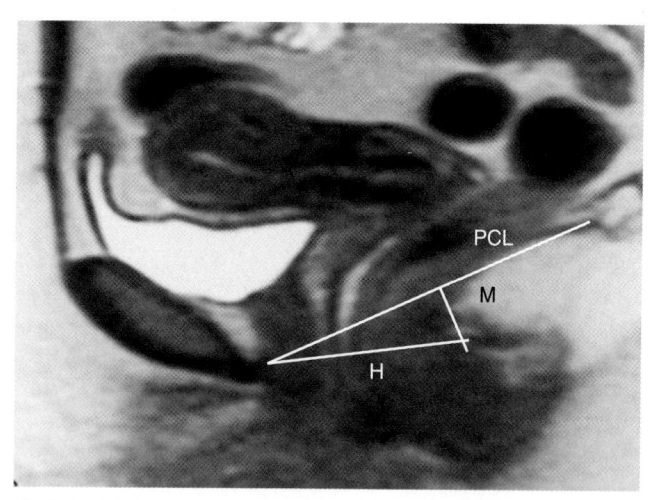

FIGURE 20-2 A normal magnetic resonance imaging scan. PCL, pubococcygeal line; H-line, width of the levator hiatus; M-line, distance from the levator plate to the pubococcygeal line.

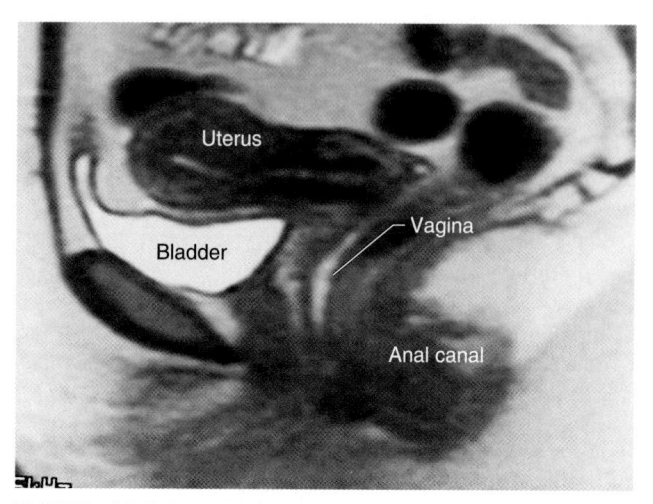

FIGURE 20-1 A normal magnetic resonance imaging scan, showing the uterus, bladder, vagina, and anal canal.

TABLE 20-1 ■ Grading of Hiatal Enlargement, Pelvic Organ Prolapse, and Pelvic Floor Descent with Magnetic Resonance Imaging

Grade	Hiatal Enlargement	Pelvic Organ Prolapse	Pelvic Floor Descent
0	<6 cm	Organ above H-line	0–2 cm
1	6–8 cm	Organ 0–2 cm below H-line	2–4 cm
2	8–10 cm	Organ 2–4 cm below H-line	4–6 cm
3	≥10 cm	Organ ≥4 cm below H-line	≥6 cm

physical examination often cannot reliably distinguish an enterocele from a high rectocele. In the past, defecography was the only available study to aid in the diagnosis of enteroceles. Enteroceles were usually identified only after repeated postevacuation straining, and opacification of the vagina was usually required to show the insinuation of small bowel loops between the rectum and the vagina.[21] In addition, voiding cystograms were performed to exclude concomitant cystocele. Until recently, dynamic contrast roentgenography and multiphasic fluoroscopic cystocolpoproctography were considered the best radiologic studies to detect organ prolapse. These studies rely on opacification with contrast material of the bladder, vagina, small bowel, and rectum. These tests may be performed with all organs opacified together, or they may be performed in phases, with each organ opacified individually before each straining phase.[4,22-24] These evaluations are invasive and time-consuming, and do not detect as many as 20% of all enteroceles.[25-27]

MRI is a much simpler and less invasive technique for the evaluation of enteroceles. Gousse and colleagues[15] compared the findings on physical examination, intraoperative findings, and MRI results in women with and without prolapse. Compared with intraoperative findings, MRI had a sensitivity of 87%, specificity of 80%, and positive predictive value of 91%. MRI was significantly superior in detecting enteroceles compared with physical examination. The images are obtained with the patient supine in the relaxed and straining state (Fig. 20-3). Neither instrumentation nor invasive procedures are needed. Similarly, Linemann and associates,[27] using MRI with opacification of organs, showed that MRI had much greater sensitivity in the detection of enteroceles compared with physical examination and dynamic cystoproctography.[27] In addition, MRI differentiated the enteroceles according to their contents (small bowel, large bowel, rectosigmoidocele, or mesenteric fat). MRI is also an excellent study that can be used to differentiate high rectoceles from enteroceles, allowing adequate surgical planning and safer planes of dissection.[14,15,18,27] Although a recent study found that multiphasic MRI with opacification of organs and multiphasic fluoroscopic cystocolpoproctography had similar detection rates for enterocele,[23] excellent images can be obtained with dynamic MRI without the use of oral or rectal contrast. Thus, the minimal information added by contrast administration does not warrant the invasiveness of organ opacification.[15,21,25] Overall, dynamic MRI is noninvasive and is superior to the other modalities in the diagnosis of enterocele.

Cystocele

A cystocele can be classified by grade according to the degree of bladder descent or by anatomic defect (central, lateral, or combination).[28] As with other forms of prolapse, high-grade cystoceles usually do not occur in isolation, and they represent a spectrum of pelvic floor dysfunction.[1,3,14] When a large vaginal mass is present, it may be difficult to differentiate a high-grade cystocele from an enterocele, vaginal vault prolapse, or a high rectocele by physical examination alone.[3-5] In addition, repair of only the cystocele, without attention to the rest of the pelvic floor, predisposes the patient to an increased incidence of enterocele, rectocele, or uterine prolapse postoperatively.[15]

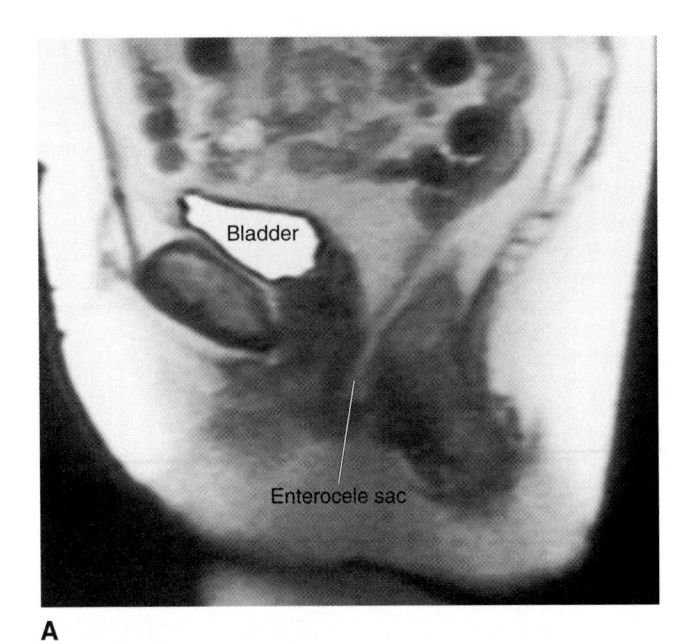

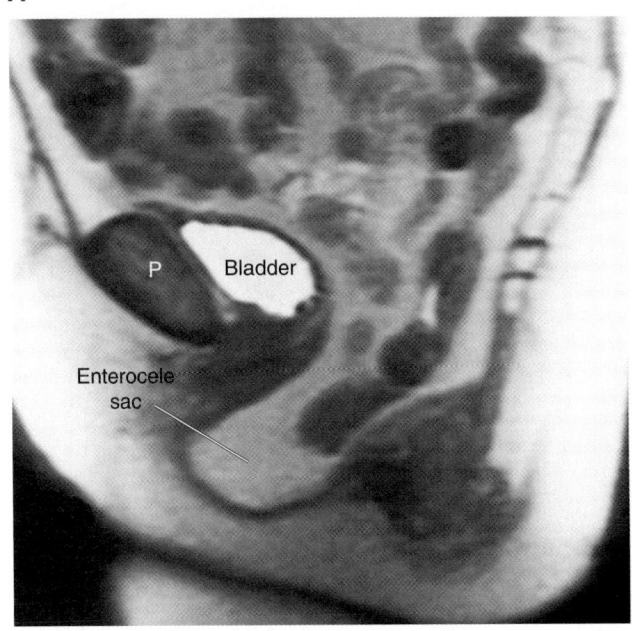

FIGURE 20-3 A, Enterocele shown with the patient relaxed. **B**, Grade 3 enterocele shown with the patient straining. A large enterocele becomes apparent when the patient strains. P, pubic bone.

The study of choice in evaluating simple, low-grade cystoceles is the voiding cystourethrogram (VCUG). Urodynamic testing should also be performed if the patient has voiding dysfunction or incontinence. VCUG and urodynamic testing should be performed in the standing position in both the relaxed and straining states. These studies are useful in determining the severity of cystocele, evaluating for urethral hypermobility and stress urinary incontinence, and documenting postvoid residual.[7] In addition, the evaluation of high-grade cystoceles should provide information on concomitant pelvic floor prolapse, urinary retention, and ureteral obstruction.

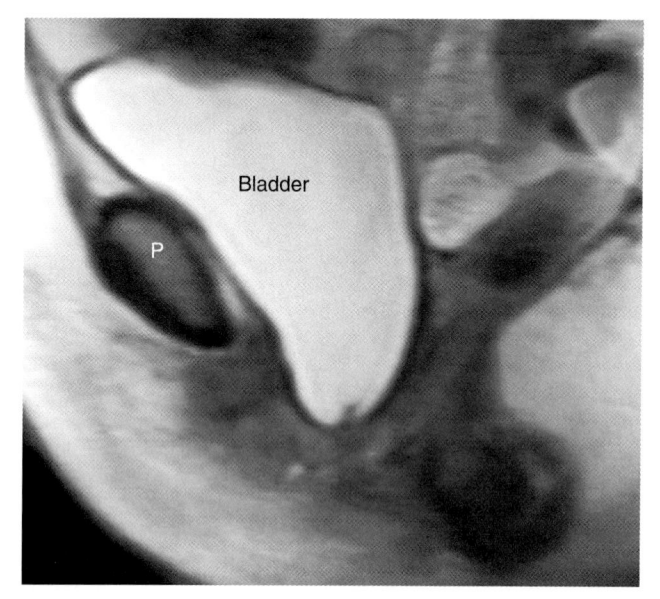

FIGURE 20-4 A grade 2 cystocele is easily seen. P, pubic bone.

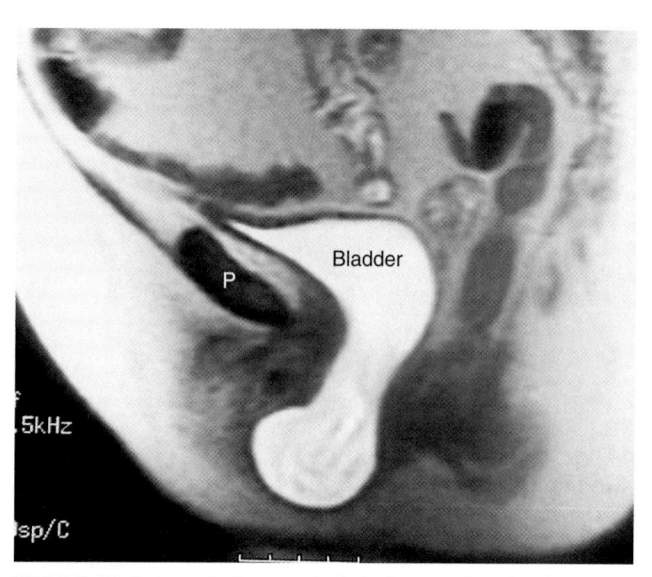

FIGURE 20-5 A grade 3 cystocele is easily seen. P, pubic bone.

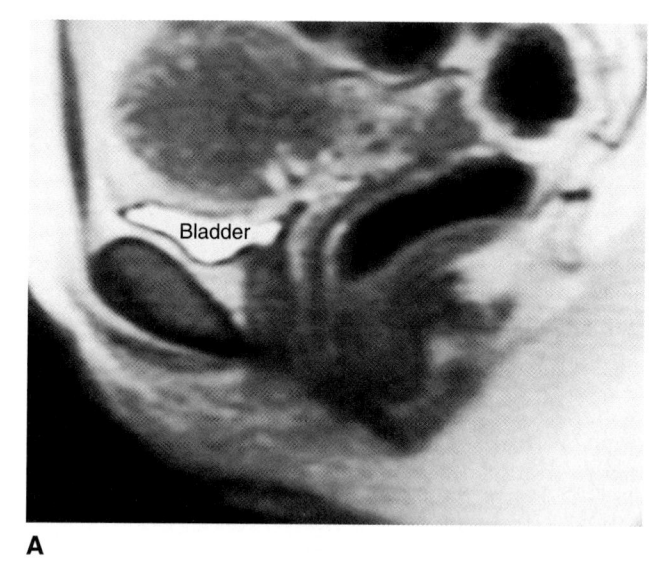

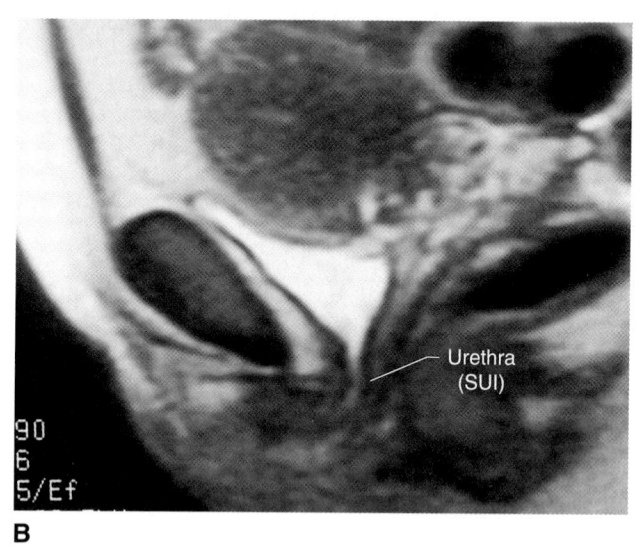

FIGURE 20-6 A, Relaxed position. **B,** Grade 1 cystocele and stress urinary incontinence shown with the patient straining.

Figures 20-4 and 20-5 show MRI scans of patients with grades 2 and 3 cystocele, respectively. Compared with intraoperative findings, MRI has a sensitivity of 100%, specificity of 83%, and positive predictive value of 97% when evaluating for cystocele.[15] In addition, MRI can be used to document the results of urethral hypermobility and postvoid urine residual tests and to evaluate ureteral obstruction and other pelvic abnormalities (Figs. 20-6 through 20-9). Gousse and associates[15] found that MRI diagnosed other types of pelvic pathology, besides prolapse, in 55 of 100 patients studied, including 3 patients with bilateral hydroureteronephrosis.

In the diagnosis of cystocele, MRI has a high degree of correlation with lateral cystourethrography, with a Spearman correlation coefficient of 0.95.[29] One disadvantage of MRI is that these studies are performed with the patient supine, without the more physiologic effect of gravity. However, MRI offers several advantages. There is no need for urethral catheterization, and the patient is not exposed to ionizing radiation. In addition, MRI provides detailed anatomic views of the three compartments of the pelvic floor at rest and during maximal pelvic strain. It also provides direct visualization of the pelvic organs for evaluation of concomitant pathology, determination of urethral hypermobility, evaluation of ureteral obstruction, and postvoid residual testing.[9,10,13-15,29]

Rectocele

Rectoceles are caused by a defect of the prerectal and pararectal fascia and the rectovaginal septum.[28] They are present in as many as 80% of asymptomatic patients who have pelvic floor dysfunction.[13] Although the diagnosis is usually made by physical examination, the reported sensitivity of pelvic examination for the diagnosis of rectocele is 31% to 80%.[3,4,6,24,30] The poor sensitivity of

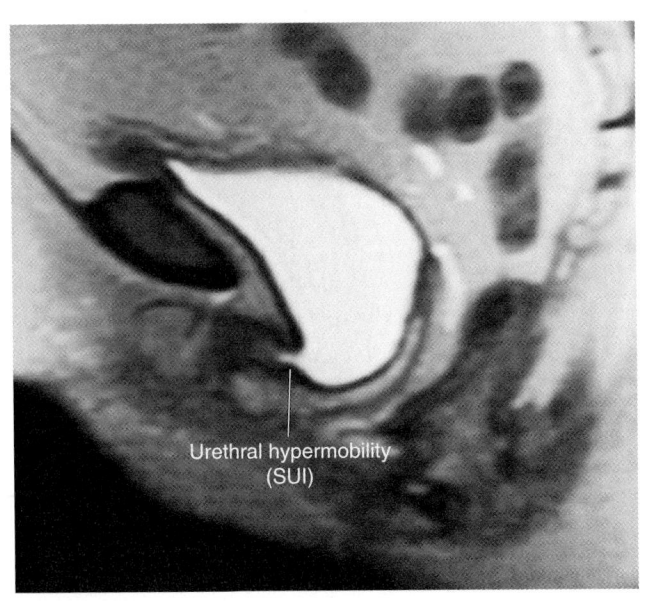

FIGURE 20-7 Urethral hypermobility and stress urinary incontinence (SUI) shown with the patient straining. Urethral hypermobility and urine leakage can be seen.

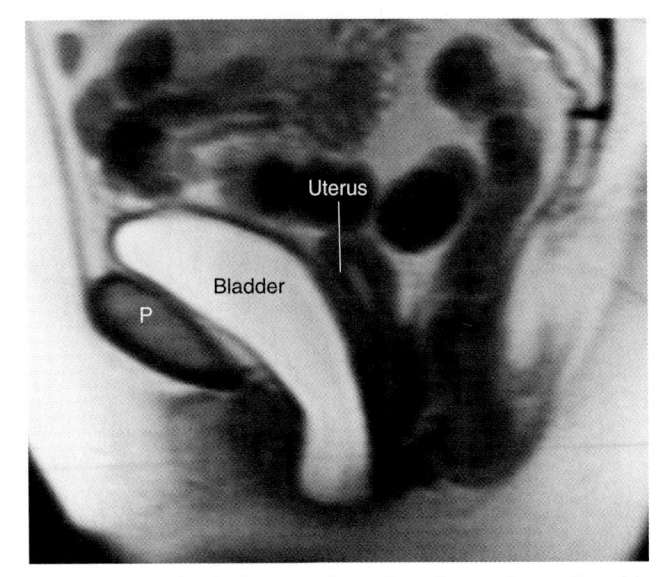

FIGURE 20-9 Grade 2 cystocele and uterine prolapse. P, pubic bone.

physical exam is due to competition among organs for space in the vagina when rectocele is accompanied by other significant prolapse.[6] In addition, it is often difficult to distinguish an enterocele from a high rectocele.

Evacuation proctography is used to diagnose enterocele, rectocele, perineal descent, and rectal intussusception.[29] Dynamic contrast roentgenography or fluoroscopic cystocolpoproctography is also used[4,22-24,30] to diagnose rectocele. The disadvantages of these techniques are their inability to visualize the soft tissue planes of the pelvic floor, their invasiveness, and their use of significant levels of ionizing radiation.

Figure 20-10 shows a rectocele diagnosed by dynamic MRI. A rectocele is easily seen when filled with gas, fluid, or gel. Although this test is highly specific, when no rectal or vaginal opacification is used, MRI can miss as many as 24% of rectoceles.[15] Tunn and colleagues[18] showed that, when rectal opacification is used during MRI, a correct diagnosis of rectocele can be made in 100% of patients, compared with intraoperative findings. Other investigators showed similar detection rates for rectocele with triphasic dynamic MRI and triphasic fluoroscopic cystocolpoproctography.[23] Therefore, to increase the ability of MRI to diagnose rectocele, rectal opacification must be used. This is usually accomplished by introducing sonographic transmission gel or gadolinium into the rectum before MRI scanning is performed. Besides the obvious disadvantage of the added invasiveness of the procedure, air introduced with the rectal agent can produce image artifacts.[15,23] Recently, upright dynamic MRI defecating proctography was described.[31] Although these studies may show greater sensitivity in detecting anorectal anomalies, their utility seems to be more pronounced in patients with disorders of defecation, including anismus and intussusception. These studies are too invasive to justify their routine use in the evaluation of rectocele.

Uterine Prolapse

Laxity of the uterosacral ligaments allows anterior movement of the cervix that leads to progressive retroversion of the uterus[28] and subsequent prolapse. The size of the uterus and the presence of concomitant uterine or ovarian pathology determine whether vaginal or abdominal hysterectomy is performed at the time of prolapse repair. Because of the need to exclude malignancy as well as the

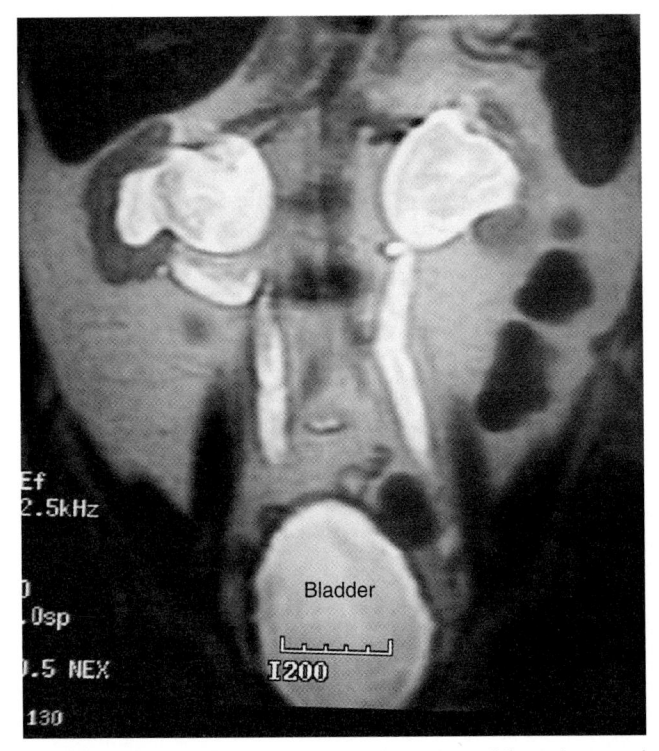

FIGURE 20-8 Grade 3 cystocele and resultant bilateral ureteral obstruction at the level of the bladder.

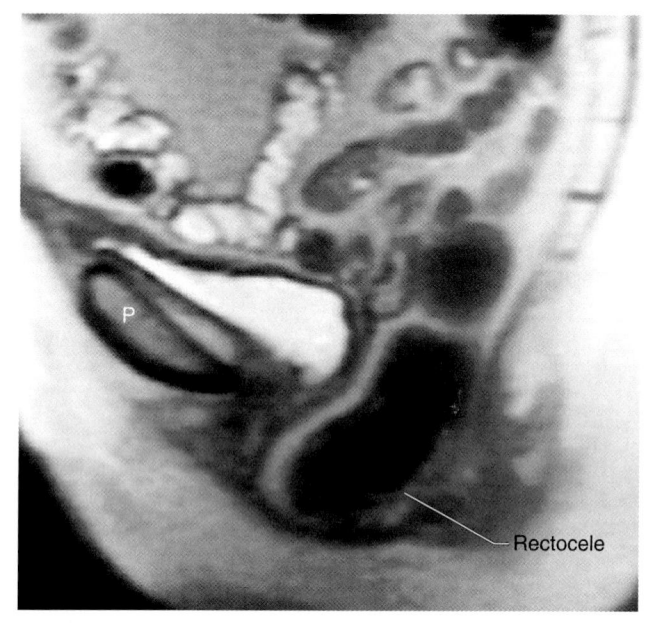

FIGURE 20-10 A rectocele is clearly seen when the patient strains. P, pubic bone.

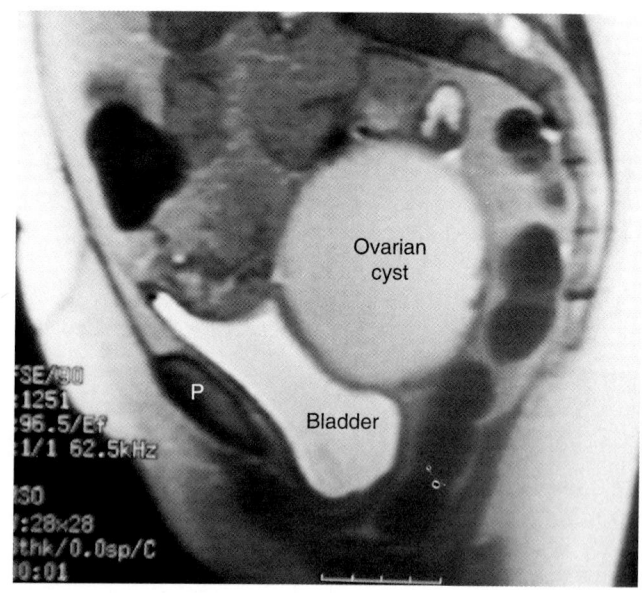

FIGURE 20-12 A large ovarian cyst in a patient with a grade 1 cystocele. P, pubic bone.

association between grade 4 uterine prolapse and insidious progressive ureteral obstruction, MRI is an excellent modality for the evaluation of uterine prolapse (Fig. 20-11). MRI is used to evaluate uterine size, position, orientation (retroversion), and pathology (e.g., fibroids, tumors, nabothian cysts) as well as ovarian pathology (cyst or mass). This information is essential for use in determining whether vaginal or abdominal hysterectomy is indicated. In addition, MRI provides information on cystocele, rectocele, urethral hypermobility, and urethral diverticula, and can be used to detect ureteral obstruction.[9,10,13-15,29] Gousse and associates[15] reported sensitivity of 83%, specificity of 100%, and a positive predictive value of 100% when comparing dynamic MRI with intraoperative findings. The findings were similar when MRI was compared with findings on physical examination alone. More importantly, MRI clearly defined the other compartments of the pelvic floor and diagnosed uterine or ovarian pathology (Figs. 20-12 and 20-13) in 30 of 100 patients evaluated.[15]

OTHER PATHOLOGY

Pelvic Masses

MRI shows excellent results in the evaluation of pelvic cystic and solid masses. It provides excellent information on uterine masses, such as fibroids, carcinoma, and

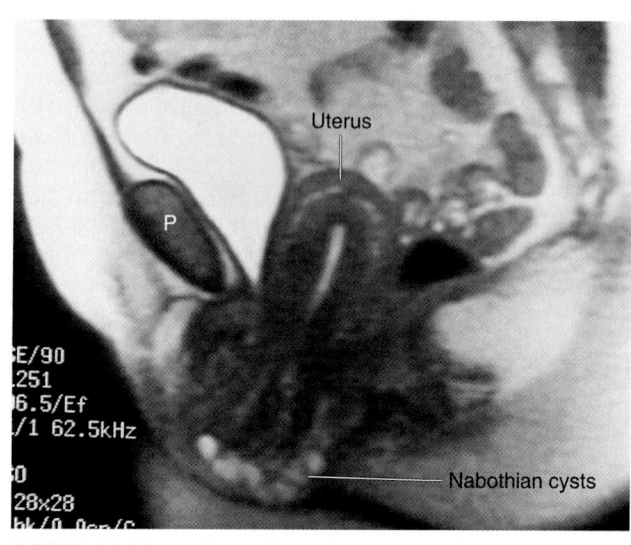

FIGURE 20-11 Uterine prolapse. The bladder, urethra, and cervix are clearly seen. Cervical nabothian cysts are seen as areas of high attenuation in the cervix. P, pubic bone.

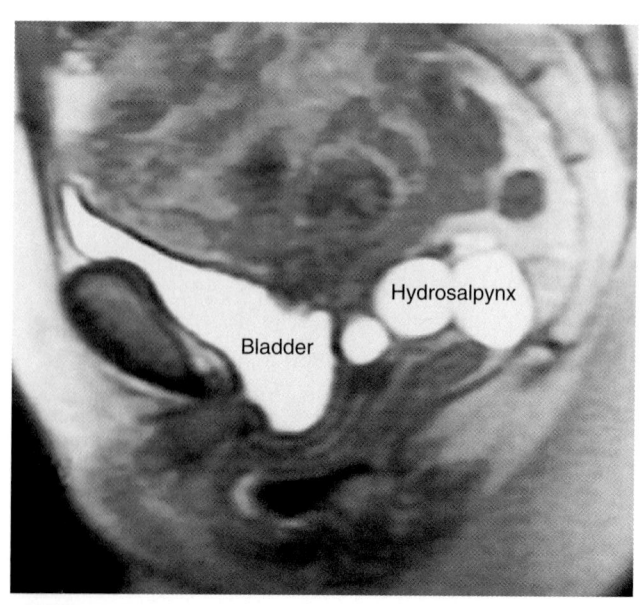

FIGURE 20-13 Hydrosalpinx in a patient with a grade 1 to 2 cystocele.

ovarian cysts (simple or complex) and solid masses. MRI also shows hydrosalpinx and other abnormalities of the fallopian tubes as well as nabothian cysts of the cervix and cysts of Bartholin's gland. MRI can also be used to evaluate endometriosis because the size and extent of endometriomas as well as pelvic organ involvement can be easily evaluated. It also provides excellent visualization of urethral cystic or solid masses as well as urethral diverticuli. For these reasons, MRI should be considered in the evaluation of all women with pelvic pain.

Urethral Diverticula

MRI has had a dramatic effect on the diagnosis of urethral diverticulum. Because most patients have non-specific lower urinary tract symptoms and the pathognomonic presentation of postvoid dribbling, urethral pain, a tender periurethral mass, and expression of pus from the urethra is uncommon, these patients often undergo extensive evaluation and treatment before a correct diagnosis is established.[32,33]

Until recently, the gold standard for the evaluation of urethral diverticula was positive pressure urethrography with a double balloon catheter (PPU).[34] This test is labor-intensive and requires specific expertise. Therefore, VCUG has been substituted in the diagnosis of diverticula. Several studies show that MRI is superior to both VCUG and PPU. Therefore, it is now the imaging modality of choice when the diagnosis of urethral diverticulum is suspected[35-38] (Figs. 20-14 and 20-15). MRI provides information on the location, number, extent (simple vs. saddlebag), and size of diverticula. Endoluminal MRI, performed with either a vaginal or a rectal coil, may provide even better image quality than simple MRI.[38]

CONCLUSION

Pelvic floor relaxation is a generalized condition that involves all of the compartments of the pelvic floor. The diagnosis of all components of pelvic prolapse is essential for surgical planning as well as for preventing surgical failure, recurrent prolapse, and reoperation. Vaginal crowding as a result of competition for space among the multiple organs that descend into the vagina makes the diagnosis of pelvic dysfunction by physical examination alone difficult.

Because pelvic floor dysfunction is usually generalized, the compartments of the pelvic floor are best imaged simultaneously. Various studies have shown MRI evaluation of normal subjects, enhancing the current understanding of normal pelvic anatomy.[39-41] On the other hand, the use of MRI to analyze the pelvic floor musculature has contributed greatly to the current understanding of pelvic floor dysfunction.[19,42-44]

MRI is the best imaging study available to evaluate pelvic floor dysfunction and to differentiate between cystocele, enterocele, rectocele, and vault and uterine prolapse. It also provides a thorough multiplanar evaluation of the pelvic contents, including the uterus, ovaries, ureters, kidneys, and pelvic floor or levator muscles. This evaluation is unavailable with any other imaging modality that uses fluoroscopy alone.[10,12-16,18,19] Although MRI is currently the best available technique for the evaluation of pelvic floor prolapse, upright dynamic MRI in an open-configuration system or even three-dimensional reconstruction for virtual imaging of the urinary tract and pelvic floor might be used for evaluation of pelvic floor dysfunction in the future.[19,44]

REFERENCES

1. Maglinte DD, Kelvin FM, Fitzgerald K, et al: Association of compartment defects in pelvic floor dysfunction. AJR Am J Roentgenol 172:439–444, 1999.
2. Safir MH, Gousse AE, Rovner ES, et al: 4-Defect repair of grade 4 cystocele. J Urol 161:587–594, 1999.
3. Kelvin FM, Maglinte DD: Dynamic cystoproctography of female pelvic floor defects and their interrelationships. AJR Am J Roentgenol 169:769–774, 1997.

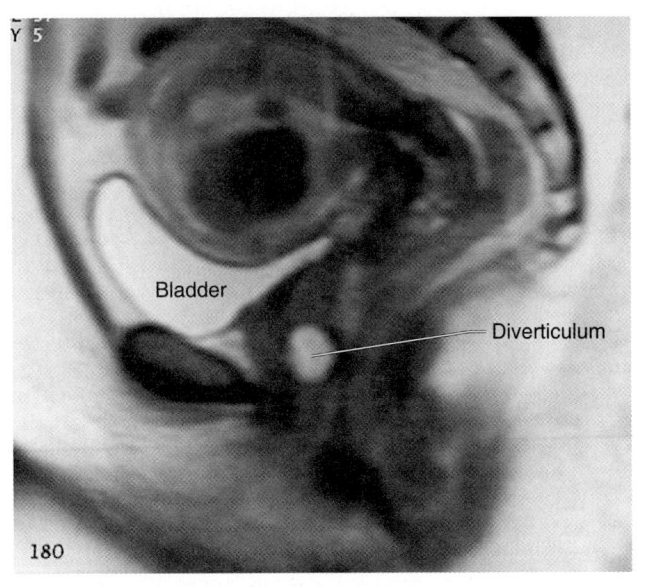

FIGURE 20-15 Sagittal view of a urethral diverticulum with signal intensity similar to that of the bladder.

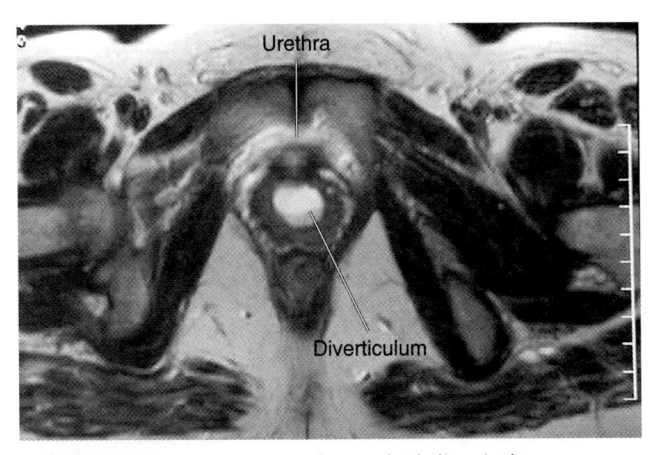

FIGURE 20-14 Coronal view of a urethral diverticulum seen as a structure with high signal intensity.

4. Kelvin FM, Hale DS, Maglinte DD, et al: Female pelvic organ prolapse: Diagnostic contribution of dynamic cystoproctography and comparison with physical examination. AJR Am J Roentgenol 173:31–37, 1999.
5. Stovall DW: Transvaginal ultrasound findings in women with chronic pelvic pain. Obstet Gynecol, 95 (4 suppl 1):S57, 2000.
6. Siproudhis L, Ropert A, Vilotte J, et al: How accurate is clinical examination in diagnosing and quantifying pelvirectal disorders? A prospective study in a group of 50 patients complaining of defecatory difficulties. Dis Colon Rectum 36:430–438, 1993.
7. Raz S, Erickson D, Sussman E: Operative repair of rectocele, enterocele and cystocele. Adv Urol 5:121–144, 1992.
8. Klutke C, Golomb J, Barbaric Z, et al: The anatomy of stress incontinence: Magnetic resonance imaging of the female bladder neck and urethra. J Urol 143:563–566, 1990.
9. Yang A, Mostwin JL, Rosenshein NB, Zerhouni EA: Pelvic floor descent in woman: Dynamic evaluation with fast MR imaging and cinematic display. Radiology 179:25–33, 1991.
10. Goodrich MA, Webb MJ, King BF, et al: Magnetic resonance imaging of pelvic floor relaxation: Dynamic analysis and evaluation of patients before and after surgical repair. Obstet Gynecol 82:883–891, 1993.
11. Strohbehn K, Ellis JH, Strohbehm JA, DeLancey JO: Magnetic resonance imaging of the levator ani with anatomic correlation. Obstet Gynecol 87:277–285, 1996.
12. Ozasa H, Mori T, Togashi K: Study of uterine prolapse by magnetic resonance imaging: Topographical changes involving the levator ani muscle and the vagina. Gynecol Obstet Invest 34:43–48, 1992.
13. Lienemann A, Anthuber C, Barron A, et al: Dynamic MR colpocystorectography assessing pelvic-floor descent. Eur Radiol 7:1309–1317, 1997.
14. Comiter CV, Vasavada SP, Barbaric ZL, et al: Grading pelvic floor prolapse and pelvic floor relaxation using dynamic magnetic resonance imaging. Urology 54:454–457, 1999.
15. Gousse AE, Barbaric ZL, Safir MH, et al: Dynamic half Fourier acquisition single shot turbo spin-echo magnetic resonance imaging for evaluating the female pelvis. J Urol 164:1606–1613, 2000.
16. Rouanet JP, Mares P, Courtieu C, Maubon A: Static and dynamic MRI of the normal and pathological female pelvic floor. J Gynecol Obstet Biol Reprod 164:1606–1613, 2000.
17. Lienemann A, Sprenger D, Jansen U, et al: Functional MRI of the pelvic floor: The methods and reference values. Radiologie 45:458–464, 2000.
18. Tunn R, Paris S, Taupitz M, et al: MR imaging in posthysterectomy vaginal prolapse. Int Urogynecol J Pelvic Floor Dysfunct 11:87–92, 2000.
19. Healy JC, Halligan S, Reznek RH, et al: Patterns of prolapse in women with symptoms of pelvic floor weakness: Assessment with MR imaging. Radiology 203:77–81, 1997.
20. Busse RF, Riederer SJ, Fletcher JG, et al: Interactive fast spin-echo imaging. Magn Reson Med 44:339–348, 2000.
21. Weidner AC, Low VHS: Imaging studies of the pelvic floor. Obstet Gynecol Clin North Am, 25:825–848, 1998.
22. Takano M, Hamada A: Evaluation of pelvic descent disorders by dynamic contrast reontography. Dis Colon Rectum 43:205–212, 2000.
23. Kelvin FM, Maglinte DDT, Hale DS, Benson JT: Female pelvic organ prolapse: A comparison of triphasic dynamic MR imaging and triphasic fluoroscopic cystocolpoproctography. AJR Am J Roentgenol 174:81–84, 2000.
24. Altringer WE, Saclarides TJ, Dominguez JM, et al: Four-contrast defecography: Pelvic "floor-oscopy." Dis Colon Rectum 38:695–699, 1995.
25. Brubaker L, Retzky S, Smith C, Saclarides T: Pelvic floor evaluation with dynamic fluoroscopy. Obstet Gynecol 82:863–868, 1993.
26. Hock D, Lombard R, Jehaes C, et al: Colpocystodefecography. Dis Colon Rectum 36:1015–1021, 1993.
27. Linemann A, Anthuber C, Baron A, Reuser M: Diagnosing enteroceles using dynamic magnetic resonance imaging. Dis Colon Rectum 43:205–212, 2000.
28. Raz S, Stothers L, Chopra A: Vaginal reconstructive surgery for incontinence and prolapse. In Walsh PC, Retik AB, Vaughan ED, Wein AJ (eds): Campbell's Urology, ed 7. Philadelphia, WB Saunders, 1059–1094, 1998.
29. Gufler H, DeGreforio G, Allman KH, et al: Comparison of cystourethrography and dynamic MRI in bladder neck descent. J Comput Assist Tomogr 24:382–388, 2000.
30. Cundiff GW, Nygaard I, Bland DR, Versi E: Proceedings of the American Urogynecologic Society Multidisciplinary Symposium on Defecatory Disorders. Am J Obstet Gynecol 182:S1–S10, 2000.
31. Lamb GM, Jode MG, Gould SW, et al: Upright dynamic MR defaecating proctography in an open configuration MR system. Br J Radiol 73:152–155, 2000.
32. Ganabathi K, Leach GE, Zimmern PE, Dmochowski R: Experience with management of urethral diverticulum in 63 women. J Urol 152:1445–1452, 1994.
33. Romanzi LJ, Groutz A, Blaivas JG: Urethral diverticulum in women: Diverse presentations resulting in diagnostic delay and mismanagement. J Urol 164:428–433, 2000.
34. Davis HJ, Cian LG: Positive pressure urethrography: A new diagnostic method. J Urol 75:753, 1956.
35. Neitlich JD, Foster HE, Glickman MG, Smith RC: Detection of urethral diverticula in women: Comparison of a high resolution fast spin echo technique with double balloon urethrography. J Urol 159:408–410, 1998.
36. Daneshgari F, Zimmern PE, Jacomides L: Magnetic resonance imaging detection of symptomatic noncommunicating intraurethral wall diverticula in women. J Urol 161:1259–1262, 1999.
37. Blander DS, Broderick GA, Rovner ES: Magnetic resonance imaging of a "saddle bag" urethral diverticulum. Urology 53:818–819, 1999.
38. Blander DS, Rovner ES, Schnall MD, et al: Endoluminal magnetic resonance imaging in the evaluation of urethral diverticula in female. Urology 57:660–665, 2001.
39. Fielding JR, Dimanli H, Schreyer AG, et al: MR-based three-dimensional modeling of the normal pelvic floor in women: Quantification of muscle mass. AJR Am J Roentgenol 174:657–660, 2000.
40. Goh V, Halligan S, Kaplan G, et al: Dynamic MR imaging of the pelvic floor in asymptomatic subjects. AJR Am J Roentgenol 174:661–666, 2000.
41. Myers RP, Cahill DR, Kay PA, et al: Puboperineales: Muscular boundaries of the male urogenital hiatus in 3D from magnetic resonance imaging. J Urol 164:1412–1415, 2000.
42. Hjartardottir S, Nilsson J, Petersen C, Lingman G: The female pelvic floor: A dome—not a basin. Acta Obstet Gynecol Scand 76:567–571, 1997.
43. Tan IL, Stoker J, Zwamborn AW, et al: Female pelvic floor: Endovaginal MR imaging of normal anatomy. Radiology 206:777–783, 1998.
44. Stenzl A, Kölle D, Eder R, et al: Virtual reality of the lower urinary tract in women. Int Urogynecol J Pelvic Floor Dysfunct 10:248–253, 1999.

CHAPTER 21

Endoscopy in Benign Pelvic Floor Dysfunction

JOHN J. KLUTKE ■ CARL G. KLUTKE

Endoscopic examination of the bladder and urethra has a wide range of diagnostic and therapeutic indications. Endoscopy of the lower urinary tract is a simple and minimally invasive procedure that should be mastered by clinicians who are interested in pelvic floor dysfunction. In contrast to magnetic resonance imaging and computed tomography, urethrocystoscopy provides a wealth of diagnostic information at minimal expense. This chapter describes the endoscopic appearance of many common pathologic conditions of the lower urinary tract and focuses on the urethroscopic and cystoscopic findings in women.

INDICATIONS

Endoscopy is indicated to exclude a foreign body or malignancy in the lower urinary tract. Specific indications include sterile hematuria or pyuria, unexplained irritative voiding symptoms (e.g., frequency, urgency, dysuria), and recurrent urinary tract infection. Endoscopy is probably not necessary as part of the routine evaluation of incontinence.[1] It does not identify which type of incontinence is present, nor does it reliably assess the dynamic function of the outlet.[2,3] Endoscopy is indicated in the evaluation of incontinence when the basic evaluation is nonspecific (e.g., when urodynamic studies do not reproduce the patient's symptoms). Endoscopy is also indicated in the evaluation of unexplained bladder or pelvic pain, in cases of suspected fistula, or to exclude operative injury of the urinary tract. A clinician who treats patients with pelvic floor dysfunction will encounter many therapeutic indications for endoscopy, including delivery of periurethral bulking agents, placement of ureteral stents, and extraction of foreign bodies.

EQUIPMENT

The clinician can choose between two configurations of equipment, depending on the clinical situation. A urethroscope is a simple device that is suited to rapid office evaluation of the urethra. A rigid 0-degree telescope is contained in a thin sheath that has no break or fenestration, allowing distension of the urethra with gas or liquid. The end-on view given by the 0-degree telescope is ideal for evaluating the urethra and bladder neck. The urethroscope is a simple, self-contained unit. It is small, thin, and comfortable for the patient, but lacks the wider applicability of the rigid cytoscope. A rigid cytoscope consists of a telescope, a bridge, and a sheath. The bridge contains ports that allow the passage of ureteral stents or cystoscopic instruments. Water or saline is used as a distension medium, and various telescopes can be interchanged. The angled field of view provided by a 30-degree or 70-degree telescope allows complete evaluation of the bladder and urethra. A 120-degree telescope may be useful for visualizing the trigone in cases of procidentia.

Flexible cystoscopes are also widely available and have many applications.[4] The flexible cystoscope is as accurate for diagnosis as a rigid cystoscope.[5] It may be better tolerated by the patient when cystoscopy is performed without anesthesia.[6]

Endoscopy is simplified with the use of a video monitor. The monitor provides a distraction for the patient as well as an easy way to record the procedure. Still exposures are best taken through the endoscope. An adapter is used to attach the camera to the eyepiece.

Technique

Endoscopic evaluation follows an orderly sequence. The mucosa of the urethra and bladder is easily abraded, and careful inspection of the urethral mucosa should be made on the first pass of the lubricated endoscope into the bladder. Lubrication with lidocaine gel minimizes discomfort during the evaluation. The endoscope is advanced beyond the urethrovesical junction and into the bladder, with care taken to avoid contact between the tip of the endoscope and the opposing bladder wall, which can leave a circular imprint of hyperemia. The bladder is inspected for foreign bodies and mucosal lesions. Inspection of the trigone and both uretheral orifices follows. The endoscope is then withdrawn to the level of the bladder neck. With the bladder neck displayed, the patient is asked to squeeze the pelvic muscles. This squeezing normally results in closure of the bladder neck around the endoscope. After the patient relaxes the pelvic floor muscles, she is asked to cough, and the clinician observes the resultant downward mobility of the bladder neck. The endoscope is slowly withdrawn from the urethra, and the urethra is inspected for diverticula while digital pressure is placed on the anterior vaginal wall. Cystoscopy is considered a clean procedure. Between procedures, equipment can be sterilized with activated dialdehyde solution (Cidex, manufactured by Johnson and Johnson in New Brunswick, New Jersey). Although urinary tract infection is the most common complication of endoscopic evaluation, the true incidence of bacteriuria with the procedure is unknown; a range of 2% to 18% is reported in the literature.[7-9] In the absence of a cost analysis showing otherwise, it is prudent to give antibiotic prophylaxis at the time of the procedure.

NORMAL ENDOSCOPIC FINDINGS

The urethra appears as a potential space with pink to white epithelium. The urethra collapses around the tip of the endoscope and opens into the bladder (Fig. 21-1). Once the endoscope is inside the bladder, reference can be made to the bladder apex, superior surface, anterolateral surfaces, bases of the posterior surface, and the bladder neck, or most inferior part. An air bubble will float to the top of the bladder, and is a useful reference point. The bladder epithelium is uniformly pale white to pink and translucent, with submucosal vessels apparent. The trigone is delineated by the ureteral orifices, the interureteric ridge, and the urethrovesical junction. It is found on the posterior wall of the bladder, just beyond the vesicourethral junction. The randomly interlaced detrusor musculature lies beneath the epithelium and, at low volumes, may give the mucosal lining a wrinkled appearance (Fig. 21-2). The urethra is an estrogen-sensitive organ.[10,11] A transition from the hormonally sensitive stratified squamous epithelium of the urethra to the transitional epithelium of the bladder occurs in the bladder neck. Squamous metaplasia often extends into the trigone, and appears as a "cake-icing" membrane overlying the bladder epithelium (Fig. 21-3). Although this appearance is sometimes known as pseudomembranous, or granular, trigonitis, this condition is very prevalent in normal women, and does not warrant biopsy.[12,13] The appearance and location of the ureteral orifices vary widely. The intramural portion of the ureter is seen coursing cephalad from each orifice. The interureteric ridge is a horizontal fold at the apex of the trigone. After one ureteral orifice is located, the interureteric ridge is a useful landmark that leads to the contralateral ureteral orifice.

PATHOLOGIC CONDITIONS

Ectopic Ureter

An ectopic ureter inserts outside the normal anatomic location on the interuretetric ridge. The condition is almost always synonymous with a duplicated collection

FIGURE 21-1 Normal appearance of the urethra. (From Klutke JJ, Klutke CG: Endoscopy in benign pelvic floor dysfunction. In Investigation and Conservation Treatment of Pelvic Floor Dysfunction. Rome, Casa Editrice Scientifica Internazionale, 1999.)

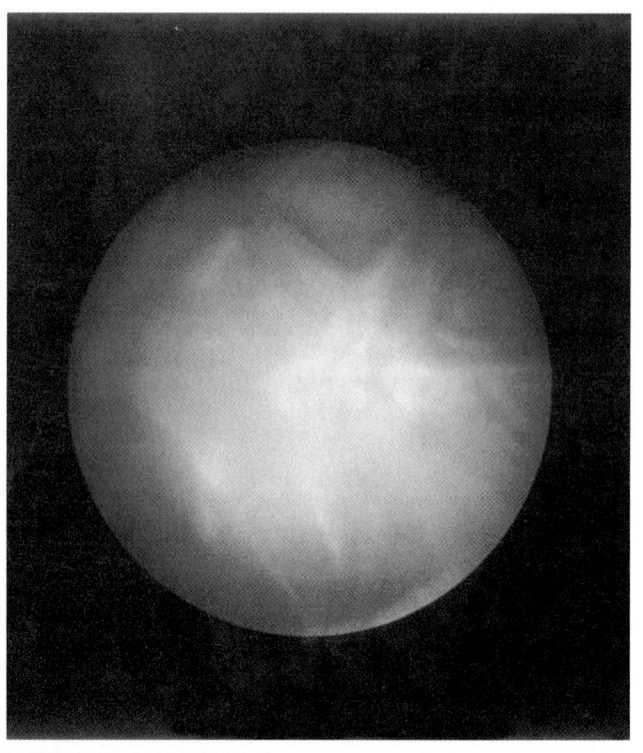

FIGURE 21-2 Trabeculated appearance of the mucosa in the normal, undistended bladder.

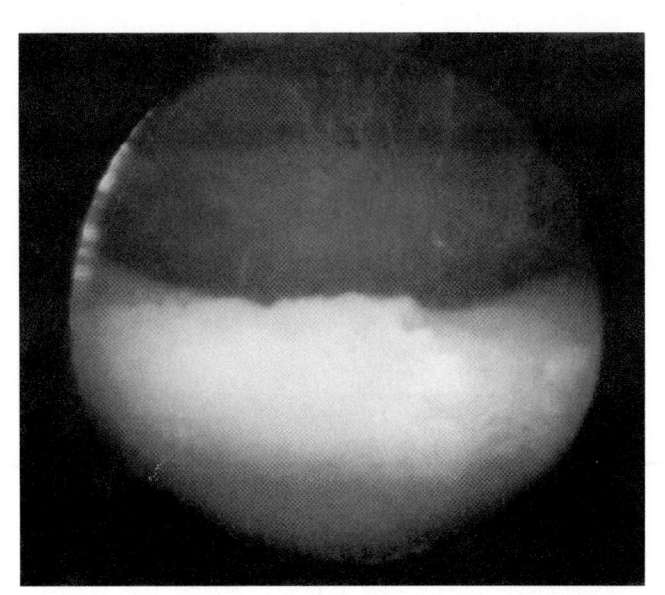

FIGURE 21-3 Squamous metaplasia with a "cake-icing" appearance at the trigone. (From Klutke JJ, Klutke CG: Endoscopy in benign pelvic floor dysfunction. In Investigation and Conservation Treatment of Pelvic Floor Dysfunction. Rome, Casa Editrice Scientifica Internazionale, 1999.)

system in women. The prevalence of a duplicated collecting system is 0.9%, making it the most common structural abnormality encountered by the endoscopist.[12] An ectopic ureter may insert anywhere more caudally on the trigone, bladder neck, urethra, or vagina, following the course of the mesonephric duct. Incontinence can occur if the ectopic ureter bypasses the sphincteric mechanism by entering the urethra distal to the bladder neck.

Extrinsic Compression

The distended bladder presses against adjacent structures. A deformation of the inner bladder surface often results from the uterus and cervix. A tumor in an organ adjacent to the bladder can indent on and deform its mucosal surface. Uterine fibroids are very prevalent in women, and often account for this effect. The appearance of a fibroma pressing from outside against a distended bladder can lead the endoscopist to mistakenly assume that a tumor is arising within the bladder. Bimanual examination of the pelvic organs to confirm the pathology is helpful.

Urethritis

Patients with urethritis have voiding symptoms referable to the urethra. Passage of an endoscope is exquisitely painful. Urethritis is present when the urethral mucosa is bright red. Coarse, irregular mucosal fronds may be seen at the bladder neck. The bladder mucosa and trigone appear normal.

Urethral Diverticula

The incidence of urethral divertcula is 1% to 5%.[14–16] In addition to a mass effect, patients may have recurrent urinary tract infection or vaginal pain after the diverticulum becomes infected. Cases of urethral carcinoma arising in a diverticulum have been reported.[17]

Endoscopy has a high false-negative rate. It should be performed if excision is planned because multiple diverticula are commonly present and may be identified preoperatively. The communication of the diverticulum into the urethra may be noted, and knowledge of its location is important to ensure complete removal. Diverticula are usually found posteriorly on the distal urethra. A plume of pus is sometimes noted, and can be traced to the mouth of the diverticulum. This effect can be enhanced by using two fingers placed in the vagina to gently squeeze or "milk" the vagina against the endoscope as the endoscope is withdrawn.

Solid Urethral Tumors

Leiomyomata occasionally arise from the smooth muscle fibers of the urethra.[18] Endoscopy shows a regular bulge that deforms the urethral lumen. Transvaginal palpation of the mass against the endoscope precisely locates the origin of the tumor and is useful in planning surgical excision. Solid tumors in the vagina should usually be removed for biopsy, even if the patient is asymptomatic.

Condyloma acuminata are common vulvar lesions that often involve the external urethral meatus and distal urethra. Although lesions usually involve the distal urethra, the squamous epithelium of the urethra extends onto the bladder trigone, and finger-like lesions projecting into the bladder neck may be condyloma. Condyloma of the bladder itself is rare.

Ureterocele

A ureterocele is a cystic dilation of the intravesical part of the ureter (Fig. 21-4). The ureterocele can be ectopic in location, with the ureteral orifice in the bladder neck or urethra. Ectopic ureteroceles are usually associated with a duplicated collecting system. When the ureteral orifice is located normally, the ureterocecle is referred to as simple or orthotopic. Ureteroceles vary from small lesions to large cysts that fill the bladder. The reported incidence varies widely, from 1 in 4000 to as many as 1 in 500 autopsies.[19,20] The abnormality may arise because of stenosis of the opening of the ureter into the bladder, and some ureteroceles cause ureteral obstruction at the ureterovesical junction. Ureteroceles may also be associated with reflux, secondary urolithiasis, and ascending infection. Clinically significant ureteroceles usually occur in children, and ureterocele is the most common cause of urinary tract obstruction in girls.[21] A small ureterocele noted incidentally in an adult woman is usually not clinically signficant.

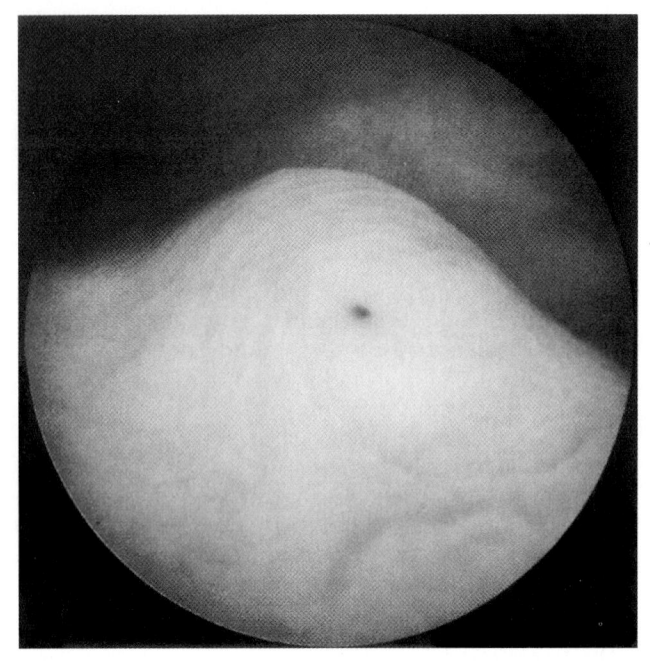

FIGURE 21-4 A simple ureterocele in the normal location on the trigone. (From Klutke JJ, Klutke CG: Endoscopy in benign pelvic floor dysfunction. In Investigation and Conservation Treatment of Pelvic Floor Dysfunction. Rome, Casa Editrice Scientifica Internazionale, 1999.)

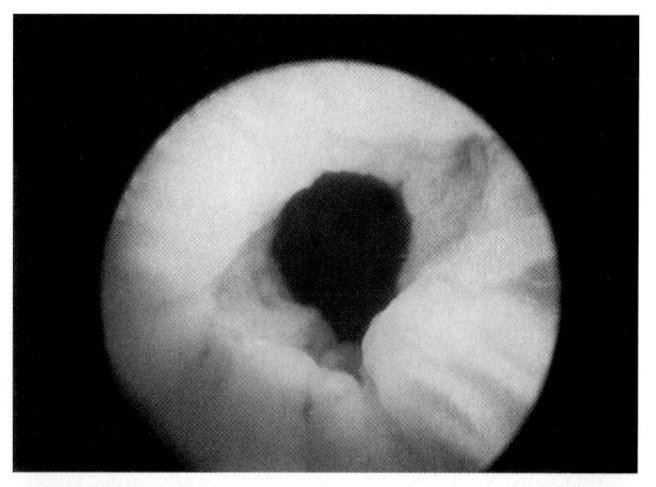

FIGURE 21-5 An open patent fibrotic proximal urethra in a patient with severe intrinsic urethral dysfunction (From Klutke CG: Endoscopic evaluation of the female lower urinary tract. In Raz [ed]: Female Urology, 2nd ed, 1996, p 147.)

Anatomic Stress Urinary Incontinence

Endoscopic findings characterize the mobility of the bladder neck with straining. The presence or absence of mobility is an important distinction in patients with stress urinary incontinence. To assess mobility, the endoscopist positions the endoscope just distal to the urethrovesical junction. When bladder neck mobility is excessive, the proximal urethra projects urine toward the observer when the patient coughs and strains. This finding is often referred to as funneling, and confirms the findings on physical examination and cotton swab testing. Such mobility of the bladder neck is often observed in normal, continent women, and is not a specific feature of stress urinary incontinence.[22] However, the lack of mobility with straining in a patient with stress urinary incontinence is a red flag in the diagnosis because a suspension procedure may fail.[23]

Intrinsic Sphincter Deficiency

Intrinsic sphincter deficiency is incontinence that occurs when the urethra loses its ability to coapt. Patients with this condition may have an open, scarred urethra on endoscopy (Fig. 21-5). This appearance is called a drainpipe or pipe stem urethra. It is probably a severe form of intrinsic sphincter deficiency. An open bladder neck is not necessarily a pathologic finding.[24,25] Endoscopic diagnosis does not detect true intrinsic sphincter deficiency in 44% of cases.[26] Endoscopic findings that suggest intrinsic sphincter deficiency should be considered in the context of other information.

Urethrovesical and Vesicovaginal Fistulas

The appearance of the bladder and urethra may be deceptive in patients with fistulas. A small fistula is often difficult to locate, especially after inflammation subsides. Locating one fistula endoscopically does not exclude other fistulas, nor does it exclude injury of the upper urinary tract. Most bladder fistulas in the United States occur after hysterectomy and usually occur near the adjacent vaginal cuff. These fistulas are found endoscopically at the posterior wall of the bladder, superior to the trigone. A probe or guidewire placed into the bladder through the fistula from the vagina can simplify the evaluation.

Endoscopy is important in determining the location of the fistula, especially in relation to the ureteral orifices. Ureteral stents can be placed if the lesion impinges on the trigone. The evaluation also determines whether inflammation is present at the margins of the fistula, an important consideration in timing surgical repair. Biopsy is often warranted to exclude malignancy.

Vesicoenteric Fistula

A vesicoenteric fistula may occur in regional enteritis, diverticulitis, or gastrointestinal cancer. Endoscopic evaluation usually shows an area of inflammation that is sometimes referred to as a herald patch because it pinpoints the site of the fistula (Fig. 21-6). Fecal matter or gas issuing into the bladder may be noted. The fistulous tract is not always seen, and oral charcoal can be administered to the patient before evaluation to help locate the tract. As with vesicovaginal and urethrovaginal fistulas, biopsy is often necessary to exclude cancer.

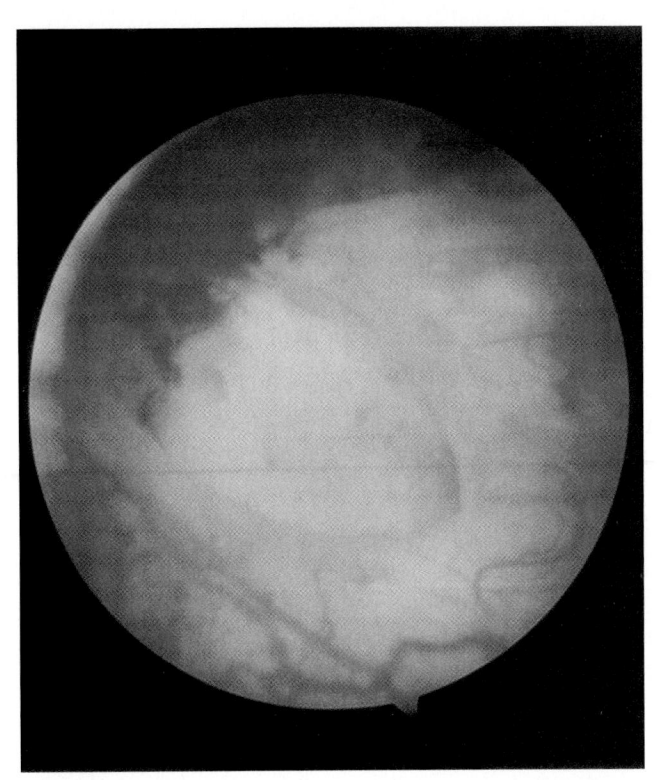

FIGURE 21-6 Endoscopic view of a vesicovaginal fistula with a well-epithelialized tract. (From Klutke JJ, Klutke CG: Endoscopy in benign pelvic floor dysfunction. In Investigation and Conservation Treatment of Pelvic Floor Dysfunction. Rome, Casa Editrice Scientifica Internazionale, 1999.)

Cancer

Bladder cancer is the eighth most common cancer in women.[27] A clinician with a busy practice treating women with benign pelvic floor disease may see one or two cases each year. Lesions may be sessile or polypoid. If abnormal lesions are noted on endoscopy, biopsy should be performed by a qualified specialist to exclude malignancy. Metastatic cancer may also be seen in the bladder or urethra, but usually only in cases of advanced disease. Endoscopy rarely detects cervical cancer at an early stage (stage I or II).[28] Findings in metastatic cancer range from bullous edema to biopsy-positive lesions involving the bladder mucosa.

Interstitial Cystitis

Interstitial cystitis is a debilitating condition characterized by suprapubic pain and irritative voiding symptoms in the absence of an apparent cause. Like any disease that lacks well-defined characteristics, the incidence is unknown. Interstitial cystitis has few, if any, objective features. Endoscopy is mandatory for making the diagnosis, although a patient with interstitial cystitis may not show the classic findings. The role of endoscopic evaluation of the bladder and urethra is primarily to exclude other disease.

During evaluation, the bladder is distended beyond the normal cystometric capacity. This technique is called hydrodistension, and is done for both therapeutic and diagnostic reasons.[29] Characteristic findings are often seen during or after hydrodistension of the bladder. Obviously, distending the bladder in patients with interstitial cystitis would be expected to be very painful, so the evaluation is done with regional or general anesthesia. Two distinctive endoscopic abnormalities are defined. The first is Hunner's ulcer, a velvety red patch on the mucosal surface of the bladder that contains congested blood vessels surrounding a granulating base (Fig. 21-7).[30] The second abnormality is reduced bladder capacity, which is often found in patients with interstitial cystitis.[31] Glomerulations are also frequently described in patients with interstitial cystitis.[32] These are pinpoint hemorrhages that are seen after distension, presumably as a result of ruptured submucosal blood vessels. It is not clear if they characterize the bladder in interstitial cystitis or occur as a result of overdistension.[33]

Abnormal cytoscopic findings in interstitial cystitis can resemble those seen in cystitis caused by radiation, viral or tuberculous infection, or chemotherapy (e.g., cyclophosphamide).[33] Therefore, bladder biopsy must be performed before the diagnosis of interstitial cystitis can be established. Biopsy specimens should be taken, even in the absence of an apparent endoscopic abnormality, to exclude carcinoma in situ, a malignant condition with subtle endoscopic findings that can mimic interstitial cystitis. Biopsy is performed after bladder distension to minimize the possibility of bladder rupture.

Endometriosis

The bladder is an uncommon site for endometriosis. When present, it involves the peritoneal surface, unless

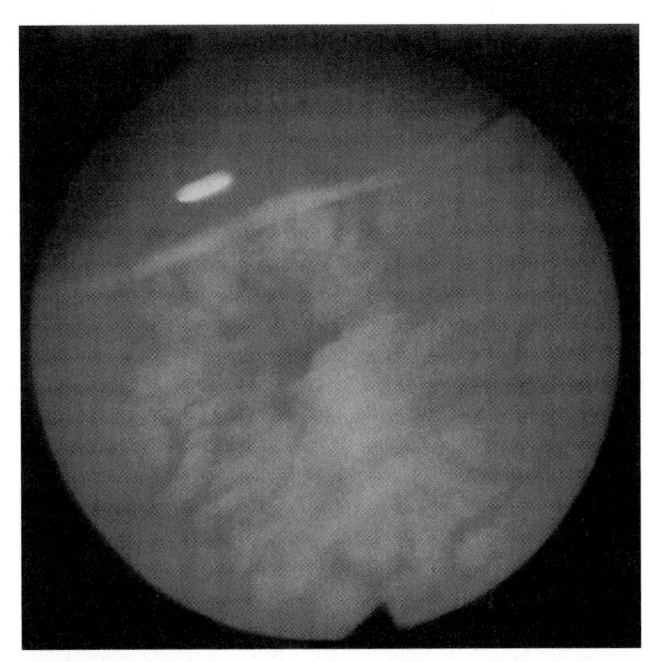

FIGURE 21-7 Hunner's ulcer with central erythema in a typical location, near the dome of the bladder. (From Klutke JJ, Klutke CG: Endoscopy in benign pelvic floor dysfunction. Investigation and Conservation Treatment of Pelvic Floor Dysfunction. Rome, Casa Editrice Scientifica Internazionale, 1999.)

the interior of the bladder was previously contaminated with endometrial cells. Rarely, invasion of the muscularis and involvement of the bladder mucosa occurs. These lesions may change during the menstrual cycle. The appearance of mucosal endometriotic implants is variable, and biopsy is required for diagnosis.

Intraoperative Endoscopy

Occasionally, intraoperative endoscopy has a role as an adjunct to operative procedures in which the structures of the lower urinary tract are at risk for injury.[34] With abdominal procedures such as colposuspension, the conventional transurethral route for endoscopy is less desirable because of the additional time required to drape and reposition the patient. Transvesicular cystoscopy is preferable to direct visualization through a bladder incision in these cases because a much smaller cystotomy is required. The cystotomy is made through a retroperitoneal approach to the superior surface of the bladder. The endoscope is introduced into the bladder, and methylene blue is administered intravenously to verify that ureteral efflux occurs. A small-diameter telescope is used alone, without the sheath, and a purse-string closure with absorbable suture prevents leakage during the evaluation, and closes the cystotomy. The bladder is drained for 3 days postoperatively.

The incidence of bladder injury in retropubic urethroplexy is not well documented, but it is probably less than 1% when performed by experienced surgeons. The use of intraoperative endoscopy to exclude injury is recommended as an adjunct rather than a routine. The procedure may be especially useful to verify suture placement on repeated urethropexy when extensive retropubic scarring is encountered.

Periurethral Bulking

Periurethral collagen injection is used to restore coaptation in the intrinsically defective urethra.[35] Endoscopy is an integral part of the procedure, and is done to verify placement of the bulking agent in the proper location at the bladder neck and proximal urethra. Several endoscopic devices have been designed for transurethral delivery of the agent. A long needle passes through the length of the endoscope to penetrate the urethral mucosa at the proximal urethra. Care is taken to prevent the bulking agent from escaping through the penetration site into the urethra. This possibility is decreased with the use of the paraurethral route. An 18-gauge spinal needle is placed at the 9 o'clock position, just lateral to the external urethral meatus. The paraurethral injection is best accomplished with a 0 endoscope with an unbeaked sheath. The needle is slowly advanced parallel to the urethra with simultaneous endoscopic display of the bladder neck. When the needle tip approaches the submucosa at the bladder neck, movement of the needle is apparent on the endoscopic display. It is important to avoid penetrating the bladder or urethral mucosa. If penetration occurs, the procedure is terminated and attempted at a later date. After the bulking agent is injected and coaptation of the urethral mucosa is verified, the procedure is repeated at the 3 o'clock position of the external meatus.

REFERENCES

1. Fantl JA, Newman DK, Colling J, et al: Urinary incontinence in adults: Acute and chronic management. Clinical Practice Guideline, No. 2, 1996 Update. Rockville, MD: U.S. Department of Health and Human Services. Public Health Service, Agency for Health Care Policy and Research. AHCPR Publication No. 96-0682, March 1996.
2. Scotti RJ, Ostergard DR, Guillaume AA, Kohatsu KE: Predictive value of urethroscopy as compared to urodynamics in the diagnosis of genuine stress urinary incontinence. J Reprod Med 35:772–776, 1990.
3. Versi E: The significance of an open bladder neck in women. Br J Urol 68:42–43, 1991.
4. Pope AJ, Wickham JEA: A user's guide to flexible cystoscopes. Br J Urol 68:10–14, 1991.
5. Clayman RV, Reddy P, Lange PH: Flexible fiberoptic and rigid rod lens endoscopy of the lower urinary tract: A prospective controlled comparison. J Urol 131:715–716, 1984.
6. Flannigan GM, Gelister JSK, Noble JG, et al: Rigid vs. flexible cystoscopy: A controlled trial of patient tolerance. Br J Urol 62:537–540, 1988.
7. Manson A: Is antibiotic prophylaxis indicated after outpatient endoscopy? J Urol 140:316–317, 1988.
8. Richards B, Bastable JRG: Bacteriuria after outpatient cystoscopy. Br J Urol 49:561–564, 1977.
9. Hares MM: A double blinded trial of half strength poly Bactrim soluble GU bladder irrigation in cystoscopy. Br J Urol 53:62–67, 1981.
10. Elia G, Bergman A: Estrogen effects on the urethra: Beneficial effects in women with genuine stress urinary incontinence. Obstet Gynecol Surv 48:509–513, 1993.
11. Bergman A, Karram MM, Bhatia NN: Changes in urethral cytology following estrogen administration. Gynecol Obstet Invest 29:211–213, 1990.
12. Wiener DP, Koss LG, Sablay B, et al: The prevalence and significance of Brunn's nests, cystitis cystica and squamous metaplasia in normal bladders. J Urol 122:317–318, 1979.
13. Tyler DE: Stratified squamous epithelium in the vesical trigone and urethra: Findings correlated with menstrual cycle and age. Am J Anat 111:319–320, 1962.
14. Andersen MJF: The incidence of diverticula in the female urethra. J Urol 98:96–99, 1967.
15. Davis BL, Robinson DG: Diverticula of the female urethra: Assay of 120 cases. J Urol 104:850–852, 1970.
16. Hoffman M, Adams W: Recognition and repair of urethral diverticula. Am J Obstet Gynecol 92:106–108, 1965.
17. Patanaphan V, Prempree T, Sewchand W, et al: Adenocarcinoma arising in female urethral diverticulum. Urology 22:259, 1983.
18. Elia G, James W, Ballard CA, Bergman A: Diagnostic considerations in coexisting bladder and urethral leiomyomata: A case report. J Reprod Med 40:670–672, 1995.
19. Campbell M: Ureterocele: A study of 94 instances in 80 infants and children. Surg Gynecol Obstet 93:705–708, 1951.
20. Uson AC, Lattimer JK, Melicow MM: Ureteroceles in infants and children: Report based on 44 cases. Pediatrics 27:971–975, 1961.

21. Coplen DE, Duckett JW: The modern approach to ureteroceles. J Urol 153:166–171, 1995.
22. Bergman A, McCarthy TA, Ballard CA, Yanai J: Role of the Q-tip test in evaluating stress urinary incontinence. J Reprod Med 32:273–276, 1987.
23. Bergman A, Koonings PP, Ballard CA: Negative Q-tip test as a risk factor for failed incontinence surgery in women. J Reprod Med 34:193–195, 1989.
24. Versi E, Cardozo LD, Studd JW, et al: Distal urethral compensatory mechanisms in women with an incompetent bladder neck who remain continent, and the effect of menopause. Neurourol Urodynam 9:579–581, 1990.
25. Chapple CR, Helm CW, Blease S, et al: Asymptomatic bladder neck incompetence in nulliparous females. Br J Urol 64:357–359, 1989.
26. Bovier FE, Pritchett TR, Kornman JD: Correlation of the cystoscopic appearance and functional integrity of the female urethral sphincteric mechanism. Urology 44:250–255, 1994.
27. Silverberg E, Boring CC, Squires TS: Cancer statistics. Ca Cancer J Cun 40:9–26, 1990.
28. Lindell LK, Anderson B: Routine pretreatment evaluation of patients with gynecologic cancer. Obstet Gynecol 69:242–247, 1987.
29. Bumpus HC: Interstitial cystitis: Its treatment by overdistention of the bladder. Med Clin North Am 13:1495–1499, 1980.
30. Hunner GL: A rare type of bladder ulcer. JAMA 70:203–212, 1918.
31. Parsons CL: Interstitial cystitis: Clinical manifestations and diagnostic criteria in over 200 cases. Neurourol Urodynam 9:241–247, 1990.
32. Walsh A: Interstitial cystitis. In Harrison JH, Gittes RF, Perlmutter AD, et al (eds): Campbell's Urology, ed 4. Philadelphia, WB Saunders, 1978, pp 693–707.
33. Hanno PM, Wein AJ: Medical treatment of interstitial cystitis (other than DIMSO-50/Elmiron). Urology 29:22–25, 1987.
34. Klutke JJ, Klutke CG, Hsieh G: Bladder injury after Burch retropubic urethropexy: Is routine cystoscopy necessary? Tech Urol 4:145–147, 1998.
35. McGuire EJ, Appell R: Transurethral collagen injection for urinary incontinence. Urology 43:413–415, 1994.

CHAPTER 22

Urodynamic Investigations

STEPHEN H. GARNETT ■ PAUL ABRAMS

The term *urodynamic studies* (UDS) was first used in the 1950s when the development of electronics enabled the simultaneous recording of bladder pressure and urine flow during voiding.[1] Urodynamic studies moved from a research to a clinical tool with the increasing appreciation of the need for information on the function and not simply the structure of the lower urinary tract when evaluating micturition disorders. The development of microchip technology enabled the computerization of UDS, which has in turn allowed the development of ambulatory studies. More recently there has been increasing emphasis on standardization of techniques and quality control as UDS have become central to the evaluation of interventions for disorders of the lower urinary tract.[2]

The value of UDS lies in the fact that symptoms of lower urinary tract dysfunction are often misleading, a situation famously summarized as "the bladder is an unreliable witness."[3] Studies have repeatedly shown the superiority of UDS over symptoms alone in diagnostic accuracy,[4-6] and the improved success rates for interventions when directed by UDS.[7]

The aims of UDS are to reproduce the patient's symptoms and to provide a pathophysiologic explanation for them. These aims must be borne in mind at all times during the urodynamic investigation because findings are relevant only when related to symptoms. Urodynamic investigations range from the simple and noninvasive to the complex and invasive and the clinician must decide which study is most appropriate to each patient. The invasive studies carry a small risk of introducing infection (around 2% to 3% in most good units), but routine antibiotic prophylaxis is not given except for special cases.[8] Invasive studies should not be performed in the presence of urinary tract infection. In patients with high spinal cord lesions, autonomic dysreflexia is a recognized, if uncommon, complication of cystometry; these patients require additional monitoring and immediate emptying of the bladder with or without the addition of an antihypertensive if symptoms of hypertension develop.[9]

The widely accepted standardization of both technique and terminology developed by the International Continence Society (ICS)[10] has facilitated comparison and interpretation of results and advanced improvements in the quality of UDS. It is important that high-quality data are derived from such studies to maximize the information available for analysis. In addition, all traces should be labeled with a zeroed scale and all cystometry should have frequent coughs recorded to check accuracy of pressure readings.[11]

Before any study, the procedure should be explained to the patient, a detailed medical history obtained, and a physical examination performed. The patient should be asked to complete a frequency–volume chart before the study because it gives important information on functional bladder capacity and average filling volumes.

UROFLOWMETRY

Urine flow studies are the simplest and only noninvasive urodynamic technique available at present. Urine flow is a product of the interaction between expressive forces (detrusor contraction and any abdominal straining) and urethral resistance, and as such it is a reflection of a number of variables. Thus uroflowmetry is not a diagnostic study, but a useful, rapid, and inexpensive screening tool. It should be remembered, however, that a low uroflow does not necessarily imply bladder outlet obstruction (BOO) and conversely a normal uroflow does not exclude it. The simplest flow study involves the clinician timing a patient's void and recording the voided volume to calculate an average flow rate. However, since von Garrelts developed his electronic flowmeter[12] in 1956, flowmeters have improved so that they now provide a graphic recording of flow rate against time. Urine flow is described with respect to flow rate and flow pattern, as shown in Figure 22-1.

Flow rate is the volume of fluid expelled per urethra per unit time, expressed in milliliters per second (mL/s).

Indications for Uroflowmetry

Flow studies are a useful screening tool, especially for bladder outlet obstruction, and are commonly combined with a measurement of the postvoid residual urine.

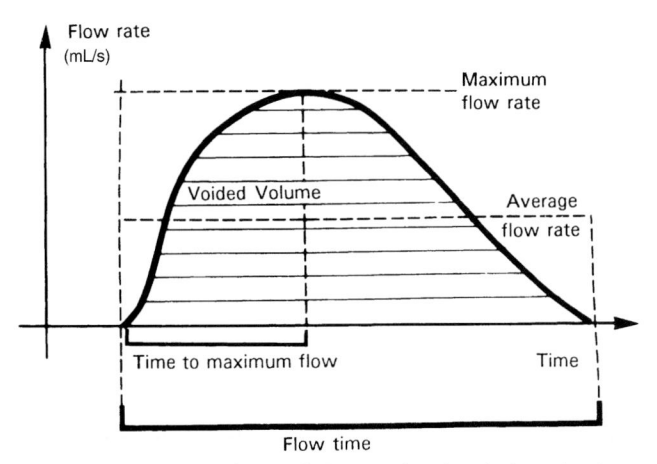

FIGURE 22-1 Terminology relating to the description of urinary flow.

All men with symptoms suggestive of BOO should be screened with flow studies. Neurologically normal children with possible functional outlet obstruction (dysfunctional voiding) should be screened with flow studies, as should women for whom stress incontinence surgery is planned. In the latter group flow studies can provide evidence of detrusor voiding function, and reduced flow rates may give rise to postoperative voiding problems. In older women with recurrent urinary tract infection, flow studies can be used to exclude relative outlet obstruction that results in residual urine.

Equipment

The three basic types of flowmeter are based on methods used to measure volume of urine voided.

- The weight transducer, or gravimetric, method operates by measuring the weight of the urine voided.
- The rotating disk method has a spinning disk onto which the urine falls, tending to slow the rotation of the disk. The disk is kept spinning by a servomotor, and the varying power needed to keep the rotation constant is proportional to urine flow rate.
- The electronic dipstick, or capacitance, method involves the use of a capacitance dipstick inserted into the urine collection vessel. The capacitance changes as the urine accumulates and is proportional to volume.

Modern commercially available flowmeters should have acceptable accuracy (<5% error rate), but it is good practice to check the performance of the flowmeter regularly with a flow–calibration device.

Interpretation of Uroflowmetry

It is essential to know the volume voided in order to interpret flow rate and flow pattern because they can vary considerably even in the same individual at different volumes. Flow rates are greatest and most reliable in volumes between 200 mL and 400 mL, and Q_{max} tends to be constant over this range. Readings from voids less than 150 mL are unreliable, and for volumes over 400 mL detrusor contractile efficiency decreases.[13–15] Interpretation of flow pattern is also influenced by the paper speed of the flowmeter printout, and a speed of 0.25 cm/sec best facilitates this. In a normal flow study, the flow curve is bell shaped and maximum flow is reached in the first 30% of the trace and within 5 seconds from the start of flow.

To use flows as a screening tool, "normal" values must be defined, and the simplest way to do this is to set minimum acceptable flow rates for groups according to age and sex.[7] Several nomograms that plot flow rate against voided volume have been constructed for different patient groups, and these can be used to facilitate interpretation[16–18] (Fig. 22-2).

In men with suspected bladder outlet obstruction, a maximum flow rate of less than 10 mL/sec correlates with a 90% probability that BOO will be diagnosed via pressure–flow studies; however, if flow rate is 10 mL/s to 15 mL/s, the incidence of BOO falls to 71% or lower.[19]

Abnormal Flow Patterns

Abnormal flows can be classified as steady flows or fluctuating flows. Diagnoses can be made only by cystometry, but they can be suggested by the following flow curves.

Steady

Detrusor Instability (Detrusor Overactivity). Typically, this instability produces a flow rate with a high Q_{max} reached in an abnormally fast time. This situation is thought to be due to the bladder neck being open before micturition begins, with only the urethral striated sphincter required to relax to permit voiding.

Bladder Outlet Obstruction. Obstructed flow curves have a low Q_{max} with reduced average flow and the average flow is greater than half the maximum flow rate. Q_{max} is usually obtained relatively quickly, but then flow rate slowly trails off, causing a prolonged void. In men,

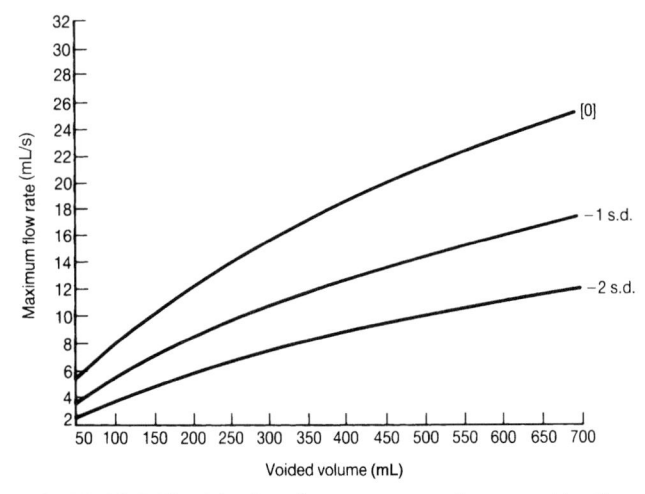

FIGURE 22-2 The Bristol uroflow nomogram for men older than 55 years, constructed from 286 flow measurements from 123 asymptomatic men.

obstructed flows may be constrictive (e.g., urethral stricture) or compressive (e.g., benign prostatic obstruction). In women BOO is uncommon, seen in only 4% of referrals for UDS.[20]

Fluctuating

Straining. Use of abdominal or diaphragmatic muscle to increase urine flow makes the trace irregular, with characteristic slow changes in flow.

Urethral Overactivity. In patients with suprasacral neurologic lesions (typically high spinal cord injury) involuntary contraction of the intraurethral striated muscle at the time of voiding, detrusor–sphincter dyssynergia, gives rise to an interrupted irregular trace with rapid changes in flow rate. An identical trace is seen in neurologically normal patients (usually children) due to involuntary intermittent contractions of the pelvic floor, or dysfunctional voiding.

Detrusor Underactivity. This instability is common in patients with a neurologic lesion, especially multiple sclerosis. The poorly sustained detrusor contraction produces a slowly varying, often interrupted flow trace. This underactivity may be seen in the absence of a known neurologic lesion, often giving a symmetric trace with a low Q_{max}.

Artifacts

Most modern uroflowmeters will automatically identify Q_{max} as the highest point on the flow curve and give a printout of various parameters, including Q_{max}. Care must be exercised when reading the printout, and the trace itself should always be inspected for artifacts because they often cause erroneous values to be given by the flowmeter[21] (Fig. 22-3).

FILLING CYSTOMETRY

The method by which the pressure–volume relationship of the bladder is measured during bladder filling is filling cystometry. To simplify interpretation of the filling study, it is helpful to consider bladder and urethral functions separately. Bladder storage function should be assessed in terms of bladder sensation, detrusor activity, bladder compliance, and bladder capacity. The urethra is assessed in terms of competency. In normal function, the detrusor muscle is relaxed during filling and the urethra is contracted. The detrusor cannot be underactive and the urethra cannot be overactive during filling. Thus in terms of filling abnormalities, the detrusor may be normal or overactive and the urethra may be normal or incompetent.

Cystometry depends on the accurate measurement of pressure, from which bladder function is derived. Pressure measurement is subject to many potential artifacts and therefore careful attention to cystometric technique is important. Further, it should be understood that the technique itself might affect the results.

Basic Concepts

The conventional cystometrogram (CMG) involves artificial bladder filling via a catheter with a specified liquid and recording the filling rate(s). Simultaneously, intravesical (p_{ves}) and abdominal pressures (p_{abd}) are recorded and detrusor pressure (p_{det}) is derived. Intravesical pressure is recorded from a catheter in the bladder and abdominal pressure is taken to be the pressure surrounding the bladder, usually estimated from a rectal or vaginal catheter. Detrusor pressure is the component of intravesical pressure created by forces, both active and passive, in the bladder wall. It is estimated by subtracting abdominal pressure from intravesical pressure.

$$p_{det} = p_{ves} - p_{abd}$$

The measuring of both abdominal and intravesical pressures together is important because it allows the investigator to determine whether changes in intravesical pressure are due to contraction of the bladder alone. Without the measurement of abdominal pressure, it

FIGURE 22-3 The upper trace shows a "squeezing" artifact. The lower trace shows a smooth, "obstructed" curve after the patient has been instructed not to hold the penis during voiding. T_{100}, time to completed void; T_Q, total flow time; T_{Qmax}, time to max flow; Q_{max}, max flow rate; Q_{ave}, mean flow rate; V_{comp}, complete voided volume.

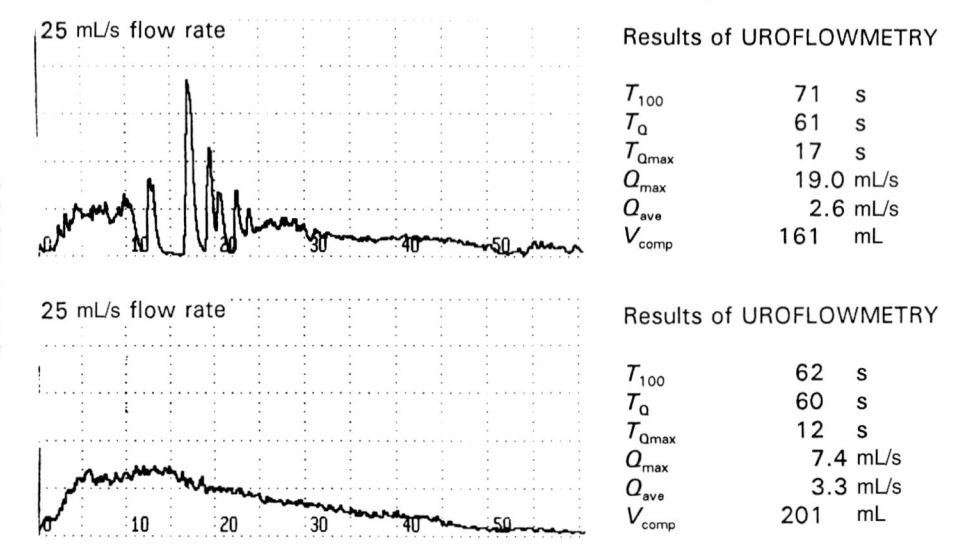

Results of UROFLOWMETRY

T_{100}	71	s
T_Q	61	s
T_{Qmax}	17	s
Q_{max}	19.0	mL/s
Q_{ave}	2.6	mL/s
V_{comp}	161	mL

Results of UROFLOWMETRY

T_{100}	62	s
T_Q	60	s
T_{Qmax}	12	s
Q_{max}	7.4	mL/s
Q_{ave}	3.3	mL/s
V_{comp}	201	mL

would be impossible to exclude the effect of abdominal straining.

Pressure Measurement

Early cystometry relied on a simple water column with a catheter placed in the bladder to measure pressure. Modern urodynamic equipment uses transducers for accurate pressure measurement. Transducers convert changes in pressure into changes in electrical voltage, which are then amplified and recorded. There are two types of pressure transducer in widespread use in urodynamic investigations:

- The external strain gauge transducer is mounted on a stand and connected to the patient by a water-filled tube, which allows transmission of pressure waves to a diaphragm connected to a strain gauge. These transducers are relatively inexpensive and robust. They measure pressure according to their position in relation to the bladder.
- The catheter tip transducer is mounted on a catheter and uses the same principle as the external strain gauge transducer, but it has the diaphragm and strain gauge sited on the catheter. These transducers are relatively more expensive, but eliminate the problems associated with a fluid-filled pressure line and offer good measures of rapid changes in pressure. They measure pressure according to their position in the bladder. Catheter-mounted transducers are essential for ambulatory UDS.

All transducers require zeroing to atmospheric pressure before use.

Technique

Urodynamic investigations should take place in a dedicated room that affords privacy and warmth. The procedure should be explained to the patient, a medical history recorded, and a physical examination performed. An initial free flow is obtained (or self-catheterization performed if this is usual for the patient). At this stage, the postvoid residual urine can be assessed by either catheterization or ultrasound. If a large residual volume is suspected, it should not be drained because this can create filling artifacts.

The bladder is catheterized urethrally, except for some children and certain special cases. Urethral catheterization is aided by local anaesthetic gel application, which does not affect the study. A separate catheter is used to assess abdominal pressure, usually per rectum although the vagina may be used (or occasionally the stomach or abdominal stomata). When using external strain gauge transducers, the transducer must be linked to the patient by a fluid-filled tube (manometer tubing). Because this tubing is used to transmit pressure changes, the walls should not be elastic; yet if they are too rigid, it will be difficult to maneuver. Generally, sterile saline is used as the fluid medium.

Two catheter lumens are required for the bladder: one for filling and one for pressure measurement. Six French-gauge dual-lumen catheters do not cause obstruction, although they may affect urethral function. Alternatively, an epidural catheter can be used to measure pressure, and it is passed into the bladder with an 8-Fr filling catheter. This procedure is straightforward in women, but the epidural catheter needs to be "railroaded" into the bladder via the eyehole of the filling catheter in men. It should then be disengaged from the filling catheter and further advanced into the bladder. In men the catheters are taped to the penis, taking care not to obstruct the urethra on the underside, and in women the catheters are taped to the inner thigh close to the urethral meatus. After filling, the 8-Fr catheter is removed for voiding studies.

The rectal catheter can be constructed easily from manometer tubing covered at the rectal end by a finger cot cut from a disposable plastic glove.[22] The finger cot, which protects from blockage by feces, should have a small cut in it to allow the escape of excess air or fluid when the catheter is flushed. The catheter is introduced using lubricant and passed to about 10 cm from the anal verge.

At this stage the lines and transducer chambers are flushed with fluid and air bubbles are excluded. Strain-gauge transducers are zeroed to atmospheric pressure at this point, but catheter-mounted transducers must be zeroed before being placed in position.

Pressure recording is started and the patient asked to cough to ensure equal pressure transmission from both lines. If the cough is not transmitted equally then the lines should be flushed again and the equipment checked to ensure no air bubbles or loose connections are present. The bladder is filled with saline or radio-opaque contrast medium at room temperature. The once popular CO_2 gas cystometry is not recommended[23,24] and is now rarely used. Men are usually filled standing and women sitting, although some patients may need to be filled supine to accommodate physical incapacity. A peristaltic pump is used to infuse the filling fluid and the filling rate must always be recorded.

The rate of filling has considerable influence on the results; and the faster the bladder is filled, the lower the bladder compliance (see Klevmark[25]) and the greater the chance of provoking involuntary detrusor contractions.[26] Most filling is at a "medium" rate between 10 mL/min and 100 mL/min, typically 50 mL/min. In children and patients with neuropathic bladder disorders, the filling rate should be very slow (<10 mL/min) because faster filling may produce artifactual bladder activity.[27] The physiologic bladder filling rate can be estimated by the formula, [Body Mass (Kg)/4] in mL/min.

The patient is asked to inform the investigator of any bladder sensations, but not to void until "permission" is given. The investigator should note the volumes at which the first sensation of bladder filling, the normal desire to void, and a strong desire to void occur. Any abnormal sensation, such as urgency, must be recorded on the trace and most modern systems have event markers for this. The bladder should be filled until the patient is comfortably full. Regular coughs during filling ensure the quality of pressure transmission.

It is important to remember that the aim of the investigation is to reproduce the patient's symptoms and to find a pathophysiologic explanation for them. With this in mind, there should be a continuous dialogue with the patient throughout the study because, as mentioned, urodynamic findings are relevant only when related to symptoms.

The filling cystometrogram should assess:

- Bladder sensation
- Detrusor activity
- Bladder compliance
- Urethral function
- Bladder capacity

Bladder Sensation

As Wyndaele notes,[28] the investigator should note the filling volume at which the following sensations occur:

- First sensation of bladder filling, when the patient is first aware of his or her bladder filling
- Normal desire to void, the feeling that leads the patient to pass urine at the next convenient moment although voiding could be delayed
- Strong desire to void, the persistent desire to void *without* the fear of leakage

Bladder sensation may be normal, increased, reduced, or absent. Pain or urgency (the persistent desire to void *with* a fear of leakage) are abnormal sensations.

Detrusor Activity

During filling detrusor activity may be normal or increased (overactivity). Normal detrusor function allows bladder filling with little or no change in pressure, and no involuntary phasic contractions occur despite provocation. Detrusor overactivity is a urodynamic observation characterized by involuntary detrusor contractions during the filling phase. These contractions may be spontaneous or provoked. There is no lower limit of pressure rise for an involuntary contraction, but it is difficult to interpret changes of less than 5 cm H_2O (Fig. 22-4).

There are certain recognized patterns of detrusor overactivity (DO):

- *Phasic DO* is defined by the characteristic wave form.
- *Unsuppressable DO* is seen when a detrusor contraction occurs at cystometric capacity and results in voiding that cannot be suppressed. There may or may not be associated sensations.

Sustained high-pressure detrusor contractions may be seen in patients with spinal cord injury. Detrusor overactivity incontinence is incontinence due to an involuntary contraction.

Detrusor overactivity should be qualified according to cause:

- *Neurogenic DO* when there is a relevant neurologic condition (detrusor hyper-reflexia)
- *Idiopathic DO* when there is no clear cause (detrusor instability)

In some patients DO is provoked by certain stimuli such as changing position, coughing, hand washing, or running water.[29] The person taking the medical history should enquire about such stimuli so that if spontaneous DO is not seen during filling provocation, known

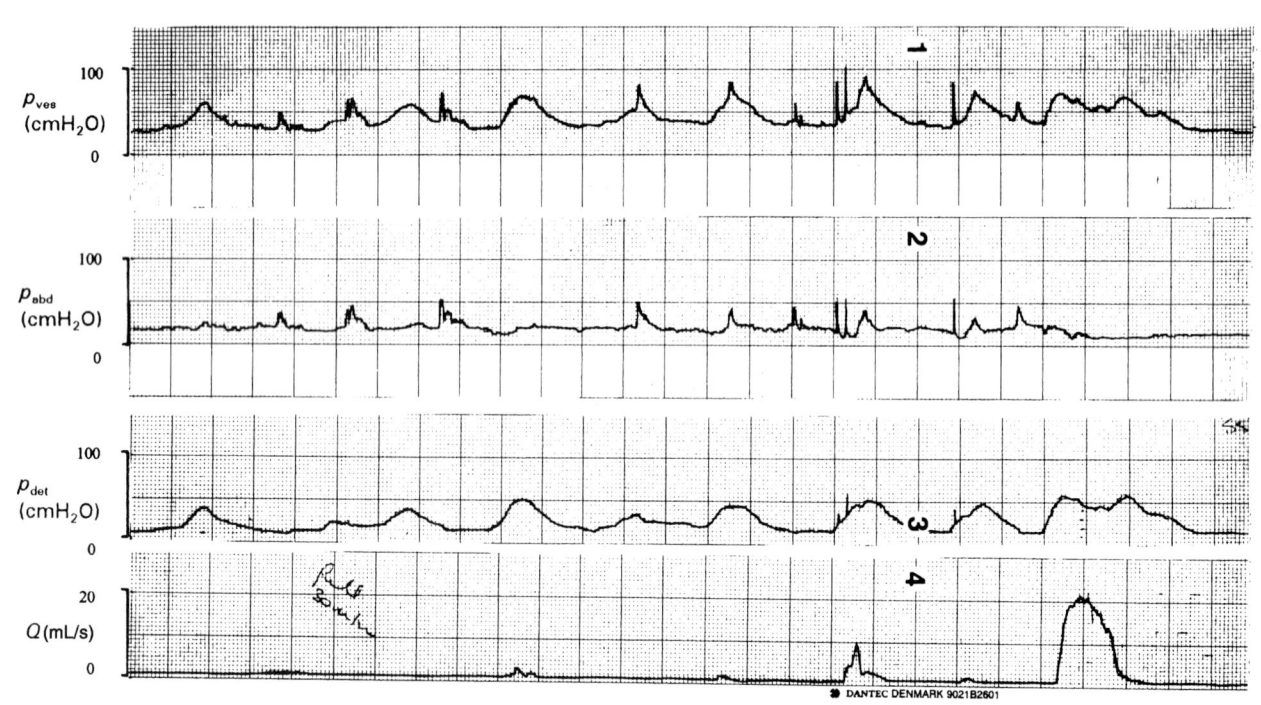

FIGURE 22-4 Detrusor overactivity. A multichannel trace showing multiple involuntary phasic detrusor contractions, four of which cause leakage seen on the flow rate trace. A normal void occurs at the end of the recording. P_{ves}, intravesical pressure; P_{abd}, abdominal pressure; P_{det}, detrusor pressure; Q, flow rate.

provocative stimuli can be tried. It is important to ask whether any DO observed correlates to the patient's usual symptoms because DO might be an artifact of the investigation. Phasic DO may not be accompanied by any sensation, in which case it is probably not clinically significant. Typically, however, phasic DO gives rise to the symptom of urgency and may lead to urge incontinence.

Bladder Compliance

Bladder compliance describes the relationship between change in bladder volume and change in detrusor pressure in terms of the increase in bladder volume per centimeter of water increase in pressure (mL/cm H_2O) (Fig. 22-5).

In normal bladder function there should be little change in intravesical pressure from empty to full. Normal compliance is greater than 40 mL/cm H_2O. To calculate compliance, the measurements should be taken of the detrusor pressure before filling starts and the detrusor pressure at cystometric capacity (or immediately before the start of any detrusor contraction that causes significant leakage).

The observation of reduced bladder compliance during conventional filling is often related to relatively fast bladder filling. If bladders are filled at physiologic rates, then there is little or no pressure change.[25]

Urethral Function

During the filling phase the urethral closure mechanism may be normal or incompetent.

- Normal urethral function maintains a positive urethral closure pressure during filling even in the presence of increased abdominal pressure, although DO may overcome it. The normal closure pressure decreases immediately prior to micturition to allow flow.
- Incompetent urethral function allows leakage of urine in the absence of a detrusor contraction. This leakage may be due to intravesical pressure exceeding resting intraurethral pressure (genuine stress incontinence, GSI, also known as urodynamic stress incontinence) or an involuntary fall in urethral pressure (urethral relaxation incontinence.)

Genuine stress incontinence is demonstrated by asking the patient to cough or perform a Valsalva test. (See section on abdominal leak-point pressures.)

If symptoms of stress incontinence are present but no leak is seen by the time the bladder is full, the filling catheter should be removed and the cough repeated. If no leak is seen, the female patient is asked to separate her legs widely and cough again. Stress incontinence may also be provoked in both men and women by exercises such as jumping up and down or jogging on the spot. When performing standard urodynamics without imaging, the external urethral meatus must be observed during these provocations.

Bladder Capacity

In examining patients with reduced or absent sensation, the investigator should refer to the frequency–volume chart for guidance on how much to fill the bladder. Otherwise, the maximum cystometric capacity is the volume at which the patient feels he or she can no longer delay micturition.

Quality Control During Cystometry

All cystometric equipment should be checked and calibrated regularly. The pump used for filling should be checked for accuracy of filling rate by using a stopwatch and measuring cylinder. The urodynamic pressure recording machinery should be calibrated with reference to the manual. All fluid-filled systems should be "primed" at the start of the study by flushing with fluid to exclude air. Zeroing and then raising the manometer tubing 100 cm and confirming that the pressure reading is now 100 cm H_2O will indicate the calibration of the pressure transducers. During the study, regular coughs, every minute, are requested from the patient to confirm acceptable and equal pressure transmission through the abdominal and intravesical lines. The cough spikes on the cystometrogram should be equal for p_{ves} and p_{abd} with a rapid rise and fall. There should be minimal change in the detrusor pressure line. If this is not the case, the lines must be reflushed and inspected for loose connections or possible loss of correct position.

These procedures will help to reduce measurement artifacts, but some "physiologic" artifacts may cause confusion. In particular, rectal contractions occur relatively frequently during urodynamic studies. When interpreting a cystometrogram, it is essential to refer to the abdominal and intravesical pressure lines and not to rely simply on the subtracted detrusor pressure (Fig. 22-6).

Ambulatory Studies

Catheter-mounted transducers and computerization of equipment have allowed the development of ambulatory urodynamic studies (AUDS). In these studies

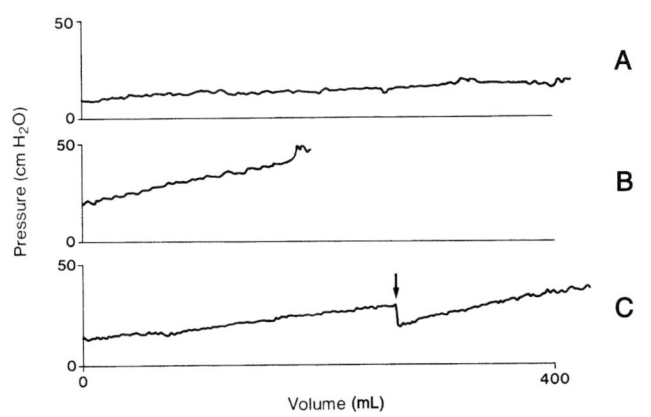

FIGURE 22-5 Various responses to filling. **A,** Normal cystometrogram. **B,** Constantly reduced compliance. **C,** Reduced compliance due to fast filling. When the infusion is stopped (*arrow*), the pressure falls immediately, only to rise again when the infusion is restarted.

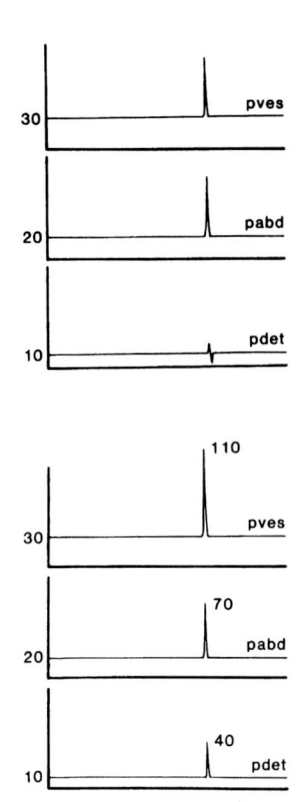

FIGURE 22-6 Quality control. Upper traces show good subtraction of a single cough with a small artifact on the p_{det} trace. Lower traces show inadequate subtraction, which requires an equipment check. P_{ves}, intravesical pressure; P_{abd}, abdominal pressure; P_{det}, detrusor pressure.

catheter-mounted transducers are connected to a portable microprocessor that is worn over the shoulder, allowing the patient to move around. This freedom of movement allows the patient to reproduce the activities that cause incontinence or other symptoms. Ambulatory urodynamic studies are used when conventional urodynamics fail to provide an explanation for the patient's symptoms.[30]

Typically, three micturition cycles are recorded: resting, ambulant, and exercise cycles. The equipment has an event marker facility for the patient to record symptoms such as urgency. Interpretation of AUDS can be difficult and is time-consuming. Objective recording of urine loss is difficult and requires the wearing of a pad that is able to electronically detect leakage. During voiding, recording equipment should be connected to flowmeters to allow synchronous pressure–flow studies.

Ambulatory studies are most frequently used to provide diagnoses for unexplained incontinence, but have generated much interesting data on bladder function in general. AUDS have confirmed that poor compliance seen on conventional cystometry is an artifact of bladder filling speed and during AUDS low compliance is replaced by phasic detrusor overactivity. Interestingly, AUDS on normal (*asymptomatic*) individuals have shown a 30% incidence of detrusor overactivity.

PRESSURE–FLOW STUDIES

With the technical advances that allowed accurate cystometry came the possibility of accurate measurement of intravesical pressure and urine flow rate during voiding. The importance of pressure–flow studies lies in the limitations of uroflowmetry: Flow is a result of the interaction between the expressive forces of the bladder or abdomen and the resistance of the bladder outlet. A low flow rate may be associated with a high voiding pressure or with a weak voiding pressure. A normal flow does not exclude bladder outlet obstruction.

At the completion of filling, when cystometric capacity is reached, the filling catheter is removed, pressure transmission is checked with a cough, and permission to void is given. For normal voiding the patient should ideally be left in private; when imaging (video) studies are being performed, however, this is not possible. The patient voids into a flowmeter while intravesical pressure and abdominal pressure are recorded simultaneously. The patient is asked to void to completion. At the completion of voiding, another cough is used to confirm the lines have remained in position.

Definitions

The following definitions[10] apply to each of the pressure curves:

- *Premicturition pressure* is the pressure recorded immediately before the initial isovolumetric contraction.
- *Opening pressure* is the pressure recorded at the onset of urine flow. There is a delay of 0.5 to 1 second in the recording of flow caused by the time it takes for urine to reach the flowmeter.
- *Opening time* is the time that elapses from the initial rise in detrusor pressure to the onset of flow. This interval is the initial isovolumetric contraction period.
- *Maximum pressure* is the maximum value of the measured pressure.
- *Pressure at maximum flow* is the minimum pressure recorded at maximum measured flow rate.
- *Closing pressure* is the pressure measured at the end of measured flow.
- *Minimal voiding pressure* is the minimum pressure during measurable flow.
- *Flow delay* is the time interval between a change in bladder pressure and the corresponding change in measured flow. (Fig. 22-7)

Again, for ease of interpretation, detrusor activity and urethral function should be considered separately. Detrusor activity may be normal, underactive, or acontractile. The normal detrusor contracts under voluntary control to empty the bladder completely with a normal flow rate. The underactive detrusor contraction is of reduced strength or duration and results in either prolonged bladder emptying or a failure to achieve complete emptying. Acontractile function is inability to demonstrate bladder contraction during the urodynamic study.

Detrusor contractility as represented by detrusor pressure is affected by outlet resistance. For instance,

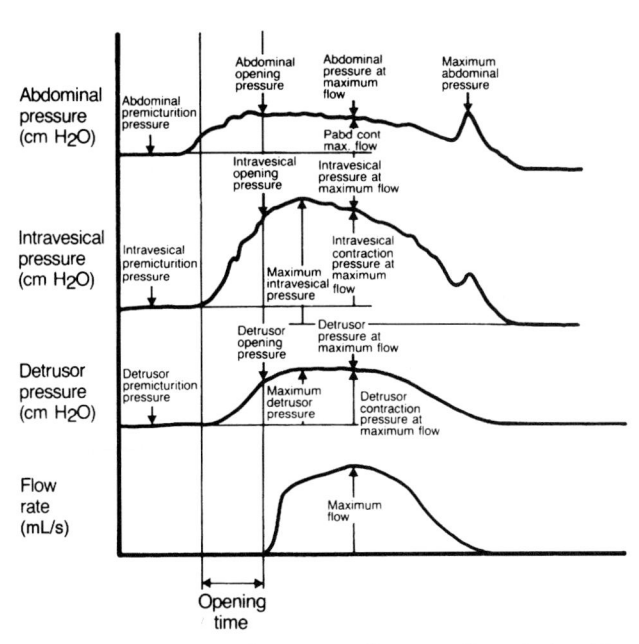

FIGURE 22-7 Diagram of a pressure–flow recording of micturition with nomenclature recommended by the International Continence Society. P_{abd}, abdominal pressure.

a normal detrusor contraction will be recorded as a high-pressure contraction if there is significant outlet resistance, as there is with BOO. In women with low urethral resistance, a normal contraction may produce only a small pressure change.

During voiding, urethral function can be normal or obstructive. A normal urethra opens to allow the bladder to be emptied and is relaxed throughout voiding. Urethral obstruction is usually due to mechanical obstruction, but may be secondary to urethral overactivity. Urethral overactivity can be due to one of the following conditions:

- *Dysfunctional voiding* is characterized by an interrupted flow rate due to involuntary intermittent contractions of the pelvic floor in neurologically normal patients (usually children).
- *Detrusor sphincter dyssynergia (DSD)* occurs in patients with neurologic disabilities when involuntary intermittent contractions of the intraurethral striated muscle cause an interrupted flow.
- *Nonrelaxing sphincter obstruction* occurs in patients with a neurologic lesion and is characterized by a nonrelaxed, partly obstructed urethra, causing a reduced urine flow. This type of obstruction is seen, for example, in patients who have spina bifida and patients who have had radical pelvic surgery (e.g., Wertheim's hysterectomy).

Mechanical Urethral Obstruction

Bladder outlet obstruction can occur at any site from the bladder neck to the external urethral meatus, but is it most often a result of benign prostatic obstruction in the male. All urethral obstruction leads to increased voiding pressures. Various nomograms have been constructed,[19,31] to plot flow rate against detrusor pressure. Working back from studies of men who had had successful surgery for BOO has made it possible to define areas on these nomograms that correspond to proven BOO. Further, by calculating the relationship between pressure and flow from these nomograms, it is possible to produce an equation to diagnose BOO without reference to the nomogram. This calculation gives the Bladder Outlet Obstruction Index, or BOOI.[32]

$$BOOI = P_{det}Q_{max} - 2Q_{max}$$

If the BOOI is greater than 40, then BOO exists; if it is below 20, then no BOO exists. In the range from 20 to 40, the result is equivocal (Fig. 22-8).

This work relates to BOO in the male. Little research has been done on defining detrusor and bladder outlet

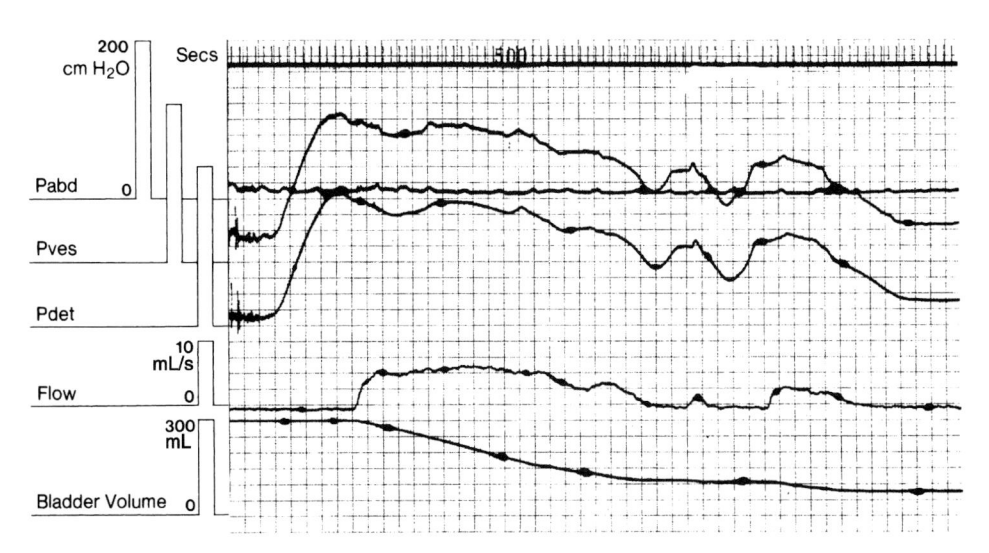

FIGURE 22-8 Pressure–flow study of urination by a 62-year old man with bladder outlet obstruction. P_{abd}, abdominal pressure; P_{ves}, intravesical pressure; P_{det}, detrusor pressure.

function during voiding in women. This lack is in part because the principle clinical problems in women are filling-phase abnormalities: urethral incompetence (stress incontinence) and detrusor overactivity. Moreover, the therapeutic maneuvers to improve voiding function in women (e.g., urethral dilatation and intermittent catheterization) tend to be relatively safe and complication free.

A Bladder Contractility Index (BCI) and a Bladder Voiding Efficiency (BVE) index have also been described,[32] allowing further definition of voiding function.

$$BCI = p_{det}Q_{max} + 5Q_{max}$$

$$BVE = (voided\ vol/total\ bladder\ capacity) \times 100$$

Artifacts During Pressure–Flow Studies

The pressure–flow void should always be compared with the initial free flow. Voiding or slippage of the urethral catheter can occur, and it gives a typical pressure trace. The environment in which the study is performed may make it difficult for some patients to void, especially if they are being observed by others. Overfilling of the bladder also makes normal voiding difficult. Detrusor overactivity may give a misleading trace; the premicturition pressure may be very high, giving the appearance of obstruction.

URETHRAL PRESSURE PROFILOMETRY

The *urethral pressure profile (UPP)* measures the intraluminal pressure along the length of the urethra with the bladder at rest. Two techniques are employed; the most widely used is the Brown and Wickham technique,[33] which measures the pressure required to perfuse a catheter at a constant rate as it is withdrawn through the urethra. The catheter has two opposing eyeholes, 5 cm from the tip, through which the perfusion fluid escapes into the urethra or bladder. Catheter tip transducers can also be used, but there is a rotational effect depending on the position the transducer faces: Pressure is highest if it is anterior facing and lowest if posterior facing, so the transducer should point laterally.

In each technique the catheter is slowly withdrawn through the urethra by an automatic pulling device set to 1 mm/sec. The occlusive pressure of the urethral walls is thus measured (Fig. 22-9).

Maximum urethral pressure is the maximum pressure of the measured profile. *Maximum urethral closure pressure (MUCP)* is the difference between the maximum urethral pressure and the intravesical pressure. *Functional profile length* is the length of the urethra along which the urethral pressure exceeds intravesical pressure.

The static UPP is performed with the patient supine and with the bladder empty or filled with a specified volume. A stress UPP has been described in which the UPP is measured during periods of intermittent stress

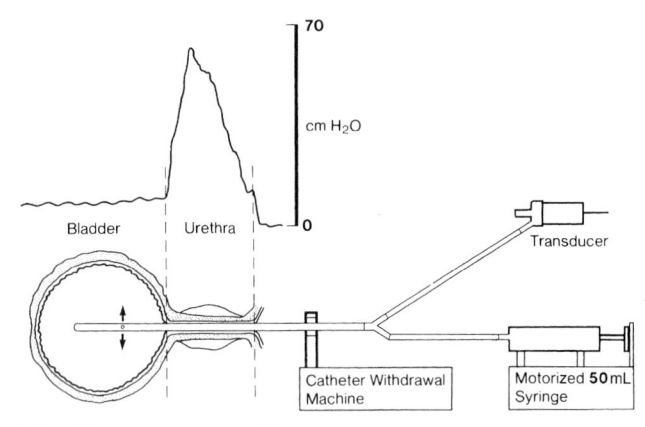

FIGURE 22-9 Brown and Wickham technique.

(coughing). However, the stress UPP is technically difficult to perform and is rarely used now.

The UPP has significant limitations: It cannot diagnose stress incontinence and many women with low UPPs are continent, and vice versa. It cannot be used to diagnose BOO. In postprostatectomy incontinence, however, there is a close association between sphincter damage and reduced maximum urethral closure pressure. In women with unexplained incontinence, measurement of MUCP for 2 minutes may show urethral instability. In patients being considered for urinary undiversion, the MUCP can indicate whether an artificial urinary sphincter or bladder neck suspension is necessary. In women with genuine stress incontinence, a very low MUCP (<20 cm H_2O) is associated with poor surgical outcome and these women require more "obstructive" surgery to ensure continence. In women with idiopathic urethral sphincter overactivity (Fowler's syndrome), the MUCP is usually abnormally high (>100 cm H_2O).

REFERENCES

1. Perez L, Webster G: The history of urodynamics. Neurourol Urodyn 11:1–21, 1992.
2. Lewis P, Abrams P: Urodynamic protocol and central review of data for clinical trials. in lower urinary tract dysfunction. Br J Urol 85 (suppl 1):20–31, 2000.
3. Bates C, Whiteside C, Turner Warwick R: Synchronous urine pressure flow cystourethrography with special reference to stress and urge incontinence. Br J Urol 42:714–723, 1970.
4. Jarvis G, Hall S, Stamp S, et al: An assessment of urodynamic investigation in incontinent women. Br J Obstet Gynaecol 87:873–896, 1980.
5. Powell P, Shepherd A, Lewis P, et al: The accuracy of clinical diagnosis assessed urodynamically. Proc 10th meeting ICS, Los Angeles, 1980, pp 3–4.
6. James M, Jackson S, Shepherd A, et al: Pure stress leakage symptomatology: Is it safe to discount detrusor instability? Br J Obstet Gynaecol 106:1255–1258, 1999.
7. Abrams P: The principles of urodynamics. In Abrams P: Urodynamics, 2nd ed. London, Springer-Verlag, 1997.
8. Dajani A, Bisno A, Chung K, et al: Prevention of bacterial endocarditis: Recommendations of the American Heart Association. JAMA 264:2919–2922, 1990.

9. Trop C, Bennett C: Autonomic Dysreflexia and its urologic implications: A review. J Urol 146:1461–1469, 1991.
10. Abrams P, Blaivas J, Stanton S, et al (ICS Committee on Standardisation of Terminology): The standardisation of terminology of lower urinary tract function. Scand J Urol Nephrol Suppl 114:5–19, 1988.
11. Lewis P, Abrams P: Urodynamic protocol and central review of data for clinical trials in lower urinary tract dysfunction. Br J Urol 85 (suppl 1):20–31, 2000.
12. Garrelts B von: Analysis of micturition. A new method of recording the voiding of the bladder. Acta Chir Scand 112: 326–340, 1956.
13. Siroky M, Olssen C, Krane R: The flow rate nomogram: I. Development. J Urol 122:665–668, 1979.
14. Marshall V, Ryall R, Austin M, et al: The use of urinary flow rates obtained from voided volumes less than 150 mL in the assessment of voiding ability. Br J Urol 55:28–33, 1983.
15. Drach G, Layton T, Bottaccini M: A method of adjustment of male peak urinary flow rate for varying age and volume voided. J Urol 128:960–962, 1982.
16. Siroky M, Olssen C, Krane R: The flow rate nomogram: II. Clinical correlations. J Urol 123:208–210, 1980.
17. Haylen B, Parys B, Anyaegbunam W, et al: Urine flow rates in male and female urodynamic patients compared with Liverpool nomograms. Br J Urol 65:483–487, 1990.
18. Kadow C, Howells S, Lewis P, et al: A flow rate nomogram for normal males over the age of 50. Proceedings of the 15th Annual Meeting of the International Continence Society, London 1985, 138–139.
19. Lim C, Abrams P: The Abrams-Griffiths Nomogram. World J Urol 13:34–39, 1995.
20. Massey J, Abrams P: Obstructed voiding in the female. Br J Urol 55:28–33, 1988.
21. Grino P, Bruskewitz R, Blaivas J, et al: Maximum urinary flow rate by uroflowmetry: Automatic or visual interpretation. J Urol 149:339–341, 1993.
22. Abrams P: Urodynamic Technique. In Abrams P, Urodynamics, 2nd ed. London, Springer-Verlag,1997.
23. Torrens M: A comparative evaluation of carbon dioxide and water cystometry and sphincterometry. Proceedings of the 7th Annual Meeting of the International Continence Society, Portoroz, Slovenia, 7:103–104, 1977.
24. Wein A, Hanno P, Dixon D, et al: The reproducibility and interpretation of carbon dioxide cystometry. J Urol 120:205–206, 1978.
25. Klevmark B: Motility of the urinary bladder in cats during filling at physiological rates. 1. Intravesical pressure patterns studied by a new method of cystometry. Acta Physiol Scanda 90:565–577, 1974.
26. Webb R, Styles R, Griffiths C, et al: Ambulatory monitoring of bladder pressures in patients with low compliance as a result of neurogenic bladder function. Br J Urol 64:150, 1989.
27. Thomas D: Clinical urodynamics in neurogenic bladder dysfunction. Urol Clin N Am 6:237–253, 1979.
28. Wyndaele J: Normality in urodynamics studied in healthy adults. J Urol 161:899–902.
29. Papa Petros P, Elmsten U: Tests for detrusor instability in women. Acta Obstet Gynecol Scand 72:661–667, 1993.
30. Swithinbank L, James M, Shepherd A, et al: The role of ambulatory urodynamic monitoring in clinical urological practice. Neurourol and Urodyn 18:3:215–222, 1999.
31. Schafer W: Basic principles and clinical application of advanced analysis of bladder voiding function. Urol Clin N Am 17:553–566, 1990.
32. Abrams P: Bladder outlet obstruction index, bladder contractility index and bladder voiding efficiency: Three simple indices to define bladder voiding function. Br J Urol 84:14–15, 1999.
33. Brown M, Wickham J: The urethral pressure profile. Br J Urol 41:211–217.

CHAPTER 23

Urodynamic Evaluation

EDWARD J. McGUIRE ■ PAUL ABRAMS

ELECTROMYOGRAPHIC STUDIES

Early studies of the electromyographic (EMG) activity of the external anal and urethral sphincter and pelvic floor muscles were usually of the interference pattern type. These studies broadly showed the guarding reflex and relaxation, or lack of relaxation, of the external sphincter and pelvic floor at the time of urination.[1,2] Studies in male patients with spinal cord injury showed lack of proper coordination and sequencing of detrusor and external sphincter responses to bladder filling in patients with suprasacral spinal cord lesions. Later, similar studies in female patients showed similar findings. The normal relationship between the external urethral sphincter–pelvic floor musculature complex and the bladder is maintained by a complex, multilevel neural network. However, overall, the relationship is reciprocal in that when the external sphincter and pelvic floor are active, the detrusor is not, and vice versa.[3-5]

Detrusor activity seems to be inhibited by suprasacral brain stem influences that drive the alpha motor neuron activity that produces pelvic floor and external sphincter contractility. The brain stem "centers" appear to control and direct the proper sequence of external sphincter and bladder responses to filling, including storage and micturition responses, through descending bulbospinal tracts. Bladder filling is associated with increased EMG activity from the pelvic floor and external sphincter, and that activity, in turn, is associated with detrusor motor inhibition. On the other hand, micturition seems to be initiated and sustained by relaxation of the external sphincter and pelvic floor musculature.[6] Loss of brain stem effects on lower urinary tract function driven by sacral cord activity interferes with the coordination and sequence of the detrusor and external sphincter responses, although a semblance of normal activity is maintained. Thus, detrusor–sphincter dyssynergia in patients with suprasacral spinal cord injury is associated with lack of guarding reflex responses to filling in the external sphincter and pelvic floor. At some point, a bladder contraction ensues, and is followed quickly by external sphincter contractile activity and then by partial inhibition of the bladder. This partial inhibition is followed by detrusor contraction. This kind of discoordinate activity may go on repetitively.[5,6] The nature of this activity suggests that reciprocal inhibition occurs locally within the sacral spinal cord, but is normally controlled by supraspinal centers.

The reciprocal relationship underpins our ability to affect detrusor activity by electrical stimulation of the external urethral sphincter, anal sphincter, pelvic floor, or posterior tibial nerve and sacral roots. The activity of the pelvic floor muscles has a direct effect, and probably an indirect effect as well, on detrusor excitability and the volume threshold that prompts a micturition reflex response. Very early studies (e.g., Caldwell[7]) in patients with mixed incontinence treated with direct electrical stimulation of the anal sphincter showed a dramatic effect on detrusor contractile incontinence and a much less dramatic effect on urethral urinary incontinence. More recent studies led to efforts to use peripheral neural stimulation to inhibit detrusor activity, and finally, to modulate bladder and urethral behavior by stimulation of the sacral roots.[8-11]

ELECTROMYOGRAPHIC DATA AND PELVIC FLOOR DYSFUNCTION

The use of EMG techniques is largely restricted to the study of detrusor–sphincter dyssynergia, which is seen in patients with lesions between the sacral cord centers and the brain stem, and possibly also to the study of a syndrome of urinary retention that is associated with EMG abnormalities in young women. This syndrome was described by Fowler and Kirby in 1985 and 1986.[12,13] There appears to be a relationship between pelvic floor musculature activity, which can be assessed by EMG techniques, and urinary stress continence. Prolapse of the vagina may be related as well.[14-17] Smith and associates[18] studied women with stress incontinence, and compared EMG findings in that group with those in normal control subjects. Fiber density was higher in patients with stress incontinence, those with stress incontinence and vaginal prolapse, and those with prolapse alone, when compared with normal control subjects. This finding suggests that denervation and reinnervation had occurred in the affected patients. Snooks and associates[19] found prolonged pudenal latency in patients with urinary stress incontinence. In a later study, in addition to increased pudendal latency, Snooks and associates[20] found increased fiber density in 14 multiparous women, suggesting that occult pudendal neural damage was incurred at the time of childbirth. How these findings are actually related to stress incontinence of various types, or to prolapse, is not clear.[21] Neural conduction times provide little information about function. DeLancey[22] showed that significant direct injury to the levator musculature may be incurred by childbirth, and some of these changes appear irreversible. Thus, single-fiber or isolated EMG studies in patients with a clinical diagnosis of stress incontinence have little value with respect to the etiology of incontinence syndromes or prolapse.[21]

VIDEO URODYNAMICS

This study, perhaps first described by Hodgkinson[23] and later by Bates and colleagues,[24] is probably the best single method to evaluate bladder function. Clearly, it is the best method to evaluate urethral function and dysfunction. As noted by Blaivas,[25] the combined use of video imaging and recording of bladder pressure, urethral pressure, flow rate, voiding urethral profilometry, and leak-point pressure testing provides precise information under visual control, which is unobtainable with any other method or combination of methods. Video urodynamic studies allow the precise diagnosis of intrinsic sphincter dysfunction and permit the detection of vesicoureteral reflux and urethral leakage. Incontinence or reflux complicates the determination of altered compliance in the absence of video monitoring. Bladder diverticula are seen immediately on video study, and are often the cause of unexplained urinary retention in men and women. The characterization of micturition and urethral sphincter function is also possible only with video dynamic studies, as is the characterization of anterior vaginal prolapse in the upright position (Fig. 23-1).

EVALUATION OF THE BLADDER

The objectives are to characterize bladder morphology (trabeculation, cellule formation, diverticula, and bladder position), determine the presence of vesicoureteral reflex, and define bladder behavior during filling. These studies involve the determination of bladder compliance and, if a detrusor contraction is elicited, the behavior of the bladder and urethra during detrusor contractility. A low-compliance bladder can cause vesicoureteral reflux and urethral leakage, but here, the expulsive force is detrusor pressure and not abdominal pressure, as it is in patients with true stress incontinence. This is a subtle,

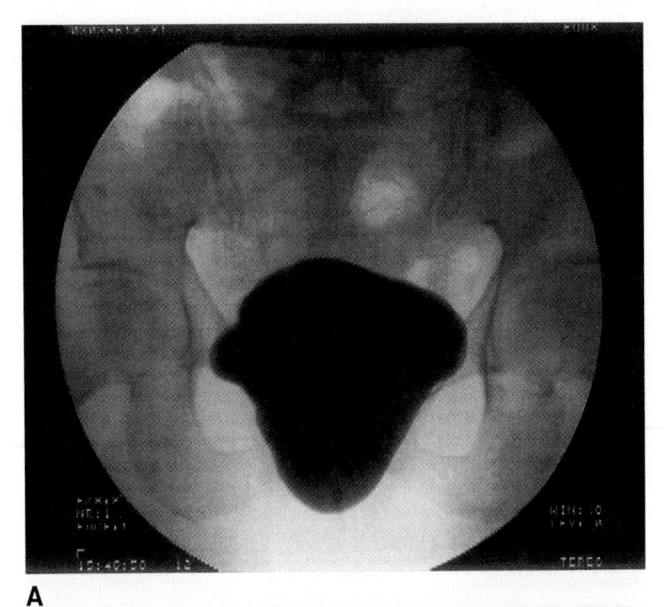

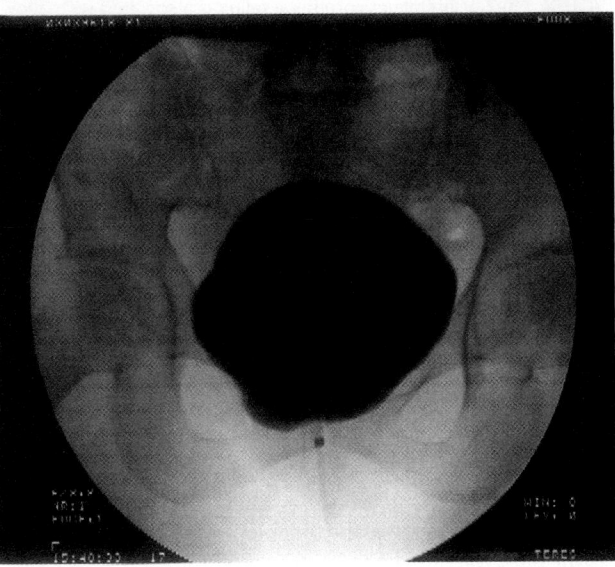

FIGURE 23-1 An upright video image obtained during urodynamic testing shows a central cystocele that is 3 cm distal to the introitus on pelvic examination. This is combined with lateral detachment of vaginal fornices from the arcus tendineus fascia pelvis. The central cystocele is narrow. The lateral detachment is more pronounced on the left than on the right, but is very broad. **A**, During straining. **B**, At rest.

but easily identified condition that may be mistaken for classic stress incontinence (Fig. 23-2).

Leakage from the urethra or vesicoureteral reflux makes the bladder pressure–volume curve (or bladder compliance) look normal or more normal. In patients with vesicoureteral reflux or large bladder diverticula, compliance testing is inaccurate (Fig. 23-3).

EVALUATION OF PROLAPSE

Careful pelvic examination with Pelvic Organ Prolapse-Quantification (POP-Q) scoring is the basic examination, but the position used for the pelvic examination

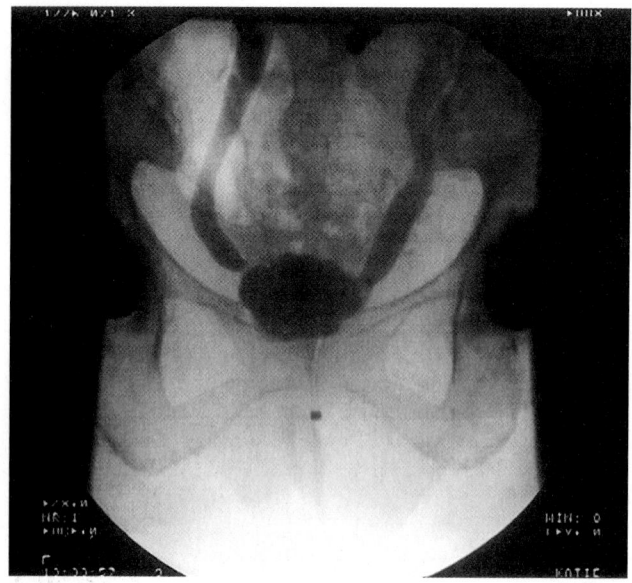

FIGURE 23-2 Bilateral vesicoretheral reflux is associated with a low-compliance bladder. This patient also had severe incontinence, especially when upright or with effort. The expulsive force is detrusor pressure, not abdominal pressure. There is nothing wrong with the sphincter.

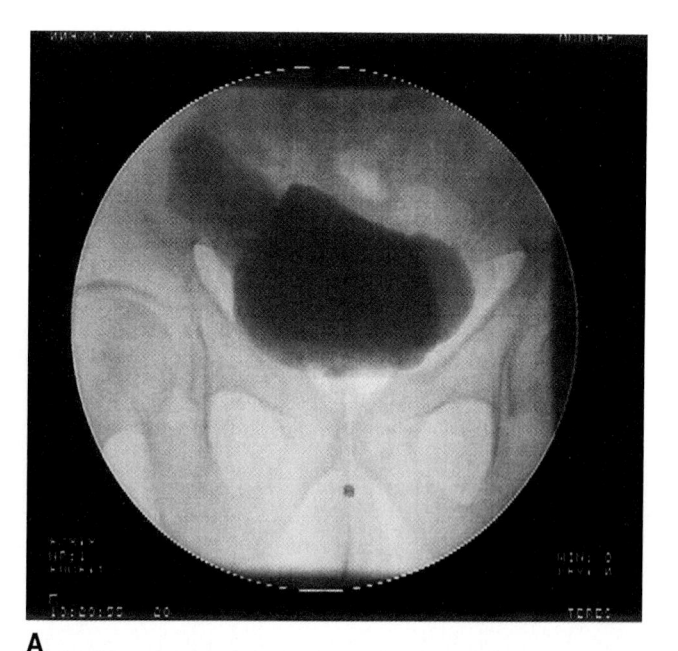

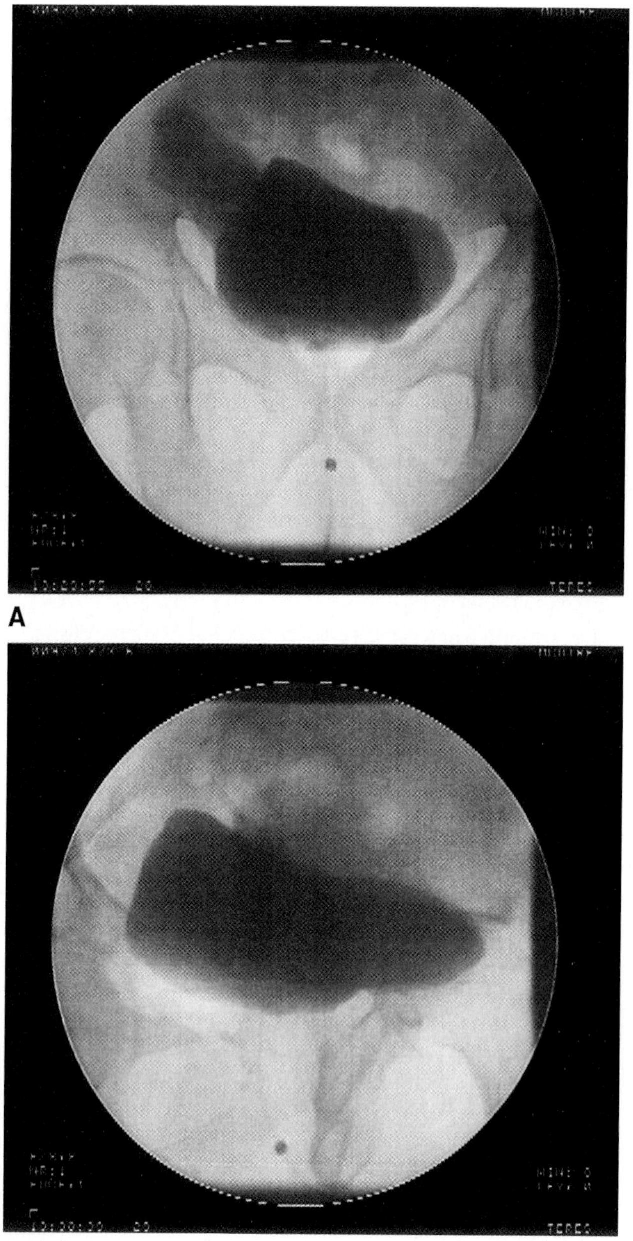

FIGURE 23-3 A, Anterior-posterior view; **B,** Oblique view; A large acquired bladder diverticulum involving most of the bladder dome is seen. The pressure–volume curve was normal and did not suggest obstruction, although a congenital bladder neck obstruction produced the large diverticulum.

can lead to underestimation of the degree of prolapse.[26] Fluoroscopy allows definition of the defect through which the bladder herniates and characterization of the size of a cystocele. It also permits detection of central defects and lateral detachment of the vagina from the arcus tendineus fascia pelvis. In addition, it shows failure of previous suspension procedures on one or both sides (Fig. 23-4 A–C). Perhaps more valuable, however, is the finding that a visible palpable prolapse does not involve the bladder. It is not uncommon to encounter patients with a "cystocele" in whom a vault prolapse, an enterocele, or a rectocele is the problem. Video urodynamic studies are particularly useful in distinguishing between a cystocele and an anterior enterocele, a distinction that can be difficult on the basis of physical examination alone.

ASSESSMENT OF URETHRAL FUNCTION

Assessing urethral function is the best use of the video urodynamic technique. Flurourodynamics lead to the description of intrinsic sphincter dysfunction and proximal urethral failure, and the observation of congenital absence of proximal urethral function in patients with myelodysplasia, and acquired proximal sphincter loss in type III stress incontinence.[27-30] Isolated loss of internal sphincter function (with severe incontinence) also occurs in some patients after abdominal perineal resection for rectal carcinoma and occasionally after radical hysterectomy, but not after complete sacral rhizotomy.[31] In persons with poor function or failure of the proximal urethra, leakage occurs at very low to low abdominal pressures, regardless of the function of the midurethral high-pressure zone and the volitional external sphincter.[32]

Video urodynamic studies allow the precise measurement of closing pressure in the proximal urethra because the pressure sensor can be placed according to operator preference (Fig. 23-5). Video observation facilitates leak-point pressure testing when leakage is driven by detrusor pressure or abdominal pressure because it allows the precise moment of leakage to be determined.

Urethral mobility that is best seen in the oblique projection is precisely characterized by video urodynamics

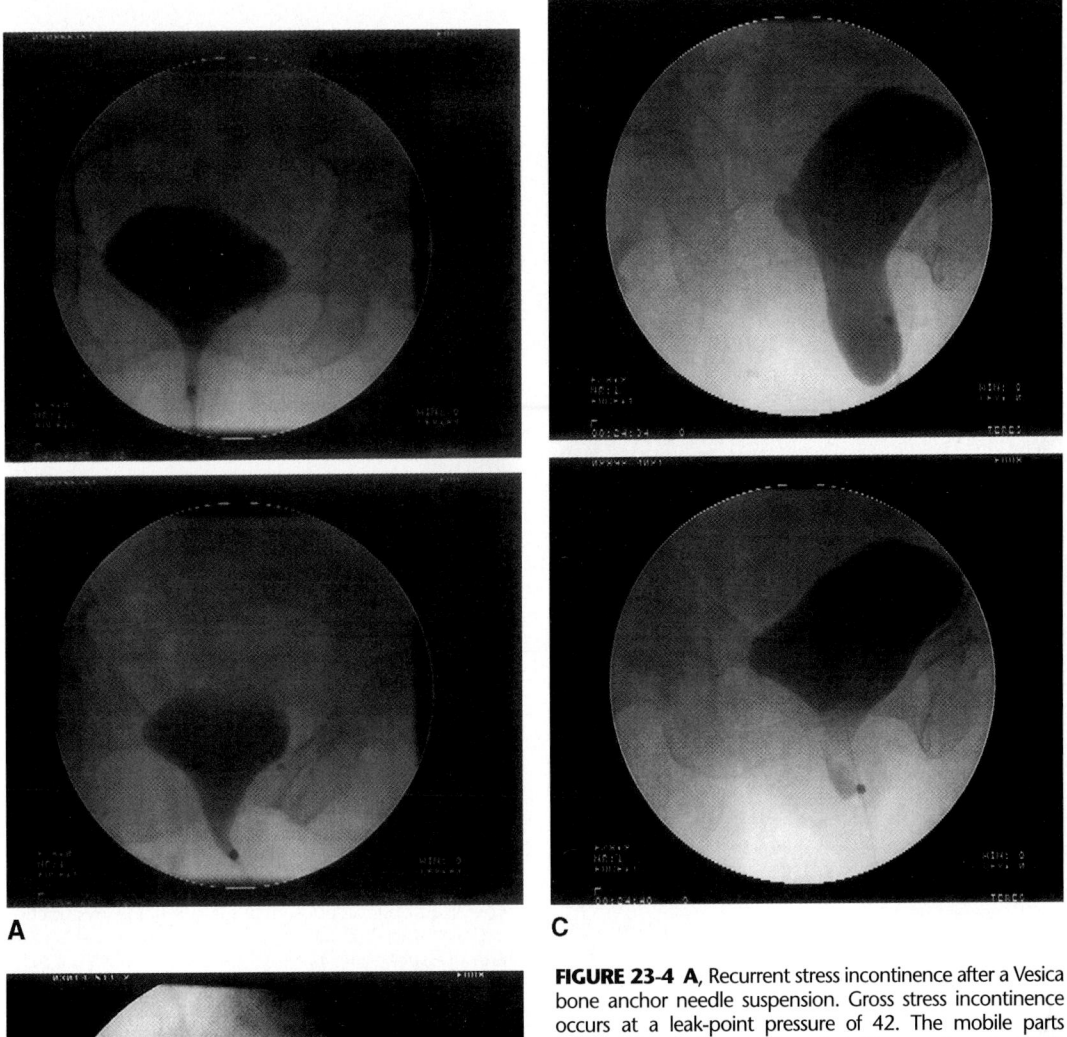

FIGURE 23-4 A, Recurrent stress incontinence after a Vesica bone anchor needle suspension. Gross stress incontinence occurs at a leak-point pressure of 42. The mobile parts include the urethra and central trigone. A cystocele is present, but can be completely reduced with a standard sling procedure. Anterior-posterior view (*top*) and oblique view (*bottom*) shown. **B,** Recurrent stress urinary incontinence after a retropubic suspension. There is mobility of the bladder base, with a broad-based cystocele that has some lateral detachment (worse on the patient's right) and gross urethral mobility. **C,** This study shows a more complex situation, with a central cystocele, but little or no motion of the urethra with straining (*top*). However, the urethra, with the prolapse reduced on pelvic examination, seems much more mobile than shown here. This may be the result of organ competition for the narrow introitus, and the cystocele may support the urethra as it herniates. In this situation, we would perform a urethral suspension on the basis of the pelvic examination findings and the possibility of organ competition for the introitus. Resting view shown at bottom.

(Fig. 23-6). Although these techniques are less well developed, rectal and anal sphincter pressure measurements and studies of rectal accommodation responses and defecation are facilitated by video imaging.

URETHRAL FUNCTION ASSESSMENT

The assessment of urethral function is an area of controversy. Practitioners in urogynecology and urology espouse different methods for the evaluation of urethral function.

URETHRAL PRESSURES

Fluid perfusion systems have been used for many years to determine urethral resistance to egress of the perfusate. The values obtained have been called urethral pressures, even though they are not really urethral pressures. Methods used to measure the urethral pressure profile vary widely, and have never been standardized in terms of catheter size, perfusion aperture type and configuration, inflow rate, inflow pressure, or speed of withdrawal. Even more fundamental is a lack of data

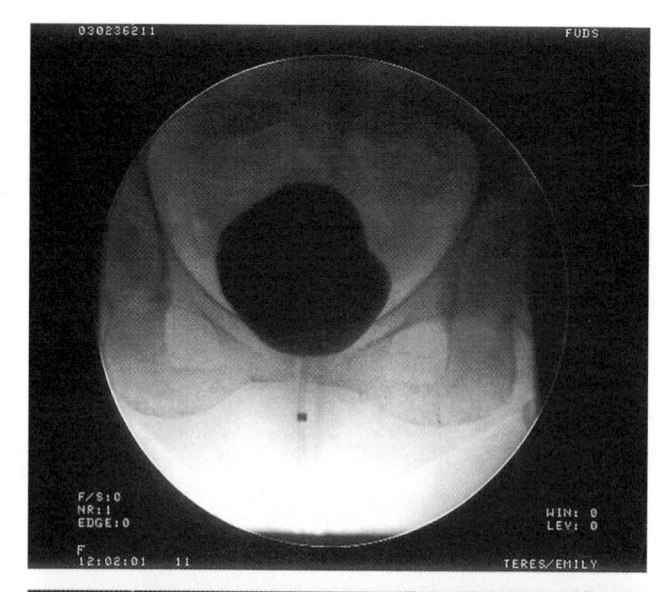

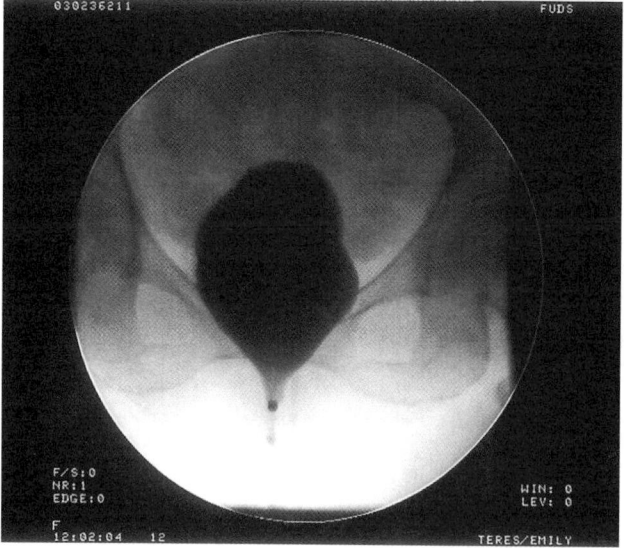

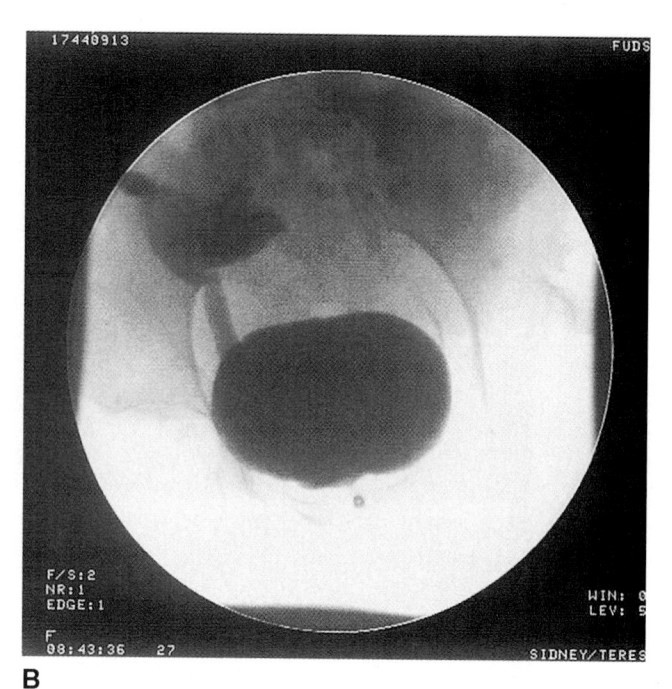

FIGURE 23-5 A, Severe stress incontinence that is a combination of type II (mobility) and intrinsic sphincter dysfunction (leak-point pressure, 36). The radio-opaque marker is seen in the midurethral high-pressure zone. **B,** Vesicoureteral reflux into a pelvic kidney in a young woman with myelodysplasia who had a sling procedure and myectomy. The radio-opaque marker is seen in the proximal urethra, where the pressure recorded by the perfusion system is 15 cm H_2O. This position is immediately under the sling. Reflux into the right pelvic kidney is primary, and is not related to pressure. This is a competent internal sphincter mechanism produced by the sling procedure.

that describe the relationship between urethral resistance to fluid perfusion and resistance by the urethral sphincter to a fluid bolus held in the bladder and acted on by either of two expulsive forces (detrusor pressure and abdominal pressure). Systems have been developed to compensate for the problems seen with perfusion systems, including membrane catheters and microtip pressure transducers. However, these systems are subject to artifacts of position, urethral motion, and patient position.

Collectively, we have made the assumption that "pressure" recorded with these devices is related to urethral function; however, this assumption has not been proven. The most common definition of stress urinary incontinence, "a condition characterized by involuntary urinary leakage when P_{ves} (bladder pressure) exceeds P_{ura} (urethral pressure)," is not technically correct. There is no way to measure P_{ura} during stress. Urethral "pressure" measured by currently available techniques does not correlate with function or, more precisely, with the ability of the urethra to resist abdominal pressure as an expulsive force acting on a bolus of bladder urine. Lose[33] noted that urethral pressure profile values did not allow the diagnosis of stress incontinence to be made, did not change predictably with treatment, and were unrelated to the severity of urinary loss. Dynamic pressure tracings and pressure transmission ratios have all of the problems associated with urethral "pressures," and are often irreproducible in the same patient.[34] In 1987, Sand and colleagues[35] suggested that a "low-pressure urethra" was the reason why a standard retropubic suspension procedure was unsuccessful in some patients. These authors measured maximal urethral closing pressure, which they defined as P_{ura} minus P_{ves}. As such, urethral "pressure" is the numeric value of the hydraulic pressure that is required to allow fluid to flow into the urethra from an aperture in a urethral closing pressure profile catheter minus the pressure recorded in the bladder at the same time. As a result, low-pressure urethra became established as a risk factor for failure of a suspension procedure to

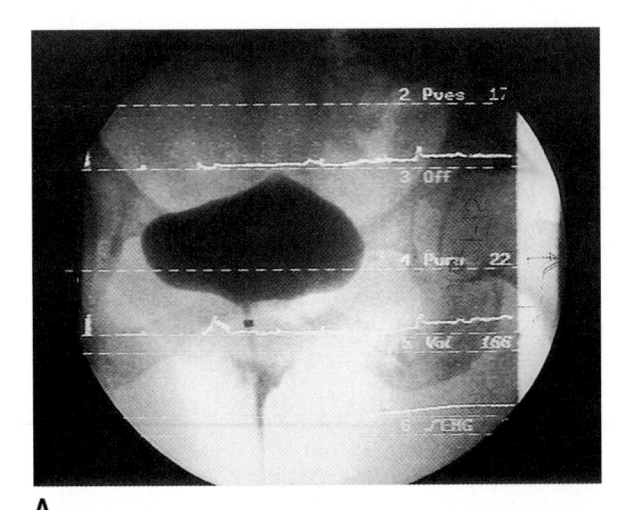

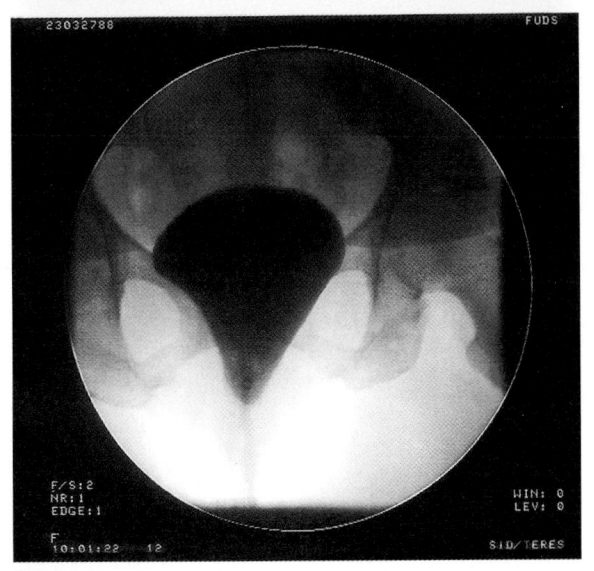

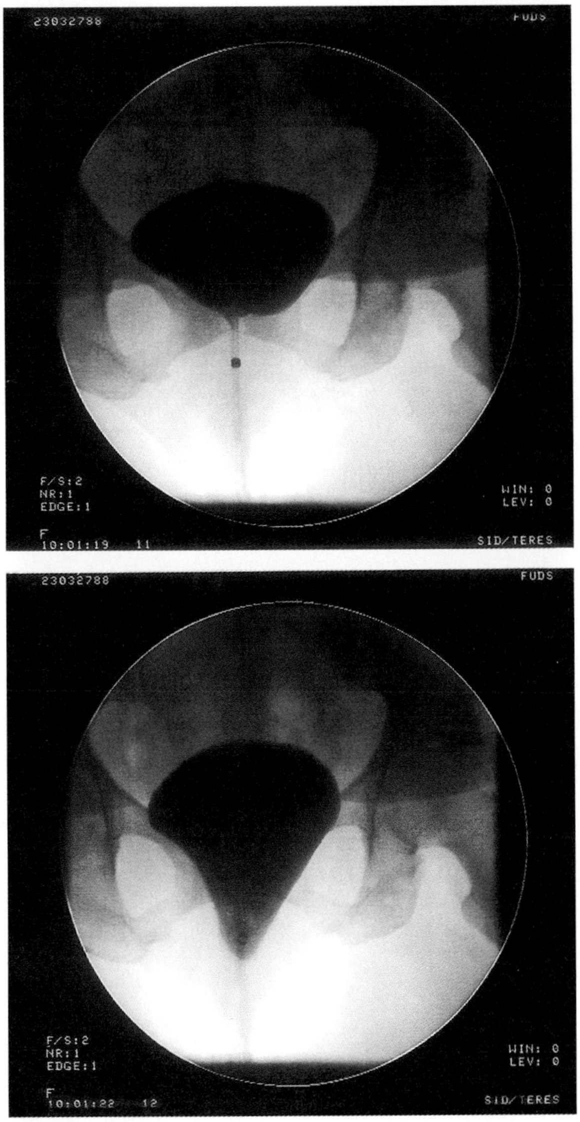

FIGURE 23-6 **A,** Severe stress incontinence with very little mobility. The leak-point pressure is 17. **B,** Some urethral mobility and a grade 4 cystocele are seen, but leakage is easily demonstrated, despite good function of the external sphincter and a peak urethral closing pressure of 65. Leak-point pressure is 38, indicating severe stress incontinence, which is a combination of hypermobility and intrinsic sphincter dysfunction.

cure stress incontinence. A tacit assumption was made that a low-pressure urethra was different from a mobile or hypermobile urethra. Therefore, a low-pressure urethra became the equivalent of intrinsic sphincter dysfunction, which was considered a variant of urethral dysfunction. This variant is characterized by poor closure of the urethra, as measured by maximal urethral closing pressure, as opposed to a mobile urethra, which is associated with a normal maximum urethral closing pressure, or at least one greater than 20 cm H_2O.

Other than real concerns about urethral pressure profile data and assumptions made about urethral function based on those data, other workers have not found that a low-pressure urethra is a common finding in patients who undergo unsuccessful suspension procedures. In addition, in prospective studies, a low-pressure urethra was not a risk factor for failure of suspension procedures.[36,37] Moreover, many studies show that urinary pressure profile data do not correlate with video urodynamic data or with data on vesical pressure at the instant of leakage recorded during continuous ambulatory monitoring studies.[38] Currently, urinary pressure profile data cannot be related specifically to urethral function.

LEAK-POINT PRESSURES

Detrusor leak-point pressures were first described in patients with myelodysplasia. As used in these patients with fixed outlet resistance and a decentralized bladder, the detrusor pressure required to induce leakage, which was generated simply by volume, was measured. This finding was related to upper-tract disease in a convincing way; if the detrusor pressure at leakage was 40 cm H_2O or greater, the risk of upper-tract deterioration was 100% if no treatment was initiated. On the other hand, patients with detrusor pressures at leakage of less than 40 cm H_2O had no such risk. Similar measurements were made over time in patients with spinal cord injury and other conditions, but these measurements involved the precise characterization of detrusor pressure as an expulsive force. In all of these studies, the higher the detrusor pressure required to induce leakage, the higher the risk of serious bladder, ureteral, and renal complications. In patients with meningomyelocele, these data on the interaction of detrusor pressure with the outlet occurred in the face of severe incontinence driven by abdominal pressure in association with congenital absence of function of the internal sphincter, which was common in these children (Fig. 23-7). A later study showed that the detrusor pressure required to induce leakage in patients with myelodysplasia was completely different from the abdominal pressure required to do the same thing.[38] This finding suggested that urethral resistance to detrusor pressure was determined by different factors than resistance to abdominal pressure. For example, a normal urethra does not leak when exposed to fairly high abdominal pressure (≤180 or 190), although a detrusor pressure of 40 to 50 is enough to induce leakage in patients with detrusor instability, even when they try vigorously to stop such leakage.

In several studies, Griffiths[39] and Schafer[40] determined that the detrusor pressure at the time of leakage was a reflection of urethral resistance and was not related to the

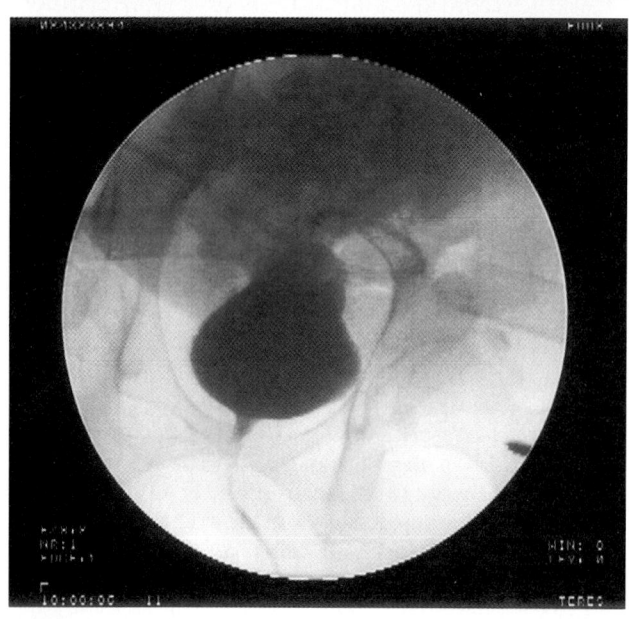

FIGURE 23-7 An open nonfunctional bladder outlet in a 7-year-old child with myelodysplasia who was treated with a vesicostomy for bladder dysfunction, recurrent infections, and pyelonephritis. We perfused the bladder to determine the detrusor pressure at which leakage occurred across the urethra; this pressure was 65. The bladder outlet was always open from the first moment of filling. These data suggest that the vesicostomy was performed for upper-tract dysfunction related to high leak-point pressure; the open bladder neck indicates severe stress incontinence. Thus, closure of the bladder outlet with a sling or a similar method must be combined with bladder augmentation to create a safe, low-pressure, continent lower urinary tract.

strength or power of the detrusor contraction. Thus, if urethral resistance is high enough, very high pressure can develop briefly in a very bad bladder. On the other hand, if urethral resistance at the time of voiding is very low, no measurable pressure might develop in a very good bladder. This concept is also directly applicable to abdominal pressure as an expulsive force. At the instant of leakage, the abdominal pressure that induces leakage is proportional to urethral resistance at that moment. In loose terms, if minimal abdominal pressure causes leakage, then urethral resistance must be low, and if higher abdominal pressures are required, then the urethra must be stronger. These findings have some implication with respect to the type of urethral dysfunction and the best options for treatment. Abdominal leak-point pressures obtained with video urodynamic imaging provide a very good idea of the relative strength of the urethra. In addition, this testing provides an assessment of the degree of urethral mobility and the existence of bladder prolapse. A firm diagnosis of stress incontinence can be made with video urodynamic studies and leak-point pressure testing. If leakage is associated with low leak-point pressures, prospective studies show that suspension operations do not work well, and in this case, slings are a much better choice.[41,42]

PROBLEMS WITH LEAK-POINT PRESSURE TESTING

Obviously, a cystocele or other vaginal prolapse can interfere with accurate leak-point pressure testing. The prolapse protects the urethra from abdominal pressure as an expulsive force because the pressure tends to be dissipated in the prolapse. The prolapsing segment may actually compress the urethra.[8] Reduction of a prolapse sharpens the diagnostic process.

Catheter size also makes a difference in leak-point pressure testing. The original leak-point pressure data were obtained with a triple-lumen 10 Fr urodynamic catheter. No studies have been done to determine leak-point pressure with various catheters controlled by video urodynamic observation.

BLADDER VOLUME

Very small and very large bladder volumes affect leak-point pressure testing. No leakage may occur when bladder volume is very small, because the bolus of urine in the bladder is insufficient to allow abdominal pressure to act. At large and very large bladder volumes, a definite detrusor component operates and leak-point pressure testing is unreliable. The best volume range for leak-point pressure testing is 200 to 250 mL.

REFERENCES

1. Kawakami M: Electromyographic investigation of the human external sphincter muscle of anus. Jpn J Physiol 4:196, 1954.
2. Maizels M, Firlit CF: Pediatric urodynamics: A clinical comparison of surface vs. needle pelvic floor/external sphincter electromyography. J Urol 125:518, 1980.
3. Fam BA, Rossier AB, Blunt K, et al: Experience in the urologic management of 120 early spinal cord injury patients. J Urol 119:485, 1978.
4. Perkash I: Detrusor-sphincter dyssynergia and dyssynergic responses: Recognition and rationale for early modified transurethral sphincterotomy in complete spinal cord lesions. J Urol 120:469, 197.

5. Blaivas JG, Sinha HP, Zayed AA, et al: Detrusor-external sphincter dyssynergia: A detailed electromyographic study. J Urol 125:542, 1981.
6. McGuire EJ, Brady S: Detrusor-sphincter dyssynergia. J Urol 121:783, 1979.
7. Caldwell KPS: The electrical control of sphincter incompetence. Lancet 2:174, 1963.
8. Fall M: Intravaginal electrical stimulation in urinary incontinence: An experimental and clinical study. Medical aspects (thesis). Gotab, Kungalv, 1977.
9. Siegel SW, Catanzaro F, Dijkema HE, et al: Long-term results of a multicenter study on sacral nerve stimulation for treatment of urinary urge incontinence, urgency-frequency, and retention. J Urol 56:87, 2000.
10. Everaert K, DeRidder D, Baert L, et al: Patient satisfaction and complications following sacral nerve stimulation for urinary retention, urge incontinence and perineal pain: A multicenter evaluation. Int Urogynecol J Pelvic Floor Dysfunction 11(4):231, 2000.
11. Walsh IK, Thompson T, Loughridge WG, et al: Non-invasive antidromic neurostimulation: A simple effective method for improving bladder storage. Neurourol Urodynam 20(1):73, 2001.
12. Fowler CJ, Kirby RS: Abnormal electromyographic activities (decelerating burst and complex repetitive discharges) in the striated muscle of the urethral sphincter in 5 women. Br J Urol 57:67, 1985.
13. Fowler CJ, Kirby RS: Electromyography of the urethral sphincter in women with urinary retention. Lancet 1:1455, 1986.
14. Anderson R: A neurogenic element to genuine urinary stress incontinence. Br J Urol 91:41, 1984.
15. Allen R, Hosker G, Smith A, et al: Pelvic floor damage and childbirth: A neurophysiological study. Br J Obstet Gynaecol 97:770, 1990.
16. Deindl FM, Vodusek DB, Hesse U, et al: Activity patterns of pubococcygeal muscles in nulliparous patients. Br J Urol 72:46, 1993.
17. Diendl FM, Vodusek DB, Hesse U, et al: Pelvic floor activity patterns: Comparison of nulliparous continent and stress incontinent women. A kinesiological EMG study. Br J Urol 73:413, 1994.
18. Smith AR, Hosker GL, Warrell DW: The role of partial denervation of the pelvic floor in aetiology of genitourinary prolapse and stress incontinence of urine: A neurophysiological study. Br J Obstet Gynaecol 96:24, 1989.
19. Snooks SJ, Badinoch DF, Tiptaft RC, et al: Perineal nerve damage in genuine stress incontinence. Br J Urol 57:422, 1985.
20. Snooks SJ, Sash M, Mathers SE, et al: Effect of vaginal delivery in the pelvic floor: A 5-year follow up. Br J Surg 77:1358, 1990.
21. Fowler CJ: Clinical neurophysiology. In Stauton SL, Monga AC (eds): Clinical Urogynecology. London, Churchill-Livingstone, 2001, p 161.
22. DeLancey JOL: Personal communication, 2001.
23. Hodgkinson CP: Stress urinary incontinence. Am J Obstet Gynecol 108:1141, 1970.
24. Bates CP, Whiteside CL, Turner-Warwick RT: Synchronous cine pressure flow to cysto urethrography with special reference to stress and urge incontinence. Br J Urol 42:714, 1970.
25. Blaivas JG: Personal communication, 2001.
26. Bump RC, Mattiasson A, Bo K, et al: The standardization of terminology of female pelvic organ prolapse and pelvic floor dysfunction. Am J Obstet Gynecol 175:10, 1996.
27. McGuire EJ, Lytton B, Pepe V, et al: Stress urinary incontinence. Obstet Gynecol 47:255, 1976.
28. Woodside JR, McGuire EJ: Urethral hypotonia after suprasacral spinal cord injury. J Urol 121:783, 1979.
29. English SF, Amundsen CL, McGuire EJ, et al: Bladder neck competence at rest in women with incontinence. J Urol 161:578, 1999.
30. McGuire EJ, Wagner FC Jr: Effects of sacral denervation on bladder and urethral function. Surg Gynecol Obestet 144:343, 1977.
31. McGuire EJ: Neurovesical dysfunction after abdominal perineal resection. Surg Clinics North Am 60:1207, 1980.
32. Nitti VW, Coombs AJ: Correlation of Valsalva leak point pressure with subjective degree of incontinence in women. J Urol 155:281, 1996.
33. Lose G: Urethral pressure measurement. Acta Obstet Gynecol Scand 166:39, 1997.
34. Swift SE, Rust PF, Ostergard DR: Intrasubject variability of the pressure-transmission ratio in patients with genuine stress incontinence. Int Urogynecol J Pelvic Floor Dysfunction 7(6):312, 1996.
35. Saud PK, Bowen LW, Panganiban R, et al: The low pressure urethra as a factor in failed retropubic urethroplasty. Obstet Gynecol 85:399, 1982.
36. Saud PK, Winkler H, Blackhurst DW, et al: A prospective randomized study comparing modified Burch retropubic urethropexy and suburethral sling for the treatment of genuine stress incontinence in a low pressure urethra. Am J Obstet Gynecol 182:30, 2000.
37. Maher CF, Dwyer PL, Carey MP, Moran PA: Colposuspension or sling for low urethral pressure stress incontinence. Int Urogynecol J Pelvic Floor Dysfunction 10(6):384, 1999.
38. McGuire EJ, Fitzpatrick CC, Wan J: Clinical assessment of urethral sphincter function. J Urol 150:1452, 1993.
39. Griffiths DJ: Assessment of detrusor contraction strength or contractibility. Neurourol Urodynam 10:1, 1991.
40. Schafer W: Principles and clinical application of advanced urodynamic analysis of voiding functions. Urol Clin North Am 17:553, 1990.
41. Masson DB, Govier FE: Modified Pereyra bladder neck suspension in patients with intrinsic sphincter deficiency and bladder neck hypermobility: Patient satisfaction with a mean follow up of 4 years. Urology 55:217, 2000.
42. Kondo A, Kato K, Gotoh M, et al: The Stamey and Gittes procedure: Long term follow up in relation to incontinence types and patient ages. J Urol 160:756, 1998.

CHAPTER 24

Electrodiagnosis

SIMON PODNAR ■ DAVID B. VODUŠEK ■ CLARE J. FOWLER

Electrophysiologic methods record bioelectrical potentials that are generated by excitable cell membranes. When applied in a clinical setting to recordings from nerves and skeletal muscle, these tests are often referred to as clinical neurophysiologic investigations.

Clinical neurophysiologic methods are well established and have been used in clinical practice for nearly half a century. When applied to pelvic floor disorders (encompassing urologic and urogynecologic patients with lower urinary tract and sexual dysfunction as well as proctologic patients with anorectal problems), the methods are referred to as uroneurophysiologic.

Neurophysiologic techniques have been applied to the pelvic floor mostly for research, but they have been proposed for everyday diagnostics in selected patients. The World Health Organization (WHO) Consensus on Incontinence stated that electrophysiologic assessment is useful in selected patients with suspected peripheral nervous system lesions, such as lower motor neuron lesions, in patients with multiple system atrophy, and in women with urinary retention.[1]

This chapter describes clinically useful and established tests that are of diagnostic value in individual patients. Concentric needle electromyography (CNEMG) and bulbocavernosus reflex (BCR) testing are discussed in detail. Other tests that are not considered of clinical value in the diagnosis of individual patients are briefly mentioned. For more detailed descriptions of these "promising" or "investigational" clinical neurophysiologic tests, refer to other reviews.[1,2]

ELECTRODIAGNOSTIC TESTS IN THE ASSESSMENT OF PATIENTS

General Remarks

A diagnostic test should be considered when the information that it may provide will significantly affect further treatment or clarify the prognosis.

Electrophysiologic tests are an extension of the clinical neurologic examination. They are helpful in evaluating patients in whom a nervous system lesion is suspected; however, they are not screening tests. They document clinically diagnosed nervous system lesions, provide data on the physiologic integrity of the nervous structures, and help to localize lesions and determine their type and severity (Table 24-1). In some patients with pelvic floor disorders, these data should be relevant for prognosis and may affect decisions about therapeutic and surgical interventions.

Other physiologic tests (e.g., urodynamic testing, manometric testing, tumescence measurements) to evaluate pelvic organ disorders test function, whereas electrophysiologic methods show the characteristics of neurologic lesions. As a result, the two types of test can be complementary rather than exclusive. Similarly, electrophysiologic tests complement imaging studies (ultrasound, computed tomography, magnetic resonance imaging) of the anal region, lower urinary tract, and other pelvic systems or regions. Imaging studies show morphologic abnormalities (e.g., anal sphincter tears, abnormal position of the bladder neck) that may cause or contribute to sacral dysfunction. Imaging studies may also show structural changes in the spinal canal, pelvis, or other structures. However, electrodiagnostic tests also have limitations (Table 24-2).

Clinical Assessment before Electrodiagnostic Testing

Some patients with pelvic floor disorders should be referred to specialists who can perform a focused clinical examination of the anogenital region. To document and quantify symptoms and obtain additional data, functional investigations (e.g., urodynamic studies, anorectal manometry) and imaging studies may be considered. If, in the course of such assessment, a neurologic lesion was suspected or if the patient belonged to one of the selected groups (discussed later), electrodiagnosis would be considered.

A focused history of the patient's symptoms must be taken first, including questions about urinary, anorectal, and sexual function. A history of low back pain radiating to the legs, and numbness and tingling on the posterior of thighs, buttocks, and in the perineal region point to cauda equina lesion. Older patients should be asked about general slowness, disordered gait, tremor, and

TABLE 24-1 ■ Unique Information Provided by Electrophysiologic Tests*

Information Provided by Test	Structure	Method	Finding
Integrity preserved	Lower motor neuron	CNEMG	Absent denervation activity Continuous firing of motor unit potentials during relaxation
	Upper and lower motor neurons	CNEMG	Dense interference pattern on voluntary activation
	Sacral reflex arc	CNEMG	Dense interference pattern on reflex activation (touch)
		Sacral reflex response	Brisk bulbocarvenosus reflex of normal latency
	Somatosensory pathways	Pudendal somtaosensory evoked potential	Normal shape and latency of responses
Localization of lesion	Root vs. plexus or nerve	CNEMG	Paravertebral denervation activity in neighboring myotomes
		SNAP	Normal (penile) SNAP with impaired (penile) skin sensation
Severity of lesion	Complete vs. partial	CNEMG	Profuse denervation activity Absent motor unit potentials
	Severe vs. moderate	Sacral reflex response	Absent bulbocarvenosus reflex
Type of lesion	Conduction block vs. axonotmesis	CNEMG	Absent or sparse denervation activity
	Axonotmesis vs. neurotmesis	CNEMG	Appearance of nascent motor unit potentials after complete muscle denervation

*This information is not provided by other pelvic floor tests. The absence of abnormality on clinical neurologic and appropriate electrodiagnostic testing (see Method column) is considered proof of preserved integrity of the neural structures, and other causes of pelvic floor dysfunction should be sought. On the other hand, the finding of an abnormality on a neurophysiologic test in an appropriate clinical setting supports and documents the clinical diagnosis of a neurogenic lesion. Electrodiagnostic tests often provide information about the lesion's severity, localization, and type (mechanism). These factors are critical for the assessment of prognosis.
CNEMG, concentric needle electromyography; SNAP, sensory nerve action potential.

TABLE 24-2 ■ Limitations of Electrodiagnostic Tests

Limitations	Causes	Comments
Uncomfortable		No significant risks
Difficult localization	Multiple lesions	Proximal lesion "masks" distal lesion on CNEMG, and distal lesion "masks" proximal lesion on SNAP
	Proximal peripheral sacral lesions	Paravertebral muscles are absent in the lower sacral segments
Timing of study	Few abnormalities seen before several weeks after injury Less pronounced pathologic signs after a few months	
Tests do not reflect the function of the entire structure studied	Low correlation with function	No electrophysiologic parameter is validated to measure weakness

CNEMG, concentric needle electromyography; SNAP, sensory nerve action potential.

autonomic dysfunction (e.g., orthostatic hypotension) to reveal extrapyramidal disorder. For research purposes, use of standardized questionnaires for anorectal,[3,4] urinary[5] and sexual[6,7] function is recommended.

As a minimum, a brief neurologic examination should be performed to look for signs of pyramidal and peripheral nervous system lesions, especially in the lower limbs, and also for extrapyramidal and cerebellar signs. Examination of the anogenital region includes assessment of anal sphincter tone, sensation of touch and pinprick in the perineal and perianal area, and eliciting of the BCR and anal reflex. If electrophysiologic tests are to be performed, the patient should be given a detailed explanation of the aims and methods of electrodiagnostic evaluation.

INNERVATION OF THE PELVIC STRUCTURES

The nervous system is divided into two motor systems (somatic and autonomic) and the somatosensory system. Within a particular anatomic system, we can distinguish central and peripheral parts. The central part includes the motor and sensory pathways in the central nervous system (brain and spinal cord). The central nervous system also contains an interneuronal system at different levels, important in neural "integrative functions" (e.g., spinal interneurons in the bulbocavernosus reflex arc[8]).

The motor system comprises an upper motor neuron (i.e., all neurons that participate in supraspinal motor control), a lower motor neuron (innervating muscles and glands), and muscle. Cell bodies of the upper motor neurons lie in the motor cortex and other gray matter (nuclei) of the brain, including some brainstem nuclei, and connect directly or via interneurons to the lower motor neurons of the spinal cord. The lower motor neurons lie either in the anterior horns of the gray matter of the spinal cord (somatomotor nuclei) or in the lateral horns of the spinal cord (autonomic nuclei). The first innervate skeletal muscle and the latter innervate smooth muscle and glands.

The somatosensory system can be divided into a peripheral part (receptors and sensory input into the spinal cord) and a central part (ascending pathways in the spinal cord and above). Sensory fibers from the skin and those accompanying axons from alpha motor neurons are called somatic afferents. Those accompanying autonomic (parasympathetic or sympathetic) fibers are called visceral afferents.

Somatic Lower Motor Neurons of the Sacral Spinal Cord

The alpha motor neurons of the sphincter (Onuf's) nucleus are somewhat smaller than those that innervate the skeletal muscles of the limb and trunk. Like other motor neurons, which innervate striated muscle, they lie in the anterior horn of the spinal cord. Their axons are of large diameter and myelinated to allow rapid conduction of impulses and travel to the periphery in the pudendal nerves. Within the muscle, the motor axon tapers and then branches to innervate muscle fibers. Each motor neuron innervates a number of muscle fibers—this constitutes the motor unit (MU). The innervation of healthy muscle is such that fibers of the same MU are unlikely to be adjacent but are scattered throughout the muscle. The diameter of the muscle area innervated by each sacral alpha motor neuron (MU territory) is probably smaller than that of the corresponding area in limb or trunk muscles.[9]

Primary Sensory Neuron

Sensory receptors are the most peripheral part of the somatic and autonomic sensory neurons. Receptors code mechanical or chemical stimuli into bioelectrical activity (changes in the electrical potentials of the neural membrane) that enters the sensory system, including the peripheral axon, cell body within the spinal ganglion and the central axon of the peripheral sensory neuron. In the spinal cord, the central axon branches with segmental branches contributing in the reflex arc and central branches conveying sensory information to the brain. Both somatic and visceral parts of the sensory system are organized in this way.

The simplified model of the neuromuscular system includes the autonomic system, which is divided into sympathetic and parasympathetic parts.

PHYSIOLOGIC PRINCIPLES OF ELECTRODIAGNOSTIC TESTING

An excitable membrane and transmission of information along it through traveling action potentials are characteristic of nerve and muscle cells. This bioelectrical activity is the substrate of function of the nervous tissue (i.e., transmission of information) and precedes the function of the muscle (i.e., contraction). This bioelectrical activity makes electrodiagnosis possible.

To obtain information about the bioelectrical activity of muscle, nerve, spinal roots, spinal cord, and brain, recordings from these structures are necessary. All clinical neurophysiologic recordings are extracellular. The electrodes may be near (i.e., intramuscular needle or wire electrodes) or distant from the source of bioelectrical activity (i.e., surface electrodes applied over the skin). The spread of electrical field through tissues from the generators obeys physical laws. From muscle, both the ongoing (spontaneous) and elicited (willfully, reflexly, by nerve depolarization) activity can be recorded. From most of the other nervous structures (e.g., nerves, spinal roots, spinal cord), spontaneous bioelectrical activity is not recorded during electrophysiologic testing. To explore these structures, stimulation (electrical pulses, and less often, magnetic or mechanical stimuli) is applied, and the propagated bioelectrical activity is recorded at some distance.

The electrophysiologic responses obtained on stimulation are compound action potentials produced by populations of biologic units (e.g., neurons, axons, muscle fibers, MUs).

CLASSIFICATION OF ELECTRODIAGNOSTIC TESTS

A functional classification of the electrophysiologic tests consists of four steps (Fig. 24-1): (1) Tests evaluating the somatic motor system (electromyography—EMG, terminal motor latency measurements, and motor evoked potentials—MEPs). (2) Tests evaluating the sensory system (sensory neurography, somatosensory evoked potentials—SEPs). (3) Methods assessing reflexes. (4) Tests assessing functioning of the sympathetic and parasympathetic autonomic nervous systems. Such a "logical" classification is preferable to a historical method of classification.

ELECTRODIAGNOSTIC TESTS THAT ARE OF DIAGNOSTIC VALUE IN INDIVIDUAL PATIENT

Electromyography

Kinesiologic Electromyography

The aim of EMG in the kinesiologic domain is to assess patterns of individual muscle activity or inactivity during defined maneuvers. These EMG recordings show the

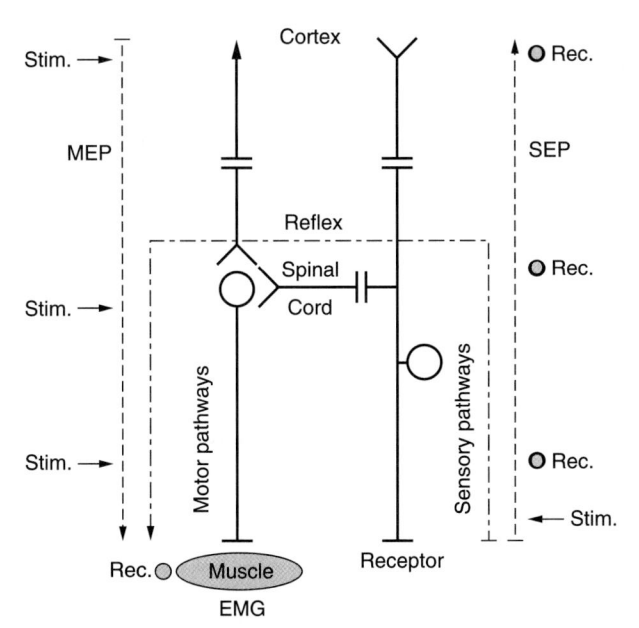

FIGURE 24-1 Components of the somatic sensory and somatic motor systems and the electrodiagnostic tests that evaluate them. Arrows on the motor (*left*) side indicate different stimulation sites (Stim) (from above) of motor cortex, spinal roots, and peripheral nerves (terminal motor latency test). Small circles on the sensory (*right*) side indicate different recording sites (Rec) (from below) from peripheral nerve (sensory nerve action potential, SNAP), spinal roots/cord, and somatosensory cortex. (For SNAP recording, both distal stimulation and proximal recording[82] or reverse[83] could be used.) In addition, concentric needle electromyography (CNEMG) and single-fiber electromyography (SFEMG) assess the lower motor neuron and muscle. Kinesiologic EMG evaluates the integrity of upper motor neuron and neurocontrol reflex arcs (From Vodušek DB: Evoked potential testing. Urol Clin North Am 23:427, 1996, p 428, Fig. 2). MEP, motor evoked potential; SEP, somatosensory evoked potential.

behavior of pelvic floor muscles during bladder (or rectum) filling and voiding (or emptying). It is usually not called "kinesiologic EMG," but the unspecified use of the term EMG for the diagnostic purposes discussed later might disorient the reader.

Various types of surface or intramuscular (needle or wire) electrodes can record the kinesiologic EMG signal. Bioelectrical activity is typically sampled from one intramuscular detection site. Since single motor unit potentials (MUPs) need not be analyzed, they can be recorded with a less sophisticated apparatus than other types of EMG, even if intramuscular electrodes are used for recording. There is no accepted standardized technique. When surface electrodes are used, there are problems with validity of the signal (e.g., artifacts, contamination from other muscles). With intramuscular electrodes in large pelvic floor muscles, there are questions about whether the whole muscle is properly represented by the sampled muscle.

The normal (kinesiologic) sphincter EMG shows continuous activity of MUPs at rest, which may be increased voluntarily or reflexly. Such activity of "low-threshold" MUPs[10] has been recorded for up to 2 hours[11] and even after subjects have fallen asleep during the examination.[12] This activity can also be recorded in many but not all detection sites of the levator ani,[13] and deeper parts of the external anal sphincter (EAS) muscle.[14] The urethral sphincter, EAS, and pubococcygeus muscles can sustain voluntarily activation for only approximately 1 minute.[13] On voiding, disappearance of all EMG activity in the urethral sphincter precedes detrusor contraction. In central nervous system disorders, however, detrusor contractions may be associated with increased sphincter EMG activity.[15,16] This detrusor–sphincter dyssynergia can be easily demonstrated by kinesiologic EMG performed as a part of urodynamic assessment.[17] Neurogenic uncoordinated sphincter behavior must be differentiated from voluntary contractions that may occur in poorly compliant patients. The pubococcygeus relaxes during voiding. The pelvic floor muscle contractions of non-neuropathic voiding dyssynergia may be a learned abnormal behavior that may occur in women with dysfunctional voiding.[18]

The pubococcygeus in the normal woman shows similar activity patterns to the urethral sphincters and the EAS at most detection sites—continuous activity at rest, some (but not invariable) increase of activity during bladder filling, and reflex increases in activity during any activation maneuver (e.g., talking, deep breathing, coughing). In health, the muscles on both sides act in unison,[13] but in disease, the patterns of activation and the coordination between the two sides may be lost.[19]

Little is known about the normal activity patterns of different pelvic floor muscles (sphincter urethrae, urethrovaginal sphincter, the EAS muscle, different parts of the levator ani, etc.). It is generally assumed that they all act in a coordinated fashion ("as one muscle") but differences have been shown even between the intra- and periurethral sphincters in normal women.[20] Coordinated behavior is frequently lost in abnormal conditions, as has been shown for the levator ani, the urethral sphincter, and the EAS.[21]

Any diagnostic value of kinesiologic EMG apart from polygraph urodynamic recordings to assess detrusor–sphincter coordination is not yet established.

The finding of voluntary and reflex activation of pelvic floor muscles is indirect proof of the integrity of respective neural pathways and should also be a part of a CNEMG examination, although the latter is performed primarily to diagnose a lower motor neuron lesion (discussed later).

Concentric Needle EMG

The aim of CNEMG testing is to differentiate abnormally from normally innervated striated muscle. Although EMG abnormalities are detected as a result of different lesions and diseases, there are in principle only two standard manifestations: (1) disease of the muscle fibers themselves and (2) changes in their innervation.

The concentric needle electrode consists of a central insulated platinum wire that is inserted through a steel cannula and the tip ground to give an elliptical area of 580×150 μm. This electrode records activity from approximately 20 muscle fibers, but the number of MUs actually recorded depends on both the local arrangement of muscle fibers in the pickup area and the level of muscle activity.

For the CNEMG examination, an advanced EMG system, which has the facility for quantitative template-based MUP analysis (multi-MUP) and interference pattern (IP) analysis (turn/amplitude) is ideal. The common amplifier filters setting for CNEMG is 5 Hz to 10 kHz, and must be checked if MUP parameters are to be measured, but they must be identical to those set when reference values were compiled.

Because of easy access, sufficient muscle bulk, and relative ease of examination, the EAS is the most practical muscle for CNEMG of the pelvic floor.[14,22] To examine the subcutaneous part of the EAS muscle, the needle is inserted about 1 cm from the anal orifice, to a depth of 3 to 6 mm. For the deeper part of the EAS muscle, 1- to 3-cm deep insertions are made at the anal orifice, at an angle of approximately 30 degrees to the anal canal axis (Fig. 24-2).[22] For MUP and IP analysis, both parts of the EAS can be sampled and data pooled because a systematic examination showed identical results.[14] For kinesiologic assessment, however, the muscles must be examined separately.[14]

Left and right EAS muscles should be examined by needle insertions into the middle of the anterior and posterior halves. The needle is angled backward and forward in a systematic manner (through two insertion sites on each side).

CNEMG examination of the EAS muscle can be divided into observation of insertion activity, of abnormal spontaneous activity, assessment of MUPs, and assessment of IP. In addition, the number of continuously active MUPs during relaxation should be observed, as well as MUP recruitment on reflex and voluntary activation.

In normal muscle, needle movement elicits a short burst of insertion activity as a result of mechanical stimulation of excitable membranes. This is recorded at a gain of 50 μV per division, which is also used to record pathologic denervation activity (sweep speed 5 to 10 ms/division). Absence of insertion activity with appropriately placed needle electrode usually means complete atrophy of the muscle (e.g., after complete conus medullaris or cauda equina lesion).[22]

Immediately after an acute complete denervation, all MU activity ceases and (apart from insertion activity) electrical silence is noted. Ten to twenty days later, insertion activity becomes more prominent and prolonged, and abnormal spontaneous activity appears in the form of short biphasic spikes (fibrillation potentials) and biphasic potentials with prominent positive deflections (positive sharp waves; Fig. 24-3). This type of activity is referred to as "denervation activity" and originates from denervated single muscle fibers.

With axonal reinnervation after complete denervation, nascent MUPs appear first and are short, low amplitude, biphasic, and triphasic, soon becoming polyphasic, serrated, and prolonged.

In partially denervated muscle, some MUPs remain and mingle eventually with abnormal spontaneous activity (after 10 to 20 days). Because the MUPs in sphincter muscles are also short and mostly biphasic or triphasic, as are fibrillation potentials, considerable EMG experience is needed to differentiate one from another. In this situation, examination of the bulbocavernosus muscle is particularly

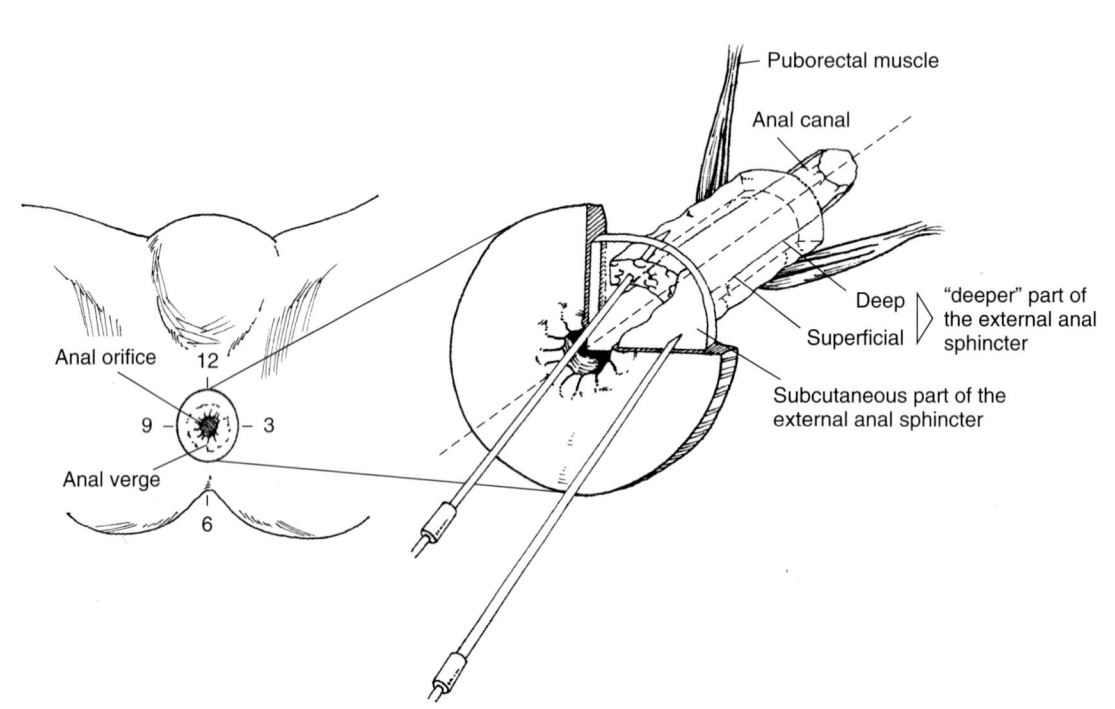

FIGURE 24-2 A method of systematic needle electrode insertion into the external anal sphincter (EAS) muscle. Needle insertions into the subcutaneous and the deeper parts of the EAS are shown on the right. Left and right halves of EAS are examined separately with two skin penetrations (for the anterior and posterior parts, respectively). With systematic movement of the needle, at least four sites in each subcutaneous or deeper part of the EAS are thus analyzed (Reprinted from Vodušek DB, Fowler CJ, Deletis V, Podnar S: Clinical neurophysiology of pelvic floor disorders. In Ambler Z, Nevšimalova S, Kadanka Z, Rossini PM [eds]: Clinical Neurophysiology at the Beginning of the 21st Century. Clin Neurophysiol (suppl 53):220, 2000, p 222, Fig. 1 with permission from International Federation of Clinical Neurophysiology.

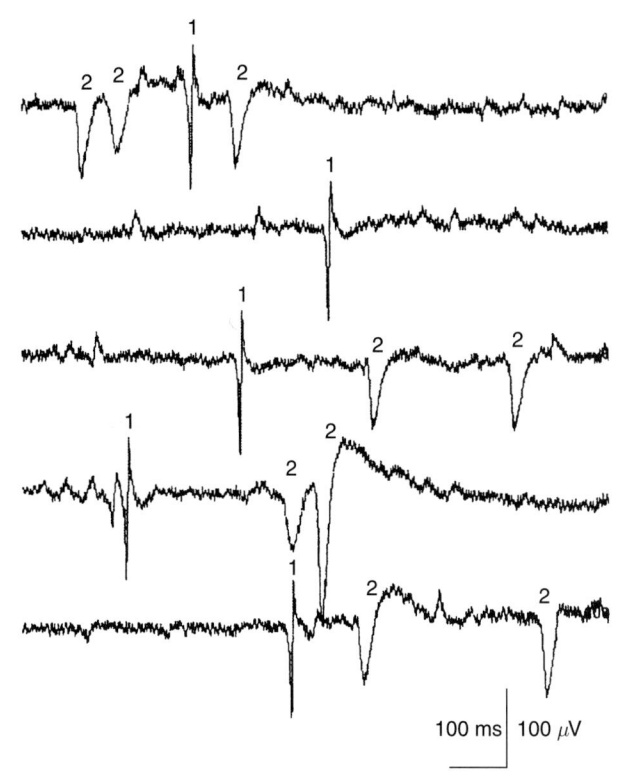

FIGURE 24-3 Electromyographic (EMG) activity during relaxation in the right half of the "deeper" part of the external anal sphincter (EAS) muscle. EMG examination was performed (using a standard concentric EMG needle) in a 56-year-old man 3 weeks after traumatic fracture of both pubic bones. Distinct pathologic spontaneous activity is seen in the form of short biphasic spikes (fibrillation potentials, 1) and biphasic potentials with prominent positive deflections (positive sharp waves, 2). Absence of continuously active motor units (MUs) points to possibility of acute complete denervation of the EAS muscle, which should be verified by attempts for maximal voluntary contractions and reflex activation. The ultimate proof of the complete muscle denervation is absence of its compound motor action potential (CMAP) on stimulation of the pudendal nerve and recorded with needle electrode.

useful as it lacks ongoing activity of low-threshold MU during relaxation (in contrast to sphincter muscles).[1]

In long-standing partially denervated muscles, peculiar abnormal activity called simple or complex repetitive discharges appears, caused by repetitive firing of groups of potentials. The activity may be provoked by needle movement, muscle contraction, and so on, or may occur spontaneously, rhythmically. This activity is sometimes found in urethral sphincters of patients without other evidence of neuromuscular disease, and indeed without lower urinary tract problems, although in such cases it is not prominent.

A type of repetitive discharge activity, called decelerating bursts (DBs) and complex repetitive discharges (CRDs), can be found in the external urethral sphincter muscles of some young women. The CRDs sound like a helicopter over the loudspeaker on the EMG system. However, DBs produce the myotonic sound similar to underwater recordings of whales. This activity may be so abundant that it causes involuntary muscle contraction and urinary retention.[23]

In contrast to limb muscles, where electrical silence is present on relaxation, in sphincter muscles, some MUPs are continuously firing. Additional sphincter MUPs can be activated reflexly or voluntarily. There are two MUP populations with different characteristics: reflexly or voluntarily activated high-threshold MUPs, which are larger than continuously active low-threshold MUPs. As a result, to increase the accuracy of MUP sampling, standardzation of activity level was suggested (for a template based multi-MUP analysis: 3–5 MUPs on a single muscle site).[10]

In partially denervated sphincter muscle, there is a loss of MUs, but the loss is difficult to quantify. Because EAS muscle contraction cannot be assessed concomitantly (in contrast to limb muscles), the reduction of the number of activated MUs and the increase in their firing rate (both expected following partial denervation) have been little studied.

Changes due to collateral reinnervation are reflected by prolongation of the waveform of the MUPs (Fig. 24-4), which may have small, late components ("satellites"). In newly formed axon sprouts and end plates, transmission is insecure, which may be reflected in MUPs as instability ("jitter" and "blocking" of individual components). Over time, if no further denervation occurs, the reinnervating axonal sprouts increase in diameter so that activation of all parts of the reinnervated MU becomes nearly synchronous, which increases the amplitude and reduces the duration of the MUPs. This phenomenon may be different in sphincter muscles in ongoing degenerative disorders, such as multiple system atrophy (MSA), where long-duration MUPs remain a prominent feature of MUs.[24] Less pronounced increase

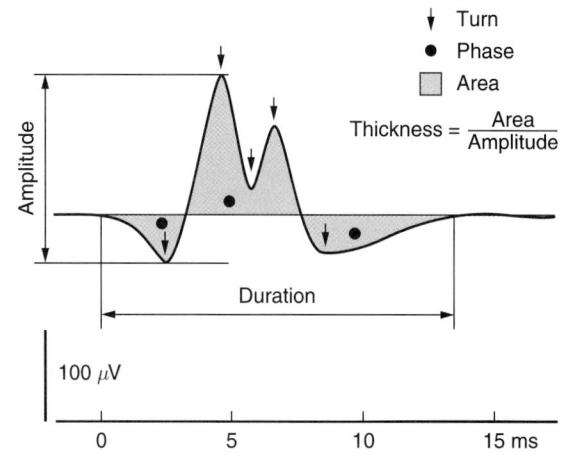

FIGURE 24-4 The motor unit potential (MUP) parameters. Amplitude is the voltage difference (μV) between the most positive and most negative point of the MUP trace. The MUP duration is the time (msec) between the first deflection and the point at which MUP waveform finally returns to the baseline. The number of MUP phases (*small circles*) is defined by the number of times the potential crosses the baseline, and it can be counted as "number of baseline crossings plus one." Turns (*arrows*) are defined as changes in direction of the MUP trace that are larger than specified amplitude (100 μV) but not crossing the baseline. MUP area measures the integrated surface of the MUP waveform (*shaded*). Rise time of the negative peak measures the time (msec) of negative upstroke of the main MUP phase. Duration of the negative peak measures the duration (msec) of the main negative MUP phase, including the satellite potentials. In addition, thickness (thickness = area/amplitude) and size index (size index = 2 * log (amplitude (mV)) + area/amplitude) parameters are automatically calculated from these "primary" MUP parameters by advanced EMG systems.

in MUP amplitude on reinnervation might also be due to a less efficient fusion of individual muscle fiber potentials in muscles with short spike components of MUPs such as sphincter (and facial) muscles.

MUP Analysis

Three techniques are available to systematically examine individual MUPs.

The first MUP analysis technique follows an algorithm similar to that used by Buchthal, who carried out the first EMG assessments.[25] They measured MUP duration and amplitude from paper records of EMG activity; nowadays the same principle is used, but the MUPs are automatically analyzed on the screen. Using this modified "manual-MUP" analysis the highest number of MUPs (≤10) can be obtained from the EAS muscle site at low levels of activity. At higher levels of activation, the baseline becomes unsteady. It takes 2 to 3 minutes for each site to be analyzed. This technique is demanding for the operator because reproducible MUPs must be identified, the one with the smoothest baseline chosen, and in most cases the duration cursors set manually. The technique is subject to bias, especially the determination of MUP duration.[26]

The introduction of the trigger and delay unit led to its widespread use for individual MUP analysis.[27] On applying this technique, during a constant level of EMG activity the trigger unit is set on a steadily firing MUP. The triggered MUP is averaged until the baseline becomes smooth, which takes about 1 minute. The number of MUPs at each site depends on the version of the technique used. In some systems only the highest amplitude MUP can be triggered, which enables sampling of only 1 to 3 MUPs from each examination site. Single-MUP analysis is time-consuming, provides fewer MUPs than the previously described technique, and is biased toward high-amplitude and high-threshold MUPs. Furthermore, it is susceptible to personal bias.[26]

The recent and sophisticated CNEMG techniques are available only on advanced EMG systems, such as the template-operated "multi-MUP" analysis.[28] Here the operator only indicates—during the appropriate level of the crisp EMG activity—when the computer takes the previous (last) 4.8-sec period of the signal. (Crisp EMG activity can be recognized by a characteristic sound over loudspeaker and indicates that the needle electrode is near muscle fibers.) From that signal, MUPs are automatically extracted, quantified, and sorted into one to six classes, which represent consecutive discharges of a particular MUP. MUP classes are then averaged and presented (Fig. 24-5). Cursors are set automatically with a computer algorithm that, in addition to certain amplitude deflection, demands the minimum angle of the MUP trace toward the baseline.[28] After acquisition, the operator edits the MUPs. Thus, one to six MUPs can be obtained from each examination site.[26,28,29]

Multi-MUP analysis is the fastest and the easiest to apply of the three mentioned quantitative MUP analysis techniques. It can be applied at continuous activity during sphincter muscle relaxation, as well as at slight to moderate levels of activation.[10,26] The multi-MUP technique has (like single-MUP analysis) difficulties with highly unstable or polyphasic MUPs. It often fails to sample them, sorts the same MUP to several classes (recognizes it as different MUPs, duplicates), cuts prolonged MUPs into two, or distorts them by averaging. The MUPs with unsteady baselines (unclear beginning or end) must be recognized and deleted.[29]

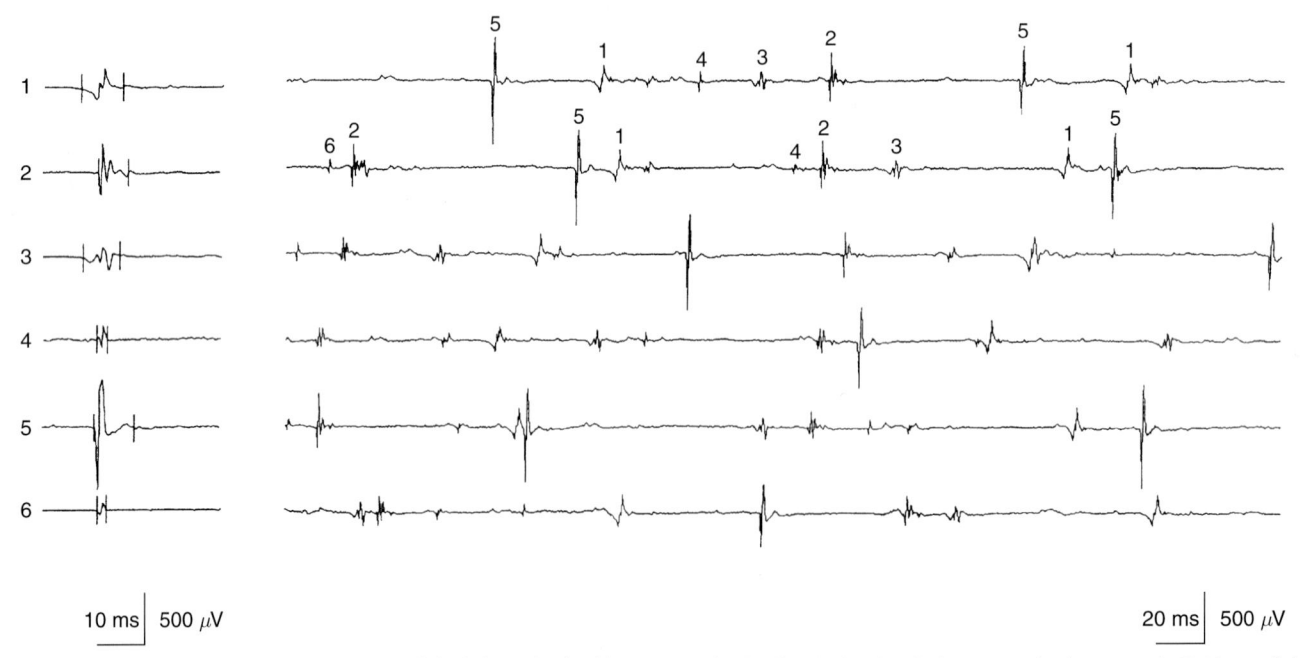

FIGURE 24-5 Slight voluntary contraction of the left urethral sphincter muscle. EMG examination (using a standard concentric EMG needle) of a 51-year-old woman was performed 10 years after cauda equina compression by a herniated intervertebral disk. *Right side of the figure* shows the original recording. At this level of activity computer-assisted (multi-MUP) analysis collected six motor unit potentials (*left column*). Altogether 15 MUPs were collected in the left half of the urethral sphincter muscle (mean amplitude 405 μV, duration 6.6 ms, area 438 μVms, and 33% MUP polyphasicity). Note that different sweep speeds were used in the MUP sample (*left column*) and the original signal.

Multi-MUP technique samples slightly fewer MUPs per muscle than the manual MUP does.[26]

In the small half of the sphincter muscle, collecting 10 MUPs is a minimal requirement on using single-MUP analysis. Using manual-MUP and multi-MUP techniques sampling of 20 MUPs (standard number in limb muscles) from each part of the EAS presents no problem in healthy control subjects[9] and most patients.[26]

Analysis made from the same taped EMG signal, using reference data for mean values and outliers showed similar sensitivity of manual-MUP, single-MUP, and multi-MUP analysis for detecting neuropathic changes in the EAS muscle of patients with chronic sequels after cauda equina or conus medullaris lesions.[26,30] Normative data obtained from the EAS muscle by standardized EMG technique using multi-MUP analysis have been published.[9]

MUP Parameters

A number of MUP parameters are used in the diagnosis of neuromuscular disease (see Fig. 24-4). Traditionally, amplitude and duration were measured and the number of phases was counted.[25]

Amplitude is the voltage (μV) difference between the most positive and most negative point on the MUP trace (see Fig. 24-4). The amplitude of MUPs is largely determined by the activity of the muscle fibers that are closest (within a 0.5-mm radius) to the recording electrode, where in the normal MU it is unlikely to find more than 2 to 3 muscle fibers.[31]

The MUP duration is the time (msec) between the first deflection and the point when MUP waveform finally returns to the baseline (see Fig. 24-4). It depends on the number of muscle fibers of particular MU within 2- to 3-mm diameter and is little affected by the proximity of the recording electrode to the nearest fiber.[31] The difficulty with duration measurement is in defining the beginning and end of MUP. Using manual positioning of duration cursors depends on amplifier gain: At higher gain, MUPs seem longer.[32] It is unclear whether to include satellite potentials into MUP duration. Satellite potentials are defined as part of MUP starting at least 3 ms after the end of main part of the MUP.[32] Although in 1986 a group of leading experts agreed not to include them in measurement,[32,33] their exclusion might reduce the sensitivity of MUP analysis, at least in MSA (unpublished personal data).

The number of MUP phases is defined by the number of times the potential crosses the baseline. It is counted as "number of baseline crossings plus one" (see Fig. 24-4).[32,34] Either the number of phases or the percentage of polyphasic MUPs can be determined. MUPs are usually called polyphasic when they have at least four phases (mono-, bi-, tri-, and polyphasic). Related to the number of phases is the number of turns. A turn is defined as a change in direction of the MUP trace, which is larger than specified amplitude but not crossing the baseline (see Fig 24-4). Number of turns is the MUP parameter particularly sensitive to reinnervation changes in small muscles such as the EAS (unpublished personal data).[9]

With computer analysis, a number of further MUP parameters is available. Thus, MUP area, rise time of negative peak, and duration of negative peak can be measured (see Fig 24-4).[9,28]

In addition, thickness (thickness = area/amplitude)[35] and size index (size index = 2*log (amplitude (mV)) + area/amplitude)[36] can be automatically calculated by advanced EMG systems. Development of these derived parameters resulted from studies aimed at finding MUP changes that would differentiate better between normal and myopathic (thickness),[35] or normal and neuropathic muscles (size index).[36] Thickness can be imagined as a base of the triangle, which presents a simplified MUP (its surface being area and its height being amplitude).[35] Myopathic MUPs are indeed distinguished from normal MUPs by their shortness on performing qualitative EMG (diminished thickness in myopathy). Size index can be seen as a "normalized" thickness—in contrast to thickness, it does not depend on the electrode's position. It has two parts, of which the first (logarithm of amplitude) increases, and thus counteracts the second (area/amplitude = thickness) that decreases on the electrode approach to the muscle fibers.[36] There has so far been no formal study comparing the sensitivity and specificity of individual MUP parameters for differentiating normal from pathologic sphincter muscles.

IP Analysis

In addition to continuous firing of low-threshold MUPs in sphincters, additional high-threshold MUPs are recruited voluntarily and reflexly.[10] By such maneuvers, the amount of recruitable MUs is estimated. Normally, MUPs should intermingle to produce a dense IP on the oscilloscope screen when muscle is contracted well, and during a strong cough.

The IP can be assessed using a number of automatic quantitative analyzes, the turn/amplitude (T/A) analysis being the most popular.[37,38,39] On applying T/A analysis, with the needle electrode in focus, subjects contract muscle voluntarily or reflexly by coughing. Examinator selects 0.5-sec time epochs of the crisp EMG signal to be analyzed.

A number of IP parameters can be measured automatically from the EMG signal: number of turns/second, amplitude/turn,[38] % activity, number of short segments (NSS), and envelope (Fig. 24-6).[39] Turns are defined as every minimum or maximum of the signal where it changes direction (i.e., constitutes a peak or trough) and the signal amplitude changes by at least 100 μV compared to the preceding and subsequent turns. Turns are counted (turns/sec; N/sec) and amplitudes between turns measured (amplitude/turn; μV).[38] The envelope (μV) is determined as the peak-to-peak amplitude that is exceeded by only 1% of peaks and 1% of troughs in the analyzed time epoch.[39] In addition, parts of the EMG signal with sharp activity (containing MUPs) are determined and counted (number of short segments, NSS; N), and percentage of time with such sharp activity within the whole time epoch is determined (% activity).[39] Samples with positive values of all IP parameters are accepted for further analysis (0 values of IP parameters are interpreted as being caused by either weak contraction or needle electrode outside the muscle). From these parameters, three plots can be produced: amplitude versus turn,[38] NSS versus % activity, and envelope versus % activity.[39] For the EAS muscle, normative clouds for these plots are available.[9] On applying T/A analysis during maximal contraction of the EAS,

FIGURE 24-6 The interference pattern (IP) parameters: number of turns/second, amplitude/turn, percent activity, number of short segments (NSS), and envelope. Turns are defined as every minimum or maximum of the signal where it changes direction (i.e., constitutes a peak or trough) and the signal amplitude changes by at least 100 μV compared to the preceding and subsequent turns. Turns are counted (N/sec) and amplitudes per turn measured (μV). The envelope (μV) is the peak-to-peak amplitude that is exceeded by only 1% of peaks and by only 1% of troughs in the analyzed time epoch. Parts of the EMG signal with sharp activity containing MUPs (*underlined*) are determined and counted (number of short segments, NSS) and percentage of time with such sharp activity within the whole time epoch is determined (% activity).

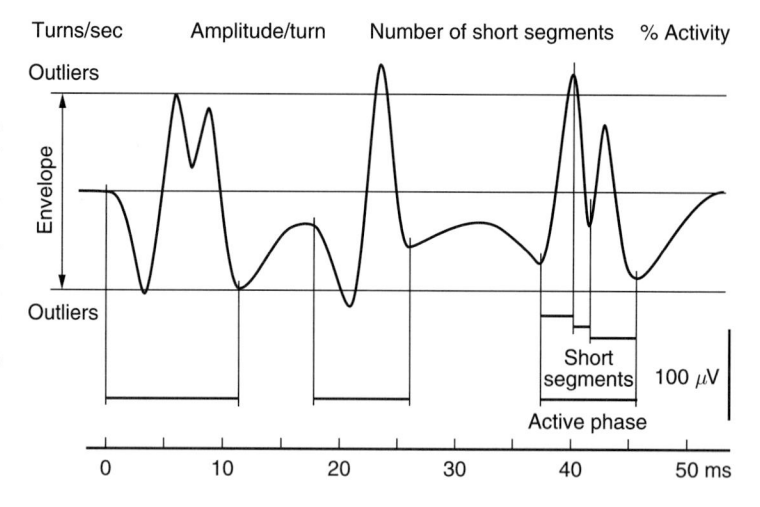

displacement of the needle electrode by a contralateral buttock is occasionally a problem, especially in muscular men.[9]

Sampling of IPs using T/A analysis is even faster than multi-MUP analysis (2 to 3 min per muscle). However, sensitivity of IP analysis for detecting neuropathic changes in the EAS muscle of patients with chronic sequels after cauda equina or conus medullaris damage is only about half of sensitivities of MUP analysis techniques.[26]

In summary, template-based multi-MUP analysis is sensitive (equally to traditional MUP analysis techniques),[26] fast (5 to 10 min per muscle), easy to apply, less prone to personal bias, and, technically, represents a clinically useful technique.[9] In the EAS muscle, its use is further facilitated by the availability of common normative data, which are unaffected by age, gender,[9] number and characteristics of vaginal deliveries,[29] mild chronic constipation,[40] or the part (the subcutaneous and the deeper) of the muscle examined.[14] All these make multi-MUP analysis the technique of choice for quantitative analysis of the EAS reinnervation.

Single-Fiber EMG

The aim of single-fiber EMG (SFEMG) testing is similar to CNEMG—to differentiate normal from abnormal striated muscle. The SFEMG electrode has similar external proportions to a concentric needle electrode, being made of a steel cannula 0.5 to 0.6 mm in diameter with a beveled tip. However, instead of having the recording surface at the tip, a fine insulated platinum or silver wire embedded in epoxy resin is exposed through an aperture on the side 1 to 5 mm behind the tip. The platinum wire forms the recording surface and has a diameter of 25 μm. It will pick up activity within a hemispheric volume 300 μm in diameter. This is much smaller than the volume of muscle tissue from which a concentric needle electrode records, which has an uptake area of 1-mm diameter. Because of the arrangement of muscle fibers in a normal MU, an SFEMG needle will record only 1 to 3 single muscle fibers from the same MU. When recording with an SFEMG needle, the amplifier filters are set so that low-frequency activity is eliminated (500 Hz–10 kHz). Thus, the contribution of each muscle fiber appears as a short biphasic positive-negative action potential.

The SFEMG parameter that reflects MU morphology is the fiber density, which is the mean number of muscle fibers belonging to an individual MU per detection site. To assemble this data, recordings from 20 intramuscular detection sites are necessary.[41] The normal fiber density for the EAS is less than 2.0.[42-44] Changes with age have been reported, showing women to have significantly greater fiber density than men.[44,45]

The SFEMG electrode is also most suitable to record any instability of MUPs, although it is not routinely performed in pelvic floor muscles for diagnostic purposes. The instability is revealed as "jitter," which is defined as the variability with consecutive discharges of the interpotential interval between two muscle fiber action potentials belonging to the same MU. It may be increased not only in diseases affecting neuromuscular transmission but also by recent reinnervation.

Fiber density is increased in reinnervated muscle. The technique has been particularly applied to sphincter muscles to correlate increased fiber density findings to incontinence.[46] Due to its technical characteristics, an SFEMG electrode is able to record even small changes that occur in MUs due to reinnervation, but it is less suitable to detect changes due to denervation itself (i.e., abnormal insertion and spontaneous activity).

SFEMG versus CNEMG

Quantified CNEMG provides the same information on reinnervation changes in muscle as the SFEMG parameter of fiber density,[47,48] but in addition, CNEMG shows pathologic spontaneous activity. In muscle after severe partial denervation, the areas of fibrosis are "silent" to EMG exploration, and the results are based only on the remaining MUP activity. The remaining innervated muscle is easier to establish with CNEMG, which records from a larger volume of tissue. Furthermore, CNEMG examination can be extended in the same diagnostic session from, for example, lumbar and upper sacral myotomes to the lower sacral myotomes after a cauda equina lesion. A concentric electrode can be used at the same diagnostic session for recording evoked direct and reflex muscle responses.

Use of concentric needles is the method of choice in routine examination of skeletal muscle and is generally available in a clinical neurophysiology laboratory, whereas single-fiber needles are not so widely used. As a consequence, SFEMG, although an established electrodiagnostic technique, is not recommended for clinical neurophysiologic evaluation of patients with pelvic floor dysfunction.

Sacral Reflexes

The term *sacral reflex* refers to electrophysiologically recordable responses of perineal/pelvic floor muscles to (electrical) stimulation of sensory fibers in the urogenitoanal region. Two reflexes—the anal and the BCR—are commonly clinically elicited in the lower sacral segments; both have the afferent and the efferent limbs of their reflex arc in the pudendal nerve and are centrally integrated at the S2–S4 cord levels. Electrophysiologic correlates of these reflexes have been described.

Measurements of latencies and amplitudes of reflex responses and evoked potentials, including sympathetic skin responses, relate not only to conduction in peripheral and central neural pathways but also to transmission across synapses and within networks of central nervous system interneurons. Therefore, conduction may be affected by factors that are not apparent from a simplified anatomic model. These factors may or may not have something to do with the putative neurogenic condition of the patient. For example, changes in the threshold, amplitude, and latency of the BCR occur as a consequence of changes in the physiologic state of the bladder,[49] and differ in pathologic conditions (i.e., suprasacral spinal cord lesions).[50] The changes represent an indicator of "central integrative" function, if the stimulus is kept constant.

The aim of electrophysiologic testing of sacral reflexes is to assess integrity of the sacral (S2–S4) spinal reflex arc and to evaluate excitation levels of sacral spinal cord motor neurons.

It is possible to use electrical,[51,52] mechanical,[53,54] or magnetic[55] stimulation. Whereas the latter two modalities have been applied only to the penis and clitoris, electrical stimulation can be applied at various sites: to the dorsal penile nerve, to the dorsal clitoral nerve, perianally, and (using a catheter-mounted ring electrode) at bladder neck/proximal urethra.[56] In clinical practice, electrical and mechanical stimulation of the penis or clitoris can be used, so this will be discussed in some detail.

The sacral reflex evoked on the dorsal penile or the clitoral nerve stimulation was shown to be a complex response, often comprising two components. The first component, with latency of about 33 msec, is the response that has been most often called the BCR. It is stable, does not habituate, and based on variability of single motor neuron latency reflex discharges, is thought to be an oligosynaptic reflex. The second component has a similar latency to the sacral reflexes evoked by stimulation perianally or from the proximal urethra. The variability of single motor neuron reflex responses within this component is much larger, as is typical for a polysynaptic reflex.[8] The second component is not always demonstrable as a discrete response. The two components of the reflex may behave somewhat differently in control subjects and in patients. In normal subjects, it is usually the first component that has a lower threshold; in patients with partially denervated pelvic floor muscles, the first reflex component cannot be obtained with single stimuli, but on strong stimulation the later reflex component does occur. This can cause confusion because very delayed reflex responses may be recorded in patients, by investigators not recognizing the possibility that it is an isolated second component of the reflex. The situation can be clarified by using double stimuli that facilitate the reflex response and may show the first component.[57]

Sacral reflex responses recorded with needle or wire electrodes can be analyzed separately for each side of the EAS or each bulbocavernosus muscle. This is important because unilateral or asymmetrical lesions are common. However, unilateral stimulation of the penis is not really possible because in patients with sensory loss (and probably also in normal subjects) the application of stronger stimulus leads to electrical spread. Mechanical stimulation (light touch or pinprick) of the perianal area on each side, with needle detection from the subcutaneous EAS muscles of each side (left and right) during the CNEMG, allows a separate testing of afferent (sensory) pathways of the lower sacral reflex arc (in addition to motor). In the authors' laboratories testing of BCR on electrical stimulation is performed in conjunction with a CNEMG if no brisk reflex response is present on mechanical stimulation of perianal or perineal region and recording from the EAS muscle.

Standardization of the technique has been proposed.[1] It was recommended that surface stimulation electrodes be placed on the penis or clitoris, 10 single, 0.2-ms long stimuli be applied at supramaximal intensity at intervals of 2 sec = 0.5 Hz. Settings for recording of BCR by concentric needle or surface electrodes placed into or over the EAS or bulbocavernosus muscle in men are use of filters, 10 Hz—10 kHz; sweep speed, 10 ms/div; and gain, 50 to 1000 µV/div. Onset latency is proposed as the only parameter measured.[1]

Sacral reflex responses on stimulation of the dorsal penile and clitoral nerve have been said to be of value in patients with cauda equina and other lower motor neuron lesions, although it is recognized that a reflex with a normal latency does not exclude the possibility of an axonal lesion in its reflex arc. Sacral reflex responses to stimulation of penis have been proposed for evaluation of neurogenic erectile dysfunction,[51] but have low sensitivity[58] and specificity.[59] In patients who have diabetes and suspected neurogenic impotence, the nerve conduction studies performed in limbs are more sensitive in revealing peripheral neuropathy than sacral reflex latencies.[60]

Abnormally short reflex latency of BCR suggests either the abnormally low position of conus medullaris[61] or a suprasacral cord lesion.[62]

Mechanical stimulation has been used to elicit BCR in both sexes and found to be a robust technique.[53] Either a standard commercially available reflex hammer or a customized electromechanical hammer can be employed.

Such stimulation is painless and can be used in children or patients with pacemakers in whom electrical stimulation is often contraindicated. The latency of the mechanically elicited BCR is comparable to the electrically elicited BCR. Differences are caused by the somewhat longer pathway for mechanically evoked stimulation (stimulates receptors instead of peripheral nerve) as well as by variability in the time course of the mechanical stimulation device.[54]

Sacral reflex testing should be a part of the diagnostic battery, of which CNEMG exploration of the pelvic floor muscles is the most important part. Electrophysiologic assessment of sacral reflexes is a more quantitative, sensitive, and reproducible way of assessing the S2–S4 reflex arcs than any of the clinical methods. The results, however, should be interpreted with caution, and the clinician should always be mindful of the clinical context.

Pudendal Somatosensory Evoked Potentials

The pudendal somatosensory evoked potentials (SEPs) are easily recorded after electrical stimulation of the dorsal penile or clitoral nerve.[63,64] As a rule, this response is of highest amplitudes at the central recording site (Cz-2 cm: Fz of the International 10 to 20 electroencephalography System) and is highly reproducible.[65] Amplitudes of the P40 measure 0.5 to 12 µV. The first positive peak at 41 ± 2.3 msec (P1 or P40) is usually clearly defined in healthy subjects using a stimulus 2 to 4 times stronger than sensory threshold current strength.[66] Later negative ($\approx$55 ms) and then further positive waves are interindividually variable in amplitude and expression and have little known clinical relevance.

Pudendal SEP recordings were used in patients with neurogenic erectile dysfunction, spinal cord lesions, multiple sclerosis, and diabetes. Such measurements were also measured in patients with neurogenic bladder dysfunction due to multiple sclerosis. It has, however, been shown that the tibial cerebral SEPs are more often abnormal than the pudendal SEPs, and only in exceptional cases is the pudendal SEPs abnormal but the tibials normal, suggesting an isolated conus involvement.[67]

A study that looked at the value of the pudendal SEPs for detecting relevant neurologic disease when investigating urogenital symptoms found it to be of lesser value than clinical examination for signs of spinal cord disease in the lower limbs (i.e., lower limb hyperreflexia and extensor plantar responses).[68] However, in some situations, such as when a patient has loss of bladder or vaginal sensation, it is reassuring to be able to record a normal pudendal SEP. The method as such is valid and robust, but its clinical value seems to be minor.

Cerebral SEPs on penile or clitoral stimulation were reported as a possibly valuable intraoperative monitoring method in patients with cauda equina or conus at risk of a surgical procedure.[69]

ELECTRODIAGNOSTIC TESTS THAT HAVE NO DIAGNOSTIC VALUE IN INDIVIDUAL PATIENTS

Neurophysiology of the Sacral Motor System

Motor Nerve Conduction Studies

Recording of the muscle response (compound motor action potential, CMAP, or M-wave)[33] on electrical stimulation of its motor nerve is the routine method of functional evaluation of distal parts of limb nerves. By stimulating the nerve at two levels, motor nerve conduction can be calculated, which is the most appropriate test for distinguishing between lesions of myelin and axons causing motor weakness. However, the technique requires access to the nerve at two well-separated points for stimulation and measurement of the distance between them, a requirement that cannot be met in the pelvis. Thus the only electrophysiologic parameter that can be measured also in the pelvic floor is the pudendal nerve terminal motor latency (PNTML). Latency measurements measure the fastest conducting fibers but give little or no information about the loss of biologic units (e.g., axons), which is more important. They, however, depend less on irrelevant biologic and technical factors and are therefore the more applicable parameter also in evoked potential and reflex studies. On the other hand, the amplitude of the compound potential correlates with the number of activated biologic units. (A conduction block and pathologic dispersion of conduction velocities within a neural pathway also affect amplitudes.) They are thus the more relevant physiologic parameter, but unfortunately they depend on many poorly controllable technical factors and are therefore variable. M-wave amplitudes of EAS or other pelvic floor muscles on stimulation of the pudendal nerves have unfortunately not proved contributory.

PNTML can be measured by recording with a concentric needle electrode from the bulbocavernosus, the EAS, or the urethral sphincter muscles in response to bipolar stimulation placed on the perianal or perineal surface. The PNTML from the perineal muscles obtained by this means are between 4.7 and 5.1 msec[52] and similar latencies have been obtained for the same technique of stimulation and recording from EAS.[70]

The more widely employed technique of obtaining PNTML relies on stimulation with a special surface electrode assembly fixed on a gloved index finger—the "St. Mark's electrode."[71] This consists of a bipolar stimulating electrode fixed to the tip of the gloved finger with the recording electrode pair placed 8 cm proximally on the base of the finger. The finger is inserted into the rectum and stimulation is performed close to the ischial spine. With this stimulator, the PNTML for the anal sphincter MEP is typically around 2 ms. The differences in latencies obtained by the perineal and transrectal techniques have not been explained, but PNTML as measured by the St. Mark's electrode seems to be curiously short. After stimulation of peripheral nerves with much thicker and faster motor nerve fibers (e.g., ulnar), terminal latencies over the 8-cm distance are around 3 ms.

Even the residual time itself (i.e., time obtained by extrapolation of the nerve conduction velocity to zero distance—time for transmission along the distal axon branches and neuromuscular junction) is longer in the ulnar nerve than the PNTML as measured by the St. Mark's electrode.[72] Because of its slower conduction, the residual time might be longer in the pudendal nerve, so it seems unlikely that the PNTML test evaluates conduction along the last 8 cm of the pudendal nerve. Stimulation of pelvic floor muscles near their neuromuscular points seems a more likely explanation.

Prolongation of the PNTML measured by the St. Mark's electrode was found in women with stress urinary incontinence,[73] women immediately[74] and 5 years[75] after vaginal delivery, but other studies did not show such changes after vaginal delivery.[44] Prolongation was found also in patients with pelvic floor prolapse.[76] This prolongation was taken as a sign of damage to the pudendal nerve and has lead to the term pudendal nueropathy, used particularly by coloproctologists. Some workers less familiar with theoretical principles of clinical neurophysiology equate a prolongation of PNTML with pelvic floor denervation. This, however, is mistaken, because prolonged latency is a poor measure of denervation, as already explained. What type of abnormality this latency prolongation indicates is unclear because there have not been any relevant morphologic studies, but it may be that unlike in the carpal tunnel syndrome where conduction slowing is in the main trunk, in patients with neurogenic lesions affecting the innervation of the pelvic floor, damage to the nerve occurs distally at sites where the motor nerve is branching within the muscle.

Delays of PNTML in patient groups, even when present, were short: ~ 0.1 to 0.3 ms, and it is unlikely that these represent a functionally relevant change. Timing of reflex responses such as are involved with the recruitment of MUs on coughing or sneezing (i.e., maneuvers that cause stress incontinence) are in the order of magnitude of tens of ms.

We found PNTML unhelpful for diagnosis in individual patients with pelvic floor disorders. Elicitability of a CMAP in pelvic floor muscles (using the perianal stimulation) may be helpful in patients with combined upper and lower motor lesions in whom no MUP activity can be recorded since the presence of CMAP excludes complete peripheral (axonal) lesion.

Anterior Sacral Root (Cauda Equina) Stimulation

Transcutaneous stimulation of deeply situated nervous tissue became possible with the development of special electrical and magnetic stimulators. When applied over the spine roots at the exit from the vertebral canal these can be stimulated, and there have been reports of these techniques applied to the sacral roots.[56,77,78]

Electrical or magnetic stimulation depolarizes underlying neural structures in a nonselective fashion, and concomitant activation of several muscles innervated by lumbosacral segments occurs. Responses from gluteal muscles may contaminate attempts to record from the sphincters and lead to error.[79] Thus, surface recordings from sphincter muscles are inadvisable.

Recording of MEP with magnetic stimulation has been less successful than with electrical stimulation, at least with standard coils, and large stimulus artifacts often occur. Positioning of the ground electrode between the recording electrodes and the stimulating coil may decrease the artifact.[80]

Showing a perineal MEP on stimulation over lumbosacral spine and recorded with a CNEMG electrode is sometimes helpful, but an absent response must be evaluated with caution. The clinical value of the test has yet to be established.

Assessment of Central Motor Pathways

Using magnetic or electrical stimulation, it has been shown to be possible to stimulate the motor cortex and record a response from the pelvic floor. Magnetic stimulation is not painful and cortical electrical stimulation is nowadays used only for intraoperative monitoring. The aim of these techniques is to assess conduction in the central motor pathways.

By electrical stimulation over the motor cortex of healthy subjects, MEPs in the EAS,[79,81] the urethral sphincter,[81] and the bulbocavernosus[79] muscles were reported. The mean latencies were 30 to 35 ms if no facilitatory maneuver was used. If, however, stimulation is performed during a period of slight voluntary contraction of the muscle of interest, the latencies of MEPs shortened significantly (for up to 8 ms), as has been shown in limb muscles.

By applying stimulation both over the scalp and in the back (at level L1) and subtracting the latency of the respective MEPs, a central conduction time (i.e., time of conduction in central motor pathways from the motor cortex) could be obtained. Central conduction times of approximately 22 msec without and about 15 msec with the facilitation (i.e., slight voluntary contraction) have been reported.[77]

Substantially longer central conduction times have been found in patients with multiple sclerosis and spinal cord lesions than in healthy controls.[78] However, since all those patients had clinically recognizable cord disease, the diagnostic contribution of the technique remains doubtful.

A well-formed sphincter MEP with a normal latency in a patient with a functional disorder or a medicolegal case may occasionally be helpful, but there is no established clinical use for this type of testing.

Neurophysiology of the Sacral Sensory System

Electroneurography of the Dorsal Penile Nerve

Electroneurography of the dorsal penile nerve is used to assess sensory nerve conduction of lower sacral segments. Theoretically, normal amplitude sensory nerve action potential (SNAP) of dorsal penile nerves in an insensitive penis distinguishes a lesion of sensory pathways proximal to the dorsal spinal ganglion (cauda equina, central pathways) from a lesion distal to ganglion.

By placing a pair of stimulating electrodes across the penile glans and a pair of recording electrodes across the base of the penis a SNAP can be recorded (with amplitude of approximately 10 μV). The sensory conduction velocity of the dorsal penile nerve has been reported as 27 m/s, and if the penis was stretched by a weight, the calculated velocity increased to approximately 33 m/s. The method was claimed to be helpful in diagnosing neurogenic erectile dysfunction caused by sensory penile neuropathy,[82] but the problems of measuring the conduction distance poses considerable practical difficulties and the test is now rarely used.

More practical seems to be the method of stimulating the pudendal nerve by St. Mark's electrode transrectally and recording from the penis.[83]

Electroneurography of Dorsal Sacral Roots

SNAPs on stimulation of dorsal penile and clitoral nerve may be recorded intraoperatively when the sacral roots are exposed. This has been helpful in preserving roots relevant for perineal sensation in spastic children undergoing dorsal rhizotomy and possibly decreasing the incidence of postoperative voiding dysfunction.[84]

At the level of lower thoracic and upper lumbar vertebrae, low-amplitude (<1 μV) spinal SEPs can be recorded with surface electrodes. They are monophasic negative potentials with a mean peak latency of about 12.5 ms[66] and are probably caused by postsynaptic activity in the spinal cord. Responses using surface electrodes are often unrecordable in obese healthy men[77] and in many women.

With epidural electrodes, sacral root potentials on stimulation of the dorsal penile nerve could be recorded only in 13 and cord potentials in 9 of 22 subjects; latencies of these spinal SEPs were 11.9 ± 1.8 ms,[85] substantiating the results obtained by surface recording.[66]

No use of such recordings out of the operating room has been established.

Cerebral SEPs on Electrical Stimulation of Urethra, Bladder, and Anal Canal

Cerebral SEPs on electrical stimulation of urethra, bladder, and anal canal are claimed to be more relevant to neurogenic bladder dysfunction than the pudendal SEP, as the A delta sensory afferents from bladder and proximal urethra, which convey impulses from these regions, accompany the autonomic fibers in the pelvic nerves (discussed earlier).

Cerebral SEPs can be obtained on stimulation of the bladder urothelium. When making such measurements it is of utmost importance to use bipolar stimulation in the bladder or proximal urethra because otherwise somatic afferents are depolarized. These cerebral SEPs have maximum amplitude over the midline (Cz-2 cm: Fz), but even so they may be of low amplitude (1 μV and less) and variable configuration, making it difficult to identify the response in some control subjects. The typical latency of the most prominent negative potential (N1) is approximately 100 ms.[86]

After stimulation of the anal canal, cerebral SEPs with a slightly longer latency than those obtained on bladder and urethra have been reported. It is not possible to record this response from all control subjects. The rectum and sigmoid colon have also been stimulated, and cerebral SEPs of two types recorded. One was similar in shape and latency to pudendal SEPs, and the other to SEPs recorded on stimulation of bladder/posterior urethra.[87]

No clinical usefulness of such recordings has been established.

Autonomic Nervous System Tests

All of the neurophysiologic methods for evaluation of the pelvic floor disorders discussed so far assess the thicker myelinated fibers only, whereas the autonomic nervous system, the parasympathetic part in particular, is the most relevant for sacral organ function. Local involvement of the sacral nervous system (e.g., trauma, compression) usually involves somatic and autonomic fibers simultaneously. However, some local pathologic conditions cause isolated lesions of the autonomic nervous system (mesorectal excision of carcinoma or radical prostatectomy). Methods that assess the parasympathetic and sympathetic systems directly would thus be very helpful. Information on parasympathetic bladder innervation can to some extent be obtained by cystometry; however, this is a test of overall organ function and usually cannot locate the lesion.

Sympathetic Skin Response

The sympathetic nervous system mediates sweat gland activity in the skin, and changes in sweat gland activity lead to changes in skin resistance. On stressful stimulation a potential shift can be recorded with surface electrodes from the skin of palms and soles, and has been reported to be a useful parameter in assessment of neuropathy involving unmyelinated nerve fibers. The sympathetic skin response (SSR) can also be recorded from perineal skin and the penis. The SSR is a reflex that consists of myelinated sensory fibers, a complex central integrative mechanism, and a sympathetic efferent limb (with postganglionic nonmyelinated C fibers).[88] The stimulus used in clinical practice is usually electrical pulse delivered to the upper or lower limb (to mixed nerves), but the genital organs can also be stimulated. The latencies of SSR on the penis after stimulation of a median nerve at the wrist have been reported between 1.5 and 2.3 sec and could be obtained in all normal subjects with a large variability.[89,90] The responses rapidly habituate, and they depend on a number of endogenous and exogenous factors including skin temperature, which should be at least 28 °C. Only an absent SSR can be considered abnormal.

There is no consensus on the clinical value of SSR testing in sacral dysfunction.

Corpus Cavernosum EMG

Electrodiagnostic tests of sacral parasympathetic nerve function (e.g., for corpus cavernosum EMG, also called spontaneous cavernosal activity)[91] would in principle constitute the most definitive indicator of neurogenic sacral organ involvement. Further research to validate this and other potentially useful methods such as detrusor EMG will clarify their place in both research and diagnostics; at present, these tests cannot be suggested for patient diagnosis.

PATIENTS FOR WHOM ELECTRODIAGNOSTIC TESTS ARE VALUABLE

Parkinsonism

Neuropathic changes can be recorded in the sphincter muscles of patients with multiple system atrophy (MSA).[15,24,34,48,92] MSA is a progressive neurodegenerative disease that is often (particularly in its early stages) mistaken for Parkinson's disease. Urinary incontinence in both sexes and erectile dysfunction in men are early features of the condition, often present for some years before the onset of typical neurologic features.[93] Autonomic failure causing postural hypotension and cerebellar ataxia causing unsteadiness and clumsiness may be additional features. The disease is usually (in 80% of patients) unresponsive to antiparkinsonian treatment. As a part of the neurodegenerative process, loss of motor neurons occurs in Onuf's nucleus so that partial but progressive denervation of the sphincter and the bulbocavernosus muscles occurs,[15] and recorded MUPs show changes of reinnervation.[24,92]

Sphincter EMG is valuable in distinguishing between idiopathic Parkinson's disease and MSA,[24,92] but it may not be sensitive in the early phase of disease,[15] and not specific after 5 years of parkinsonism.[94] Prolonged duration of MUPs,[24,92] abnormal spontaneous activity,[34] as well as diminished number of continuously active low-threshold MUs and IP abnormalities[95] are described markers for degeneration of Onuf's nucleus in patients with MSA. The changes of chronic reinnervation may be found in other parkinsonian syndromes, such as progressive supranuclear palsy (PSP).[96] Chronic reinnervation changes can also be demonstrated as an increase in fiber density on SFEMG.[48] In contrast to previous reports, a recent study did not show significant differences between two small groups of patients with MSA and Parkinson's disease.[97] This might be a consequence of excluding late components from MUP duration, which was made also in another study that did not find MUP analysis useful.[34] In a small number of patients with MSA or primary autonomic failure, the EAS muscle CNEMG was reported sensitive and specific for men, but nonspecific for women, in supporting a diagnosis of MSA.[98]

Kinesiologic EMG performed during urodynamic testing can be also valuable for patients with Parkinson's disease[15] and for patients who have MSA[16] document loss of coordination between detrusor and urethral sphincter muscles (detrusor–sphincter dyssynergia).

CNEMG, including observation of denervation activity[34] and quantitative MUP analysis,[24,92] is clearly indicated in patients with suspected MSA, particularly in the early stages of the disease.[94] If this test is normal in the first few years of the disease but the suspicion of the disease persists, it might be of value to repeat the test.[15]

Cauda Equina and Conus Medullaris Lesions

Lesions to the cauda equina or conus medullaris are an important cause of pelvic floor dysfunction. Usually the neural tissue damage is caused by compression within the spinal canal due to disk protrusion, spinal fractures, epidural hematomas, tumors, congenital malformations, and so on. Unfortunately, damage to the cauda equina still occurs as a result of surgery, mainly on lumbar disks.

Symptoms depend very much on the etiology of the lesion. In cases of disk protrusion, spinal fractures, and epidural hematomas, presentation is often dramatic. Acute severe back pain radiating to legs, associated by numbness and tingling in the legs (particularly the posterior aspects of the thighs), buttocks, and perineal region are noted first. Urinary retention with overflow incontinence and later severe constipation follow. In disk protrusion history of previous back pain with sciatica, in spinal fractures the history of trauma, and in epidural hematomas a history of coagulation disorder (or anticoagulation therapy) is often present. With tumors, the presentation of the cauda equina lesion is much more insidious.

After detailed clinical examination of the perineal region (with particular emphasis on perianal sensation), CNEMG of the EAS muscle (and sometimes bulbocavernosus muscle) and evaluation of BCR (when absent clinically) are electrophysiologic tests that must be considered. Neurophysiologic assessment is useful to determine the sequels of the lesion, and in insidious cases for reaching the diagnosis.

Generally stated, detection of pathologic spontaneous activity by CNEMG has good sensitivity and specificity to show moderate and severe partial denervation, and complete denervation, of pelvic floor muscles 3 weeks or more after injury to the cauda equina or conus medullaris. Traumatic lesions to the lumbosacral spine or particularly to the pelvis (see Fig. 24-3) is probably the only acquired condition in which complete denervation of the perineal muscles can be observed.[26] Most lesions (including trauma), however, cause partial denervation. CNEMG of the bulbocavernosus muscles is of particular importance a few weeks after partial denervation in the lower sacral myotomes to detect fibrillation potentials.

CNEMG (MUP analysis) can show changes of reinnervation, which appear months after injury.[26] After a cauda equina lesion, the MUPs are likely to be prolonged and polyphasic,[99] and other MUP parameters are also increased.[26] Similar marked changes are seen in patients with lumbosacral myelomeningocele.

BCR is useful in evaluation of subjects with cauda equina or conus medullaris lesions to assess the integrity of the reflex arc. In patients with a tethered cord syndrome measurement of BCR latency can be of additional value, as a very short reflex latency in this clinical situation supports the possibility of the abnormally low position of the conus medullaris.[61]

Urinary Retention in Women

For many years it was said that isolated urinary retention in young women was due to psychogenic factors or was the first symptom of onset of multiple sclerosis. However, CNEMG in this group showed that many such patients have profuse complex repetitive discharges (CRDs) and decelerating burst (DB) activity in the urethral sphincter muscle.[100]

Why this activity occurs is not known but in the syndrome described by one of the authors, it was associated with polycystic ovaries.[101] Typically, patients with this syndrome are premenopausal, and the condition has its maximum incidence in women younger than 30 years. This pathologic spontaneous activity endures during micturition and may cause obstruction to flow.[18] The disorder of sphincter relaxation apparently leads to secondary changes in detrusor function—either instability or failure of contractility can occur.

Because CNEMG detects both changes of denervation and reinnervation (e.g., with a cauda equina lesion), as well as this peculiar abnormal spontaneous activity, it can be argued that this test is mandatory in women with urinary retention.[18,100] It should be carried out before stigmatizing a woman as having "psychogenic urinary retention."

PATIENT GROUPS IN WHOM ELECTRODIAGNOSTIC TESTS ARE OF RESEARCH INTEREST

Neurophysiologic techniques have been important in research, and substantiated hypotheses that a proportion of patients with sacral dysfunction, such as stress urinary and idiopathic fecal incontinence, have involvement of the nervous system,[71,73] established the function of the sacral nervous system in patients with suprasacral spinal cord injury,[102] and showed consequences of particular surgeries.[103] However, in individual patients from these groups, electrodiagnostic tests are unlikely to be contributory.

Primary Muscle Diseases

There are only few reports of pelvic floor muscle EMG in generalized myopathy. In skeletal muscle, the typical features of myopathy are small, low-amplitude polyphasic MUPs recruited at mild effort. Such changes have not been reported in the pelvic floor, even in patients with known generalized myopathy.[104] Pelvic floor muscle involvement on histology in limb-girdle muscular dystrophy in a nulliparous woman has been reported, but CNEMG of her urethral sphincter was reported as normal.[105] Myopathic involvement was reported in the puborectalis and the EAS in patients with myotonic dystrophy.[106] Such reports are so far only of research interest.

Urinary Incontinence

Because of the suspected role of denervation in the genesis of genuine stress incontinence (GSI), EMG techniques have been used to look at the extent of nerve damage after childbirth and in the assessment of women with GSI. SFEMG was used to measure fiber density in the EAS and an increase was shown in women with urinary GSI.[107] The relationship of GSI, genitourinary prolapse, and partial denervation of the pelvic floor was studied. Using SFEMG (fiber density) pubococcygeus was found to be partially denervated or reinnervated in women with GSI, genital prolapse, or both. Age-related denervation or reinnervation changes were found, too.[108] Using a CNEMG to examine pubococcygeus after childbirth, significant increase in MUP duration was found following vaginal delivery.[109] The changes were most marked in women who had urinary incontinence 8 weeks after delivery and who had had a prolonged second stage and given birth to heavier babies.

In a recent study of the EAS muscle that used advanced MUP and IP analysis techniques, three of five IP parameters differed between the parous and nulliparous women, but no significant difference was found in any of nine evaluated MUP parameters.[29] On multiple linear regression analysis, the number of deliveries was related to several MUP and IP parameters: the time elapsed since last delivery to MUP, and slight stress urinary incontinence to IP parameters. A group of parous women with (slight) GSI had less neuropathic MUP parameters than those without had. It was concluded that vaginal delivery is related to EAS muscle CNEMG abnormalities, but these are minor and seem not to indicate loss of sphincter function. This study casts some doubt on the common preconception[74] that significant damage to peripheral innervation of the EAS occurs even during uncomplicated deliveries.[29] On examination of the urethral sphincter muscle, significantly more fibrillation potentials, fewer MUPs, a higher percentage of polyphasia, and less maximum voluntary electrical activity were found on CNEMG in a group of women with GSI than were found in controls. On muscle biopsy the patient group had lower skeletal muscle and a higher connective tissue content.[110] Despite these findings, the role of the urethral sphincter CNEMG in subjects (particularly women) with urinary incontinence has not been proved. Although CNEMG of this muscle seems the logical choice in patients with urinary incontinence possibly of neurogenic origin, only a small amount of (pathologic) muscle tissue remains in many incontinent parous women.[110] This finding would be expected and will not affect therapeutic considerations, which rely primarily on a generalized involvement of the pelvic floor innervation (as shown by CNEMG of the EAS muscle). Thus, examination of the urethral sphincter often may not provide relevant additional information to that already obtained by CNEMG of the EAS muscle, in this clinical situation.

On kinesiologic EMG performed as a part of urodynamic evaluation in stress-incontinent patients, the patterns of pubococcygeus muscle activation as well as coordination between the two sides may be lost.[19]

In the individual incontinent patient without signs or symptoms of a neurologic condition, the contribution of neurophysiologic testing is not expected to be helpful or necessary.

Anal Incontinence

Anal incontinence of unknown cause is a clinical condition for which CNEMG of the EAS has been suggested as useful,[111] as a rule after an anal ultrasound examination to exclude structural lesions of the sphincter mechanism. In such patients, clinical and electrophysiologic signs of a more generalized (i.e., MSA, etc.), or proximal (i.e., cauda equine or conus medullaris), involvement of the lower sacral myotomes should be looked for. In a subgroup of patients in whom no cause of anal incontinence can be established (i.e., idiopathic anal incontinence) diminished number (absence) of continuously firing low-threshold MUs during relaxation was noted as the only electrophysiologic abnormality (unpublished personal data).

There is no consensus on the usefulness of neurophysiologic testing in patients with anal incontinence and normal findings on clinical neurologic examination.

Chronic Constipation

Constipation is a heterogeneous syndrome[4,112] that is common in the general population if loose diagnostic criteria are applied (17.5%)[113] but rarer with more stringent criteria (2%).[114] Applying electrophysiologic techniques—SFEMG (fiber density)[73,115] and semiquantitative[112,116] or manual-MUP quantitative[117] CNEMG—several studies showed EMG changes in the EAS muscles of severely constipated subjects, although this is not a universal finding.[112,116] Injury to the pelvic floor innervation in constipated patients was attributed to repeated straining. In a recent study using advanced MUP and IP analysis, no abnormalities were demonstrable in the EAS muscles of patients with a history of mild chronic constipation.[40]

Radiographic methods are more useful in the diagnosis of chronic constipation. They show both main mechanisms of constipation: prolonged colonic transit (using radiographic markers) and obstructed defecation (abnormal movement patterns of pelvic floor during defecation). Evaluation of the second condition may be helped using kinesiologic EMG, as, for instance, in patients with nonrelaxing puborectalis syndrome (a subtype of obstructed defecation) in whom continuous contraction of the puborectalis muscle during defecation was demonstrated.[21,118] Such kinesiologic EMG testing, however, has been neither much routinely applied nor so far standardized. As a consequence, at the moment, it cannot be recommended as an established method for evaluation of severely constipated patients.

Erectile Dysfunction

Neurophysiologic techniques were extensively used in research that substantiated the hypothesis that a proportion of patients with erectile dysfunction have involvement of the nervous system. Several electrodiagnostic techniques were proposed. Sensory penile neuropathy was claimed to be the cause of erectile dysfunction by testing the sensory conduction velocity of the dorsal penile nerve[82]; testing of BCR to electrical stimulation of the dorsal penile nerves has been proposed also.[51] However, the sensitivity and specificity of this technique were poor because many patients with probable neurogenic erectile dysfunction had reflex latencies within the normal range.[58] Conversely, patients with hereditary motor and sensory demyelinating neuropathy (HMSN I) with normal bladder and sexual function had delayed sacral reflex responses.[59] Findings in diabetics with suspected neurogenic erectile dysfunction showed limb conduction studies were more sensitive in showing peripheral neuropathy than BCR latencies.[60] Pudendal SEP recordings have also been used in patients with neurogenic erectile dysfunction due to spinal cord lesions,[58] multiple sclerosis,[119] and diabetes,[60] but they were found to be of no greater value than clinical examination to detect spinal cord disease.[120]

Autonomic function tests were proposed to be more sensitive than measuring somatic parameters of the sacral nervous system, and SSR recording in limbs was claimed to be more informative than BCR and pudendal SEP testing in patients with organic erectile dysfunction.[121] Recording SSR from the penis was reported to be even more informative[90] because it assesses local afferent innervation.

Penile smooth muscle is an obvious target for electrophysiologic recordings in patients with erectile dysfunction,[122] but EMG of this muscle is controversial, particularly as regards the source and nature of the signal.[91]

The Consensus on Erectile Dysfunction recently stated that neurophysiologic testing (CNEMG and BCR) is helpful in only very selected patients suspected to have a neurogenic condition on the basis of the clinical neurologic examination.[123]

Diseases of the Central Nervous System

As a part of urodynamics, kinesiologic tests are often useful in patients with CNS signs who have a pelvic floor disorder. Electrodiagnostic tests of conduction performed in patients with "central" lesions are only very occasionally indicated. CNEMG is not indicated in central lesions unless segmental spinal cord (conus medullaris) involvement is suspected.[1]

CONCLUSION

Several electrophysiologic tests have been proposed for evaluation of the pelvic floor, the sphincter muscles, and their motor and sensory innervation. Although all tests mentioned in this chapter continue to be of research interest, the CNEMG is of definite usefulness in everyday routine diagnostic evaluation of selected groups of patients with pelvic floor dysfunction, those with atypical parkinsonism, or those with traumatic lesions. Probably the only group of patients in whom the sacral dysfunction should be considered an indication for CNEMG are young women with urinary retention.

New computer-assisted techniques of CNEMG analysis are expected to improve the usefulness of the test as a diagnostic method to show neuropathic pelvic floor muscle involvement. Further research into and experience with other discussed neurophysiologic tests will reveal their contribution to clinical assessment of individual patients, which is unknown.

REFERENCES

1. Fowler CJ, Benson JT, Craggs MD, et al: Clinical neurophysiology. In Abrams P, Cardozo L, Khoury S, Wein A (eds): Incontinence. Plymouth, UK, Health Publication, 2002, pp 389–424.
2. Vodušek DB, Fowler CJ: Clinical neurophysiology. In Fowler CJ (ed): Neurology of Bladder, Bowel and Sexual Dysfunction. Boston, Butterworth-Heinemann, 1999, p 109.
3. Jorge JM, Wexner SD: Etiology and management of fecal incontinence. Dis Colon Rectum 36:77, 1993.
4. Agachan F, Chen T, Pfeifer J, et al: A constipation scoring system to simplify evaluation and management of constipated patients. Dis Colon Rectum 39:681, 1996.
5. Donovan JL, Badia X, Naughton M, Gotoh M: Symptom and quality of life assessment. In Abrams P, Cardozo L, Khoury S, Wein A (eds): Incontinence. Plymouth, UK, Health Publication, 2002, p 267.
6. O'Leary MP, Fowler FJ, Lenderking WR, et al: A brief male sexual function inventory for urology. Urology 46:697, 1995.
7. Rosen RC, Riley A, Wagner G, et al: An international index of erectile function (IIEF): A multidimensional scale for assessment of erectile dysfunction. Urology 49:822, 1997.
8. Vodušek DB, Janko M: The bulbocavernosus reflex: A single motor neuron study. Brain 113:813, 1990.
9. Podnar S, Vodušek DB, Stålberg E: Standardization of anal sphincter electromyography: Normative data. Clin Neurophysiol 111:2200, 2000.
10. Podnar S, Vodušek DB: Standardisation of anal sphincter EMG: Low and high threshold motor units. Clin Neurophysiol 110:1488, 1999.
11. Chantraine A, Leval J, Onkelinx A: Motor conduction velocity in the internal pudendal nerves. In Desmedt JE (ed): New Developments in Electromyography and Clinical Neurophysiology, vol 2. Basel, Karger, 1973, p 433.
12. Jesel M, Isch-Treussard C, Isch F: Electromyography of striated muscle of anal urethral sphincters. In Desmedt JE (ed): New Developments in Electromyography and Clinical Neurophysiology, vol 2. Basel, Karger, 1973, p 406.
13. Deindl FM, Vodušek DB, Hesse U, et al: Activity patterns of pubococcygeal muscles in nulliparous continent women. Br J Urol 72:46, 1993.
14. Podnar S, Vodušek DB: Standardization of anal sphincter electromyography: Uniformity of the muscle. Muscle Nerve 23:122, 2000.
15. Stocchi F, Carbone A, Inghilleri M, et al: Urodynamic and neurophysiological evaluation in Parkinson's disease and multiple system atrophy. J Neurol Neurosurg Psychiatry 62:507, 1997.
16. Sakakibara R, Hattori T, Uchiyama T, et al: Urinary dysfunction and orthostatic hypotension in multiple system atrophy: Which is the more common and earlier manifestation? J Neurol Neurosurg Psychiatry 68:65, 2000.
17. Chancellor MB, Kaplan SA, Blaivas JG: Detrusor-external sphincter dyssynergia. In Bock G, Whelan J (eds): Neurobiology of Incontinence. Chichester, John Wiley, 1990, p 195.
18. Deindl FM, Vodušek DB, Bischoff C, et al: Dysfunctional voiding in women: Which muscles are responsible? Br J Urol 82:814, 1998.
19. Deindl F, Vodušek DB, Hesse U, et al: Pelvic floor activity patterns: Comparison of nulliparous continent and parous urinary stress incontinent women. A kinesiological EMG study. Br J Urol 73:413, 1994.
20. Chantraine A, De Leval J, Depireux P: Adult female intra- and peri-urethral sphincter-electromyographic study. Neurourol Urodynam 9:139, 1990.
21. Mathers SE, Kempster SAS, Swash M, et al: Constipation and paradoxical puborectalis contractions in anismus and Parkinson's disease: A dystonic phenomenon? J Neurol Neurosurg Psychiatry 51:1503, 1988.
22. Podnar S, Rodi Z, Lukanović A, et al: Standardization of anal sphincter EMG: Technique of needle examination. Muscle Nerve 22:400, 1999.
23. Fowler CJ, Kirby RS, Harrison MJG: Decelerating bursts and complex repetitive discharges in the striated muscle of the urethral sphincter associated with urinary retention in women. J Neurol Neurosurg Psychiatry 48:1004, 1985.
24. Palace J, Chandiramani VA, Fowler CJ: Value of sphincter EMG in the diagnosis of multiple system atrophy. Muscle Nerve 20:1396, 1997.
25. Buchthal F: Introduction to Electromyography. Copenhagen, Scandinavian University Press, 1957.
26. Podnar S, Vodušek DB, Stålberg E: Comparison of quantitative techniques in anal sphincter electromyography. Muscle Nerve 25:83, 2002.
27. Czekajewski J, Ekstedt J, Stålberg E: Oscilloscopic recording of muscle fiber action potentials: The window trigger and delay unit. Electroencephalogr Clin Neurophysiol 27:536, 1969.
28. Stålberg E, Falck B, Sonoo M, et al: Multi-MUP EMG analysis: A two-year experience in daily clinical work. Electroencephalogr Clin Neurophysiol 97:145, 1995.
29. Podnar S, Lukanović A, Vodušek DB: Anal sphincter electromyography after vaginal delivery: Neuropathic insufficiency or normal wear and tear? Neurourol Urodynam 19:249, 2000.
30. Stålberg E, Bischoff C, Falck B: Outliers: A way to detect abnormality in quantitative EMG. Muscle Nerve 17:392, 1994.
31. Nandedkar S, Sanders D, Stålberg E, Andreassen S: Simulation of concentric needle EMG motor unit action potentials. Muscle Nerve 11:151, 1988.
32. Stålberg E, Andreassen S, Falck B, et al: Quantitative analysis of individual motor unit potentials: A proposition for standardized terminology and criteria for measurement. J Clin Neurophysiol 3:313, 1986.
33. AAEE glossary of terms used in clinical electromyography. Muscle Nerve 10 (suppl 8):G1, 1987.
34. Schwarz J, Kornhuber M, Bischoff C, et al: Electromyography of the external anal sphincter in patients with Parkinson's disease and multiple system atrophy: Frequency of abnormal spontaneous activity and polyphasic motor unit potentials. Muscle Nerve 20:1167, 1997.
35. Nandedkar S, Barkhaus P, Sanders D, et al: Analysis of the amplitude and area of the concentric needle EMG motor unit action potentials. Electroencephalogr Clin Neurophysiol 69:561, 1988.
36. Sonoo M, Stålberg E: The ability of MUP parameters to discriminate between normal and neurogenic MUPs in concentric EMG: Analysis of the MUP "thickness" and the proposal of "size index." Electroencephalogr Clin Neurophysiol 89:291, 1993.

37. Willison RG: Analysis of electrical activity in healthy and dystrophic muscle in man. J Neurol Neurosurg Psychiatry 27:386, 1964.
38. Stålberg E, Chu J, Bril V, et al: Automatic analysis of the EMG interference pattern. Electromyogr Clin Neurophysiol 56:672, 1983.
39. Nandedkar SD, Sanders DB, Stålberg EV: Automatic analysis of the electromyographic interference pattern: Part II. Findings in control subjects and in some neuromuscular diseases. Muscle Nerve 9:491, 1986.
40. Podnar S, Vodušek DB: Standardization of anal sphincter electromyography: Effect of chronic constipation. Muscle Nerve 23:1748, 2000.
41. Stålberg E, Trontelj JV: Single Fiber Electromyography: Studies in Healthy and Diseased Muscle, ed 2. New York, Raven Press, 1994.
42. Neill ME, Swash M: Increased motor unit fiber density in the external anal sphincter muscle in ano-rectal incontinence: A single fiber EMG study. J Neurol Neurosurg Psychiatry 43:343, 1980.
43. Vodušek DB, Janko M: SFEMG in striated sphincter muscles. Muscle Nerve 4:252, 1981.
44. Jameson JS, Chia YW, Kamm MA, et al: Effect of age, sex and parity on anorectal function. Br J Surg 81:1689, 1994.
45. Laurberg S, Swash M: Effects of aging on the anorectal sphincters and their innervation. Dis Colon Rectum 32:737, 1989.
46. Snooks SJ, Badenoch DF, Tiptaft RC, et al: Perineal nerve damage in genuine stress incontinence. Br J Urol 57:422, 1985.
47. Vodušek DB, Janko M, Lokar J: EMG, single fiber EMG and sacral reflexes in assessment of sacral nervous system lesions. J Neurol Neurosurg Psychiatry 45:1064, 1982.
48. Rodi Z, Vodušek DB, Denišlič M: External anal sphincter electromyography in the differential diagnosis of parkinsonism. J Neurol Neurosurg Psychiatry 60:460, 1996.
49. Dyro FM, Yalla SV: Refractoriness of striated sphincter during voiding: Studies with afferent pudendal reflex arc stimulation in male subjects. J Urol 135:732, 1986.
50. Sethi RK, Bauer SB, Dyro FM, et al: Modulation of the bulbocavernosus reflex during voiding: Loss of inhibition in upper motor neuron lesions. Muscle Nerve 12:892, 1989.
51. Ertekin Ç, Reel F: Bulbocavernosus reflex in normal men and patients with neurogenic bladder and/or impotence. J Neurol Sci 28:1, 1976.
52. Vodušek DB, Janko M, Lokar J: Direct and reflex responses in perineal muscles on electrical stimulation. J Neurol Neurosurg Psychiatry 46:67, 1983.
53. Dystra D, Sidi A, Cameron J, et al: The use of mechanical stimulation to obtain the sacral reflex latency: A new technique. J Urol 137:77, 1987.
54. Podnar S, Vodušek DB, Tršinar B, et al: A method of uroneurophysiological investigation in children. Electroencephalogr Clin Neurophysiol 104:389, 1997.
55. Loening-Baucke V, Read NW, Yamada T, et al: Evaluation of the motor and sensory components of the pudendal nerve. Electroencephalogr Clin Neurophysiol 93:35, 1994.
56. Vodušek DB: Evoked potential testing. Urol Clin North Am 23:427, 1996.
57. Rodi Z, Vodušek DB: The sacral reflex studies: Single versus double pulse stimulation. Neurourol Urodynam 14:496, 1995.
58. Tackmann W, Vogel P, Porst H: Somatosensory evoked potentials after stimulation of the dorsal penile nerve: Normative data and results from 145 patients with erectile dysfunction. Eur Neurol 27:245, 1987.
59. Vodušek DB, Zidar J: Pudendal nerve involvement in patients with hereditary motor and sensory neuropathy. Acta Neurol Scand 76:457, 1987.
60. Vodušek DB, Ravnik-Oblak M, Oblak C: Pudendal versus limb nerves electrophysiologic abnormalities in diabetics with erectile dysfunction. Int J Impot Res 2:37, 1993.
61. Hanson PH, Rigaux P, Gilliard C, et al: Sacral reflex latencies in tethered cord syndrome. Am J Phys Med Rehabil 72:39, 1993.
62. Bilkey WJ, Awad EA, Smith AD: Clinical application of sacral reflex latency. J Urol 129:1187, 1983.
63. Haldeman S, Bradley WE, Bhatia N: Evoked responses from the pudendal nerve. J Urol 128:974, 1982.
64. Haldeman S, Bradley WE, Bhatia N, et al: Cortical evoked potentials on stimulation of pudendal nerve in women. Urology 6:590, 1983.
65. Guérit JM, Opsomer RJ: Bit-mapped imaging of somatosensory evoked potentials after stimulation of the posterior tibial nerves and dorsal nerve of the penis/clitoris. Electroencephalogr Clin Neurophysiol 80:228, 1991.
66. Vodušek DB,: Pudendal somatosensory evoked potential and bulbocavernosus reflex in women. Electroencephalogr Clin Neurophysiol 77:134, 1990.
67. Rodi Z, Vodušek DB, Denišlič M: Clinical uro-neurophysiological investigation in multiple sclerosis. Eur J Neurol 3:574, 1996.
68. Delodovici ML, Fowler CJ: Clinical value of the pudendal somatosensory evoked potential. Electroencephalogr Clin Neurophysiol 96:509, 1995.
69. Vodušek DB, Deletis V, Abbott R, et al: Prevention of iatrogenic micturition disorders through intraoperative monitoring. Neurourol Urodynam 9:444, 1990.
70. Pedersen E, Klemar B, Schroder HD, et al: Anal sphincter responses after perianal electrical stimulation. J Neurol Neurosurg Psychiatry 45:770, 1982.
71. Kiff ES, Swash M: Normal proximal and delayed distal conduction in the pudendal nerves of patients with idiopathic (neurogenic) faecal incontinence. J Neurol Neurosurg Psychiatry 47:820, 1984.
72. Brown FW: The Physiological and Technical Basis of Electromyography. London, Butterworth, 1984.
73. Snooks SJ, Barnes PR, Swash M, et al: Damage to the innervation of the pelvic floor musculature in chronic constipation. Gastroenterology 89:977, 1985.
74. Snooks SJ, Swash M, Setchell M, et al: Injury to the pelvic floor sphincter musculature in childbirth. Lancet 2:546, 1984.
75. Snooks SJ, Swash M, Mathers SE, et al: Effect of vaginal delivery in the pelvic floor: A 5-year follow-up. Br J Surg 77:1358, 1990.
76. Benson T, McClellan E: The effect of vaginal dissection on the pudendal nerve. Obstet Gynecol 82:387, 1993.
77. Opsomer RJ, Caramia MD, Zarola F, et al: Neurophysiological evaluation of central-peripheral sensory and motor pudendal fibers. Electroencephalogr Clin Neurophysiol 74:260, 1989.
78. Eardley I, Nagendran K, Lecky B, et al: The neurophysiology of the striated urethral sphincter in multiple sclerosis. Br J Urol 67:81, 1991.
79. Vodušek DB, Zidar J: Perineal motor evoked responses. Neurourol Urodynam 7:236, 1988.
80. Jost WH, Schimrigk K: A new method to determine pudendal nerve motor latency and central motor conduction time to the external anal sphincter. Electroencephalogr Clin Neurophysiol 93:237, 1994.
81. Thiry AJ, Deltenre PF: Neurophysiological assessment of the central motor pathway to the external urethral sphincter in man. Br J Urol 63:515, 1989.

82. Bradley WE, Lin JTY, Johnson B: Measurement of the conduction velocity of the dorsal nerve of the penis. J Urol 131:1127, 1984.
83. Amarenco G, Kerdraon J: Pudendal nerve terminal sensitive latency: Technique and normal values. J Urol 161:103, 1999.
84. Deletis V, Vodušek DB, Abbott R, et al: Intraoperative monitoring of dorsal sacral roots: Minimizing the risk of iatrogenic micturition disorders. Neurosurgery 30:72, 1992.
85. Ertekin Ç, Mungan B: Sacral spinal cord and root potentials evoked by the stimulation of the dorsal nerve of penis and cord conduction delay for the bulbocavernosus reflex. Neurourol Urodynam 12:9, 1993.
86. Hansen MV, Ertekin Ç, Larsson LE: Cerebral evoked potentials after stimulation of the posterior urethra in man. Electroencephalogr Clin Neurophysiol 77:52, 1990.
87. Loening-Baucke V, Read NW, Yamada T: Further evaluation of the afferent nervous pathways from the rectum. Am J Physiol 25:G927, 1992.
88. Arunodaya GR, Taly AB: Sympathetic skin response: A decade later. J Neurol Sci 129:81, 1995.
89. Opsomer RJ, Pesce FR, Abi Aad A, et al: Electrophysiologic testing of motor sympathetic pathways: Normative data and clinical contribution in neuro-urological disorders. Neurourol Urodynam 12:336, 1993.
90. Daffertshofer M, Linden D, Syren M, et al: Assessment of local sympathetic function in patients with erectile dysfunction. Int J Impot Res 6:213, 1994.
91. Colakoglu Z, Kutluay E, Ertekin Ç: The nature of spontaneous cavernosal activity. BJU Int 83:449, 1999.
92. Eardley I, Quinn NP, Fowler CJ, et al: The value of urethral sphincter electromyography in the differential diagnosis of parkinsonism. Br J Urol 64:360, 1989.
93. Beck RO, Betts CD, Fowler CJ: Genitourinary dysfunction in multiple system atrophy: Clinical features and treatment in 62 cases. J Urol 151:1336, 1994.
94. Libelius R, Johansson F: Quantitative electromyography of the external anal sphincter in Parkinson's disease and multiple system atrophy. Muscle Nerve 23:1250, 2000.
95. Gilad R, Giladi N, Sadeh M: Quantitative EMG of sphincter ani in normal individuals and multiple system atrophy. Clin Neurophysiol 110:S94, 1999.
96. Vallderiola F, Valls-Solè J, Tolosa ES, et al: Striated anal sphincter denervation in patients with progressive supranuclear palsy. Mov Disord 9:117, 1995.
97. Giladi N, Simon ES, Korczyn AD, et al: Anal sphincter EMG does not distinguish between multiple system atrophy and Parkinson's disease. Muscle Nerve 23:731, 2000.
98. Ravits J, Hallett M, Nilsson J, et al: Electrophysiological tests of autonomic function in patients with idiopathic autonomic failure syndromes. Muscle Nerve 19:758, 1996.
99. Fowler CJ, Kirby RS, Harrison MJG, et al: Individual motor unit analysis in the diagnosis of disorders of urethral sphincter innervation. J Neurol Neurosurg Psychiatry 47:637, 1984.
100. Fowler CJ, Kirby RS: Electromyography of the urethral sphincter in women with urinary retention. Lancet 1:1455, 1986.
101. Fowler CJ, Christmas TJ, Chapple CR, et al: Abnormal electromyographic activity of the urethral sphincter, voiding dysfunction, and polycystic ovaries: A new syndrome? BMJ 297:1436, 1988.
102. Koldewijn EL, van Kerrebroeck PhEV, Bemelmans BLH, et al: Use of sacral reflex latency measurements in the evaluation of neural function of spinal cord injury patients: A comparison of neuro-urophysiological testing and urodynamic investigations. J Urol 152:463, 1994.
103. Liu S, Christmas TJ, Nagendran K, et al: Sphincter electromyography in patients after radical prostatectomy and cystoprostatectomy. Br J Urol 69:397, 1992.
104. Caress J, Kothari M, Bauer S, et al: Urinary dysfunction in Duchenne muscular dystrophy. Muscle Nerve 19:819, 1996.
105. Dixon PJ, Christmas TJ, Chapple CR: Stress incontinence due to pelvic floor muscle involvement in limb-girdle muscular dystrophy. Br J Urol 65:653, 1990.
106. Herbaut AG, Nogueira MC, Panzer JM, et al: Anorectal incontinence in myotonic dystrophy: A myopathic involvement of pelvic floor muscles (letter). Muscle Nerve 5:1210, 1992.
107. Anderson R: A neurogenic element to urinary genuine stress incontinence. Br J Urol 91:41, 1984.
108. Smith ARB, Hosker GL, Warrell DW: The role of partial denervation of the pelvic floor in aetiology of genitourinary prolapse and stress incontinence of urine: A neurophysiological study. Br J Obstet Gynaecol 96:24, 1989.
109. Allen R, Hosker G, Smith A, et al: Pelvic floor damage and childbirth: A neurophysiological study. Br J Obstet Gynaecol 97:770, 1990.
110. Hale DS, Benson JT, Brubaker L, et al: Histologic analysis of needle biopsy of urethral sphincter from women with normal and stress incontinence with comparison of electromyographic findings. Am J Obstet Gynecol 180:342, 1999.
111. Aanestad O, Flink R: Interference pattern in perineal muscles: A quantitative electromyographic study in patients with faecal incontinence. Eur J Surg 160:111, 1994.
112. Vaccaro CA, Cheong DM, Wexner SD, et al: Pudendal neuropathy in evacuatory disorders. Dis Colon Rectum 38:166, 1995.
113. Drossman DA, Sandler RS, McKee DC, et al: Bowel patterns among subjects not seeking health care: Use of a questionnaire to identify a population with bowel dysfunction. Gastroenterology 83:529, 1982.
114. Johanson JF, Sonnenberg A, Koch TR: Clinical epidemiology of chronic constipation. J Clin Gastroenterol 11:525, 1989.
115. Fink RL, Roberts LJ, Scott M: The role of manometry, electromyography and radiology in the assessment of intractable constipation. Aust N Z J Surg 62:959, 1992.
116. Vaccaro CA, Wexner SD, Teoh TA, et al: Pudendal neuropathy is not related to physiologic pelvic outlet obstruction. Dis Colon Rectum 38:630, 1995.
117. Bartolo DCC, Jarratt JA, Read NW: The cutaneo-anal reflex: A useful index of neuropathy? Br J Surg 70:660, 1983.
118. Jorge JM, Wexner SD, Ger GC, et al: Cinedefecography and electromyography in the diagnosis of nonrelaxing puborectalis syndrome. Dis Colon Rectum 36:668, 1993.
119. Kirkeby HJ, Poulsen EU, Petersen T, Dorup J: Erectile dysfunction in multiple sclerosis. Neurology 38:1366, 1988.
120. Betts CD, Jones SJ, Fowler CG, et al: Erectile dysfunction in multiple sclerosis: Associated neurological and neurophysiological deficits, and treatment of the condition. Brain 117:1303, 1994.
121. Kunesch E, Reiners K, Müller-Mattheis V, et al: Neurological risk profile in organic erectile impotence. J Neurol Neurosurg Psychiatry 55:275, 1992.
122. Stief CG, Kellner B, Hartung C, et al: Computer-assisted evaluation of the smooth-muscle electromyogram of the corpora cavernosa by fast Fourier transformation. Eur Urol 31:329, 1997.
123. Lundberg PO, Brackett NL, Denys P, et al: Neurological disorders: Erectile and ejaculatory dysfunction. In Jardin A, Wagner G, Khoury S, et al (eds): Erectile Dysfunction. Plymouth, UK, Health Publication, 2000, p 593.

CHAPTER 25

Investigation of Disorders of Anorectal Function

FRANÇOIS MION ■ HENRI DAMON ■ LUC HENRY

Anal incontinence and constipation are the most common functional disorders of the anorectal system. Often, these symptoms are integrated with others that involve dysfunction of the anterior and median segments of the pelvic floor. Both the history and the findings on clinical examination contribute to accurate diagnosis and adequate management. However, functional investigations and imaging techniques may be needed in difficult cases. Transanal ultrasonography, perineal electrophysiology, anorectal manometry, and dynamic imaging of the pelvic organs may alter therapeutic management. This chapter focuses on the techniques and clinical use of transanal ultrasonography (TAU), anorectal manometry, and defecography. See Chapter 24 for a description of the methods used for electrodiagnosis.

TRANSANAL ULTRASONOGRAPHY

TAU with a high-frequency probe was first described during the late 1980s.[1] This noninvasive method allows an accurate study of the anal sphincter. It now plays an important role in the diagnostic workup of functional anorectal diseases.

Technical Requirements and Method for Anal Ultrasonography

TAU is mainly performed with a rigid 360-degree rotating probe. Most studies are currently done with the Bruel & Kjaer (Copenhagen, Denmark) ultrasound system, equipped with a 7- to 10-MHz transducer and a rigid sonolucent plastic cone. Flexible echoendoscopes or linear probes may also be used.[2]

To reduce the risk of infection, a condom covers the end of the probe, with coupling gel applied on both sides of the condom.

TAU is performed without bowel cleansing or sedation. The patient is usually placed in the left lateral position, although Frudinger and colleagues[3] recommended the prone position. Endovaginal insertion of the probe is an alternate route.[4,5] Three-dimensional reconstruction of the anal canal is possible,[6] but its usefulness must be shown.

TAU can be performed in all cases, except in patients with tight anal stenosis (because the external diameter of the probe is 17 mm) or painful proctologic diseases, such as perineal abscess.

The anal canal is examined downward from the rectal end. Three radial scans are systematically obtained: an upper scan, at the level of the puborectalis muscle; a median scan, where both the internal and external sphincters are present; and a lower scan, where only the subcutaneous external sphincter can be seen.

Normal Anal Ultrasonographic Anatomy

Successive circumferential hyperechoic or hypoechoic rings are present around the intra-anal probe (Fig. 25-1):

1. The first hyperechoic ring around the probe corresponds to the submucosa.
2. The second hypoechoic ring is the internal sphincter, which varies in thickness from 1.5 to 3 mm.
3. The third hyperechoic ring, which is usually heterogeneous, represents the external sphincter. It may be difficult to identify, and may appear hypoechoic relative to the longitudinal muscle of the rectum, which may be seen in some cases.
4. The puborectalis muscle is seen as the upper limit of the anal canal, and forms a U-shaped sling behind the anorectum. It is slightly hyperechoic and heterogeneous (Fig. 25-2).
5. The superficial transverse perineal muscles can be seen converging at the central point of the perineum. They appear as two transverse hypoechoic bands, and must not be misinterpreted as anterior defects.
6. Perianal and ischiorectal fat is represented by the heterogeneous, slightly hypoechoic area seen around the sphincteric structures.

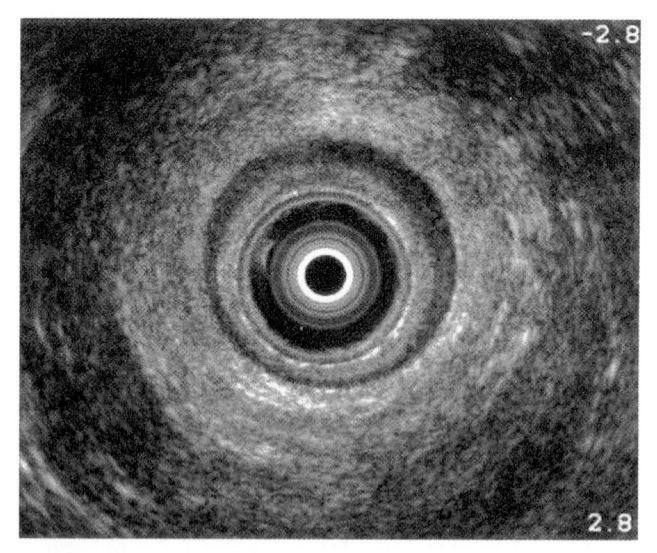

FIGURE 25-1 A transanal ultrasonography scan obtained at the median level of the anal canal in a normal patient. The hypoechoic ring represents the internal anal sphincter, and the larger hyperechoic and heterogeneous ring adjacent to it represents the external anal sphincter.

The structural anatomy of the external sphincter varies according to sex: in women, the anterior and superior parts are incomplete. Therefore, this finding can be misinterpreted as an anterior sphincter defect.[7]

Clinical Applications of Transanal Ultrasonography

Anal Incontinence

TAU is useful for the diagnosis of internal and external sphincter defects, primary degeneration of the internal sphincter, and anorectal anomalies.

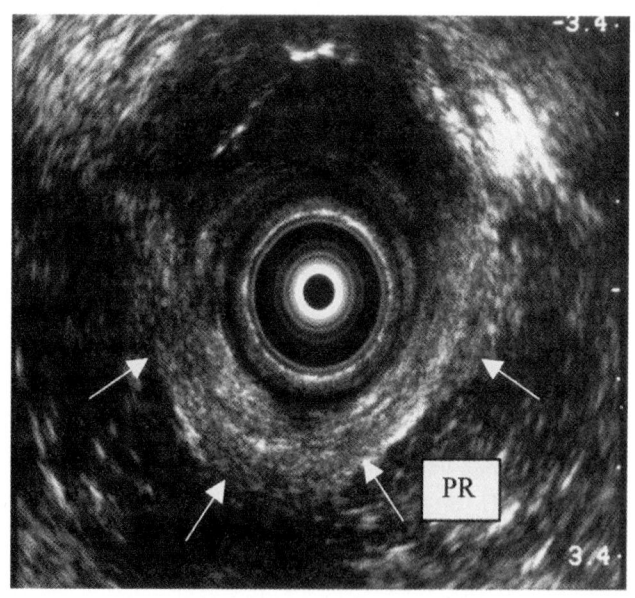

FIGURE 25-2 A transanal ultrasonography scan obtained at the upper level of the anal canal in a normal patient. The internal sphincter is seen as a thin internal hypoechoic ring, and the puborectalis muscle (PR) appears as a U-shaped hyperechoic sling that is open anteriorly (*arrows*).

Internal sphincter defects are identified by a clear rupture of the internal hypoechoic ring, which is easily seen on TAU (Fig. 25-3). Its significance has been validated in patients undergoing elective internal sphincterotomy.[8] Interobserver agreement is excellent for the diagnosis of internal sphincter defect.[9]

External sphincter defects are hypoechoic and slightly heterogeneous areas within the concentric slings of the external sphincter (Fig. 25-4). They are sometimes more difficult to assess than internal defects. TAU diagnosis of external sphincter defects has been validated with electromyography and histology.[10,11] TAU has replaced electromyography for the mapping of external sphincter defects because it is much less invasive and has similar efficacy. Its sensitivity and specificity are greater than 80%. Recent studies suggest that TAU may yield a false-positive diagnosis of sphincter defects.[12]

The high prevalence of sphincter defects detected by TAU (<65% of patients with anal incontinence and 20%–40% of continent women) leads to questions about their clinical significance.[13] The size of the lesions is probably important to assess, and the most relevant measurement appears to be their radial size.[6] Large defects (>90 degrees) and possibly combined defects of the internal and external sphincters are the most clinically relevant.[14]

TAU may help to differentiate between traumatic and nontraumatic causes of anal incontinence.

Vaginal delivery induces approximately 35% of anal sphincter defects. Sultan and colleagues[15] were the first to show this noxious effect: the first vaginal delivery produces a higher rate of sphincter defects, and the use of forceps increases the risk. Others confirmed these findings.[16,17] Postobstetric anal lesions are mainly anterior defects of the external sphincter. These lesions are not always associated with postpartum clinical signs of anal incontinence, but may contribute to symptoms in postmenopausal women.

Proctologic surgery is often responsible for anal sphincter lesions: surgical treatment of anal fistula is a

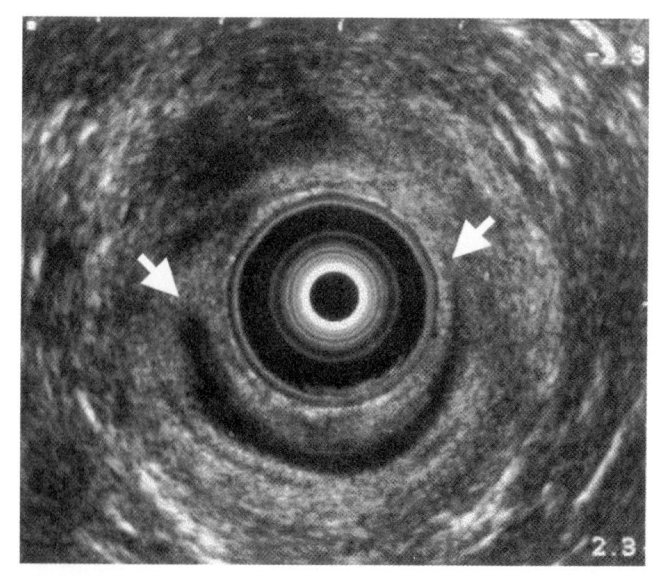

FIGURE 25-3 Transanal ultrasonography scan of an anterior defect of the internal anal sphincter. The extremities of the ruptured muscle are shown by *arrows*. The radial size of this defect is nearly 180 degrees.

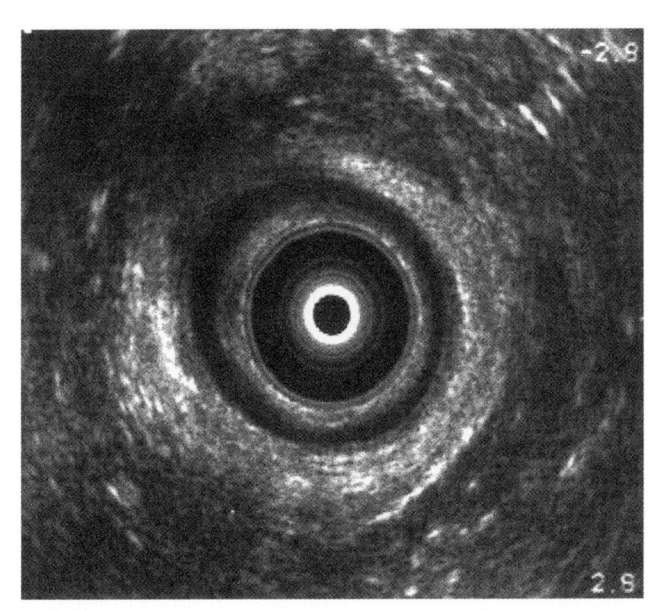

FIGURE 25-4 Transanal ultrasonography scan of a left anterior defect of the external anal sphincter. The internal sphincter is intact, as shown by the regular hypoechoic ring. The defect of the external sphincter is represented by a hypoechoic area within the hyperechoic external ring. Its radial size is nearly 70 degrees.

classic cause of sphincter defects.[13] Anal dilation produces an almost characteristic echographic finding, with fragmentation of the internal sphincter.[18] Recent studies show the high prevalence of anal sphincter lesions after hemorrhoidectomy, fistulectomy, or ileoanal anastomosis.[19] Left colectomy or rectal anterior resection may lead to internal sphincter defects.[20]

Sexual abuse is a rare and poorly documented cause of anal incontinence. Multiple internal sphincter disruptions have been described after anal rape.[21] On the other hand, consensual anoreceptive intercourse does not seem to significantly damage the anal sphincter.[22]

Vaizey and colleagues[23] described primary degeneration internal sphincter syndrome, which is characterized by passive fecal incontinence, low anal pressure at rest, and a thin, hyperechoic internal sphincter on TAU. According to these authors, this syndrome of unknown cause may represent up to 4% of cases of nontraumatic anal incontinence. The diagnosis of congenital anal anomalies leading to fecal incontinence has also greatly benefited from the emergence of TAU.[24]

Anal Suppurations

Although magnetic resonance imaging is probably the best method for studying complex fistulas, intrasphincteric suppurations may be studied with TAU. Fistulas are seen as hypoechoic lines that may be enhanced by the injection of oxygenated water, and abscesses appear as hypoechoic areas.[25,26] Sometimes the internal orifice of the fistula can be identified. TAU normally does not show suprasphincteric or extrasphincteric projections of fistulas because of the limited focal length of the probe.

The role of TAU in the diagnosis of other functional perineal diseases, such as chronic pelvic pain and pelvic floor disorders, has not been validated adequately.

Practical Uses of Transanal Ultrasonography in Diagnosis and Treatment

If anal incontinence persists for 12 weeks after delivery, TAU may be recommended. Fynes and colleagues[27] suggested performing a prophylactic cesarean procedure for the second delivery in women with a significant sphincter defect. In patients with no clinical symptoms of anal incontinence, systematic TAU does not seem useful.

In patients with anal incontinence, TAU is mandatory. Its excellent diagnostic value for detecting anal sphincter defects determines whether surgical sphincter repair is indicated. Usually, TAU is part of the diagnostic workup, in association with manometry and electrophysiologic studies.

TAU is a simple, rapid, and noninvasive imaging technique for assessing anal sphincter anatomy. Its major clinical indication is anal incontinence and possibly some forms of fistula in ano. Prospective studies are needed to determine its usefulness in patients with other pelvic floor disorders.

ANORECTAL MANOMETRY

Functional testing of anorectal physiology was developed during the early 1960s.[28,29] Anorectal manometry allows a better understanding of the physiology of continence and defecation. Its role in the diagnostic workup of diseases of the pelvic floor is now clearly delineated.

Technical Requirements for Anorectal Manometry

A manometric assembly line includes a catheter (which comes in direct contact with the patient), pressure transducers, a recording system to store the digitized signals, and software to allow analysis of the recordings.

Several types of catheters are used to measure pressure within the rectum and anal canal. These include perfused catheters with side openings; perfused catheters with sleeve; air- or water-filled balloon catheters; and probes equipped with solid-state microtransducers.

Perfused catheters with side openings are the most commonly used, and single-use probes are commercially available. These probes are thin, flexible, and well tolerated. They allow multiple recordings to be obtained at different sites in both the longitudinal and transversal axes. These catheters have two main disadvantages. (1) They record pressure in only one direction, and thus do not take into account the asymmetry of pressures within the anal canal. (2) The water infused in the rectum or anal canal may induce abnormal reflexes.[30]

Because of the very low compliance of modern pressure transducers (<0.05 μL/100 mm Hg), the catheter perfusion system determines the compliance of the entire system. Polyvinyl (or silicone) catheters with an inner diameter of 0.6 to 0.8 mm are usually adequate. Standard pneumohydraulic low-compliance perfusion pumps (e.g., Arndorfer or Dentsleeve manometric pump) are usually recommended. However, for routine anorectal manometry, simpler perfusion systems such as UroKit 4 (Medtronic) and a pressure cuff inflated to 300 mm Hg give reliable results, with rates of pressure increase constantly higher than 300 mm Hg/sec for pressures ranging from 100 to 250 mm Hg (personal data). These systems are much less expensive than dedicated pneumohydraulic pumps, and provide an excellent way to prevent infection because they are disposable between each patient, or at least every day.

Perfused sleeve catheters provide a nonradial measurement of pressures along the anal canal. They cannot differentiate between internal and external sphincter activities, but may be useful for prolonged recordings, because they span the length of the anal canal and thus limit the risks of migration of the probe.[31]

Balloon catheters also provide a signal that is the sum of all pressures exerted on the probe from each direction. Positioning of the probe in the rectum and anal canal is simple and reproducible. The absence of water perfusion in the anal canal limits artifacts. However, the size of the balloons modifies anal sphincter resting tone because of distension of the anus, and limits the number of site recordings in the anal canal to two. Furthermore, latex balloons must be changed between uses to allow for decontamination of the catheter. This tedious process can be overcome by performing the tests with a condom covering the inserted length of the probe.

Finally, probes with microtransducers eliminate the measurement errors induced by hydraulic transmission, and they are easy to insert because of their small radial size (<5 mm). As with perfused catheters, measured pressures are radial and thus depend on the positioning of the transducers. The clinical use of these probes is limited by their relative fragility, their cost, and the need for disinfection with products such as glutaraldehyde.

Several computerized polygraphs are now commercially available. Some are dedicated to anorectal manometry, and others add software for urodynamic studies or other measurements of digestive motility. Automatic analyses of the recordings are provided, but systems that allow for complete manual control of the produced data are preferred.

Pressure Units

Most results obtained in anorectal laboratories or reported in the literature are expressed in millimeters of mercury (mm Hg) or centimeters of water (cm H_2O), which are units of length, not pressure. The international system pressure unit is the Pascal (Pa), and the results of anorectal manometry may be conveniently expressed in hecto- or kilo-Pascals (hPa or kPa), with 1 kPa = 9.87 cm H_2O or 7.5 mm Hg.

Routine Anorectal Manometric Studies

Pressure recordings should be made in at least three sites simultaneously: the rectum, upper anal canal (which is more representative of the activity of the internal sphincter), and lower anal canal (which is more representative of the activity of the external striated anal sphincter).

Study of the Resistive Compartment of Anorectal Physiology: The Anal Sphincter

Baseline closure pressure of the anal canal at rest can be measured with rapid or step-by-step pull-through, which gives the pressure profile of the anal canal. Another way to perform this study is to average the pressure in the upper and lower anal canal for 10 to 30 minutes. This averaged pressure is probably more relevant to physiology because it causes less stimulation of anal receptors than the pull-through technique.[32] Anal pressure at rest may cause spontaneous pressure variations in the form of ultraslow waves (with a frequency of 3 cycles/min) in constipated patients with anal hypertonia.[33] Between 70% and 80% of the resting pressure of the anal canal is related to internal sphincter muscle activity.

Low anal pressures at rest are seen in patients with fecal incontinence, and suggest internal sphincter dysfunction, which is usually associated with soiling.

The length of the anal canal or of the high-pressure zone can be determined during a rapid pull-through examination performed with an automatic puller that maintains a constant speed (usually 10 mm/sec).[34]

Six or eight radial perfused catheters and an automatic puller can be used to perform vector manometry of the anal canal. This test uses computerized calculation to reconstruct the pressure profile of the anal canal in three dimensions as well as to calculate the asymmetry index (Fig. 25-5).[35] The asymmetry index may be increased in patients with anal sphincter defects, indicating the need for morphologic tests, such as TAU.

Anal pressures measured during voluntary squeeze depend on the muscular activity of the striated external sphincter. The maximal amplitude of the pressure variation from the baseline pressure and the duration of squeeze pressure are measured. The anal asymmetry index during voluntary squeeze can be determined by vector manometry, as described earlier. The cough reflex is another way to test the external sphincter. The increase of abdominal pressure in relation to cough is accompanied by a reflex contraction of the external sphincter, and thus by an increase in anal pressure.

Variations in anal pressure during strain are recorded: normal relaxation of the external sphincter during a defecation attempt decreases anal pressure (Fig. 25-6). Anismus, or abdominoperineal asynchronism, is an abnormal condition found in patients with outlet obstruction (dyschezia), and is shown by an increase or a lack of decrease in anal pressure during straining.[36] During straining, intrarectal pressure readings reflect intra-abdominal pressure, and thus the quality of the abdominal wall contraction (Fig. 25-7).

The conditions of anorectal manometry may lead to a false-positive diagnosis of anismus. Ideally, patients should sit on a commode and be left alone to proceed to a real straining effort.

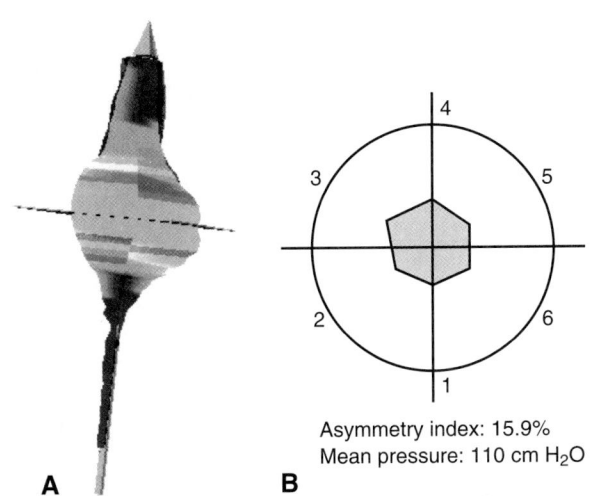

FIGURE 25-5 (**A**) Three-dimensional representation of anal pressures as obtained with vector manometry. (**B**) Representation of a cross-section of the high-pressure zone, showing the vector volume and calculated anal asymmetry index.

Asymmetry index: 15.9%
Mean pressure: 110 cm H$_2$O

- Rectal contraction (rectorectal reflex). This short-lived contraction is meant to allow stools to proceed to the anal canal and is part of the so-called sampling reflex.
- Relaxation of the internal anal sphincter (rectoanal inhibitory reflex). The decrease in anal pressure observed is proportional in amplitude and duration to the intensity of the stimulus. This reflex is present in the newborn, and its absence is the manometric landmark of Hirschsprung's disease.[37]
- Contraction of the external anal sphincter (rectoanal excitatory reflex). The pressure increase observed in the lower part of the anal canal is proportional in amplitude and duration to the intensity of the stimulus. This contractile reflex is acquired during childhood and depends on the conscious perception of rectal distension.[38]

The test of expulsion of a filled rectal balloon may be used to confirm anismus: the patient is asked to expel a rectal balloon inflated with 50 to 80 mL air. Again, this test should be performed as physiologically as possible.

Study of the Rectoanal Reflexes

This part of the manometric study is performed with a rectal balloon mounted on a catheter. Rapid distension of this balloon with small amounts of air (10–60 mL) induces the following changes (Fig. 25-8):

Study of the Capacitive Compartment of Anorectal Physiology: The Rectal Reservoir

The conscious rectal sensitivity threshold is measured by inflating a latex balloon in the rectum. The threshold corresponds to the smallest distension volume that elicits a conscious sensation (5–40 mL in healthy volunteers). This threshold may be significantly increased in constipated patients.[32]

With larger distension volumes (≤400 mL), it is possible to test the volumes that induce the first need to defecate and the urgent need to defecate. Once again, these volumes may be significantly increased in constipated patients (especially those with a megarectum), or decreased in incontinent patients with a small rectum (e.g., ulcerative colitis).

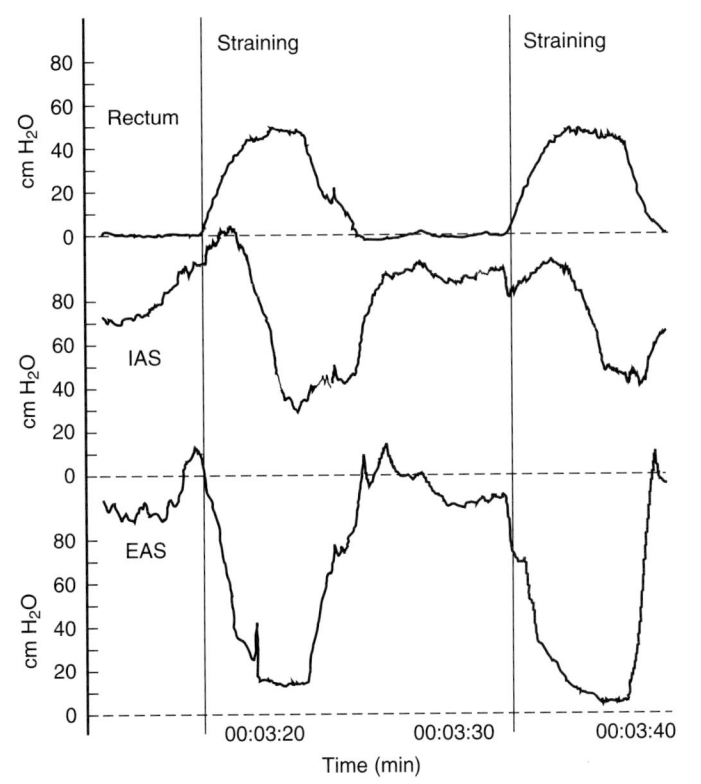

FIGURE 25-6 A straining effort is physiologically associated with a pressure decrease in the anal canal, corresponding to relaxation of the internal (IAS) and external anal sphincters (EAS).

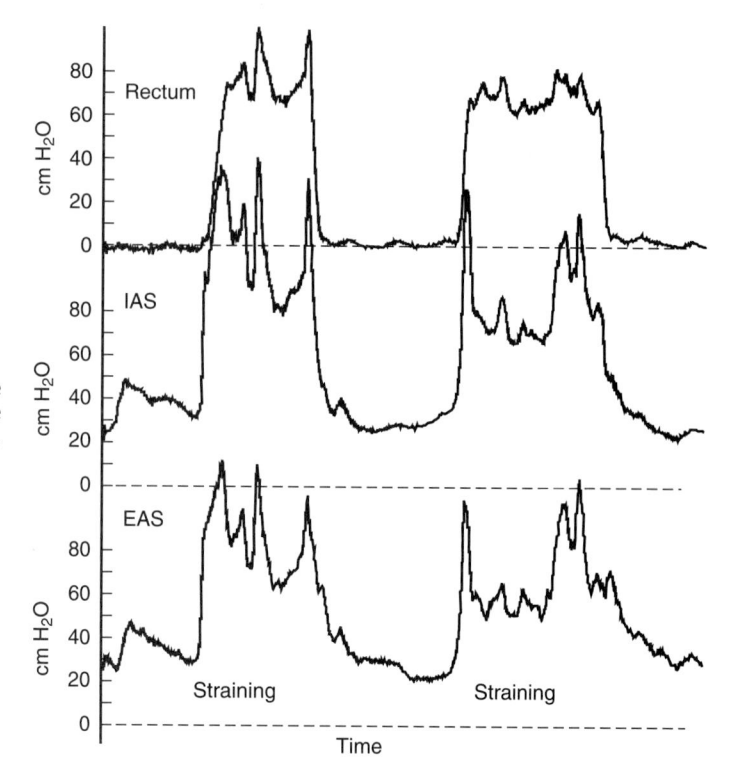

FIGURE 25-7 In a patient with anismus, anal canal pressure increases during a straining effort. The measured pressure in the rectum reflects the increase in intra-abdominal pressure. IAS, internal anal sphincter; EAS, external anal sphincter.

The distension volume that causes a painful sensation can be used to determine the rectal pain threshold. This threshold is lower in patients with irritable bowel syndrome.[39]

The study of rectal compliance is performed with a latex balloon mounted on a manometric catheter that is placed in the rectum. The balloon is inflated with air at increments of 30 to 60 mL. The slope of the pressure–volume curve allows calculation of compliance ($\Delta V/\Delta P$). Maximal compliance is the ratio of the maximal tolerable volume and the corresponding measured pressure (Fig. 25-9). The latex balloon should have infinite compliance[40]; otherwise, the compliance of the balloon should be measured outside of the rectum and subtracted from the values obtained in the rectum.

Rectal compliance may be increased in patients with megarectum or rectal atonia. It is decreased when fibrosis of the rectal wall is present, as in inflammatory bowel disease.

Indications for Anorectal Manometry

Constipation

In patients with constipation, the major role of manometry is to exclude Hirschsprung's disease, especially in children. The rectoanal inhibitory reflex can be tested, even in the newborn. Manometry is especially useful in

FIGURE 25-8 Rectoanal reflexes. Rapid inflation of an intrarectal balloon with decreasing volumes of air initiates a rectal contraction, relaxation of the internal sphincter, and brief contraction of the external sphincter. The amplitudes of the rectoanal reflexes are proportional to the distending volume.

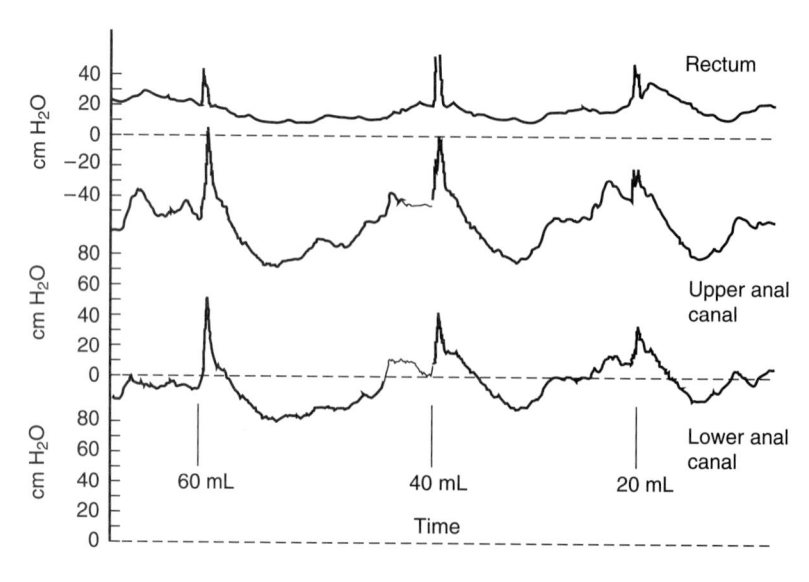

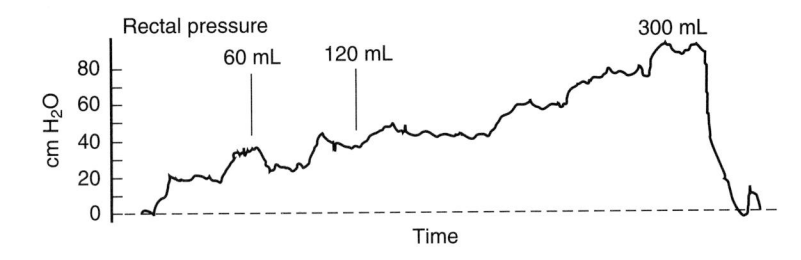

FIGURE 25-9 The rectal pressure–volume curve obtained by progressive inflation of an infinitely compliant rectal balloon. The slope of the curve yields the rectal compliance. The ratio of maximal tolerable volume over maximal pressure gives the maximal compliance.

short forms of aganglionosis, in which radiology and pathology may miss the diagnosis.

Anismus is a common finding in constipated adults and children. Other abnormalities that may be found include anal hypertonia, impaired rectal sensation, increased rectal capacity, and compliance. These findings should be used to guide biofeedback training.

Incontinence

A weak resting anal pressure may indicate dysfunction of the internal sphincter, whereas a low pressure increase during squeezing indicates external sphincter dysfunction. We showed (unpublished data) that a low anal asymmetry index on vector manometry can exclude a significant sphincter defect.

Impaired rectal sensation, decreased rectal compliance, and decreased length of the anal canal may also be found associated with fecal incontinence. These findings can be used to guide biofeedback treatment.[41]

Abnormalities of the rectoanal reflexes (especially loss of proportionality between the intensity of the stimulus and the amplitude and duration of the rectoanal inhibitory reflex), impaired rectal sensation, or the absence of anal contraction during voluntary squeeze may indicate central neurologic disease (e.g., multiple sclerosis, spinal cord lesion).[42]

Descending perineum syndrome, which is often associated with anal incontinence, is characterized by three manometric abnormalities: anal contraction during straining, decreased rectal compliance, and low anal squeeze pressures.[43] A solitary rectal ulcer, which may be part of descending perineum syndrome, may have a similar manometric appearance.

Thus, manometry remains an important tool in the functional evaluation of the rectoanal complex. Its diagnostic value for the management of anal incontinence and constipation was recently confirmed.[44]

RADIOGRAPHIC STUDY OF THE PELVIC FLOOR

Defecography, first described by Mahieu and associates,[45] allowed the description and understanding of rectal evacuation disorders. It remains the gold standard radiologic technique in males. However, the frequent association in women between anorectal dysfunction and disorders of the anterior and median perineum led to technical improvements that included marking of the vaginal cavity, bladder,[46] and pelvic loops of the small bowel. These changes led to the introduction of a complete dynamic examination of the pelvic organs, the pelvic viscerogram.

Technique

A barium paste with a consistency approximating that of normal stool is prepared at least 1 hour before the start of the examination. This paste is made of a mixture of 250 mL barium sulfate (Micropaque, Guerbet, Aulnay-sous-Bois, France), 125 mg cornstarch, and 150 mL water, and cooked on a gentle fire. After the paste cools, 300 mL is put aside for rectal filling and 10 mL is placed in the bottom of a 20-mL syringe, which is then filled with 10 mL liquid barium sulfate, and used for vaginal marking.

Ninety minutes before the start of the examination, the patient is asked to swallow 200 mL barium sulfate, to obtain marking of the small bowel pelvic loops.

After meticulous perineal asepsis is performed on the patient in the supine position, a small catheter is inserted in the bladder, which is filled with 200 mL water-soluble contrast medium with 300 mg/mL iodine (Telebrix 30, Guerbet). The bladder catheter is left in place during the examination to allow precise marking of the bladder neck.

Vaginal marking is then performed by injection of the contents of the 20-mL syringe prepared as described earlier. The liquid phase marks the vaginal walls, and the solid phase molds the vaginal cavity.

The patient is then turned to the left lateral position, and the distal sigmoid colon and rectum walls are marked with 60 mL Micropaque. A manual injector is used to fill the rectum with 200 to 300 mL barium paste. The amount of injected paste used is determined by the patient's feeling of rectal fullness or pain, or by anal reflux of paste.

Radiologic views are then obtained from a lateral exposure, with the patient sitting on a commode to facilitate retrieval of the evacuated products. The following exposures are obtained:

- At rest
- During squeezing (voluntary anal contraction)
- During straining (Valsalva maneuver)
- Three or four exposures are obtained
- During rectal evaluation

These views may be replaced by videoscopic or rapid-sequence recording (3 images/sec).

After the urinary catheter is withdrawn, one or two images are taken during micturition and one is taken during straining after bladder emptying. If micturition is impossible under fluoroscopic control, the patient can go to the toilet before obtaining the last exposure.

Two measurements are obtained to show the mobility of pelvic organs within the bone frame:

1. The distance between the rectoanal junction and the ischial tuberosities
2. The distance between the bladder neck and the lower edge of the pubic symphysis

Normal Results of Pelvic Viscerogram (Fig. 25-10)

At Rest

At rest, small bowel lies above the pelvic organs. Listed from top to bottom and front to back, respectively, they are the bladder, vagina, and rectum. The anal canal is closed, and the rectoanal angle is 60 to 105 degrees.[47] The rectoanal junction projects at the level of the ischial tuberosities, or no more than 15 mm below them.[48] The bladder neck faces the lower edge of the pubic symphysis, and is usually hidden behind the posterior edge of the femoral diaphysis. The vagina is vertical and is in close contact with the bladder and rectum.

During Voluntary Squeeze

During voluntary squeeze, the bladder neck and rectoanal junction move 20 to 25 mm up from their resting position, and the rectoanal angle closes by 20 to 25 degrees.

During Straining

During straining, the bladder neck and rectoanal junction move down 5 to 40 mm from their resting position, and the rectoanal angle opens by 20 to 25 degrees (to approximately 130 degrees). The upper segment of the anal canal is open, with a mean width of 17 ± 4 mm.

During Rectal Evacuation

Qualitative, quantitative, and morphologic assessment of rectal evacuation must be performed.

- **Qualitative assessment.** The straining effort does not need to be significant. Rectal evacuation progresses smoothly, without digital or other maneuvers, and the call to stool sensation disappears when the rectum is empty.
- **Quantitative assessment.** The complete process of rectal evacuation does not exceed 20 to 30 seconds. The rectoanal angle opens to 140 degrees,[45] and no rectal residue is left at the end of evacuation.
- **Morphologic assessment.** The rectum empties without anterior or downward deformation. However, anterior deformation of less than 2 cm of the anterior wall is considered physiologic, and is often observed in healthy volunteers and asymptomatic subjects.[49,50]

- **Mobility of pelvic organs.** During straining, small bowel pelvic loops remain above the ischial tuberosities. The bladder neck remains above the lower edge of the pubic symphysis, and does not move more than 15 mm down from its resting position. The bladder base remains above the horizontal line that passes by the bladder neck. The vagina remains in close contact with the anterior wall of the rectum, and follows its movements. Vaginal fornices are at the level of the median part of the rectum.

Micturition

Exposures are obtained during micturition to evaluate the urethral morphology. The diameter of the urethra is regular from the bladder neck down to the meatus. The speed and quality of bladder emptying are evaluated, as well as the absence of residual urine. These images may be difficult to obtain because of psychological blocking of micturition, which is much more common than with defecation.

Straining after Defecation and Micturition

During straining, the cul-de-sac of Douglas remains above the ischial tuberosities.

Abnormal Findings on Pelvic Viscerogram

Functional, positional, and morphologic disorders of the pelvic organs can be detected by pelvic viscerogram. These radiologic signs may explain some of the clinical symptoms of dyschezia and anal incontinence.

Functional Abnormalities

Functional abnormalities are usually found in association with anismus or a solitary ulcer of the rectum. The following radiologic features may be found:

- Paradoxical closure of the rectoanal angle during straining and defecation
- Marking of the puborectalis muscle on the posterior wall of the rectoanal junction, appearing as a rounded, anteriorly convex deformation
- Decreased rectal evacuation rate[51,52]

Recently, Faucheron and Dubreuil[51] described a radiologic feature of rectal akinesia that included nearly complete motionlessness of the rectum and rectoanal junction during straining and squeezing as well as a decreased rectal evacuation rate.

Positional Abnormalities

In patients with a descending perineum, the rectoanal junction is in is a normal position at rest; however, on straining, it descends 30 mm or more below the ischial tuberosities.[48] The descended perineum is a permanent extension of the rectoanal junction 30 mm or more beyond the lower edge of the ischial tuberosities.

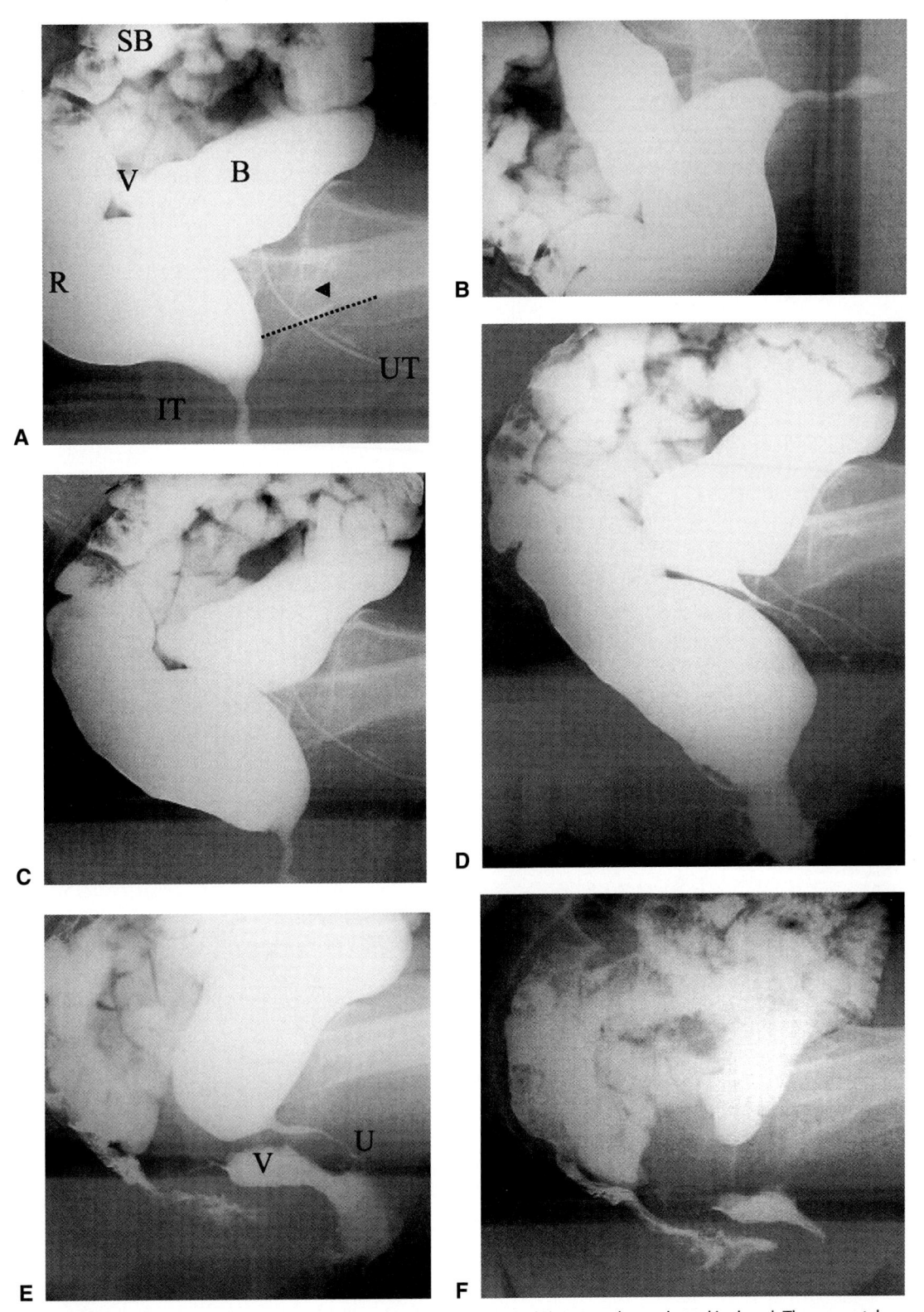

FIGURE 25-10 A pelvic viscerogram obtained in a normal patient. (**A**) At rest, the anal canal is closed. The anorectal junction lies above the lower edge of the ischial tuberosities (IT). The urethrovesical junction, well identified by the urinary tube (UT), is located above the inferior margin of the pubic symphysis (*arrowhead*). This location corresponds to the posterior edge of the femoral diaphysis (*dotted line*). (**B**) During squeezing, the anorectal junction and urethrovesical junction move up, and the anorectal angle closes. (**C**) On straining, the anorectal junction and urovesical junction move down less than 3 cm from their resting position, and the anorectal angle opens. (**D**) During defecation, the opening of the anal canal is less than 2 cm wide. The rectum is in line with the anal canal. (**E**) During micturition after defecation, the urethrovesical junction remains above the posterior edge of the femoral diaphysis. (**F**) During a straining effort after micturition and defecation, the bladder and rectum are empty. A small physiologic supra-anal rectal prolapse can be seen. Small bowel loops stay above the pelvic organs, and the anterior rectal wall stays in close contact with the vagina. B, bladder; R, rectum; SB, small bowel; U, urethra; V, vagina.

These abnormalities are usually observed in patients with descending perineum syndrome; dyschezia, anal bleeding, and mucous discharge as a result of mucosal rectal prolapse; pelvic pain; urinary and anal incontinence; and vaginal prolapse.

Morphologic Abnormalities

Rectal Prolapse

Rectal prolapse is downward sliding of all or part of the layers of the rectal wall, leading to invagination within the rectal lumen or anal canal. Several types are described[53]:

- Anterior or circular mucosal prolapse. At defecography, the folds are less than 3 mm deep. This type of mucosal prolapse is rarely symptomatic, and is frequently associated with other pelvic floor disorders.
- Internal mucosal and muscular prolapse remains in the rectum or slides down within the anal canal. Intrarectal internal prolapse is seen in up to 40% to 50% of normal subjects.[49,54] The intra-anal type is found in 35% of women with genital prolapse. During defecography, this prolapse usually appears at the end of rectal evacuation. It develops from the anterior rectal wall and is associated with a low rectal exclusion pocket (serosa-coated ring pocket of rectal prolapse) of variable volume,[55] which can be misinterpreted as an anterior rectocele (Fig. 25-11). The prolapse may be reduced during squeezing maneuvers. During the examination, it is important to note whether the patient has an associated incomplete rectal evacuation or a feeling of incomplete rectal emptying. In these cases, the prolapse is the likely cause of the patient's symptoms.
- Complete external rectal prolapse (or procidentia) is usually obvious from the history or clinical examination. In some cases, a pelvic viscerogram can be used to show rectal prolapse and associated abnormalities (Fig. 25-12). Exteriorization of the prolapse is most likely to occur during straining while in the squatting position. At the end of rectal evacuation, the anal canal is grossly dilated and deformed by the circumferential descent of the rectum. The liquid barium that is injected before the paste allows visualization of a rectal mucography, with its circular folds extending beyond the anal margin. The cul-de-sac of Douglas and its contents may form an enterocele within the prolapse (Fig. 25-13). This complete prolapse is not corrected by simple squeezing maneuvers, and usually, manual reduction is needed. At the end of the radiologic examination, simple inspection of the anal margin confirms the diagnosis.

Enterocele

Enterocele is abnormal descent of the contents of the cul-de-sac of Douglas, mainly small bowel. This peritoneal structure may also contain sigmoid colon or epiploic structures. Some authors[55] suggest that peritoneocele is a more appropriate term for this abnormality.

These abnormalities are seen in women only, frequently after hysterectomy.[46,56] The clinical diagnosis is often difficult, and pelvic viscerogram is the most sensitive technique to disclose these abnormalities. The radiologic diagnosis is based on a loss of contact between the rectum and the vagina, with different structures visible between them:

- Small bowel loops
- Sigmoid colon
- A radiologic transparency punctuated by small air bubbles, corresponding to a digestive structure without barium

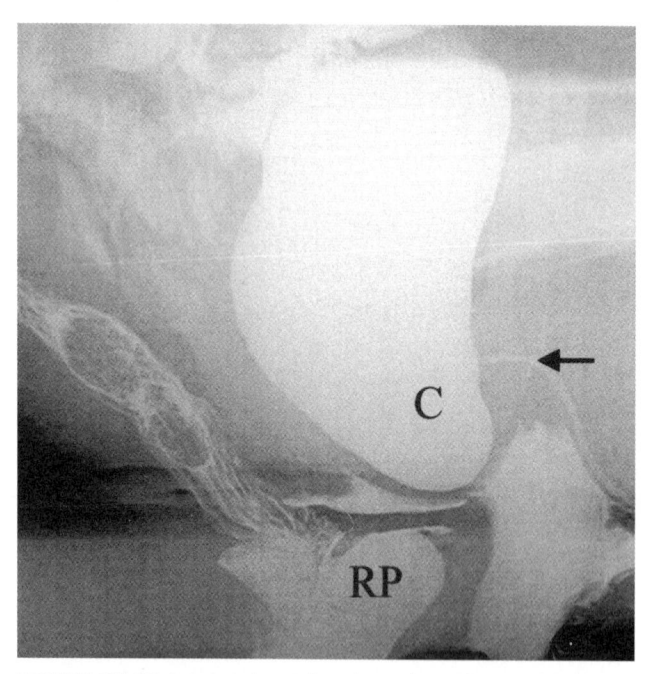

FIGURE 25-11 Intra-anal rectal prolapse in a 38-year-old woman with anal and stress urinary incontinence. At the end of evacuation, the serosa-coated ring pocket of the prolapse (RP) may be misinterpreted as a small anterior rectocele. Pathologic descent of the bladder neck (*arrow*) and bladder base are seen. C, cystocele.

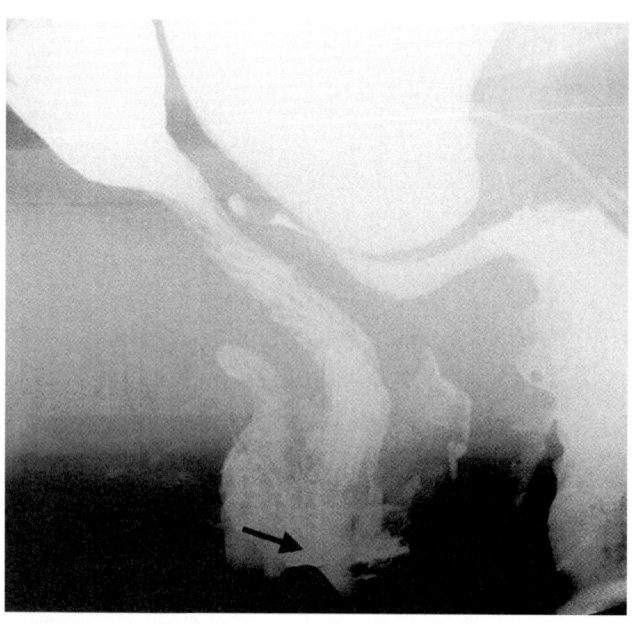

FIGURE 25-12 External rectal prolapse in a 62-year-old woman with anal and stress urinary incontinence. The tip of the rectal prolapse emerges at the anal verge (*arrow*).

- A radiologic transparency without bubbles, corresponding to epiploic structures

These peritoneoceles are never present from the start, when the rectum and bladder are full, but often appear after rectal evacuation, or more rarely, after micturition. At this stage, the patient is asked whether she has a sensation of complete rectal evacuation, while the empty rectum is deformed or pushed back by the enterocele.

Some authors divide enterocele into three types[55]:

1. Rectal enterocele, which is associated with an internal prolapse or a complete rectal prolapse
2. Vaginal enterocele, which is directed toward the vagina (posterior colpocele)
3. Septal enterocele, in which the hernial sac has an intermediate position

These types may occur at the same time in up to 50% of cases[55] (see Fig. 25-13).

Rectocele

Rectocele is a deformation of the lower part of the anterior rectal wall toward the vagina. In some cases, the deformation involves the posterior or lateral rectal walls. It is uncommon in men. Clinically, rectocele is suspected in patients with dyschezia or fecal incontinence. Patients with rectocele-inducing dyschezia often use digital endovaginal maneuvers to obtain rectal evacuation.[57] Anal incontinence associated with rectocele may correspond to late, uncontrolled evacuation of the rectocele contents after the passage of stool.[58] Urinary stress incontinence is less common[57] (Fig. 25-14).

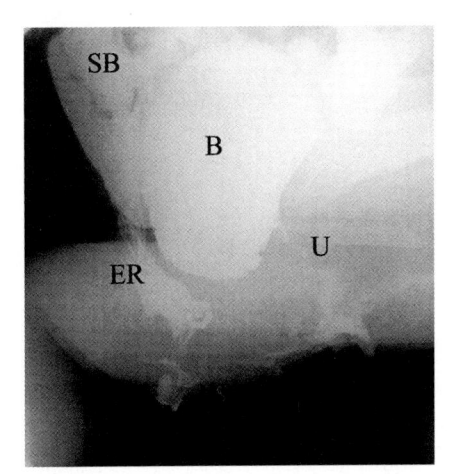

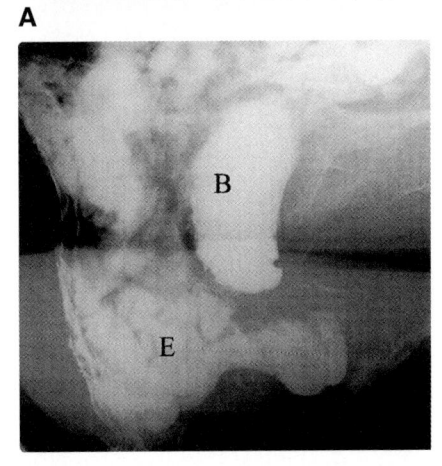

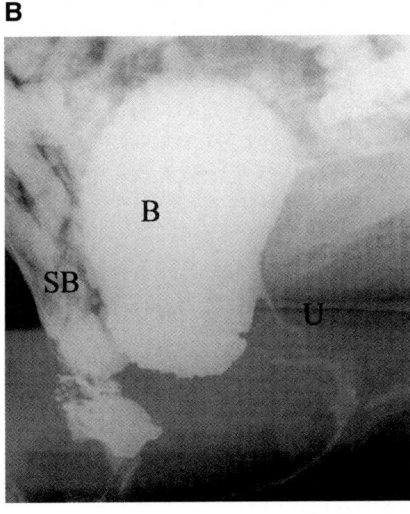

FIGURE 25-13 A large enterocele in a 73-year-old woman with recurrent genital prolapse and stress urinary incontinence 6 years after hysterectomy and Burch retropubic urethropexy. (**A**) After defecation and during micturition, the small bowel loops are in the normal position. (**B**) After partial bladder voiding, the small bowel loops are lower. The forceful straining that is necessary to obtain micturition in this case shows an intra-anal rectal prolapse. (**C**) After nearly complete bladder emptying, a large enterocele develops posteriorly, toward the intrarectal prolapse, and anteriorly, to form a posterior colpocele. B, bladder; E, enterocele; ER, empty rectum; SB, small bowel; U, urethra.

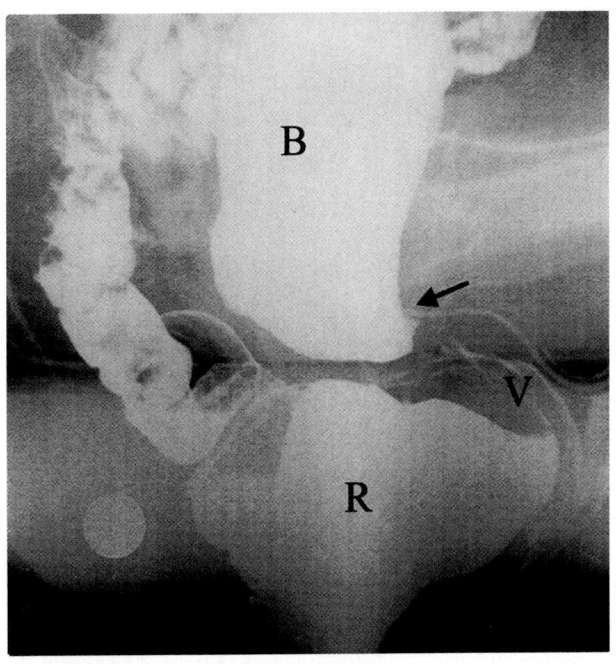

FIGURE 25-14 A large anterior rectocele in a 71-year-old woman with difficult rectal evacuation and genital prolapse, but no urinary symptoms. The rectocele may play a role in sustaining and limiting the descent of the bladder neck (*arrow*) that may prevent symptoms of stress urinary incontinence. B, bladder; R, rectocele; V, vagina.

Clinically and radiologically, the differential diagnosis between an anterior rectocele and the serosa-coated ring pocket of an internal rectal prolapse is often difficult. If this distinction is accepted, then true isolated anterior rectocele is relatively rare.

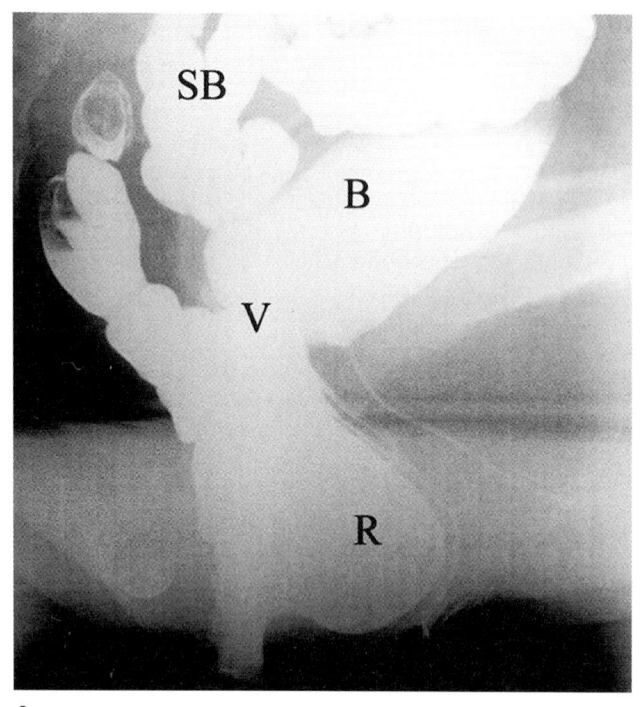

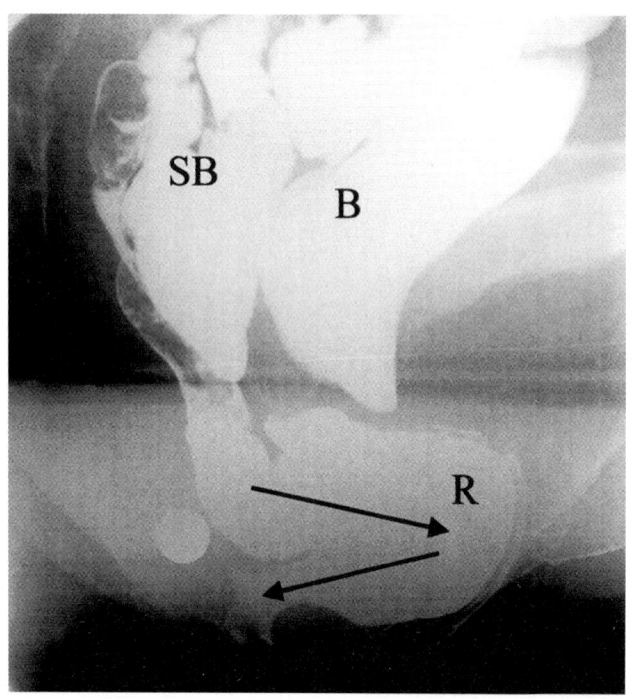

Radiologically, progressive deformation of the anterior wall of the rectum during unsuccessful straining efforts can be seen on fluoroscopy. The increase in intra-abdominal pressure is directed forward rather than downward.

Small anterior rectoceles are found in up to 80% of asymptomatic subjects.[49,50] Their size, measured as the distance between the extended line of the anterior border of the anal canal and the tip of the rectocele, is always less than 3 cm.

A symptomatic rectocele is usually larger than 3 cm, and retains the barium paste unless digital pressure is applied to the vagina or perineum.[59] A very large rectocele may create a closed anorectal angle; when this occurs, its pathogenic role in dyschezia is evident (Fig. 25-15).

No significant association between rectocele and other pelvic floor disorders has been described, except for descending perineum syndrome.[60,61]

The main value of pelvic viscerogram in this setting is the objective finding of rectocele and associated abnormalities, such as enterocele, preoperatively.[62]

Other Abnormalities

Pelvic viscerogram can be used to show other pelvic floor disorders, such as vaginal vault prolapse, uterine prolapse, trigonocele (i.e., descent of the trigone below the level of the bladder neck), and bladder neck descent (≥15 mm beyond the inferior border of the pubic symphysis). A discussion of these disorders and their significance is beyond the scope of this chapter.

Conclusion

Pelvic viscerogram is more sensitive than clinical examination for the detection of pelvic floor disorders.[46] The observed abnormalities must be interpreted with regard to clinical symptoms, especially when surgical treatment is planned. So far, dynamic magnetic resonance imaging has not shown any superiority compared with pelvic viscerogram in the detection of pelvic floor abnormalities such as rectocele, enterocele, or rectal prolapse.[63–66]

FIGURE 25-15 A large rectocele in a 71-year-old woman with anal incontinence, dyschezia, and a posterior colpocele. (**A**) During rectal evacuation, a bulge is seen in the rectal anterior wall. (**B**) At the end of defecation, barium is trapped in a large rectocele. Further evacuation is prevented because the lower rectum and the initial portion of the anal canal are oriented in opposite directions (*arrows*). B, bladder; R, rectocele; SB, small bowel; V, vagina.

REFERENCES

1. Law PJ, Bartram CI: Anal endosonography: Technique and normal anatomy. Gastrointest Radiol 14:349–353, 1989.
2. Meyenberger C, Bertschinger P, Zala GF, et al: Anal sphincter defects in fecal incontinence: Correlation between endosonography and surgery. Endoscopy 28:217–224, 1996.
3. Frudinger A, Bartram CI, Halligan S, et al: Examination techniques for endosonography of the anal canal. Abdom Imaging 23:301–303, 1998.
4. Sandridge DA, Thorp JM: Vaginal endosonography in the assessment of the anorectum. Obstet Gynecol 86:1007–1009, 1995.
5. Poen AC, Felt-Bersma RJ, Cuesta MA, et al: Vaginal endosonography of the anal sphincter complex is important in the assessment of faecal incontinence and perianal sepsis. Br J Surg 85:359–363, 1998.
6. Gold DM, Bartram CI, Halligan S, et al: Three-dimensional endoanal sonography in assessing anal canal injury. Br J Surg 86:365–370, 1999.

7. Sultan AH, Kamm MA, Hudson CN, et al: Endosonography of the anal sphincters: Normal anatomy and comparison with manometry. Clin Radiol 49:368–374, 1994.
8. Sultan AH, Kamm MA, Nicholls RJ, et al: Prospective study of the extent of internal anal sphincter division during lateral sphincterotomy. Dis Colon Rectum 37:1031–1033, 1994.
9. Gold DM, Halligan S, Kmiot WA, et al: Intraobserver and interobserver agreement in anal endosonography. Br J Surg 86:371–375, 1999.
10. Law PJ, Kamm MA, Bartram CI: A comparison between electromyography and anal endosonography in mapping external anal sphincter defects. Dis Colon Rectum 33:370–373, 1990.
11. Deen KI, Kumar D, Williams JG, et al: Anal sphincter defects: Correlation between endoanal ultrasound and surgery. Ann Surg 218:201–205, 1993.
12. Sentovich SM, Wong WD, Blatchford GJ: Accuracy and reliability of transanal ultrasound for anterior anal sphincter injury. Dis Colon Rectum 41:1000–1004, 1998.
13. Karoui S, Savoye-Collet C, Koning E, et al: Prevalence of anal sphincter defects revealed by sonography in 335 incontinent patients and 115 continent patients. Am J Roentgenol 173:389–392, 1999.
14. Fynes MM, Behan M, O'Herlihy C, et al: Anal vector volume analysis complements endoanal ultrasonographic assessment of postpartum anal sphincter injury. Br J Surg 87:1209–1214, 2000.
15. Sultan AH, Kamm MA, Hudson CN, et al: Anal-sphincter disruption during vaginal delivery. N Engl J Med 329:1905–1911, 1993.
16. Rieger N, Schloithe A, Saccone G, et al: A prospective study of anal sphincter injury due to childbirth. Scand J Gastroenterol 33:950–955, 1998.
17. Damon H, Henry L, Bretones S, et al: Postdelivery anal function in primiparous females: Ultrasound and manometric study. Dis Colon Rectum 43:472–477, 2000.
18. Nielsen MB, Rasmussen OO, Pedersen JF, et al: Risk of sphincter damage and anal incontinence after anal dilatation for fissure-in-ano: An endosonographic study. Dis Colon Rectum 36:677–680, 1993.
19. Felt-Bersma RJ, van Baren R, Koorevaar M, et al: Unsuspected sphincter defects shown by anal endosonography after anorectal surgery: A prospective study. Dis Colon Rectum 38:249–253, 1995.
20. Farouk R, Duthie GS, Lee PW, et al: Endosonographic evidence of injury to the internal anal sphincter after low anterior resection: Long-term follow-up. Dis Colon Rectum 41:888–891, 1998.
21. Engel AF, Kamm MA, Bartram CI: Unwanted anal penetration as a physical cause of faecal incontinence. Eur J Gastroenterol Hepatol 7:65–67, 1995.
22. Chun AB, Rose S, Mitrani C, et al: Anal sphincter structure and function in homosexual males engaging in anoreceptive intercourse. Am J Gastroenterol 92:465–468, 1997.
23. Vaizey CJ, Kamm MA, Bartram CI: Primary degeneration of the internal anal sphincter as a cause of passive faecal incontinence. Lancet 349:612–615, 1997.
24. Emblem R, Diseth T, Morkrid L: Anorectal anomalies: Anorectal manometric function and anal endosonography in relation to functional outcome. Pediatr Surg Int 12:516–519, 1997.
25. Law PJ, Talbot RW, Bartram CI, et al: Anal endosonography in the evaluation of perianal sepsis and fistula in ano. Br J Surg 76:752–755, 1989.
26. Poen AC, Felt-Bersma RJ, Eijsbouts QA, et al: Hydrogen peroxide-enhanced transanal ultrasound in the assessment of fistula-in-ano. Dis Colon Rectum 41:1147–1152, 1998.
27. Fynes M, Donnelly V, Behan M, et al: Effect of second vaginal delivery on anorectal physiology and faecal continence: A prospective study. Lancet 354:983–986, 1999.
28. Schuster MM, Hendrix TR, Mendeloff AL: The internal sphincter response: Manometric studies on its normal physiology, neural pathways, and alteration in bowel disorders. J Clin Invest 42:196–207, 1963.
29. Lawson JON, Nixon HH: Anal canal pressure in the diagnosis of Hirschsprung's disease. J Pediatr Surg 2:544–552, 1967.
30. Meunier PD, Gallavardin D: Anorectal manometry: The state of the art. Dig Dis 11:252–264, 1993.
31. Dent JA: A new technique for continuous sphincter pressure measurement. Gastroenterology 71:263–267, 1976.
32. Meunier P, Marechal JM, de Beaujeu MJ: Rectoanal pressures and rectal sensitivity studies in chronic childhood constipation. Gastroenterology 77:330–336, 1979.
33. Ducrotté P, Denis P, Galmiche JP, et al: Motricité anorectale dans la constipation idiopathique: Etude de 200 patients consécutifs. Gastroenterol Clin Biol 9:10–15, 1985.
34. Nivatvongs S, Stern HS, Fryd DS: The length of the anal canal. Dis Colon Rectum 24:600–601, 1981.
35. Braun JC, Treutner KH, Dreuw B, et al: Vectormanometry for differential diagnosis of fecal incontinence. Dis Colon Rectum 37:989–996, 1994.
36. Read NW, Timms JM, Barfield LJ, et al: Impairment of defecation in young women with severe constipation. Gastroenterology 90:53–60, 1986.
37. Meunier P, Marechal JM, Mollard P: Accuracy of the manometric diagnosis of Hirschsprung's disease. J Pediatr Surg 13:11–15, 1978.
38. Molander ML, Frenckner B: Electrical activity of the external anal sphincter at different ages in childhood. Gut 24:218–221, 1983.
39. Meunier P: L'intestin hypersensible. Gastroenterol Clin Biol 14:33C–36C, 1990.
40. Krogh K, Ryhammer AM, Lundby L, et al: Comparison of methods used for measurement of rectal compliance. Dis Colon Rectum 44:199–206, 2001.
41. Guillemot F, Bouche B, Gower-Rousseau C, et al: Biofeedback for the treatment of fecal incontinence: Long-term clinical results. Dis Colon Rectum 38:393–397, 1995.
42. Bardoux N, Leroi AM, Touchais JY, et al: Difficult defecation and/or faecal incontinence as a presenting feature of neurologic disorders in four patients. Neurogastroenterol Motil 9:13–18, 1997.
43. Touchais JY, Ducrotte P, Weber J, et al: Relationship between results of radiological pelvic floor study and anorectal manometry in patients consulting for constipation. Int J Colorectal Dis 3:53–58, 1988.
44. Diamant NE, Kamm MA, Wald A, et al: American Gastroenterological Association technical review on anorectal testing techniques. Gastroenterology 116:735–760, 1999.
45. Mahieu P, Pringot J, Bodart P: Defecography: I. Description of a new procedure and results in normal patients. Gastrointest Radiol 9:247–251, 1984.
46. Hock D, Lombard R, Jehaes C, et al: Colpocystodefecography. Dis Colon Rectum 36:1015–1021, 1993.
47. Goei R, van Engelshoven J, Schouten H, et al: Anorectal function: Defecographic measurement in asymptomatic subjects. Radiology 173:137–141, 1989.
48. Dubreuil AE, Denies L, Salicru B: Etude de la dynamique périnéale en défécographie: Périnée normal, descendant en poussée et descendu au repos. Bull Fr Coloproctol 3:15–19, 1991.
49. Shorvon P, McHugh S, Diamant NE, et al: Defecography in normal volunteers: Results and implications. Gut 30:1737–1749, 1989.

50. Bartolo DCC, Bartram CI, Ekberg O, et al: Proctography: Symposium. Int J Colorect Dis 3:67–89, 1988.
51. Faucheron JL, Dubreuil A: Rectal akinesia as a new cause of impaired defecation. Dis Colon Rectum 43:1545–1549, 2000.
52. Karlbom U, Nilsson S, Pahlman L, et al: Defecographic study of rectal evacuation in constipated patients and control subjects. Radiology 210:103–108, 1999.
53. Pigot F, Faivre J: Troubles de la statique ano-recale. Gastroenterol Clin Biol 21:17–27, 1997.
54. Wald A, Caruana BJ, Freimanis MG, et al: Contribution of evacuation proctography and anorectal manometry to evaluation of adults with constipation and defecatory difficulty. Dig Dis Sci 35:481–487, 1990.
55. Bremmer S, Mellgren A, Holmström B, et al: Peritoneocele: Visualization with defecography and peritoneography performed simultaneously. Radiology 202:373–377, 1997.
56. Delest A, Cosson M, Douterlant C, et al: Elytrocèle: Etude rétrospective de 134 dossiers. Facteurs favorisants et comparaison des voies d'abord abdominale et périnéale. J Gynecol Obstet Biol Reprod 25:464–470, 1996.
57. Vilotte J, Merrouche M, Sobhani I, et al: Dyschésie féminine, association fonctionnelles et troubles de la statique pelvienne. Presse Med 23:886–890, 1994.
58. Rex DK, Lappas JC: Combined anorectal manometry and defecography in 50 consecutive adults with fecal incontinence. Dis Colon Rectum 35:1040–1045, 1992.
59. Kelvin FM, Maglinte DDT: Dynamic cystoproctography of female pelvic floor defects and their interrelationships. Am J Roentgenol 169:769–774, 1997.
60. Yoshioka K, Matsui Y, Yamada O, et al: Physiologic and anatomic assessment of patients with rectocele. Dis Colon Rectum 34:704–708, 1991.
61. Mellgren A, Bremmer S, Johanson C, et al: Defecography: Results of investigation in 2816 patients. Dis Colon Rectum 37:1133–1141, 1994.
62. Van Dam JH, Ginai AZ, Gosselink MJ, et al: Role of defecography in predicting clinical outcome of rectocele repair. Dis Colon Rectum 40:201–207, 1997.
63. Delemarre JB, Kruyt RH, Doornbos J, et al: Anterior rectocele: Assessment with radiographic defecography, dynamic magnetic resonance imaging, and physical examination. Dis Colon Rectum 37:249–259, 1994.
64. Healy JC, Halligan S, Reznek RH, et al: Dynamic MR imaging compared with evacuation proctography when evaluating anorectal configuration and pelvic floor movement. Am J Roentgenol 169:775–779, 1997.
65. Vanbeckevoort D, Van Hoe L, Oyen R, et al: Pelvic floor descent in females: Comparative study of colpocystodefecography and dynamic fast MR imaging. J Magn Reson Imaging 9:373–377, 1999.
66. Matsuoka H, Wexner SD, Desai MB, et al: A comparison between dynamic pelvic magnetic resonance imaging and videoproctography in patient with constipation. Dis Colon Rectum 44:571–576, 2001.

CHAPTER 26

Diagnostic Evaluation of Erectile Dysfunction

FARSHAD SHAFIZADEH ■ ALBERT C. LEUNG ■ ARNOLD MELMAN

In 1992 a National Institutes of Health Consensus Panel defined erectile dysfunction (ED) as the inability to achieve or maintain an erection sufficient for satisfactory sexual function.[1] Data from the Massachusetts Male Aging Study indicate that the prevalence of erectile dysfunction of any degree is 39% in 40-year-old men and up to 67% in those aged 70 years.[2] Based on these data, erectile dysfunction will affect more than 25 million men from 40 to 70 years of age by the year 2005.[3]

Prior to the 1970s, erectile dysfunction commanded little clinical interest. Impotence was believed to be primarily a psychological disorder. The treatment usually consisted of empiric testosterone injection and psychotherapy and it was often ineffective. In the early 1970s, however, a new era of therapy for erectile dysfunction was initiated with the development of biological inert, flexible silicone and an effective penile prosthetic implant.[4-6] In the early 1980s, intercavernous injection of vasoactive drugs became another therapeutic option for erectile dysfunction.[7,8] Vacuum therapy was introduced by the end of 1980s and became the third form of therapy for erectile dysfunction.[9] The recognition of prostaglandin E_1 (PGE_1) as a possible therapy and the approval of intracavernous injection of PGE_1 by the US Food and Drug Administration (FDA) in 1996 were significant advances in the diagnosis and treatment of ED.[10,11] For the first time the US government legitimized, and paid for, the treatment of ED. Soon thereafter the FDA gave approval for intraurethral alprostadil and oral sildenafil.[12,13] The latter, along with its extensive promotional campaign, has allowed the discussion and treatment of ED to leave sports-page advertising and enter the world of everyday communications. Its ease of use and acceptance by the public has promulgated the concept that can it be used not only as a therapeutic tool but for primary diagnosis as well. This concept was put forth at the WHO international conference held in Paris in July 1999.[14] Today's era of managed care coupled with the availability of highly effective yet nonspecific treatment options have raised questions regarding the need for sophisticated diagnostic tests.

At the present time, the availability, effectiveness, and ease of administration of oral medication as first-line therapy for ED has diminished the need to diagnose the cause of the problem. Moreover, Viagra (sildenafil citrate), the only oral agent approved by the FDA for treating erectile dysfunction, is particularly successful in treating men with psychological (i.e., normal end-organ) causes of ED. The issue of treatment without evaluation is compounded by the cost (of diagnostic tests, physician's fees, time lost from work) and time (multiple visits to the office) needed to establish an accurate diagnosis. During an era of increased pressure by government agencies and insurance payers to limit medical costs, as well as the simple absence of resources in developing countries, there are further demands to offer a "goal-directed" (i.e., limited, rapid, and cheap) approach to treatment. Thus, the question is, what evaluation, if any, is necessary to establish a psychological cause of erectile dysfunction in a man seeking treatment for the problem when current available therapies to create an erection are so successful?

The answer is contingent on several factors that are independent of the physician's therapeutic ability to create penile rigidity. Both LoPiccolo[15] and Mohr and Beutler[16] emphasize that formulation of the best treatment plan is the primary purpose of the diagnostic assessment. The prognosis of the effects of therapy as determined by assessment of the patient and sexual partner is of paramount importance in the specific recommendation for therapy. That raises the question, how can one assess the prognostic application of a therapy in goal-directed treatments if absolutely no assessment is done of the patient and sexual partner? Furthermore, as many as 25% of men who present themselves to the urologist's office want only information, not therapy, for their problem. They will not use therapy of any type offered to them. Those men will drop from the therapy program and will be viewed as treatment failures if follow-up questioning is done.

The goal of this chapter is to formulate a scheme for urologists interested in diagnosing and treating erectile dysfunction. The interaction of conscious and unconscious stimuli from the brain (i.e., the psychological effect) on erection and the patient's (and partner's) need for treatment, preference of treatment, and satisfaction with the treatment must be taken into consideration.

PATHOPHYSIOLOGY OF ERECTILE DYSFUNCTION

Normal sexual function in the male involves libido, initiating erection, orgasm with ejaculation, and a refractory period. Sexual response in the male can be divided into the behavioral, erectile, and ejaculatory phases. For normal erectile function to ensue, three vascular events must occur: an increase in arterial flow into the penis via patent cavernosal arteries, sinusoidal relaxation and filling of the corpora cavernosa, and a decrease of venous flow out of the corpora. Functional impairment of arterial inflow or inadequate restriction of outflow, or both, can result in erectile dysfunction. More recently, it has become obvious that a failure of local control mechanisms that regulate the relaxation and contraction of the corporal smooth muscle may be significantly abnormal in most cases of erectile dysfunction. Failure of regulation of local relaxatory neurotransmitters, such as nitric oxide, or the excess of neurotransmitters that result in smooth muscle contraction, such as adrenergic neurotransmitters and endothelin, may account for many causes of erectile dysfunction.

CLASSIFICATION OF ERECTILE DYSFUNCTION

There are numerous reasons for a man not to have a rigid erection. In general, erectile dysfunction is summarized into two major classes: psychogenic and organic. In an important study, LoPiccolo[15] determined the etiology of erectile failure in 63 men independently evaluated for the degree of psychological and organic impairment. That evaluation followed complete psychological, vascular, hormonal, neurologic, and Nocturnal Penile Tumescence (NPT) determinations. Three clinicians separately reviewed the clinical and psychological data and each arrived at a score ranging from 0 (purely psychological) to 4 (purely organic). The results showed that the vast majority of men had combinations of problems of organic and psychological etiology. In fact, in that group, only 10 of the men were diagnosed with a purely psychogenic and 3 with a purely organic etiology. In a similar study in which the patients were referred to a urologist's office, the breakdown in diagnosis was 28.8% pure organic, 39.7% pure psychogenic, 25.1% mixed, and 6.4% unknown.[16] The implication is that even men with clear physical causes of their erectile dysfunction have psychological issues that can cloud the results of medical therapy. LoPiccolo emphasizes that erectile failure is a continuum with a small percentage of men with a pure state at the extreme ends and the majority with mixed conditions in the center.[15]

In a new study reported by Lee and colleagues,[17] the authors sought to identify the number of men with psychopathology in a group referred to their institution's Urology Department for ED. The prevalence of significant psychiatric disease was as high as 33% (40/120); 37.5% of that group suffered from major depression and 10% were schizophrenic. The report highlights the need to identify the psychological issues during the focused history taking. The identification of depression, schizophrenia, and drug and alcohol abuse requires that those problems be treated before an effort is made to correct the ED.

Recently, the advent of self-administered tests to categorize the presence of ED by symptom score has come into vogue. The prominent use of the brief sexual function inventory and the use of the International Index of Erectile Function (IIEF)[18] during the Viagra trials has promulgated the use of such devices not only to test the effect of therapies on the erectile condition but to describe the erectile condition based on the patient's observations of his erectile capacity. The question is whether men with psychogenic erectile dysfunction are good observers of their erectile capacity or whether they tend to minimize their erectile capacity for a range of reasons. That question was addressed in a report by Davis-Joseph and colleagues,[19] who studied the accuracy of a formal history of sexual function and general physical examination to establish a diagnosis for the cause of ED. The study included 45 men with a mean age of 57 years. Most important, 20% of men initially diagnosed with organic ED because of their history were eventually classified as having normal erectile capacity after multidisciplinary testing. Others have also studied this under-reporting of erectile capacity. Ackerman and Carey[20] note that the affect associated with ED, such as performance concerns and apprehension, can lead to interference and distraction from erotic cues. Barlow[21] has shown that men with ED underestimate the amount of erection response and decreased their erection response when demands to obtain an erection were made on them.

The organic cause could be neurogenic, endocrinologic, vascular, pharmacologic, or iatrogenic. Currently, the organic cause of erectile dysfunction is considered the most common cause. Box 26-1 lists the classification of erectile dysfunction and the most common functional failure associated with each class.

BOX 26-1	Classification of Erectile Dysfunction
ETIOLOGY	**FUNCTIONAL**
Neurogenic	Failure to initiate or maintain
Endocrinologic	Failure to fill
Arteriogenic	Failure to fill (slow initiation and early detumescence)
Venogenic	Failure to achieve rigidity or penetration and maintain
Psychogenic	Failure to achieve detumescence (priapism)
Pharmacologic	
Iatrogenic	

MODALITIES OF TESTING FOR ERECTILE DYSFUNCTION

In general, two levels of diagnostic workup exist to evaluate erectile dysfunction. The first-level approach, initially suggested by Lue,[22] is the "patient's goal-directed method." This approach is a streamlined process that consists of a medical and psychosexual history, physical examination, and hormonal and laboratory testing followed by a choice of therapeutic trial with oral medications, vacuum pump device, or intracavernous injections. Subsequent diagnostic workup and treatment planning is based on several factors that include patient response, clinical findings, and patient persistence.

The second level of diagnostic workup, which involves a more detailed approach, is directed to identify the cause of the dysfunction, thereby allowing men who have a possibly reversible problem to receive definitive therapy. This evaluation entails one or more of the following tests: psychologic consultation, nocturnal penile tumescence testing, advanced neurologic testing, and functional arterial and venous studies. Figure 26-1 shows the algorithm for initial evaluation of a patient with erectile dysfunction. The age, marital status, and partner status, as well as concomitant medical disease, also influence the treatment approach.

Medical and Psychosexual History

Just as it is for any other disease, a thorough medical and social history and physical examination is essential to evaluation of a man with erectile dysfunction. Since erectile dysfunction is often multifactorial, a good history and a

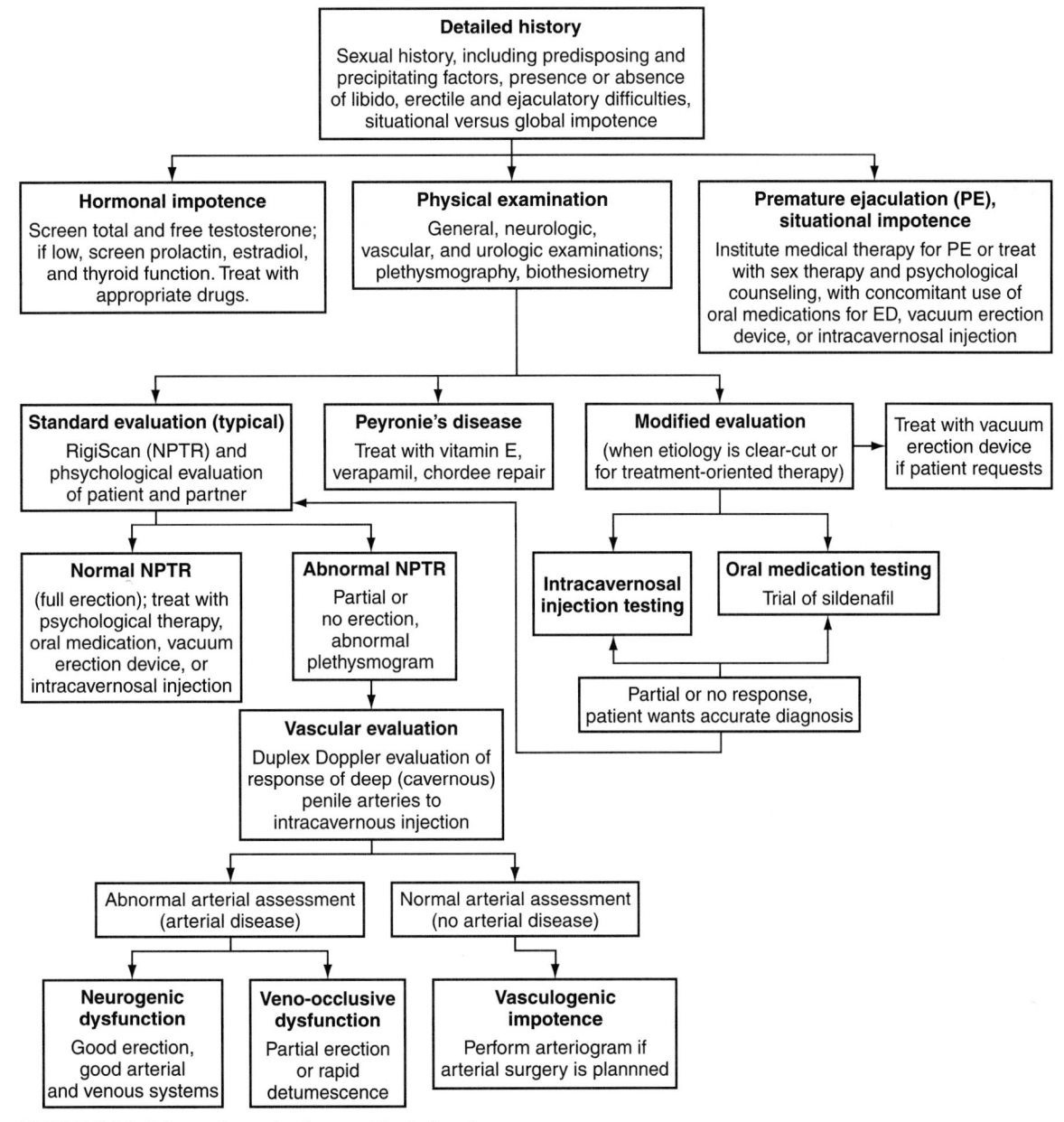

FIGURE 26-1 Schema for evaluating erectile dysfunction.

complete physical examination can help determine whether the dysfunction is a result of anatomic, psychogenic, endocrinologic, neurogenic, or vascular abnormalities.

When taking the history, a priority is to gain an accurate understanding of the patient's actual problem. An important goal is to identify during which phase of the male sexual response the patient's problem occurs (Box 26-2). Many men who claim they are impotent do not have an erectile problem but instead suffer dysfunction in one of the other four phases of sexual response. Often the sexual history provides the most helpful information in directing further evaluation and treatment. An adequate psychosocial history includes the duration of impotence, level of libido, and complete inventory of sexual partners. The presence of morning erection, intermittency, and any psychological conflict may help determine whether the dysfunction is mainly psychogenic or organic. In fact, the sexual history items with the greatest predictive power are those regarding early morning erection and erectile quality.[23]

Problems with libido are usually related to depression, life stress, marital dissatisfaction, or hormonal abnormalities. Patients with these problems should undergo screening for total and free testosterone, prolactin, estradiol, and thyroid-stimulating hormone (TSH). The psychological disorders are occasionally the sole primary cause of erectile dysfunction and early recognition allows the physician to dismiss further costly workup. When an overt psychological or marital problem is identified during the history, the patient should be referred to an appropriate professional for treatment after a complete physical examination. The patient should be questioned as to whether he is experiencing nocturnal, masturbatory, or situational loss of erection. A positive response usually suggests a reversible psychogenic etiology (Box 26-3), although vascular steal syndrome is a possibility.

The history should also reveal conditions that may be causing organic dysfunction (Table 26-1). Since atherosclerosis is the primary cause of impotence in 70% of men with organic dysfunction, conditions that predispose to atherosclerotic diseases (e.g., hypertension, hyperlipidemia, hypertriglyceridemia, diabetes, and smoking) should be identified during the history taking. Most organic, nonreversible causes of erectile dysfunction begin to develop after age 50, and prevalence increases with each decade.

Some drugs are commonly known to precipitate erectile dysfunction. Table 26-2 lists several classes of drug and their influence on sexual function. Drugs that interfere with hormonal, monoaminergic, and cholinergic mechanisms are frequently associated with impaired sexual desire,

BOX 26-3 Reversible Causes of Erectile Dysfunction

PSYCHOGENIC CAUSES
- Depression
- Anxiety
- Marital discord
- Ejaculatory problems

SOCIAL CAUSES
- Drugs, smoking, alcohol abuse

ORGANIC CAUSES

Arterial Insufficiency

Chordee

Hormonal Abnormalities
- Hypotestosteronemia
- Hypothyroidism
- Hyperthyroidism
- Hyperprolactinemia

Medications
- Beta blockers
- Alpha blockers
- Tricyclic Antidepressants

TABLE 26-1 ■ Conditions Associated with Erectile Dysfunction

Disease State	Basis of Erectile Dysfunction
Diabetes	Psychogenic factors
	Neurogenic: loss of fibers
	Arterial and venous: small vessel disease
	Myopathy
	Endothelial dysfunction
	Hormonal
Peyronie's disease	Loss of elastin and increased collagen formation
	Venous insufficiency
Aging	Decrease in sexual desire
	Takes longer to achieve erection
	Need for more direct physical stimulation
	Decreased response to visual stimulation
	Diminished penile rigidity
	Rapid detumescence post orgasm
	Reduced quality of orgasm
	Prolonged refractory period
	Reduced force of emission and ejaculation or premature ejaculation
Uremia	Atherosclerosis
	Peripheral neuropathy
	Medications and dialysis
	Endocrine problems
Alcohol use	Acute use: Behavioral changes (CNS depression) and temporary erectile dysfunction that may be related to dopamine
	Chronic use: abnormal endocrine function due to increased aromatization of androgens
	Development of peripheral neuropathy
	Behavioral and psychiatric changes
AIDS & Erection	Autonomic neuropathy
	Hormonal (hypogonadotropic hypogonadism)

BOX 26-2 Phases of the Male Sexual Response

Libido
Erection
Orgasm
Ejaculation
Refractory period

TABLE 26-2 ■ Medications Causing Erectile Dysfunction

Drug Type	Associated Side Effects
Antidepressants	Decreased libido, erectile dysfunction, and ejaculatory inhibition; serotonergic and anticholinergic properties of the heterocyclic antidepressant medications
Antipsychotics (neuroleptics)	Decreased libido, erectile dysfunction and ejaculatory inhibition ± priapism Decreased libido due to hyperprolactinemia resulting from dopamine-receptor antagonism in the pituitary and hypothalamus Erectile dysfunction and ejaculatory impairment are also characteristic of neuroleptics with high anticholinergic and œ-adrenergic activities
Antihypertensives	Act at the central level like œ-adrenergic receptor agonists (e.g., clonidine) Act at the peripheral level like methyldopa Direct action at the corporal level (intracellular calcium channel regulations) Drop in systemic blood pressure (perfusion pressure to coroporeal space)
Diurectics	Spironolactone: blocks testosterone synthesis and competitively binds to androgen receptor Hydrochlorothiazide: decreases libido, gynecomastia, mastodynia
Cardiovascular drugs	Digoxin: effect due to elevated level of estrogen and reduced testosterone due to similarity of chemical structure of digoxin and sex steroids; induces erectile difficulties via blockade of the Na+,K+-ATP-ase pump, resulting in a net increase in intracellular calcium and subsequent increased tone in the corporeal smooth muscle Antihyperlipidemic: enhances hepatic metabolism of androgens Beta blockers: propranolol at high doses may impair libido Atenolol may have lesser incidence of ED than propanolol
Drug of abuse	Alcohol: chronic use leads to abnormal endocrine function due to increased aromatization of androgen, development of a peripheral autonomic neuropathy, and behavioral changes Tobacco: vasoconstriction, endothelial damage, direct corporeal smooth muscle damage, atherosclerosis Cocaine: diffuse arteriosclerotic changes at the arterial bed as a result of endothelial toxicity
Antiandrogens	Blocks androgen synthesis Finasteride: 5% incidence of ED Estrogen, spironolactone, ketoconazole, and digoxin lower serum testosterone
Miscellaneous drugs	Metoclopramide: effect through CNS dopamine-receptor antagonist, which is similar to neuroleptics, leading to hyperprolactinemia Anticonvulsants: increases hepatic enzyme induction, leading to increased androgens metabolism Opioids: effects by reducing testosterone levels Nonsteroidal anti-inflammatory agent (e.g., indomethacin): inhibits prostaglandin formation Barbiturates: increased hepatic P-450 microsomal enzyme induction, thereby leading to increased metabolism of hormones

arousal, or ejaculation. As a general rule, drugs that potentiate the action of dopamine or antagonize serotonin have stimulatory effects and those that enhance serotonergic activity or diminish dopaminergic activity interfere with sexual functions. Noradrenergic pathways in the brain may inhibit penile erection. Inhibition of adrenergic activity in the central nervous system appears to depress male sexual behavior. Drug regiments that increase peripheral adrenergic tone have been correlated with erectile failure, whereas those that decrease postsynaptic alpha-1-adrenergic receptor activity are associated with priapism. For example, chronic treatments with amphetamine and cocaine, which indirectly increase alpha-1-adrenergic receptor activity, have been associated with erectile dysfunction. In contrast, a variety of drugs with alpha-1-adrenergic antagonist activity, as is the case with some antipsychotics, have been reported to cause priapism. Drugs that have adrenergic or cholinergic actions frequently impair ejaculatory functions of older men. Some patients are more vulnerable because of underlying medical conditions such as vascular, neurologic, and hormonal disorders.

Physical Examination

Every patient should have a complete physical examination with primary attention toward sexual and genital development as well as identification of vascular, endocrinologic, or neurologic abnormalities. Palpation of the penis should be done routinely to identify fibrosis or plaque formation (chordee, Peyronie's plaque). Gynecomastia and small, soft testes may suggest an endocrine abnormality (e.g., hypogonadism, hyperprolactinemia) or certain genetic diseases (e.g., Klinefelter's syndrome, Kallmann's syndrome).

A careful neurologic examination is important for a patient with a history suggestive of peripheral or central neuropathies such as diabetes or hypertension. A vascular examination should also be routine in the initial examination of a patient with erectile dysfunction. Any abnormality in distal pulses may suggest peripheral vascular disease and therefore a possible vascular cause of erectile dysfunction.

Biothesiometry and plethysmography are often part of the initial physical examination. Biothesiometry is a rapid, simple test that identifies the loss of penile sensation secondary to unexpected neurologic disease or natural aging.[24] Plethysmography is a simple, accurate, reproducible, diagnostic screening test that identifies diminished penile blood flow. When the history suggests arterial disease and plethysmographic results are abnormal, the diagnosis can be firmly established with duplex ultrasonography, intracorporal injection, or both. These modalities will be discussed in detail later.

We have evaluated patients by careful history, physical examination, psychologic evaluation, and RigiScan monitoring followed by additional testing and found that history and physical examination alone had 95% sensitivity but only a 50% specificity in diagnosis of organic erectile dysfunction. Therefore, a multifaceted comprehensive approach is required to fully evaluate and diagnose erectile dysfunction.[19]

Psychometry and Psychological Interview

Early psychological explanations of erectile dysfunction focused on anxiety as a predominant cause. It was hypothesized that anxiety states were incompatible with sexual arousal, thereby resulting in inhibited sexual responding.[25,26] Subsequently, Masters and Johnson's revolutionary sex therapy techniques were developed based on the hypothetical causes of sexual dysfunction, such as performance anxiety, negative attitudes about sex, and early sexual trauma.[27] Since that time, researchers and clinicians have proposed other factors such as depression, anxiety, psychosocial stress, and conflict in marital relations.[21,28]

Psychological stimuli can inhibit penile erection by two mechanisms: direct inhibition of the spinal erection center by the brain as an exaggeration of the normal suprasacral inhibition[29] and excessive sympathetic outflow or elevated peripheral catecholamine levels. Clinically, compared to normal controls, higher levels of serum norepinephrine have been reported in patients with psychogenic erectile dysfunction. Predisposing personality disorders also have been described as a cause of psychogenic erectile dysfunction.[30]

In obtaining psychometry and psychological history, the primary goals are to differentiate between primary versus secondary, constant or situational, and partner-specific dysfunction. Structured interviews focusing on presenting symptoms have shown promise as generalized screening instruments indicating that further organic assessment is needed or that a psychological etiology can be safely assumed (Box 26-4).[31,32] There are several different self-reported questionnaires developed for the assessment of patients with erectile dysfunction. Although there is some overlap of questions asked in different instruments, each questionnaire has a slightly different focus, reflecting the purpose for which the instrument was developed. The advantage of a standardized questionnaire is that it might detect information that the clinician or investigator might otherwise overlook. For example, it is not uncommon for a man to complain of impotence when it is not the primary problem. Some men may complain of impotence while the main problem is premature ejaculation.

The International Index of Erectile Function (IIEF) is a 15-item self-reported inventory questionnaire that was specifically designed to assess erectile dysfunction in response to pharmacologic intervention.[18] It measures erectile function, orgasmic function, libido, and satisfaction. It is simple, highly reliable, and available in many languages. The norms for this instrument are under development.

A similar instrument is the Brief Male Sexual Function Inventory (BMSFI) developed in a urologic context by O'Leary and colleagues.[33,34] It is brief (11 questions), easy to use, and also available in multiple languages. It measures drive, erectile function, ejaculation, and satisfaction. Many of the items in this instrument are the same as those in the International Index of Erectile Function. There is minimal evidence to recommend use of one of these instruments over the other. The norms for this instrument are also under the development.

A problem facing the nonpsychiatric physician in the evaluation of a patient with erectile disorder is the comorbidity of sexual disorders and certain psychiatric syndromes.[35,36] Although various treatment approaches may reverse erectile failure in psychiatric patients, the clinician would not want to miss an underlying treatable and possibly fatal psychiatric disease such as major depressive disorder and panic disorder. Both of these disorders have high suicide rates. Numerous studies have demonstrated that general physicians underdiagnose psychiatric disorders such as depression and anxiety disorders.[37,38] Although several questionnaires have been developed for the diagnosis of common psychiatric disorders, such as the Minnesota Multiphasic Personality Inventory (MMPI), they are often too comprehensive to be a useful screening instrument. The primary psychiatric conditions that the physician needs to screen for in diagnosing erectile dysfunction are depression and anxiety disorder. Recent research suggests that two questions are sufficient for brief screening of depression. The questions are (1) During the past month, have you often been bothered by feeling down, depressed, or hopeless? (2) During the past month,

---

BOX 26-4 Standardized Questionnaire for Preliminary Assessment of Erectile Dysfunction

1. Chief complaint
2. Accurate description of erectile abnormality
   - Problem initiating or maintaining erection
   - Duration of erection
     - Erection lost before or during coitus
     - Loss of erection associated with ejaculation
     - Positional differences (missionary vs. side-to-side, upright, or female-superior)
3. Duration of problem
   - Intermittent or situational
   - Traumatic event at onset (e.g., death of family member [widower's syndrome], accident, argument, loss of job)
4. Change in erectile deficit (e.g., plateauing, worsening, improving)
5. History of premature ejaculation
6. History of penile or pelvic trauma or back pain
7. Penis straight or curved when erect
8. Morning, night, or masturbatory erections
9. Libidinal status
10. Social history
    - Alcohol abuse
    - Drug abuse
    - Cigarette smoking
11. Personal or family history of medical or psychiatric diseases
    - Hypertension
    - Diabetes
    - Coronary artery disease
    - Depression
    - Anxiety
12. Paresthesias (including change in penile sensation)
13. Change in strength, gait, loss of balance
14. Symptoms of claudication
15. Patient's perception of causes of problems/patient's goal in seeking appointment

have you often been bothered by little interest in or pleasure from doing things? These questions, along with anxiety scales, can be added to the IIEF questionnaire.[39]

Evaluating the patient's partner is an important adjunct to psychosocial evaluation. In our many years of experience, we have found that the best treatment results are achieved by considering information from an interview with the patient's sexual partner.[40,41] Although some men refuse to involve their partners in the evaluation, the partners themselves generally are cooperative and pleased to be part of the process.[40] These interviews are essential not only to confirm the patient's history and the possible role of marital conflict, but also to identify the combined goals of the couple. Such an interview often helps determine the type of therapy that best suits the patient and his partner. Often the information obtained from the partner and the patient are contradictory. The partner's interview, therefore, can modify or confirm the initial diagnosis and can also influence the recommended treatment. If for no other reason than to increase the accuracy of history taking, partner interviews seem invaluable.[40]

If considerable marital discord is suspected based on the psychosocial history, the physician might consider referral for counseling in addition to treatment to correct the erectile problems. Rapid tools for the detection of marital discord include the Locke Wallace Marital Adjustment Test, a 15-item questionnaire, and the longer instrument, the Dyadic Adjustment Scale.[42]

Diagnostic Testing

Nocturnal Penile Tumescence Testing

Although taking the history and performing the physical examination are essential to the diagnosis of erectile dysfunction, a firm diagnosis based solely on these two modalities has been a matter of contention.[43] Nocturnal Penile Tumescence (NPT) testing has been developed since 1970 primarily to help distinguish psychogenic and organic causes of impotence.

The association between sleep and erection was documented as early as 1940.[44] Sleep-related erection or nocturnal penile tumescence is a cycle of erections associated with rapid eye movement (REM) sleep in all potent men. The mechanism responsible for these erections is presumed to rely on neurovascular responses similar to those of erotically induced erections. Therefore, patients who have a normal NPT are presumed to have a normal capacity for spontaneous erotically induced erection. The NPT study consists of a nocturnal monitoring device that measures the number of erections, maximal penile rigidity, circumference, and duration of each erectile episode.[45] The patient is awakened during maximum tumescence to measure axial rigidity; a device is applied to the penile tip and shaft where upon it measures the force required to buckle the penis. A buckling resistance of 500–550g is considered minimum for vaginal penetration. This study is also performed in conjunction with electroencephalography, electro-oculography, and electromyography, as well as breathing and movement monitoring.

However, this sleep monitoring NPT study is considered unreliable by some sleep physiologists who believe that severely fragmented and disturbed sleeps render this study uninterpretable.

Although NPT is a noninvasive test, it has several limiting factors: (1) the mechanism of nocturnal penile tumescence is assumed to rely on neurovascular responses similar to erotically induced erection, although this is not fully elucidated and some believe that the results correlate poorly with actual sexual performance reported by the patients[46]; (2) parameters found during NPT may not correlate with clinical findings such as comparison of tumescence and rigidity (i.e., patient may have sufficient tumescent but not have enough penile rigidity for vaginal penetration); (3) no standard has been established, therefore interpretation varies among investigators; and (4) some sleep disturbances, such as apnea and motor agitation, as well as some psychological diseases, such as depression and anxiety, can falsely affect NPT results.

There are several studies attempting to standardize the NPT. Cilurzo suggests the following as normal parameters for NPT: four to five erectile episodes per night with mean duration of greater than 30 minutes and an increase in circumference of greater than 3 cm at base and 2 cm at the tip with greater than 70% rigidity at the base and the tip.[47] Due to the cost of the NPT test, the RigiScan, which is a simpler device, was introduced in 1985. The RigiScan is used in the patient's home and monitors rigidity, tumescence, and number and duration of erections during sleep. However although it is easier to use, the RigiScan presents similar limitations to those of the original methods used for an NPT study. To increase its viability the RigiScan test is performed for three consecutive nights to ensure a minimum of one REM sleep by the subject.

Endocrine Testing

Androgens influence libido and sexual behavior. Possible hormonal regulation of the sacral parasympathetic cord nuclei and of neurons in the hypothalamus and limbic system have been suggested by the demonstration of androgen receptors in these sites. Patients with castrated levels of testosterone, however, can achieve erections in response to visual sexual stimulation. This observation suggests that the neurovascular mechanisms that control erection are functional in the presence of low levels of androgens. On the other hand, it has been shown that hypogonadal men have decreased nocturnal penile erectile activity that responds to androgen replacement,[48,49] whereas exogenous testosterone therapy reportedly has little effect on potency in impotent men with borderline low testosterone levels.[50,51] The major endocrinologic disorders associated with impotence are hypogonadotropic hypogonadism, hypergonadotropic hypogonadism, and hyperprolactinemia (Box 26-5).[52,53] Potency is not restored in approximately half of these patients despite the normalization of serum testosterone levels. This implies some degree of antagonism by prolactin to the peripheral action of testosterone. Erectile complaints may also be associated with both the hyper- and hypothyroid

> **BOX 26-5** **Endocrinologic Causes of Erectile Dysfunction**

States Causing Hypogonadotropic Hypogonadism (↓ LH & ↑ FSH)

GONADOTROPIN-RELEASING HORMONE (GnRH) DEFICIENCY

- Hypothalamic lesions (tumors, encephalitis, granulomas, craniopharyngioma)
- Prader-Willi syndrome (massive obesity, neonatal hypotonia, hyperphagia, mental retardation)
- Alström's syndrome (obesity, nephropathy, hypertriglyceridemia, hyperuricemia, acanthosis nigricans, hypogonadotropic hypogonadism)
- Familial hypoprolactinemia (see below as well), hemochromatosis, neurosarcoma, myotonic dystrophy, aging

PITUITARY DISORDERS (GONADOTROPIN DEFICIENCY)

- Isolated LH deficiency (Pasqualini syndrome, eunuchoidism, absent secondary sexual characteristics, oligospermia)
- Tumors (functioning and nonfunctioning)
- Pituitary infarction
- Empty sella syndrome
- Hemochromatosis

STATES CAUSING HYPERGONADOTROPIC HYPOGONADISM (↑ LH & ↓ FSH)

TESTICULAR DISORDERS (PRIMARILY GONADAL FAILURE)

- Impaired Leydig cell activity
  Inborn errors of testosterone biosynthesis
  - 3-beta-hydroxysteroid dehydrogenase (male or female pseudohermaphrodism, adrenal insufficiency)
  - 17-alpha-hydroxylase deficiency (male pseudohermaphrodism, hypogonadism, sexual infantism, hypertension, hypokalemic alkalosis)
  - 17-20-desmolase deficiency
  - 17-beta-hydroxysteroid oxidoreductase deficiency
  Leydig cell hypoplasia
  Testicular unresponsiveness (possible LH failure)
  Androgen-resistant states and enzyme defects
  - Testicular feminization (absence of androgen receptors)
  - Incomplete androgen sensitivity (Reiffenstein's syndrome)
  - 5-alpha-reductase deficiency (pseudovaginal perineal scrotal hypospadius/familial incomplete male pseudohermaphrodism)

- Undescended testes, acquired bilateral torsion of testes, orchitis
- Seminiferous tubule dysgenesis (Klinefelter's syndrome)
- Pure gonadal dysgenesis (46XX, 46XY)

STATES CAUSING HYPERPROLACTINEMIA (INCIDENCE 1%–5%)

HYPOTHALAMIC DISEASE
Tumors (craniopharyngioma), granulomas

PITUITARY DISORDERS
Tumors (functioning: microadenoma or macroadenoma; acromegaly)

DRUGS
Alpha-methyl dopa
Reserpine
Phenothiazine (e.g., chlorpromazine)
Butyrophenones (haloperidol)
Verapamil
Cocaine
Cimetidine
Opioids

MISCELLANEOUS DISORDERS
Primary hypothyroidism
Diabetes
Chronic renal failure
Cirrhosis
Chest wall lesions (neurogenic mechanisms)
Stress ideopathic

MISCELLANEOUS

SYSTEMIC DISEASE

- Liver diseases (up to 75% incidence of ED)
- Thyroid diseases (ED in less than 2%)
- Chronic renal failure
- Sickle disease, sickle cell anemia (trait and disease)
- Nutritional disorders (protein malnutrition, zinc deficiency)
- Estrogen excess

AUTOIMMUNE DISEASE

- AIDS
- Polyglandular autoimmune disease (multiple endocrine failure)

---

state. Hyperthyroid states are commonly associated with diminished libido and less often with erectile dysfunction. In hypothyroid states, impotence has been reported and may be secondary to associated low testosterone secretion and elevated prolactin levels.

The incidence of endocrinopathy as the cause of erectile dysfunction has been reported to be close to 1.7% in the latest large series.[54] Indications for obtaining endocrine studies are controversial.[55] Some suggest that routine endocrine testing with its high cost may add no information to a complete history and physical examination. Endocrine testing has been recommended in patients without clinical evidence of hypogonadism.[51] On the other hand, despite the amount of money spent to find very few patients with endocrine disease, some argue that finding the occasional cases of primary or secondary hypogonadism or hyperprolactinemia justifies the expense. For this reason, most physicians routinely perform a minimal endocrine screening on every patient who presents with erectile dysfunction.

The endocrine studies for evaluation of men with erectile dysfunction are targeted toward the hypothalamic–pituitary–testicular axis. These assays are serum testosterone, prolactin, and luteinizing hormones. Serum-free testosterone hormone is measured in patients with decreased testosterone-binding globulin, namely, those with obesity, acromegaly, and hypothyroidism.

Typically, patients who report diminished desire, with or without erections, and those with clear clinical evidence of hypogonadism benefit the most from endocrine testing. Frequently, patients with hyperprolactinemia supply a clue: They have protean symptoms of malaise aside from loss of libido and erectile dysfunction. And abnormally high prolactin level (>22 ng/mL) can lower testosterone secretion by inhibiting secretion of luteinizing hormone–releasing hormone by the hypothalamus and thereby result in impotence.[56]

A reasonable approach is to obtain a serum testosterone level during the initial evaluation of a patient with erectile dysfunction. If the initial testosterone level is 500 ng/dL or higher, there is no need for further evaluation or endocrine therapy; however, if the initial level is below 500 ng/dL, and especially if the testosterone is less than 300 ng/dL, it is advisable to repeat the test and obtain serum-free testosterone, luteinizing hormone, and prolactin levels simultaneously.[57] This is to differentiate primary from secondary hypogonadism. Only men with clearly documented primary hypogonadism are candidates for testosterone replacement therapy.

Neurologic Evaluation of Impotence

Erectile dysfunction is a common complaint of patients with many neurologic diseases. Peripheral neuropathies, cauda equina syndrome, pelvic and pudendal nerve lesions, spinal cord trauma, Parkinsonism, Alzheimer's disease, multiple sclerosis, and cerebrovascular insufficiency are common causes of impotence. Vascular abnormalities, certain drugs, and psychological disorders associated with disturbance of neurologic or neuromuscular function can also be associated with impotence.[58] Penile erection is under the regulation of the autonomic system, and a host of neurotransmitters have been implicated in erectile physiology. Erection is controlled by both the sympathetic and parasympathetic nerves, with the sympathetic nervous system inhibiting erections while the parasympathetic system contains excitatory pathways. Nonetheless, neither a cholinergic nor an adrenergic neurotransmitter system is entirely responsible for the control of erection.[59,60] Sexual stimuli result in neurologic impulses via somatic and autonomic motor tracts to the erectile apparatus, generating tumescence. Studies suggest the importance of the reticular activating system, a region that facilitates connections among the spinal cord, cerebellum, hypothalamus, rhinencephalon, and cerebral cortex in the integration of physiologic sexual function.[61] Experiments demonstrate that erections can be generated with stimulation of the lateral, dorsolateral, hypothalamic, medial preoptic, and anterior hypothalamic regions, and lesions placed experimentally in these areas are associated with impotence.[62] The extraspinal peripheral pathways travel to the penis from sympathetic and parasympathetic regions. The sympathetic nerves travel in the inferior mesenteric and superior hypogastric plexus through the hypogastric nerve to the pelvic plexus and through the cavernous nerve to the penis. Numerous studies suggest that the motor control of erection is exerted via both sympathetic and parasympathetic nerve fibers, and that neither a cholinergic nor an adrenergic neurotransmitter system is solely responsible for erectile function. Apomorphine SL activates the hypothalamic-hippocampal oxytocinergic pathway through D2 dopamine receptor stimulation in the paraventricular nucleus (PVN). Activation of PVN results in increased parasympathetic outflow and nitric oxide release, eventually leading to corporal muscle relaxation and erection. While approved in Europe, apomorphine SL is still pending approval from the FDA. More thorough understanding and knowledge of the microneuroanatomy of the penis can refine nerve-sparing techniques during urologic operations so that the risk of impotence as a complication can be lessened.

The neurologic evaluation serves to identify a neurologic component and the nature and location of the underlying neuropathology. Neurologists commonly employ certain diagnostic tests in the evaluation of erectile dysfunction. Nocturnal penile tumescence and rigidity testing has been the most common test to differentiate psychogenic from organic impotence, although it cannot determine the exact cause of impotence. Differentiating neurogenic and psychogenic impotence from vascular causes can be achieved by the intracavernosal injection of smooth muscle relaxants such as papaverine or PGE_1. A rigid erection following the injection is believed to be in support of neurogenic impotence. Both the NPT testing and the erectile response to intracavernosal pharmacotherapy assess the autonomic efferent component indirectly.[63] When neurogenic impotence is suspected, tests are available to confirm the diagnosis or to localize the lesion in the nervous system. These tests include dorsal penile nerve conduction velocity, bulbocavernous reflex and urethroanal reflex responses, and pudendal somatosensory evoked response, although abnormalities identified through these tests may not correlate with the ability to achieve an erection. The bulbocavernous reflex response can be assessed by stimulating the dorsal penile nerve and recording over the perineum or rectal sphincter, since the penile nerve conduction velocity can be measured indirectly by stimulating the proximal and distal shaft of the penis. Penile biothesiometry simply measures the sensory function or vibration perception threshold of the penis and can be used as an initial screening test. The procedure involves using a portable handheld electromagnetic vibration device that has a fixed vibration frequency but a variable vibration amplitude; it is placed on the lateral penile shaft bilaterally and the glans penis. The patient is then asked to inform the examiner when he first senses vibration as the amplitude of vibration is slowly increased and when he senses the disappearance of vibration as the amplitude is slowly decreased. Although no tests can directly measure the autonomic component of erectile function, testing of the autonomic cardiovascular reflexes suggests that abnormal reflexes are associated with aging and organic impotence, indicating the equal importance of autonomic dysfunction in the etiology of erectile failure.[64] Cystometrography and tests of certain vascular functions regulated by the autonomic nervous system—including blood pressure and pulse response to cold, sympathetic skin responses to electrical stimulation, and orthostatic measurements of blood pressure and pulse—have been suggested as ways of identifying autonomic neuropathy in impotent patients.[65]

Studies have shown that delayed stimulus conduction and processing along peripheral and sacral neural pathways are related to patient age to a significant degree.

Collagen infiltration, arteriosclerotic malnutrition, and progressive peripheral neuropathy are possible causes for the age-related decrease in penile sensitivity and sexual activity, and peripheral neuropathy along with sacral neurologic disturbances are responsible for much of the decrease in penile sensitivity.[66] Herbert has shown that sexual activity of rhesus monkeys depends on dorsal penile nerve (sensory) function. Thus, sensory deficit may be an important cause of erectile dysfunction.[67]

The peripheral and central pudendal nerve afferent pathways can be assessed through somatosensory evoked potential testing, by recording the evoked potential waveforms (EEG) overlying the sacral cord and cerebral cortex. Klausner and Batra have shown that pudendal nerve somatosensory evoked potential testing is a valuable procedure in evaluating patients with possible pudendal afferent pathway dysfunction, and the test is significantly correlated with neurological history and physical examination.[68] This study measures latency values, time of stimulation to the first replicated spinal response, that are prolonged or not recordable in patients who possess lesions in the ascending neuronal pathways. Since first described by Haldeman and colleagues, somatosensory evoked potential testing has evolved into a promising tool in the evaluation of neurogenic impotence.[69] Patients with positive neurologic and physical findings should undergo the test based on the significant correlation as reported by Klausner and Batra.[68] Somatosensory evoked potential testing can be most useful as an objective measurement of the presence, location, and nature of afferent penile sensory dysfunction in patients with abnormal neurologic screening results.[63]

The integrity of the corporeal nerves and concentration of neurotransmitters have been studied in evaluating neurogenic impotence. Electron microscopic findings demonstrate degeneration or loss of Schwann's cells and nerve axons in the corporeal tissue of impotent patients. Furthermore, a decrease in the intracorporeal vasoactive intestinal peptide concentration is detected in insulin-dependent diabetics when compared to nondiabetic and psychogenic patients with erectile dysfunction. In vivo and in vitro studies emphasize the adverse effect of hyperglycemia and accumulation of glucose metabolites on nerve and endothelium cells, and neuropathy and angiopathy can be considered crucial factors in the etiology of impotence in diabetic men.[70] Other reports demonstrate that intracorporeal amounts of vasoactive intestinal peptidergic, cholinergic, and adrenergic nerves are decreased in the penis of diabetic patients, although Melman and colleagues report that cavernous myelinated and unmyelinated nerve fibers are unaltered in impotent diabetic patients.[71] Nitric oxide synthase may be of diagnostic value in neurogenic impotence through cavernosal biopsy specimen studies.[72]

Pharmacotesting

In 1982 Ronald Virag noted during the course of vascular reconstruction that infusion of papaverine into the hypogastric artery produced erection.[73] Subsequently in 1983, work by others who studied the pharmacorelaxing property of different agents resulted in the development of combined pharmacoinjection therapy.[74] Bennett and colleagues first described the clinical efficacy of trimix: papaverine, phentolamine, and PGE_1.[75] In July 1995, Upjohn Company (Kalamazoo, Michigan) received Food and Drug Administration approval to market injectable PGE_1 (Caverject) specifically for the diagnosis and treatment of erectile dysfunction. This agent is the most popular agent for intracavernous injection (ICI) therapy secondary to its safety.

Pharmacotesting consists of intracavernous injection and visual rating of the subsequent erection. It is the most used diagnostic procedure for erectile dysfunction. It is simple, safe, minimally invasive, and cost effective, and it can be performed without monitoring equipment. Even though a standard intercavernous test dosage has never been established for any agent, a common approach is to inject 5 micrograms of alprostadil in the first dose, increasing the dose in the same or subsequent session up to 40 micrograms if the patient fails to respond. A positive response merely reflects an intracavernous pressure equal to or greater than 80 mm Hg, whereas the maximum erectile response as determined by the systemic blood pressure can be much higher. A positive test therefore implies psychogenic impotence, presumably excluding significant venous or arterial pathology.[76] However, Pescatori and coworkers have shown that a patient can have mild arterial insufficiency even if he responds well to the intracavernous injection of vasoactive drugs.[77] In their study, 41% of responders had gradient more than 24 mm Hg between systemic and cavernous systolic blood pressure. Conversely, a negative erection may also be due to excessive adrenergic constrictor tone secondary to anxiety.[78,79] Kim and Oh demonstrated that the level of norepinephrine in penile blood during the test is higher in patients with psychogenic erectile dysfunction than in healthy controls or patients with vascular erectile dysfunction.[80] Moreover, in the psychologic group, the norepinephrine level appeared significantly higher in nonresponders than in responders. Up to 25% of the nonresponders may show predominance of psychological factors.

The most feared complication of pharmacotesting is prolonged erection, or priapism. The group most prone to a prolonged erection are younger patients with nonvascular erectile dysfunction and a better baseline erectile function.[81] Therefore, the dosage for initial testing should be adapted to the characteristics of the patients and lowered in those with suspected neurogenic or psychological dysfunction. Three different vasoactive agents are used for pharmacotesting: papaverine, papaverine-phentolamine, and prostaglandin (PGE_1). In a multicenter study comparing papaverine, papaverine-phentolamine, and PGE_1, PGE_1 emerged as the most accurate diagnostic drug, with an overall erection rate of 74% and a prolonged erection rate of only 0.1%.[82]

Vascular Investigation of Erectile Dysfunction

The penis is a specialized vascular organ that exists in either the flaccid or the erect position. The complex hemodynamic alterations associated with normal erection require precise modulation of neural pathways and the integrity of penile smooth muscle of both the supplying blood vessels and the corporal trabeculae. In the flaccid state, the corporal smooth muscle of cavernous arteries, helicine arterioles, and corpora are tonically contracted, limiting the inflow of blood to the corpora to a small amount that enters the penis for nutritional purposes at a flow of about 5 mL/min.[83] To obtain a penile erection, four physiologic events are necessary: intact neural innervation, intact arterial supply, appropriately responsive corporal smooth muscle, and intact veno-occlusive mechanics. On arrival of sexual stimuli generated peripherally or centrally, neurotransmitters from nonadrenergic, noncholinergic (NANC) nerves are generated at corporal smooth muscle cells. This leads to relaxation of vascular and corporal smooth muscle cells, initiating the cascade of events that lead to penile erection. Functional impairment of either arterial inflow or inadequate restriction of venous outflow may result in erectile dysfunction.[84] It has become obvious that a failure of the local control mechanisms that regulate the relaxation and contraction of the corporal smooth muscle may be significantly abnormal in most cases of erectile dysfunction. The failure of regulation of local relaxatory neurotransmitters or endothelin may account for many causes of erectile dysfunction.

The incidence of vascular disease as the primary cause of erectile dysfunction is estimated to be between 10% and 20%. This incidence also increases with age secondary to increased risk of atherosclerosis. Aside from atherosclerosis, other vascular diseases that affect medium to small blood vessels can affect erectile function; among them are systemic lupus erythematosus (SLE) and polyarteritis nodosa. Erectile dysfunction can also be a prominent finding in Leriche's syndrome, which involves a thromboembolic occlusion of the aorta or the iliac arteries. The hallmark symptom of this disease is intermittent claudication of the thighs, buttocks, or calf muscles.

Arterial Inflow Investigation

The inflow blood supply to the penis arises from the internal pudendal arteries, terminal branches of the hypogastrics. The internal pudendal arteries trifurcate and form the arteries to the bulbous urethra, the cavernous arteries, and the dorsal arteries of the penis. The deep artery enters the medial crus and runs the entire length of the penis. It provides the main blood supply to the corpora cavernosa. Similarly, the dorsal artery passes over the medial aspect of the crus beneath Buck's fascia and travels the entire length of the corpora to the glans. It gives off several circumflex branches to the mid-dorsal corpora cavernosa. The blood supply to the glans is supplied by the urethral arteries traveling within the corpora spongiosum and is separate from the cavernosal blood supply. However, a report by Puech-Leao describes several variations in the vascular pattern of penile vasculature.[85] For example, one dorsal artery might be responsible for most of the blood flow to both corpora.

Several noninvasive and invasive techniques have been developed to assess the arterial blood supply to the penis: penile blood pressure, penile brachial index, selective interpudendal pharmacoangiography, Doppler sonography, color duplex Doppler ultrasound, radionuclide washout of penile blood, and the injection of intracorporal vasoactive agents such as papaverine or trimix.

Penile Artery Pressure and Penile Brachial Index

In 1971 Gaskell described a noninvasive test of penile arterial inflow; he used a photometer to quantify the absorption of light by the pigment oxyhemoglobin in the glans penis.[86] An occlusive cuff at the base of the penis was slowly loosened, and the pressure at which oxyhemoglobin became measurable in the glans then indicated the penile systolic blood pressure.

Abelson used the Doppler stethoscope to measure penile blood pressure in flaccid state.[87] Based on his observation, penile systolic blood pressure in flaccid state should not be less than 30 mm Hg below the brachial systolic blood pressure. Since then Penile Brachial Index has been developed. It is a simple, noninvasive, and usually inexpensive test. The standard method of measuring the penile artery pressure involves an 8- to 10-MHz Doppler ultrasound probe and an occlusive 2.5 to 3 cm wide blood pressure cuff placed around the base of the penis.[88,89] Simultaneous brachial artery pressure is compared to either the highest penile pressure or the mean of all vessels in which systolic pressures can be elicited, and a score called Penile Brachial Index (PBI) is calculated. Most authors have considered a score lower than 0.6 as diagnostic of vasculogenic erectile dysfunction. Metz reports a mean PBI in a group of potent men with a median age of 54 of 0.86 ± 0.08.[89] The predictive value of a positive test was 91% and that of a negative test only 72%. Michal and colleagues modified the PBI test with a dynamic component by adding lower extremity and pelvic musculature exercises, with Doppler stethoscope; auscultation is being performed before and after exercise.[90] A decrease in the ratio of penile systolic pressure <0.15 indicates pelvic steal syndrome or significant penile inflow disease.[91]

The shortcomings that reduce the accuracy of this test include variation in penile artery supply (as reported by Puech-Leao), variation in penile size (occasionally making measurement even with a small cuff difficult), arterial spasm, lack of a significant pressure drop with small vessel disease, and uncertainty about whether the cavernous or dorsal artery is being auscultated.[92] Subsequent reviews comparing the PBI values of normal and impotent patients reveal some overlap, and pressures were inadvertently obtained from the dorsal artery not reflecting the central cavernous arteries.[93]

Strain-gauge plethysmography has been suggested as a more accurate, reproducible, and easier technique than the Doppler probe.[94] In this method, the pulsations of all vessels entering the penis are recorded in a more objective and less time-consuming manner than with the standard Doppler technique. Strain-gauge plethysmography has a reported specificity of 100% and accuracy of 95%. The primary drawback of the method is that the penis is measured at rest when the blood flow is at a minimum rather than at maximal flow.

Color Duplex Doppler Testing

In 1985 Lue and colleagues introduced the technique of high-resolution sonography and quantitative Doppler spectrum analysis to evaluate dynamic changes in cavernous arterial flow after intracorporal injection of papaverine.[95] A 10-MHz duplex scanner combined with a pulsed 4.5-MHz range-gated Doppler subsystem allows simultaneous imaging and flow measurements of cavernous arteries. This test provides an objective, minimally invasive evaluation of a suboptimal or equivocal erectile response to an intracavernous vasoactive agent (in a neurologically normal man). The original parameter used to infer the integrity of penile circulation was cavernous peak systolic velocity (PSV). Subsequently, other Doppler parameters such as end diastolic arterial velocity, systolic rise time (from the start of systolic velocity to the maximum value), and cavernous artery acceleration (peak flow velocity over systolic rise time) have been added to define penile inflow disease better. Lue and colleagues proposed that an adequate response in the cavernous arteries should produce a >0.7-mm post-injection arterial diameter, and >25-cm/s PSV. They found that cavernous arteries that did not dilate by 75% suggested arterial disease. However, other investigators found no correlation between percentage changes in arterial diameter dilation and clinical response.[96-98] On the other hand, subsequent studies show that the cavernous arterial diameters normally decrease from the proximal to distal penis and that measurement of cavernous arterial lumens actually exceeds ultrasound resolution of the 7- to 10-MHz probes. Thus arterial diameters are considered much less significant than arterial dynamics. Results of several studies, including the groups at University of California–San Francisco, Baylor University series, and Harvard Medical School, reported normal subjects with mean PSV of 34.8 cm/s to 47 cm/s; however, each of these groups concurred that a peak systolic velocity <25 cm/s suggests severe penile arterial insufficiency.[99] When penile angiography was compared to duplex Doppler examinations of the same patients, PSV <25 cm/s was consistently associated with severe arterial disease. In a report from the Mayo Clinic series, PSV <25 cm/s had a sensitivity of 100% and specificity of 95% in patients with abnormal pudendal arteriography.[100,101] A PSV of 35 cm/s or more was consistently associated with normal penile arteriograms. The Mayo Clinic group has recommended that arteriography should not be performed on patients with good clinical response to vasodilating injection with bilateral peak systolic velocities >30 cm/s and arterial dilation to 0.7 mm.

Venous Impotence: Evaluation and Treatment

The penis is a complex vascular organ that requires the coordination of vascular, neural, and hormonal factors to achieve penile erection sufficient for coitus. Penile erection and detumescence are principally vascular events coordinated by the relaxation and contraction of arterial and corporeal smooth muscle. Such events contribute to the establishment of sufficient intracavernosal pressure for penile rigidity, determined by the retention of blood inside the corpora cavernosum, which can be compromised by venous outflow resistance dysfunction. The venous system of the erectile apparatus include the superficial system draining the penile skin to the saphenous veins, the deep dorsal vein of the penis draining the glans penis and corpora cavernosa to the periprostatic venous plexus of Santorini, and the cavernous and urethral veins draining to the internal pudendal veins (Fig. 26-2).[102] The veno-occlusive mechanism works through the relaxation of corporeal (trabecular) smooth muscle, which allows compression of the relaxed muscle against the tunica albuginea, thereby closing the emissary veins. The emissary veins receive blood from the subalbugineal venules that drain the endothelium-lined lacunar spaces, and ultimately open into the deep dorsal vein or circumflex veins. Incomplete occlusion of the emissary veins can be secondary to insufficient relaxation of the corporeal smooth muscle, leading to venous leakage and erectile dysfunction. The tone of the corporeal smooth muscle, either impaired relaxation or heightened contractility, is therefore a major determinant of erectile function.

Since first described by Ebbehoj and Wagner in 1979, the diagnosis of veno-occlusion dysfunction as a cause of impotence has received increasing attention. The failure to retain blood in the corpora during tumescence can be secondary to macroanatomical, pharmacologic, cellular, or biochemical abnormalities that adversely affect the tone of the corporeal smooth muscle.[103] Wespes and Schulman hypothesize that abnormalities in the normal regulation between collagen synthesis and degradation contribute to trabecular structural alterations and fibrosis.[104] An increase in the collagen content or stiffness of erectile tissue as seen in aging can contribute to organic impotence. Excessive connective tissue is proposed to be responsible for a higher likelihood of venous leakage, since a critical ratio of corporeal smooth tissue to total erectile

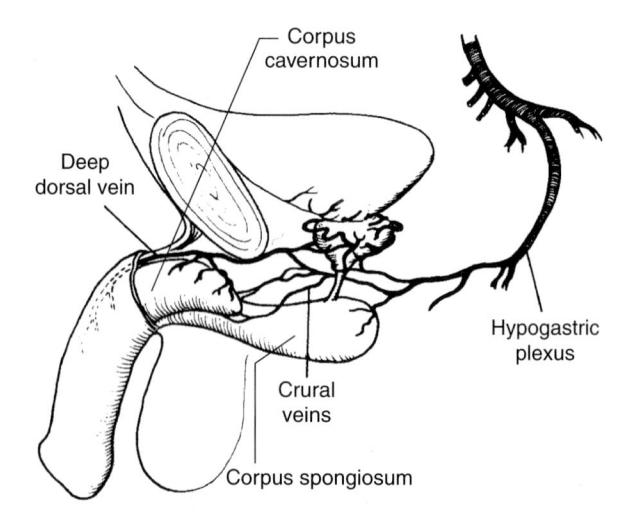

FIGURE 26-2 Longitudinal view of the primary deep veins that drain the corpora. The deep dorsal vein is usually a single vein that is fed by the circumflex and emissary veins and by numerous smaller veins from the corpora. (Adapted from Melman A: Neural and vascular control of erection. In Rosen RC, Leiblum SR [eds]: Erectile Disorder, Assessment and Treatment. New York: The Guilford Press, 1992, pp 55–71.)

tissue may be necessary for successful veno-occlusion.[52,105] Other studies suggest that the primary erectile abnormality lies not at the level of collagen content or distribution but rather at the level of the corporeal smooth muscle cells since patients with venous leakage or arterial lesions have a decreased amount of smooth muscle fibers in the corpora.[52,106] Incomplete closure of the emissary veins secondary to the thickened tunica albuginea can be the cause of venous impotence in Peyronie's disease. Since sufficient corporeal smooth muscle relaxation is necessary for erectile potency, much research has focused on the neurotransmitters or neuromodulators and improved intracavernous pharmacotherapy that can restore muscle tone. However, modulation of corporeal smooth muscle tone is unlikely to benefit patients who have localized or general fibrosis, such as Peyronie's disease and postpriapismic fibrosis, and congenital venous enlargement. Overall, Lue has proposed five types of venous impotence: (1) large veins draining the corpora, which can be congenital; (2) enlarged venous channels caused by tunica albuginea distortion, as occurs with aging; (3) failure of cavernous smooth muscle relaxation secondary to fibrosis or gap junction dysfunction; (4) inadequate neurotransmitters release; and (5) abnormal communication between the cavernosum and the spongiosum or glans.[107]

The diagnosis of venous incompetence is established by first confirming that the patient has erectile dysfunction, perhaps by performing RigiScan analysis and penile plethysmography (pulse volume recording) as baseline studies and to rule out arterial insufficiency. RigiScan monitors nocturnal penile tumescence and rigidity by measuring penile circumference and radial rigidity through loops connected to a microcomputer that is strapped to the patient's thigh. Normal parameters are an increase in circumference at the tip of the penis of 2 cm or more and an increase in circumference at the base of the penis of 3 cm or more. Rigidity, a function of displacement of the loop tightened around the penis, of 55% or more is generally regarded as the normal value.[65] Intracavernous pharmacotesting can also serve as a treatment trial to assess the quality of erectile function. The pharmacologic erection can be induced with an intracavernous injection of Trimix (papaverine; phentolamine; and PGE_1) or PGE_1. Papaverine is a phosphodiesterase inhibitor that prolongs the action of intracellular cyclic adenosine monophosphate (AMP) and causes vascular smooth muscle relaxation. If erection is not achieved, the test should be considered inconclusive and other diagnostic tests should be sought. Penile plethysmography measures volume changes with each pulsatile expansion of the penis, with attention to the amplitude, acceleration phase, and presence of a dicrotic notch after a pneumatic cuff that contains a sensitive transducer is applied at the penile base and inflated to mean systolic pressure. Duplex sonography has been proposed as a minimally invasive initial diagnostic test of vasculogenic impotence and a valuable indirect test in detecting venous leakage.[108,109] The advantages of penile duplex ultrasound are the ability to visualize penile anatomy, measure arterial flow velocity (peak systolic velocity), assess arterial compliance and pharmacologic response, and evaluate venous efflux. Studies suggest that a maximum peak systolic velocity of more than 25 cm/s to 30 cm/s along with a end diastolic velocity of greater than 5 cm/s to 7 cm/s is diagnostic of venous leakage,[110,111] although Kropman and colleagues conclude that end diastolic velocity of patients with negative reactions to intracavernous pharmacologic stimulation is not a good indicator of pathologic venous leakage.[108] Nonetheless, pharmacocavernosometry and cavernosography remain the gold standard in demonstrating venous leakage. Cavernosometry measures changes in intracorporeal pressures at different rates of perfusion with the use of a smooth muscle relaxant and cavernosography is used to visualize penile venous drainage during erection through contrast agent perfusion. During the procedure, one corpus is cannulated using a 19-gauge butterfly needle and attached to a Sarns infusion pump, while a 23-gauge butterfly needle is placed into the ipsilateral side and connected to a strain gauge. Then 30 mg of papaverine is injected and after 10 minutes, warm normal saline is infused in increments of 50 mL/min up to 200 mL/min or until an erection occurs. If rigidity occurs, the saline is infused at a rate sufficient to keep the penis rigid and the pressure greater than 90 mm Hg to 100 mm Hg. If no rigidity results, iothalamate meglumine 43% is injected at 23.6 mL/min with a Harvard infusion pump. The study is done with fluoroscopy, then cavernosography is performed by obtaining anteroposterior and various oblique view radiographs at frequent intervals. The combination of inability to generate penile rigidity with saline infusion after papaverine administration and the demonstration of contrast medium in the glans, corpus spongiosum, or deep crural veins is diagnostic of cavernous leak.[111] Other studies use the maintenance flow rate and induction flow rate as diagnostic criteria in the assessment of cavernosometry. *Induction flow rate* is the lowest rate required to induce an erection; *maintenance flow rate* is the lowest rate needed to maintain an erection, and it is a more reliable and reproducible parameter and of more diagnostic value.[112] When the maintenance flow rate exceeds a certain value or when the intracorporeal pressure simply fails to reach a certain level despite increase in the flow rate, venous leakage can be diagnosed as the cause of impotence. The actual site of venous leakage can be manifested as shunts from the corpora cavernosa to the spongiosum or glans, or as leakage into the dorsal, crural, or pudendal veins (Figs. 26-3 and 26-4).[113] Since veno-occlusive dysfunction can be attributed to the underlying corporeal smooth muscle or alteration in the fibroelastic components of the trabecula, electromyography is also a possible diagnostic screening tool, and biopsies of the erectile tissue can be used to perform microscopic or ultrastructural histologic studies to evaluate abnormalities of the smooth muscles, neurotransmitters, and fibroelastic fibers. Treatment of veno-occlusive dysfunction has been controversial[114] and includes vacuum constriction devices, radiographic insertion of detachable balloons and coils, penile prosthesis placement, and venous ligation. Treatment of venous leakage aims to entrap blood within the corpora cavernosum by preventing venous outflow. Vacuum constriction devices achieve this objective by retaining blood distal to the constriction

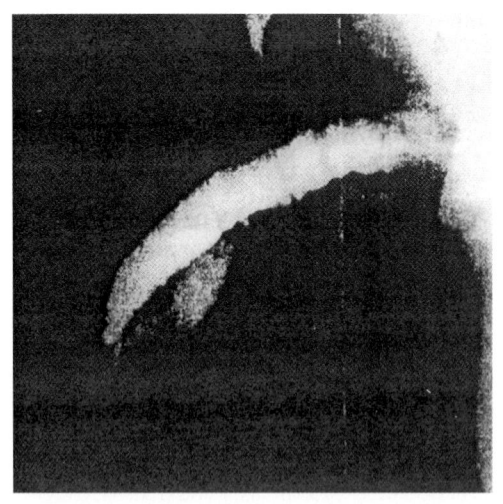

FIGURE 26-3 Standard cavernosogram after injection of papaverine (30 mg). There is no flow of contrast into the venous draining system. (From Melman A: Evaluation and management of erectile dysfunction. Surg Clin North Am 86(5):965, 1988.)

ring and site of venous leakage. Studies have reported that vacuum tumescence devices are superior to intracavernous pharmacotherapy in treating severe veno-occlusive dysfunction.[115] Patients first presenting with venous impotence may be more suited to a trial of such noninvasive devices. Penile prosthesis placement is a treatment option for general erectile dysfunction and is not specific for venous impotence. However, if the prosthesis is removed secondary to complications such as postoperative infection or even gangrene, the patient is rendered impotent due to corporeal destruction and fibrosis depending on how the rods are placed during corporeal dilation. Penile venous outflow can also be restricted through embolization of the veins draining into the pelvis by using occlusive balloons and coils.

Dynamic infusion cavernosometry and cavernosography with vasoactive drugs can yield information on various sites of venous leakage, and Shabsigh and colleagues demonstrate that the majority of patients have more than one leakage site, with the deep dorsal and cavernous veins being the most common combined sites.[116] But despite the ability of many investigators to identify the presence and sites of leakage from the corpora cavernosa, uniform success rates through venous ligation have not been achieved. While some investigators report improvement in approximately 80% of patients, others report a success rate of only 20%, possibly representing poor follow-up or relapse upon longer follow-up.[117] The surgical approach is limited to ligating or cauterizing the dysfunctional veins as diagnosed by cavernosometry and cavernosography. However, a shift to the perineal crural veins occurs if the dorsal venous system is ligated. The low success rate of venous ligation and relapse can be attributed to the failure to diagnose concomitant arterial insufficiency, underlying smooth muscle defect or compliance difficulties, and the development of collateral circulation. Some patients who underwent reoperation developed a significant increase in the number of veins draining from the corpora, and Kerfoot and colleagues demonstrated that a corporospongiosal shunt is the most common site of recurrent leakage.[118] Studies suggest that more extensive ligation, including the cavernous, crural, and deep dorsal venous systems, may yield better success by avoiding relapse from secondary veins[119]; nonetheless, Lue reports that the long-term results of venous ligation for impotence are approximately 60% at best.[120] Defects in the cavernous smooth muscles (not the veins themselves) most likely explain the limited success of venous ligation. To treat veno-occlusive dysfunction better, the physiology of the corporeal smooth muscle must be further delineated and the pathognomonic changes identified.

Angiography/Arteriography in the Evaluation of Impotence

Although numerous diagnostic tests (e.g., RigiScan analysis, penile plethysmography, penile brachial index, duplex sonography, and pulsed Doppler analysis) are available in the evaluation of impotence, angiography remains the gold standard in assessing vasculogenic erectile dysfunction. RigiScan results are most useful when nocturnal tumescence and rigidity is demonstrated but the patient experiences total absence of erection during sexual activity. This finding suggests psychogenic erectile dysfunction, but an abnormal RigiScan finding does not provide substantive information regarding the cause. Other limitations of nocturnal penile tumescence studies include uncertainty about a normal standard for rigidity, false-negatives in the absence of REM sleep, and the absence of nocturnal tumescence in some patients who are suffering from depression, anxiety, or sleep apnea. *Penile brachial index* is the penile systolic pressure divided by the brachial systolic pressure, and may serve as a noninvasive test of vasculogenic impotence. An 8.0- to

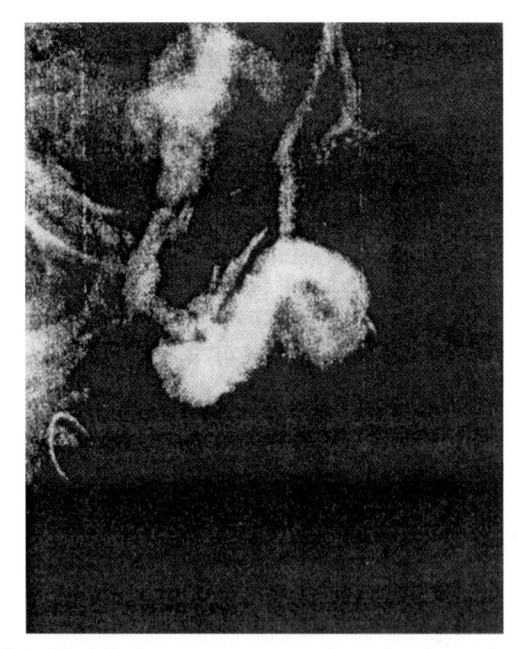

FIGURE 26-4 Drainage of contrast into draining veins after injection of papaverine (30 mg). This is a positive study. (From Melman A: Evaluation and management of erectile dysfunction. Surg Clin North Am 86(5):965, 1988.)

10.0-mHz Doppler ultrasonic probe and an occlusive 2.5 to 3.0 cm wide blood pressure cuff placed around the penile base are usually employed to measure penile artery pressure. However, a normal penile brachial index cannot rule out significant arterial lesions since measurements are usually obtained on a flaccid penis, and arteries with the highest blood flow in this state contribute little to the corpora cavernosa during erection. Furthermore, pressure readings can be altered secondary to inappropriate cuff fit, and sensitivity and specificity of the penile brachial index are never scientifically documented.[121] Although high-resolution duplex ultrasonography with pharmacologic stimulation has recently become a popular noninvasive and low-cost test that provides a functional assessment of the cavernous arteries, the procedure is operator-dependent and can provide inaccurate results if significant variations, such as arterial branching and collaterals, exist in the penile anatomy.[122] Thus, despite the invasive nature of angiography, it remains the preferred test for penile arterial evaluation and is necessary in patients being considered for penile revascularization.[123]

Penile angiography is performed with nonionic contrast medium and intracavernous papaverine injection, providing optimal visualization of the arterial tree. After the common femoral artery is punctured, a catheter is placed in the proximal hypogastric artery, 60 mg of papaverine is injected into the patient's corpus cavernosum in order for him to obtain an erection, and selective hypogastric angiograms are performed. However, nonopacification of the penile vasculature may result from inappropriately dilated arteries. Sympathetic influences may inhibit sinusoidal relaxation and may interfere with the smooth muscle relaxants, and because angiograms are performed under local anesthesia, its invasive nature can create anxiety in the patient and ultimately incomplete cavernous smooth muscle relaxation.[121] Spinal anesthesia can be used since sympathetic blockade causes cavernous tissue relaxation and tumescence. Angiography performed in a patient with isolated or concomitant venous leakage may yield erroneous findings secondary to the escape of smooth muscle relaxants from the corpora. The timing of the papaverine injection is also critical; measurements during the latent and tumescent phases will be higher than those obtained during full erection because the high intracavernous pressure in the erect phase reduces flow and compresses the deep penile arteries.[124] Thus, parameters should be measured during early tumescence, usually 3 to 5 minutes after papaverine administration. Because papaverine cannot be metabolized in the penile tissue, priapism can be a complication after full erection and close monitoring is required to prevent ischemia to the cavernosal tissue. It has also been reported that a penile arteriovenous shunt is induced by vasodilators during angiography.[125] Despite these potential shortcomings, angiography remains the standard by which other tests should be evaluated. Nonetheless, the invasiveness of the procedure should limit its use in select cases of pelvic injury, in young healthy patients suspected of having isolated arterial disease, or when surgical repair such as revascularization is being considered.[124] When an arterial lesion is suspected, the patient's risk factors (e.g., atherosclerosis, hypertension, hyperlipidemia, and diabetes) and potential for a long-lasting cure should be considered and evaluated before proceeding to angiography because continuing atherosclerosis secondary to such risk factors yields disappointing long-term arterial bypass results.[111]

Penile angiography is particularly useful in evaluating variant anatomy. In a selective internal pudendal angiography study in 195 impotent men, Rosen and colleagues found that the internal pudendal artery is variable in its origin, arising independently from the main hypogastric trunk, as a branch of the anterior division of the hypogastric trunk, or from the inferior gluteal artery.[126] An accessory pudendal artery was present in 7% of the patients, arising from the anterior division of the hypogastric, and provided the major arterial flow to the common penile artery. In an autopsy study, Breza and colleagues found an accessory pudendal artery in 7 of 10 cadavers; and it arose from the obturator artery in 4, the inferior vesical artery in 3, and the superior vesical artery in 1 man.[127] Another autopsy study by Martinez-Pineiro and colleagues revealed anatomical variations in the penile arterial distribution in more than half of 12 cadavers, with an accessory pudendal artery providing additional blood supply in more than a quarter of the systems.[128] Thus, an accessory pudendal artery may exist and should be considered if distal penile arteries cannot be visualized, since the accessory artery may be the dominant source of blood supply. Bilateral angiograms should always be obtained because of the prevalence of unilateral or asymmetric disease. It is also imperative to obtain angiograms prior to penile revascularization so that the detailed anatomy and integrity of the vessels can be assessed and anastomosis optimally performed.

CONCLUSION

In conclusion, ED is a very common and complex disorder with multi-factorial etiologies including psychological, hormonal, neurological, and vascular origins. Advancements in diagnostic techniques and technological imaging have made possible more detailed and effective investigations into the causes of ED. This in turn has allowed physicians to counsel patients more effectively in regards to treatment and therapeutic options. However, due to their limitations, side effects, and ever-increasing medical costs, such investigations into the causes of ED may not always be warranted. Additionally, with the recent discovery and understanding of the molecular and physiologic basis of erection, very effective oral agents have been developed, making the treatment of ED easier regardless of its cause.

Recognizing ED as a symptom of a progressive disease and its association with one or more underlying medical disorders is essential. To that end, we are required to use a multi-disciplinary approach to evaluate and to utilize the appropriate diagnostic tools to determine the underlying cause of ED in each individual patient.

REFERENCES

1. NIH Consensus Development Panel on Impotence. NIH Consensus Conference. JAMA 270:83, 1993.
2. Feldman HA, Goldstein I, Hatzichristou DG, et al: Impotence and its medical and psychosocial correlates: Results of the Massachusetts Male Aging Study. J Urol 151:54, 1994.
3. Melman A, Gingell C: The epidemiology and pathophysiology of erectile dysfunction. J Urol 161:5, 1999.
4. Pearman, RO: Treatment of organic impotence with implantation of a penile prosthesis. J Urol 97:716, 1976.
5. Small MP, Carrion H, Gordon JA: Small-Carrion penile prostheses: New implant for management of impotence. Urology 5:479, 1975.
6. Furlow WL: Surgical management of impotence using the inflatable penile prosthesis: Experience with 36 patients. Mayo Clin Proc 51:325, 1976.
7. Virag R: Intracavernous injection of papaverine for erectile failure. Lancet 2:938, 1982.
8. Brindley GS: Cavernosal alpha-blockade: A new technique for investigating and treating erectile impotence. Brit J Psychiat 143:332, 1983.
9. Witherington R: Vacuum constriction device for management of erectile impotence. J Urol 133:190, 1985.
10. Adaikan PG, Kottegoda SR, Ratnam SS: A possible role for prostaglandin E1 in human penile erection. In: Abstract Book, Second World Meeting on Impotence. Prague, Czechoslovakia, 1986.
11. Linet OJ: Long-term safety of intracavernosal alprostadil in men with erectile dysfunction. New Engl J Med 334:873, 1996.
12. Padma-Nathan H, Hellstrom WJG, Kaiser FE, et al: Treatment of men with erectile dysfunction with transurethral alprostadil. N Engl J Med 336:1, 1997.
13. Goldstein I, Lue TF, Padma-Nathan H, et al: Oral sildenafil in the treatment of erectile dysfunction. N Engl J Med 338:1397, 1998.
14. Jardin A, Wagner G, Khoury S, et al (eds): Erectile Dysfunction. Plymouth, England, UK, Health Publications, 2000.
15. LoPiccolo J: Psychological evaluation of erectile dysfunction. In Carson, CC, Kirby RS, Goldstein I (eds): A Textbook of Male Erectile Dysfunction. Oxford, england, Isis Medical Media, 1999.
16. Mohr D, Beutler L: Erectile dysfunction: A review of diagnostic and treatment procedures. Clin Psychol Rev 10:123, 1990.
17. Lee JC, Surridge D, Morales A, Heaton JPW: The prevalence and influence of significant psychiatric abnormalities in men undergoing comprehensive management of organic erectile dysfunction. Int J Impot Res 12(1):47–51, 2000.
18. Rosen R, Riley A, Wagner G, et al: An international index of erectile dysfunction (IIEF): A multidimensional scale for assessment of erectile dysfunction. Urology 49:822, 1997.
19. Davis-Joseph JB, Tiefer L, Melman A: Accuracy of the initial history and physical examination to establish the etiology of erectile dysfunction. Urology 45:498, 1995.
20. Ackerman MD, Carey MP: Psychology's role in the assessment of erectile dysfunction: Historical precedents, current knowledge, and methods. J Consult Clin Psychol 63:862, 1995.
21. Barlow D: Causes of sexual dysfunction: The role of anxiety and cognitive interference. J Consult Clin Psychol 54:140, 1986.
22. Lue TF: Impotence: A patient's goal-directed approach to treatment. World J Urol 8:67, 1990.
23. Ackerman MD, D'Attilio JP, Antoni MH, et al: The predictive significance of patient-reported sexual functioning in RigiScan sleep evaluation. J Urol 146:1559, 1991.
24. Newman H, Melman A: Impotence testing and age. Sex Disab 8:175, 1987.
25. Wolpe J: Psychotherapy by reciprocal inhibition. Stanford, Stanford University Press, 1958.
26. Lazarus A: The treatment of chronic frigidity by systematic desensitization. J Nerv Ment Dis 136:272, 1963.
27. Master W, Johnson V: Human sexual inadequacy. Boston: Little Brown, 1970.
28. Meisler AW, Carey MP: Depressed affect and male sexual arousal. Arch Sex Behav 20:541, 1991.
29. Steers WD: Neural control of penile erection. Semin Urol 8:66, 1980.
30. Hartman U: Psychological subtypes of the erectile dysfunction: Result of statistical analysis and clinical practice. World J Urol 15:56, 1997.
31. Segraves RT, Schoenberg HW: Use of sexual history to differentiate organic from psychogenic impotence. Arch Sex Behav 16:125, 1987.
32. Abel GG, Becker JU, Cunningham-Ather J, et al: Differential diagnosis of impotence in diabetes. Neurol Urodynamics 1:57, 1982.
33. O'Leary MP, Fowler FJ, Lenderking WR, et al: A brief male sexual function inventory for urology. Urology 46:697, 1995.
34. O'Leary MP: Clinical trials in sexual dysfunction. Int J Impot Res 10:S7, 1998.
35. Othmer E, Othmer SC: Evaluation of sexual dysfunction. J Clin Psychiatry 48:191, 1987.
36. Lineadal E, Stefansson JG: The life time prevalence of psychosexual dysfunction among 55 to 57 year olds in Iceland. Soc Psychiatry Psychiatr Epidemiol 2:91, 1993.
37. Kessler D, Lloyd K, Lewis G, Grar DP: Cross-sectional study of symptom attribution and recognition of depression and anxiety in primary care. BMJ 318:436, 1999.
38. Weiler E, Bisserbe JC, Maier W, Lecrubier Y: Prevalence and recognition of anxiety syndromes in five European primary care settings: A report from the WHO study on psychological problems in general health care. Br J Psychiatry 34:18, 1998.
39. Melman A, Levine S, Sachs B, et al: Psychological issues in diagnosis and treatment. In Jardin A, Wagner G, Khoury S, et al (eds): Erectile dysfunction. Plymouth, England, Health Publications, 2000, p 407.
40. Tiefer L, Melman A: Interview of wives: A necessary adjunct in the evaluation of impotence. Sex Disab 6:167, 1983.
41. Ehrensaft MK, Condra M, Morales A, et al: Communication patterns in patients with erectile dysfunction and their partners. Int J Impot Res 6:25, 1994.
42. Spanier BG: Measuring dyadic adjustment: New scales for assessing the quality of marriage and similar dyads. J Marital Fam Ther 24:15, 1976.
43. Hatch JP, DeLaPena AM, Fischer JG: Psychometric differentiation of psychogenic and organic erectile disorders. J Urol 138:781, 1987.
44. Harverson HM: Genital and sphincter behavior of the male infant. J Gen Psychol 56:95, 1940.
45. Kessler WO: Nocturnal penile tumescence. Urol Clin North Am 15:81, 1988.
46. Condra C, Morales A, Surridge DH: The unreliability of nocturnal penile tumescence recording as an outcome measurement in the treatment of organic impotence. J Urol 135:280, 1986.
47. Cilurzo P, Canale D, Turchi P: The RigiScan system in the diagnosis of male sexual impotence. Arch Ital Urol Androl 64:2, 1992.

48. Buvat J, et al: Endocrine screening in 1,022 men with erectile dysfunction: Clinical significance and cost-effective strategy. J Urol 158:1764, 1997.
49. Cunningham GR, et al: Principles and Practice of Endocrinology and Metabolism. Philadelphia, JB Lippincott, 1995.
50. Schiavi RC, White D, Mandeli J, Levine AC: Effect of testosterone administration on sexual behavior and mood in men with erectile dysfunction. Arch Sex Behav 26:231, 1997.
51. Morales A, Johnston B, Heaton JP, Lundie M: Testosterone supplementation for hypogonadal impotence: Assessment of biochemical measures and therapeutic outcomes. J Urol 157:849, 1997.
52. Nehra A, Goldstein I, Pabby A, et al: Mechanisms of venous leakage: A prospective clinicopathological correlation of corporeal function and structure. J Urol 156(4):1320–1329, 1996.
53. Tserotas K, Merino G: Andropause and the aging male. Arch Androl 40:87, 1998.
54. Johnson AR, Larow JP: Is routine endocrine testing of impotence in men necessary? J Urol 147:1542, 1992.
55. Kim YC, Buvat J, Carson CC, et al : Endocrine and metabolic aspects including treatment. In Jardin A, Wagner G, Khoury S, et al (eds): Erectile dysfunction. Plymouth, England, Health Publications, 2000, pp 207–240.
56. Akpunonu B, Mutgi AB, Federman DJ, et al: Routine prolactin measurement is not necessary in the initial evaluation of male impotence. J Gen Int Med 9:336, 1994.
57. Maatnan TJ, Montague DK: Routine endocrine screening in impotence. Urology 27:499, 1986.
58. Report of the Therapeutics and Technology Assessment Subcommittee of the American Academy of Neurology: Assessment: Neurological evaluation of male sexual dysfunction. Neurology 45:2287–2292, 1995.
59. Benson GS, McConnell JA, Lipshultz LI, Corriere JN, et al: Neuromorphology and neuropharmacology of the human penis. J Clin Invest 65:506–513, 1981.
60. Melman A, Henry D: The possible role of catecholamines of the corpora in penile erection. J Urol 121:419–421, 1979.
61. Bors E, Comarr AE: Neurologic disturbances of sexual function with special reference to 529 patients with spinal cord injury. Urol Survey 10:191–222, 1960.
62. Melman A: Neural and vascular control of erection. In Rosen RC, Leiblum SR (eds): Erectile Disorders: Assessment and Treatment. New York, The Guilford Press, 1992, pp 55–71.
63. Padma-Nathan H: Neurologic evaluation of erectile dysfunction. Urol Clin North Am 15:77, 1988.
64. Nisen HO, Larsen A, Lindstrom BL, et al: Cardiovascular reflexes in the neurological evaluation of impotence. Br J Urol 71:199, 1993.
65. Sharlip ID: Evaluation and nonsurgical management of erectile dysfunction. Urol Clin North Am 25:647–659, 1998.
66. Bemelmans BLH, Meuleman EJH, Anten BWM, et al: Penile sensory disorders in erectile dysfunction: Results of a comprehensive neuro-urophysiological diagnostic evaluation in 123 patients. J Urol 146:777, 1991.
67. Herbert J: The role of the dorsal nerves of the penis in the sexual behavior of the male rhesus monkey. Physiol Behav 10:293, 1973.
68. Klausner AP, Batra AK: Pudendal nerve somatosensory evoked potentials in patients with voiding and/or erectile dysfunction: Correlating test results with clinical findings. J Urol 156:1425, 1996.
69. Haldeman S, Bradley WE, Bhatia NN, Johnson BK: Pudendal evoked responses. Arch Neurol 39:280, 1982.
70. Bemelmans BLH, Meuleman EJH, Doesburg WH, et al: Erectile dysfunction in diabetic men: The neurological factor revisited. J Urol 151:884, 1994.
71. Melman A, Henry DP, Felten DL, O'Connor B: Effect of diabetes upon penile sympathetic nerves in impotent patients. South Med J 73:307, 1980.
72. Brock G, Nunes L, Padma-Nathan H, et al: Nitric oxide synthase: A new diagnostic tool for neurogenic impotence. Urology 42:412, 1993.
73. Virag R, Legman M, Zwang G, et al: Utilization de l'érection passive dans l'exploration de l'impuissance d'origine vasculaire. Contracep Fertil Steril 7:707, 1979.
74. Zorgniotti AW, et al: Auto-injection of the corpus cavernosum with a vasoactive drug combination for vasculogenic impotence. J Urol 141:323, 1989.
75. Benett AH, Carpenter AJ, et al: An improved vasoactive drug combination for a pharmacological erection program. J Urol 146:1564, 1991.
76. Virag R, Frydman D, et al: Intercavernous injection of papaverine as a diagnostic and therapeutic method in erectile failure. Angiology 35:79, 1984.
77. Pescatori ES, Hatzichristou DG, et al: A positive intercavernous injection test implies normal veno-occlusive but not necessarily normal arterial function: A hemodynamic study. J Urol 151:1209, 1994.
78. Buvat J, Buvat HM, et al: Is intracavernous injection of papaverine a reliable screening test for vascular impotence? J Urol 135:476, 1986.
79. Meuleman EJH, et al: The value of combined papaverine testing and duplex scanning in men with erectile dysfunction. Int J Impot Res 2:87, 1990.
80. Kim SC, Oh MM: Norepinephrine involvement in response to intracorporeal injection of papaverine in psychogenic impotence. J Urol 147:1530, 1992.
81. Lomas GM, Jarow JP: Risks factors for papaverine-induced priapism. J Urol 147:1280, 1994.
82. Porst H: Diagnostic use and side-effect of vasoactive drugs: A report on over 200 patients with erectile failure. Int J Impot Res 2:222, 1990.
83. Wagner G: Aspects of genital physiology and pathology. Sem Neurol 12:87, 1992.
84. Christ GJ: The penis as a vascular organ: The importance of corporeal smooth muscle tone in the control of erection. Urol Clin North Am 22:727, 1995.
85. Puech-Leao P: Second World Meeting on Impotence. Prague, Czechoslovakia, 1986.
86. Gaskell P: The importance of penile blood pressure in cases if impotence. Can Med Assoc J 105:104, 1971.
87. Abelson D: Diagnostic value of the penile pulse and blood pressure: A Doppler study of impotence in diabetics. J Urol 113:636, 1975.
88. Lane RJ, Appleberg M, Williams W: A comparison of two techniques for the detection of the vasculogenic component of impotence. Surg Gynecol Obstet 155:230, 1982.
89. Metz P, Christensen J, Mathiensen FR, Ostri P: Ultrasonic Doppler pulse wave analysis versus penile blood pressure measurement in the evaluation of arteriogenic impotence. VASA 12:363, 1983.
90. Michal V, Kramar R, Pospichal J: External iliac "steal syndrome." J Cardiovasc Surg 19:355, 1978.
91. Goldstein I: Vasculogenic impotence: Role of the pelvic steal test. J Urol 128:300, 1982.
92. Reiss H: Doppler auscultation difficulties in the cavernous artery of the penis. Urology 26:222, 1985.

93. Schwartz AN: A comparison of penile brachial index and angiography: Evaluation of corpora cavernosa arterial inflow. J Urol 143:510, 1990.
94. Doyle DL, Yu J: Comparison of Doppler and strain-gauge plethysmography to detect vasculogenic impotence. Can J Surg 29:338, 1986.
95. Lue TF, Hricak H, Marich KW, Tanagho EA: Vasculogenic impotence evaluated by high resolution ultrasonography and pulsed Doppler spectrum analysis. Radiology 155:777, 1985.
96. Collins JP, Lewandowski BJ: Experience with intracorporeal injection of papaverine and duplex ultrasound scanning for assessment of arteriogenic impotence. Br J Urol 59:84, 1987.
97. Benson CB, Vickers MA: Sexual impotence caused by vascular disease: Diagnosis with duplex sonography. Am J Roentgenol 153:1149, 1989.
98. Benson CB, Aruny JE, Vickers MA: Correlation of duplex sonography with arteriography in patients with erectile dysfunction. Am J Roentgenol 160:71, 1993.
99. Shabsigh R, et al: Comparison of penile duplex ultrasonography with nocturnal penile tumescence monitoring for the evaluation of erectile impotence. J Urol 143:924, 1990.
100. Quam JP, et al: Duplex and color Doppler sonographic evaluation of vasculogenic impotence. Am J Roentgenol 153:1141, 1989.
101. Lewis RW, King BF: Dynamics of color Doppler sonography in the evaluation of penile erectile disorders. Int J Impot Res 6:A30, 1994.
102. Lue TF, Tanagho EA: Physiology of erection and pharmacological management of impotence. J Urol 137:829, 1987.
103. Ebbehoj J, Wagner G: Insufficient penile erection due to abnormal drainage of cavernous bodies. Urology 13(5):507–510, 1979.
104. Wespes E, Schulman C: Venous impotence: Pathophysiology, diagnosis and treatment. J Urol 149:1238–1245, 1993.
105. Moreland RB, Nehra A: Pathophysiology of erectile dysfunction: A molecular basis. In Carson CC, Kirby R, Goldstein I (eds): Textbook of Erectile Dysfunction. Oxford, Isis Medical Media, 1999, p 105.
106. Lerner SE, Melman A, Christ GJ: A review of erectile dysfunction: New insights and more questions. J Urol 149:1246–1255, 1993.
107. Lue TF: Erectile dysfunction associated with cavernous and neurological disorders. Editorial. J Urol 151:890, 1994.
108. Kropman RF, Schipper J, Oostayen JA, et al: The value of increased end diastolic velocity during penile duplex sonography in relation to pathological venous leakage in erectile dysfunction. J Urol 148:314, 1992.
109. Merckx LA, DeBruyne RMG, Goes E, et al: The value of dynamic color duplex scanning in the diagnosis of venogenic impotence. J Urol 148:318, 1992.
110. Vale JA, Feneley MR, Lees WR, Kirby RS: Venous leak surgery: Long-term follow-up of patients undergoing excision and ligation of the deep dorsal vein of the penis. Br J Urol 76:192–195, 1995.
111. Melman A: Evaluation and management of erectile dysfunction. Surg Clin North Am 68:965–981, 1988.
112. Kromann-Andersen B, Nielsen KK, Nordling J: Cavernosometry: Methodology and reproducibility with and without pharmacological agents in the evaluation of venous impotence. Br J Urol 67:517, 1991.
113. Melman A: The urologic treatment of male sexual dysfunction. In Veith F (ed): Current Critical Problems in Vascular Surgery. St. Louis, Quality Medical Publishing, 1992, p 332.
114. Blackard CE, Borkon WD, Lima JS, Nelson J: Use of vacuum tumescence device for impotence secondary to venous leakage. Urology 41:225, 1993.
115. McMahon CG: Nonsurgical treatment of cavernosal venous leakage. Urology 49:97, 1997.
116. Shabsigh R, Fishman IJ, Toombs BD, Skolkin M: Venous leaks: Anatomical and physiological observations. J Urol 146:1260, 1991.
117. Rossman B, Mieza M, Melman A: Penile vein ligation for corporeal incompetence: An evaluation of short-term and long-term results. J Urol 144:679, 1990.
118. Kerfoot WW, Carson CC, Donaldson JT, Kliewer MA: Investigation of vascular changes following penile vein ligation. J Urol 152(3):884–887, 1994.
119. Kim ED, McVary K: Long-term results with penile vein ligation for venogenic impotence. J Urol 153:655, 1995.
120. Lue TF: Penile venous surgery. Urol Clin North Am 16:607–611, 1989.
121. Rajfer J, Canan V, Dorey FJ, Mehringer CM: Correlation between penile angiography and duplex scanning of cavernous arteries in impotent men. J Urol 143:1128, 1990.
122. Lopez JA, Espeland, Jarow JP: Interpretation and quantification of penile blood flow studies using duplex ultrasonography. J Urol 146:1271, 1991.
123. Wahl S, Rubin M, Bakal C: Radiologic evaluation of penile anatomy in arteriogenic impotence. Int J Impot Res 9:93, 1997.
124. Mueller SC, Lue TF: Evaluation of vasculogenic impotence. Urol Clin North Am 15:65, 1988.
125. DeHoll JD, Angle FA, Steers WD: Vasodilator induced arteriovenous shunt during penile arteriography for impotence. J Urol 158:2240, 1997.
126. Rosen MP, et al: Arteriogenic impotence: Findings in 195 impotent men examined with selective internal pudendal angiography. Radiology 174:1043, 1990.
127. Breza J, Aboseif SR, Orvis BR, et al: Detailed anatomy of penile neurovascular structures: Surgical significance. J Urol 141:437, 1989.
128. Martinez-Pineiro L, Julve E, Martinez-Pineiro JA: Topographical anatomy of the penile arteries. Br J Urol 80:463–467, 1997.

PART IV

CONSERVATIVE TREATMENT: TECHNIQUES

CHAPTER 27

Lifestyle Interventions

DIANE KASCHAK NEWMAN

Behavior modification is a treatment option for persons with urinary incontinence (UI) and overactive bladder (OAB). Changing a person's behavior, environment, or lifestyle can mitigate or reduce symptoms (urine leakage or incontinence, urgency, frequency, and nocturia).[1] Behavior modification involves learning new skills and strategies for preventing urine loss and other symptoms and it has a growing body of clinical research. In the United States, therapies have been combined to include interventions called behavioral treatments.

The 1992 U.S. Agency for Health Care Policy and Research (AHCPR) published the clinical practice guideline called Urinary Incontinence in Adults, which recommends behavioral treatments as first-line interventions.[2] This guideline defines behavioral interventions as a group of therapies used to modify stress, urge, or mixed urinary incontinence by changing the person's bladder habits or by teaching new skills. The interventions include lifestyle changes (e.g., cessation of smoking, weight reduction, elimination of dietary bladder irritants, adequate fluid intake, bowel regulation, moderation of physical activities, and exercises), toileting programs (e.g., habit training and prompted voiding); and bladder retraining; pelvic muscle training or rehabilitation (using methods such as biofeedback, vaginal weights, and pelvic muscle electrical stimulation). A great deal of research on the role of lifestyle changes in relation to UI and OAB relies on clinical information only, however, and does not assess the actual effect of applying or deleting the behavior in question on these conditions. A common complaint of behavioral treatments is that the outcome reflects the combination of treatments rather than the result from a single intervention.

This chapter outlines the current research as well as clinical practice on the use of behavioral therapies, specifically lifestyle and self-care practices. Self-care practices such as adequate fluid management, elimination of dietary irritants, cessation of smoking, bowel regulation, and moderation of exercise and weight reduction are ways to prevent or reduce UI, but they are not actively promoted (Box 27-1). Research shows that it is possible to prevent incontinence in community dwelling elderly women.[3] If clients learn to alter certain habits through self-care practices, further treatments may not be necessary. This chapter targets the behaviors that, if altered, can have positive effects on bladder function.

LIFESTYLE FACTORS

Smoking

Increased intra-abdominal pressure may promote the development of UI and urinary urgency, particularly in women. This increased pressure exists with conditions that include pulmonary diseases such as asthma, emphysema, and chronic coughing such as seen in smokers. Smoking in particular increases the risk of developing all forms of UI, and stress UI in particular; the level of risk depends on the number of cigarettes smoked. There may be several causes of the increased risk of stress UI in smokers. Compared with nonsmokers, smokers have stronger, more frequent and more violent coughing, which may lead to earlier development of damage to the urethral sphincteric mechanism and vaginal supports.[4] Violent and frequent prolonged coughing can increase downward pressure on the pelvic floor, causing repeated stretch injury to the pudendal and pelvic nerves. Smoking is also the most important etiological factor in bladder cancer.[5] In addition, elements of tobacco products may have antiestrogenic hormonal effects, which may influence collagen synthesis. Nicotine contributes to large phasic bladder contractions, as shown in animal studies through the activation of purinergic receptors; nicotine seems to affect the human bladder similarly.[6,7] There may also be an association between nicotine and increased detrusor contractions.

Bump[8] showed that women who previously smoked had a 2.2-fold increase and those who currently smoked have a 2.5-fold increase in stress UI. The risk of UI in women caused by cigarette smoking was estimated to be 28%. This study indicates that the risk of genuine stress UI is positively correlated with both the current intensity of cigarette consumption and the degree of lifetime exposure to cigarette smoking. The increased prevalence of stress incontinence in smokers is independent of other risk factors such as older age, parity, obesity, and hypoestrogenism. There is research indicating that smoking

269

> **BOX 27-1** | **Patient Education Tool: Controlling Incontinence and Overactive Bladder Symptoms**
>
> **Adequate Fluid Intake.** Individuals with urinary symptoms often limit their intake of fluids so that they will not have to urinate often. Individuals with overactive bladder who have a high fluid intake (>2400 cc/day) may show a reduction in incontinent episodes and voiding frequency by lowering their fluid intake. Incontinent persons with low fluid intakes (<1500 cc/day) may benefit from increasing their fluid intake. Reducing fluid intake after 6 P.M. (or 2 or 3 hours before bedtime) and concentrating fluid intake during morning and afternoon hours may decrease nighttime incontinence.
>
> **Smoking Cessation.** Nicotine is irritating to the detrusor muscle, causing bladder contractions and urgency. A smoker's repeated and chronic coughing may cause urinary leakage. Smoking cessation may help to decrease urine leakage.
>
> **Dietary Modification.** Individuals with incontinence and overactive bladder may benefit from caffeine reduction. Significant rise in detrusor pressure with bladder filling has been demonstrated with caffeine. This is especially true for persons who drink large amounts of coffee or tea and complain of urinary frequency with urge incontinence. Caffeine is found in milk chocolate, soft drinks, over-the-counter medications, and is used as a flavoring agent in many baked goods and processed foods, although it may not be listed on the product label. The US Food and Drug Administration has listed that more than 1000 drugs that are bought off the shelf in US pharmacies and drug stores contain caffeine. Tapering caffeine intake slowly may prevent migraine headaches ("withdrawal"). The effect of other foods and beverages on the bladder is not understood but elimination of one or all of the following items may improve bladder control.
>
> - Alcoholic beverages
> - Citrus juices and fruits
> - Beer and wine
> - Highly spiced foods
> - Carbonated beverages
> - Sugar and honey
> - Milk and milk products
> - Corn syrup
> - Soft drinks with caffeine, tea, coffee, even decaffeinated tea and coffee
> - Artificial sweetener (aspartame)
>
> It is recommended that eliminating these foods one by one may reduce UI in some individuals and identify the foods that contribute more to the symptoms.
>
> **Maintaining Optimal Weight.** Weight-reduction programs for moderately and morbidly obese women may reduce urinary symptoms such as urgency and frequency of incontinence because of reduced pressure on the bladder.
>
> **Bowel Regularity.** Constipation and difficulty with defecation (straining during bowel movements) causes increased pressure on the bladder, leading to overactive bladder. Individuals should keep regularity through increased intake of fiber and fluids and regular exercise. A successful way to increase fiber is by using a "special bran recipe." Mix together 1 cup applesauce, 1 cup coarse unprocessed wheat bran, and 3/4 cup prune juice. Refrigerate mixture and take 2 tablespoons of the mixture every day. Take the mixture in the evening for a morning bowel movement. Increase the bran mixture by 2 tablespoons each week until bowel movements are regular. Always drink one large glass of water with the mixture.
>
> Adapted from Newman, DK: Managing and Treating Urinary Incontinence, Baltimore, Health Professions Press, 2002, pp 105–110. Copyright Clearance Center.

can cause symptoms of urge incontinence and urgency and frequency. One case-control study of 80 incontinent and 80 continent women established a strong statistical relationship between cigarette smoking and urinary incontinence.[9] This study indicates that incontinent smokers are more often prone to urge UI, whereas nonsmoking incontinent women experienced more stress UI. Nuotio and colleagues[10] showed a correlation between smoking and urinary urgency in a population-based survey of 1059 women and men aged 60 to 89 years. A large cross-sectional study evaluated multiple risk factors, including smoking, for incontinence in pregnant women.[11] Smokers were more likely to report incontinence than nonsmokers. In a survey of 2128 middle aged and elderly men who smoked or formerly smoked, Koskimaki and colleagues showed an increased risk of lower urinary tract symptoms (LUTS).[12] Symptoms included incomplete bladder empting and hesitancy, daily frequency, nocturia, urgency, and urge incontinence. The effects of smoking on lower urinary tract symptoms are probably mediated through the development of benign prostatic hypertrophy (BPH). Use of tobacco products by men may increase accumulation of androgens in the prostate gland. The study also found that the risk of lower urinary tract symptoms in men decreased after cessation of smoking, disappearing after 40 years.

No data have been reported about whether smoking cessation by women resolves incontinence. Bump[8] did not demonstrate a decreased risk of incontinence if the woman stopped smoking. So once this anatomical and neuromuscular damage occurs, it is probably irreversible. Nevertheless, strategies to discourage women from smoking should be implemented. At the very least, women should be educated on the relationship between smoking, UI, and OAB.

Obesity

Obesity is an independent risk factor for the development of stress and mixed UI in women.[13-17] Excessive body weight, specifically measured by sagittal abdominal diameter, affects bladder pressure. The stress UI with obesity may be secondary to increases in intra-abdominal pressure on the bladder and greater urethral mobility. Also, obesity may impair blood flow or nerve innervation to the bladder. Body mass index (BMI) is considered an objective and accurate method of assessing individual weight status. It is calculated by dividing weight in kilograms by the square height in meters. A woman with a BMI of ≤ 29 is considered at normal or low weight; a woman with a BMI of ≥ 30 is obese.

Elia, Dye, and Scariati[13] reported on 540 women who responded to a questionnaire and whose BMI status was obtained. The association between BMI and UI was statistically significant. Mommsen and Foldspang[16] reported on 2589 women in Denmark who responded to a mailed questionnaire. Body mass index was found to correlate with urge UI in women who reported having one or more episodes of cystitis. Poor personal hygiene in obese women may lead to an infectious process. Mommsen also found a relationship between stress UI and an increased BMI.[16] Dwyer, Lee, and Hay[18] found that women with genuine stress UI or with detrusor instability have a higher mean BMI than the general population of the same age. Roe and Doll[19] reported on 6139 (53% response rate) respondents to a postal survey on incontinence status. Significantly more respondents with UI had a higher mean BMI when compared with continent respondents. This association was more prevalent in obese women than men. Brown and colleagues[20] studied 2763 women who completed questionnaires about prevalence and type of incontinence as part of a randomized trial of hormone therapy. A higher BMI and higher waist-to-hip ratio were found to be predictors of stress UI and also of mixed UI when the major component was stress. This study found that the prevalence of at least weekly stress UI increased by 10% per 5 units BMI. Hojberg and colleagues[11] found that a BMI >30 and smoking were possible risk factors for pregnant women.

Weight loss is an acceptable treatment for morbidly obese women. Research has shown that stress UI symptoms decrease in morbidly obese women who undergo extreme weight loss after gastric bypass surgery.[21,22] At this time, there is little information on whether weight loss resolves incontinence in women who are moderately obese. Subak and colleagues[23] reported on moderately obese women who were on a weight loss program, who were experiencing four or more UI episodes per week and who had BMIs between 25 and 45. Among women achieving a weight loss of >5%, six out of six had a >50% reduction in UI frequency, compared with one in four women with <5% weight loss. There was a 60% decrease in use of absorbent pads following weight loss. No change was observed in voiding frequency or nocturia. This study showed improvement in UI with as little as 5% loss from baseline weight.

Obese women should lose weight prior to surgery to improve the technical ease, increase the durability, and decrease the failure rate of the surgery.[18] Maintaining normal weight through adulthood may be an important factor in the prevention of UI. Given the high prevalence of both incontinence and obesity in women, weight reduction should be recommended as part of the conservative management and behavior modification for obese women suffering from UI. This may be a reasonable and achievable goal for many women.

Dietary Habits

Persons can decrease urine leakage, urgency, and frequency through modification of certain dietary habits, which include fluid management, intake restriction of bladder irritants, and bowel regulation.

Fluid Management

Individuals with UI and OAB symptoms may subscribe to either a restrictive or excessive fluid intake behavior. It is important to teach the client that adequate fluid intake is necessary to eliminate irritants from the bladder and prevent UI. Underhydration may play a role in the development of urinary tract infections (UTIs), and it decreases the functional capacity of the bladder.[24] Surveys of community-residing elders report self-care practices that include the self-imposed restrictions of fluid intake because they fear UI, urinary urgency, and urinary frequency.[25-27] Adequate fluid intake is very important for older adults who already have a decrease in their total body weight and are at increased risk for dehydration. Institutionalized clients are chronically dehydrated since most require assistance to eat and drink. Although drinking less liquid does result in less urine in the bladder, the smaller amount of urine may be more highly concentrated and irritate the bladder mucosa. Highly concentrated (dark yellow, strong smelling) urine may cause urgency and frequency. It can also encourage bacteria to grow, which can lead to an infection. In addition, inadequate fluid intake is a risk factor for constipation, another problem common in older adults.

However the research showing the relationship of quantity of fluid intake to urinary symptoms is inconclusive. In a geriatric population, there appears to be a strong relationship between evening fluid intake, nocturia, and nocturnal voided volume.[28] Nygaard and Linder[29] surveyed teachers and questioned their voiding habits at work, allotted breaks, and bladder complaints including UTIs and incontinence. Teachers who drank less while working to decrease their voiding frequency had a twofold higher risk of UTI than those who did not report self-imposed fluid restriction. There was no association between UTI and either voiding infrequently at work or the mean number of voids at work. Fitzgerald and colleagues[30] surveyed women who worked for a large academic center. Of the 1113 women surveyed 21% ($N = 232$) reported UI at least monthly. Incontinent women were significantly older and had a higher BMI than continent women. The strategies women in this study used to avoid urinary symptoms was limiting fluids and avoiding caffeinated beverages. Wyman and colleagues[31] reported a positive relationship between fluid intake and severity of UI in women older than 55 years with stress UI. However, this study showed no correlation in women with detrusor instability. In a randomized trial,[24] 32 women were assigned to one of three groups: increase fluid intake by 500 cc over baseline, decrease by same amount, or maintain baseline level. The authors reported that 20 women who had fewer incontinent episodes at the end of the trial attributed this to drinking more fluids. Women in this study noted that it was easier to limit daily intake than to increase it.

The recommended daily fluid intake is 1500 mL, but many feel that a more appropriate intake is 1800 mL to 2400 mL per day. To be adequately hydrated, older clients must consume at least 1500 mL to 2000 mL per day of liquids.[32] The fluid intake formula is based on body weight in kilograms (2.2 pounds = 1 kilogram) and implies a positive health status (e.g., no fluid restrictions), modest physical activity, and stable environment temperature (e.g., hot versus cold temperature environments).[33] There are three steps in calculations:

1. For the first 10 kg of body weight, the fluid requirement is 100 mL/kg, or 1000 mL.
2. For the second 10 kg, the fluid requirement is 50 mL/kg, or 500 mL.
3. For weight over 20 kg, the fluid requirement is 20 mL/kg, or 200 mL.

Many clients, especially women who are dieting, may drink excessive fluids up to a total of 4000 mL/day. If they are experiencing UI, they should decrease their fluid intake.

The timing of fluid may be important in persons who have problems with nocturia. Aging causes an increase in nocturia, defined as the number of voids recorded from the time the individual goes to bed with the intention of going to sleep to the time the individual wakes with the intention of rising. Nocturia is an average of more than 2 nocturnal voids per night. Nocturia is caused by excessive passage of large volumes of urine (polyuria). Aging is associated with changes in the renal and hormonal systems involved in the conservation of water and sodium. As a consequence there is increased nocturnal urine production. Chronic medical conditions such as congestive heart failure, venous stasis with peripheral edema, hypoglycemia and excess urine output, and obstructive sleep apnea, as well as diuretics and evening/nighttime fluid consumption are causes of nocturnal poyluria. During the night, there is a lower level of physical activity and body fluid moves more quickly from one part of the body to another, causing an increase in the amount of urine in the bladder. To decrease nocturia precipitated by drinking fluids primarily in the evening or with dinner, the person should be instructed to reduce fluid intake after 6 P.M. and shift intake toward the morning and afternoon (Box 27-2).

Influence of Bladder Irritants

The type of fluid or food is important. Caffeine is a xanthine derivative, a natural diuretic and bladder irritant. It acts similarly to thiazide diuretics. Caffeine is a central nervous system stimulant that reaches peak blood concentrations within 30 to 60 minutes after ingestion and has an average half-life of 4 to 6 hours. Caffeine can cause a significant rise in detrusor pressure leading to urinary urgency and frequency following caffeine ingestion.[34] Caffeine has an excitatory effect on the detrusor muscles.[35]

More than 80% of the US adult population consumes caffeine in the form of coffee, tea, or soft drinks daily. In the United States, average caffeine consumption is estimated at approximately 200 mg daily, which is equivalent to two 6-oz cups of brewed coffee.[36] Caffeine occurs naturally in coffee beans, tealeaves, and cocoa beans. The concentration of caffeine in products such as coffee depends on the preparation (e.g., instant contains 65 mg to 110 mg and brewed contains 80 mg to 135 mg). Caffeine is found in liquids such as sodas (e.g., Mountain Dew, Pepsi, Coca-cola) and foods and candy that contain milk chocolate (e.g., 7 mg in 10 ounces of milk chocolate). Carbonated drinks that are identified as "caffeinated colas" have been associated with an increased risk of stress urinary incontinence.[37] Additionally, the U.S. Food and Drug Administration (FDA) has listed more than 1000 over-the-counter drugs that contain caffeine, which is usually listed on the label of the products. Some over-the-counter drugs (e.g., Excedrin, Anacin) and prescription medications (e.g., Darvon compound, Fiorinal) contain caffeine.[38] Nutritional supplements, puddings, and cakes that contain cocoa are favorite foods and daily staples in institutionalized settings. However, cocoa is also a source of caffeine.

Alcohol also has a diuretic effect. Alcohol causes a release of antidiuretic hormone from the posterior pituitary.[34] Anecdotal evidence suggests that eliminating dietary factors such as artificial sweeteners (aspartame) and certain foods (e.g., highly spiced foods, citrus juices, and tomato-based products) may promote continence.[39]

BOX 27-2 Patient Education Tool: Preventing Nighttime Voiding and Incontinence

As you get older, your kidneys make more urine at night when you are asleep. Since your bladder has more urine, you need to get up more often to void.

WHAT CAN I DO TO CUT DOWN ON THE AMOUNT OF URINE AT NIGHT?
Limit your fluids in the evening. Stopping evening fluids with the completion of the evening meal, commonly at 6 P.M. can help. But remember to maintain adequate non-caffeinated fluid intake (6 to 7 8-ounce glasses) during the day.

WHAT DRINKS OR FOODS MAY BE IRRITATING?
Beverages that contain caffeine and alcohol are more irritating. So eliminate all caffeinated and alcoholic beverages in the afternoon and especially in the evening. Do not drink these beverages after 6 P.M. Remember that even decaffeinated drinks (tea, coffee, soda) have some caffeine and should be avoided. Chocolate has caffeine; chocolate ice cream, pudding, or cake as an evening snack may worsen your nighttime problem.

WHAT ELSE CAN I DO?
As you age, your body starts to retain water (called edema) in the lower legs and ankles. To decrease this swelling, lie down on your left side for $1^1/_2$ to 2 hours in the late afternoon or early evening. When watching TV or after lunch, prop your legs on a stool or chair. Then proceed with regular evening activities for a few hours before bedtime. This will cause you to excrete some of the excess water before retiring so that it is not such a load on your bladder throughout the night.

Try not to use a bedpan or urinal unless you are afraid of falling on the way to the bathroom. Get out of bed to urinate to help your bladder empty more fully.

Adapted from Newman, DK: Managing and Treating Urinary Incontinence, Baltimore, Health Professions Press, 2002. Copyright Clearance Center.

In a study by Tomlinson and colleague, UI decreased (63% decrease in urine leakage) when caffeine consumption was reduced from 900 mL to 480 mL.[40] Arya and colleagues[41] found that women ($N = 20$) with higher caffeine intake (361 mg to 607 mg per day) had a 2.4-fold increased risk for detrusor instability than women ($N = 10$) with a low caffeine intake (110 mg to 278 mg per day). There was also a correlation between current smoking and caffeine intake. Bryant, Dowell, and Fairbrother[42] conducted a prospective randomized trial of persons with symptoms of urgency, frequency, and urge UI who routinely ingested 100 mg or more of caffeine per day. Both groups were taught bladder training but the intervention group was also instructed to reduce caffeine intake to <100 mg/day. Significant improvement in urgency (61% decrease), in voiding frequency (35% decrease), and urine leakage (55% decrease) was seen in the treatment group when compared to the baseline. Tomlinson[40] showed that 34 women with symptoms of UI (mostly mixed) who decreased caffeine intake (from 900 mg/day to 480 mg/day) also decreased episodes of daily urine loss also (from 2.33 to 1.0 per day).

Even though current research is not conclusive, clients with UI and OAB should be assessed for amount of caffeine intake. They should be advised about the possible adverse effects caffeine may have on the detrusor muscle and the possible benefits of reduction of caffeine intake.[43] The client should be instructed to switch to caffeine-free beverages and foods or eliminate them and see if urinary urgency and frequency decrease. If they continue to consume caffeine, clients with incontinence and OAB should take no more than 100 mg/day to decrease urgency and frequency. The client should be taught to restrict caffeine through behavior modification. Instructions should include encouraging the client to gradually replace caffeinated beverages or foods with noncaffeinated ones. Since caffeine crosses the blood-brain barrier and can reduce blood flow to the brain, a sudden withdrawal from caffeine can cause headaches, nervousness, nausea, and muscular tension.

Because fluid intake and type of liquid consumed can be contributing factors to incontinence and OAB symptoms, request that the client keep a Bladder Record or Voiding Diary, noting type and amount of daily intake (Fig. 27-1). This diary can be used to measure effectiveness of interventions.

Bowel Regularity

Because chronic constipation and straining can contribute to stress UI and pelvic organ prolapse, dietary changes should assist persons who have constipation and strain at stool. Constipation is defined as having fewer than 3 stools per week. It is estimated that at least 17% of the adult population is constipated at some point in their lives. Usually a client's definition of constipation is considerably broader, however, and includes straining at stool, painful defecation, dry hard stools, small stools, and incomplete or infrequent stool evacuation. Studies of severely constipated women who have strained at stool over a prolonged period have demonstrated changes in pelvic floor neurological function.[44] Lubowski and colleagues[45] report that denervation of the external anal sphincter and pelvic floor muscles may occur in association with a history of excessive straining on defecation. Many believe that if these are lifetime habits, they may have a cumulative effect on pelvic floor and bladder function.

There is very little research that assesses the effect of regulating bowel function on incontinence and OAB. Spence-Jones and colleagues[46] found that straining excessively at stool was significantly more common in women with stress UI and in women with prolapse than in women who experienced neither condition. Moller, Lose, and Jorgensen[47] reported an almost uniform positive association between straining at stool and constipation and lower urinary tract symptoms in women ($N = 487$) 40 to 60 years of age. Moller felt that chronic constipation and repeated straining efforts induced progressive neuropathy in the pelvic floor.

Because research suggests that chronic constipation and straining may be risk factors for the development of incontinence and OAB, self-care practices that promote bowel regularity should be an integral part of any treatment program. Treatment of elderly patients can significantly improve lower urinary tract symptoms, which include urgency and frequency.[48] Suggestions to reduce constipation include the addition of fiber to the diet, increased fluid intake, regular exercise, external stimulation, and establishment of a routine defecation schedule. Improved bowel function can also be achieved by determining a schedule for bowel evacuation so that the client can take advantage of the "call to stool," or the urge to defecate. The schedule should be determined by the client's bowel elimination pattern and previous time pattern for defecation. The client should be advised never to ignore the feeling that the bowel needs to be emptied. Also ensure that the client has adequate time to toilet. Normal defecation requires relaxation of the pelvic floor muscle, particularly of the anal sphincter, adequate rectal tone, and sensation of rectal filling. Normal sensation of rectal filling is key to providing motivation and a learned response, and it underlines the cognitive component of normal defecatory function.[39] These cognitive and behavioral components suggest that in some cases constipation is a learned or conditioned response. The bowel is relatively quiet at night. Therefore, the optimal time to schedule defecation is in the morning and after a meal, preferably breakfast. The gastrocolic reflex, the mass propulsion of material through the large intestine after a meal is strongest on an empty stomach. The peristalsis created by this reflex propels feces to the descending colon and rectum. Sufficient time should be set aside to allow undisturbed visits to the bathroom. The urge to have a bowel movement should not be ignored.

Combining fluid management, elimination of bladder irritants, and regulation of bowels may yield the maximum benefit. Dougherty and colleagues[49] conducted a randomized, controlled trial that incorporated reduction of caffeine consumption, adjusting the amount and timing of intake of fluids, and making dietary changes to promote bowel regularity, which were termed "self-monitoring activities." Women in the intervention group also received bladder training and biofeedback-assisted pelvic muscle exercises. Two hundred eighteen women

Name_____   Date_____

INSTRUCTIONS

- Column 1- Place a check next to the time you urinated in the toilet.
- Column 2- Place a check next to the time you have an accident, large or small.
- Column 3- Place a check next to the time you change your WET PADS.
- Column 4- Note a reason why you may have had an accident, like sneezing, coughing, lifting something heavy, "couldn't make it to the bathroom," etc.
- Column 5- Make a check for every 8 oz or 1 glass of fluid you drink and indicate if it contains caffeine.

TIME INTERVAL	Column 1 URINATED IN TOILET	Column 2 HAD AN ACCIDENT	Column 3 CHANGED WET PAD	Column 4 REASON FOR ACCIDENT	Column 5 THE FLUID I DRANK
6-8 AM					
8-10 AM					
10-12 NOON					
12-2 PM					
2-4 PM					
4-6 PM					
6-8 PM					
8-10 PM					
10-12 MID					
OVERNIGHT					

COMMENTS:_____

FIGURE 27-1 Bladder record.

with stress, urge, or mixed UI were randomized and 178 completed one or more follow-ups. At 2 years the intervention group's UI severity decreased by 61%. Self-monitoring and bladder training accounted for most of the improvement.

Physical and Occupational Stressors

Another lifestyle behavior associated with triggering stress UI in young, healthy women is physical exertion. Urinary incontinence is commonly seen among elite athletes,[50] women in the military, and some dancers particularly during training.[51] High-impact physical activities increase the downward force on the pelvic floor muscles and overwhelm an otherwise healthy continence mechanism. Sports such as gymnastics and basketball create a sudden increase in intra-abdominal pressure, causing stress UI. Repeated mechanical overload from repetitive physical activities can adversely affect pelvic floor tissue. Also, UI may be secondary to pelvic floor muscle fatigue. Defects or injury of supporting pelvic structure can lead to pelvic organ. It is disturbing that when UI occurs during exercise, women will either stop the activity or change the type of exercise in which they engage.

Nygaard[52] examined 144 elite nulliparous athletes (mean age 19.9 years). A total of 40 athletes (28%) reported urine loss while participating in their sport, two thirds describing it as frequent. Overall, an estimated one third of women experience at least one episode of urine loss during participation in their sport. Activities most likely to provoke incontinence included jumping, (e.g., basketball), running, and making impact on the floor as gymnasts do with dismounting or after flips. Urine loss appeared not to be severe and quantity was small; only one athlete reported wearing an absorbent perineal pad. Thyssen and colleagues[51] questioned elite athletes ($N = 291$, average age 22.8 years) in eight sports including professional ballet. A total of 51.9% had urine loss while participating in their sport or in daily life situations. The activities most likely to produce urine loss were jumping and running. Reported self-care measures included use of an absorbent pad or panty shield to contain the urine and restriction of fluid intake.

There is little information on whether strenuous exercise or activity causes incontinence later in life. In a study of women who had been Olympians approximately 25 years earlier, those who competed in gymnastics or track and field were not more likely to report daily or weekly incontinence than Olympians who had competed in swimming.[53]

There is increasing information about the relationship between occupational (workplace) stressors and UI, as well as pelvic organ prolaspe.[54] Women in blue-collar jobs (e.g., factory, sales) usually have limited rest breaks and access to a bathroom. Many of these jobs require heavy lifting and bending, walking, or standing, which places the women at greater risk for UI, urgency, and frequency.

Jorgensen, Heiin, and Gyntelberg[55] reported that Danish nursing assistants, who are exposed to frequent heavy lifting, were 1.6-fold more likely to undergo surgery for pelvic organ prolapse or UI than women in the general population. Fitzgerald and colleagues[30] surveyed women who worked for a large academic center. Of the 1113 women surveyed, 21% ($N = 232$) reported UI at least monthly. Incontinent women were significantly older and had a higher BMI than continent women. Women in this study used self-care practices such as using absorbent products, limiting fluids, and so on.

Several studies have reported on the relationship between UI and military training and activities. Women in the military have physically demanding roles and the presence of UI can interfere with lifestyle as well as ability to perform assigned duties. Davis and Goodman[56] noted that in U.S. Airborne Infantry School, 6 weeks of training could include daily 4-mile runs, pull-ups, sit-ups, push-ups, and high-impact aerobics with significant jumping. In this group, 9 nulliparous trainees developed stress incontinence and pelvic floor defects, including cystourethroceles, during airborne training. Sherman, Davis, and Wong[57] found that 27% ($N = 450$) of US female army soldiers (average age 28.5 years) experienced problematic UI, with 19.9% saying they leaked significantly during training tests. However, only 5.3% felt that urine leakage had a significant impact on their regular duties. This may due to the fact that 30.7% women stated that they took precautions such as voiding prior to training, wearing "extra-thick" pads, and limiting fluid intake. A very disturbing finding in this study was that 13.3% of women restricted fluid intake while participating in strenuous field training. A third study[58] looked at women flying in high-performance combat aircraft. Aircrews who fly in high-gravity aircraft perform an M-1 maneuver, which is a modified Valsalva with an isometric contraction of the lower extremities. This movement may place women pilots at risk for urine loss due to increased intra-abdominal pressure and increased gravity load. Results of a questionnaire of aircrew ($N = 274$) indicated that 26.3% had experienced urine loss at some time. However, pilots did not have higher UI rates than women in other positions (e.g., navigators and weapon system operators). In this study, as in others, crew positions, vaginal delivery, and age were found to be significant risk factors.

CONCLUSION

Although research showing the effectiveness of changes in certain lifestyle behaviors on urinary incontinence (stress, urge, or mixed), urgency, and frequency may not be conclusive, many health care providers frequently recommend alterations in lifestyle and behavior. Individuals who have sufficient knowledge about these lifestyle measures can incorporate them readily into their daily routines if they are cognitively and functionally capable and motivated. Staff in institutionalized health care settings can incorporate these measures in routine medical and nursing care. Research on lifestyle behaviors has been increasing in the last two decades. The resultant knowledge has shaped public health agendas (e.g., use of tobacco warnings in the United States), developed preventive services, and evaluated the efficacy of medical practice and health services. Lifestyle changes and behavior modification are integral to clinical management of UI and OAB. Health care providers need to understand the efficacy, as well as the limitations, of these interventions.

REFERENCES

1. Nygaard I, Bryant C, Dowell C, Wilson PD: Lifestyle interventions for the treatment of urinary incontinence in adults. Cochrane Incontinence Group, Cochrane Database of Systematic Reviews, No. 2, 2002.
2. Fantl JA, Newman DK, Colling J, et al: Urinary Incontinence in Adults: Acute and Chronic Management Clinical Practice Guideline, No 2, Update, Rockville, MD: US Department of Health and Human Services. Public Health Service, Agency for Health Care Policy and Research, AHCPR Publication No. 96-0682, 1986.
3. Association of Women's Health, Obstetric and Neonatal Nurses: Evidence-based clinical practice guideline, Continence for Women, Washington, DC, 2000.
4. Bump RC, McClish DM: Cigarette smoking and pure genuine stress incontinence of urine. A comparison of risk factors and determinants between smokers and nonsmokers. Am J Obstet Gynecol 170(2):579–582, 1994.
5. Cohen SM, Johansson SL: Epidemiology and etiology of bladder cancer. Urol Clin North Am 19:421–428, 1992.
6. Koley B, Koley J, Saha JK: The effects of nicotine on spontaneous contractions of cat urinary bladder in situ. Br J Pharmacol 83:347–355, 1984.
7. Ruggieri MR, Whitmore KE, Levine RM: Bladder purinergic receptors. J Urol 144:176–181, 1990.
8. Bump RC, McClish DM: Cigarette smoking and urinary incontinence. Am J Obstet Gynecol 167(5):1214–1218, 1992.
9. Tampakoudis P, Tantanassis T, Grimbizis G, et al: Cigarette smoking and urinary incontinence in women—a new calculative method of estimating the exposure to smoke. Eur J Obstet Gyneco Reprod Biol 63:17–30, 1995.
10. Nuotio M, Jylha M, Koivisto AM, Tammela TLJ: Association of smoking with urgency in older people. Eur Urol 40:206–212, 2001.
11. Hojberg K-E, Salvig JD, Winslow NA, et al: Urinary incontinence: Prevalence and risk factors at 16 weeks of gestation. Br J Obstet Gynaecol, 106:842–850, 1999.
12. Koskimaki J, Hakama M, Huhtala H, Tammela TLJ: Association of smoking with lower urinary tract symptoms. J Urol 159:1580–1582, 1998.
13. Elia G, Dye TD, Scariati PD: Body mass index and urinary symptoms in women. Int Urogynecol J 12:366–369, 2001.

14. Brown JS, Seeley DG, Fong J, et al: Urinary incontinence in older women: Who is at risk? Obstet Gynecol 87:715–721, 1996.
15. Burgio KL, Matthews KA, Engel BT: Prevalence, incidence and correlates of urinary incontinence in healthy, middle-aged women. J Urol 146:1255–1259, 1991.
16. Mommsen S, Foldspang A: Body mass index and adult female urinary incontinence. World J Urol 19:319–322, 1994.
17. Diokno AC, Brock BM, Herzog AR, Bromberg J: Medical correlates of urinary incontinence in the elderly. Urology 36:129–138, 1990.
18. Dwyer PL, Lee ETC, Hay DM: Obesity and urinary incontinence in women. Br J Obstet Gynecol 95:91–96, 1988.
19. Roe B, Doll H: Lifestyle factors and continence status: Comparison of self-report data from a postal survey in England. J WOCN 26(6):312–319, 1999.
20. Brown JS, Grady D, Ouslander JG, et al: Prevalence of urinary incontinence and associated risk factors in postmenopausal women. Obstet Gynecol 94(1):66–70, 1999.
21. Bump RC, Sugerman H, Fantl JA, McClish DM: Obesity and lower urinary tract function in women: Effect of surgically induced weight loss. Am J Obstet Gynecol 166:392–399, 1992.
22. Deitel M, Stone E, Kassam HA, et al: (1988) Gynecologic-obstetric changes after loss of massive excess weight following bariatric surgery. J Am Coll Nutr 7(2):147–153, 1988.
23. Subak LL, Johnson C, Whitcomb E, et al: Does weight loss improve incontinence in moderately obese women? Int Urogynecol J 13:40–43, 2002.
24. Dowd TT, Campbell JM, Jones JA: Fluid intake and urinary incontinence in older community-dwelling women. J Community Health Nurs 13(3):179–186, 1986.
25. Engberg SJ, McDowell BJ, Burgio KL, et al: Self-care behaviors of older women with urinary incontinence. J Obstet Gynecol Neonatal Nurs 21(8):7–14, 1995.
26. Johnson TM, Kincade JE, Bernard SL, et al: Self-care practices used by older men and women to manage urinary incontinence: Results from the national follow-up survey on self-care and aging, J Am Geriatr Soc 48(8):894–902, 2000.
27. Thomas AM, Morse JM: Managing urinary incontinence with self-care practices. J Gerontol Nurs 17(6):9–14, 1991.
28. Griffiths DJ, McCracken PN, Harrison GM, Gormley EA: Relationship of fluid intake to voluntary micturition and urinary incontinence in geriatric patients. Neurourol Urodyn 12:1–7, 1993.
29. Nygaard IE, Linder M: Thirst at work—an occupational hazard? Int Urogynecol J Pelvic Floor Dysfunct 8(6):340–343, 1997.
30. Fitzgerald S, Palmer MH, Berry SJ, Hart K: Urinary incontinence: Impact on working women. AAOHN J 48(3):112–118, 2000.
31. Wyman JF, Elswick RK, Wilsom MS, Fantl JA: Relationship of fluid intake to voluntary micturitions and urinary incontinence in women. Neurourol Urodyn 10:463–473, 1991.
32. Kayser-Jones J, Schell ES, Porter C, et al: Factors contributing to dehydration in nursing homes: Inadequate staffing and lack of professional supervision. J Am Geriatr Soc 47:1187–1194, 1999.
33. Wells, TJ: Nursing management. In O'Donnel PD (ed): Urinary Incontinence. St Louis, Mosby, 1997, pp 439–433.
34. Creighton SM, Stanton SL: Caffeine: Does it affect your bladder? Br J Urol 66:613–614, 1990.
35. Lee JG, Wein AJ, Levin RM: The effect of caffeine on the contractile response of the rabbit urinary bladder to field stimulation. Gen Pharmacol 24(4):1007–1011, 1993.
36. Lamarine RJ: Selected health and behavioral effects related to the use of caffeine. J Community Health 19(6):449–466, 1994.
37. Dalloso HM, McGrother CW, Matthews RJ, and the Leicestershire MRC Incontinence Study Group. The association of diet and other lifestyle factors with overactive bladder and stress incontinence: A longitudinal study in women. BJU Intl 92:69–77, 2003.
38. Newman DK: The Urinary Incontinence Sourcebook, 2nd ed. Chicago, Lowell House, 1999.
39. Newman DK: Managing and Treating Urinary Incontinence. Baltimore, Health Professions Press, 2002.
40. Tomlinson BU, Dougherty MC, Pendergast JF, et al: Dietary caffeine, fluid intake and urinary incontinence in older rural women. Int Urogynecol J Pelvic Floor Dysfunct 10:22–28, 1999.
41. Arya LA, Myers DL, Jackson ND: Dietary caffeine intake and the risk for detrusor instability: A case-control study. Obstet Gynecol 96(1):85–89, 2000.
42. Bryant CM, Dowell CJ, Fairbrother G: Caffeine reduction eduction to improve urinary symptoms. Br J Nurs 11(8):560–565, 2002.
43. Gray M: Caffeine and urinary continence, J WOCN 28:66–69, 2001.
44. Snooks SJ, Barnes PRH, Setchell M, Henry MM: Damage to the innervation of pelvic floor musculature in chronic constipation. Gastroenterol 89:977–981, 1985.
45. Lubowski DZ, Swash M, Nicholls RJ, Henry MM: Increase in pudendal nerve terminal motor latency with defaecation straining. Br J Surg 75:1095–1097, 1988.
46. Spence-Jones C, Kamm MA, Henry MM, Hudson CN: Bowel dysfunction: A pathogenic factor in uterovaginal prolapse and urinary stress incontinence. Br J Obstet Gynecol 101:147–152, 1994.
47. Moller LA, Lose G, Jorgensen T: Risk factors for lower urinary tract symptoms in women 40 to 60 years of age. Obstet Gynecol 96(3):446–451, 2000.
48. Charach G, Greenstein A, Rabinovich P, et al: Alleviating constipation in the elderly improves lower urinary tract symptoms. Gerontology 47:72–76, 2001.
49. Dougherty MC, Dwyer JW, Pendergast JF, et al: A randomized trial of behavioral management for continence with older rural women. Res Nurs Health 25:3–13, 2002.
50. Nygaard IE, Thompson F., Svengalis SL, Albright JP: Urinary incontinence in elite nulliparous athletes. Obstet Gynecol 84(2):183–187, 1994.
51. Thyssen HH, Clevin LS. Olesen L, Lose G: Urinary incontinence in elite female athletes and dancers. Int Urogynecol J 13:15–17, 2002.
52. Nygaard I: Prevention of exercise incontinence with mechanical devices. J Reprod Med 40:89, 1995.
53. Nygaard IE: Does prolonged high-impact activity contribute to later urinary incontinence? A retrospective cohort study of female Olympians. Obstet Gynecol 90(5):718–722, 1997.
54. Palmer MH, Fitzgerald S, Berry SJ, Hart K: Urinary incontinence in working women: An exploratory study. Women Health 29(3):67–80, 1999.
55. Jorgensen S, Heiin HO, Gyntelberg F: Heavy lifting at work and risk of genital prolapse and herniated lumbar disc in assistant nurses. Occup Med 44:47–49, 1997.
56. Davis GD, Goodman M: Stress urinary incontinence in nulliparous female soldiers in airborne infantry training. J Pelvic Surg 2(2):68–71, 1996.
57. Sherman RA, Davis GD, Wong MF: Behavioral treatment of exercise-induced urinary incontinence among female soldiers. Mil Med 162:690–694, 1997.
58. Fischer JR, Berg PH: Urinary incontinence in United States Air Force female aircrew. Obstet Gynecol 94(4):532–536, 1999.

CHAPTER 28

Pelvic Floor Muscle Exercises

JULIA H. HERBERT

There is no muscle in the body whose form and function is more difficult to understand than the levator ani.
—Dickinson (1889)

For more than half a century, health professionals have researched the effects of exercises for the pelvic floor muscles in the prevention and treatment of urinary incontinence, bowel dysfunction, and sexual dysfunction in both men and women. Today, pelvic floor muscle training is the most commonly recommended type of physical therapy for women with stress incontinence of urine.[1] This chapter discusses the background of these exercises, describes suggested exercise regimens (protocols), and considers the clinical effectiveness of this therapy.

HISTORY

Exercises for the pelvic floor muscles, or levator ani, have been described by many authors over the last 50 years. The most famous is probably Arnold Kegel, an American obstetrician and gynecologist. Kegel began his work in 1932, and published his clinical experiences in the late 1940s and early 1950s. His work is still often referenced in current publications.

"Kegeling" is a common pastime in the United States, and many patients and clinicians in other countries call pelvic floor muscle exercises "Kegel" exercises. Kegel[2] described specific exercises for the pelvic floor muscles, and he stated that these exercises are distinct from haphazard general exercise. He described four stages in the successful use of pelvic floor exercises to treat stress incontinence:

1. Identification of the pubococcygeus by digital palpation
2. Instruction of the patient in exercises of the pubococcygeus designed to develop its supportive and sphincteric function
3. Correct contractions. These are always more important than strong contractions; this is pointed out to every patient
4. Continuation of therapy beyond the disappearance of symptoms, until the conditioned reflex control is firmly established, as it exists in normal women

Although these principles were written more than half a century ago, many of them are still applied to pelvic floor muscle training. However, considerable disagreement persists about the content, frequency, and effectiveness of training programs.

ROLE OF THE PELVIC FLOOR COMPLEX

The muscular part of the pelvic floor complex is often referred to as the pelvic floor, but the anatomic name is the levator ani. The pelvic floor complex is actually a combination of muscles and fascia attached to the pelvic bones. The muscular portion is divided into deep and superficial perineal muscles, and the latter group includes the external anal sphincter. The muscle fibers are attached to the bony pelvis with a network of endopelvic fascia.

Support

The main function of the pelvic floor muscles is to provide postural support to the pelvic organs; consequently, type I, or slow-twitch, fibers are predominant. In healthy muscle, these fibers have high endurance and low contraction speed, and are resistant to fatigue. However, to respond to sudden changes in intra-abdominal pressure, the pelvic floor muscles also contain type II, or fast-twitch, fibers that contract strongly and quickly to provide short bursts of activity.

According to Gilpin and associates,[3] within the pelvic floor, the distribution of fiber types is approximately 70% slow-twitch fibers and 30% fast-twitch fibers. These authors also noted a decrease in type II fibers in the periurethral and perianal area in women with symptoms of genitourinary prolapse or urinary stress incontinence. This finding suggests that changes in pelvic floor muscle function are associated with prolapse and incontinence.

Urinary Stress Incontinence

During periods of increased intra-abdominal pressure, the pelvic floor muscles are believed to act as a type of platform or hammock, as described by DeLancey.[4] The hammock of muscles under the urethra allows the increased intra-abdominal pressure to compress the urethra against this resistance, preventing urine leakage. Recognizing the role of the endopelvic fascia, Petros and Ulmsten[5] proposed the integral hypothesis based on the view that the pelvic floor is a single functional unit. If a part of the structure is weakened (e.g., the pubourethral ligament), then the hammock has lost some of its original function and cannot perform efficiently. The integral theory also suggests that obstruction of the urethra is caused by both sphincter activity and compression of the urethra as a result of contraction of the pelvic floor muscles.

Dougherty[6] postulated that the effects of pelvic floor muscle training on the symptoms of stress incontinence are the result of muscle hypertrophy. Muscle hypertrophy accounts for most gains achieved by skeletal muscle; however, Dougherty also suggests that neuromuscular coordination is at least as important as hypertrophy for the successful treatment of stress incontinence. In 1998, Miller and colleagues[7] described a study of older women (mean age, 68 years) who had symptoms of mild to moderate stress incontinence. The intervention group was taught the technique of intentionally contracting the pelvic floor muscles before and during a cough ("The Knack"). In a relatively short time (1 week), the results showed a significant reduction in urine loss when the women used "The Knack" compared with coughing without precontraction of the pelvic floor.

Urinary Urge Incontinence

The role of the pelvic floor muscles in urge incontinence is less clear. Therapy is usually based on improving pelvic floor muscle function, in particular, the ability to sustain a contraction, and then using the improved muscle function in a bladder retraining program. Reflex inhibition of a detrusor contraction may be possible by producing a voluntary contraction of the striated muscles of the pelvic floor and activating the perineodetrusor inhibitory reflex, as described by Mahony and colleagues.[8]

Fecal Incontinence

The mechanism for maintaining continence of fecal material (liquid, solid, and gas) relies on an intact and functioning internal anal sphincter. However, the external anal sphincter, which forms part of the superficial pelvic floor muscles, also contributes to this mechanism. The role of the external anal sphincter is considered particularly important during sampling, when the internal sphincter relaxes (rectoanal inhibitory reflex) and the rectal contents enter the upper part of the anus. When this occurs, continence is believed to be preserved by contraction of the external anal sphincter; there is some debate as to whether this is a reflex or voluntary response.[9] The deepest part of the external anal sphincter is intimately related to the posterior fibers of the levator ani, which form the puborectalis. This muscle maintains the anorectal angle and contributes to the continence mechanism. To postpone the sensation to defecate and remain continent, the external anal sphincter must have endurance (type I fibers) and be able to sustain a voluntary contraction.

PELVIC FLOOR MUSCLE TRAINING PROGRAMS

Although many authors have conducted research on pelvic floor muscle training programs, there is little consensus as to what constitutes an effective program. In a review of 43 randomized trials in women with symptoms or urodynamic diagnoses of stress, urge, or mixed urinary incontinence, marked variations were noted in the content of the exercise programs.[1]

Basic Principles

Kegel[2] recommended performing as many as 300 to 400 pelvic floor muscle contractions daily, but gave little information about the intensity of each contraction. As described by Bø,[10] the two main principles of strength training for skeletal muscles are overload and specificity. Specificity is particularly important in relation to the pelvic floor muscles because approximately 30% of women have difficulty performing a correct contraction on the first attempt. The pelvic floor is surrounded by many larger groups of muscles, such as the quadriceps and glutei. Women often incorrectly contract these muscle groups when attempting to contract the pelvic floor muscles. Another common mistake is to produce a Valsalva, or bearing-down, maneuver. Bø[10] also describes the importance of instructor-conducted exercises in establishing the correct action of the pelvic floor muscle and maintaining motivation to continue with the exercise program.

In addition to the muscle group being exercised, specificity concerns the type of training used in relation to the dysfunction and symptoms.[11] For example, in a case of urinary stress incontinence, the function required of the pelvic floor muscles is to assist the urethral closure pressure provided by the urethral sphincter, the resting tone of the levator ani, and mucosal coaptation. This requires a quick maximum voluntary contraction of the pelvic floor muscles; therefore, in this case, the training program must emphasize type II fibers. During contraction of the pelvic floor muscles, motor units are recruited in order of increasing size, with type I fibers recruited at low intensity and type II fibers recruited only at high intensity. Therefore, the training program must include high-intensity exercises. Type II fibers fatigue rapidly because of the rapid depletion and slow replacement of adenosine triphosphate. For this reason, the exercise program should allow relaxation between contractions. The contribution of type I fibers should not be overlooked; they are responsible for maintaining the postural position of the pelvic floor, from which type II fibers can then function effectively.

If the pelvic floor muscle dysfunction is related to fecal incontinence, training must emphasize the external anal sphincter and puborectalis. Focusing on the anal sphincter and posterior muscle fibers, to the extent of using anal rather than vaginal or external electrodes to provide biofeedback to assist muscle training, is considered more effective than conventional pelvic floor exercises.[12] For this reason, some clinicians call exercises for bowel dysfunction sphincter exercises.

Coactivation of Abdominal Muscles

Traditionally, pelvic floor muscle exercises are practiced in isolation, without activity of the abdominal or hip muscles. However, Sapsford and colleagues[13] describe how this practice has been challenged by a number of authors, who noted activity in the rectus abdominis in association with pelvic floor muscle contraction and palpable coactivation of the abdominal muscles during functional activities, such as raising the head and shoulders. Sapsford and colleagues[13] showed that the rectus abdominis, obliquus internus abdominis, obliquus externus abdominis, and transversus abdominis are all coactivated with maximal contraction of the pelvic floor muscles. An additional study (Sapsford and colleagues[13]) described in the same report also showed that the reverse occurs, in that pubococcygeal electromyographic activity increased in response to isometric contractions of the abdominal muscles. These authors suggested that this activity could be used for therapeutic effect, by encouraging submaximal deep abdominal isometric contractions to enhance pubococcygeal training. The study also considered the effect of altering the position of the lumbar spine during exercise, and concluded that a neutral or extended position is preferable.

Although the studies were conducted on small numbers of subjects (7 and 2, respectively), this report raises questions about the traditional technique for teaching isolated pelvic floor muscle contractions, in which movement of other muscle groups is restricted, and suggests that clinicians should expect abdominal activity, and not avoid it, during pelvic floor muscle exercises.

Who Teaches Pelvic Floor Exercises?

The content of a program of pelvic floor muscle training may vary considerably from one researcher or clinician to another. In the analysis of Hay-Smith,[1] specific parameters of training programs were examined. In most of the trials considered in this analysis, women were individually taught how to correctly contract their pelvic floor muscles. Some women were taught in groups (three trials), and others did not state how the training was provided. In one trial, the specific aim was to compare group exercise with individualized training. The clinicians involved in these studies were physiotherapists, nurses, nurse practitioners, or clinical nurse specialists, although more than one fourth of the reports did not state who taught the exercises. Surprisingly, only 16 of the 43 trials that were analyzed stated that vaginal palpation was performed to verify that voluntary pelvic floor muscle contractions were done correctly before training began.

Frequency of Exercises

Most trials stated that a daily home program of exercise was used. Daily training programs varied significantly, with some requiring participants to exercise for a specific length of time each day (e.g., 5 minutes twice daily), perform a specific number of contractions each hour (e.g., 5), perform a specific number of contractions each day (e.g., 50), or repeat contractions a specific number of times each day (e.g., 12 contractions three times daily). In half of the trials, the total number of contractions per day could be calculated; the number varied from 36 to 200.

Work–rest Phase

Again, there appears to be little consensus about the work–rest phase in pelvic floor muscle training. Most of the studies considered in this analysis mentioned the use of both slow (sustained) and fast (rapid) contractions, although the times stated for the work phase varied from 4 seconds to 30 to 40 seconds, with few studies stating the rest phase. Only one fourth of the studies described assessing the pelvic floor before the exercise program began. Clearly, if the muscle function is not evaluated before the start of the exercise program, meeting the basic principle of specificity is difficult, and the program cannot be tailored to overload the muscle.

One trial described use of "The Knack," which is a voluntary contraction of the pelvic floor muscles before an increase in intra-abdominal pressure, as the entire muscle training program.[7] Five other trials included "The Knack" with other pelvic floor muscle exercises.

The gradation, or progression of exercises is also considered important,[11] because the function of the pelvic floor at the beginning of a training program may vary considerably from one person to another. Exercises may be progressed by increasing the duration of the contraction or the number of repetitions, or by grading the contraction technique. Bø[10] addressed this issue by using an intensive training program. The intensive exercise group attended a 45-minute class once a week, in groups of 10 to 12. This class included the use of sustained contractions, lasting 6 to 8 seconds, with three or four fast contractions performed during the sustained contraction. The contractions were performed in different positions, with the legs abducted. The instructor provided strong verbal encouragement during the training sessions. The women were also encouraged to perform the intensive pelvic floor contractions, in sets of 8 to 12, three times daily at home. Miller and colleagues[11] approach the gradation process differently, describing five levels of progression. The first two levels aim to improve participants' ability to identify the pelvic floor muscles. Next are two levels of strength training, and finally, a maintenance program that is performed once or twice a week.

Length of the Training Program

Hay-Smith and colleagues[1] reported that the total length of time given for pelvic floor muscle training varied from 1 week[7] to 6 months.[10] However, more than one third of the trials used a training period of 12 weeks. Any changes in muscle function during the first 6 weeks of training are likely to be caused by more effective recruitment of motor units and increased frequency of excitation. The increase in strength caused by muscle hypertrophy is a much longer process.[6,10] The American College of Sports Medicine[14] recommends that, in general, the time for strength training for striated muscle fibers should be at least 5 months, with the potential for further improvements after this time.

ADVERSE EFFECTS OF PELVIC FLOOR MUSCLE EXERCISES

Often, research trials do not report adverse effects of pelvic floor muscle training programs. The analysis by Hay-Smith and associates[1] noted that the few adverse events associated directly with exercising the pelvic floor muscles were usually minor and reversible. Examples include pain during contraction, discomfort during exercises, and a desire to avoid being continually occupied with the problem.

EFFECTIVENESS

Most research studies clearly show that pelvic floor exercises significantly benefit those who are well motivated and able to comply with an exercise regimen. Furthermore, this effect can be sustained for up to 8 years.[6] Unfortunately, although various authors report significant improvement or cure, because of the wide variation in outcome measures used, it is difficult to compare results. In addition, many different exercise regimens appear to be effective,[1] raising questions about which elements, or combinations of elements, are most effective. Some trials use questionable exercise regimens that are not based on accepted physiologic principles of strength training.

Recent trials have begun to address issues of quality of life. Hay-Smith and colleagues[1] suggested that the development of broad outcome measures that are important to women are vital to future research programs.

CONCLUSION

Over the last half century, much research has been carried out with regard to pelvic floor muscle exercises. Unfortunately, there is little consensus as to the content of an effective exercise program, with many authors ignoring the basic principles of muscle strength training. In addition, there is uncertainty about the effect of combining pelvic floor exercises with other modalities, such as biofeedback and neuromuscular stimulation.[1] Finally, few researchers have considered the effect of an exercise program on quality of life.

REFERENCES

1. Hay-Smith EJC, Bø K, Berghmans LCM, et al: Pelvic floor muscle training for urinary incontinence in women: Cochrane review. In The Cochrane Library, issue 1. Oxford, Update Software, 2001.
2. Kegel AH: Progressive resistance exercise in the functional restoration of the perineal muscles. Am J Obstet Gynecol 56:238–249, 1948.
3. Gilpin SA, Gosling JA, Smith ARB, et al: The pathogenesis of genitourinary prolapse and stress incontinence of urine: A histological and histochemical study. Br J Obstet Gynecol 96:15–23, 1989.
4. DeLancey JOL: Structural support of the urethra as it relates to stress urinary incontinence: The hammock hypothesis. Am J Obstet Gynecol 170:1713–1720, 1994.
5. Petros PE, Ulmsten UI: An integral theory and its method for the diagnosis and management of female urinary incontinence. Scand J Urol Nephrol Suppl 153:1–93, 1993.
6. Dougherty MC: Current status of research on pelvic muscle strengthening techniques. J Wound Ostomy Continence Nurs 25(2):75–83, 1998.
7. Miller JM, Ashton-Miller JA, DeLancey JO: A pelvic muscle precontraction can reduce cough-related urine loss in selected women with mild SUI. J Am Geriatr Soc 46(7):870–874, 1998.
8. Mahony DT, Laferte RO, Blais DJ: Incontinence of urine due to instability of micturition reflexes: Part I. Detrusor reflex instability. Urology 15(3):229–239, 1980.
9. Jorge JMN, Wexner SD: Etiology and management of fecal incontinence. Dis Colon Rectum 36:77–97, 1993.
10. Bø K: Techniques. In Schussler B, Laycock J, Norton P, Stanton S (eds): Pelvic floor re-education: Principles and practice. London, Springer-Verlag, 1994, pp 134–139.
11. Miller J, Kasper C, Sampselle C: Review of muscle physiology with application to pelvic muscle exercise. Urol Nurs 14:92–97, 1994.
12. Norton C, Hosker G, Brazzelli M: Biofeedback and/or sphincter exercises for the treatment of faecal incontinence in adults: Cochrane review. In The Cochrane Library, issue 1. Oxford, Update Software, 2001.
13. Sapsford RR, Hodges PW, Richardson CA, et al: Co-activation of the abdominal and pelvic floor muscles during voluntary exercises. Neurourol Urodynam 20:31–42, 2001.
14. American College of Sports Medicine (ACSM): The recommended quantity and quality of exercise for developing and maintaining cardiorespiratory and muscular fitness in healthy adults. Med Sci Sports Exerc 22:265–274, 1990.

CHAPTER 29

Electrical Stimulation

ALAIN P. BOURCIER ■ KWANG TAE PARK

Electrical stimulation, or electrostimulation, has been used in medical practice and physical medicine in the form of functional (electrical) prostheses developed to improve gait. Electrical currents are applied therapeutically to stimulate muscle contraction, usually through activation of nerves that supply muscles. Electrical stimulation was first used in the management of urinary incontinence in 1952, when Bors[1] described the influence of electrical stimulation on the pudendal nerves, and in 1963, when Caldwell[2] developed electrodes that were permanently implanted into the pelvic floor and controlled by radiofrequency. Since this time, many investigators around the world have used this therapy. Alexander and Rowan,[3] using an "electric pessary," and Suhel,[4] who introduced an integrated appliance (automatic vaginal stimulator), provided new methods for nonimplantable perineal stimulation.

Godec and associates[5] first described the use of non-implanted stimulators specifically for bladder inhibition. Initial work in animals indicated the potential of this therapy, and early clinical experience in Europe supported its likely efficacy. Much confusion surrounds electrical stimulation, and some is the result of inconsistent nomenclature. Commonly used terms include functional electrical stimulation and neuromuscular electrical stimulation. Further confusion has arisen because of the wide range of stimulators, probes, and applications used. It can be difficult to understand the different methods and techniques used for electrostimulation. These techniques include the following:

- Long-term (chronic, weak) electrical stimulation
- Short-term (acute, strong) electrical stimulation
- Acute maximal functional electrical stimulation
- Maximum pelvic floor stimulation

Over the last 10 years, many techniques have been introduced for clinical use, but many experts disagree about fundamental issues. Problems include a lack of consistency in the types of electrical stimulation used, disagreement about the parameters used to treat incontinence, and contradictions in the results obtained. On the other hand, a substantial body of research attests to the efficacy of this treatment. This chapter provides a physiologic explanation of the mechanisms of treatment, recommendations for its practical use, and an international overview of the clinical findings.

BASIC PRINCIPLES AND MECHANISM OF ACTION

Electrical stimulation is an effective treatment for stress incontinence and urge incontinence. This technique uses natural pathways and the micturition reflexes (Fig. 29-1), and its efficacy relies on a preserved reflex arc, with complete or partial integrity of the pelvic floor muscle innervation.[6] Based on animal experiments, direct stimulation of afferent or efferent fibers appears to be the most important mechanism to enhance the reflex response (Figs. 29-2 and 29-3).

The mechanism of electrical stimulation for stress and urge incontinence is urethral closure by contraction of the pelvic floor muscle fibers and reflex inhibition of detrusor contraction. Urethral closure occurs by direct stimulation. Closure of the urethra by electrical stimulation of the pudendal nerve is caused mainly by direct stimulation of the pudendal nerve efferent, which supplies the striated paraurethral and pelvic floor muscles and is supported by activation of hypogastric efferents to the smooth paraurethral muscles.[7,8]

Bladder inhibition is accomplished through three mechanisms:

1. Activation of afferent fibers within the pudendal nerve by activation of the hypogastric nerve at low intravesical pressure, corresponding to the filling phase
2. Direct inhibition of the pelvic nerve within the sacral cord at high intravesical pressure
3. Supraspinal inhibition of the detrusor reflex[9,10]

Electrical stimulation is commonly used in the treatment of urinary incontinence and pelvic floor dysfunction to improve the function of the urethral sphincteric mechanism, levator ani muscles, and external anal sphincter. These muscles have fast and slow twitch fibers: the slow twitch fibers could be important in developing sustain tone to occlude the urethra, whereas the fast twitch could be involved in pelvic reflex contraction.

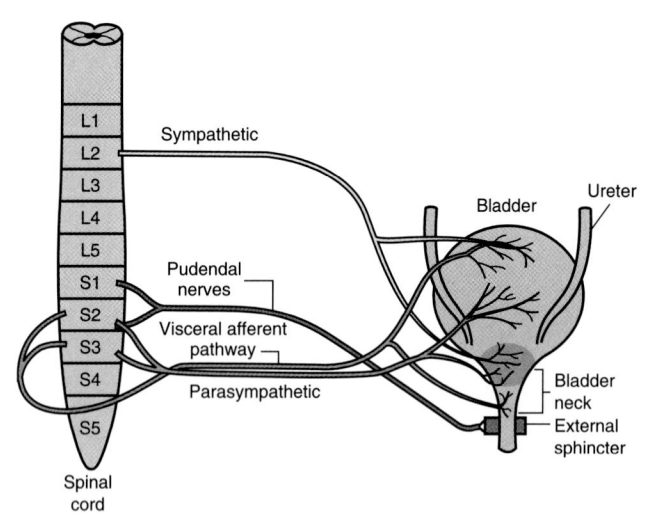

FIGURE 29-1 Electrical stimulation mechanisms. Pudendal nerve stimulation can cause a direct pelvic floor contraction, and, through the spinal cord, a reflex pelvic nerve stimulation, which results in inhibition of bladder activity.

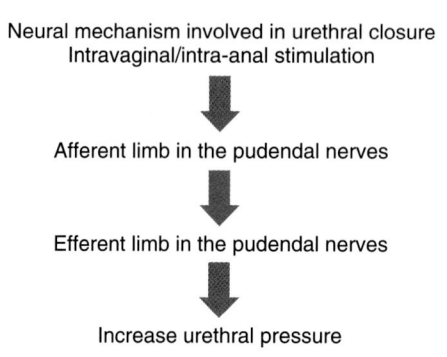

FIGURE 29-3 The neural mechanisms involved in the increase of urethral pressure. Urethral closure is provided by direct stimulation.

Electrical stimulation may simply increase the bulk of the levator ani muscles and the proportion of fast-twitch fibers and thus the ability of muscles to respond to a sudden increase in intra-abdominal pressure. The stimulus may increase the number and strength of slow-twitch fibers, improving resting urethral closure. In principle, defective control of the urinary bladder, resulting in urge incon-tinence, is caused by a central nervous dysfunction that affects central inhibitory control of the micturition reflex. Appropriate electrical stimulation may restore the inhibition effect.[11]

Threshold intensity varies inversely with fiber diameter. Any pulse configuration can provide nerve activation, and many stimulation waveforms have been used to cause neural excitation.[9,11] These include biphasic capacitively coupled pulses, monophasic square pulses, biphasic square pulses, and monophasic capacitively coupled spike pulses. Short square-wave pulses (200–1000 msec) are the most effective. To minimize electrochemical reactions at the electrode–mucosa interface, biphasic or alternating pulses are recommended.[12]

The size and position of the electrodes are of utmost importance to the response. Small electrodes and high charge densities are necessary to avoid tissue damage, which is presumably dependent on the generation of heat and formation of toxic products through electrochemical reactions. Heat production correlates to the amount of energy delivered and the electrochemical reactions to the electrical charge transferred by each pulse. The use of a low frequency further reduces energy consumption. Bidirectional pulses should reduce electrochemical reactions. Moreover, intermittent stimulation helps to avoid harmful effects by decreasing total energy.[13]

The effects of electrical stimulation on urethral closure and detrusor inhibition are optimal with different stimulation parameters: 20 to 50 Hz and 5 to 10 Hz. The sacral afferent nerves, particularly the autonomic nerves of the pelvic organs, are poorly myelinated (A delta) or unmyelinated (C) fibers, which conduct current at a slow rate of 5 to 20 Hz. Thus, in the treatment of bladder instability and hyper-reflexia, low-frequency stimulation is applied to the pudendal nerve afferents through probes. In both forms of electrical stimulation, the frequencies are chosen based on the clinical diagnosis. In mixed incontinence, two strategies are used. One strategy involves the use of a compromise setting of approximately 20 Hz; the other involves delivering both low-frequency and high-frequency stimuli.[14]

Low frequencies (1–5 Hz) generate twitch contractions, allowing little sustained tension to develop in the muscle. Slow-twitch muscle fibers have a natural firing rate of 10 to 20 Hz, whereas fast-twitch fibers fire at 30 to 60 Hz. Current frequencies of greater than 40 Hz may cause undue fatigue and should be avoided. In a healthy muscle, at frequencies of approximatively 30 Hz, muscle contractions usually become fused or tetanized, so that a smooth contraction is apparent. Current frequencies of 10 to 40 Hz that last approximately 250 to 500 msec activate fast and slow motoneurons. At high frequencies, the muscle weakens rapidly because of neuromuscular transmission; at lower frequencies, less fatigue occurs. Chronic stimulation may increase the relative number of slow-twitch fibers, probably by helping to transform fast-twitch fibers to slow units, which can sustain the contraction longer. Stimulation recruits muscle fibers in a less predictable order than that of a voluntary contraction (i.e., type two fibers may be recruited before type one).[15] Long-term electrical stimulation[16,17] induces nearly complete transformation of fast-twitch to slow-twitch fibers

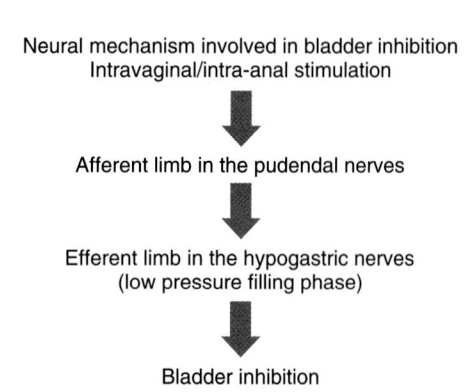

FIGURE 29-2 The neural mechanisms involved in bladder inhibition.

that have a high energy capacity. Frequencies of 10 to 60 Hz induce such transformation, which occurs after almost 30 days of electrical stimulation. Most patients have some relapse after 30 days, possibly as a result of the reverse process associated with immobilization or inactivity. During the "on" time, the stimulation delivers a train of individual pulses of prescribed amplitude, duration, and frequency. The length of the "off" time defines the recuperative period for the stimulated muscles.[18]

The length of the "off" time defines the recuperation period for stimulation. The ratio of stimulation time to rest time is called the duty cycle. A typical duty cycle is approximately 1:2. The patient's diagnosis and degree of muscle weakness should be considered when identifying a suitable duty cycle for initiation of the electrical stimulation program.[18] In case of weakness or neurologic impairment, a ratio of 1:3 may be appropriate.[19] As muscle strength or endurance improves, the ratio of on-to-off time may be decreased. Most commercially available devices allow adjustment of the time that the stimulus takes to reach peak intensity and return to zero intensity. In order to reduce the problem of discomfort, the amplitude of the stimulus (intensity) is progressively delivered, allowing the patient to become accustomed to the stimulation as it increases from no perceptible levels to sensory and finally motor thresholds. Most electrical stimulators introduced in the last decade provide constant voltage or constant current that maintains the same current waveform, regardless of changes in impedance. Great individual variations in the stimulus can be tolerated without incurring unpleasant sensations. This difference is related to impedance.

Variant technology is a new attempt to overcome methodologic limits and avoid problems, such as discomfort and muscle fatigue, that occur with "conventional" electrostimulation.[20] The main characteristics of variant technology are:

- Optimization of the stimulation waveform
- Synchronization to adjust energy
- Automatic energy control and structure of the double-channel electrode

The need to change the parameters is guided by the different situations encountered in everyday practice, such as differences in connective tissue,[21,22] hormonal changes associated with the menstrual cycle,[23] and anatomic differences in patients of different ethnic groups.[24]

This concept is fundamentally different and is not based on constant voltage or current, but on an energy variation method. It involves appropriate trade-off of each parameter that determines stimulation energy and various stimulation phases. In electrostimulation, the maximum output energy per pulse can be described as follows:

$$\text{Energy} = V_m \times Q \, [\text{mJ/pulse}]$$

where V_m is maximum voltage and Q is charge.

The interest of the method is changing voltage, V_m, whenever stimulated. This approach is fundamentally different from setting the voltage into maximum stimulation intensity. Therefore, to change the energy in this formula, the method of changing response charge is effective.

$$Q = 2V_m : Z_s \times t \, [\mu C/\text{pulse}]$$

where t is pulse width and Z_s is approximately resistance only.

Hence, response charge is proportional to pulse width. Because the number of action potentials per person differs, the ion charge Q that controls cell pumping must be different as well. According to the formula, ion charge Q, which differs, must be adjusted by variable factors, such as V_m and pulse width. Therefore, the method used to change duty is the method that achieves the same effect as changing V_m with pulse width.

In the variant method, electrostimulation is described as an energy summation of variant vector addition or subtraction from the double-channel system.

As shown in the first variant formula, energy per pulse is modified by changing the supplied voltage and electric charge. The electric charge is changed according to supplied voltage and pulse width. Supplied voltage is proportional to the duty and intensity of the current. The intensity of the current is related to the skin resistance of the vagina or anus, and duty is proportional to frequency and pulse width. As discussed earlier, the energy per pulse determines the treatment cycle through phases, units, and sessions. This innovative technology[20] is characterized by hundreds of stimulation programs that can be used to meet various requirements.

Other methods of electrical stimulation include faradism and interferential therapy. Faradism is similar to maximal stimulation: short bursts of cycled stimulation are given to produce a pelvic floor contraction, and the patient is instructed to perform a voluntary contraction. Interferential therapy involves setting up two competing currents (two interfering medium-frequency currents) that produce low-frequency stimulation in the area of interest. Interference current[25] is produced by mixing two or three independent circuits of alternating current with pulses of 3000 to 5000 Hz. When the currents from these circuits interact within the tissues, an amplitude-modulated beat is produced. Interferential therapy can be applied with four electrodes[26] or with a bipolar technique, in which case the amplitude-modulated current is produced electronically and supplied to the body with two electrodes.

Different application techniques have been proposed. With the bipolar technique,[27] one electrode is placed over the anus and the second is located inferior to the symphysis pubis and held in place by a small sandbag. Pudendal nerve stimulation has been used to treat stress incontinence[28] and hyper-reflexia.[14] Another important variation is the use of external electrodes and implanted (sacral) electrodes to deliver the electrical current.

Transcutaneous electrical stimulation of acupuncture points (Fig. 29-4) may be used to inhibit detrusor activity. Surface electrodes are placed bilaterally over both tibial nerves or both common peroneal nerves.[29] Percutaneous

FIGURE 29-4 Transcutaneous electrical stimulation of the peripheral nerves may facilitate inhibition of detrusor activity, with specific parameters: intensity of 5 to 8 V, frequency of 10 Hz, and intensity of 10mA adjustable.

stimulation of peripheral S2 and S3 afferents by way of the posterior tibial nerve modulates unstable detrusor activity. Posterior tibial nerve stimulation[30] is performed with a 34-gauge needle inserted 5 cm cephalad to the medial malleolus (Fig. 29-5). Transcutaneous electrical stimulation of the peripheral nerves may facilitate inhibition of detrusor activity with specific parametersm such as intensity of 5 to 8 V, frequency of 2 to 10 Hz, and pulse width of 5 to 20 msec.

Significant evidence shows denervation of the pelvic floor in women with pelvic floor dysfunction, mainly as a result of vaginal childbirth or other pelvic trauma, surgery, or aging. Pudendal nerve latency is prolonged by vaginal delivery[31,32] and vaginal surgery for prolapse.[33] Patients with urinary incontinence or pelvic organ prolapse have longer pudendal nerve latency periods than continent control subjects.[34] Histologic evidence of denervation was seen in biopsy specimens taken from the pubococcygeus at surgery for genital prolapse or stress incontinence.[33] To improve urethral closure, innervation of the pelvic floor must exist. No effect can be expected in patients with complete lower motor neuron lesions. If the muscles are completely denervated, physiotherapy is unlikely to be effective. However, any surviving muscle fibers will be hypertrophied. After denervation injury, such as occurs after pelvic surgery or vaginal childbirth, electrical stimulation may be used to recondition muscle and facilitate sprouting of surviving motor axons. These abnormalities are potentially reversible, or at least treatable, because the nerve supply is not completely disrupted.[15] Because electricity has been used to stimulate denervated muscle for many years,[35-37] electrical stimulation could be used to produce reinnervation or electrical reorganization of the pelvic floor. Although the reason for stimulating denervated muscle appears logical, findings on the efficacy of such treatment are contradictory.

There is no unanimity of opinion about the ultimate degeneration of denervated muscle fibers. Therefore, when discussing the therapeutic technique, particular attention must be paid to the following requirements:

- Duration of the impulse should be as short as possible, yet long enough to elicit a contraction
- The rest period between successive stimuli should be at least four to five times longer than the duration of the stimulus
- The increase should be as steep as possible to avoid stimulation of intact axons
- The intensity of the stimulus must be sufficient to achieve a moderately strong contraction, but should avoid causing the patient unnecessary discomfort[20]

Stimulation to enhance motor control, whether it is called a facilitation technique or a muscle re-education program, provides a tremendous amount of sensory information to the central nervous system, through a variety of sensory modalities and afferent pathways, for both automatic and conscious processing. Therefore, electrical stimulation may improve reinnervation after partial denervation by enhancing sprouting of surviving motor axons.

CLINICAL PRACTICE

Different types of electrical stimulation include office therapy and the home treatment program.[38,39]

Office therapy is also called the outpatient program or in-clinic treatment. With this approach, a stationary device (Fig. 29-6) with a wide range of electrical parameters is used in the office or clinic under the control of the therapist. The system can be modified to suit the needs of each patient. Devices with microcomputers allow the caregiver to change the stimulation parameters (e.g., waveform, pulse width, frequency) based on patient history and urodynamic data.

Many probes are available (Figs. 29-7, 29-8, and 29-9), including a standard two-ring vaginal probe; a tampon two-ring vaginal probe; an inflatable (expandable) intravaginal probe; an intra-anal probe; disposable probes; and a two-channel vaginal and anal insertion

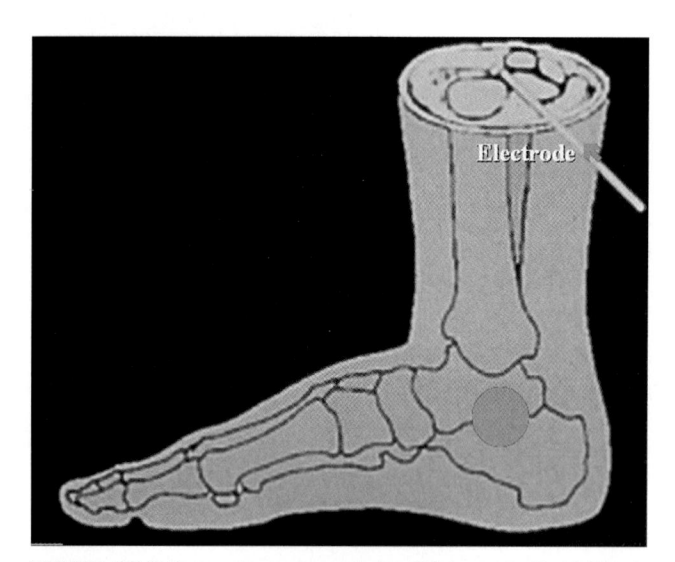

FIGURE 29-5 Transcutaneous posterior tibial nerve stimulation is performed with a needle inserted 5 cm cephalad to the medial malleolus.

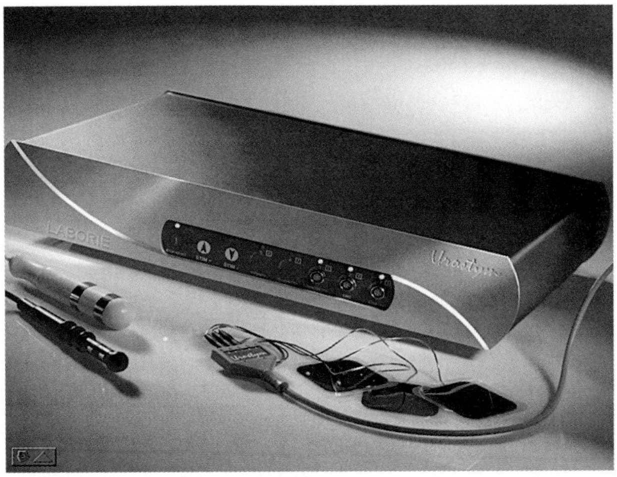

FIGURE 29-6 A stationary device with a wide range of electrical parameters is used to provide electrical stimulation in the office or clinic under the control of a therapist (Courtesy Laborie, Inc.).

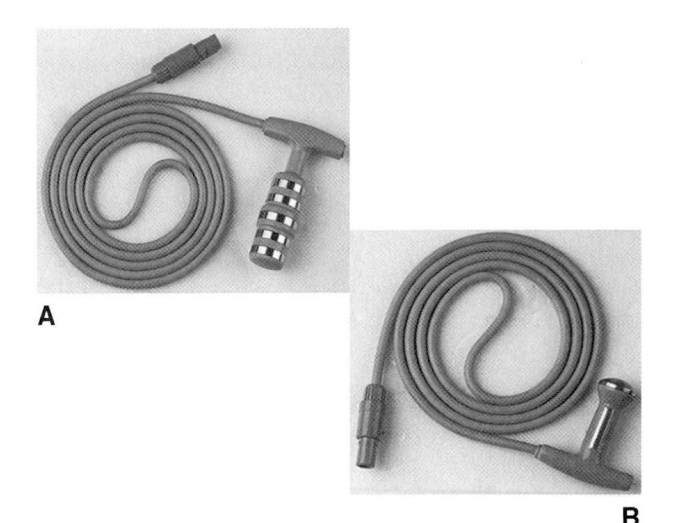

FIGURE 29-8 Other types of probes. **A**, The reference electrode is inserted in the middle of the vaginal probe. **B**, An anal probe (HMT Inc.) with lateral electrodes.

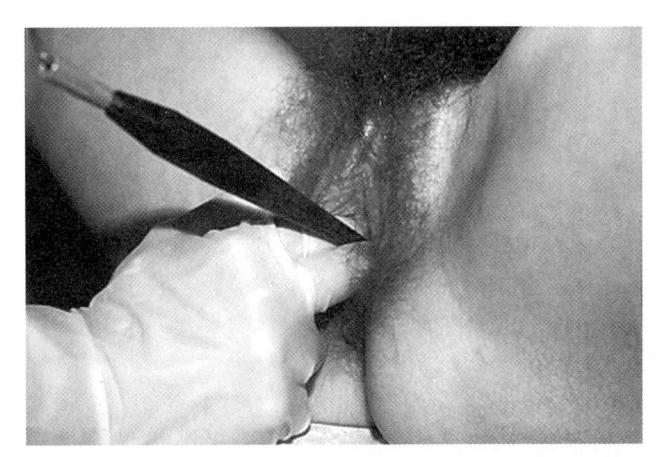

probe. Special conditions that affect the choice of probe include:

- Vaginal size (depth of 4–12 cm) and shape (e.g., atresia or gaping vagina)
- Vaginal angle (10–45 degrees) and quality of the levator ani (thin or thick fibers)
- Type and degree of vaginal wall descent

Accurate assessment of individual anatomic differences allows the therapist to select the appropriate electrodes to obtain the most effective results.

The home treatment program is also called home care, and used for patients who received previous instruction in the use of these stimulator devices. Different types of stimulation units are used. One type consists of a separate box that contains the electronic components and a battery. The box is connected to a probe. Another type consists of a fully integrated unit, with the electronic circuit and battery contained within the plug. However, most units are battery-powered stimulators that provide stimulus output. Most systems use 9 to 12 V batteries. With both forms of electrical stimulation, the frequency is chosen based on the clinical diagnosis, as discussed earlier.

Low frequencies (10–20 Hz) are used for urge incontinence, and high frequencies (35–50 Hz) are used for stress incontinence. Short-term maximal stimulators are one-channel, battery-powered units that emit either continuous or intermittent biphasic pulses of 10 to 100 Hz at a pulse width of 0.5 to 1 msec. Some stimulators have controls that are used to adjust frequency, duty cycle, and timing. The stimulus and intensity of the current are also adjustable, and all of these systems allow easy graduation in the intensity of contraction.

Some equipment allows the use of a combination of office therapy and a home treatment program (Fig. 29-10). The unit that the patient uses at home can be connected to a computer (Fig. 29-11). RT software and an RS serial cable can be used to integrate the home and office systems.

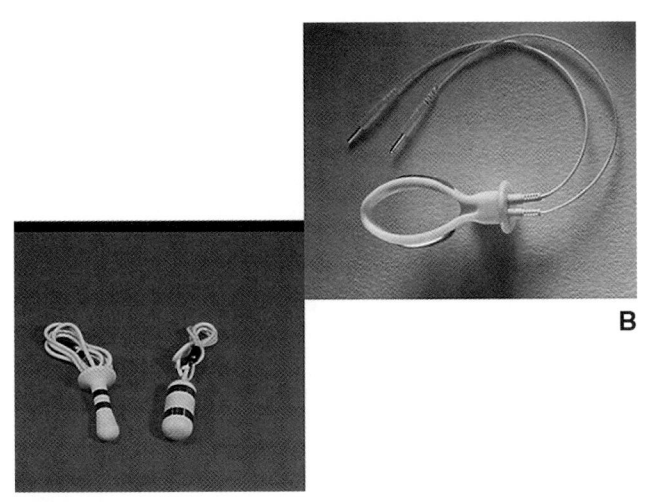

FIGURE 29-7 Probes used in current practice. **A**, A tampon two-ring vaginal probe (right) and an intra-anal probe (left). **B**, A probe designed specifically for patients with a wide vaginal introitus.

FIGURE 29-9 During a severe relaxation of the pelvic floor, a monopolar electrode is used. The patient is in lithotomy position with one leg well supported. The therapist, after a proper application of this probe, stimulates the pubococcygeus on each side of the vagina.

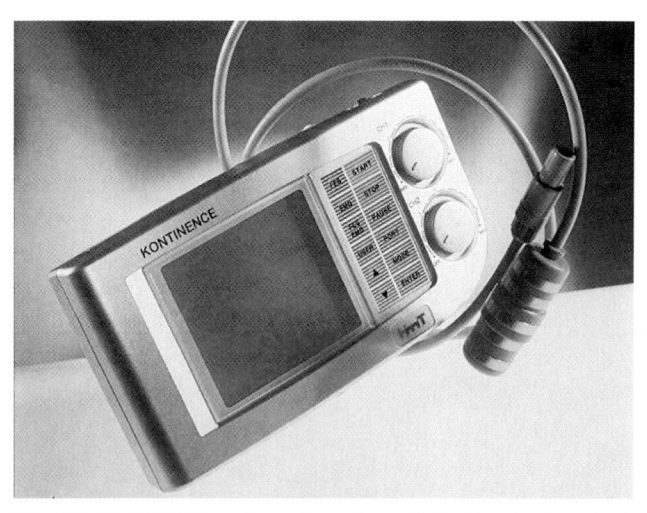

FIGURE 29-10 Different equipment used in the treatment of patients who receive a combination of office therapy and a home treatment program. (Courtesy InCare Medical Product PRS.)

Selection of Patients

Therapeutic stimulation is recommended for women with urinary incontinence and pelvic floor dysfunction[40] who underwent unsuccessful pelvic floor muscle training as a first-line treatment. Pelvic floor electrical stimulation is one of nonsurgical approaches when treating urinary incontinence. The stimulation increases the urethral resistance by strengthening the pelvic floor muscles as well as decreasing the detrusor contractions in case of overactive bladder.

Electrical stimulation must be performed in conjunction with a pelvic floor training program (stress incontinence) or bladder drill (urge incontinence).

The main contraindications to electrical stimulation are as follows:

1. Demand heart pacemakers
2. Pregnancy, if the risk of pregnancy exists
3. Post-volume residual (PVR) >100 mL
4. Obstruction of the urethra, a fixed and radiated urethra, or a heavily scarred urethra
5. Bleeding
6. Urinary tract infection or vaginal discharge
7. Complete peripheral denervation of the pelvic floor
8. Severe genital prolapse with complete eversion of the vagina

There are a few strict contraindications (1, 2, 6, 7), and there is general agreement that a patient with pelvic floor disorder associated with other conditions (4, 5, 8) will not respond to treatment. Although patients with severe genital prolapse are poor candidates, mild prolapse is not a significant problem. A patient with severe urinary incontinence due to sphincteric incompetence is considered a nonresponder for electrical stimulation, although some investigators reported improvement and some success in this group.[41,42]

Many patients will not accept treatment with vaginal or anal probes because of ethical and religious beliefs. These concerns must be taken into account before this therapy is advocated. This issue is especially relevant when home treatment is being considered, because some patients will not agree to insert the device themselves and some will refuse this type of treatment altogether. Functional, anatomical, and attitudinal barriers are more common in frail elderly people. Cognitively or functionally impaired subjects require a participating caregiver. In the elderly, home care treatment could be performed by a nurse or a physical therapist.

Patients with mild to moderate incontinence are the best candidates for this treatment, regardless of age. Because of the slight discomfort and embarrassment that may occur during stimulation, motivated patients of any age are the best candidates for this therapy. For unmotivated patients, however, another technique may be recommended (e.g., electromagnetic stimulation [see Chapter 30]).

Clinical Results

One major problem in reviewing the literature on incontinence is the lack of data on the pretreatment status of patients, particularly when noninvasive forms of therapy are studied.[15] The interpretation of data may be limited because patients often are not classified urodynamically. Nonimplanted stimulators are effective in treating urinary incontinence: overall, an improvement or cure rate of approximately 50% is common. No serious morbidity is reported with this type of therapy. Side effects that are common with drug therapy (e.g., anticholinergics, alpha-adrenergics) do not occur with electrical stimulation. Many stimulation devices and protocols have been used to treat the same condition, such as 20 minutes of maximal stimulation with vaginal and buttock electrodes, performed under general anesthesia,[43] and 6 months of low-intensity stimulation at 10 Hz with vaginal electrodes.[44]

Since 1977, more than 30 international English language studies have been cited in the literature. These studies are difficult to compare, and we recommend reading the articles to obtain the details of each study.

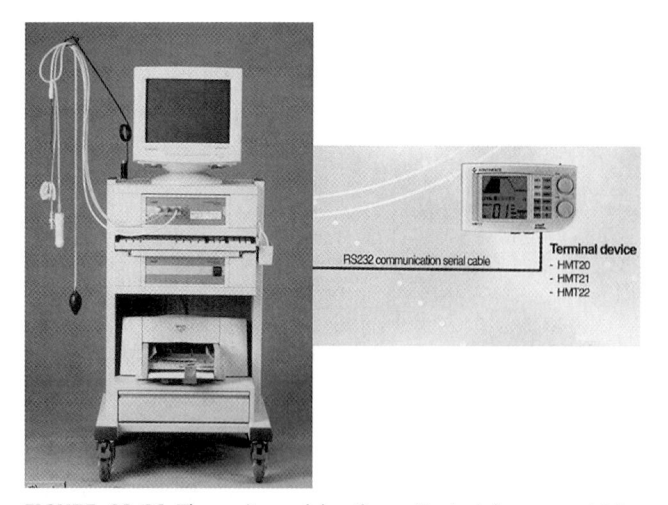

FIGURE 29-11 The unit used by the patient at home could be connected to a stationary device. (Courtesy HMT Inc.)

Here, we discuss important studies that include a large number of patients or include randomized clinical trials.

Eriksen and Eik-Nes[45] performed a study of chronic stimulation with a dual vaginal–anal electrode in 55 patients. They found an initial response rate of 68%, with 47% of the overall group becoming dry. The objective response was an improved stress profile. Kralj[46] studied the influence of the type of idiopathic urge incontinence on the efficient outcome of treatment with acute maximal electrical stimulation. Eighty-eight female patients were divided into motor urge ($n = 40$) and sensory groups ($n = 48$). Both groups underwent vaginal stimulation for 20 minutes. Of the 40 patients in the motor urge group, 55% were cured and 20% showed improvement, whereas 25% showed no change. Of the 48 patients in the sensory group, 87.5% were cured and 12.5% showed improvement.

Bent and associates[47] conducted a study with 45 patients with genuine stress incontinence ($n = 14$), detrusor instability ($n = 10$), and mixed incontinence ($n = 21$), and assessed the applicability of electrical stimulation and patient response to short-term electrical home therapy. Treatment was administered for 15 minutes twice daily for 6 weeks. Treatment consisted of biphasic stimulation at 20 Hz for urge and at 50 Hz for genuine stress incontinence. The ratio of the duty cycle was 2 seconds "on" and 4 seconds "off." Subjective results showed improvement in 71% of patients with genuine stress incontinence, 70% of patients with urge incontinence, and 52% of patients with mixed incontinence. The pressure–transmission ratio improved in four patients, and urethral pressure profiles improved in five patients with genuine stress incontinence. Bladder capacity during cystometry improved in only one patient with detrusor instability.

The report of Sand and colleagues[48] is the only published placebo-controlled study of electrical stimulation. This study showed unquestionable superiority of the treatment arm. Fifty-two women with genuine stress incontinence were enrolled (treatment group, $n = 35$; placebo group, $n = 17$). The treatment group underwent 12 weeks of stimulation twice daily and current was delivered via a single vaginal electrode. The parameters used were: 50 Hz with a pulse width of 0.3 msec. Intensity varies from 0 mA to 100 mA and duty cycle was 5 seconds "on" and 10 seconds "off." The placebo group received sham electrical stimulation with output limited to 1 mA. The number of episodes of incontinence decreased significantly in the treatment group, as measured by both daily ($P = 0.04$) and weekly ($P = 0.009$) leakage as well as the pad test. Subjective assessment of frequency of urine loss showed significant improvement in the treatment group.

Luber and Wolde-Tsadik[49] performed a prospective randomized controlled study to evaluate the effect of electrical stimulation on urinary incontinence. They used a sample of 54 patients who had genuine stress incontinence. Patients in the treatment group ($n = 20$) underwent treatment for 15 minutes twice daily for 12 weeks with vaginal electrode stimulation at a frequency of 50 Hz and pulse duration of 2 msec. The placebo group ($n = 24$) underwent sham electrical stimulation with no current in the patient circuit. Subjective cure and improvement rates at 3 months were 25% and 29.2% in the treatment and sham treatment groups, respectively. Rates of objective cure (negative stress test results on urodynamic studies) were 15% of treatment group and 12% of control group. Subjective cure was improvement in 25% in the treatment group and 29% in the control group.

Bourcier and Juras[39] conducted a study to establish the effectiveness of two different modalities: home treatment, consisting of daily application for 20 minutes twice daily for a 6-week period; and office therapy, consisting of twice weekly treatment administered in the clinic for an average of 12 sessions. Of the 95 patients included in the study, 50 received home treatment and 45 received office therapy. Twelve patients had undergone a hysterectomy, and six had previously undergone colposuspension. All were evaluated with urodynamic tests. Home treatment consisted of daily application for 20 minutes twice daily for a 6-week period. Patients with urge incontinence received biphasic capacity coupled pulses with a continuous current of 20 Hz at a pulse width of 0.75 msec. Patients with genuine stress incontinence received biphasic square pulses of 50 Hz at a pulse width of 1 msec. Current intensity was 0 to 90 mA or 0 to 24 V.

During the first follow-up period (3 months), 71% of patients in the office therapy group reported subjective improvement, as did 51% of patients in the home treatment group. During the late follow-up period (6 months), 85 patients were studied (7 patients in the home treatment group and 3 in the office therapy group withdrew).

Of the patients who participated in late follow-up, 47 patients were in the office therapy group (28 patients with genuine stress incontinence and 19 with urinary incontinence) and 38 patients were in the home treatment group (23 patients with genuine stress incontinence and 15 with urinary incontinence).

The cure rate was approximately 50%. This study shows that both office therapy and home treatment are effective forms of treatment for patients with genuine stress incontinence or urinary incontinence. In addition, this treatment has no side effects. The results show a higher degree of improvement with office therapy than with home treatment. The number of patients who did not continue physiotherapy is much higher in the group with urge incontinence (43%) than in the group with genuine stress incontinence (15%). Patients with urge incontinence had less motivation to continue with therapy and also had a higher degree of psychological factors (e.g., chronic depression, psychosomatic disturbances, hysterical personality), which included reluctance to cooperate actively with treatment. Many factors (age, severity of incontinence) are less crucial than previously thought, but the single factor that is consistently associated with positive outcome is greater motivation and/or compliance with the intervention.[50]

Laycock and Jerwood[51] conducted a randomized trial comparing electrical stimulation with interferential therapy with sham electrical stimulation in 30 women with genuine stress incontinence (treatment group, $n = 15$; placebo group, $n = 15$). The placebo group was treated for 30 minutes (10 minutes at 1 Hz, 10 minutes at a 10–40 Hz sweep, and 10 minutes at 40 Hz). Patients in the treatment group had an average of 10 sessions with perineal body and symphysis pubis electrodes, with treatment administered at the maximum acceptable intensity. The placebo group underwent sham electrical stimulation with no current in the patient circuit. In both groups, the results of the pad test were reduced, but a significantly greater reduction in urine loss occurred in the treatment group ($P = 0.0085$). Perineometry showed a significant increase in strength in the treatment group only. The assessment of muscle strength involves digital palpation (power is graded from 0 to 5) as well as use of a perineometer. This device, when connected to a manometer, registers changes in pressure to a voluntary pelvic floor muscle contraction. Sensitivity depends on the device. Frequency of voids decreased significantly in the treatment group only. The authors reported subjective cure or improvement in 33.3% of the electrical stimulation group versus 27.3% of the sham electrical stimulation group, but did not state the time of assessment.

Brubaker and colleagues[52] compared electrical stimulation with sham electrical stimulation in women with urodynamically proven detrusor instability, and found a significant reduction in detrusor overactivity in the electrical stimulation group only. This prospective double-blind, randomized control trial included 121 women who had genuine stress incontinence (n = 60), urge incontinence (n = 28), and mixed incontinence (n = 33). The study had two groups: treated group (n = 61) and placebo controlled group (n = 60) with sham electrical stimulation. Patients underwent 8 weeks of treatment, which was administered twice daily for 20 minutes. Electrical stimulation was administered twice daily with a vaginal probe at 20 Hz with a pulse duration of 0.1 msec with 2 seconds "on" and 4 seconds "off." The output was 0–100 mA; in the placebo group, sham electrical stimulation was characterized by no current in patient circuit. Objective cure was reported in 49% of patients in the treatment group who had detrusor instability, and no change was observed in genuine stress incontinence in either group. The authors found no significant change in the number of women who had genuine stress incontinence on urodynamic testing at 2 months.

On the basis of the various above studies, it appeared that there were considerable variations in electrical protocols but there is a trend in favor of active stimulation over placebo stimulation, specially for patients with overactive bladder. The results in the electrical protocols are demonstrated in the following:

- Post-treatment follow-up and drop out of 6 weeks[43] to 7 years.[53] Follow-up periods were variable, with the shortest time being 6 weeks[43] and the largest 7 years.[53] The most commonly used outcome measures included a voiding diary,[48] a self-assessment[43,48] and urodynamic evaluation.[17,43]
- Frequency and pulse width. The most commonly used frequency was 20[52] to 50 Hz,[49] with some trials reporting the use of 35 Hz.[44] Pulse width ranges from 0.08[54] to 100 msec.[52]
- Duration of treatment. The length of treatments was also variable, from one single 20-minute treatment to treatments lasting several months. The shortest treatment was 10 sessions,[55] and the longest treatment was 6 months.[56] Medium-length treatment periods were based on twice-daily stimulation for 8 to 12 weeks.
- Type of current waveform. Berghmans[57] reported the use of alternating biphasic and rectangular pulses at a frequency of 10 to 40 Hz.

The First International Consultation on Incontinence[58] recommended further high-quality randomized control trials, with long-term follow-up, to investigate all aspects of the use of electrical stimulation in the treatment of urinary incontinence. The second report[59] concludes, "There is a lack of consistency in electrical protocols that implies a lack of understanding of the physiological principles of rehabilitating urinary incontinence through electrical stimulation. There are many differences in clinical application that have not yet been investigated. It seems likely to continue until the infinite variation of stimulation parameters available to researchers and clinicians is narrowed by further investigation into the biologic rationale underpinning electrical stimulation."

CONCLUSION

A number of methods have been used to stimulate the striated muscles of the pelvic floor, including the levator ani, external urethral sphincter, and external anal sphincter. Correction of continence with electrical stimulation has been achieved with various techniques, with results showing both increased urethral closure pressure and bladder inhibition. Electrical stimulation is indicated for patients who are not strongly motivated to perform pelvic floor exercises, for those with weak pelvic floor muscle activity, and for those with contraindications to surgery (genuine stress incontinence) or medication (urinary incontinence). Electrical stimulation is an effective mode of therapy for urinary incontinence and pelvic floor dysfunction. As the use of electrotherapy grows due to advances in technology, it is necessary that health care professionals carefully analyze innovative applications and demand a demonstration on the efficacy of this therapy.

REFERENCES

1. Bors E: Effect of electrical stimulation of the pudendal nerves on the vesical neck: Its significance for the function of cord bladders. J Urol 167:925, 1952.
2. Caldwell KP: The electrical control of sphincter incompetence. Lancet 2:174–175, 1963.
3. Alexander S, Rowan D: Electrical control of urinary incontinence by radio implant: A report of 14 patients. Br J Surg 55:358–364, 1968.
4. Suhel P: Adjustable nonimplantable electrical stimulation for correction of urinary incontinence. Urol Int 31:115–123, 1976.
5. Godec C, Cass AS, Ayala G: Bladder inhibition with functional, electrical stimulation. Urology 6:663–666, 1975.
6. Fall M, Lindstrom S: Electrical stimulation: A physiologic approach to the treatment of urinary incontinence. Urol Clin North Am 18(2):393–407, 1991.
7. Fall M, Erlandson BE, Carlsson CA, Lindström S: The effect of intravaginal electrical stimulation on the feline

urethra and urinary bladder. Scand J Urol Nephrol 44:19–30, 1978.
8. Erlandson BE, Fall M, Carlsson CA, Linder L: Mechanisms for closure of the human urethra during intravaginal electrical stimulation. Scand J Urol Nephrol 44 (suppl):49–54, 1978.
9. Fall M, Lindstrom SHG: Inhibition of overactive bladder by functional electrical stimulation. In Appell RA, Bourcier AP, La Torre F (eds): Pelvic Floor Dysfunction: Investigations and Conservative Treatment. Rome, Casa Editrice Scientifica Internazionale, 1999, pp 267–272.
10. Vodusek DB, Light JK, Libby JM: Detrusor inhibition induced by stimulation of pudendal nerve afferents. Neurourol Urodynam 5:381–389, 1986.
11. Sundin T, Carlsson CA: Reconstruction of severed dorsal roots innervating the urinary bladder: An experimental study in cats. Studies on the normal afferent pathways in the pelvic and pudendal nerves. Scand J Urol Nephrol 6:176–184, 1972.
12. Plevnik S, Janez J, Vrtacnick P, et al: Short-term electrical stimulation: Home treatment for urinary incontinence. World J of Urology 4:24–26, 1986.
13. Crago PE, Peckham PH, Mortimer JT, Van der Meulen JP: The choice of pulse duration for chronic electrical stimulation via surface, nerve and intramuscular electrodes. Ann Biomed Eng 2:252, 1974.
14. Lindstrom S, Fall M, Carlsson CA, Erlandson BE: The neurophysiologic basis of bladder inhibition in response to intravaginal electrical stimulation. J Urol 129:405–407, 1983.
15. Mantle J: Physiotherapy for Incontinence. In Cardozo L, Staskin D (eds): Textbook of Female Urology and Urogyneacology. London, Isis Medical Media, 2001, pp 351–358.
16. Bazed MA, Thüroff JW, Schmidt RA: Effect of chronic electrostimulation of the sacral roots on the striated urethral sphincter. J Urol 128:1357, 1982.
17. Eriksen BC, Eik-Nes SH: Long-term electrostimulation of the pelvic floor: Primary therapy in female stress incontinence. Urol Int 44:90–95, 1989.
18. Eriksen BC: Urinary incontinence: Electrical stimulation. In Besnon JT (ed): Female Pelvic Floor Disorders, Investigations and Management. New York, Norton Medical Books WW Norton, 1992, pp 219–231.
19. Laycock J, Plevnik S, Senn E: Electrical stimulation. In Schüssler B, Laycock J, Norton P, Stanton S (eds): Pelvic Floor Re-education: Principles and Practice. London, Springer-Verlag 1994, pp 143–153.
20. Bourcier AP: New variant technology. Pelvic Floor Rehabilitation Workshop, Seoul National University Hospital, Seoul, Korea. June 16, 2001, pp 1–7.
21. Keane DP, Bayley AJ, Abrams P, Sims TJ: Analysis of collagen status in premenopausal nulliparous women in genuine stress incontinence. Br J Obstet Gynecol 104:994–998, 1997.
22. Makinen J, Sonderstrom KO, Kuohoma P, Hirvonen T: Histological changes in the vaginal connective tissue of patients with and without uterine prolapse. Arch Gynecol 239:17–20, 1986.
23. Van Geelen JM, Doesburg WH: Urodynamics studies in the normal menstrual cycle: The relationship between hormonal changes during the menstrual cycle and the urethral pressure profile. Am J Obstet Gynecol 41:384–392, 1981.
24. Zaccharin RF: A "Chinese anatomy": The pelvic supporting tissue of the Chinese and occidental female compared and contrasted. Aust N Z Obstet Gyencol 17:1, 1997.
25. Kloth LC: Interference current. In Nelson RM, Curier DP (eds): Clinical Electrotherapy, ed 2. Norwalk, Appleton & Lange, 1991, p 221.
26. Olah KS, Bridges N, Denning J: The conservative management of patients with symptoms of stress incontinence: A randomized, prospective study comparing weighted vaginal cones and interferential therapy. Am J Obstet Gynecol 162:87, 1990.
27. Laycock J, Green RJ: Interferential therapy in the treatment of incontinence. Physiotherapy 74:161, 1988.
28. Laycock J: Interferential therapy in the treatment of genuine stress incontinence. In Proceedings of the 18th Annual Meeting of the International Continence Society. Neurourol Urodynam 7:268–269, 1988.
29. McGuire EJ: Treatment of motor and sensory detrusor instability by electrical stimulation. J Urol 129:78, 1983.
30. Fynes M, Cleaver S, Murray C, et al: Evaluation of the effect of posterior tibial nerve stimulation in women with intractable urge urinary incontinence. In Proceedings of the 31st Annual Meeting of the International Continence Society. Neurourol Urodynam 20:116, 2001.
31. Sultan AH, Kamm MA, Hudson CN: Pudendal nerve damage during labour: Prospective study before and after childbirth. Br J Obstet Gynaecol 101:22–28, 1994.
32. Benson JT, McCellan EJ, Pillai-Allen AV: Bulbocavernosus reflex study in asymptomatic females (abstract). Int J Urogynecol 4(6):403, 1993.
33. Smith ARB, Hosker GL, Warrell DW: The role of pudendal nerve damage in the aetiology of genuine stress incontinence in women. Br J Obstet Gyencol 96:29–32, 1989.
34. Gilpin SA, Gosling JA, Smith ARB, Warrell DW: The pathogenesis of genitourinary prolapse and stress incontinence of urine: A histological and histochemical study. Br J Obstet Gynaecol 96:15–23, 1989.
35. Cummings JP: Electrical stimulation of denervated muscles. In Gersh MR (ed): Electrotherapy in Rehabilitation. Philadelphia, FA Davis, 1992, p 269.
36. Spielholz NI: Electrical stimulation of denervated muscle. In Nelson RM, Curier DP (eds): Clinical Electrotherapy, ed 2. Norwalk, Appleton & Lange, 1991, 121.
37. Cole BG, Gardiner PF: Does electrical stimulation of denervated muscle continued after reinnervation, influence of recovery of contractile function? Exp Neurol 85:52, 1984.
38. Bourcier AP: Office therapy and home care perineal stimulation. Urodynam Neurourodynam Continence 2:83–85, 1992.
39. Bourcier AP, Juras JC: Electrical stimulation: Home treatment versus office therapy. Eighty-ninth Annual Meeting of American Urological Association, San Francisco, May 14–19, 1994. J Urol 151(5):1171, 1994.
40. Bourcier AP, Mamberti-Dias A, Susset J: Functional electrical stimulation in uro-gynecology. In Appell RA, Bourcier AP, La Torre F (eds): Pelvic Floor Dysfunction: Investigations and Conservative Treatment. Rome, Casa Editrice Scientifica Internazionale, 1999, pp 259–266.
41. Sand PK: Pelvic floor stimulation treatment of the low pressure urethra. Int J Urogynecol 4(6):403, 1993.
42. Bourcier AP: Evaluation and nonsurgical management: Biofeedback and electrical stimulation. In Blaivas J, Karraum M (eds): Proceedings of the Second International Seminar on Female Urology and Urogynecology, Bal Harbour, June 26–28. Yardley, PA, Fusion Medical Education LLC, 2003, pp 1–8.
43. Shepherd AM, Tribe E, Bainton D: Maximum perineal stimulation: A controlled study. Br J Urol 56:644–646, 1984.
44. Knight S, Laycock J, Naylor D: Evaluation of neuromuscular electrical stimulation in the treatment of genuine stress incontinence. Physiotherapy 84(2):61–71,1998.
45. Eriksen BC, Eik-Nes SH: Long-term electrostimulation of the pelvic floor: Primary therapy in female stress incontinence. Urol Int 44:90–95, 1989.

46. Kralj B: Treatment of idiopathic urge incontinence with functional electrical stimulation. Proceedings of the International Uro Gynecological Association 18th Annual Meeting, Nîmes, France, 1993, p 323.
47. Bent AE, Sand PK, Ostergard DR, Brubaker LT: Transvaginal electrical stimulation in the treatment of genuine stress incontinence and detrusor instability. Int Gynecol J 4:9–13, 1993.
48. Sand PK, Richardson DA, Statskin DR, et al: Pelvic floor electrical stimulation in the treatment of genuine stress incontinence: A multicenter, placebo-controlled trial. Am J Obstet Gynecol 173:72–79, 1995.
49. Luber KM, Wolde-Tsadik G: Efficacy of functional electrical stimulation in treating genuine stress incontinence: A randomised clinical trial. Neurourol Urodynam 16:536–540, 1997.
50. Lagro-Jansen ALM, Debryune FMJ, Smith AJA, Van Weel C: The effects of treatment of urinary incontinence in general practice. Fam Pract 9:284–289, 1992.
51. Laycock J, Jerwood D: Does pre-modulated interferential therapy cure genuine stress incontinence? Physiotherapy 79:553–560, 1993.
52. Brubaker L, Benson T, Bent A, et al: Transvaginal electrical stimulation for female urinary incontinence. Am J Obstet Gynecol 177:536–540, 1997.
53. Bourcier A, Juras J: Pelvic floor rehabilitation: A seven year follow-up. Proceedings of the Abstract Books of the International Continence Society 24th Annual Meeting, Prague. 1994, pp 43–44.
54. Blowman C, Pickels C, Emery S, et al: Prospective double-blind control trial of intense physiotherapy with and without stimulation of the pelvic floor in the treatment of genuine stress incontinence. Physiotherapy 77:661–664, 1991.
55. Henella SM, Hutchins CJ, Robinson P, Macvicar J: Non operative method in the treatment of female genuine stress incontinence of urine. J Obstet Gynecol 9:222–225, 1989.
56. Bo K, Talseth T, Holme I: Single blind, randomized controlled trial of the pelvic floor exercises, electrical stimulation, vaginal cones and no treatment in management of genuine stress incontinence in women. BMJ 318(7182):487–493, 1999.
57. Berghmans LCM, Van Waalwijk V, Van Doorm ESC, et al: Efficacy of extramural physical therapy modalities in women with proven bladder overactivity: A randomized clinical trial. Neurology and Urodynamics 19(4):496–497, 2000.
58. Wilson PD, Bo K, Bourcier A, et al: Conservative management in women. In Abrams P, Khoury S, Wein A (eds): Incontinence. Plymouth, Plymbridge, 1999, pp 579–636.
59. Wilson PD, Bo K, Hay-Smith J, et al: Conservative treatment in women. In Abrams P, Cardozo L, Khoury S, Wein A (eds): Incontinence. Plymouth, Plymbridge, 2001, pp 571–624.

CHAPTER 30

Extracorporeal Electromagnetic Stimulation Therapy

ROGER P. GOLDBERG ■ NIALL T. M. GALLOWAY ■ PETER K. SAND

ELECTROMAGNETIC STIMULATION: SCIENCE AND MEDICAL APPLICATIONS

The therapeutic potential of magnetic energy has been a subject of long-standing interest within both conventional and alternative medical practice. Many devices that use either permanent magnets or changing magnetic fields claim a wide variety of clinical benefits, some real and others disproved. For diagnosing and treating bladder and pelvic floor dysfunction, extracorporeal magnetic stimulation of the sacral nerve roots continues to evolve as a noninvasive treatment for incontinence and other lower urinary tract disorders, and an alternative to transcutaneous electrical neuromodulation. The conduction characteristics of magnetic energy confer several practical advantages for its use as a noninvasive treatment alternative. Moreover, its clinical application may provide theoretical insight into the neurobiology of the pelvic floor and lower urinary tract. This chapter examines the use of extracorporeal electromagnetic stimulation for managing urinary incontinence, bladder disease, and other pelvic floor dysfunction, and describes the history of the therapeutic application of electromagnetic energy.

Background

In the 18th century, an Italian physician and astronomer named Galvani first used a battery made of copper and iron to trigger the twitch of a frog's leg. Since then, the relationship between electrical charge and magnetism has been explored and understood with ever-increasing depth. In the most basic terms, the movement of any particle or electric current generates a surrounding circular magnetic field. Conversely, exposing an electric conductor (whether a metallic object or human tissue) to a changing magnetic field induces the flow of electrical current through a shift of electrons. Electromagnetic radiation consists of both electric and magnetic waveforms that travel in tandem at right angles to one another, across a variety of frequencies.

Many generations after Galvani and Faraday, these classic findings have found widespread application throughout the modern world. Electromagnetic fields are a ubiquitous feature of the high-tech landscape, in the form of electrical power lines, cellular phones, and personal technology devices. In the medical realm, magnetic resonance imaging is the most familiar application of electromagnetic energy, which is considered the safest and most precise technique for modern diagnostic imaging. Electromagnetic fields that are generated to stimulate the peripheral and central nervous systems share the same fundamental components, and no adverse effects have been reported.[1]

Pulsed electromagnetic fields, rather than continuous fields, are most commonly used for the stimulation of human tissue. These fields are generated by high-voltage electric currents applied to a surface stimulation coil. At the tissue level, electrical eddy currents are induced by a flow of ions establishing differences in voltage between two spatial points. If the voltage gradient is sufficiently strong and the change of field is rapid, membrane depolarization occurs, establishing an action potential along adjacent peripheral nerve tissue.[2] In the pelvis, stimulation of the lumbosacral roots initiates this sequence of events, leading to nerve depolarization, stimulation of the motor end plates, and ultimately, pelvic floor muscle contraction. Thus, in contrast to electrical stimulation, which directly stimulates the nerve,[3] magnetic stimulation is a vehicle that secondarily generates ion flow and eddy currents to which nerve tissue is particularly sensitive. Despite this distinction, no differences appear to exist between electrical and magnetic stimulation in the nature of the eventual nerve depolarization and the movement of action potentials along the axon.[4]

Early commercial magnetic stimulation units operated in a single-pulse mode. These units were followed by repetitive stimulators.[5] Conventional stimulators deliver pulses of less than 100-μsec duration, at frequencies of 20 to 50 Hz. The depth of magnetic field penetration, or focal length, is proportional to the diameter of the stimulating coil. The strength of the induced electrical field decreases exponentially with distance from the core. The spatial distribution of the maximum magnetic field reflects the size and shape of the stimulating coil, usually a hollow-centered "doughnut," in contrast to the "bull's-eye" field that is created by electrical stimulation. Most extracorporeal pelvic floor stimulation units use concave saddle-shaped coils. Advanced iron-core coils have been developed to eliminate the need for external cooling systems while the sacral nerve roots and pelvic floor are stimulated at frequencies of up to 50 Hz for extended periods.[6] Recent design modifications allow for a focal depth of up to 6 cm and a bull's-eye-shaped stimulating field, enhancing the ability to target deeper pelvic structures.

Perhaps the single most important feature of magnetic energy, distinguishing it from electrical current, is that its conduction is unaffected by tissue impedance. Electrical stimulation requires relatively high voltages at the skin to compensate for decay as the current traverses soft tissue and bone.[7] As a result, transvaginal and transrectal probes are used for more direct application of the energy source to the pelvic floor nerves and musculature. Although these devices have proven effective in many patients, the inconvenience and occasional discomfort associated with probe insertion, particularly in the setting of vaginal atrophy, stenosis, or prolapse, tends to limit compliance with therapy. In contrast, the strength of the electromagnetic field (measured in teslas) decreases predictably with the inverse square of the distance from the source of the electromagnetic field, regardless of the tissue density encountered along that distance. This indifference of magnetic field transmission to tissue density confers major advantages for its clinical application, because establishing a current at the nerve root level requires relatively little current to be generated at the body surface. Thus, deep structures, such as the lumbar roots, brachial plexus, and sciatic and femoral nerves, can be magnetically stimulated without patient discomfort. Additionally, extracorporeal magnetic stimulation produces minimal heat at the target tissue level, while maintaining eddy current densities estimated at more than 12.7 $\mu A/mm^{-2}$.

Effects on Human Tissue

In 1965, Bickford and Fremming[8] reported on the stimulation of peripheral nerves with a sinusoidal magnetic field, provoking muscle contradictions. Single-pulse stimulation of peripheral nerves was later shown to trigger muscle action potentials[9] caused by electrical depolarization within the field. Since that time, magnetic fields have been clinically applied to both central and peripheral nerves. For example, transcranial electromagnetic stimulation with 1.5 to 2.0 tesla has been used as an alternative to electroconvulsive therapy for the treatment of depression and to trigger seizure activity during ablation neurosurgery. Extracorporeal magnetic innervation has been used peripherally to alleviate pain syndromes, improve neuromuscular function in patients with chronic progressive multiple sclerosis, and trigger electrical osteogenesis in patients with hypoplastic bone disorders, with modest success. Along the cervical spine, magnetic stimulation of the phrenic nerves has been used in critical care settings to assess diaphragmatic contractility in ventilator-dependent patients. This treatment was as effective as electrical stimulation, but less painful.[10]

ELECTROMAGNETIC STIMULATION OF THE PELVIC FLOOR

Magnetic pulses can facilitate the stimulation of autonomic and somatic nerve pathways in the pelvic floor, without the use of electrodes.[11] As reported by Opsomer and associates[12] and several investigators since then,[13,14] magnetic fields applied to the S2–S4 nerve roots trigger motor evoked potentials in the pelvic sphincter muscles and toe flexors, with a latency of 25 to 30 msec.[15] Single-pulse magnetically evoked motor potentials may provide a useful alternative to conventional electrical stimulation for nerve conduction and latency studies.[16] For therapeutic application, it was first reported in 1995 that high-frequency, or continuous, magnetic stimulation of S3, delivering up to 20 pulses/sec, produces clinically useful stimulation of the pelvic floor musculature, increased pressure in the anal canal,[17] and contraction of the external sphincter. Extracorporeal magnetic innervation technology has been incorporated into a commercial product, the NeoControl Pelvic Floor Therapy System (Neotonus, Atlanta, GA), which has been approved by the US Food and Drug Administration for the treatment of urinary incontinence in women. Clinical trials are underway to assess the utility of electromagnetic innervation for fecal incontinence, sexual dysfunction, postpartum pelvic floor rehabilitation, interstitial cystitis, postprostatectomy urinary incontinence, and fecal incontinence. Preliminary results show significant efficacy for treating chronic pelvic pain syndrome in men. At 3 months, the 62% response rate was significantly greater than the rate of 13% in patients treated with placebo ($P = 0.05$).[18]

Extracorporeal electromagnetic stimulation does not require any probes, skin preparation, or physical or electrical contact with the skin surface. The patient sits fully clothed on a chair that contains an electromagnet controlled by an external power source. Optimal coil position can be mapped by visual confirmation of toe flexion or anal contractions. Alternatively, for research purposes, objective measurement may be obtained from surface electromyographic recordings of the lateral foot or the anal sphincter. The amplitude of the pulsating current can be adjusted to achieve an appropriate field volume and induce a nerve impulse. Maximal response of the pudendal nerve for detrusor inhibition appears to occur after stimulation 10 cm below the iliac crest and 5 cm lateral to the midline.[19] In clinical practice, treatment is typically performed for 6 to 10 weeks before patient response is evaluated. This time frame is similar to that associated with most other forms of pelvic rehabilitation.

The precise action of magnetic stimulation on the sacral nerve roots, pelvic floor, and continence mechanism is not fully understood. The term neuromodulation implies an overall retraining of nerve activity, and magnetic stimulation likely acts through several neurologic pathways that contribute to coordinated micturition. Pelvic floor afferents, autonomic efferents, and somatic motor fibers play a role in supplying the pelvic floor musculature and striated sphincters,[20] although the relative importance of each component, with respect to the efficacy of pelvic floor stimulation, remains unclear. Furthermore, the neuromuscular structure of the pelvic floor can vary widely between individual patients, specifically with respect to the amount of functional muscle mass present and the order or disorder of activity among the resident population of motor units. For example, inducing contractions within a pelvic floor that is characterized by severely atrophic muscles requires higher thresholds, and will likely be limited by a lower ceiling of maximum therapeutic potential, compared with a case of mildly weakened pelvic musculature. The composition of nerve fibers targeted by extracorporeal magnetic stimulation may also differ widely between individual patients. For example, animal models have shown that after spinal injury, the afferent neurons within the sacral micturition reflex arc undergo a transformation from predominantly larger myelinated fibers to small, unmyelinated C-fibers. Thus, in different clinical scenarios, magnetic neuromodulation may act on significantly different populations of both nerve units and muscle fibers. As a result, the clinical efficacy of electromagnetic stimulation varies accordingly.

Magnetic Neuromodulation for Bladder Overactivity

In broad terms, detrusor instability appears to result from imbalances between facilitative and inhibitory signals within the voiding reflex.[21] Suppression of involuntary detrusor activity by neuromodulation may be explained by at least two effects on the autonomic balance. These are activation of pudendal nerve afferents blocking parasympathetic detrusor motor fibers through the spinal reflex arc and activation of inhibitory hypogastric sympathetic neurons. These effects may occur alone or in combination.[22] The relative importance of parasympathetic stimulation versus sympathetic inhibition is uncertain. Some investigators argue that parasympathetic efferent fibers innervating the bladder are not activated by S3 magnetic stimulation because they are unmyelinated and small, with a relatively high tissue membrane capacitance, compared with myelinated alpha afferents and somatic motor fibers.[4,19] Stimulation of sympathetic fibers, particularly those that maintain smooth muscle tone within the intrinsic urethral sphincter, is probably an important secondary mechanism of action.

Modulation of somatic nerve activity also appears to play a role. Stimulation of pudendal nerve afferent branches probably creates an inhibitory spinal reflex through vesicoinhibitory pathways at the S3 nerve root, similar to the putative effect of electrical stimulation. Additionally, activation of S3 somatic motor efferents that supply the striated external sphincter may promote detrusor relaxation by improving external urethral sphincter tone. Diminished urethral sphincter tone, with funneling of urine into the proximal urethra, causes a reflex detrusor contraction in some animal models. Finally, repetitive maximal contraction of the levator muscle complex may act as a passive Kegel exercise, and facilitate transformation of fast-twitch to slow-twitch striated muscle fibers.[23] The combined effects on both the autonomic and somatic reflex arcs, and reconditioning skeletal muscle to a stronger, more efficient baseline, probably account for the efficacy of pelvic floor stimulation in the treatment of detrusor overactivity.

Clinically, continuous magnetic stimulation has shown efficacy in the treatment of bladder overactivity and urge incontinence. The effect of functional magnetic stimulation on detrusor hyper-reflexia was examined by Sheriff and colleagues[15] in patients after spinal cord injury. Magnetic stimulation successfully inhibited the involuntary contractions that characterize detrusor hyper-reflexia, lowering the magnitude of bladder contractions while increasing bladder capacity and compliance.

McFarlane and associates[19] assessed the immediate effect of magnetic stimulation in 12 patients during bladder contractions associated with idiopathic detrusor instability. Involuntary detrusor contractions were repetitively provoked by rapid infusion of saline into the bladder, and the immediate effect of stimulation of the S3 nerve root was assessed. Stimulation of the S3 nerve root during unstable detrusor contractions stronger than 15 cm H_2O had a suppressive effect in all 12 patients at varying stimulation strengths. The degree of suppression varied directly with the intensity of magnetic stimulation. Furthermore, magnetic stimulation eliminated the subjective sensation of urgency in all cases. Residual suppression of involuntary contractions persisted for up to 70 seconds in three patients; however, longer-term outcomes were not reported. These authors concluded that sacral magnetic stimulation acutely suppressed idiopathic detrusor instability. In another study, normal voiding was suppressed and bladder relaxation occurred after magnetic stimulation of the sacral nerve roots initiated during urination.[24] Finally, Yamanashi and colleagues[25] reported subjective improvement in six of eight women with urge incontinence, as measured by bladder volume at first desire to void ($P = 0.02$), maximum cystometric capacity ($P = 0.02$), nocturia ($P = 0.03$), episodes of daytime leaking ($P = 0.03$), and quality-of-life scores ($P = 0.02$). Objectively, bladder overactivity resolved during cystometry in two of six women with known detrusor instability.

Magnetic Neuromodulation and Voiding Function

Stimulation of the pelvic nerve carrying parasympathetic innervation to the detrusor, at least in theory, could be expected to promote detrusor contraction, and perhaps micturition, in an areflexic bladder.[4] Magnetic stimulation of the sacral roots has been evaluated in this clinical setting. In dogs with neuropathic bladders after pelvic ganglionectomy, Shafik[26] showed significantly increased vesical pressure after intermittent sacral magnetic stimulation, raising the possibility of improved evacuation. Intravenous injection of atropine prevented the vesical response to sacral magnetic stimulation, suggesting a primary role of cholinergic pathways. Although this author suggested a potential role for electromagnetic therapy in the treatment of patients after spinal cord injury, clinical efforts to trigger human micturition by sacral magnetic stimulation have had limited success. Brodak and colleagues[4] evaluated magnetic stimulation in the treatment of 11 patients with spinal cord injury, and elicited a detrusor response in seven of nine responders. However, the contraction strength at maximum magnetic stimulation averaged only 12 cm H_2O, which is insufficient for bladder emptying. More recently, Lin and colleagues[27] evaluated the efficacy of magnetic stimulation for promoting micturition of the acontractile bladder in humans. Using sacral and suprapubic stimulation, the authors reported a mean change in bladder pressure (P_{ves}) of 24.4 and 16.5 cm H_2O, respectively. Clinically, 17 of 22 patients with spinal cord injury were able to void. The increased vesical pressure was not likely to be an artifact of elevated intra-abdominal pressure, because neither abdominal muscle contraction nor rectus muscle electromyographic activity appears to increase during sacral magnetic stimulation.[28]

Magnetic Neuromodulation for Stress and Mixed Incontinence

A prospective multicenter observational study was conducted to evaluate extracorporeal magnetic enervation for the treatment of stress urinary incontinence. Biweekly treatments, each lasting 20 minutes (10 minutes at 5 Hz and 10 minutes at 50 Hz), were administered for 6 consecutive weeks. No control group was included in the study design. Early results were reported on 50 patients who were evaluated for more than 3 months. Within the initial sample, 17 (34%) were dry, 16 (32%) were not using more than one pad daily, and 17 (34%) were using more than one pad daily. Pad use was reduced from 2.5 to 1.3 ($P = 0.001$), and the mean number of episodes of daytime leakage decreased from 3.3 to 1.7 ($P = 0.001$). Among 69 women with stress incontinence, subjective improvement was reported in 77% after 6 weeks of twice-weekly therapy, with 56% reporting no leakage. Pad use was reduced from 2.3 daily at baseline to 0.5 daily ($P < 0.05$), and mean pad weight decreased from 4.5 to 0.5 oz ($P < 0.05$). Daily episodes of leakage declined from 2.5 to 0.8 daily ($P < 0.05$), and quality-of-life scores improved significantly. No differences from baseline were found in pad weight. These findings compare favorably with those reported for electrical stimulation, for which cure rates for stress urinary incontinence range from 8% to 90%.[25,29] However, notably, 17% of women in this sample reported more episodes of incontinence at 2 weeks, compared with their pretreatment survey. At the 18-week visit, 22% reported overall worsening of symptoms. Long-term follow-up of 47 patients who completed more than 6 months of follow-up was reported.[30] At 6 months, 13 women (28%) were completely dry and 25 (53%) were using one pad or less daily. Pad use was decreased in 33 women (70%), and the number of pads used daily remained significantly lower (2.2 vs. 1; $P < 0.005$) within the cohort.

The risk factors that predict success of extracorporeal electromagnetic stimulation were evaluated in this same study group with a case–control retrospective analysis.[31] Successful response to therapy was statistically linked to the absence of four risk factors: (1) previous hysterectomy, (2) previous anti-incontinence procedures, (3) incontinence lasting more than 10 years, and (4) the use of drugs known to cause incontinence. Among patients who met these criteria, 69% had greater than 50% improvement at 2 weeks and 57% had greater than 50% improvement at 18 weeks after treatment. In this subgroup, complete cure was achieved in 44% at 2 weeks and in 43% at 18 weeks.

Other factors may affect the success of extracorporeal magnetic stimulation. Brodak and associates[4] observed that body habitus may influence treatment outcome. The most significant detrusor responses occur in thin patients, presumably because a shorter distance is traversed by the magnetic field, from the stimulating coil to the sacral nerve roots. The same investigators studied the effect of bladder volume on the efficacy of sacral magnetic stimulation in 11 patients with spinal injury.[4] Bladder volume was increased in 100-mL increments until either detrusor instability was observed or a maximum volume of 400 mL was reached. The effect of magnetic stimulation was recorded at these various bladder volumes. No detrusor response was seen at bladder volumes of less than 200 mL; in contrast, seven patients had contractions at volumes greater than 200 mL, although five of these contractions were less than 10 cm H_2O. The authors concluded that the detrusor response to stimulation dampened with increasing bladder volume.

The most effective treatment parameters for extracorporeal magnetic innervation have yet to be determined, including pulse width, number of pulse cycles, and duration of therapy. Protocols reported for the treatment of stress incontinence include cycles of 1 minute on and 30 seconds off, for 15 to 30 minutes, twice weekly for 6 to 8 weeks. However, systematic comparisons of different treatment regimens have not been reported.

Urodynamic Correlates

Most consistently, threshold levels of sacral magnetic stimulation have been shown to elevate urethral pressure. Yamanashi and associates[25] showed a 16% increase in maximum urethral closure pressure after stimulation, compared with the prestimulation level ($P = 0.03$). Women treated with a sham device showed no change in urethral pressure. In another study by the same investigators,[2] 23 patients with incontinence (both stress and urge) showed a 21% increase in maximum urethral closure pressure ($P = 0.04$) and a 34% increase in maximum intraurethral pressure. In patients with stress incontinence who were analyzed separately, mean urethral closure pressure increased by 18%. The effect of magnetic stimulation on urethral pressure appears to be nearly identical to that of electrical stimulation. In fact, when magnetic stimulation and electrical stimulation were applied separately to the same pudendal nerve of the same dog, the same increase in urethral pressure resulted.[2]

In some patients, maximum bladder capacity appears to increase after extracorporeal magnetic innervation. McFarlane and associates[19] showed increases in cystometric filling volume after magnetic stimulation of S3. Similarly, Yamanashi and associates[25] showed increased bladder volumes at first and maximum cystometric capacity, during stimulation of patients with urge incontinence. On the other hand, one prospective study[32] did not identify significant alterations in urodynamic parameters, including urethral pressure, functional urethral length, and cystometric capacity, after sacral magnetic stimulation. This may be related to the use of different equipment and stimulation parameters.

FUTURE CHALLENGES

Whether magnetic stimulation can produce sustained alterations in neuromuscular activity within the pelvic floor remains a question for future studies to address. Whereas a significant number of patients show an immediate response to electrical stimulation of S3, achieving long-term neuromodulation poses a more formidable clinical challenge. McFarlane and associates[19] showed residual suppression of detrusor overactivity for more than 1 minute after magnetic innervation. Yamanashi and colleagues[25] later found that maximum urethral closure pressure remained significantly greater than pre-stimulation pressures for up to 15 minutes after a functional continuous magnetic stimulation session. In clinical series, individual patients with long-term improvement have been reported,[28] and observational follow-up of a treated cohort of incontinent women was recently obtained by a telephone survey, at a mean of 2.9 years (range, 1.4–3.5).[33] In 50 of 59 women who were reached for follow-up, subjective improvements were found in stress leakage, nocturnal leakage, and perceived volume of urine leaked. Pad usage was significantly less than baseline (1.1 vs. 3.1; $P < 0.001$), and 70% of respondents rated the treatment as effective. Although the study design was uncontrolled and susceptible to recall bias, these results suggest that extracorporeal magnetic innervation may have a sustained effect.

In its current form, magnetic neuromodulation has practical and technical limitations. The need for repeated office-based treatment sessions is a logistical barrier for some women. In addition, in contrast to electrical stimulation units, the current technology lacks portability. Finally, because the depth and width of magnetic field penetration are proportional to coil diameter, current technology remains best suited for stimulation of a field, rather than a narrowly focused target, such as a pinpoint source of pelvic pain.

No medical conditions appear to pose a particular hazard to patients receiving extracorporeal magnetic stimulation. Concern about the induction of ventricular fibrillation was addressed in animal models by several investigators, with no cases induced in dogs using field strengths of up to 2.4 tesla.[34] The risk of triggering epileptic foci was a topic of theoretical concern during the early use of transcranial magnetic stimulation, but has not been an issue in its clinical application. Perhaps the strongest evidence supporting the safety of magnetic stimulation is the absence of adverse effects from magnetic resonance imaging, which uses strong and continuous electromagnetic field exposure throughout the body.

CONCLUSION

Extracorporeal magnetic stimulation is used to stimulate peripheral nerves in a manner similar to electrical stimulation, with several important clinical advantages. Because magnetic energy conducts through tissue layers with minimal attenuation, transcutaneous stimulation of deep anatomic structures, such as sacral nerve roots, is possible with minimal patient discomfort. The mechanisms that explain the clinical efficacy of this technique have not been fully outlined, but magnetic stimulation appears to induce reflex inhibitory effects on the detrusor muscle through both afferent and efferent stimulation of sacral nerves and through both autonomic and somatic pathways, similar to electrical sacral nerve stimulation.[21] Prospective clinical follow-up has shown subjective and objective improvement after 6 weeks of treatment with extracorporeal magnetic innervation. Six months after therapy, pad use remained significantly reduced in 70% of patients, frequency of episodes of leakage decreased from 3.0 to 1.7, and up to 28% of women remained completely dry. Urodynamically, increased urethral pressure and maximum cystometric capacity appear to correlate with clinical efficacy. Perhaps most importantly, improved Incontinence Quality of Life[35] scores are significantly associated with fewer episodes of leakage, fewer pad changes, and reduced urinary frequency after extracorporeal magnetic innervation therapy.[36]

Extracorporeal magnetic stimulation provides a useful alternative for patients who do not respond to drug therapy, are poor surgical candidates, or lack the agility to manage electrical stimulation devices. Ongoing clinical experience with sacral magnetic stimulation and future technical modifications may continue to increase the applicability of this technique as a noninvasive and effective treatment for a wide range of lower urinary tract and pelvic floor disorders.

REFERENCES

1. Jalinous R: Technical and practical aspects of magnetic nerve stimulation. J Clin Neurophysiol 8:10–25, 1991.

2. Ishikawa N, Suda S, Sasaki T, et al: Development of a noninvasive treatment system for urinary incontinence using a functional continuous magnetic stimulator (FCMS). Med Biol Eng Comput 36:704–710, 1998.
3. Barker AT: An introduction to the basic principles of magnetic nerve stimulation. J Clin Neurophysiol 8:26–37, 1991.
4. Brodak PP, Bidair M, Joseph A, et al: Magnetic stimulation of the sacral roots. Neurol Urodynam 152:533–540, 1993.
5. Nielson JF, Klemar B, Kiilerich H: A new high frequency magnetic stimulator with an oil-cooled coil. J Clin Neurophysiol 12(5):460–467, 1995.
6. Appell R, Bourcier AP, Torre F: Pelvic Floor Dysfunction: Investigations and Conservative Treatment. Rome, Casa Editrice Scientifica Internazionale, 1999.
7. Hallett M, Cohen LG: Magnetism: A new method for stimulation of nerve and brain. JAMA 262:538–541, 1989.
8. Bickford RG, Fremming BD: Neuronal stimulation by pulsed magnetic fields in animals and man. Digest of the 6th International Conference on Medicine and Electronics Biology and Engineering, Tokyo 1965, p 112.
9. Polson MJR, Barker AT, Freeston IL: Stimulation of nerve trunks with time-varying magnetic fields. Med Biol Eng Comput 20:243–244, 1982.
10. Laghi F, Harrison MJ, Tobin MJ: Comparison of magnetic and electrical phrenic nerve stimulation in assessment of diaphragmatic contractility. J Appl Psychol 80:1731–1742, 1996.
11. Evans BA: Magnetic stimulation of the peripheral nervous system. J Clin Neurophysiol 8:77–84, 1991.
12. Opsomer RJ, Guerit JM, Wese FX, Van Cangh PJ: Pudendal cortical somatosensory evoked potentials. J Urol 135:1216–1218, 1986.
13. Eardley I, Nagendran K, Kirby RS, Fowler CJ: A new technique for assessing the efferent innervation of the human striated urethral sphincter. J Urol 144:948–951, 1990.
14. Jost WH, Schimrigk K: A method to determine pudendal nerve motor latency and central motor conduction time to the external sphincter. Electroencephalogr Clin Neurophys 93:237–239, 1994.
15. Sheriff MK, Shah PJ, Fowler C, et al: Neuromodulation of detrusor hyper-reflexia by functional magnetic stimulation of the sacral roots. Br J Urol 78:39–46, 1993.
16. Bemelmans BLH, Van Kerrebroeck PEV, Notermans LHS, et al: Motor evoked potentials from the bladder on magnetic stimulation of the cauda equina: A new technique for investigation of autonomic bladder innervation. J Urol 147:658–661, 1992.
17. Craggs MD, Sheriff MKM, Shah PJR, et al: Responses to multi-pulse magnetic stimulation of spinal nerve roots mapped over the sacrum in man. J Physiol 483:127, 1995.
18. Patel A, Rowe E, Laverick L: A prospective randomized, placebo-controlled, double-blinded study of electromagnetic therapy in the treatment of chronic pelvic pain syndrome in men. Poster Presentation, International Bladder Symposium, Washington, DC, March 8–11, 2001.
19. McFarlane JP, Foley SJ, DeWinter P, et al: Acute suppression of idiopathic detrusor instability with magnetic stimulation of the sacral nerve roots. Br J Urol 80:734–741, 1997.
20. Craggs MD, McFarlane JP, Foley SJ, et al: Detrusor relaxation following suppression of normal voiding reflexes by magnetic stimulation of the sacral nerves. J Physiol 53:501P, 1997.
21. Schmidt RA, Jonas U, Oleson KA, et al: Sacral nerve stimulation for the treatment of refractory urinary urge incontinence. J Urol 162(2):352–357, 1999.
22. Linsstrom S, Fall M, Carlsson CA, Erlandson BE: The neurophysiological basis of bladder inhibition in response to intravaginal electrical stimulation. J Urol 129:405–410, 1983.
23. Kralj B: Conservative treatment of female stress urinary incontinence with functional electrical stimulation. Eur J Obstet Gynecol 85:53–56, 1999.
24. Craggs MD, McFarlane JP, Knight SL, et al: Detrusor relaxation of the normal and pathological bladder. Br J Urol 79 (suppl 4):58–59, 1997.
25. Yamanashi T, Yasuda K, Suda S, et al: Effect of functional continuous magnetic stimulation for urinary incontinence. J Urol 163:456–459, 2000.
26. Shafik A: Magnetic stimulation: A novel method for inducing evacuation of the neuropathic rectum and urinary bladder in a canine model. Urology 54(2):368–372, 1999.
27. Lin VW, Wolfe V, Frost FS, Perkash I: Micturition by functional magnetic stimulation. J Spinal Cord Med 20(2):218–226, 1997.
28. Shafik A: Effect of magnetic stimulation on the contractile activity of the rectum in the dog. Eur Surg Res 30:268–272, 1998.
29. Sand PK, Richardson DR, Staskin SE, et al: Pelvic floor stimulation in the treatment of genuine stress incontinence: A multicenter placebo-controlled trial. Am J Obstet Gynecol 173:72–79, 1995.
30. Galloway NTM, El-Galley RES, Sand PK, et al: Update on extracorporeal magnetic innervation therapy for stress urinary incontinence. Urology 56:82–86, 2000.
31. Sand P, Appell R, Bavendam T, et al: Factors influencing success with extracorporeal magnetic innervation (ExMI) treatment of mixed urinary incontinence. Abstract accepted for presentation at the International Bladder Symposium, Washington, DC, November 1999.
32. Galloway NTM, El-Galley RES, Sand PK, et al: Extracorporeal magnetic innervation therapy for stress urinary incontinence. Urology 53(6):1108–1111, 1999.
33. Carlan SJ, Bhullar A: Follow-up of patients who underwent extracorporeal magnetic innervation therapy for urinary incontinence: 2.9 years after initial treatment. Poster presentation, International Bladder Symposium, Washington, DC, March 8–11, 2001.
34. McRobbie DM, Foster MA: Cardiac response to pulsed magnetic fields with regard to safety in NMR imaging. Phys Med Biol 30:695–702, 1985.
35. Wagner TH, Patrick D, Bavendam TG: Quality of life in persons with urinary incontinence: Development of a new measure. Urology 47(1):67–72, 1996.
36. Bavendam T, Braddon L, Carlan S, et al: Impact of extracorporeal magnetic innervation on quality of life in the treatment of stress urinary incontinence. Abstract presentation, American Urological Association, Atlanta, GA, April 2000.

CHAPTER 31

Biofeedback Therapy

ALAIN P. BOURCIER ■ KATHRYN L. BURGIO

Biofeedback is a term for external psychophysiological feedback, physiological feedback, or augmented proprioception. The basic approach is to provide individuals with information about the physiological activities in their bodies, including their brains. The field that deals most directly with information processing and feedback is *cybernetics*.[1,2] Biofeedback can be defined as the use of monitoring equipment to measure internal physiological events, or various body conditions of which the person is usually unaware, to develop conscious control of body processes. Biofeedback is a process that uses instruments to detect, measure, and amplify internal physiological responses to provide the individual with feedback of those responses.[3,4] The field of biofeedback has a rich and fascinating history. For several decades, only the voluntary musculoskeletal system mediated by the central nervous system (CNS) was considered responsive to instrumental learning or operant conditioning. The autonomic nervous system (ANS) was believed to function automatically and even unconsciously. By the 1970s, research had demonstrated that autonomic responses were modifiable and researchers began to investigate the specificity and patterning of learned visceral responses and cognitive mediating strategies for producing visceral changes. Many of the early studies were primarily psychophysiological, examining the effects of feedback on specific physiological systems.[5-10]

The most common modalities of biofeedback involve electromyography (EMG), manometry, thermal measurement, electroencephalography (EEG), electrodermal feedback, and respiration rate. Recently several medical teams have employed biofeedback devices that are partially or totally placed inside the body. These include sensors (EMG, pressure sensors) for detecting and measuring the activity of anal or urinary sphincters and pelvic floor muscles. Techniques have been developed to measure activity of the detrusor muscle for treatment of urinary incontinence and of the anal canal for treatment of fecal incontinence and constipation. This chapter describes treatment of pelvic floor dysfunction. (For information about biofeedback and the management of diseases of colon and rectum, see Chapter 34).

One aim of physical therapy has always been to assist patients by improving their physiologic self-regulation within their natural environment.[11] Biofeedback is a very specific treatment that can restore bladder control by teaching patients to modulate the mechanisms of continence. Biofeedback has now gained several potential applications for urologic conditions, having been successfully used for patients with urologic disorders such as detrusor instability, detrusor sphincter dyssynergia, and enuresis. Also, behavioral therapy can be used in combination with pharmacologic therapy to provide an excellent response with minimal side effects.

A major reason for high interest in biofeedback is that the patient is actively involved in treatment. There are many practical applications of biofeedback in the treatment of lower urinary tract disorders. This chapter presents various methods of biofeedback and describes their use in clinical practice.

BIOFEEDBACK METHODS

Biofeedback makes physiologic change possible by means of operant conditioning or trial-and-error learning, in which a response is learned and performed depending on whether that response is followed by reinforcement. For biofeedback to be useful, four conditions must be met.[12] First, there must be a readily detectable and measurable response, such as bladder pressure or pelvic floor muscle activity. Second, there must be variability in that response, detectable change as opposed to total paralysis. Third, there must be a perceptible cue such as the sensation of urgency that indicates to the patient when control should be performed. Fourth, because biofeedback is based on learning, it requires the active involvement of a motivated patient. Of particular importance is the patient's ability to modify bladder function through operant conditioning. In the application of biofeedback to the treatment of urinary incontinence, the concepts of neurophysiology of voiding and learning and conditioning are combined to accomplish the clinical objective of voluntary control of bladder function.[13,14] The different methods of biofeedback are described next.

Cystometric Biofeedback

During cystometrograms, bladder pressure readings were available to his patients and may have provided a mechanism for feedback that allowed them to acquire better control. He referred to his method as inhibitory re-educative training, but he clearly described a form of intervention that would now be termed biofeedback. Other authors have described similar methods.[15]

The original technique for biofeedback in the management of idiopathic detrusor instability was described by Cardozo and colleagues.[16] After an initial explanation, the patient's detrusor pressure was measured cystometrically and recorded on a chart recorder. A voltage-to-frequency converter was connected to the detrusor-pressure strain-gauge amplifier. This emitted an auditory signal rather like a siren. Alternatively, for patients who exhibited confusing rectal contractions during the treatment sessions, the auditory feedback could be transferred to the intravesical-pressure strain gauge. The gain and frequency range were adjusted to suit the individual patient, but once a baseline tone was decided upon, the note emitted through the loudspeaker increased in pitch as the detrusor pressure rose and decreased as it fell. A mirror was positioned in such a way that the patient could observe the detrusor (or intravesical) pressure tracing. Female patients attended four to eight 1-hour sessions during which the bladder was filled two or three times using 0.9% saline prewarmed to body temperature. When detrusor contractions occurred, they could be heard and seen, and these signals were associated with the symptoms of urgency and urge incontinence. The women were instructed to attempt to control the pitch of the auditory signal by deep breathing, general relaxation, tightening certain muscle groups, or by any other means they found helpful. As patients learned to control their detrusor pressure during supine cystometry, provocative maneuvers such as erect cystometry, laughing, coughing, and running the water taps were employed.[17]

Burgio and colleagues[18] used a similar technique of bladder biofeedback in a behavioral training program for older men and women with urge incontinence. During training sessions, patients observed bladder pressure during retrograde filling and practiced keeping bladder pressure low. Cystometric biofeedback requires the use of transurethral bladder catheter and a rectal pressure monitor for the suppression of the uninhibited contractions (Figs. 31-1 and 31-2). The bladder catheter measures increases in intravesical pressure indicative of uninhibited contractions. The rectal catheter measures and subtracts the intra-abdominal pressure. Artificial filling of the bladder necessary for this technique of biofeedback represents more accurately the conditions under which continence must be achieved during regular daily activities. Although this concept appears to be clinically relevant, filling of the bladder requires catheterization with its associated discomfort and a small degree of risk. Such therapy could be proposed using urodynamics equipment with the biofeedback program included.

Pelvic Floor Muscle Biofeedback

Several approaches have been taken to measuring pelvic floor muscle activity to provide biofeedback: including urethral, vaginal, or anal feedback using manometry or electromyography. An important technical issue is the quality of the signal source used for feedback. As early as the 1940s, Kegel[19,20] developed and used the perineometer, an instrument that consisted of an intravaginal balloon attached to an external pressure gauge, which registered the pressure exerted by the pubococcygeus muscles. It was the first biofeedback device for pelvic floor muscle training. This method uses manometry

FIGURE 31-1 During cystometric biofeedback, bladder pressure readings are available to the patients and may provide feedback that allows them to acquire better control. The rectal catheter measures and subtracts the intra-abdominal pressure. The patient is requested to produce a voluntary pelvic floor contraction when she feels the strong urge to void.

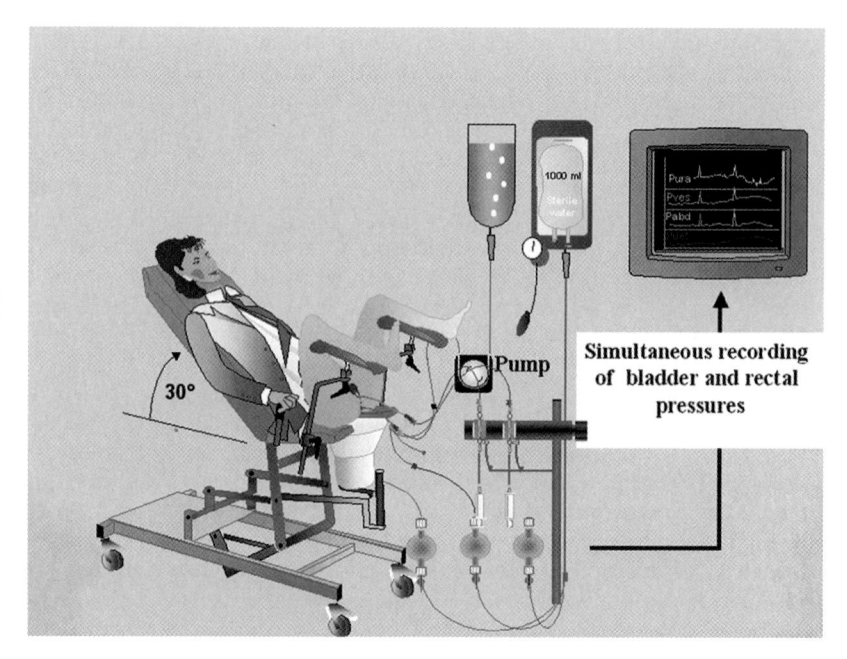

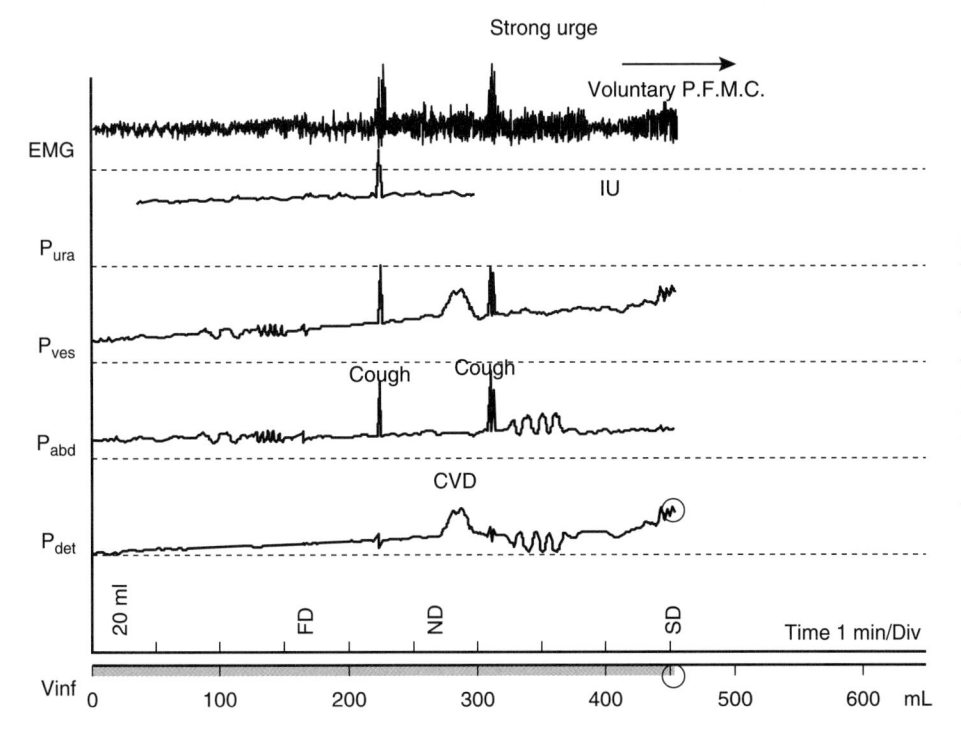

FIGURE 31-2 When detrusor contractions occur they can be seen on the monitor. These signals are associated with symptoms of strong urgency. The patient is requested to produce a voluntary maximum pelvic floor muscle contraction (PMFC) to control the detrusor pressure. EMG, electromyogram; P_{ura}, urethral pressure; P_{ves}, vesical pressure; P_{abd}, intra-abdominal pressure; P_{det}, detrusor pressure; V_{inf}, infusion volume in mL.

(pressure) biofeedback by means of an intravaginal or intrarectal device. An advantage of pressure manometry (Fig. 31-3) is that as the patient contracts her pelvic floor muscles the device produces a resistive pressure that may give additional feedback to the patient (Fig. 31-4).

Following the vaginal manometry method, EMG emerged for recording pelvic floor muscle activity. Different signal sources have been used but EMG activity has evolved as the preferred signal source for many types of biofeedback therapy.[21-23] Electromyographic activity of pelvic floor muscle contractions has become a common signal source for the treatment of urinary incontinence.[24] Vaginal EMG is recorded via surface electrodes in the vaginal introitus or via a vaginal probe (Fig. 31-5) with electrodes embedded. The vaginal probe is easy to insert and remove and most of the time it is comfortable.

Biofeedback of the urethral or anal sphincter or pelvic floor muscles is used in the management of urinary incontinence and voiding difficulties. The external anal sphincter and the external urethral sphincter have similar innervation via branches of the pudendal nerves. Although there are conflicts in the literature about the issue of correspondence between the anal and urethral sphincters, several studies indicate that these muscles act

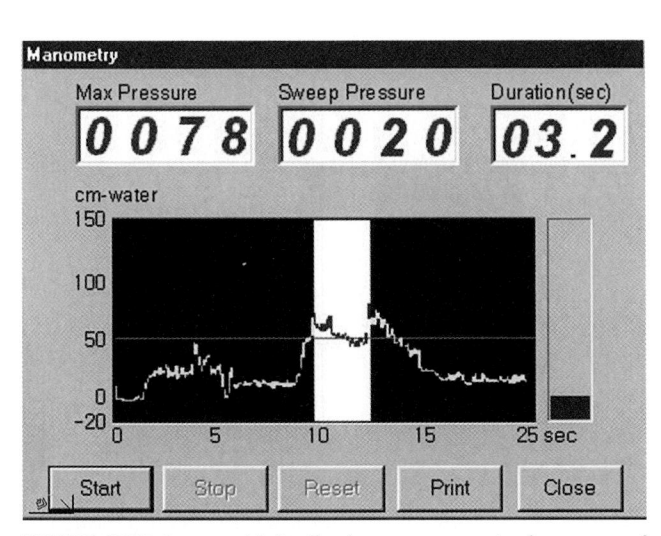

FIGURE 31-3 Pressure biofeedback uses manometry by means of an intravaginal or intrarectal device.

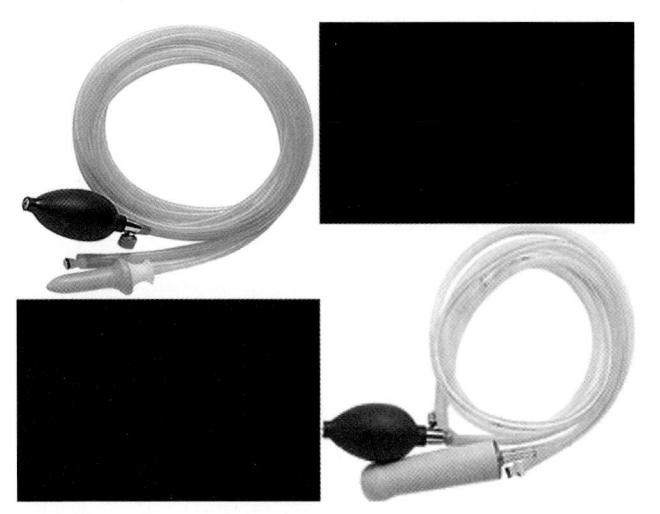

FIGURE 31-4 An advantage to using pressure manometry is the fact that, as the patient contracts her pelvic floor muscles, the device produces a resistive pressure that gives feedback. Biofeedback may involve anal (*top*) or vaginal (*bottom*) manometric probes using pressure with information produced in visual and/or auditory form.

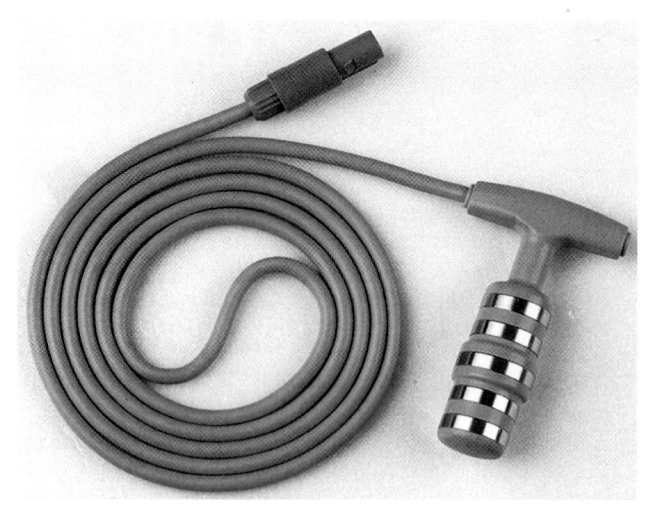

FIGURE 31-5 Vaginal EMG. The vaginal probe is easy to insert and remove and most of the time it is comfortable.

in concert[25] and data indicate that training and controlling the anal sphincter results in urinary sphincter activity that corresponds in magnitude.[26] Anal sphincter activity can be measured by pressure balloons located by the external anal sphincter (for manometry) or by surface electrodes placed around the anus at the 10 o'clock and 2 o'clock positions. Electromyographic activity can be measured also by electrodes embedded in a rectal probe.

The EMG instruments are designed to detect the weak electrical signals generated during muscle contraction. Surface electrodes are electrically conductive pathways in contact with the skin (abdominal muscles) or mucosa (vaginal or anal).

Continuous monitoring of the EMG signal is important to be sure that there is no undetected signal interference and that electrode placement provides an appropriate EMG signal. Correct placement of surface electrodes is fundamental to detect and measure a signal accurately.

The three common signal sources (bladder pressure, anal sphincter pressure, and vaginal EMG) are significantly altered by increases in intra-abdominal pressure. Simultaneous measurement of abdominal activity should be done with all biofeedback therapy techniques. Intra-abdominal pressure can be measured easily using an internal rectal balloon. Electromyographic activity of the rectus abdominis muscles can be determined by surface electrodes. The abdominal muscle activity is displayed via two active electrodes placed 3 cm apart just below the umbilicus. A ground electrode is placed on a convenient bony prominence, such as the iliac crest.[12,27,28] EMG biofeedback training has a twofold purpose: to increase the activity of weak muscle groups and to promote relaxation of spastic or tense muscles.

EQUIPMENT AND CLINICAL PRACTICE

Biofeedback equipment has become sophisticated and expensive. Biofeedback devices are often chosen on the basis of cost and ease of application. There are two basic types of equipment designed to suit the setting in which biofeedback is implemented: (1) the outpatient clinic, where the patient is trained using a comprehensive clinic system and (2) the individual's home, where a smaller unit is used, generally on a more frequent basis. If possible, one should select a unit with multiple choices for visual displays. This unit should also have capabilities for simultaneous monitoring and display of abdominal muscle activity. Abdominal muscle activity should be monitored simultaneously with pelvic floor muscles so that patients can learn to contract pelvic floor muscles selectively. These measurements can be accomplished through a two-channel system.

Home training biofeedback units, because of a lower price, are limited to one channel for biofeedback. Other units have less flexibility but have an advantage in providing two channels, which allow for a maintenance program (Fig. 31-6). Once the initial biofeedback program has been completed, maintenance can be done using home care biofeedback monitors. The new trend is to interface the home unit with an existing diagnostic system (Fig. 31-7) and these units are readily transferable from the office setting to the home training unit. Multichannel systems (Fig. 31-8A) allow pressure and electromyographic measurements as well as abdominal measurements, thereby providing the clinician with multiple methods of biofeedback.

Another approach to biofeedback for urinary incontinence[18] combines bladder pressure and pelvic floor musculature biofeedback in a procedure that provides simultaneous visual feedback of bladder, external anal sphincter, and intra-abdominal pressures. Using three-channel biofeedback, patients are taught to contract and relax pelvic floor muscles selectively without increasing bladder pressure or intra-abdominal pressure. In our practice,[29,30] we use a microcomputer-based system with a wide range of parameters (Fig. 31-8B) that allows us to regulate the treatment according to the specific requirements of the patient, specifically in daily activities. The

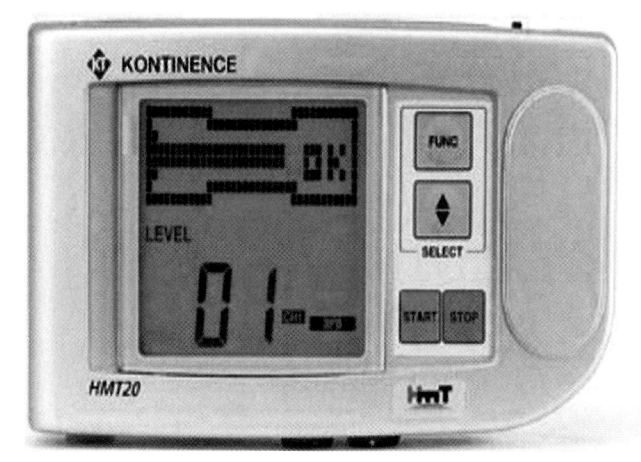

FIGURE 31-6 A dedicated biofeedback home care unit (HMT Inc.) allows the patient to get a perfect visual scale that displays performance.

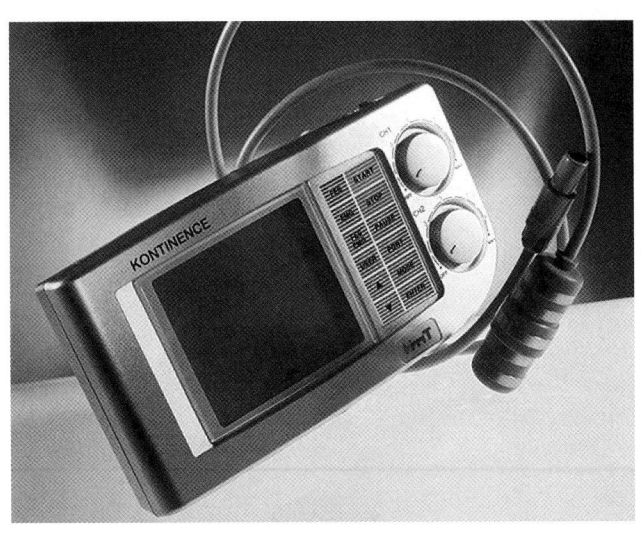

FIGURE 31-7 The new trend is to interface the home unit with a diagnostic system. The hand-held unit with a microcomputer provides a graphic display and can be connected to a unit in the office or clinic (HMT Inc.)

system records simultaneous measurements of EMG activity of pelvic floor muscles, rectus abdominis muscles, and other skeletal muscles (gluteal, adductors, etc.).

In clinical practice, we currently use pelvic floor therapy systems, which include products for home-based and office-based treatments and provide the most comprehensive and advanced platforms for treatment of pelvic floor dysfunction. Most of the equipment now available ensure effective treatment outcomes for most patients. The most important features are adjustable color and screen configuration; session graphs with summary of data; audio and visual goal-setting; annotated markers; templates; and animation. Using such equipment, it is possible to provide more "enjoyable" exercise programs (various levels of difficulty) and to conduct statistical analyses.

Biofeedback Technique

According to the patient's main complaint, the clinical procedures of biofeedback therapy can be divided into three groups: pelvic floor relaxation, genuine stress incontinence, and urge incontinence. These categories include most patients treated for lower urinary tract disorders in an outpatient biofeedback laboratory. The following sections describes the clinical procedures for a program of pelvic floor muscle training with biofeedback, which requires four stages: (1) awareness of pelvic floor musculature, (2) muscle strengthening, (3) reflex or automatic contraction, and (4) use of new skills in activities of daily life.

Stage 1: Awareness of the Pelvic Floor Musculature

The initial step in treatment is to help the patient identify the pelvic floor muscles. It is important to test contractility and to know how the patient contracts the pelvic floor muscles when instructed to squeeze around

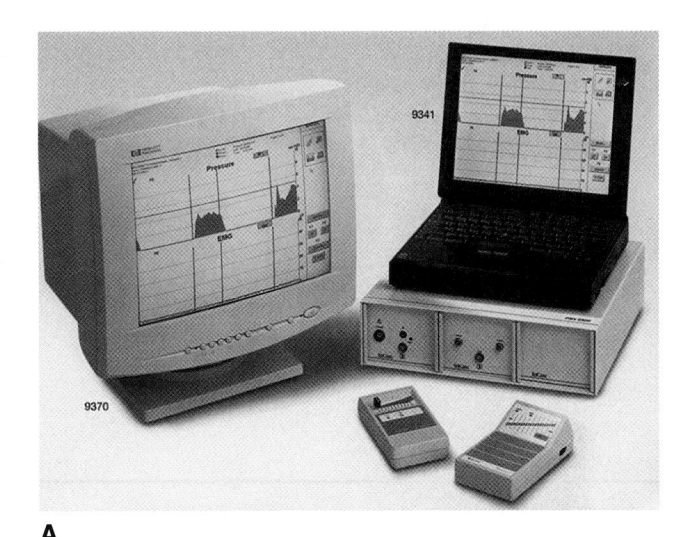

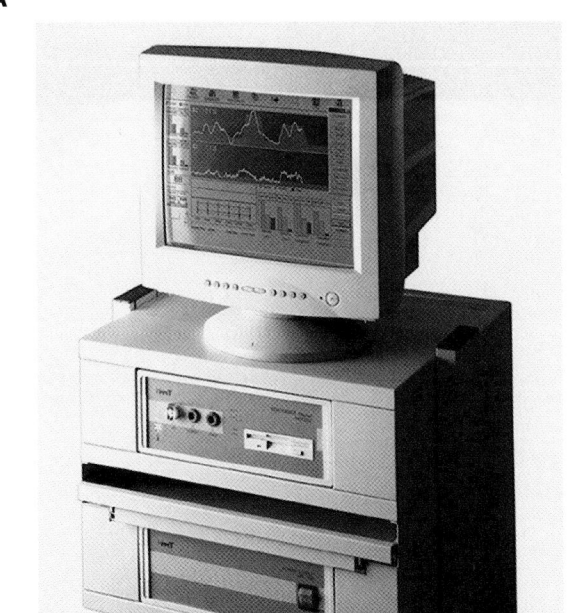

FIGURE 31-8 Multichannel systems (**A**, Hollister-Incare Inc.; **B**, HMT Inc.) allows pressure and electromyographic measurements as well as abdominal measurements. All these devices can also be used for electrical stimulation.

the examining fingers. Very often the contraction is performed incorrectly (Fig. 31-9). Instead of lifting up with the muscles, the patient is observed to be bearing down, which is counterproductive because it increases intra-abdominal and therefore bladder pressure.[30,31] This response has been referred to as a "reversed perineal command"[32] or a "paradoxical perineal command." The frequency of such incorrect contraction is about 22% in women after childbirth and it decreases to about 10% in women around menopause. Bump and colleagues[33] reported that 50% of women were unable to perform a voluntary pelvic floor muscle contraction following brief verbal instruction and as many as 25% mistakenly performed a Valsalva maneuver.

It seems clear that patients who bear down in this way must be identified before being asked to practice

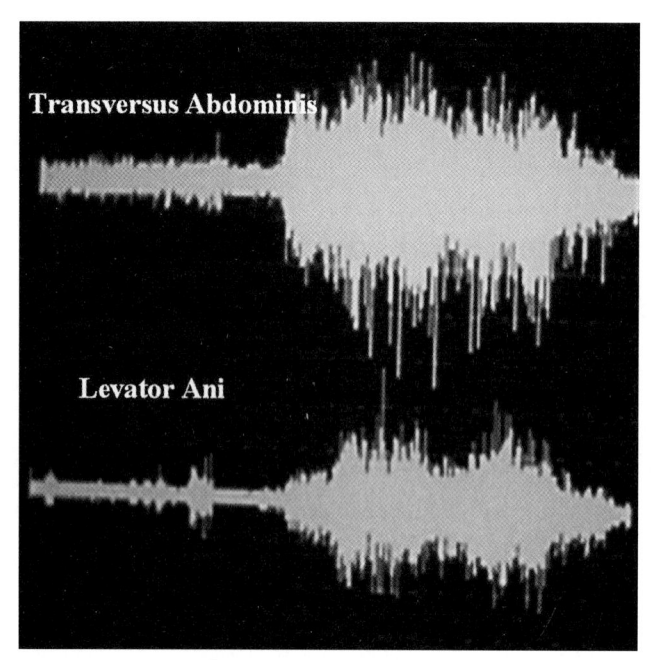

FIGURE 31-9 Recordings of both the levator ani muscles (*bottom*) and the transversus abdominis muscle (*top*). The "pusher" is squeezing the vaginal hiatus and strongly contracting the abdominal muscles.

Kegel exercises at home, or the efforts will be futile. In addition, women might increase vaginal wall descent or worsen urinary incontinence by increasing intra-abdominal pressure. Besides the group of patients who are unable to perform a proper voluntary pelvic floor contraction, it seems very rare to perform a voluntary pelvic floor contraction without a co-contraction of the abdominal muscles. Research suggests that it is not possible to maximally contract the pelvic floor muscle without co-contraction of transverse abdominal muscle (*transversus abdominis*). Contraction of this muscle can be observed as a pulling in of the abdominal wall with no movement of the pelvis. This is mainly observed in women who regularly practice sports. In that case, these patients demonstrate abdominal recruitment due to general physical activities making these muscles very strong. This is probably why Bo[34] suggests that co-contraction of the other related muscles (e.g., glutei and hip abductors) should be minimized so that the pelvic floor muscles are targeted and contraction of them is not masked by strong contraction of other muscle groups.

During the initial biofeedback session, it is also common to observe patients perform pelvic muscle contractions accompanied by the contraction of synergistic muscles such as adductors (pressing the knees), or gluteal muscles (squeezing the buttocks). This natural substitution of the stronger muscles for the weakened or minimally perceived motor response can also have negative consequences.

An instrumentation system allows multiple measurements and modalities to be displayed on a monitor and stored in a computer database (Fig. 31-10). Feedback must be relevant in order to enhance learning and to focus on agonist (levator ani muscles) and antagonist muscles (abdominal muscles). Patients should be able to recognize that the proper muscles are being used appropriately. Therapy is first concentrated on the inhibition of the antagonist muscles and decreasing activity of surrounding muscles, while increasing the response of the agonist. Since the aim of performing the contraction is to contract the pelvic floor muscles correctly, the proprioceptive signals generated by the substituting muscles can easily be misinterpreted as originating from the pelvic floor rather than from the antagonist muscles represented by strong abdominal muscles. When the substituting muscles contract, their afferents can mask low-intensity sensory signals that may be generated by the weakened pelvic floor muscles. This faulty maneuver perpetuates the substitution pattern and delays the development of increased awareness of the isolated pelvic floor muscles. During the initial session, this pattern occurs quite often as the patient attempts to contract her pelvic floor muscles by moving the upper part of her abdomen, even rising off the table. When instructed to relax the abdominal muscles or the surrounding muscles (adductors/gluteal), the substitution of the interfering muscles may be detected by the biofeedback equipment. An abdominal substitution pattern used when attempting to "hold back" leads to a false maneuver of pushing down, which causes a rise in intra-abdominal pressure. With such recruitment, the contraction would only maximize a rise of intra-abdominal pressure, resulting in an increase in EMG abdominal signals.

To minimize inappropriate tensing, it is helpful to train patients to keep these muscles relaxed when trying to prevent urine loss. For this purpose, patients are instructed to breathe evenly and to relax abdominal muscles. During the training sessions, the patient is also asked to place one hand on her lower abdomen to palpate the faulty abdominal contraction.

Biofeedback therapy provides the patient with better volitional control over skeletal muscles such as levator ani and urinary sphincter, heightened sensory awareness of the pelvic floor area, and decreased muscle antagonist contractions.

Stage 2: Muscle Strengthening

The pelvic floor muscles hold the pelvic organs like a hammock, providing support as well as stabilization. Normally, when the woman is erect, the levator ani muscles, together with the respective fasciae, contribute to the support of the vaginal canal, the urethra, and the rectum. In patients with pelvic relaxation, this normal muscular support is lost. The levator ani hiatus is wider and the levator plate is weakened and relaxed. When the pubococcygeal portions of the levator ani sling contract, they shorten lengthwise, gaining thickness and lessening the pelvic floor aperture transversely, thus reducing the anteroposterior diameter considerably.[35] A tonic contraction of the levator ani maintains a high position of the vesical neck and may compensate for an increase in intra-abdominal pressure. The levator ani support[36] is provided predominantly by slow-twitch fibers, which are responsible for maintaining static muscle tone. During stressful events, phasic fast-twitch fibers provide a rapid

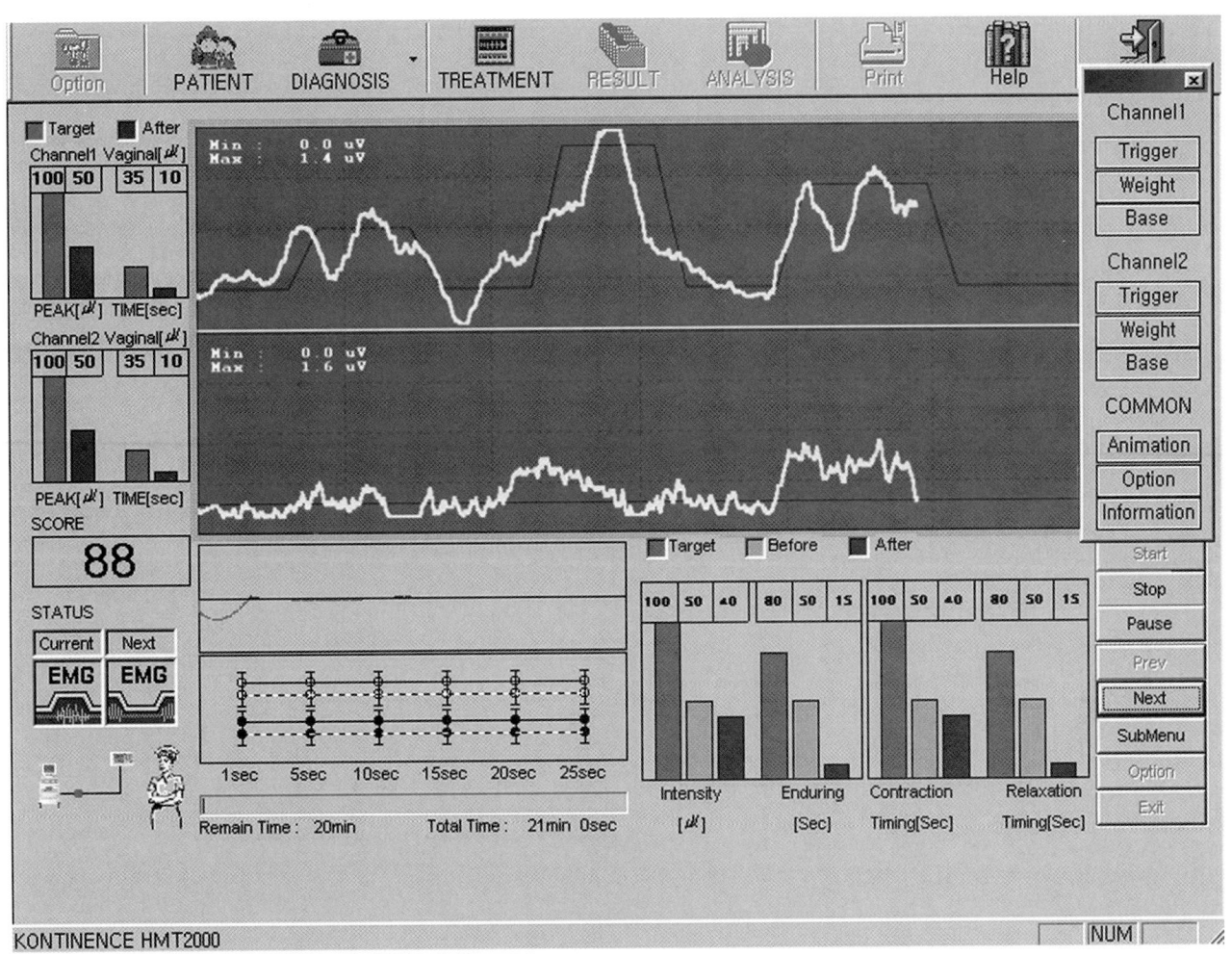

FIGURE 31-10 Recordings of both the levator ani muscles (*top*) and the abdominal muscles (*bottom*). During the hold maneuver, the patient could not sustain the contraction for more than 3 seconds and uses the abdominal muscles (co-contraction).

forceful contraction.[37,38] When muscles have weakened, there is little perception of the contraction because the intensity of the proprioceptive feedback to the brain is relative to the amplitude of the muscle contraction. Muscle strength can be improved through a program of pelvic floor muscle exercise.

In planning a pelvic floor muscle exercise program it is important to follow these basic guidelines: Patients should be selected according to grades of the pelvic floor muscles; a trained therapist should be present to give proper instruction in the level of contraction; the exercise program should be tailored to the individual; body positions should be modified after several sessions; and types of contraction should be alternated.

During exercise sessions, it is very important to recruit fast-twitch fibers by fast contractions to develop strength and slow-twitch fibers by slow contractions to increase endurance.[37] Regular strength training increases the number of activated motor units, frequency of excitation, and muscle volume. To induce hypertrophy, both fast- and slow-twitch fibers should be contracted. To achieve these objectives, a successful pelvic floor muscle training (PFMT) program must include rapid forceful contractions, sustained maximal voluntary contractions, and fast contractions superimposed on the end of each prolonged contraction. Effective strength training relies on specificity (co-contraction of other groups of muscles such as glutei and hip adductors should be minimized) and overload (increasing length and duration of contractions and reduction of rest periods).

The only anatomic relationship between the levator ani and the other pelvic floor muscles is provided by the obturatus internus. The puboccygeal segment of the levator ani originates in the tendinous arch, a thickening of the obturator fascia; the iliococcygeus begins at a membranous insertion to the inner surface of the obturator internus at the tendinous arch of the levator ani.[39] This anatomic consideration of the voluntary or reflex contraction of the levator ani and obturator internus is important in setting up the protocol of a PFMT program. This endopelvic connection to the tendinous arch may assist the levator ani in support because it limits the descent of the pelvic organs during increased intra-abdominal pressure. It could be postulated that in patients with weakening and stretching of the levator ani, even in those with partial denervation, some muscular components such as the obturator internus might be recruited in the early stages of pelvic floor exercises.

If there is a major weakness of the pelvic floor muscles, contraction of the gluteus maximus can also produce an overflow of activity into the levator ani.

Different exercises may be proposed to such a patient. The "flick contraction" exercise is performed by contracting and relaxing the levator ani as tightly as possible for 1 second. An average of 3 sets of 12 contractions during the session is recommended. The "hold contraction" exercise is performed by lifting and pulling up the levator ani and then holding the contraction for at least 6 seconds. As control improves, the time of this sustained contraction can be extended to 10 or 12 seconds. Patients are instructed to contract their muscles with 3 sets of 8 slow maximal contractions sustained for 6 to 8 seconds each. Effective strength training relies on overload (i.e., increasing resistance to, frequency, or duration of muscle contraction). The "intensive contraction" exercise involves the recruitment of levator ani muscles with other groups of muscles in different positions, controlling the levator ani in increments to the point of maximum tension.

The treatment sessions are essentially training sessions that aim to increase the strength and endurance of the pelvic floor muscles. Because biofeedback requires effort, the sessions should not overtax the patient. In general, the initial sessions are shorter than subsequent sessions, and if the patient's performance begins to deteriorate, it is recommended that the session be interrupted because muscle fatigue leads to muscle compensation. It is thought that pelvic floor muscle training and exercise is most useful if conducted in a variety of positions including sitting and standing, rather than restricted to the traditional supine positions. Training periods of at least 20 weeks have been recommended, but it is important to assess patients individually to determine the degree of pelvic floor muscle weakness to prevent adverse effects caused by muscle fatigue.

Stage 3: Reflex (Automatic) Contraction

In normal situations, with increased intra-abdominal pressure, the rectum, uterus, and upper vagina are pushed downward and backward. The levator plate tenses and rises owing to reflex muscular contraction. Sudden increases in intra-abdominal pressure are transmitted to the urethra. Sudden changes in abdominal pressure elicit a reflex contraction of the levator ani muscles. It has been suggested that a strong, fast, well-timed voluntary pelvic floor muscle contraction[40] will clamp the urethra, preventing urethral descent and leakage during an abrupt intra-abdominal pressure.[34] It has been claimed that the downward pressure from the abdominal viscera has to be offset by the strength of the urogenital diaphragm, and the forward pressure of the pelvic floor increases the tendency to visceral protrusion. This active element, owing to a striated muscle effect, allows improved pressure transmission, but also promotes greater efficiency of the pelvic floor reflex by active means. In pelvic floor disorders, female patients may lose this reflex muscle contraction, and one of the goals of biofeedback therapy is to enable patients to "relearn" this reflex.[41]

The teaching process aims to demonstrate how the levator ani muscles must be contracted before and during increased intra-abdominal pressure, particularly with strenuous effort during heavy physical activity. During the learning process of the reflex contraction (Fig. 31-11), called the "stress strategy" or "the perineal blockage before stress technique," the levator ani must be contracted before any rise of intra-abdominal pressure.[42] At the end of this process, women must be conscious of a constant contraction of the levator ani and can use the technique of perineal blockage before physical stress. This skill of using pelvic floor muscle contraction to prevent stress leakage has also been called "the knack."[43]

In the treatment of stress urinary incontinence, De Lancey posits that a quick strong pelvic floor muscle contraction will clamp the urethra, increasing urethral pressure and preventing leakage during an abrupt or sustained increase in intra-abdominal pressure.[44] DeLancey also suggests that an effective contraction of the pelvic floor muscle may press the urethra against the pubic symphysis, creating a mechanical pressure rise.[45] The "reflex contraction" is a feed-forward loop since it may precede the bladder pressure rise by 200 to 250 milliseconds.[40]

Pelvic floor muscle strength and control are also important to the control of urge incontinence.[18] Patients with urge incontinence are taught "urge strategies" to prevent loss of urine during detrusor contractions. Patients with urge incontinence typically report that they rush to the toilet when they experience a sensation of urgency to void. Voluntary pelvic floor muscle contraction to control urge has been shown to be effective in the management of urge incontinence.[18,46,47] Godec and colleagues[48] inhibited reflex contraction of the detrusor muscle with an electrically stimulated contraction of the pelvic floor muscle. Reflex inhibition of detrusor contractions may accompany repeated voluntary pelvic floor contractions.[49] Patients are taught a more effective pattern of responding to urgency. They are told not to rush to the toilet because this movement increases abdominal

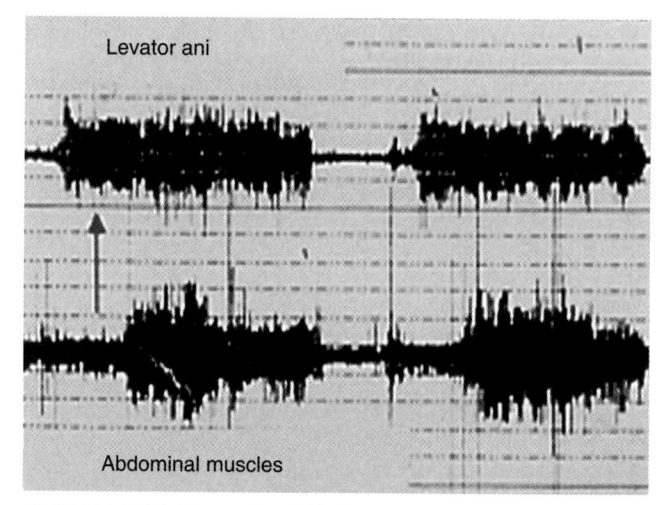

FIGURE 31-11 The perineal blockage before stress technique, or the knack. During the learning process of the reflex contraction the levator ani (*top*) must be contracted before any increase in intra-abdominal pressure occurs (*bottom*).

pressure on the bladder, increasing the likelihood of incontinence.[50] Instead, they are encouraged to pause, sit down if possible, practice relaxing, and contract the pelvic floor muscles maximally several times in an effort to diminish urgency, inhibit detrusor contraction, and prevent urine loss. When urgency subsides, they then proceed at a normal pace to the toilet.[18,46]

Stage 4: Use of New Skills in Daily Activities

Urinary stress incontinence and pelvic organ prolapse are primarily related to erect posture. We may assume that erect posture and a constant increase in intra-abdominal pressure alter female urethrovesical function. In the vertical position, the urethra leaves the bladder at the point of maximum combined intra-abdominal pressure and gravity force. We can assume a certain relationship between pelvic floor support and intra-abdominal pressure. A pelvic floor muscle reflex occurs with a sudden increase in intra-abdominal pressure. On the basis of this concept we developed the applied biofeedback technique, referring to EMG of the levator ani combined with synergistic and antagonistic muscle activity in a standing position.

The evolution of women's professional and business activities and stressful environments represent high-risk factors for pelvic floor relaxation. The intra-abdominal pressure in the standing position is two or three times greater than that in the supine position. Without a treatment protocol implemented in a standing position, especially with movement, neuromuscular re-education is pointless. This method is based on the relationship between pelvic floor muscle control and rise in intra-abdominal pressure. It consists of pelvic floor muscle contraction during the abrupt increase of the intra-abdominal pressure that occurs during standing and exercising.[41,51]

In our practice,[30,31,53] we use office equipment that allows patients to assume different positions as they learn to use the pelvic floor muscles to prevent incontinence. The trainer helps patients change their reactions by establishing targets and assisting them to develop new habits and modify their physical activities. The simulation of daily activities is a very important stage in which selected "home stress" or a physical task is used to access the patient's ability to perform a real-life activity. In general, one should start with easy tasks and progressively make the activities more difficult and more functional. It is optimal for patients to be standing when they perform these exercises (Fig. 31-12).

Successful recovery of the ability to perform daily activities without incontinence is most likely when the pelvic floor muscle strength is combined with a refined control of the functional activity. For this purpose, we use equipment[41] including a video monitor connected to a computerized unit (see Fig. 31-8B), which monitors EMG activity of muscle groups. We ask the patient to perform various tasks, very similar to domestic activities, such as carrying a baby basket or lifting items from the floor. The perineal blockage technique is useful in providing feedback to the active woman during exercise.[51,52] In some cases, as soon as the pelvic floor contraction is effective, we request perineal contraction

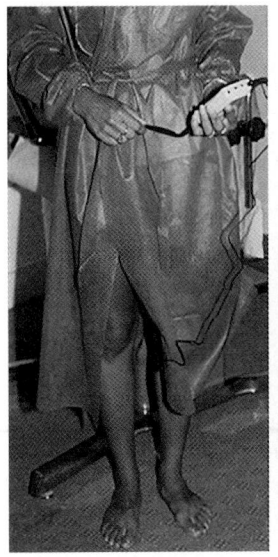

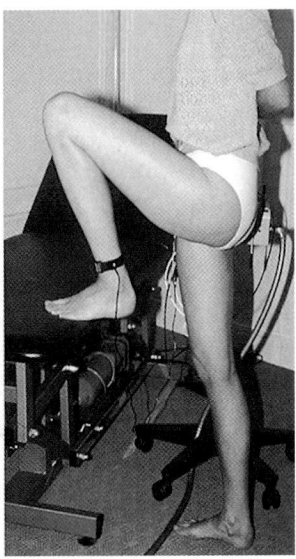

FIGURE 31-12 Applied biofeedback during exercises. A short vaginal sensor and electrode wire set for accessory muscles are used for the exercise program. The patient walks and contracts her muscles at different periods (*left*) and performs movement with the use of the knack technique (*right*).

with synergic muscles (external hip rotators, gluteal muscles, and adductor muscles) and later with antagonist muscles (*rectus abdominis*). If the patient has some difficulty in performing these exercises, we suggest that she practice in different positions, such as lying and sitting. For sportswomen,[41,52,53] we recommend using a treadmill (Fig. 31-13), which represents the opportunity to combine speed and endurance. The underlying concept is that the circumstances and precipitants of incontinence must be taken into account during treatment

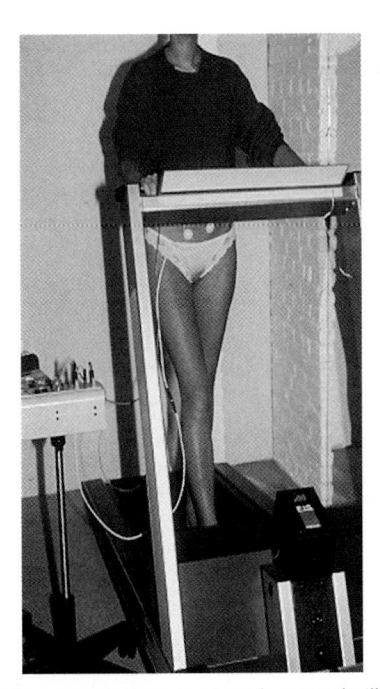

FIGURE 31-13 Applied biofeedback with a treadmill. Patient jogs for 15 minutes and parameters are selected according to the type of exercise, strength, and endurance.

sessions to provoke a reflex pelvic floor muscle contraction in response to stress. Accuracy of speed (from 2.5 mph to 6 mph) and slope (from 5% to 12%) is assumed for a precisely controlled workout. The introduction of the treadmill or other sports equipment into our program for sportswomen is one way to allow the patient to perform real physical activities in a medical environment.[52,53]

CLINICAL RESULTS

Many studies have demonstrated that treatment with biofeedback reduces incontinence. The data show clearly that the treatments are safe and effective, and they yield high levels of patient satisfaction. This chapter does not provide a comprehensive review of this literature, but rather describes selected papers that are considered important because of their large sample size or randomized clinical trial design. We recommend that readers refer to the original articles for details of each study.

Clinical Results with Bladder Biofeedback

Cardozo and colleagues[54] reported a study of 34 women between the ages of 16 and 65 years treated by bladder biofeedback. They were given an average of 5.4 sessions of cystometric biofeedback. Female patients were treated in 4 to 8 hour sessions at weekly intervals during which the bladder was filled 2 to 3 times using 0.9% saline prewarmed to body temperature. A total of 87% were cured or improved subjectively and 60% objectively. No one's condition was worsened by biofeedback. The six patients who failed to improve had severe detrusor instability, with detrusor contractions >60 cm of water and cystometric capacity <200 m. They found it impossible to inhibit detrusor activity. One of them was later found to have multiple sclerosis. Patient follow-up proved difficult, but of 11 women who were initially cured or improved, 4 remained completely cured and 2 had undergone surgery. These long-term results seem disappointing, but all the patients in the group had previously failed drug therapy.[55]

Millard and Oldenburg[56] used bladder training or bladder biofeedback or a combination of both to treat 59 women with frequency, nocturia, urgency, and urge incontinence. The women underwent urodynamic testing, which revealed detrusor instability alone in 38 women, detrusor instability and sphincter incompetence in 6, sensory urgency in 12, and sensory urgency and sphincter incompetence in 3. All patients were initially hospitalized for 5 to 14 days and then assigned to either a Frewen-type bladder training program or to a weekly outpatient biofeedback program. Millard and Oldenburg state that "biofeedback was undoubtedly the most useful of the techniques."[56] They claimed a 74% cure or major improvement rate for patients with detrusor instability. None of those with detrusor instability and urethral incompetence were cured, though 3 of them improved, with conversion to stable cystometry. Of the women with sensory urgency, 92% benefited. It is difficult to see how biofeedback could have helped them as their symptoms could not have been associated with cystometric changes. We think that patients are using their inhibition skills to abort detrusor contractions and give themselves enough time to reach the bathroom; it is difficult to separate components of treatment (bladder retraining, biofeedback).

Kjolseth and colleagues[57] assessed the outcome of biofeedback therapy (bladder filling with visual stimuli) in 15 children aged 6 to 12 years and 7 adults aged 20 to 50 years, with cystometrically proven detrusor instability. Detrusor pressure was visually conveyed to the patient during repeated bladder fillings. Patients were instructed to inhibit detrusor pressure incrementally by tensing the pelvic floor musculature. None of the children was completely cured but 9 showed a marked decrease in the number or extent of symptoms. Two children showed moderate improvement, and for 4 children the treatment failed. One adult was completely cured, 2 showed moderate improvement, and 4 remained the same. None of these patients was converted to stable bladder.

In an uncontrolled study, Burgio and colleagues[18] demonstrated an 88% reduction in incontinence episodes in elderly men with urge incontinence who participated in an average of four ½-hour biofeedback training sessions. O'Donnell[58] treated 20 male patients (>65 years old) with urge incontinence using 1-hour sessions twice weekly for 5 weeks. The mean number of incontinence episodes was decreased from 5.1 to 2.0 per day after treatment.

Clinical Results with Pelvic Floor Muscle Training

Pelvic floor muscle training (PFMT) is commonly implemented using simple verbal feedback given to the patient during palpation of the PFM by the therapist, or biofeedback involving vaginal or anal EMG probes or pressure sensors. Different trials compared PFMT with biofeedback versus PFMT alone.[47,59-67] Most of the studies investigated the effect of biofeedback for women with stress incontinence with or without detrusor instability, comparing biofeedback-assisted pelvic floor muscle training with pelvic floor training alone. Sample sizes ranged from 19 to 135.[58,60] Only three had intervention groups of more than 25 participants.[47,60,67] The most common outcome measures were self-assessment,[59,60] urodynamic testing,[60,62] voiding diary,[47,55,58,59] some measure of PFM strength[55,59] and pad test.[57,58,67] Follow-up periods were variable; all studies conducted at least one posttreatment assessment within 6 weeks to 3 months of treatment onset. One trial conducted follow-up for 2 to 3 years.[62]

There was some variation in the types of biofeedback used. Two of the studies used vaginal biofeedback,[55,56,67] and two used vaginal pressure biofeedback.[56,60] Studies gave visual biofeedback to women or both auditory and visual biofeedback. Only two of the studies gave women biofeedback devices to use at home,[59,67] the others all required clinic attendance to use biofeedback. All trials reported significant improvement in both treatment groups, but only Glavind[62] and Burgio[64] reported PFMT with biofeedback to be superior to PFMT alone.

Burns and colleagues conducted a randomized clinical trial of vaginal EMG biofeedback in treatment of urinary incontinence in a group of women with stress or mixed incontinence.[60,63] As part of this trial older women (>55 years old) were assigned to 8 weeks of biofeedback-assisted PFMT. A no-treatment control group contained 38 subjects. Biofeedback combined with daily practice resulted in a mean 61% reduction in frequency of urine losses, which was not significantly better than training without biofeedback, which resulted in a mean 59% reduction of incontinence. Both were significantly better than the mean 9% increase in incontinence demonstrated by the control group.

Burgio and colleagues treated 24 stress incontinent women, ages 29 to 64 years, for 6 weeks.[64] One group received simultaneous bladder, sphincter, and abdominal pressure feedback and the control group received verbal feedback based on vaginal palpation. All patients in both groups received comprehensive training in 100 trials across four training sessions. Cures or improvement (at least 50% reduction of incontinence) resulted for 92% of the biofeedback group and 55% of the control patients. The biofeedback group averaged 75.9% reduction in the frequency of incontinence, significantly greater than the mean 51% shown by the verbal feedback group. The authors concluded that although many patients can succeed without biofeedback, it improves the patient's ability to learn appropriate pelvic floor muscle contractions and increases the likelihood of successful outcome.

Berghmans and colleagues suggested that the group that had biofeedback improved more quickly than the group that used only pelvic floor muscle training at 6 weeks, although there was no significant differences at 12 weeks; this has not been confirmed by any other study to date.[65]

In a controlled clinical trial, Wilson and colleagues compared four groups: PFMT at home, hospital-based PFMT with biofeedback, PFMT with interferential therapy, and PFMT with faradism.[66] He reported greater symptomatic improvement in the hospital-based PFMT with biofeedback group compared with PFMT at home. In a recent study by Morkved and colleagues, 94 women with urodynamic stress incontinence were randomized to 6 months of pelvic floor muscle training with a physical therapist with or without biofeedback at home. Training with home biofeedback resulted in higher rates of objective cure, but the difference between groups was not statistically significant.[67] The authors noted that the value of the home biofeedback may be that it motivates many women and should be an option in clinical practice.

Because the mechanisms of urge incontinence are in some ways different from the mechanisms for stress incontinence, the role that biofeedback plays in treating these conditions may be different as well. The contribution of biofeedback in the treatment of urge incontinence has been examined in two studies. The first was a small, randomized study of 20 older men and women with persistent urge incontinence.[68] Patients who were trained without biofeedback responded as well to treatment as those trained with bladder-sphincter biofeedback.

Later, a larger randomized controlled trial corroborated this finding. Burgio and colleagues studied 222 older women with predominantly urge incontinence. Patients were randomly assigned to behavioral training with biofeedback, behavioral training without biofeedback, or behavioral training with a self-help booklet. Instead of biofeedback, training was done with verbal feedback based on vaginal palpation. Patients in the biofeedback group showed a 63% reduction of incontinence, which was not significantly different from the 69% reduction in the verbal feedback group.[47] These findings indicate that careful training with verbal feedback is as effective as biofeedback in the first line treatment of urge incontinence, and that biofeedback can be reserved for those cases in which women cannot successfully identify their muscles.

A single study presented long-term follow-up data.[62] At 2 years subjective cure or improvement rates were higher in the PFMT with biofeedback group than the group doing PFMT alone. The First and Second International Consultation on Continence reported that "there is some variation in biofeedback protocols that may reflect availability of biofeedback equipment and the ongoing technical developments in this area. It appears there is Level 1b evidence to suggest that PFMT with either biofeedback or intravaginal devices is more effective than PFMT alone in women with genuine stress incontinence."[69,70]

Clinical Results with Lower Urinary Tract Symptoms

Stein and colleagues evaluated the long-term effectiveness of transvaginal or transrectal EMG biofeedback in 28 patients with stress and urge incontinence.[71] Sixty percent of the patients had detrusor instability, as demonstrated by urodynamics. Biofeedback successfully treated 5 of 14 (36%) patients with stress incontinence and 9 of 21 (43%) with urge incontinence. The treatment response was durable throughout follow-up, from 3 to 36 months in all of the responding patients. The authors concluded that biofeedback is a moderately effective treatment for stress and urge incontinence and should be offered to patients as a treatment option.

Pelvic floor muscle training with biofeedback is also effective for treatment of predominantly urge incontinence. Burgio and colleagues conducted a randomized clinical trial to compare biofeedback-assisted behavioral training to drug therapy (oxybutynin chloride) for treatment of urge incontinence in ambulatory, community-dwelling older women.[46] A volunteer sample of 197 older women (55 to 92 years of age) were evaluated and randomized to four sessions (8 weeks) of biofeedback-assisted behavioral treatment, drug treatment, or a placebo control condition. Daily bladder diaries were completed by patients before, during, and after treatment. Behavioral training, which resulted in a mean 80.7% improvement, was significantly more effective than drug treatment (mean 68.5% improvement, [$P = .009$]). Similarly, a larger proportion of subjects in the behavioral group achieved at least 50% and 75% reductions of incontinence ($P = .002$, $P = .001$). Although the values for full recovery of continence (100%) followed a similar pattern, the differences were not statistically significant ($P = .07$). Several secondary outcome measures were used to assess the patients' perceptions of treatment. On every parameter, the behavioral group reported the highest perceived improvement and satisfaction with treatment progress ($P < .001$).

Wyman and colleagues compared the efficacy of bladder training, pelvic floor muscle exercise with biofeedback-assisted instruction, and combination therapy in women with genuine stress incontinence, and those with detrusor instability.[72] This was a large randomized clinical trial with three treatment groups. Women with incontinence (N = 204: 145 with urinary stress incontinence and 59 with urge incontinence due to instability) received a 12-week intervention program, including six weekly office visits and six weekly mail or telephone contacts. They were followed up immediately and after 3 months. The combination therapy group had significantly fewer incontinent episodes, better quality of life, and greater treatment satisfaction immediately after the therapy. No differences between groups were observed at 3-month follow-up. The authors concluded that combination therapy of bladder training and PFMT with biofeedback had the greatest immediate efficacy in the management of female urinary incontinence.

Clinical Results with Detrusor-Sphincter Dyssynergia

Maizels and colleagues[73] and Sugar and Firlit[74] have treated a number of children (N = 3 and N = 10) with detrusor–sphincter dyssynergia. Electromyographic surface electrodes were placed perineally and connected to the biofeedback equipment. During voiding, the children received biofeedback with instructions to relax the urethral sphincter. Feedback was provided by either direct visual observations of the EMG activity of the urethral sphincter or the intensity of the sound reflecting the intensity of the EMG activity. Recognition of the dyssynergistic contractions was subsequently easily observed and in most cases corrected.

CONCLUSION

Biofeedback is a treatment methodology that has considerable potential application for urogynecologic conditions. Using this method, pelvic floor dysfunction including incontinence, pain, and pelvic relaxation can be brought under conscious awareness, including the contraction and relaxation of skeletal and smooth muscle.

Biofeedback represents an important consideration in the initial treatment of urinary incontinence as well as pelvic floor muscle dysfunction for women of all ages. Even though surgery is usually necessary for women who suffer from severe stress urinary incontinence, biofeedback can be useful for these patients as well because they can become actively involved in their own treatment and achieve better control of the perineal area. Further, biofeedback may be used to help relieve symptoms such as urge incontinence, detrusor instability, irritative symptoms, and voiding difficulty that often arise as a result of surgery for stress incontinence. Thus, biofeedback-assisted training can be used not only as a conservative first-line therapy for stress, urge or mixed incontinence, alone or in combination with other behavioral or pharmacologic therapy, but also as a useful adjunct to surgery for urogynecologic conditions.

The Second International Consultation on Incontinence recommended that "further large, high-quality randomized control trials are required to investigate the effectiveness of biofeedback assisted pelvic floor muscle training. Two areas requiring attention are women who are not able to voluntarily contract the pelvic floor muscles and the rate of improvement in biofeedback assisted training versus pelvic floor training alone."

REFERENCES

1. Brener J: Operant reinforcement feedback and efficiency in learned motorcontrol. In Coles MGH, Donchin E, Porges SW (eds): Psychophysiology. New York, Guilford Press, 1986.
2. Ashby WR: An Introduction to Cybernetics. New York, Wiley, 1963.
3. Basmajian JV: Biofeedback: Principles and Practice for Clinicians, 2nd ed. Baltimore, Williams & Wilkins, 1978.
4. Olson RP: Definitions of Biofeedback. In Schwartz MS (ed): Biofeedback: A Practitioner's Guide. New York, Guilford Press, 1987, pp 33–37.
5. Budzinski TH: Biofeedback strategies in headache treatment. In Basmajian JV (ed): Principles and Practice for Clinicians. Baltimore, Williams & Wilkins, 1979, pp 132–152.
6. Miller NE: Learning of visceral and glandular responses. Science 168:434–435, 1969.
7. Patel C: Biofeedback-aided relaxation and mediation in the management of hypertension. Biofeed Self Regul 2:1–47, 1977.
8. Sargent JD, Green EE, Walters CD: Preliminary report on the use of autogenic feedback training of migraine and tension headaches. Psychosom Med 35:129–135, 1973.
9. Schwartz MS, Shapiro D: Learned control of cardiovascular integration in man through operant conditioning. Psychosom Med 33:57–62, 1971.
10. Surwit RS: Behavioral approaches to Raynaud's disease. Psychother Psychosom 36:224–245, 1981.
11. Keefe FJ, Surwit RS: Electromyographic feedback: Behavioral treatment of neuromuscular disorders. J Behav Med 1:13–25, 1978.
12. Burgio KL: Urinary incontinence: Biofeedback therapy. In Benson JT (ed): Female Pelvic Floor Disorders. New York, Norton Medical Books, 1992, pp 210–218.
13. O'Donnell PD: Biofeedback therapy. In Raz S (ed): Female Urology. Philadelphia, WB Saunders, 1996, pp 253–262.
14. Norgard JP, Djurhuus JC: Treatment of detrusor sphincter dyssynergia by biofeedback. Urology Int 37:236–239, 1982.
15. Willington FL: Urinary incontinence: A practical approach. Geriatrics 35:41–48, 1980.

16. Cardozo LD, Stanton SL, Hafner J: Biofeedback in the treatment of detrusor instability. Br J Urol 50 (Suppl 5A): 250–254, 1978.
17. Cardozo LD: Biofeedback in overactive bladder. Br J Urol 85 (suppl 3):24–28, 2000.
18. Burgio KL, Whitehead WE, Engel BT: Urinary incontinence in the elderly: Bladder/sphincter biofeedback and toileting skills training. Ann Inter Med. 103:507–515, 1985.
19. Kegel AH: Physiologic therapy for urinary incontinence. JAMA 146:915–917, 1951.
20. Kegel AH: Progressive resistance exercise in the functional restoration of the perineal muscles. Am J Obstet Gynecol 56:238–248, 1948.
21. Hudzinski LG: Neck musculature and EMG biofeedback in treatment of muscle contraction headache. Headache 23:86–90, 1983.
22. Dohrman RJ, Laskin DM: An evaluation of EMG biofeedback in the treatment of myofacial pain-dysfunction syndrome. J Am Dent Assoc 96:656–662, 1978.
23. Johnson HE, Hockersmith V: Therapeutic electromyography in chronic back pain. In Basmajian JV (ed): Biofeedback: Principles and Practice for Clinicians, 2nd ed. Baltimore, Williams & Wilkins, 1983.
24. O'Donnell PD, Beck C, Eubanks C: Surface electrodes in perineal electromyography. Urol 32(4):375–379, 1988.
25. Lose G, Tanko A, Colstrup H, Anderssen JT: Urethral sphincter electromyography with vaginal surface electrodes: A comparison with sphincter electromyography recorded via periurethral coaxial, anal sphincter needle, and perineal surface electrodes. J Urol 133:815–818, 1985.
26. Burgio KL, Engel BT, Quilter RE, Arena VC: The relationship between external anal and external urethral sphincter activity in continent women. Neurourol Urodyn 10:555–562, 1991.
27. O'Donnell PD, Doyle R: Biofeedback therapy technique for treatment of urinary incontinence. Urology 37(5):432–436, 1991.
28. Burns PA: Biofeedback therapy. In O'Donnell PD (ed): Urinary Incontinence. St Louis, Mosby-Year Book, 1997, pp 273–277.
29. Bourcier AP: Pelvic floor rehabilitation. Int Urogynecol J 1:31, 1990.
30. Bourcier AP: Pelvic floor rehabilitation. In Raz S (ed): Female Urology. Philadelphia, WB Saunders, 1996, pp 263–281.
31. Bourcier AP: Applied biofeedback in pelvic floor re-education. In Appell RA, Bourcier AP, La Torre F (eds): Pelvic Floor Dysfunction: Investigations and Conservative Treatment. Rome, Casa Editrice Scientifica Internazionale, 1999, pp 241–248.
32. Bourcier AP, Bonde B, Haab F: Functional assessment of pelvic floor muscles. In Appell RA, Bourcier AP, La Torre F (eds): Pelvic Floor Dysfunction. Investigations and Conservative Treatment. Rome Casa Editrice Scientifica Internazionale, 1999, pp 97–106.
33. Bump RC, Hurt G, Fantl A, Wyman J: Assessment of Kegel muscle exercise performance after brief verbal instruction. Am J Obstet Gynecol 165:322–329, 1991.
34. Bo K: Pelvic floor muscle exercise for the treatment of stress urinary incontinence. Exercise physiology perspective. Inter Uro Gynecol J 6:282–291, 1995
35. Raz S: The anatomy of pelvic floor support and stress incontinence. In Raz S (ed): Atlas of Transvaginal Surgery. Philadelphia, WB Saunders, pp 1–22, 1992.
36. De Lancey JOL: Pubovesical ligaments: A separate structure from the urethral supports. Neurourol Urodyn 8:53, 1989.
37. Dixon JS, Gosling JA: The role of the pelvic floor in female urinary incontinence. Int Urogynecol J 1:212–217, 1990
38. Dougherty MC, Bishop KR, Abrams RM, et al: The effect of exercise on the circumvaginal muscles in post partum women. J Nur Midwifery 34:8–14, 1989.
39. De Lancey JOL: Functional anatomy of the female lower urinary tract and pelvic floor. In Block G, Wheland J (eds): Neurobiology of Incontinence. London, John Wiley & Sons, pp 57–76, 1990.
40. Constantinou CE, Govan DE: Contribution and timing of transmitted and generated pressure components in the female urethra. In: Female Incontinence. New York, Allan Liss, 1981.
41. Bourcier AP, Juras JC, Jacquetin B: Urinary incontinence in physically active and sportwomen. In Appell RA, Bourcier AP, La Torre F (eds): Pelvic Floor Dysfunction: Investigations and Conservative Treatment. Rome, Casa Editrice, 1999, pp 9–17.
42. Bourcier AP: Biofeedback and electrical stimulation. In Blaivas J, Karram M (eds): Proceedings of the Second Annual International Seminar on Female Urology and Urogynecology. Yardley, PA, Fusion Medical Education LLC, 2003, pp 26–29.
43. Miller J, Ashton-Miller JA, De Lancey JOL: The knack: Use of precisely timed pelvic muscle contraction can reduce leakage in USI. Neurourol Urodyn 15,4, 1Bs 90, Proceedings of ICS Athens, 1996.
44. De Lancey JOL: Structural aspects of urethral function in the female. Neurourol Urodyn 7:509–519, 1988.
45. De Lancey JOL: Anatomy and mechanisms of structures around the vesical neck: How vesical neck position might affect its closure. Neurourol Urodyn 7:161–162, 1988.
46. Burgio KL, Locher JL, Goode PS, et al: Behavioral versus drug treatment for urge incontinence in older women: A randomized clinical trial. JAMA, 23:1995–2000, 1998.
47. Burgio KL, Goode PS, Locher JL, et al: Behavioral training with and without biofeedback in the treatment of urge incontinence in older women: A randomized controlled trial. JAMA 288:2293–2299, 2002.
48. Godec C, Cass AS, Ayala GF: Bladder inhibition with functional electrical stimulation. Urology 6:663–666, 1975.
49. Berghmans LCM, Van Doorn ESC, Nieman F, et al: Efficacy of extramural physical therapy modalities in women with proven bladder overactivity: A randomized clinical trial. Neurourol and Urodyn 19(4):496–497, 2000.
50. Glavind, Hahn L, Naucler J, et al: Urodynamic assessment of pelvic floor training. World J Urol 9:162–166, 1991.
51. Bourcier AP: Pelvic floor rehabilitation. In Raz S (ed): Female Urology. Philadelphia, WB Saunders, 1996, pp 263–281.
52. Bourcier AP, Juras JC: Nonsurgical Therapy For Stress Incontinence. In Klutke CG, Raz S (eds): The Urol Clin of North Am. Philadelphia, WB Saunders, 1995 pp 613–627.
53. Bourcier AP: Conservative treatment of stress incontinence in sportswomen. Neurourol Urodyn 9:232, 1990.
54. Cardozo LD, Abrams PD, Stanton SL: Idiopathic detrusor instability treated by biofeedback. Br J Urol 50:521–523, 1978.
55. Cardozo LD, Stanton SL: Biofeedback: A 5 year review. Br J Urol 56:220, 1984.
56. Millard RJ, Oldenburg BF: The symptomatic, urodynamic and psychodynamic results of bladder re-education programmes. J Urol 130:715–719, 1983.
57. Kjolseth D, Madsen B, Knudsen LM: Biofeedback treatment of children and adults with idiopathic detrusor instability. Scand J Urol Nephrol 28:243–247, 1994.
58. O'Donnell PD, Doyle R: Biofeedback therapy technique for treatment of urinary incontinence. Urology 37(5):432–436, 1991.

59. Castelden CM, Duffin HM, Mitchell EP: The effect of physiotherapy on stress incontinence. Age Ageing 13:235–237, 1984.
60. Burns PA, Pranikoff K, Nochajksi TH, et al: A comparison of effectiveness of biofeedback and pelvic muscle exercise treatment of stress incontinence in older community-dwelling women. J Gerontol 48:167–174, 1993.
61. Laycock J, Brown JS, Cusak C, et al: A multicentre prospective, randomized controlled group comparative study of the efficacy of vaginal cones and PFX. Neurourol and Urodyn 18(4):301–302, 1999.
62. Glavind K, Nohr SB, Walter S: Biofeedback and physiotherapy versus physiotherapy alone in the treatment of genuine stress incontinence. Inter Urogynecol J 7:339–343, 1996.
63. Burns PA, Pranikoff K, Nochakski T, et al: Treatment of stress incontinence with pelvic floor exercises and biofeedback. JAGS 38:341–344, 1990.
64. Burgio KL, Robinson JC, Engel BT: The role of biofeedback in Kegel exercise training for stress urinary incontinence. Am J Obstet Gynecol 154:58–64, 1986.
65. Berghmans LCM, Frederijs CMA, De Bie RA, et al: Efficacy of biofeedback, when included with pelvic floor muscle exercise treatment, for genuine stress incontinence. Neurourol Urodyn 15:37–52, 1996.
66. Wilson PD, Al Samarrai T, Deakin M, et al: An objective assessment of physiotherapy for female genuine stress incontinence. Br J Obstet Gynaecol 94:575–582, 1987.
67. Morkved S, Bo K, Fjortoft T: Effect of adding biofeedback to pelvic floor muscle training to treat urodynamic stress incontinence. Obstet Gynecol 100:730–739, 2002.
68. Burton JR, Pearce KL, Burgio KL, et al: Behavioral training for urinary incontinence in elderly ambulatory patients. J Am Geriatr Soc 36:693–698, 1988.
69. Wilson PD, Bo K, Bourcier A, et al: Conservative management in women. In Abrams P, Khoury S, Wein A (eds): First International Consultation on Incontinence. Plymouth, Plymbridge, 1999, pp 579–636.
70. Wilson PD, Bo K, Hay-Smith J, et al: Conservative management in women. In Abrams P, Cardozo L, Khoury S, Wein A (eds): Second International Consultation on Incontinence. Plymouth, Plymbridge, pp 573–624, 2002.
71. Stein M, Discippio W, Davia M: Biofeedback for the treatment of stress and urge incontinence. J Urol 153:641–643, 1995.
72. Wyman JF, Fantl JA, McClish DK: Comparative efficacy of behavioural interventions in the management of female urinary incontinence. Continence Program for Women Research Group. Am J Obstet Gynecol 179:999–1007, 1998.
73. Maizels M, King LR, Firlit CF: Urodynamic biofeedback: A new approach to treat vesical sphincter dyssynergia. J Urol 122:205–209, 1979.
74. Sugar EC, Firlit CG: Urodynamic biofeedback: A new approach for childhood incontinence/infection (vesical voluntary sphincter dyssynergia). J Urol 128:1253–1258, 1882.

CHAPTER 32

Bladder Retraining

GERALD J. JARVIS

No single treatment modality should be considered the first choice of treatment in the management of either the unstable bladder or the urge syndrome. Bladder retraining, sometimes termed bladder drill, is a noninvasive treatment modality that has been used not only for these two conditions but also for mixed incontinence and even stress incontinence. It has been widely studied over the last 20 to 25 years, although there is little scientific published work in the last few years. An excellent review of the subject is available in the Cochrane Library.[1]

Bladder retraining is a form of behavioral therapy in which a patient with an intact nervous system "relearns" to inhibit a detrusor contraction or a sensation of urgency. Such behavioral therapies include biofeedback, hypnotherapy, and acupuncture.

There are good reasons for holding the prior belief that behavioral methods of therapy may be of value in idiopathic urge syndromes. Although these have been a subject of review,[2] they can be summarized as follows:

- A strong emotive event in a patient's life may be the initial trigger for such urinary symptoms.
- Patients with detrusor instability have a higher neuroticism score on formal testing than the patients with genuine stress incontinence.
- There is a relationship between detrusor instability and hysterical personality trait.
- Patients with detrusor instability are more likely to have psychosexual problems than patients with genuine stress incontinence.
- Other behavioral forms of therapy, such as hypnosis, are effective methods of treatment.
- Treatment is itself associated with a strong placebo effect, which has been estimated between 4% and 47% in clinical trials.

The rationale of bladder retraining is to make a patient aware of the problem and enlist her help in treatment by using behavioral therapy in a structured regime. It is generally held that bladder drill is more effective on an inpatient basis than an outpatient basis, perhaps because patients are withdrawn from their own environment and placed in a situation where their major daily task is to concentrate on their treatment, although there is no specific randomized trial to support this common view. A frequently used treatment regime can be broken into the following components:

- Exclude pathology.
- Explain the condition to the patient.
- Explain the treatment and its rationale to the patient.
- Instruct the patient to void at set times during the day, for instance, every hour. The patient must not void between these times; she must wait or be incontinent.
- The voiding interval is increased by increments, perhaps half-hours, when the initial goal is achieved and the process is then repeated.
- The patient should have a normal fluid intake.
- The patient should keep her own input and output chart. The increasing volumes of urinary output at increasing intervals act as a reinforcement reward.
- The patient should receive praise and encouragement on reaching her daily targets.

Patients who are selected for such regimes should be physically and cognitively able, and motivated. Any variation of the regime must contain the three cardinal components, namely patient education, scheduled voiding, and positive reinforcement.[2,3]

Bladder retraining was first described in 1966 by Jeffcoate and Francis, who called it bladder discipline. Later, a series of articles by Frewen brought widespread attention to the role of bladder retraining. Evidence on efficacy is now available not only from cohort studies but also from randomized trials. Typical results note that up to 90% of patients become continent, although there is a relapse rate up to 40% within 3 years of treatment. Such relapses could be treated by reinstitution of a retraining program.

Good evidence from randomized trials indicate that bladder retraining compared with either no treatment or delayed treatment is effective. In one such study, 90% of the treatment group became continent, 83.3% of the treatment group became symptom-free, and 23.3% of the control group were both continent and symptom-free. The majority of patients with a urodynamically demonstrable unstable bladder who were rendered symptom-free also became stable on urodynamic assessment.[4] A larger study demonstrated that 12% of the treatment group became continent, and 76% had reduced their incontinence episodes by at least 50%. Overall, 55% of people reported an improvement in quality of life.[5] In both studies the improvement was maintained 6 months after the institution of retraining regimes. Other studies have shown a cure rate between 50% and 86.6% with improvement rates reported in the region of 75% to 87.3%.[6]

Several studies have compared bladder retraining regimes with pharmacological treatment. One randomized trial noted that 84% of women were subjectively continent and 76% subjectively improved following bladder retraining, compared with 56% continent and 48% symptom-free following a combination of anticholinergic therapy.[7] A further randomized trial compared bladder retraining with a 6-week course of oxybutynin and found a similar clinical cure rate (74%) with both regimes. However, the relapse rate was higher in the drug group than in the bladder retraining group, since those who maintained their bladder retraining program showed superior results.[8]

Further studies have addressed the issue of supplementing bladder retraining with drug treatment. Although the data from such studies are currently limited, there is no evidence so far that supplemental drug therapy is superior to bladder retraining alone.[1] Thus, bladder retraining appears to be equal or superior to drug treatment and may have greater long-term benefits.

There are numerous areas for future study. There is a lack of consistency in bladder retraining programs. There is a need not only to evaluate an optimal program but also, most important, to identify the optimal increment in both the voiding interval and the rate at which the voiding interval is altered following attainment of each stage of the regime. A shorter initial voiding interval, for instance, may be necessary for women with more intense frequency or with less confidence. There is clearly a popular benefit from widespread treatment in a community as opposed to a small number of patients treated in hospital, but there is a need to determine the optimum supervision in the community. There is a need for comparison between bladder retraining and other physical interventions. There is limited data, for instance, comparing bladder retraining with pelvic floor muscle retraining, estrogen replacement, and electrical stimulation.

Further evaluation is needed of the place of bladder retraining in the presence of genuine stress incontinence rather than an urge syndrome. In a comparison between bladder retraining and pelvic floor muscle training, there were similar and significant reductions in incontinence episodes and improvement in quality of life whether the patients were treated with bladder retraining alone, pelvic floor muscle training alone, or a combination of them.[9]

The quality of available studies is variable and outcome measures are inconsistent. At the current time, some studies report outcomes at between 3 and 6 months, others at 12 months following randomization, and a small number of studies have assessed symptoms up to 6 years following enrollment. The outcome measures included a subject report of cure or improvement, the keeping of a urinary diary, repeat urodynamic assessment, pad tests, and quality of life evaluation. However, even considering seven randomized controlled trials available from the literature, there were still only 259 people about whom such conclusions can be drawn.[1] There is a clear need for larger studies.

There is a need to identify factors that influence the outcome of bladder retraining regimes. The age and mobility of a patient are likely to be relevant. Wilson and colleagues offer some evidence that lower age is associated with a better outcome.[6] There is a need to explore further whether the urodynamic diagnosis is really is relevant so long as pathology has been excluded. There may be poorer results associated with isometric contractions in excess of 100 cm of water and the presence of coexisting nocturnal enuresis. There is a need to assess patient compliance.

Only a minority of studies have reported whether or not there were adverse effects associated with bladder retraining. It is perhaps to be expected that there are no adverse effects and no adverse effects reported in the literature, although the author is aware of a single patient who developed a deep venous thrombosis during an inpatient bladder retraining regime. Overall, it appears to be a safe treatment that is acceptable to patients.

CONCLUSION

Bladder retraining is an effective treatment for women with urge, stress, and mixed urinary incontinence. It is not yet clear whether the urodynamic diagnosis will specifically affect the likelihood of success. There is a lack of consistency in bladder retraining programs and an optimal regime needs to be identified. However, it is possible that regimes will need to be tailored to the individual patient.

Bladder retraining appears to have benefits similar to those of drug treatment, does not appear to be benefited by supplementary drug treatment, and may have greater long-term benefits than drug therapy. Bladder retraining appears to be largely free of adverse effects and is acceptable to patients.

There is a need for large randomized controlled trials that assess the place of bladder retraining alone and in combination and comparison with drugs and physical treatment modalities. Standardized outcome measures are necessary and they should be identified clearly in any study and should include an assessments of continence and quality of life.

REFERENCES

1. Roe B: Bladder training for urinary incontinence in adults. In *Cochrane Library*, issue 3, 2000.
2. Jarvis GJ: Investigation and management of the unstable bladder. In Bonnar J (ed): Recent Advances in Obstetrics and Gynaecology, Vol. 19. Churchill Livingstone, 1995.
3. Fantl JA, Newman DK, Colling J, et al: Urinary incontinence in adults. In Clinical Practice Guideline, No. 2, Rockville, MD, U.S. Department of Health and Human Services, Public Health Services, Agency for Health Care Policy and Research, 1996.

4. Jarvis GJ, Millar DR: Controlled trial of bladder drill for detrusor instability. Br Med J 281:1322–1323, 1980.
5. Fantl JA, Wyman JF, McClish DK: Efficacy of bladder retraining in older women with urinary incontinence. JAMA 265:306–313, 1991.
6. Wilson PD, Bo K, Bourcier A, et al: Conservative management in women. In Abrams P, Khoury S, Wein A (eds): Incontinence. 2nd ed. Plymouth, UK, World Health Organization, 2002, pp 571–624.
7. Jarvis GJ: A controlled trial of bladder drill and drug therapy in the management of detrusor instability. Br J Urol 53:365–366, 1981.
8. Columbo M, Zanetta G, Scalambrino S, et al: Oxybutynin and bladder retraining in the management of female urinary urge incontinence. Int Urogynaecol J 6:63–67, 1995.
9. Wyman JF, Fantl J, McClish DK, et al: Comparative efficacy of behavioral interventions in the management of female urinary incontinence. Am J Obstet Gynecol 179:999–1007, 1998.

Incontinence Aids: Pads and Appliances

Jean-Pierre Dentz

Urinary incontinence is observed in approximately 5% to 10% of the general population in Europe and North America. However, it is predominant in the female population, affecting an estimated 10% to 58% of multiparous and elderly women, and may affect women at any age. It is often considered an unavoidable condition. After the age of 35 years, 3 in 10 women have trouble with continence, with an average age of 46 years.[1]

Most cases of incontinence can be cured with conservative treatment or surgery, but some cases are not suitable for these procedures. Examples include minor leakage, light urine loss that occurs only with intense physical stress (e.g., playing sports), and some physical or psychological conditions (e.g., advanced age).[2]

Urinary or fecal incontinence is a significant problem for mentally disturbed, geriatric, and pediatric patients. In these frail patients, continence aids should be the only therapeutic approach. Some patients with severe dementia show improvement after participating in a rehabilitation program, but they must use pads during this period.[3]

Pads and absorbent pants are used by many incontinent women, either permanently or during retraining of the bladder and pelvic floor. Many men are reluctant to use garments that are designed principally for women, and male pads and penile devices are available for use by men who experience urinary incontinence after prostate surgery. The first adapted continence aids were distributed in the United Kingdom and Sweden in the early 1960s, and the all-in-one pads that are worn on the body were introduced around 1980.

In recent years, many new products have become available for people suffering from incontinence.[4] For example, marsupial pants that have a waterproof pouch and a T-shape to hold a pad in place led to a significant improvement in the quality of life of bedridden patients.

Because of the increasing interest in the problem of incontinence and concern about the associated cost, health authorities in many countries instituted programs to help people with this disease.[5] In the United Kingdom, health authorities defined and legalized the role of continence advisors. These practitioners have special training and are registered as either a continence advisor or a physiotherapist specializing in continence.

PATIENT EVALUATION

Urinary incontinence is involuntary loss of urine through the urethra that is severe enough to have social effects. Assessment of the incontinent patient demands a methodical approach, starting with a careful history to identify the type, duration, and severity of urinary incontinence.

History

During the history, the type of incontinence must be identified (i.e., urge, stress, or overflow) as well as the relevant precipitating factors (e.g., playing sports, pregnancy, coughing). Overflow incontinence typically occurs in patients with chronic urinary retention, with bed-wetting and permanent incontinence without the sensation of the need to void.

The patient should be asked about symptoms of frequency and urgency as well as about nocturia and the amount of fluid consumed. The history also includes the onset, duration, and evolution of leakage and associated events. The patient should also be asked to describe the severity of incontinence subjectively. The severity of leakage can be evaluated objectively with a pad test that consists of weighing the urine lost during a stress program. Finally, the patient should be asked whether incontinence results in any social restriction.

Physical Examination

Inspection of the perineum, particularly the skin around the vulva and anus, for irritation or dermatitis, vaginitis, and discharge, can give an indication of the severity of urine loss. The condition of the underwear provides additional information. Observation of the patient's mobility and dexterity provides a useful indication of the patient's ability to use continence aids.

Evaluation of Environmental and Social Factors

Disability is the change in physical condition that is caused by disease, whereas handicap is the change in social condition that is caused by the environment. The distinction between disability and handicap highlights the need to consider two types of factors in the treatment of incontinence:

1. Intrinsic factors (physical or mental disability)
2. Extrinsic (environmental) factors[6]

During the history, the examiner should attempt to assess the patient's surroundings and quality of life (e.g., living alone, in a clean room, in dirty sheets and squalor). In addition, the examiner should evaluate the patient's access to toilet facilities.

PADS AND PANTS

Leakage is determined by the rapidity of pad penetration, the durability and capacity of the pad material, the absorption capacity of the pad core and the velocity of pad saturation, and the amount of urine that escapes out of the pad (sponge effect).

The probability of urine loss increases with urine volume, but there is no lower volume limit that predicts dryness. At low volumes (≤ 350 g), shaped pads seem to prevent leakage most effectively.[7]

Criteria for Disposable Pads

It is difficult to find a perfect pad, but easy to find an adapted one. An adapted pad must have the following characteristics:

- Designed specifically to prevent urine leakage
- Soft and nonirritating
- Comfortable
- Easy to use
- Low in cost

Types of Disposable Pads

Consequently, the type of pad is chosen according to the following characteristics:

- Severity of leakage
- Frequency of leakage (nocturnal or permanent incontinence)
- Associated fecal incontinence
- Patient mobility
- Degree of disability in patient
- Manual agility and dexterity

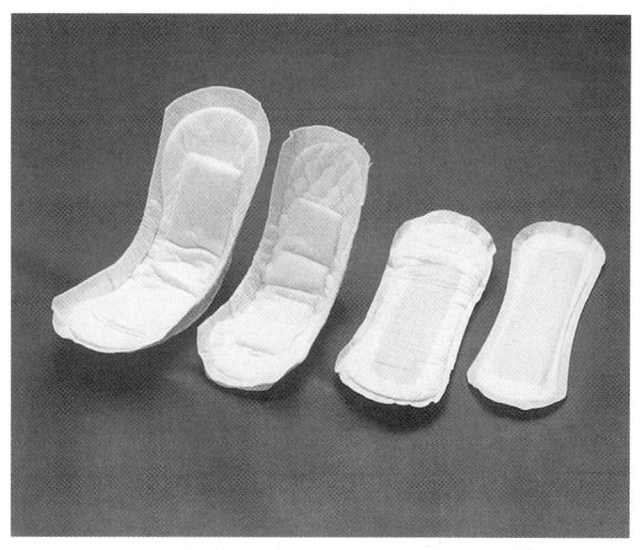

FIGURE 33-1 Incontinence pads are available in a variety of sizes and shapes. (Courtesy of Kimberly-Clark.)

Many types and sizes of pads are proposed for use by women and men (Fig. 33-1):

- Small pads for minor incontinence (50–110 g)
- Intermediate pads for medium incontinence (110–170 g)
- Large pads for severe incontinence (170–250 g)
- Penile cones or shells for male incontinence
- "Marsupial" (pouch) pants for bedridden patients
- Disposable pads and pants
- Disposable protection, including all-in-one pads and pants (Fig. 33-2)
- Disposable bed pads or undersheets (Fig. 33-3)

All disposable pads are made of three laminated layers:

1. An inner layer made of liquid-permeable soft voile
2. A middle layer with an absorbent core
3. An outer sheet made of soft, waterproof plastic

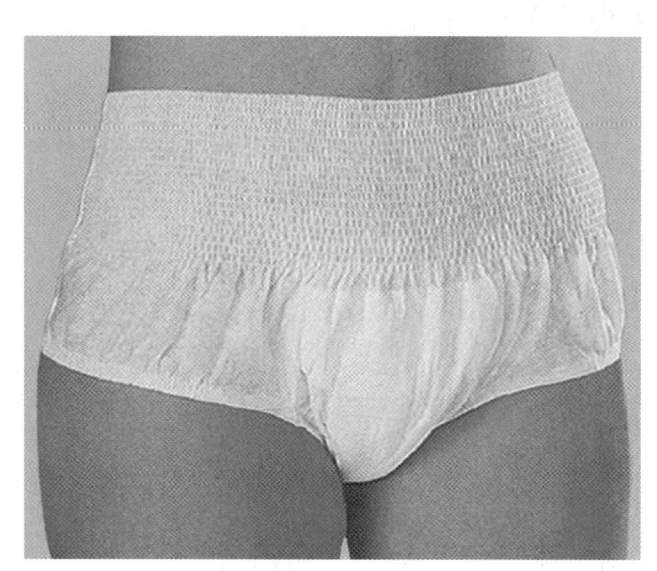

FIGURE 33-2 All-in-one pads and pants. (Courtesy of Kimberly-Clark.)

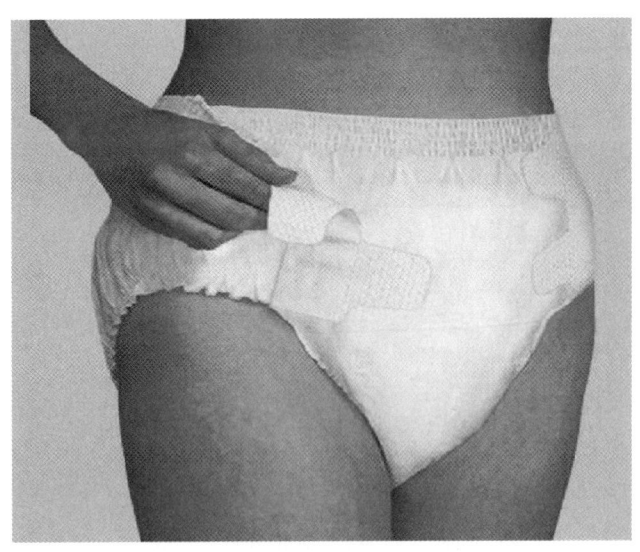

FIGURE 33-3 Disposable absorbent product. (Courtesy of Kimberly-Clark.)

Structure of the Inner Layer

The inner layer is made of permeable voile that allows fluid to transfer to the core of the pad, and stays dry when the pad is wet. The material is an airy net voile that is hypoallergenic and tolerated by the skin.

Structure of the Medium Layer

The core of the pad is typically made of absorbent pulp. The superabsorbent material is a powder that is incorporated into the core and bonds with the fibers. A chemical conversion transforms the powder into gel.[8]

Structure of the Outer Sheet

The outer layer is a sheet of soft, leakproof plastic that maintains the shape of the pad. The pads must be comfortable when wet or dry, and they must maintain an anatomic shape. Shorter, shaped pads appear to be better tolerated than longer, rectangular pads. Pads that allow accelerated penetration are usually less comfortable.

Considerations for Patients Who Use Disposable Pads

Skin tolerance may be related to the pH of the urine, but acidity is not the only factor that causes skin irritation. No studies show a significant correlation between local tolerance and discomfort in people with a high risk of dermatitis. Many patients may be unable or unwilling to express their opinion or describe their comfort level. These patients may be difficult to evaluate.[9]

After leakage occurs, patients may feel uncomfortable because of the psychological effect of the leak, regardless of whether they feel damp. One potential source of concern is odor. Some pads contain deodorizer-impregnated fibers. The most common type is neutralizing deodorizer applied to the pad.[10] An additional concern is that material impregnated with urine is an active bacteriologic medium.

Aesthetic considerations are receiving increasing attention. Pads can be used alone or with marsupial pants, which allow the patient to change pads without removing the pants. Pads can also be contained within the pants (all-in-one styles).[11,12] Pants resemble normal underwear, and small-volume pads are often better accepted by patients.[13] Shaped pads are easier to put on and take off than rectangular pads.

To comfortably fit the anatomy of the perineal body, pads of different shapes are available:

1. Rectangular (classic) pads that are rolled on and cut to the optimal length
2. Wing-folded pads
3. T-shaped, or hourglass-shaped, pads (Fig. 33-4)

The type of pad must be selected according to its size and capacity for absorbing urine. A large, costly, plastic-backed pad is not necessary when a small or medium pad will provide adequate protection. Pads are available for day and night use. Pads for night use are larger and capable of absorbing larger volumes of urine.[14]

When a specific pad is applied, the outer edges should be folded upward to create a gully to receive the urine and prevent spillage before absorption occurs (Fig. 33-5). Pads may be expensive, and patients must achieve a balance between changing the pad too often and changing it so infrequently that the skin becomes sore and chafed.

After the decision is made that a patient will use pants and pads to remain dry and comfortable, either permanently or while more active methods are being considered, the patient needs a sufficient supply of pads of the correct size.[15]

Patients need instruction for the use and care for continence aids (e.g., how to fit pads, how to launder or dispose of pants and pads).[16] Patients must also know how and where to obtain additional supplies (e.g., from a clinic, from the manufacturer, or at a pharmacy).

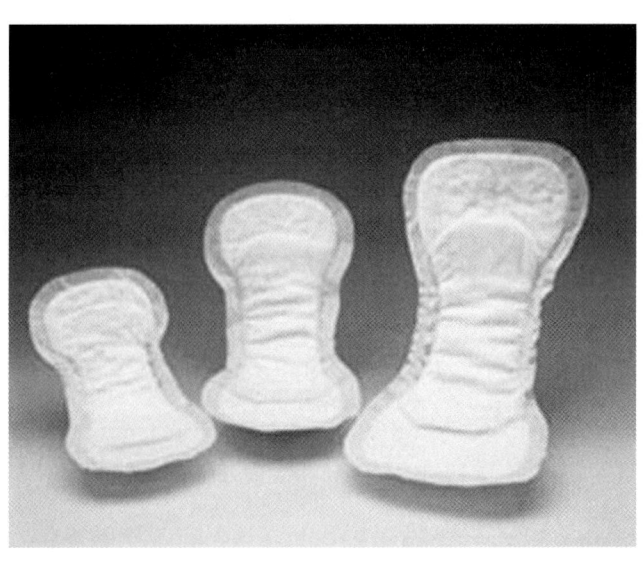

FIGURE 33-4 T-shaped pads. (Courtesy of Tena.)

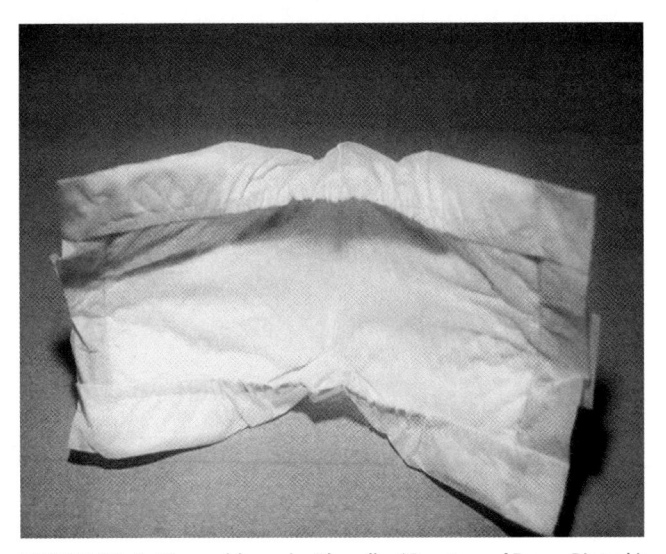

FIGURE 33-5 Disposable pad with gully. (Courtesy of Braun Biotrol.)

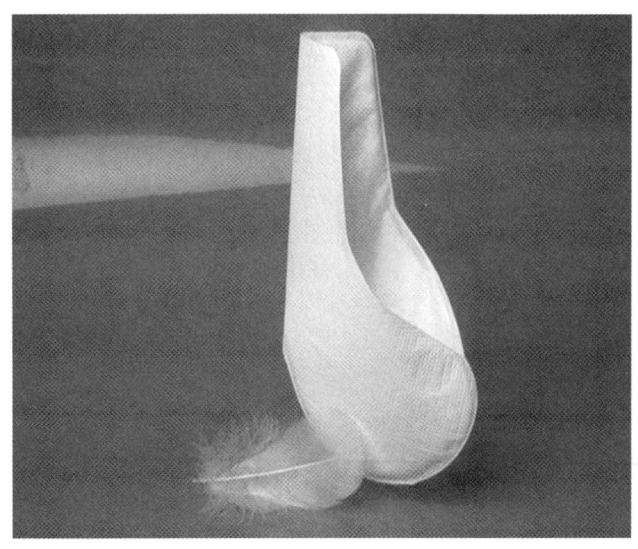

FIGURE 33-6 Penile shell. (Courtesy of Braun Biotrol.)

A useful adjunct to meet the patient's needs is a cooperation card that is carried at all times by the wearer. Staff at the clinic or physician's office should complete all necessary information so that the patient can receive the correct items. Financial considerations must not be overlooked. Although pants can be expensive, their cost is relatively low compared with the cost of the pads that would be required to replace them.[17]

Male Devices

Disposable Pads

Penile Cones and Shells

Many men with minor or intermittent incontinence use a penile shell, which is a cone-shaped absorbent device (Fig. 33-6) that attaches to the underwear with an adhesive strip. The patient places the genitals inside the shell. The core of the shell is made of pulp that includes superabsorbent powder. The absorptive capacity of the shell is approximately 250 mL.

Collecting Devices

Penile Sheath

The penile sheath consists of a condom with a distal collar that is connected to a urine-collecting bag by a tube (Fig. 33-7).

Selection. Size is a fundamental criterion in selection. Placing the sheath on a flaccid, retracted penis is not easy; keeping it in position is even more difficult. The size of the sheath must suit the diameter of the penis. If the sheath is too large, it slides and urine escapes. If it is too small, the penis becomes irritated and edema and balanitis may occur.

Sheaths are usually made of latex or silicone, and a proximal hem simplifies application on the penis. The collecting collar must be thicker than the condom to prevent spiraling (Fig. 33-8). The inner diameter of the collecting tube should allow maximal drainage.

Fixing Devices. Fixing devices include hook-and-loop (Velcro, Manchester, NH) strips and double-sided adhesive tape. Erythemas and penile stem wounds can appear on areas of irritation or may occur while adhesives are removed.

Self-adhesive Sheaths. Self-adhesive penile sheaths are available, and some types have a no-reflux valve. Other types allow no-touch installation, or application without skin contact. These sheaths are expensive, but offer improved comfort and security.

Urine-collecting Bags

Urine-collecting bags are chosen according to the patient's needs. Patients with good mobility require simple and morphologic ambulatory bags of adequate capacity. These bags are fixed to the leg with a Velcro strip. Bedridden patients require large-capacity bags that may be fixed to the bed with a hook or placed on

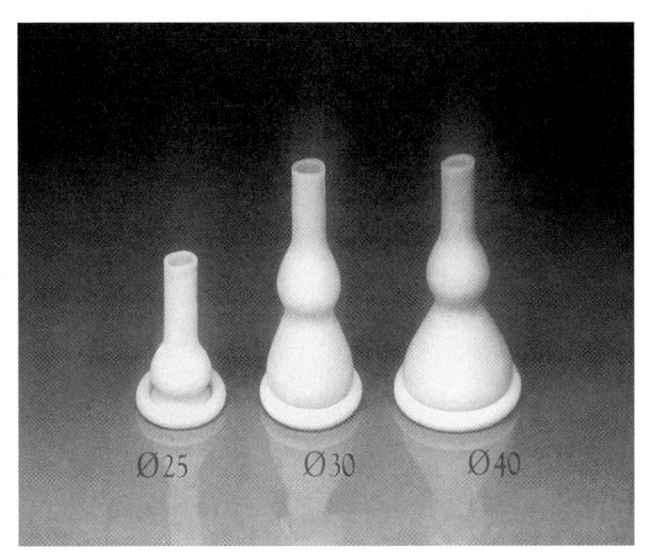

FIGURE 33-7 Penile sheaths in a variety of sizes (mm). (Courtesy of Braun Biotrol.)

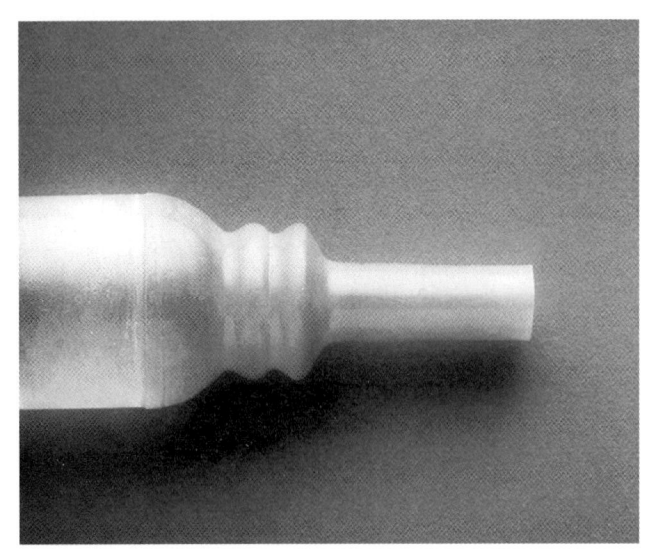

FIGURE 33-8 Collecting collar of a penile sheath.

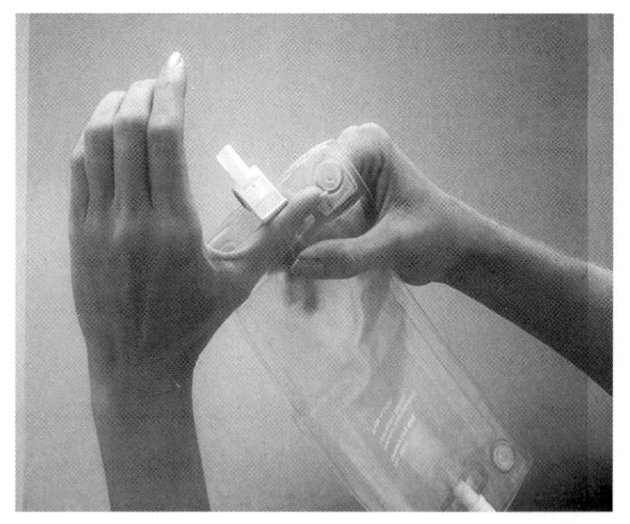

FIGURE 33-10 Valve device for emptying the collection bag. (Courtesy of Hollister.)

the floor because of their long connecting tubes (Fig. 33-9).

The capacity must be large enough to avoid the need for frequent emptying (350–700 mL for an ambulatory bag). A bag that attaches to the leg while filling seems to be the most common type, and offers the most security. The attachment to the leg must be strong and comfortable. Rubber bands and Velcro strips are the most common types.

The bag must include an emptying device, ideally one that the patient can operate with one hand (Fig. 33-10). Bags are now available with a no-reflux device that prevents collected urine from returning to the tube when pressure is applied to the bag.

The bag must be attached below the level of the bladder because gravity facilitates urine drainage. To prevent the tube from bending and clamping, the tube must be as short as possible. Collecting bags must be emptied and changed regularly to prevent the proliferation of organisms and resultant colonization and infection of the urinary lower tract.

CONCLUSION

Disposable pads and pants are not prescription items in most of Europe, but are obtained in pharmacies and supermarkets. Heath care providers are often poorly informed about available options and poorly equipped to make recommendations to their patients who have difficulty choosing the most appropriate product.

Although cost is an important consideration, the least expensive item may not be the most effective choice. Unfortunately, the most effective absorbent products are expensive for long-term use, but often provide the greatest comfort, security, and self-respect.

REFERENCES

1. Thomas TM, Plymat KR, Blannin JP, Meade TW: Prevalence of urinary incontinence. Br Med J 281:1243, 1980.
2. Resnik NM, Wetle TT, Scherr P, et al: Urinary incontinence in community dwelling elderly: Prevalence and correlates. Proceedings of the 16th Annual Meeting of the International Continence Society, Boston, MA, Sept 1986.
3. Bear M, Dwyer JW, Benveneste D, et al: Home-based management of urinary incontinence: A pilot study with both frail and independent eiders. J Wound Ostomy Continence Nurs 24(3):163, 1997.
4. Bainton D, Shepherd AM, Blannin JB: Pads and pants for urinary incontinence. Br Med J 285:419, 1982.
5. Cottenden AM: Incontinence pads: Clinical performance, design and technical properties. J Biomed Eng 10(6):506, 1988.
6. Mandelstam D: Disability and incontinence. Int Rehabil Med 4(1):3, 1982.
7. Hellstrom L, Milsom I, Larsson M, Ekelund P: Adapting incontinent patients' incontinence aids to their leakage volumes. Scand J Caring Sci 7(2):67, 1993.
8. Scandinavian Pulp, Paper and Board Committee: Fluff specific volume and absorption properties. Paper SCAN-C 33:80, 1980.

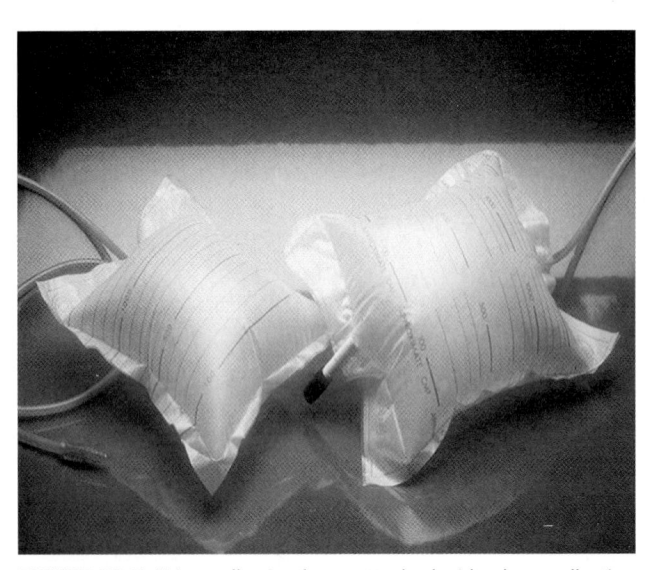

FIGURE 33-9 Urine-collecting bags, attached with a long collection tube. (Courtesy of Braun Biotrol.)

9. Davis JA, Leyden MD, Grove GL, Raynor WJ: Comparison of disposable diapers with fluff absorbent and fluff plus absorbent polymers: Effects on skin pH and diaper dermatitis. Paediatr Dermatol 6:102, 1989.
10. Fukui J, Shirai H, Ogawa A, et al: A newly designed deodorant pad for urinary incontinence. J Am Geriatr Soc 38(8):889, 1990.
11. Hay J: Incontinence pants: One system. Nurs Mirror 158(7):28, 1984.
12. Butturini E: Pants for incontinence patients. N Z Nurs J 83(9):26, 1990.
13. Clancy B, Malone-Lee J: Reducing the leakage of body-worn incontinence pads. J Adv Nurs 16(2):187, 1991.
14. Cottenden A, Ledger D: Incontinence pads: Predicting their leakage performance using laboratory tests. Neurourol Urodynam 12(3):289, 1993.
15. Shepherd AM, Blannin JP: A clinical trial of pants and pads used for urinary incontinence. Nurs Times 76(23):1015, 1980.
16. Thornburn P, Cottenden A, Brooks R, et al: Improving the performance of small incontinence pads: A study of "wet comfort." J Wound Ostomy Continence Nurs 24(4):219, 1997.
17. Tam G, Adamson M, Knox JG: A cost-effectiveness trial of incontinence pants. Nurs Times 74(29):1198, 1978.

CHAPTER 34

Pelvic Floor Re-education in Bowel Diseases

GUY VALANCOGNE ■ GUILLAUME CARGILL ■ ALAIN WATIER

Pelvic floor and anorectal re-education have an important place in the treatment of rectoanal complex dysfunctions. Indications, nonindications, and contraindications rest on a solid understanding of the anorectal physiology. Four essential points should be remembered[1,2]:

1. The complementary relationship between the "capacitive" rectal system and the "resistive" muscular system
2. The mixed muscular system: smooth and striated
3. Equally mixed innervation: motor and neurovegetative, sympathetic and parasympathetic
4. A performance that depends on the upstream digestive system

Indications and Contraindications

Stringent and accurate clinical examination, kinesitherapeutic evaluation, and functional manometric, electrophysiologic, and radiologic explorations can lead to a clear need for adapted functional re-education. Physiologic concerns include the following:

- Resistive muscular system dysfunctions, including poor quality contractions, hypocontractility, hyporesistance, hyperfatigability, and sphincter hypotonia[1,3-5]
- Abdominoperineal incompetence, especially the absence of abdominoperineal locking[1,3,4,6-9]
- Capacitive rectal system dysfunctions, including hyposensitivity, capacity and compliance reduction (e.g., incontinence, substitution reservoirs), and capacity and compliance increase (e.g., constipation)[1,10-18]
- Problems associated with rectal static, including rectocele, solitary rectal ulcer, first-degree prolapse, and more typically, descending perineum syndrome[1,4,8,19,20]
- The results of congenital anorectal defects and colorectal and anal surgeries[1,3,13,14,20]
- Encopresis[1,12,15,17,21-26]
- Pelviperineal pain[1,27]

Contraindications are rare and include local infection, pain, tears, or fistulas that do not permit the use of incontinence treatment techniques or that make the treatment of dyschesia impossible.

Hypotonia of the anal canal is not a good indication for re-education because it is essentially a smooth muscle deficiency that is, by definition, inaccessible to kinesitherapy; in this case, one should maximize use of the voluntary striated muscles.

The main contraindications to rectal re-education are inflammatory diseases. Radiation therapy is more a limitation to the possibilities of capacity and rectal compliance improvement as a result of histologic modifications of the rectal wall.

RE-EDUCATION METHODS AND TECHNIQUES

Physical Therapy

It is traditionally accepted that 50% of patients do not know how to use their perineal region. Therefore, increasing the patient's awareness of the pelviperineal region and teaching voluntary contraction and bearing down movements are essential steps. A sphincter contraction, whatever its strength, is useful and efficient only if it can be used in incontinence risk situations, such as an urge to pass gas or to defecate and during efforts such as coughing, sneezing, walking, and running. Therefore, work must be done on the quality of the contraction that must be achieved without apnea and without help from parasitic and antagonistic muscles, such as the abductors and buttocks.

The pelvic floor muscles are composed of type 1 and type 2 fibers to ensure the different tone, strength, and endurance functions. Analytic and global exercises must develop these properties.[1-3,5]

1. Type 1 tone fibers are developed through contractions done at 50% to 75% of maximum strength and held for 4 to 10 seconds. At the onset of treatment, the patient performs a series of contractions that last 4 seconds. Progression is achieved by either increasing the

number of contractions to 30 or increasing the duration of contractions to 10 seconds. The "required" duration of a contraction must be related to rectal compliance and, in particular, to the time necessary for rectal adaptation.

2. Type 2 phasic fibers are exercised through 1- to 3-second rapid contractions done at maximum intensity. Progression is achieved by increasing the number of serials until a least five successive 10-contraction serials can be completed.

These contractions are performed in various positions: lying down at first, then sitting down, standing, and finally in positions corresponding to each particular case according to the patient's profession and his or her private, gymnastic, or sports activities. The variations of circumstances are part of the automation work during efforts known as abdominoperineal locking.

The patient's motivation and participation are the most important factors in the success of re-education. Exercising at home is essential. A personal file is established for each patient and serves as a baseline to evaluate progress.

The perineal–sphincter work can be integrated into a global work: the ABDO-MG method[9] associates the voluntary abdominal work of the rectus abdominis muscles and the transverse with a rocking movement of the pelvis and an abdominal girdle reflex movement resulting from an electrostimulation triggered at the exact time as the voluntary movement, all being done during a totally free expiration without resistance through an exsufflation tube. This global movement triggers a reflex contraction of the pelvic floor muscles, which renders the method particularly interesting when the voluntary contraction is weak or done wrong.

Exercises with Digital Palpation[1,5,28]

Anal and rectal digital examinations primarily allow evaluation of the following muscle properties[29]:

- Tone, at rest, is rated as normotonic, hypotonic, or hypertonic.
- Contraction strength is rated from 0 to 5, according to international rating.
- Contraction duration or resistance should be at least 5 seconds and must be capable of lasting 10 seconds.
- Fatigability: five contractions must be completed in an identical manner.

Exercises with digital palpation are the best way to achieve muscular activity control. They are used with all the obvious precautions, and if the protocol requires it, at each session. They are particularly efficient for learning to perform the adapted movement without synkinesis or apnea. They allow work on the various types of fiber and permit the application of resistance. They are used throughout the treatment. They may be adapted depending on the clinical results, and they serve to evaluate the progression of pelvic floor re-education and facilitate the patient's participation because of their proprioceptive effect.

The stretch reflex is a muscular facilitation technique that involves the myotatic reflex that is triggered by a brief traction of the anal canal by the index finger during a rectal examination. The response precedes and improves voluntary contraction because of the recruitment of a larger number of motor units.

Contraindications to the manual technique include:

- Psychological factors related to the patient's psychological profile or history
- Anatomic factors, such as fissures, local wounds, and painful hemorrhoids
- Sociologic or cultural factors
- Age: they are rarely used with children, only used in cases of strict necessity

Biofeedback

Biofeedback is a pelvic perineal re-education technique that uses a signal that is usually visual, but may be auditory, which allows the patient with an anorectal or perineal functional anomaly to understand and correct the trouble. This signal may be made up of one or many pressure curves, of electromyographic signals, and of variable and proportional columns of the registered activity (Fig. 34-1). Last, for a child, the curve may be replaced by the concept of ludic or audiovisual graphs.[1,5,12,30–32]

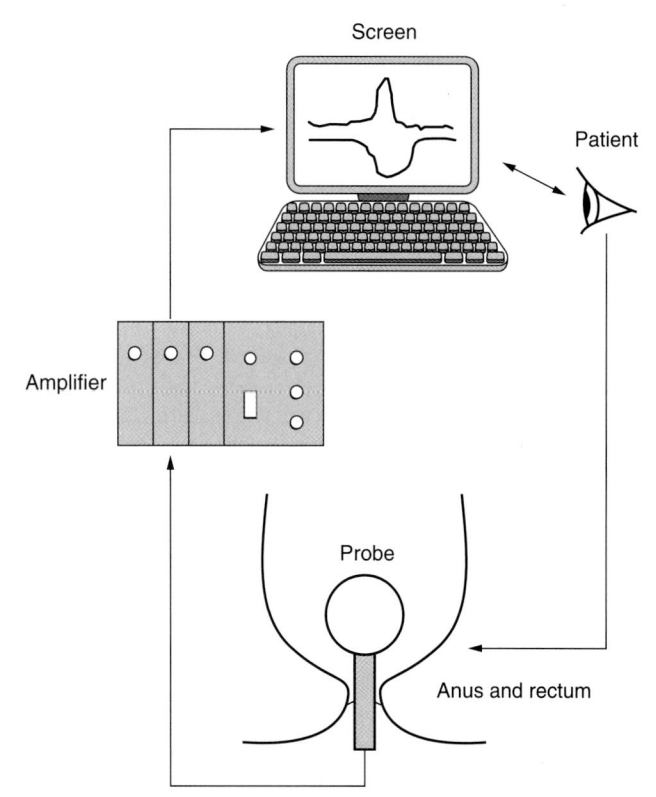

FIGURE 34-1 Principle of biofeedback. The patient observes the signal on the monitor. The re-educator comments on the signal and the abnormal findings and explains how to correct the abnormalities.

Biofeedback allows the treatment of multiple disorders (e.g., anal incontinence, sensitive disorders, evacuation disorders, anismus) with adults as well as children as soon as children are able to understand what is expected of them. Therefore, this type of treatment holds a distinctive place among the surgical and pharmacologic techniques. Only re-education and in particular biofeedback attempts to re-establish normal function, allowing normal and conscious use of the organ.

Not all types of re-education are *biofeedback*, although the term is often used for techniques that do not belong to this nomenclature. Moreover, biofeedback is not appropriate for all anorectal diseases: Re-education of the sphincter tone or voluntary contraction reinforcement belongs more to contractile gymnastics than to biofeedback.

The type of work to be accomplished must be determined through evaluation of the anomalies to be re-educated. A complete anorectal manometry is a prerequisite. In the clinical context, defecocolpocystography, electrophysiologic evaluation, and urodynamic evaluation may offer complementary information.

The technique requires a particular physical as well as psychological preparation and a specific setup. Each session is based on a rather particular exchange with the patient, especially if the child is young or has had a traumatic experience. Explanations must be simple so that the technique can correct the abnormal findings shown by the visual or auditory signal. The visualization system as well as the operator must not be traumatizing. Psychological factors are an important aspect of biofeedback re-education. Some authors even consider biofeedback an instrumental psychotherapy.

Follow-up is necessary to allow the patient to maintain the quality of the obtained results. Therefore, information must flow freely throughout the therapeutic team, which must be open to various physical and psychological dimensions related to the patient's problem.

Electrotherapy

Electrotherapy[1,5,29,33] is a controversial technique, without effect for some, efficient for others (including us); it is not in any way a passive re-education technique but an active-assistive technique, with the patient making voluntary contractions simultaneously with administration of the shocks. Electric shocks (impulses) are transmitted to the perineal sphere through external electrodes or with an anal probe. A vaginal probe may be used for women if use of an anal probe is contraindicated (e.g., there are fissures, stenosis, pain, psychological distress). Biphasic stimulation with a mean of zero and a progressive slope are used. The frequency range is 40 Hz to 100 Hz for phasic fibers and 15 Hz to 40 Hz for tonic fibers. The pulse width is on the order of µs to ms. To prevent damage to the nerves, careful consideration must be given to the level of stimulation. For this reason, anal sphincter neuropathy is systematically assessed for with a complete electrophysiologic evaluation. During this examination, one should try to find the most efficient stimulation frequency for the deficient muscle responsible for the anal insufficiency.

This type of stimulation allows a 70% return to normal continence, even when clear neuropathy is present. Delays are variable and may be long.

In protocols, electrostimulation usually follows biofeedback and manual techniques. However, muscular movements induced by stimulation are the preferred technique to increase pelvic floor awareness when voluntary contraction is weak.

Rectal Re-education

Re-education of rectal physical properties, capacity, adaptability, sensitivity, and reflex thresholds is an integral part of the rectoanal re-education.[1] The modifications demonstrated during the functional rectoanal exploration or at the initial kinesitherapeutic evaluation may be primary, as in the case of inflammatory diseases, but are more often secondary, such as the altered sensibility and urge to defecate for those with chronic constipation and reduction of the rectal capacity with incontinent patients. Re-education must be preceded by complete anorectal manometry to measure the rectal compliance, continence, and various sensitivity thresholds. These measurements are used as points of reference throughout the process of re-education.

Principles of Rectal Re-education

Rectal re-education is usually conducted in the second phase of the re-educational protocol, typically starting in the fourth or fifth session, after the kinesitherapy, biofeedback, and electrotherapy techniques are completed. The material used is the "rectal re-education balloon," which may be used alone or connected to a pressure sensor for manometric biofeedback. The balloon is inflated with air or water.

For sensitivity re-education, the principle is to conduct successive decreasing volume distensions, to teach the patient to feel volumes of ever decreasing size, until a physiologic threshold of 20 mL is reached.

Rectal capacity and compliance re-education is conducted with progressive 5-mL to 10-mL steps, dilations interrupted by rest periods, then increasing to a volume threshold of 180 mL to 200 mL.

Rectosphincteric reflex re-education is conducted with Pavlovian training: The multiplication of voluntary movements leads to access of the muscular response automaticity. The rectoanal inhibitory reflex (RAIR) evaluates the relaxation of the internal anal sphincter during rectal distension. The striated rectosphincteric reflex is a reflex contraction of the external sphincter in response to rectal dilation; it precedes the voluntary contraction and allows emergency continence.

Contraindications

Re-education should be considered only in the absence of progressive rectal pathology, for example during a colitis outbreak. Radiotherapy is either a contraindication because of bleeding or discharge, or it is a limitation because viscoelastic modifications do not allow a significant increase of the reservoir capacity.

In the postoperative period, notably after a coloanal or ileoanal anastomosis, a minimum delay of 6 to 8 weeks must be observed.

Local pathologies such as fissures and hemorrhoids are not real contraindications, but they may hinder the insertion of a balloon. Fistulas are absolute contraindications.

ANAL INCONTINENCE RE-EDUCATION

Anal Origin Incontinence Re-education

Exercises are conducted on the basis of the initial evaluation; therefore, it is difficult to standardize a protocol. Generally, three phases are evident: initiation, reinforcement, and maintenance.[1,3,5,7,9,13,28,30,34]

Initiation Phase

Generally, the first two sessions (sometimes more) are dedicated to learning contraction quality and different types of contraction.

Phasic fibers are exercised by rapid 1-second contractions, in a series of five movements that is repeated five times. Tonic contractions are maintained for 5 seconds at moderate intensity and repeated 15 to 20 times.

Exercising at home is introduced at the first session by recording in the patient's file the exercises he must practice. At this stage, the patient is asked to perform three sessions daily, alternating between exercises. During this phase, exercises are performed in the prone position.

Biofeedback is practiced during the first sessions with surface electrodes on the perineum central fibrous core and on the abdominal muscles to minimize their participation.

Electrotherapy using the same surface electrodes is involved, at this stage, only with acquisition of movement awareness.

Reinforcement Phase

The reinforcement phase constitutes the core of the sessions. Phasic contractions are conducted in series of 10 movements, repeated three times at the beginning and then progressing to five times. Tonic contractions are held for 4 seconds and progressively to 10 seconds, in series of 10 movements at the onset and then progressing to 30 movements.

These exercises are done in the prone, sitting, and standing positions, then in personal or gymnastics positions according to the patient's usual gymnastic or professional activities.

Biofeedback and electrostimulation are usually practiced with a probe. Each session addresses the two types of fiber, in variable portions as indicated by the initial evaluation.

Exercises at home are done an average of four times daily, alternating the exercises done in the prone, sitting, and standing positions.

Maintenance Phase

The maintenance phase is an excellent method of maintaining acquired results and preventing recurrences. Sessions are conducted bimonthly and then monthly to help the patient to maintain motivation and to regularly adapt exercises to keep pace with progress and to new situations.

Rectal Origin Incontinence Re-education

Rectal Capacity and Compliance Re-education

The aim of re-education is to provide the rectal reservoir a sufficient capacity, ideally approximately 200 mL; volumes of 120 mL to 180 mL usually provide a significant improvement in the quality of life.

The technique rests on progressive dilation of the rectum with balloons. It is not without risk and the biofeedback signal is as useful to the patient as to the re-educator. This technique must be preceded by the teaching of simple re-education principles. The lubricated probe is inserted, the balloon is inflated with air or liquid by means of a 50- or 60-mL syringe. The distension should be slow to avoid triggering painful sensations and rectal contraction. The first dilation is always inferior at 10 mL to 15 mL from the (B3) threshold indicated by manometry. Dilations are done progressively adding 5-mL volumes, interrupted with 1-minute rest periods, allowing rectum adaptation (Fig. 34-2). After the first 5-mL gain followed by a return to the basic value, a 10-mL gain is achieved in two 5-mL attempts and a return to the basic level ± 5 mL. The attained dilation should be held, depending on the patient, for a few seconds to 1 or 2 minutes. A second 10-mL dilation, in two 5-mL levels, is achieved, then a third, which could be repeated once or twice. The balloon is then deflated and the procedure repeated after a rest of 3 to 5 minutes. Three or four successive sequences take place during the session. The average session lasts 15 to 20 minutes, and the average gain per session is usually 10 mL to 15 mL. It is important that even if at the start of treatment, gain appears rapid, it

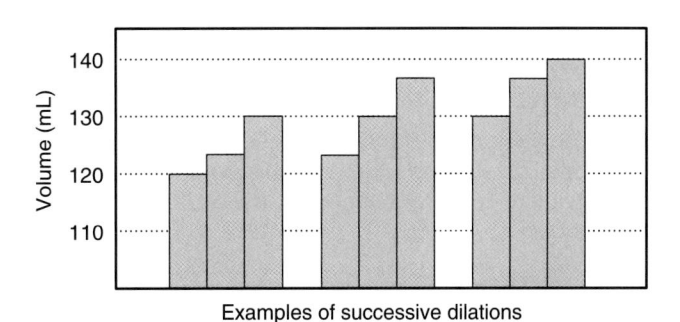

FIGURE 34-2 Rectal capacity and compliance re-education with progressive dilation with a balloon.

must remain conservative at 10 mL to 15 mL per session. It is also necessary to constantly monitor the pressure in the rectal balloon in parallel with dilations. High-pressure elevation (>6 Kpa in our practice) may result in a parietal lesion. Dilations may be uncomfortable but should not be painful. Care should be taken to advise the patient before the start of re-education of the risks and inconveniences, such as the passage of mucus and rectal bleeding. The presence of blood on the probe is possible.

Striated Recto Sphincteric Reflex Re-education

The external anal sphincter contraction reflex is acquired at childhood during the learning of stool control, when a child becomes aware of the first sensation and the first control of the urge to defecate. The reflex, defined by the threshold that is the smallest distending volume necessary to obtain a contraction, is detectable by surface EMG. This reflex deficit is responsible for urge incontinence.[1]

The principle of a re-education is Pavlovian: The multiplication of voluntary contractions in response to dilation will lead to the resurgence of an automatic response.

The material is a balloon inflated by air. The muscular response may be controlled by biofeedback with external EMG electrodes or a manometric probe.

In this protocol, the first volume distended is greater than the threshold volume determined at the functional exploration. Distending is brief and repeated many times at the same volume. As soon as the patient perceives dilation, he must respond with a brief and powerful contraction. The distended volume is then reduced by 5 mL to 10 mL in relation to the individual's progress. Because the average gain per session is 10 mL to 15 mL, it requires five to eight sessions to obtain a reflex response.

PELVIC FLOOR RE-EDUCATION AND CONSTIPATION

Dyschesia is often the result of a positive anorectal pressure gradient during defecation. It may originate from an anal canal striated muscle paradoxical contraction (dyssynergia asynchronism, anismus), rectoanal inhibitor reflex perturbation, smooth muscle hyperactivity (hypertonia), or rectal hypocontractility.[1,12,21,22]

Re-education of Constipation of Anal Origin

Striated Rectosphincteric Dyssynergia Re-education

Striated rectosphincteric dyssynergia is absence of relaxation or striated muscle paradoxical contraction (external anal sphincter or puborectalis) of the anal canal during defecation.

Objectives

The objective of re-education is fivefold:

1. Acquisition of an anal canal striated muscle relaxation during defecation
2. Reduction of straining
3. Improvement of the hygienodietary habits
4. Re-education of rectal function
5. Behavioral approach; that is, throughout the treatment, the therapist attempts to define and correct the dysfunction: Is it simply a bad habit? a behavioral problem? or the indicator of a much more serious problem?

Material

Awareness perception and re-education are achieved by biofeedback, usually with surface electrodes. This technique allows the patient to observe paradoxical sphincter contraction on the screen. The use of a balloon with pressure measurement favors a more selective approach when anal sphincter dyssynergia must be dissociated from puborectalis dyssynergia.

Methods

The first session is devoted to the explanation, in simple terms, of dyssynergia to the patient and awareness perception by biofeedback, which allows visualization of the paradoxical contraction.

The setting and the importance of general relaxation before defecation are essential elements. Therefore, they are immediately studied at the first session, then revised at every ensuing session. The real "motor" of the bowel movement is rectal contraction that is "authorized" at the central level; therefore, at least 1 minute must be allowed to trigger that physiologic movement.

Anal relaxation is also essential. Under biofeedback control, the patient must achieve the lowest possible pressure on EMG or pressure curve monitoring. The corresponding sensation is studied under biofeedback control so it is integrated and reproducible when the patient goes to the washroom.

Position Influence. The angle of the trunk and the femur must be reduced as much as possible to relax the perineal muscles. Therefore, too high a toilet bowl is maladjusted, especially for children and elderly people.

A normal defecatory maneuver is acquired through a protocol associates relaxation and defecation and helpful maneuvers to improve the technique of defecation.

Defecation-Assisting Maneuvers

The straining efforts are generally too systematic and usually too violent; they are partly responsible for rectal static problems. Only the very weak "straining-starter" remains physiologic to initiate defecation. However, if this pressure is too rapid or too strong, the myotatic reflex is triggered at the level of the puborectal muscles and the external anal sphincter, causing a striated rectosphincteric dyssynergia. Therefore, the terminal constipation re-education protocol integrates a "diaphragmatic piston" apprenticeship and a "correct straining effort" that is systematic, nonviolent, and efficient.

Work on the anorectal complex biomechanics and our studies have brought us to reconsider the defecatory modalities and to describe the piston maneuver and proper pushing techniques.[6]

Defecation-assisting maneuvers include the following:

- Inspiratory piston: a diaphragmatic inhalation followed by a 5-second apnea. The produced pressure is held with a proper orientation, in the anal canal axis, by countersupport of the abdominal transverse muscle.
- Valsalva maneuver: forcible exhalation against the closed glottis (must be minimized).
- Exhalation against resistance, with an instrument or the hand held against the mouth.

Physiologic and biomechanical studies show that resisted exhalation permits a significantly increased pressure in the rectum, an adapted orientation of straining that permits voluntary assistance to defecation and a visceral "support" in maintaining the physiologic amplitude mobility (CT-scan documented). It is a phenomenon that allows efficient action on the content (stools), while ensuring maintenance of the container (rectum) and realizing a real stool "demolding" during expulsion.

These techniques are learned during retrocontrol sessions so they can be associated with the perfect relaxation of the anal canal. In practice, the patient will be told to attempt, in the toilet, 5 to 8 "piston" trials.

Aside from exhalation against resistance maneuvers, further straining maneuvers (Valsalva maneuver) should be used with caution. In fact, the patient should attempt a straining maneuver only if he or she is certain of the presence of a stool in the rectum; the patient must be taught not to confuse a real defecatory need and a false need, particularly frequent in rectal static troubles or in functional colopathies. Usually, straining attempts are limited to four or five.

Bowel Movement Protocol

In summary, the bowel movement protocol includes the following steps:

1. The first minute in the toilet is devoted to installation and relaxation; the relaxation must be total, but also centered on the anal region.
2. The first bowel movement assistance method is the piston maneuver, during which the patient must maintain perfect relaxation, but without repeating the movement more than five to eight times.
3. In case of real need, the patient may use the proper straining technique (exhalation against resistance) and repeat it four or five times.
4. In total, the time spent in the toilet must not exceed 8 minutes. If attempts are unsuccessful, it is preferable to take a walk or perform gymnastic movements or colon massage, rather than multiply the attempts.
5. Rectal, sensitivity, and compliance re-education are usually started at the fourth session.
6. Hygiene and dietary advice for the treatment of terminal constipation is normally addressed at the first session.
7. Trials and results are noted from the second or third session in a follow-up booklet to follow results and adjust treatments.

Smooth Muscle Rectosphincteric Dyssynergia Re-education

Re-education aims to reharmonize the rectoanal inhibitory reflex (RAIR) response to rectal distension. Rectal distension with 20 mL to 30 mL should induce a reflex relaxation of the IAS. The amplitude of this reflex should be proportional to the volume of distension. This response may be out of phase or of insufficient amplitude, which may induce dyschesia. Negative manometric biofeedback with an anal pressure probe is used; the goal is for the patient to modify the synchronization and amplitude of the internal sphincter response to rectal distension. First, the patient must recognize the abnormal anal response to rectal distension, then real biofeedback work proceeds because the patient must learn to correct the sphincter response during successive balloon distensions.

Anal Canal Hypertonia Re-education

Type 1 and type 2 muscle fibers may be responsible for anal canal hypertonia. Levator ani, puborectal, and external anal sphincter striated muscle fiber hyperactivity are referred to as striated hypertonia and, when relevant, as levator hypertonia. In cases of smooth-fiber hyperactivity, it is referred to as smooth hypertonia, or anal canal hypertonia. The diagnosis is made during digital anorectal examination or with functional exploration by measuring the anal canal closing pressure.

Ideally re-education techniques act in complementarity on the whole of the hypertonia components. The techniques include the following:

- Kinesitherapy is a contraction–relaxation technique based on the principle of secondary inhibition to a long-lasting contraction (.15 to 20 seconds). In fact, beyond this duration, a gamma loop stimulation sets in and triggers a "cut-off" system or muscle relaxation. Therefore, under biofeedback the patient does long contractions followed by a short resting period.
- In manual techniques, all the necessary physical and psychological precautions are taken; they require the patients' participation and are never painful. The interventions are done in either the dorsal or lateral decubitus position, with a well-lubricated forefinger.
- Massage interventions involve stretching the anal canal by circular movements with the intent of progressively stretching muscular fibers. Transversal stretching movements go in all directions. Puborectal stretching massages use sweeping stretching movements. The contraction–relaxation technique uses the forefinger to help the contraction strength by the counterpressure effect, and then improves secondary relaxation through the finger traction-elongation effect. Massage sessions last 4 to 6 minutes to prevent irritation and secondary stiffness.
- The biofeedback is of the negative type because the patient is seeking a decrease of muscular activity. The system sensor is of the manometric type because the registration and the work concern anal canal pressure. The display of the curve on the screen is rather slow, on the average 30 seconds per screen display. The patient observing the screen accomplishes a relaxation effort in

an attempt to reduce the curve. This effort is carried out for 8 to 10 minutes.

Rectal Origin Constipation Re-education

Modifications of rectal sensitivity and compliance are generally the consequences of long-term constipation. This functional "megarectum" is characterized by an increase of the rectal capacity, to more than 250 mL, and as a consequence, a B1 rectal sensitivity threshold and a B2 need sensation, respectively, to more than 30 mL and 100 mL. These modifications are diagnosed through functional exploration or kinesitherapeutic evaluation. Rectal re-education is integrated in the constipation re-education protocol, normally starting from the fourth session.

Objective

The objective is the recuperation of the sensitivity thresholds; rectal capacity will be obtained in the long range as a result of regular rectum emptying.

Material

Material is the rectal re-education balloon, usually air distended, sometimes water distended.

Principles

Re-education is performed on an empty rectum; therefore, if necessary the patient must be asked to use a suppository or a small evacuation enema before the session. Brief distensions with decreasing volumes are used to re-educate the patient to feel ever decreasing volumes; between each distension, the balloon is completely deflated; and a pause of 3 or 4 seconds is observed (Fig. 34-3).

Protocol

Recuperation of rectum sensory threshold can be acquired by the following measures:

1. The first distensions are performed to a volume higher than the threshold evidenced at the evaluation.
2. The following distensions are performed at volumes reduced by 10-mL slices.
3. Five to eight distensions are performed at the same level so the patient can identify the new sensation.

This re-education session lasts 10 to 15 minutes. The average gain is 10 mL to 15 mL per session, therefore, with somewhat rapid progress and total recuperation in four to six sessions. To prevent recurrence, this effort must be repeated at regular intervals for many weeks.

Terminal Constipation Re-education Results

The involved population is rather large because it concerns children, sometimes very young, and adults, sometimes very old. Re-education is limited by physical, intellectual, and psychological capabilities; therefore re-education may be considered in very young children if they demonstrate a will and a capability to participate and concentrate for a few moments. Normalization of bowel movements is usually rapid with this re-education protocol: 80% to 85% of patients succeed in conserving anal canal relaxation and reducing dyschesia significantly in three to six sessions. The average pace is two sessions per week. However, this rapid recuperation must not hide the risks of recurrence. Therefore, bimonthly review sessions are indispensable; also, they facilitate behavioral and dietary follow-up. Therefore, the total number of sessions is 8 to 10. The long-term follow-up, 11.2 years in our study, shows that 66% of patients do not relapse and that 33% of them needed repeat sessions after a few months; in total, 87% no longer experience long-term terminal constipation symptoms or dyschesia.

RECTAL PROLAPSE RE-EDUCATION

Static rectal problems are the result of one or many processes, with an initial lesion of the muscular pelvic floor, mainly the perineal central fibrous core. This imbalance gradually brings lesions of ligaments and fasciae, creating an autoaggravating vicious cycle.[1,4,8]

Various rectal static troubles are described according to symptoms according to the degree and location of symptoms:

- Complete or total prolapse and mucosal prolapse that develops from the rectal wall
- The posterior vaginal wall deformity (colpocele) may be accompanied by a protrusion of the anterior rectal wall toward the vagina (rectocele)
- Elytrocele (Douglas pouch herniation)
- The solitary rectal ulcer syndrome, usually associated with an evacuation disorder
- The descending perineum syndrome, a clinical entity reflecting a progressive modification and alteration of pelvic floor dynamics[20]

In the etiology of prolapse, acquired factors such as obstetric traumas and the effects of professional and personal life events on the pelvic floor are responsible

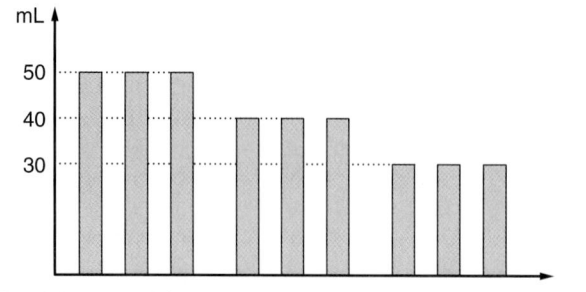

FIGURE 34-3 Brief distensions with decreasing volumes are used to re-educate the patient to feel decreasing volumes.

for hyper pressures. Also described are congenital factors such as connective tissue diseases, as well as pelvivertebral osteobiomechanic complex modifications. The prolapse may concern one or many pelvic organs. Thus, the fundamental principle of any therapeutic approach is to evaluate and to treat the cause and the aggravating factors, if possible, before treating the underlying pathology.

Re-education Principles

Indications and rate of success of re-education depend on the nature and the importance of the lesions. Re-education is not indicated for exteriorized prolapse and when the rectum suspension means are damaged, in which case surgery is indicated. On the other hand, re-education may be very efficient in first-degree static troubles: Not that anatomic troubles can be deleted, but deterioration can be limited and discomfort and malaise reduced. Finally, re-education may precede surgery and thus improve long-term results by limiting the risk of relapse.

Re-education Techniques and Protocols

Protocols are personalized and adapted, but there are three fundamental objectives. Therefore, three categories of technique (corrective, compensatory, and curative) can be discerned[1]:

1. First objective: to suppress causal and deteriorating efforts on rectal static such as rectal dyschesia and perineal hypotonicity through corrective techniques:
   - Striated rectosphincteric dyssynergia is re-educated through protocols that associate general and anal relaxation, suppression or reduction of straining during defecation, hygienodietary counseling, and behavioral therapy.
   - Perineal tonicity re-education is essential to the stability and protection of the pelvic floor. The techniques used—massage therapy, biofeedback, and electrostimulation—aim to develop and improve the type 1 fiber efficiency through low-intensity and long-duration contractions.
   - Reharmonization of the pelvic-vertebral dynamics deals with the ability of the abdominal muscles to maintain their competence, and to reinstitute the physiologic vertebral curves.[9,28,35]
2. Second objective: to transitionally compensate the fixation means deficit, and therefore, to maintain the pelvic equilibrium during the effort through compensatory techniques:
   - Abdominoperineal locking during efforts. Perineal locking is first a voluntary contraction, then progressively a reflex contraction during efforts. At the same time the abdomen contracts inward to act as a cushion during physical exercises and as a pelvic floor protector. The effort is predominantly by the abdominal transverse muscle contraction, which is essential to pelvic stability.
   - The manual counterpressure technique allows pushing back manually the prolapse in case of obstruction or during defecation; this may be a counterpressure against the anal margin to maintain the rectum prolapse or, using an intravaginal finger, to maintain the rectocele. A good number of female patients spontaneously use these manual techniques but are embarrassed doing it; they must be reassured and encouraged to use them because they reduce the obstruction and reduce straining efforts significantly.
3. Third objective: Curative techniques
   - Restoration of abdominal competence[6,7,9]: Abdominal competence is the capacity of the abdominal muscle belt to behave physiologically during an effort, that is, to contract so as to support the abdominal anterior wall. Therefore, it must be assessed at the initial re-education evaluation, according to "abdominal testing": The hand is placed on the abdomen; the test is positive when the abdomen remains relatively stable during a coughing effort; it is negative when the abdomen protrudes.

     The first phase of re-education attempts to re-establish the competence of the abdominal muscle belt in its active container and protector roles and to re-establish the perineal locking reflex during efforts. The ABDO-MG method associates an expiration without resistance through a small tube, an abdominal contraction movement, and a movement of retroversion of the pelvis.[9] The movement is accompanied by an abdominal synchronous electrostimulation. This abdominal reflex will be progressively automated during coughing or sneezing, as well as during load carrying. On the other hand, the exercise causes reflex contraction of the pelvic floor; this abdominoperineal method is practicable very shortly after childbirth, which confers it a preventive role against pelvic static troubles.
   - The abdominal hypopressure techniques are classified into three groups: the diaphragmatic aspiration techniques, the neurofacilitation techniques, and the hypopressive gymnastic exercises.[35] All generate a negative pressure quantifiable with a rectal manometric probe and will activate abdominal and perineal contraction reflexes. The hypopressive abdominal gymnastic is used mainly in the postpartum preventive framework, that is, in young women without symptoms. The tonimetric speculum permits evaluation of the voluntary contraction and basal tone of the pelvic floor muscles. Hypopressive abdominal gymnastic is intended for patients with basal hypotonia indicated by tonimetric examination.

DIETARY AND PHARMACOLOGIC TREATMENT

Abnormal colonic motility aggravates anorectal dysfunction. Constipation is an aggravating factor for terminal dyschesia and, conversely, diarrhea aggravates anal incontinence. Therefore, colonic motility must be considered in re-education. Regulation of the intestinal transit alone may notably improve the patient's clinical status. Globally, three situations may be considered: constipation, diarrhea, and irritable bowel syndrome.

Constipation

In the United States, in 1991, more than 4.5 million people had serious constipation. Women, children, and persons older than 65 years were the most affected. There are three times as many women affected by constipation as men.

Dietary fiber deficiency, liquid ingestion deficiency, lack of exercise, the ingestion of certain medicines, changes in lifestyle, and suppression of the urge to defecate are all factors predisposing to constipation. Constipation treatments depend on hygiene, adapted dietary treatment, and, in case of failure, medication.

Meals must be eaten at regular hours, in a calm environment, and with proper efficient mastication. Physical activity is advised. Often persons do not respond to their physiologic bowel movement needs. They prefer to postpone their urge to a more convenient time (sociologic defecation). The patient should set regular elimination periods. An evacuation attempt immediately after a meal is desirable to benefit from the gastrocolic reflex. The time spent in the toilet must be brief. Normal defecation should not be an exercise of straining. The social environment must respect the tranquility and the privacy of toilets.

Fiber is part of all balanced diets. In North America, most people consume only 10 g to 15 g of fiber a day, whereas the recommended consumption is approximately 35 g/day. Many people simply ignore the importance of fiber in their diet.

Dietary fibers are, in part, vegetables partially or wholly resistant to human digestion. They are found in whole-grain cereal products, fruits, vegetables, nuts and seeds, and legumes.[1,21] Fibers are neither digested nor absorbed by the organism. Some fibers are water soluble and others not. Soluble fibers (oat bran, barley, psyllium, skinless fruits and vegetables, legumes) are easily dispersed in water and liquid and rapidly turn into a gelatin in the digestive tract. They are fermented only when they reach the colon. Insoluble fibers (whole-grain cereal products, vegetable membrane, and fruit and vegetable skins) travel through the digestive tract without major change.

Fibers favor peristalsis. They absorb water, facilitate stools softening, and produce a mass effect. As they reduce pressure in the intestine, the colon needs less effort to propel the stools. Stools are also less difficult to expel. Fiber is also influenced by bacterial flora. Colonic fermentation of dietary fiber polysaccharides leads to many changes in the colonic lumen. Unfortunately, adherence to this type of constipation treatment is only 50%, even though it is nearly 80% efficient.

It is recommended that the patient increase his or her ingestion of liquids at the same time as fibers are increased in the diet. Six to eight glasses of water must be drunk every day.

Certain medications may induce constipation. They must be identified and avoided (narcotic pain medication, antispasmodics, iron, calcium, antidepressants, etc.). Daily use of laxatives should be exceptional. Unfortunately, many persons find all kinds of reasons to use them. Stimulant laxatives must be eliminated (phenolphthalein, bisacodyl, cascara sagrada, aloe, senna). The use of mass agents or softening agents is permitted.

Diarrhea

Diarrhea is characterized by the emission of liquid stools too frequently or in too large a quantity. Diarrhea can be acute or if it lasts for longer than 1 month chronic diarrhea. Acute diarrhea is often infectious; it is treated with a diet that varies according to the intensity of the trouble and with substances to correct the water and electrolyte imbalances. Chronic diarrhea can be motor, secretory, osmotic, or exudative. Motor diarrhea is characterized by transit acceleration, and it is essentially related to intestinal dysfunction, to hyperthyroidism, and to neurologic or anatomic causes. Problems with intestinal function account for more than 80% of cases. Whatever its mechanism, chronic diarrhea affects the nutritional status, generating multiple shortcomings that must be compensated.

In cases of idiopathic inflammatory disease diarrheas (Crohn's disease, rectocolite hemorrhage, and radic enteritis), the fiber-free diet is of limited usefulness. Its efficiency affects stool volumes and numbers but not the inflammatory component.

In the situation of motor diarrhea, the use of dietary fibers may be helpful for some patients.

Irritable Bowel Syndrome

This syndrome is characterized by an abnormal bowel motility pattern and an inadequate perception of distension (viscerosensitivity) modulated by biopsychosocial factors. The physiopathology of this syndrome remains obscure, although a relationship to stress is evident. Abdominal pain with constipation, diarrhea, or sometimes alternation between diarrhea and constipation are cardinal clinical features. In the diarrhea form, the diagnosis is far from evident and justifies a digestive evaluation in search of other etiologies.

Usually the treatment relies on a good patient–doctor relationship, hygiene, proper stress management, dietary manipulations, and use of antispasmodic drugs. The efficacy of diet in this pathology has never been demonstrated. However, it is common sense, considering the intestinal hypersensitivity, to propose that the patient avoid gas-forming foods. When constipation exists, fiber intake sometimes improves the transit. Antispasmodic drugs are often helpful in this situation.

When diarrhea and constipation alternate, mucilage is particularly efficient. In diarrhea periods, it slows down the small intestine and the evacuation of the stomach, and it regulates the intestinal transit by increasing the stool consistency. Conversely, in constipation periods, it plays a regulating laxative role.

The treatment of functional diarrhea is more difficult. Antispasmodic drugs are often necessary to relieve the accompanying pain. Mucilage reduces the fecal matter and increases the stool consistency without reducing daily fecal output. The use of cholestyramine may correct bile salts malabsorption associated diarrheas. Loperamide and codeine are used as last resorts.

A biopsychosocial approach is indicated for most patients.

THE PSYCHOLOGICAL ASPECT OF ANORECTAL RE-EDUCATION

Perineal re-education is difficult to approach and especially anal sphincter re-education without referring to psychological aspects that are raised by this pathology and its treatment.[36] Multiple aspects must be considered. In the case of constipated patients, there may exist a certain obsessional note. A certain psychorigidity may also be observed.

Patients afflicted with an irritable bowel syndrome are often "stressed" patients, fragile and sometimes depressive. Physical or sexual abuses may be found in more than 40% of these patients, especially if they have anismus.

Depression often accompanies anal incontinence. It is the result of the patient's embarrassment about his or her trouble and the difficulty to talk about it. It is also related to the social consequences of the disease. Of course, when incontinence is associated with dyschesia or severe constipation, psychological troubles may develop as a result.

The repercussion of anorectal dysfunction on psychological function is all the more comprehensible because it concerns an organ that is important in our relational life (cleanliness), thus it affects the psychological development during childhood. The psychological and phantasmagoric intricacies with the urogenital sphere are equally important.

Therefore, at every stage of treatment, it is important to consider this dimension of the disease. The initial interview, in addition to the physical aspects of the disease, will search for psychological troubles that could be explored further by evaluation scales or quality-of-life questionnaires. By doing so, the patients will often realize the psychological repercussion of their disease and the importance of dealing with it. Sometimes the patient, feeling that his or her distress is suspected, will voluntarily reveal an underlying suffering that must be heard. In such circumstances, it is sometimes permissible to propose, aside from the anorectal pathology assumption, an associated psychological assessment. This double approach can only be beneficial to the patient.

During physical examination we must also consider the fact that the patient exposes part of the anatomy that is sometimes judged shameful. The local examination must be conducted as it would be with a person who had a history of sexual violence or abuse so as to prevent further psychological injury. This is necessary because further physiological explorations will follow, and re-education will be more difficult if we have not put the patient at ease. The same precautions are to be taken for anorectal manometry.

All these gestures are to be accompanied by a reassuring dialogue and attentive listening to the patient's complaint.

One must willingly postpone a working session (exploration or re-education) to deal with the patient's psychological distress. Reference for psychological support and use of psychotropic drugs is useful in some cases.

Among the techniques to treat patients for their functional abnormalities as well as their psychological troubles, psychosomatic relaxation must be mentioned. This technique may be useful to improve intestinal troubles sometimes associated with perineal pathologies (irritable bowel syndrome, motor diarrhea). It is also useful to modify the body image. It is especially important in treatment of certain troubles such as anal sphincter hypertonia. In fact in the latter case, relaxation practiced with control of the sphincter tone normally allows a significant reduction of the anal tone. So, it is possible in teaching the patient the relaxation technique to facilitate defecation follow a brief session.

The relaxation exercises associated with biofeedback must be distinguished from the exercises conducted in the framework of psychotherapy. In psychotherapy they are preceded and followed by a discussion aiming to find the causes of an underlying psychological problem. It is sometimes interesting and necessary to associate both therapies, the patient learning to relax more rapidly and more deeply, increasing the chances of success of re-education while alleviating the underlying psychological problem.

In our minds, this corporal approach integrates rather well with the treatment of perineal problems. Yoga techniques are less indicated because they associate stress management and breathing exercises that are sometimes difficult to integrate in treating anismus and other defecatory problems.

In some cases, anorectal exploration and treatment reveals a severe underlying psychiatric disease that will require more complex interventions. It would be preferable to await improvement of the patient's psychic condition before undertaking re-education.

The examination and treatment of the patient with perineal problems should be undertaken by informed and trained personnel capable of assuming the physical and psychological care of the patient. Regular contact between the re-educator and the psychotherapist is a must.

REFERENCES

1. Valancogne G: Rééducation en coloproctologie. Paris, Masson, 1993, pp 1–19.
2. Shafik A: A new concept of the anatomy of the anal sphincter mechanism and the physiology of defecation: XXXI. Straidynia: An etiopathologic study. J Clin Gastroenterol 10:179–184, 1988.
3. Valancogne G: La rééducation des déficits ano-rectaux dans le post-partum. Kinésith Scient (373):21–25, 1997.
4. Villet R, Buzelin JM, Lazorthes F: Les Troubles de la Statique Pelvi-périnéale de la Femme. Paris, Vigot, 1995.

5. Pelissier E, Lopez S, Mares S: Rééducation Vésico-sphinctérienne et Ano-rectale. Paris, Masson, 1992.
6. Valancogne G: Rééducation périnéologique et pressions dans l'enceinte manométrique abdomninale. Abstracts of the Congrès of SIFUD. Lyon, 2001.
7. Richardson C, Hodges P: Therapeutic Exercise for Spinal Segmental Stabilization. Edinburgh, Churchill Livingstone, 1999, pp 41–54.
8. Beco J: Comprendre la fonction en regardant l'image: L'échographie en périnéologie. In Odyssée (ed): La Périnéologie Comprendre un Equilibre et le Préserver. Viviers, Belgigue, 1994, pp 42–55.
9. Guillarme L: Intérêts d'une Rééducation Abdominale Spécifique dans les Dysfonctionnements Abdomino-pelviens et Périnéux Secondaires à la Grossesse et à la Chirurgie Abdominale. St Etienne, Mémoire D.U. Université J.Monnet, 1992.
10. Valancogne G, Louis D: Apport de l'exploration fonctionnelle ano-rectale en coloproctologie. Rev Fr Gastroenterol 25(252):1382–1389, 1989.
11. Ahran P: Données physiologiques et physiopathologiques sur la motricité rectale du canal anal chez les enfants. C R Soc Biol 165(3):651, 1971.
12. Emery Y, Descos L, Meunier P, et al: Constipation terminale par asynchronisme abdomino-pelvien: Analyse des données étiologiques, cliniques, manométriques et des résultats thérapeutiques après rééducation par biofeedback. Gastroenterol Clin Biol 12:6–11, 1988.
13. Arhan P, Devroede G, et al: Idiopathic disorders of fecal continence in children. Pediatrics 71:774–779, 1983.
14. Meunier P: Physiopathologie des dysfonctionnements de la motricité du tube digestif terminal. Thèse de doctorat en biologie humaine, faculté de Lyon, no. 56, 1985, pp 130–163.
15. Meunier P, Marechal JM, Jaubert de Beaujeu M: Rectoanal pressure and rectal sensitivity: Studies in chronic childhood constipation. Gastroenterology 77:330–336, 1979.
16. Benninga MA, Buller HA, Heymans HSA, et al: Is encopresis always the result of constipation? Arch Dis Child 71:186–193, 1994.
17. Eren S, Wagner Y, Heldenberg D, Golan M: Studies of manometric abnormalities of the rectoanal region during defecation in constipated and soiling children: Modification through biofeedback therapy. Am J Gastroenterol 83(8):827–831, 1988.
18. Swanwick T: Encopresis in children: A cyclical model of constipation and faecal retention. Br J Pract 14(353):514–516, 1991.
19. Mahieu PHG: La défécographie: Technique de la défécation et de ses désordres fonctionnels. Paris, EMC Radiodiag IV, 33480 A10,11–1988, p 12.
20. Henry MM, Swash M: Coloproctology and the pelvic floor. London, Butterworths, 1985, pp 242–243.
21. Valancogne G, Louis D: Les constipations terminales de l'enfant. Kinésith Scient (362):30–38, 1996.
22. Clayden GS: Reflex anal dilatation associated with severe chronic constipation in children. Arch Dis Child 63:832–836, 1988.
23. Loening-Baucke V: Abnormal recto-anal sphincter response in chronically constipated children. J Pediatr 100:213–218, 1982.
24. Valancogne G: L'encoprésie de l'enfant. Kinésith Scient (362):39–45, 1996.
25. Hatch TF: Encopresis and constipation in children. Pediatr Clin North Am 35(2):257–280, 1988.
26. Levine MD, Mazonson P, Bakow H: Behavorial symptom substitution in children cured of encopresis. Am J Dis Child, no. 134, 1990.
27. Fulpin J: Douleurs abdominales récidivantes et asynchronisme abdomino-pelvien. Thèse doctorat en médecine, Université Claude Bernard, Lyon, UER Grange Blanche, no. 411, 1990.
28. Caufriez M: Thérapies manuelles et instrumentales en urogynécologie, tome II. Bruxelles, Maïté, 1989, p 199.
29. Valancogne G, Galaup JP: La rééducation pendant la grossesse et dans le post-partum. Rev Fr Gynecol Obstet 88(10):498–508, 1993.
30. Norton C, Kamm MA: Outcome of biofeedback for faecal incontinence. Br J Surg 86(9):1159–1163, 1999.
31. Loening-Baucke V: Abnormal recto-anal sphincter response in chronically constipated children. J Pediatr 100:213–218, 1982.
32. Loening-Baucke V: Biofeedback treatment of chronic constipation and encopresis in childhood: Long-term outcome. Pediatrics 96(1):105–110, 1995.
33. Grosse D, Valancogne G: Les techniques d'électrostimulations dans la rééducation périnéo-sphinctérienne. Kinésith Scient (373):25–32, 1997.
34. Bouchoucha M, Faye A, Arsac M: Importance de la mesure du temps de transit colique dans la prise en charge de l'incontinence anale idiopathique. Gastroenterol Clin Biol 24(2):A106, 2000.
35. DeGasquet B: L'incontinence urinaire d'effort chez les multigestes. Dossier Obstet 94 (220):46–55.
36. Deniker F: La constipation: Approche psycho-pathogénique. JAMA Suppl 160, 1988.

CHAPTER 35

Pelvic Floor Re-education in Urogynecology

SYLVAIN MEYER ■ GUNNAR LOSE

To date, few objective clinical comparative studies with large numbers have been carried out to assess the effectiveness of conservative treatments.
—*Concluding sentence of the introduction to the chapter on conservative management of urinary incontinence in women, published in the consensus book from the First International Consultation on Incontinence, Monaco, June 1998*[1]

Incontinence, including stress, urge, and mixed urinary types, is becoming recognized as a worldwide problem, especially in countries with high socioeconomic levels, in which women are living approximately 20 years longer than they were 30 to 40 years ago. Physiologic aging of the urethrovesical unit occurs between the ages of 15 and 80 years, with the loss of about 1 fiber daily of the 30,000 to 35,000 fibers present in the striated urethral sphincter.[2,3] Furthermore, the urethrovesical unit can be injured by one or more vaginal births, leading to further development of fecal and stress urinary incontinence and decreased quality of vaginal sexual response, with or without accompanying uterovaginal prolapse.[4,5]

Over the last 15 years, patients and physicians have shown increasing interest in conservative treatments. In almost all countries in which incontinence treatments are practiced, these are now accepted as a safe initial therapeutic measure for use before surgical treatment is considered. Surgery can be avoided in an estimated one third of patients who have stress incontinence.

The indications for conservative treatment have been extended to other pelvic floor problems. These techniques are prescribed in women with the following symptoms:

■ Genuine stress urinary incontinence
■ Urge incontinence
■ Mixed (i.e., urge and stress) incontinence
■ Pelvic floor rehabilitation after vaginal delivery
■ Fecal incontinence
■ Sexual difficulties

Different techniques of pelvic floor re-education have been described, and are prescribed daily by a wide variety of specialists, such as gynecologists, urologists, neurologists, internists, and general practitioners, as well as by physiotherapists trained in pelvic floor re-education.

TECHNIQUES OF PELVIC FLOOR RE-EDUCATION AND THEIR MODE OF ACTION

Pelvic Floor Muscle Training (PFMT)

PFMT has a long history. It was originally described in 1948 by Kegel, who reported successful treatment of urinary incontinence in 64 women who were trained with a perineometer to control the intensity of contraction of the perineal musculature.[6]

The pelvic floor musculature is composed mainly of slow-twitch and fast-twitch fibers that are distributed in various proportions. Striated urethral rhabdosphincter fibers consist mainly of slow-twitch fibers. Fast-twitch fibers are present only in the compressor urethrae located in the distal portion of the urethra. These slow-twitch fibers are responsible for a constant tonus that maintains closure of the urethral cylinder.

The pelvic floor musculature is connected to the urethral sphincter muscle by lateral striated muscle connections that anchor the urethral muscle to the pelvic wall. Muscle fibers are a mixed population of slow-twitch and fast-twitch fibers. Fast-twitch fibers can contract very quickly during a sudden increase in intra-abdominal pressure. The pressure increase appears first in the urethra, preceding that in the bladder by approximately 200 to 250 msec.[7]

During pelvic floor training, women are taught how to contract the pelvic floor muscles and to dissociate pelvic floor contraction from abdominal contraction. A strong, fast contraction of the pelvic floor muscles elevates the bladder neck, clamping the urethra by pressing it against the pubic symphysis.[8] Regular training increases the number of activated motor unit potentials as well as the frequency (neural adaptation) and volume (hypertrophy) of excitations.[9] A well-timed contraction of the pelvic floor muscles can prevent urethral descent, opening of the bladder neck, and escape of urine during sudden increases in intra-abdominal pressure.

Successful PFMT requires regular training after special training with a skilled physiotherapist. Many protocols have been described, and there is now a consensual trend to adopt protocols that include three sets of 8 to 12 slow-velocity maximal contractions, each sustained for 6 to 8 seconds, performed three to four times a week, and continued for at least 4 to 5 months.

The first step in pelvic floor re-education is usually a conversation with the patient about her anatomy and the problems she is experiencing. At this time, the patient should be told what she will do and experience during the pelvic floor re-education program. This conversation is followed by PFMT, which is the basic treatment with which each physiotherapist begins a re-education program.

This technique is often supplemented with the following:

- Biofeedback
- Intravaginal resistance devices
- Vaginal cones
- Electrical stimulation
- Bladder retraining

Biofeedback

Biofeedback techniques are used to increase the patient's awareness of the intensity and frequency of pelvic floor muscle contractions. Several approaches are used.

With one approach, the physiotherapist uses one or two fingers to palpate the levator muscles while assessing the patient's ability to contract the pelvic floor muscles.

Another approach is to use a special device consisting of a vaginal or anal probe with electromyographic sensors to provide the patient with information about the contractile force of the pelvic floor muscles. The contractile force is plotted on a screen on which the patient can follow her progress. The shape of the curve is analyzed, and the maximal pressure, area under the curve, and initial pressure gradient are calculated. The area under the curve is believed to represent the slow-twitch fibers of the pelvic floor muscle. The pressure gradient represents fast-twitch fibers, and the maximum pressure represents a combination of both fiber types. This method is used when the bladder is empty because the parameters are affected by bladder volume.

Different perineometer devices are used, and the pressure increase may be recorded with a traditional membrane pressure sensor, a vaginal balloon, or a water-filled perineometer.[10,11] Traditional perineometers also recorded intra-abdominal pressure during the Valsalva maneuver, which may be misinterpreted as pelvic floor contraction. Surface electromyography electrodes were developed to circumvent this problem. The vaginal surface electrode is now placed 3 cm from the introitus to allow accurate recording of pelvic floor muscle activity during contraction and provide good feedback to the patient.

The reproducibility of perineometric measurements has been studied[12] and standardized. Pelvic floor muscle strength should not be analyzed during the first session. Because of the learning process involved, the first and second pelvic floor muscle assessments are usually lower than the third; in addition, at each visit, the first value should be discarded and the mean of the next three or four contractions used.

Intravaginal Resistance Devices

Many devices (mainly air- or water-inflated balloons or perineometers) operate on the same principle: after the device is inserted into the vagina, the patient is asked to contract the pelvic floor muscles. Then the device is pulled out of the vagina with a pulley system that applies gradually increasing force.

Vaginal Cones

Vaginal cones were developed by Plevnik in 1985[13] as a new method to allow patients to train the pelvic floor musculature on a daily basis at home, without the need for a physiotherapist.

This simple concept uses a set of cones ranging from 20 to 100 g that are inserted into the vagina. When the patient stands and walks around, the cones tend to slip out of the vaginal ring, giving a "falling out" sensation that results in a pelvic floor muscle contraction. Once the patient can hold the 20-g cone in the vagina for 20 minutes on two separate occasions, the next heaviest cone is used.

This pelvic floor muscle contraction is carried out through reflex activation of the sensory afferent fibers of the pudendal and pelvic nerves. The activation occurs when vaginal wall mechanical tension receptors are activated and stimulate the pelvic floor muscles by pudendal nerve efferents mediated through an S2–S4 sacral cord reflex. This technique has the advantage of forcing the patient to contract only the pelvic floor muscles and not other groups of muscles, such as the abdominal or gluteal muscles, which are often contracted simultaneously during voluntary pelvic floor exercises.

Electrostimulation or Electrical Stimulation

Electrical stimulation is a technique of neuromuscular stimulation that is used to increase pelvic floor muscle contraction force and resistance to intra-abdominal hyperpressure. Commonly used terms include:

- Functional electrical stimulation
- Neuromuscular electrical stimulation, which is described on the basis of the type of current (e.g. faradism, interferential)
- Interferential therapy

The basic principle of this therapy is to stimulate the motor units of the pelvic floor muscles with electrical current that is applied through external (abdominal, leg, or perineal), internal (vaginal or anal), and implanted (sacral) electrodes. A wide range of currents (e.g., four-pole or two-pole applications, with electrodes of equal or unequal size), devices, parameters, and applications is used. Recent advances include the use of portable home stimulators that are prescribed after ambulatory training with skilled physiotherapists.

Currently, two main types of electrical stimulation are used:

1. Long-term, or chronic, electrical stimulation delivered below the sensory threshold for 6 to 12 hours (primarily for stress incontinence)
2. Maximal electrical stimulation, in which high-intensity stimulation is delivered just above the pain threshold for short periods (15–30 minutes) several times a week (mainly for urge incontinence)

The original technique, proposed in 1963 by Caldwell,[14] used electrodes implanted in the pelvic floor musculature to activate the urethral closure mechanism.

Current electrical stimulation techniques are believed to act by stimulating somatic efferent pathways, not by direct muscle stimulation. However, the mechanisms by which electrical stimulation acts on the pelvic floor muscles are complex, because both muscle and nerve and both motor and sensory fibers can be excited by electrical currents. Electrical stimulation must be considered general, or global, stimulation because it may not be possible to excite only a single type of neural fiber because of the anatomic proximity of the fibers. Furthermore, because of important morphologic and physiologic differences between the excitable structures, they show different sensitivity to the various parameters of electrical stimulation. Because the depolarization threshold of motor nerve fibers is much lower than that of muscle fibers, the term pelvic floor stimulation (i.e., direct muscle stimulation) is a misnomer.

Neuromuscular electrical stimulation has various physiologic effects, including the following:

- Alteration of cell membrane potentials that modify cell behavior
- Increased axonal budding
- Increased muscle bulk with hypertrophy of muscle cells and changing motor unit types (transforming fast-twitch fibers into slow-twitch fibers)
- Increased muscle strength as a result of the following:
  - Repeatedly overloading the pelvic floor muscles by repeated maximal contractions when using maximal stimulation
  - Effectively targeting and training type II fast-twitch muscle fibers when using maximum stimulation
  - Modifying the physiologic and metabolic characteristics of normal and "wounded" muscle fibers, transforming them into slow-twitch motor fibers (thus increasing endurance, albeit at the expense of strength), when using low-frequency and low-intensity chronic stimulation

Electrical stimulation of the pelvic floor produces contraction of the levator ani and, subsequently, of the external urethral sphincter (anchored by its lateral muscular attachments to the lateral levator muscle wall) and external anal sphincter. It also produces reflex inhibition of the detrusor muscle.[15]

Electrical stimulation has a therapeutic effect in patients with completely or partially intact peripheral innervation. Electrical stimulation is unlikely to be effective in patients with complete pelvic floor denervation.

Bladder Retraining

Bladder retraining, also known as bladder drill, bladder discipline, or bladder re-education, is a behavioral technique that is used to re-establish control of urinary continence and "normal" urinary habits in women. This technique was introduced in 1966 by Jeffcoate and Francis,[16] who recommended a special daily program of bladder re-education to re-establish normal bladder function.

The mechanisms of action of this technique are poorly understood, and the following hypotheses have been proposed[17–19]:

- Improved cortical inhibition of detrusor contraction
- Improved cortical facilitation of urethral closure during bladder filling
- Improved central modulation of afferent sensory impulses
- Behavior modification as a result of increased awareness of lower urinary tract function
- Increased capacity of the lower urinary tract

Extracorporeal Magnetic Innervation (ExMI)

ExMI is a new technique for pelvic floor training in incontinent women. ExMI is a completely noninvasive, painless, and effective technique that uses pulsed magnetic fields that pass through all body tissues without attenuation. ExMI is based on the classic principle of magnetic induction that was developed in 1830 by Faraday, who discovered that electric currents can be induced in a conducting medium by the application of a time-varying magnetic field.

ExMI produces a highly focused, time-varying magnetic field that penetrates deep into the perineum, stimulating innervation of the pelvic floor muscles by activating all branches of the pudendal and splanchnic nerves. These magnetic fields pass through clothing, bone, and soft tissues, creating an electrical potential that causes ion flow in the soft tissues of the pelvic floor. This ion flow causes brief depolarization of resting motor neurons. When a threshold is reached, an action potential is generated and propagates naturally down the axon through the usual Na^+ and K^+ ion fluxes. After these impulses reach the motor endplate, the pelvic floor muscles respond by contracting at a rate equal to the output pulse rate of the therapy head. Unless the output pulse rate exceeds the ability of the muscles to contract and relax, the muscles contract and relax with each pulse, resulting in constant, or titanic, contraction.

This technology, marketed as the Neocontrol Pelvic Floor Therapy System (Neotonus, Marietta, GA) is a no-touch technique because it is administered while the patient sits fully clothed on the ExMI chair. The physician determines the frequency and strength of the contractions. Each session lasts approximately 20 minutes, with about two sessions per week for 8 weeks (Figs. 35-1 and 35-2).

RESULTS

Many studies have assessed the benefits of pelvic floor re-education and can be found by searching MedLine, Excerpta Medica, and the Cochrane Urinary and Faecal Incontinence Review Group database. Of the available studies, 57 research publications were considered of sufficient quality for inclusion in the chapter on pelvic floor re-education in the World Health Organization (WHO) book on incontinence.[1] These studies met the following criteria: all were randomized, controlled, clinical, and pragmatic trials in women with stress, urge, or mixed incontinence, and were written in English, German, or Scandinavian languages. For bladder retraining, randomized, controlled studies (rare) and nonrandomized controlled trials were retained only when written in English.

No systematic review with meta-analyses (quantitative synthesis) has been done, and only two systematic reviews of physical therapies for female stress urinary incontinence have been published.[20,21] In the more recent study, Berghmans and colleagues[20] analyzed 22 randomized, controlled studies and considered only 11 to be of sufficient quality for inclusion. These authors reported the following findings:

- The benefits of pelvic floor muscle exercises in the prevention of stress urinary incontinence are not clear.
- Pelvic floor muscle exercises are effective in reducing the symptoms of stress urinary incontinence.
- Limited evidence shows the efficacy of a high-intensity versus a low-intensity regimen of pelvic floor muscle exercises.
- Biofeedback combined with pelvic floor muscle exercises is no better than pelvic floor muscle exercises alone.
- Evidence shows that electrical stimulation is superior to sham electrical stimulation.
- Limited evidence shows no difference between electrical stimulation and other physical therapies.

When the benefits or supposed benefits of these different methods for pelvic floor rehabilitation are considered, significant variations can be seen in how these techniques are taught to women and practiced by physiotherapists.

Pelvic Floor Muscles

Different publications report the use of a variety of parameters for PFMT. The length of the training period

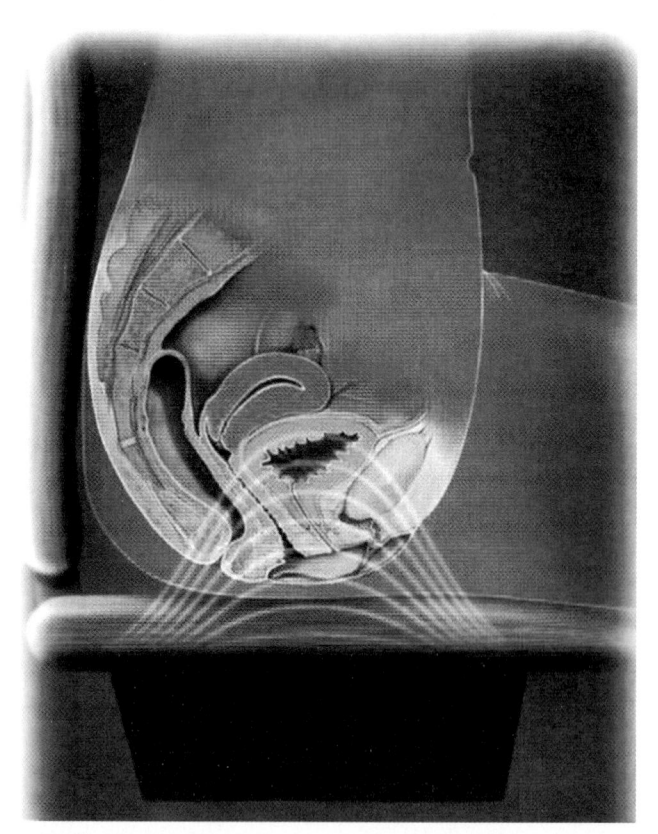

FIGURE 35-1 Principle of extracorporeal magnetic innervation. A highly focused, time-varying magnetic field penetrates deep into the perineum.

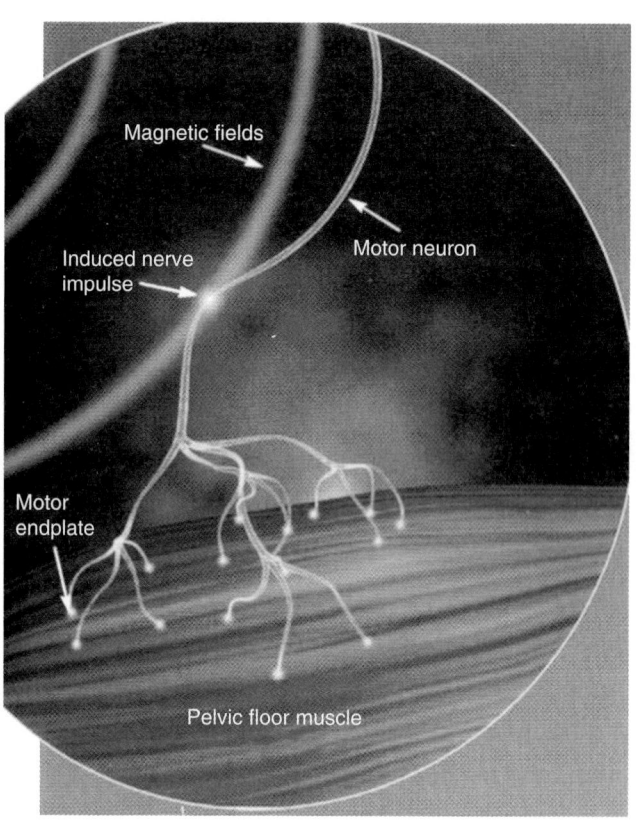

FIGURE 35-2 The magnetic field activates all of the branches of the pudendal and splanchnic nerves, inducing repetitive contractions of the pelvic floor musculature.

varies from 6 weeks[22] to 6 months,[23] programs can include hourly contractions[24] or a set of contractions repeated three times daily,[23] the number of pelvic floor contractions performed daily ranges from 36[23] to 200,[25] the length of hold varies from 3 seconds[25] to 40 seconds,[26] and training can be provided on an individual or group basis.

Before a patient begins a pelvic floor training program, a skilled physiotherapist and a practitioner with experience in treating patients with pelvic floor problems must be available to teach the correct program and control the efficacy of pelvic floor training to prevent muscle fatigue caused by overly vigorous exercise.

Near-maximal contractions seem to be the most significant factor in increasing pelvic floor strength. These contractions must be sustained for 6 to 8 seconds to recruit an increased number of motor units and fast-twitch fibers. PFMT should consist of three sets of 8 to 12 slow-velocity maximal contractions performed three to four times a week, and training is continued for up to 15 to 20 weeks.[27,28]

Compliance with such a program shows great variation from one country to another. Although Bo and colleagues[23] found an excellent compliance rate of 70% at 4 years of follow-up in a small group of 20 women, others found compliance rates of 51% at 12 months[29] and 27% at 4 years in 226 women who claimed to have performed PFMT for longer than 1 year.[30]

The expected rate of short-term cure or improvement with PFMT is 65% to 75%. It is impossible to distinguish the cure rate from the improvement rate, but symptom improvement appears to be more common than cure.

In women with stress, urge, or mixed incontinence, evidence suggests that PFMT is better than no treatment. In two studies, 68% and 74% of women undergoing PFMT reported cure or improvement compared with 5% and 3% of patients not undergoing PFMT.[29,30] Another study reported that 68% of patients undergoing PFMT achieved cure or improvement compared with 18% of control subjects.[25]

Is PFMT Alone Better Than PFMT Associated With Other Techniques?

The results in patients who underwent PFMT alone could not be compared with those in patients who underwent electrical stimulation alone because of a lack of consistency in the different trials.

Three studies reported better results with PFMT compared with electrical stimulation. The respective cure and improvement rates were 100% versus 80%, 65% versus 32%, and 64% versus 27%.[22,24,26] Other studies found the reverse, with electrical stimulation giving cure or improvement rates of 82% or 66% compared with 41% or 44% for PFMT.[31,32] Finally, another study found no significant differences in both groups,[33] whereas another found significant improvement in both groups, with PFMT showing significantly better results than electrical stimulation.[34]

PFMT and Biofeedback versus PFMT Alone

Some trials comparing the simultaneous use of biofeedback and PFMT reported equal effectiveness in providing significant improvement.[20,25,35] A single study reported that PFMT with biofeedback was superior to PFMT.[35]

PFMT with Intravaginal Resistance Devices versus PFMT Alone

Similarly, trials comparing PFMT in combination with intravaginal resistance devices with PFMT alone found a significant improvement in both groups, with no difference between the groups.[36,37]

PFMT with Electrical Stimulation versus PFMT Alone

When PFMT in combination with electrical stimulation was compared with PFMT alone, a single trial found significant improvement in both groups, identical cure and improvement rates (64%), and no significant difference between the groups.[22]

PFMT with Cones versus PFMT Alone

When PFMT in combination with cones was compared with PFMT alone, a single trial found significant improvement in both groups, with nearly identical cure rates (84.5% and 85.5%) in both groups.[38]

PFMT alone seems to be as effective as PFMT combined with biofeedback, intravaginal resistance devices, or electrical stimulation. Many physiotherapists use these other techniques as adjunct treatments for genuine stress urinary incontinence or mixed incontinence.

Biofeedback Alone

No trial has been published evaluating the benefits of biofeedback alone.

Electrical Stimulation Alone

Many stimulation protocols have been used, including different types of stimulation (from 20 minutes under anesthesia[39] to 4 months),[32] a different number of stimulation sessions or different timing of the sessions (from three times a week[22,40] to twice daily[32,41]), and the use of continuous or pulse current, using intravaginal, perineal and abdominal, or leg electrodes. Furthermore, the indications for electrical stimulation treatment included stress, mixed, and urge incontinence.

The only trial comparing electrical stimulation with no treatment found significant improvement in the patients who received electrical stimulation,[24] but there is insufficient evidence to conclude that electrical stimulation is better than no treatment.

Similarly, the results of the comparison of electrical stimulation versus sham electrical stimulation are controversial. Most studies found a significant improvement in the electrical stimulation group compared with the group who received no treatment or sham electrical stimulation. However, the rates of successful outcome varied greatly (27% vs. 0%,[22] 100% vs. 33%,[42] and 56% vs. 33%[41]), and two studies found no difference between the groups.[43,44] Although the issue of whether there is a difference in results with electrical stimulation versus sham electrical stimulation in the treatment of stress incontinence is unresolved, a single trial[43] showed increased benefit of electrical stimulation versus sham electrical stimulation in the treatment of detrusor instability.

Electrical Stimulation versus Vaginal Cones

When electrical stimulation was compared with the use of cones, both groups showed improvement, without a significant difference between them.[34,40]

Electrical Stimulation versus Anticholinergic Drugs in the Treatment of Urge Incontinence

A single trial found electrical stimulation and anticholinergic drugs equally effective in the treatment of urge incontinence.[32] Furthermore, the type of electrical stimulation seems unimportant in terms of the cure or improvement rate in women treated for genuine stress urinary incontinence. Improvement was seen in both groups of patients treated with either "acute" electrical stimulation with PFMT or "chronic" electrical stimulation and PFMT[33] or with interferential electrical stimulation with PFMT or "faradism" electrical stimulation with PFMT.[45] However, in all of these studies, there is a lack of consistency in the parameters used to treat the different types of incontinence, and it is not clear whether one protocol is more effective than another.

Bladder Retraining

Several variations are seen in the various studies of bladder retraining, from restriction of voiding between assigned toilet times to a self-scheduling regimen with no restriction of voiding if urgency becomes unbearable. Furthermore, some studies used an assigned interval of 30 minutes to 2 hours, and some included the use of adjunct therapy, such as PFMT or anticholinergic drugs.

The effects of treatment are seen within 2 weeks of beginning treatment,[19] but reported success rates in reducing urinary incontinence vary from 12% to 90%.[17,19,46] The long-term success rate (remaining continent or symptom-free) varies from from 42% to 80%.[47,48]

Bladder Retraining versus No Treatment

The bladder retraining group showed significant improvement compared with the untreated group in a population of women with detrusor instability and urge incontinence or with genuine stress urinary incontinence, detrusor instability, and mixed incontinence. A highly significant difference was seen at 6 months, with 90% of the treatment group reporting continence and 83% remaining symptom-free. In contrast, at 6 months, only 23% of the control group was continent and symptom-free.[17,46]

Significant improvement, lasting from 6 weeks to 6 months, was also seen using a standardized questionnaire. In studies that used a voiding diary to measure outcomes, cure rates ranged from 50% to 86%, and improvement rates were 75% to 87%.[49]

Bladder Retraining versus PFMT

These two techniques seem to have equal success, with cure rates of 18% versus 13% at 3 months and 16% versus 20% at 6 months, and improvement rates of 52% versus 46% at 3 months and 57% and 56% at 6 months.[18]

Bladder Retraining versus Anticholinergic Drugs

The success or improvement rate reported with bladder retraining differs from that reported with anticholinergic drug therapy. Some authors,[50] using flavoxate and imipramine, found that 84% of patients undergoing bladder retraining and 56% receiving drug treatment were continent. Other authors, using oxybutynin, found similar clinical cure rates of 74% and 73% with the two treatments[51]; however, a higher cure rate with oxybutynin was seen in women with detrusor instability alone (74% vs. 42%). Therefore, bladder retraining appears to have benefits similar to those of drug therapy, and may have long-term benefits.

Bladder Retraining in Combination with Drugs

Again, the results of studies are controversial, and further randomized, controlled trials are needed to compare the effect of bladder retraining alone and in combination with drugs.

However, studies show the following:

- No additional benefit of anticholinergic drugs[52,53]
- Additional benefit of anticholinergic drugs (i.e., terodiline)[54]
- No significant difference between bladder retraining alone (79% cure rate) and bladder retraining plus anticholinergic drugs (84% cure rate)[55]

Extracorporeal Magnetic Innervation

Because ExMI is a new technique, few trials have been published. In a study of 66 women with stress urinary incontinence, Bavendam and associates[56] reported that 80% of patients had an improved incontinence quality-of-life score, with fewer leaks, fewer pad changes, and decreased urinary frequency after ExMI therapy. In two cohorts of women with stress urinary incontinence (76 patients with short-term data at 8 weeks and 58 patients with long-term data at 24 weeks), ExMI was effective, with cure rates of 44% and 43% at 8 and 24 weeks, respectively.[57]

Another multisite prospective clinical study of ExMI found significant improvement in the symptoms of stress incontinence in 50 patients: 34% of patients were dry and 32% used no more than one pad daily. In addition, the number of episodes of leakage per day decreased from 3.3 to 1.7.[58] However, studies with longer follow-up are needed to determine the efficacy of this technique.

ANTI-INCONTINENCE DEVICES

Devices that are used to manage urinary stress incontinence work by the following mechanisms:

- External urinary collection
- Intravaginal support of the bladder neck
- Blockage of urinary leakage by occlusion at the external meatus or with an intraurethral insert

Indications for anti-incontinence devices include the following:

- Initial or long-term management of urinary incontinence
- As an adjunct to conservative therapy, such as pelvic floor training
- To postpone or avoid surgery
- After other forms of therapy are unsuccessful

These devices may allow women to resume a normal level of activity or to participate in sports without the need for surgery. Varying degrees of manual dexterity are required, depending on the type of device used.

Current external collecting devices are cumbersome and have no documented efficacy. Intravaginal devices are familiar to most women because they are similar to sanitary tampons. They are easy to use and can be worn for longer periods without being removed to allow micturition. These features make them practical for everyday use and also reduce cost. Intraurethral devices may be difficult to insert and can cause urethral irritation, urinary tract infection, hematuria, and migration to the bladder. They also must be removed to allow voiding, making them expensive for daily use. Various external occlusive devices are available, some of which can be reapplied after voiding and reused for up to 1 week. However, long-term efficacy and safety data have not been reported.

PELVIC FLOOR RE-EDUCATION TO PREVENT URINARY INCONTINENCE AFTER VAGINAL DELIVERY

Insufficient evidence is available for assessment of the efficacy of physical therapy in the prevention of urinary incontinence. The results of only three prospective randomized, controlled studies have been published (with a fourth in press), and there has been no long-term follow-up.

In one study, the authors reported no difference in the prevalence or severity of incontinence 3 months after delivery in a group of women who performed "usual" postnatal exercises compared with another group who followed a more intensive exercise program.[59] Two other studies gave contradictory results in the assessment of pelvic floor muscle strength between groups of patients who were trained postnatally. In one study, PFMT alone and PFMT plus intravaginal resistance devices gave the same results.[60] In another study, better results were obtained with PFMT and cones than with PFMT alone.[61]

More recent trials indicate significant usefulness of PFMT in the postnatal period. Morkved and Bo[62] found that pelvic floor muscle exercises, performed for 8 weeks, starting 8 weeks after vaginal delivery, significantly reduced urinary incontinence and increased pelvic floor muscle strength in the trained group. Wilson and Herbison[63] carried out a similar study by comparing the effect of physiotherapist-taught pelvic floor muscle exercises with that of standard postnatal pelvic floor muscle exercises 1 year after delivery. They found a lower prevalence of incontinence in the group of patients trained by the physiotherapist, but without any significant difference in perineometric measurements between the two groups.

In a recent randomized, controlled study beginning 3 months after delivery, a re-education program (including PFMT, biofeedback, and electrical stimulation) significantly reduced the incidence of genuine stress urinary incontinence in treated patients compared with untreated patients (19% vs. 2%). However, the different pelvic floor parameters (i.e., clinical and urodynamic findings) showed no significant differences between the two groups.[64]

PELVIC FLOOR RE-EDUCATION FOR FECAL INCONTINENCE

Recent advances in pelvic floor investigations, especially ultrasonographic endoanal examinations, emphasize the importance of anal sphincter lesions: 3% of primiparous women have clinically apparent injury to the anal sphincter after delivery, whereas endosonography shows occult anal sphincter damage in 35% of patients 6 weeks after the first delivery.[65] In another study of 43 women who had instrumental delivery, Sultan and associates[66] found that 81% of forceps deliveries and 24% of vacuum deliveries were associated with ultrasonographic anal sphincter damage. In a randomized study of 600 women, Johannson and colleagues[67] also found a significantly higher incidence of maternal injury after forceps delivery compared with vacuum delivery.

PFMT in combination with retraining is the initial conservative treatment, providing a 67% improvement in incontinence scores, with 27% of patients achieving complete cure.[68] Biofeedback is more frequently used and is reported to improve or eliminate symptoms in approximately 70% of patients with fecal incontinence.[69] In 80% of patients with fecal incontinence and a structurally normal intact sphincter, cure is achieved. The cure rate is 56% in patients with an external sphincter defect and 64% in those with an internal sphincter defect.[69] The success rate of biofeedback declines slightly with time, with a decrease from 64% to 41% reported 21 months after treatment.[70] The best results reported in patients who have fecal incontinence and are treated with biofeedback are as high as 84% and 92%.[71,72]

Electrical stimulation in combination with PFMT seems to be more effective than PFMT alone, with no significant differences found in women with fecal incontinence of idiopathic or traumatic origin.[73]

PELVIC FLOOR RE-EDUCATION FOR SEXUAL PROBLEMS

Few reports have considered the effects of pelvic floor muscle re-education in patients with reduced intensity of vaginal climax or increased time to reach climax. Although clitoral orgasm is almost never affected by vaginal delivery, the quality of vaginal climax is decreased in 18% to 25% of patients after spontaneous unassisted vaginal delivery.[74,75] The pudendal nerves are of central importance in normal sexual activity, carrying excitatory information from the perineum, parasympathetic stimuli to the clitoris, and somatic impulses to the bulbocavernosus, ischiocavernosus, and pubococcygeus muscles. During vaginal orgasm, the striated muscles around the vagina contract, thereby producing increased pressure in the vagina.[76] However, no correlation was found between decreased intravaginal pressure recordings during pelvic floor muscle contractions and the severity of the pathology. This lack of correlation can be explained by the complexity of the physiologic pathways involved in vaginal sexual climax. These pathways include mechanical receptors (mostly located in the anterior vaginal wall), normal sensory pathways to the S2–S3 dorsal roots of the medullar cord, synaptic connections to the pudendal nerves innervating the striated muscles of the pelvic floor, and finally, connections to the central nervous system.[77] These structures can be injured individually or in combination during vaginal delivery.

Originally, Kegel believed that pelvic floor muscle exercises were useful, concluding that "in a large percentage of cases, it will be found that lack of vaginal sensation and 'frigidity' can be traced to faulty development of function of the pubococcygeus muscle."[78] This assertion seemed to be confirmed by other authors who reported that the pubococcygeus muscle was "in better condition" in women who were able to achieve noncoital and coital orgasm.[79] Unfortunately, further studies did not confirm the usefulness of pelvic floor muscle re-education in improving the quality of vaginal climax, when comparing patients with and without such re-education.[80,81] More recent studies found that pelvic floor muscle re-education, coupled with biofeedback and electrical stimulation, seems to be effective in treating these problems. Ten months after vaginal delivery, the cure rate was 44% in re-educated patients; however, symptoms disappeared spontaneously in 25% of patients who did not have re-education.[82] Further randomized studies are needed to assess the usefulness of pelvic floor muscle re-education in the treatment of sexual disorders.

PELVIC FLOOR MUSCLE RE-EDUCATION AFTER SURGERY

No specific study evaluating the usefulness of pelvic floor re-education performed after anti-incontinence surgery to improve its results has been published.

CONCLUSION

Over the last 10 years, various pelvic floor re-education techniques have taken an important place in the treatment of pelvic floor symptoms, and they are now regularly prescribed by health professionals. Many factors, such as patient age and severity of incontinence, traditionally considered contraindications to such conservative forms of treatment, are no longer considered crucial. Skilled professionals can initially treat pelvic floor problems of any severity by prescribing 9 to 12 sessions of PFMT, with or without adjuncts, such as biofeedback, intravaginal resistance devices, cones, or electrical stimulation.

The factors that are most often associated with a positive outcome are the motivation and the compliance of the women using these techniques. These conservative treatments can be used without previous urodynamic evaluation. In addition, they are painless and are usually well tolerated, with minimal, treatable adverse effects. For psychological reasons, some women reject such "intimate-contact" treatments. The new ExMI technique seems to be a promising development in conservative treatment.

Systematic postdelivery re-education, now often requested by young women, also seems to be useful. This treatment encourages patients to talk about their pelvic floor problems, previously considered "unspeakable" by some women.

Before surgery is considered for the treatment of urinary or fecal incontinence, with or without simultaneous correction of uterovaginal prolapse, it seems reasonable to prescribe conservative treatments, unless they are rejected by the patient. Close collaboration with skilled physiotherapists is a prerequisite for the treatment of pelvic floor disorders.

REFERENCES

1. Wilson PD, Bo K, Bourcier A, et al: Conservative management in women. In Abrams P, Khoury S, Wein A (eds): First International Consultation on Incontinence. Plymouth, Plymbridge, 1998, pp 579–636.
2. Perruchini D, De Lancey JOL, Miller A, et al: The number and diameter of striated muscle fibres in the female urethra. ICS meeting, Yokohama, 1997. Neurourol Urodynam 16:405–406, 1997.

3. Perucchini D, De Lancey JOL, Miller JA: Regional striated muscle loss in the female urethra: Where is the striated muscle vulnerable? ICS meeting, Yokohama, 1997. Neurourol Urodynam 16:407–408, 1997.
4. Meyer S, Schreyer A, De Grandi P, Hohlfeld P: The effects of birth on urinary continence mechanisms and other pelvic-floor characteristics. Obstet Gynecol 92:613–618, 1998.
5. Meyer S, Hohlfeld P, Achtari C, et al: Birth trauma: Short and long-term effects of forceps delivery compared with spontaneous delivery on various pelvic floor parameters. Br J Obstet Gynecol 107(11):1360–1365, 2000.
6. Kegel AH: Progressive resistance exercise in the functional restoration of the perineal muscles. Am J Obstet Gynecol 56:238–248, 1948.
7. Constantinou CE, Govan DE: Contribution and timing of transmitted and generated pressure components in the female urethra. In Zinner N, Sterling AM (eds): Female Incontinence. New York, Alan R. Liss, 1981.
8. De Lancey JOL: Anatomy and mechanics of structure around the vesical neck: How vesical neck position might affects its closure. Neurourol Urodynam 7:161–162, 1988.
9. Plevnik S, Jenez J, Vrtacnik P, et al: Short-term electrical stimulation: Home treatment for urinary incontinence. World J Urol 4:24–26, 1986.
10. Ferguson KL, McKey PL, Bishop KR, et al: Stress urinary incontinence: Effect of pelvic muscle exercise. Obstet Gynecol 75:671–675, 1990.
11. Laycock J, Jerwood JA: A clinical study of the pelvic floor muscles by perineometry. Neurourol Urodynam 10:390–391, 1991.
12. Wilson PD, Herbison GP, Heer K: Reproducibility of perineometry measurements. Neurourol Urodynam 10(4):399–400, 1991.
13. Plevnik S: New method for testing and strengthening of pelvic floor muscles. In Proceedings of the 15th Annual Meeting of International Continence Society. International Incontinence Society, 1985, pp 267–268.
14. Caldwell KPS: The electrical control of sphincter incompetence. Lancet 2:174–175, 1963.
15. Laycock J, Plevnik S, Senn E: Electrical stimulation. In Schüssler B, Laycock J, Norton P, Stanton S (eds): Pelvic Floor Reeducation: Principles and Practice, London, Springer Verlag, 1994, pp 143–156.
16. Jeffcoate TNA, Francis WJ: Urgency incontinence in the female. Am J Obstet Gynecol 94:604–618, 1966.
17. Fantl, JA Wyman JF, McClish DK, et al: Efficacy of bladder training in older women with urinary incontinence. JAMA 265:609–613, 1991.
18. Wyman JF, Fantl JA, McClish DK, et al: Bladder training in older women with urinary incontinence: Relationship between outcome and changes in urodynamic observations. Obstet Gynecol 77:281–286, 1991.
19. Wyman JF, Fantl JA, McClish DK, et al: Comparative efficacy of behavioral interventions in the management of urinary incontinence. Am J Obstet Gynecol 179:999–1007, 1998.
20. Berghmans LC, Hendriks HJ, Bo K, et al: Conservative treatment of stress urinary incontinence in women: A systematic review of randomised clinical trials. Br J Urol 82(2):181–191, 1998.
21. Bo K: Physiotherapy to treat genuine stress incontinence. Int Continence Surv 6(2):2–8,1994.
22. Hofbauer VJ, Preisinger F, Nürnberger N: Der stellenwert der physiotherapie bei der weiblichen genuinen stress-inkontinenz. Z Urol Nephrol 83:249–253, 1990.
23. Bo K, Hagen RH, Kvarstein B, et al: Pelvic floor muscle exercise for treatment of female stress urinary incontinence: III. Effects of two different degrees of pelvic floor muscle exercises. Neurourol Urodynam 9:489–502, 1990.
24. Henalla SM, Hutchins CJ, Robinson P, Macvicar J: Non-operative methods in the treatment of genuine stress incontinence of urine. J Obstet Gynecol 9:222–225, 1989.
25. Burns PA, Pranikoff K, Nochajksi TH, et al: A comparison of effectiveness of biofeedback and pelvic muscle exercise treatment of stress incontinence in older community-dwelling women. J Gerontol 48:M167–M174, 1993.
26. Hahn I, Sommar S, Fall M: A comparative study of pelvic floor training and electrical stimulation for the treatment of genuine female stress urinary incontinence. Neurourol Urodynam 10:545–554, 1991.
27. Bump RC, Hurt G, Fantl A, Wyman J: Assessment of Kegel muscle exercise performance after brief verbal instruction. Am J Obstet Gynecol 165:322–329, 1991.
28. American College of Sports Medicine: The recommended quantity and quality of exercise for developing and maintaining cardiorespiratory and muscular fitness in healthy adults. Med Sci Sports Exerc 22:265–274, 1990.
29. O'Brien J, Austin M, Sdethi P, O'Boyle P: Urinary incontinence: Prevalence, need for treatment and effectiveness of intervention by nurse. BMJ 303:1308–1312, 1991.
30. Lagro-Janssen ALM, Debruyne FMJ, Smits AJA, Van Weel C: The effects of treatment of urinary incontinence in general practice. Fam Pract 9:284–289, 1992.
31. Laycock J, Jerwood D: Does pre-modulated interferential therapy cure genuine stress incontinence? Physiotherapy 79:553–560, 1993.
32. Smith JJ: Intravaginal stimulation randomized trial. J Urol 155:127–130, 1996.
33. Laycock J, Knight S, Naylor D: Prospective randomized, controlled trial to compare acute and chronic electrical stimulation in combination therapy for GSI. Proceedings of the 25th Annual Meeting of the International Continence Society. Neurourol Urodynam 14:425–426, 1995.
34. Wise BG, Haken J, Cardozo L, Plevnik S: A comparative study of vaginal cone therapy, cones + Kegel exercises, and maximal electrical stimulation in the treatment of female genuine stress incontinence. Proceeding of the 23rd Annual Meeting of the International Continence Society. Neurorurol Urodynam 12:436–437, 1993.
35. Glavind K, Nohr SB, Walter S: Biofeedback and physiotherapy versus physiotherapy alone in the treatment of genuine stress incontinence. Int Urogynecol J 7:339–343, 1996.
36. Shepherd AM, Montgomery E: Treatment of genuine stress incontinence with a new perineometer. Physiotherapy 69:113, 1983.
37. Ferguson KL, Bishop KR, Kloen P, et al: Stress urinary incontinence: Effect of pelvic muscle exercise. Obstet Gynecol 75:671–675, 1990.
38. Pieber D, Zivkovic F, Tamussino G, et al: Pelvic floor exercise alone or with vaginal cones for the treatment of mild to moderate stress urinary incontinence in premenopausal women. Int Urogynecol J 6:14–17, 1995.
39. Sheperd AM, Tribe E, Bainton D: Maximum perineal stimulation: A controlled study. Br J Urol 56:644–646, 1984.
40. Olah KS, Bridges N, Denning J, Farrar DJ: The conservative management of patients with symptoms of stress incontinence: A randomized, prospective study compared weighed vaginal cones and interferential therapy. Am J Obstet Gynecol 162:87–92, 1990.
41. Sand PK, Richardson DA, Statskin DR, et al: Pelvic floor electrical stimulation in the treatment of genuine stress incontinence: A multicenter, placebo-controlled trial. Am J Obstet Gynecol 173:72–79, 1995.

42. Blowman C, Pickles C, Emery S, et al: Prospective double blind controlled trial of intensive physiotherapy with and without stimulation of pelvic floor in the treatment of genuine stress incontinence. Physiotherapy 77:661–664, 1991.
43. Brubaker L, Benson T, Bent A, et al: Transvaginal electrical stimulation for female urinary incontinence. Am J Obstet Gynecol 177:536–540, 1997.
44. Luber KM, Wolde-Tsadik G: Efficacy of functional electrical stimulation in treating genuine stress incontinence: A randomized controlled trial. Neurourol Urodynam 16:543–551, 1997.
45. Wilson PD, Al Samarrai T, Deakin M, et al: An objective assessment of physiotherapy for female genuine stress incontinence. Br J Obstet Gynecol 94:575–582, 1987.
46. Jarvis GJ, Millar DR: Controlled trial of bladder drill for detrusor instability. BMJ 281:1322–1323, 1980.
47. Mahady LW, Begg BM: Long term symptomatic and cystometric cure of the urge incontinence syndrome using a technique of bladder re-education. Br J Obstet Gynaecol 88:1038–1043, 1981.
48. Snape J, Castelden CM, Duffin HM, et al: Long term follow-up of habit retraining for bladder instability in elderly patients. Age Ageing 15:292–298, 1989.
49. Wyman JF, Fantl JA, Mcclish DK, et al: Effect of bladder training on quality of life of older women with urinary incontinence. Int Urogynecol J 8:223–229, 1997.
50. Jarvis GJ: A controlled trial of bladder drill and drug therapy in the management of detrusor instability. Br J Urol 53:565–566, 1981.
51. Columbo M, Zanetta G, Scalambrino S, et al: Oxybutinin and bladder training in the management of female urge incontinence: A randomized study. Int Urogynecol J 6:63–67, 1995.
52. Wiseman PA, Malone-Lee J, Rai GSA: Terodiline with bladder retraining for treating detrusor instability in elderly people. BMJ 302:994–996, 1991.
53. Szonyi G, Collas DM, Ding YY, et al: Oxybutinin with bladder retraining for detrusor instability in elderly people: A randomised controlled trial. Age Ageing 24:287–291, 1995.
54. Klarskov P, Gerstenberg TC, Hald T: Bladder training and terodiline in females with idiopathic urge incontinence and stable detrusor function. Scand J Urol Nephrol 20:41–46, 1986.
55. Fantl JA, Hurt GW, Dunn LL: Detrusor instability syndrome: The use of bladder retraining drills with and without anticholinergics. Am J Obstet Gynecol 140:885–890, 1981.
56. Bavendam T, Braddon L, Carlan S, et al: Impact of extracorporeal magnetic innervation (ExMI) on quality of life in the treatment of stress urinary incontinence (abstract). American Urological Association Meeting, Atlanta, GA, April 29, 2000.
57. Sand P, Appell R, Bavendam T, et al: Factors influencing success with extracorporeal magnetic innervation (ExMI) treatment of mixed urinary incontinence (abstract). International Bladder Symposium, Washington, DC, November 4, 1999.
58. Niall T, Galloway M, Rizk E, et al: Extracorporeal magnetic innervation therapy for stress urinary incontinence. Urology 53:1108–1111, 1999.
59. Sleep J, Grant A: Pelvic floor exercises in post-natal care. Midwifery 3:158–164, 1987.
60. Dougherty MC, Bishop K, Abrams RM, et al: The effects of exercise on the circumvaginal muscles in post-partum women. J Nurse Midwifery 34:8–14, 1989.
61. Jonasson A, Larsson B, Pschera H: Testing and training of the pelvic floor muscles after chilbirth. Acta Obstet Gynaecol Scand 68:301–304, 1989.
62. Morkved S, Bo K: The effect of post-partum pelvic floor muscle exercise in the prevention and treatment of urinary incontinence. Int Urogynecol J 8:217–222, 1997.
63. Wilson PD, Herbison GP: A randomised controlled trial of pelvic floor muscle exercises to treat post-natal urinary incontinence. Int Urogynecol J 9:257–264, 1998.
64. Meyer S, Hohlfeld P, Achtari C, et al: Pelvic floor education after vaginal delivery: A randomized controlled study. Obstet Gynecol 97:673–677, 2001.
65. Sultan AH, Kamm MA, Hudson CN, et al: Anal sphincter disruption during vaginal delivery. N Engl Med 329:1905–1911, 1993.
66. Sultan AH, Kamm MA, Bartram CI, Hudson CN: Anal sphincter trauma during instrumental delivery. Int J Gynaecol Obstet 43(3):263–270, 1993.
67. Johansson RB, Rice C, Doyle M, et al: A randomised prospective study comparing the new vacuum extractor policy with forceps delivery. Br J Obstet Gynaecol 100(6):524–530, 1993.
68. Rieger NA, Wattchow DA, Sarre RG, et al: Prospective trial of pelvic floor retraining in patients with fecal incontinence. Dis Colon Rectum 40(7):821–826, 1997.
69. Norton C, Kamm MA: Outcome of biofeedback for faecal incontinence. Br J Surg 86:1159–1163, 1999.
70. Glia A, Gylin M, Akerlund JE, et al: Biofeedback training in patients with fecal incontinence. Dis Colon Rectum 41(3):359–364, 1998.
71. Patankar SK, Ferrara A, Levy JR, et al: Biofeedback in colorectal practice: A multicenter statewide, three-year experience. Dis Colon Rectum 40(7):827–831, 1997.
72. Ko CY, Tong J, Lehman RE, et al: Biofeedback is effective therapy for fecal incontinence and constipation. Arch Surg 132(8):829–833, 1997.
73. Sprakel B, Maurer S, Langer M, et al: Value of electrotherapy within the scope of conservative treatment of ano-rectal incontinence. Zentralbl Chir 123(3):224–229, 1998.
74. Meyer S, Hohlfeld P, Achtari C, et al: Birth-trauma: Short and long-term effects of forceps delivery compared with spontaneous delivery on various pelvic floor parameters. Br J Obstet Gynaecol 107(11):1360–1365, 2000.
75. Meyer S, Achtari C, Russolo A, et al: Early and late effects of spontaneous delivery on the different pelvic floor parameters in primiparae patients without pelvic floor re-education (abstract). ICS-IUGA meeting, Denver, 1999.
76. Lechtenberg R, Ohl DA (eds): Normal sexual response in sexual dysfunction: Neurologic, urologic, and gynecologic aspects. Philadelphia, Lea & Febiger, 1994, pp 21–43.
77. Sacco F, Rigon G, Sacchini D: Forceps delivery and long term follow-up urinary incontinence. Minerva Ginecol 48(9):355–358, 1996.
78. Kegel AH: Sexual functions of the pubo-coccygeous muscle. West J Surg Obstet Gynecol 60:521–534, 1952.
79. Kline-Graber G, Graber B: Diagnosis and treatment procedures of pubo-coccygeal deficiencies in women. In Lo Piccolo J, Lo Piccolo L (eds): Handbook of Sex Therapy. New York, Plenum, 1978.
80. Roughan PA, Kunst L: Do pelvic floor exercises really improve orgasmic potential? J Sex Marital Ther 7(3):223–229, 1981.
81. Chambless DL, Sultan FE, Stern TE, et al: Effect of pubococcygeal exercise on coital orgasm in women. J Consult Clin Psychol 52(1):114–118, 1984.
82. Meyer S, Megalo A, DeGrandi P, Hohlfeld P: The birth trauma: The effects of early reeducation on the different pelvic floor parameters in primipara vaginally delivered. Poster presented at the 1st International Consultation on Incontinence, Monaco 1998.

CHAPTER 36

Management of Incontinence in the Elderly

Pat D. O'Donnell ■ Alain P. Bourcier

Urinary incontinence is one of the most debilitating problems of the elderly. Urinary incontinence (UI) affects every aspect of an elderly person's life. One of the most personally devastating aspects of urinary incontinence is the self-imposed social isolation because of a constant fear of incontinence in public, which would be very embarrassing. Also, there is continuous concern about the odor of urine resulting from incontinence episodes. Such self-imposed isolation occurs at a time in an individual's life when social interaction is a critical part of the quality of life. This results in the most serious personal issue faced by the elderly, which is loss of self-esteem. The economic costs of urinary incontinence to the individual and to society are enormous, but the personal loss to the individual is by far the worst. Unfortunately, since urinary incontinence in the elderly is not a fatal disease, many people think it is part of the aging process. When the patient's survival is not an issue, medical research and therapeutic options are not pursued in the same way as they are for life-threatening diseases.

Although quality of life issues for the elderly have not inspired an aggressive approach to therapeutic options proportional to the magnitude of the problem, the immense economic impact on society of urinary incontinence in older people has created an acute awareness of the severity of the health care issue. Further research initiatives will eventually occur.

SOCIAL

Community Dwelling

The community-dwelling elderly patient with urinary incontinence presents a very different management decision to the clinician than does the chronic care patient. The quality of life for most older people is much greater if they continue to dwell in the general community than if they are in an institution. For this reason, clinicians should make every effort to facilitate the patient's remaining in a comfortable and safe community-dwelling situation.

Unfortunately, urinary incontinence is often the single factor that results in the decision to place an elderly patient in a chronic care environment. For this reason, an aggressive approach to the treatment of UI in the community-dwelling elderly should be taken to prevent institutionalization if possible. Most community-dwelling individuals perform at much higher mental and physical levels than chronic care patients do. Therefore, behavioral therapies that require significant patient participation (e.g., biofeedback therapy) become an extremely important treatment option for the community-dwelling patient. In addition, elderly community-dwelling women with stress urinary incontinence are much more likely to be considered for a surgical procedure if, beyond the ability to tolerate the operative procedure, they can care for themselves in the postoperative period if, for example, clean intermittent self-catheterization will be required. Likewise, the elderly community-dwelling man with urge UI with associated bladder outlet obstruction is much more likely than a chronic care patient to tolerate a surgical procedure for treatment of bladder outlet obstruction. As appropriate, surgical procedures should be pursued aggressively to prevent the community-dwelling patient's becoming a chronic care patient. Surgeons should be extremely careful in selecting operative procedures for community-dwelling patients in order to avoid adversely affecting the patient's quality of life. It would defeat the purpose of operative intervention if complications related to procedure resulted in converting a community-dwelling patient into a chronic care patient. Therefore, both surgical and nonsurgical treatment options for treatment of urinary incontinence in elderly community-dwelling patients should be pursued aggressively when possible so that the patient can continue living in the general community.

Chronic Care

Elderly chronic care patients tend to function mentally and physically at lower levels than community-dwelling elderly patients. A significant difference between young and old people is that usually in the former there is a single cause for incontinence while in the latter there are co-morbid conditions. Impairments of cognitive and sensory function are more common in the elderly. Therefore, urodynamic studies have great significance in the diagnostic evaluation of the elderly chronic care patient with UI. Unfortunately, the quality and completeness of the urodynamic evaluation of the elderly chronic care patient often suffers because the patient's ability to cooperate and participate is limited. Many clinicians feel that the frail elderly should not be subjected to extensive urodynamic studies because of the invasiveness of the procedures, but this is a position that all clinicians should seriously reconsider. It is always of the utmost importance that the clinician approach the treatment of urinary incontinence in the elderly patient with as much diagnostic information as is possible. Therefore, it is essential that the urodynamic laboratory develop methods and techniques for evaluation of the chronic care elderly patient that result in the least possible discomfort to the patient and provide the most clinical information possible. The clinician cannot afford to give up the most valuable source of objective information about bladder and urethral function in a patient population for which the clinical information is needed the most.

The therapeutic options available to the chronic care population are also considerably different from those for community-dwelling patients. For example, an elderly woman in chronic care with SUI who does not respond to nonsurgical therapies is much less likely to be a candidate for a surgical procedure than the community-dwelling patient. Likewise, the elderly male in chronic care with urge UI and associated bladder outlet obstruction is much less likely to be a candidate for a surgical procedure to relieve bladder outlet obstruction than the community-dwelling patient. With the rapidly increasing aging population, it is essential that surgical therapies and surgical techniques be developed that will allow safe and successful surgical treatment of voiding dysfunctions in elderly people.

1 FUNCTIONAL STATUS

Mental Status

The mental status of both the community-dwelling and chronic care–dwelling elderly patient is an extremely important consideration in the diagnosis and management of urinary incontinence. Simple assessments such as the minimental state evaluation (MMSE) is a common instrument for a clinical assessment of mental performance.[1] Multiple standardized assessments may be used for any elderly patient with urinary incontinence in the preparation of planning, evaluation, and treatment of incontinence. Almost all therapies for urinary incontinence require some degree of patient participation to be effective. For example, even pharmacologic therapy for the community-dwelling patient requires following instructions and observing possible side effects. Behavioral therapies, especially biofeedback, require significant patient participation.[2,3] In addition, surgical procedures require extensive patient involvement. Following some operative procedures, involvement by caregivers is required for a short time even in patients with good mental status.

Physical Status

Physical ability of the elderly patient is an essential consideration in the evaluation and management of urinary incontinence. A common, simple assessment of physical status is the activities of daily living (ADL) scale. Again, many standardized clinical assessments of physical functional status can be used to determine how well the patient will likely be able to participate in the evaluation and management of urinary incontinence.

The treatment of urinary incontinence in older patients must be based on as accurate a diagnosis as possible and any therapeutic option must be feasible for the patient based on his or her social and functional status. Unrealistic expectations of an elderly patient's functional ability often results in a long-term failure of therapy. Likewise, failure to recognize the capabilities of the patient can result in a conservative therapeutic approach that compromises the patient's quality of life.

PATIENT EVALUATION

Clinical Evaluation

The aims of evaluation of UI in older persons are similar to those of younger adults (see Chapter 16): identifying reversible causes, associated serious conditions, and type of established UI in order to set up individually tailored treatment plans. However, evaluation of UI in frail older persons differs from younger adults for several reasons. Urinary incontinence is frequently associated with deficits outside the urinary tract that affect mobility, mentation, manual dexterity, and motivation, which impair the ability to toilet independently.[4]

The most important part of the clinical evaluation of any patient with urinary incontinence is the voiding history and the physical examination. Unfortunately, the clinical history of many elderly patients is difficult to obtain; information is likely to be incomplete or not quite accurate. Often, the spouse or caregivers can provide the most reliable information about the patient's urinary incontinence. The physical examination is always extremely important in evaluating incontinence in older people, especially women. The vaginal examination is usually performed using only the posterior blade of the speculum in order to assess the anterior vaginal wall and urethral meatus. One objective of the physical examination of elderly women is to determine the degree of atrophic changes in the vagina and to assess the degree of pelvic organ prolapse. Prolapse related to urinary incontinence involves particularly the presence of a cystocele and prolapse at the level of the bladder neck.

The physical examination of the elderly male with urinary incontinence is usually less helpful than that of the female in the clinical management decision. The digital rectal examination of the prostate gland can indicate the size of the prostate gland and the presence of any nodules that may be suspicious for prostate cancer. The digital rectal exam is not an accurate method for assessment of the prostate's size. However, that size is probably not very important since size of the prostate has a poor correlation with the degree of bladder outlet obstruction. The examination of an incontinent person includes a functional testing that consists of digital as well as apparatus-based tests. Digital evaluation is an essential part of the pelvic floor muscles (PFM) assessment. The original evaluation was first proposed in 1982[5]; Laycock[6] later developed the P.E.R.F.E.C.T. assessment scheme (Power, Endurance, number of Repetitions, number of Fast second contractions, and Every Contraction is Timed). However, aging affects the lower urinary tract and is associated with a reduction in speed, strength, and duration of skeletal neuromuscular reactions and a decreased strength of skeletal muscle involving the PFM. Since the PFM function is easy to assess, it should be assessed routinely in elderly women with UI. The reliability of PFM strength measurement is highest in the digital examination, followed by perineometer measurements, and then by vaginal cones tests.[7]

A neurologic examination of the perineum and external genitalia is always done. However, in patients who walk with a normal gait, and have no history of stroke, insulin-dependent diabetes, back surgery for disc disease, or other obvious neurologic diseases, the likelihood of identifying a neurologic etiology of incontinence on physical examination is extremely low. However, the problem of incomplete information for diagnosis of the etiology of incontinence in elderly patients is so common that every attempt to obtain any information that might be helpful should be done to treat this complicated group of patients.

In summary,[4] history and physical examination of older and younger patients are similar, but for elderly patients greater attention is paid to comorbid conditions and to emotional, cognitive, functional, and environmental status.[4] Documentation of UI includes the following:

- Bladder diaries with focus on diurnal micturition and number of incontinent episodes
- Pad test for quantifying the severity of UI
- Postvoid residual volume estimated by catheterization or ultrasound to identify patients with values superior to 200 mL
- Urinalysis for infection, hematuria, and glycosuria
- Urodynamics testing with simple bed-cystometry (of limited value)
- Urodynamic investigation with multichannel evaluation to understand pathophysiologic mechanisms underlying UI in frail older patients; fundamental and warranted when diagnostic uncertainty may affect therapy

2 THERAPY

Geriatric Considerations in the Management of Incontinence

It is important to identify conditions that do not involve the lower urinary tract but that can exacerbate or precipitate incontinence (e.g., impaired cognition, mobility, dexterity, environment, concomitant factors, and motivation) and that might be partly or fully reversible.

Several diseases and functional factors are prevalent in geriatric patients and can prominently influence both the diagnosis and the management of urinary incontinence.[8,9] Many older patients are fit and healthy and treatment is straightforward; on the other hand, those older than 85 years may have multiple conditions that can affect the therapy. With increasing age, chronic illness becomes more common. Many diseases common in the geriatric population can affect the central and peripheral nervous systems, impair mobility, and cause cognitive deficits. The most common comorbid conditions that affect the management of urinary incontinence are:

- Neurologic: stroke, Parkinson's disease, Alzheimer's disease, dementia
- Cardiovascular: congestive heart failure, venous insufficiency
- Musculoskeletal: degenerative joint diseases of the lower extremities
- Medical: diabetes mellitus, sleep disorders, prostatic enlargement, urinary tract infections, depression, constipation

There is a close association of functional disabilities caused by impaired mobility or cognition and UI in geriatric populations, especially among frail, older people.[10] Neurologic and musculoskeletal disorders, alone or in combination, can impair mobility and interfere with independent toileting. All conservative management options used with younger adults can be used with selected frail, older, motivated people.[11]

Before prescribing drugs to treat UI in frail, older people:

- Consider drug use only as an adjunct to other conservative management strategies
- Avoid using some drugs with increased risk of side effects
- Start with low dosage and titrate slowly

Age is not a contraindication to surgery, however, in older people and especially frail or disabled older people, a trial of conservative treatment should be offered before surgery is considered. For many geriatric patients, complete cure with total dryness is an unrealistic goal.

It is necessary to consider the social supports of elderly patients when determining treatment plans. The elderly frequently depend on adult children and other caregivers (neighbors and friends) to help them comply with treatment and to provide transportation to clinics and medical facilities.

Behavioral Interventions

Behavioral therapy for treatment of urinary incontinence in older patients is one of the most common initial therapeutic management choices regardless of the social and functional status of the patient or the etiology of the incontinence.[12] Because the major objective of treatment of urinary incontinence is improved quality of life for the patient, behavioral therapy offers the least possibility of adverse effects that would lead to decreased quality of life resulting from the therapy itself.

For the community-dwelling patient, biofeedback therapy is an excellent choice because the treatment is more specific as a behavioral therapy than pelvic muscle exercises (PME). Biofeedback therapy requires much more patient participation than other behavioral therapies, but it offers the patient an excellent treatment outcome of reduced incontinence. The ideal treatment outcome in younger patients is complete continence with normal voiding. For many older patients, however, that is an unrealistic goal. The older patient can experience a significant improvement in quality of life by a reduction in the frequency of volume of involuntary urine loss of 50% or more. Therefore, failure to achieve continence does not mean that the therapy failed.[13] Biofeedback therapy is usually a much more feasible treatment option for community-dwelling patients than for chronic care patients. Although biofeedback therapy can be done in a chronic care environment, it can be extremely labor intensive if significant mental and physical impairment exist.

Pelvic muscle exercise programs are also a common initial therapy for elderly incontinence patients. Behavioral therapies including biofeedback therapy and pelvic muscle exercises can be used with both men and women with urinary incontinence. Pelvic muscle exercises are more difficult with the elderly than biofeedback because of the patient's inability to understand the therapeutic technique. When a PME program is used to UI in the elderly, it is essential that the clinician be assured that the patient is capable of understanding the PME program and is participating appropriately. Behavioral interventions have been especially designed for frail older people with cognitive and physical impairments that may affect the person's ability to learn new behaviors. For behavioral therapy to be effective, patients must be cognitively intact, be highly motivated, and have transportation for several clinic visits. Patients are taught how to do pelvic floor muscle exercises, use strategies for managing urgency, and regularly maintain bladder records. These techniques are highly effective in selected community-dwelling patients, especially women.[11]

Bladder drill procedures imposed a lengthening interval between voids to establish a normal frequency of urination and were purposed to result in normalization of bladder function. Bladder drills were often combined with anticholinergic therapy and sedatives to help cope with severe urgency. Fantl and colleagues demonstrated that older women reduced their episodes of incontinence by a mean of 57% using bladder training, whereas little improvement occurred with a no-treatment control condition. This result was achieved with only six weekly half-hour visits after the initial assessment and training visit.[13]

Evidence exists that prompted voiding is effective in the short term for improving dryness (i.e., improved continence) in nursing home residents and in some home care patients. Results, especially in the nursing homes, depend on the staff's compliance with the protocol.[4]

Because improvements are based on the ability to learn and attain skills and on conscious changes in daily behavior, behavioral treatments of patients with cognitive impairment have limited success. Little is known of the effectiveness, potential, or acceptability of combining therapies for incontinence. Ouslander and colleagues[14] studied the combined treatment of prompted voiding and oxybutynin or placebo among functionally impaired nursing home patients with detrusor instability. Neither the drug nor the placebo demonstrated clinically significant benefits when added to prompted voiding therapy in the nursing home setting.

Electrical Stimulation and Biofeedback

Electrical stimulation for treatment of urinary incontinence related to the overactive bladder in the elderly patients has been done for many years. The technique for delivering electrical stimulation has varied significantly among clinicians. Many new electrical stimulation devices are available now for the clinician to use. It is reasonable for the clinician to use the electrical stimulation device that is most suited to the practice patterns and patient population being treated. While the technique appears effective, unanswered questions remain about stimulation current and method of delivery. A relatively simple technique involves a transcutaneous electrical nerve stimulator (TENS). The surface electrodes can be placed over the S2 sensory dermatome and the continuous stimulation adjusted to the tolerance of the patient. A continuous 30-day trial of this device is a relatively simple clinical approach to electrical stimulation. The more sophisticated units should produce better results and may be a consideration if the initial TENS unit therapy program is not effective. Also, it is a reasonable to use a combination of electrical stimulation with pharmacologic and behavioral therapy.

Device-based conservative therapies for urinary incontinence have been studied very little in older persons, particularly in those who are frail. Most studies show a benefit, but do not specify whether age affects outcome. Because pelvic floor muscle training with biofeedback requires active participation of the patient, cognitive status and motivation are important selection factors. Biofeedback-assisted behavioral training has been tested in several clinical series with mean reductions of incontinence ranging from 56% to 80%. A recent randomized study of a group of older women (55 to 92 years old) with urge incontinence compared biofeedback-assisted behavioral training with standard drug therapy (oxybutynin) and demonstrated[15] that all patients had reduction of UI in early stages of treatment. Patients reported most improvement with behavioral training. In the behavioral training group only 14% of patients wanted to change to another treatment as compared to 75.5% of patients in drug therapy group who wanted to change treatments. This study showed that biofeedback-assisted behavioral training is at least as effective as oxybutynin for the treatment of urge incontinence. Biofeedback-assisted pelvic floor muscle training can effect dramatic continence improvements in cognitively intact but frail elderly. Although response in older persons can be good, it is not clear whether age affects response to biofeedback-assisted pelvic muscle exercises.

Unlike biofeedback, which requires active participation of the patient to be successful, electrostimulation is a passive therapy of the pelvic floor. Older persons may respond to electrical stimulation of the pelvic floor as well as younger persons. Electrical stimulation of the pelvic floor may have equal benefit in younger and older patients.[4]

Pharmacologic Management

Symptoms of an overactive bladder represent the most common presenting problem associated with urinary incontinence in the elderly. This is often true even in elderly women who have a significant component of stress UI. A common therapeutic approach to the overactive bladder is anticholinergic therapy. The two most common drugs used are oxybutynin and tolterodine. Although the standard dose of oxybutynin is 5 mg three times daily, the side effects of this drug in the elderly typically require a lower dose. Although oxybutynin has been effective in treating overactive bladder in elderly patients, it is tolerated very poorly in some elderly people because of the side effects. Tolterodine might represent a significant advancement in the pharmacologic therapy of the overactive bladder in the elderly because of possible side effects in this population. A dose of 2 mg of tolterodine twice daily is usually tolerated well with minimal side effects in older patients and appears to be effective in treatment of symptoms related to an overactive bladder.

Pharmacologic suppression of overactive bladder symptom appears to be the effectiveness of behavioral therapy alone in frail or institutionalized older persons. Among women older than 65 years, estrogen deficiency is universal and reviews of estrogen therapy for UI suggest there may be an effect on irritative voiding. It is possible to reserve estrogen therapy for women who have signs of atrophic vaginitis (erythema, petechiae) or very low maturation indices. Caution is required when prescribing any medication to frail elderly because of increased susceptibility to side effects. Oxybutynin and bladder-relaxant medications are clearly effective in selected geriatric outpatients and may be used as an adjunct to a toileting program in frail, older people. However, since many drugs have been associated with causing or contributing to incontinence, all current medications should be reviewed before prescribing. Drugs that can have several bothersome adverse effects include vasopressin, tricyclic antidepressants (imipramine, desipramine, amitriptyline), propantheline, and ephedrine. Such underlying conditions include dry mouth, constipation, gastroesophageal reflux, glaucoma, urinary retention and dementia.

More data must be gathered from frail elderly regarding the efficacy and risks of treating types other than urge incontinence, and studies focusing on a wide range of topics are needed.

Pads, Appliances, and Catheters

Absorbent products, which account the majority of expenditure on incontinence aids and appliances, can be classified into four categories: e.g., bedpads (underpads) and bodyworn products, each available as disposable (single-use) items and reusable (washable) variants designed to be laundered and reused many times.[4] Immunocompromised people should not use bedpads made from recycled paper because of the risk of infection.

Particular attention should be paid to the appearance, discretion, fit, and comfort of different reusable pants with integral pad for lightly incontinent women. Personal preference of users with regard to topsheet material and integral waterproofing should be considered carefully when selecting products. Reusable pants generally require less storage space than disposables. It is possible to use a mix of disposable and reusable products; some users who choose disposable pants at home prefer reusables when traveling. Selecting an appropriate pad or appliance to achieve social continence requires patient-centered consideration of effective containment of urine or feces, ease of use, discretion, and cost.[16,17]

Bladder drainage in frail older persons with difficulty emptying the bladder may be unavoidable when there is complete failure of bladder emptying, surgical treatment is not wanted by the patient or the family, or the patient prefers catheterization.[18]

When a catheter is used, it is important to determine the reason that it was introduced and to consider alternative management strategies. If the catheter is to remain in place, the patient should have an appropriate indication for its chronic use. As with all catheterized patients, bacteriuria is universal in elderly catheterized patients and it should not be treated unless there are clear symptomatic episodes (fever, anorexia) or if bacteriuria persists after catheter removal.

Surgical Intervention in Women and in Men

The surgical treatment of incontinence in the elderly is a very complex issue.[19,20] Since UI is not a fatal disorder, the risk of surgery in this group of patients is often greater than the potential benefits. Also, since the objective of incontinence therapy is improved quality of life, surgical therapy could worsen the quality of life if a serious complication occurred. However, as urologists and gynecologists become more aware of the quality of life issues involving the elderly, modifications of surgical techniques have been done to markedly decrease the risk and to ensure a high degree of success of surgery. As alternative surgical techniques are developed for treatment of bladder outlet obstruction in men and sphincteric incompetence in women, it is likely that more elderly patients with urinary incontinence will be candidates for surgical therapy. With the advent of routinely performing major surgery in elderly people safely and effectively, even in patients with multiple risk factors, we can expect surgical therapy for urinary incontinence in elderly patients to become more common.

Once the decision has been made to operate, the choice of surgical procedure is essentially the same for a given urodynamic diagnosis in an elderly women and in younger women. The goals of identifying the risk factors are to diminish the cardiopulmonary status; mobility; prevention of complications such as renal failure; and early recognition of complication.[4] Elderly women probably have long-term results from incontinence surgery similar to those in younger women. Some frail older persons benefit from surgical interventions but the preoperative evaluation is of critical importance with medical risk factors. Data are lacking about the effects of age in most studies.

Because growing numbers of elderly men with localized prostate cancer are undergoing prostatectomy or radiation therapy, the numbers of men with iatrogenic incontinence are increasing. In older men, prostate enlargement caused by benign prostate or cancer and obstruction by the prostate or stricture can cause symptoms that mimic those of overactive bladder. Thus, in many older men with overactive bladder symptoms, it is important to exclude obstruction before initiating bladder-relaxant therapy. Urinary tract infections are also common in the geriatric population, affecting 30% of frail men who live in long-term institutions. Eradication of bacteriuria in these patients has no effect on the severity of urinary incontinence. Between 50% and 75% of older men with bladder outlet obstruction have overactive bladder. If incontinence after prostatectomy (TURP) persists longer after 1 year of conservative treatment, those who are still suffering with severe urinary incontinence due to sphincter incompetence may benefit from another surgical procedure. In addition to injection of bulking agents, the main procedures are the sling procedures (fascia sling procedures, rectus fascial slings with needle suspension, bone anchored slings) and the artificial sphincter. Implantation of an artificial sphincter is the most efficacious treatment currently available for significant male urinary incontinence due to sphincter incompetence, but with a possibility of reintervention in 20% of cases.

CONCLUSION

The numerous conditions that affect the diagnosis and the management of UI in older frail patients include neurologic and cardiovascular disorders, musculoskeletal conditions, psychiatric illness, and endocrinologic diseases. Treatment depends on numerous factors, ranging from comorbidities and functional status to transportation, finances, and caregivers' preference. The therapy must be individualized and communicated clearly to older patients. The physical therapies have no side effects but are tiring for these frail old people, and medications have many adverse effects and can be bothersome and exacerbate existing conditions common in older patients.

REFERENCES

1. Resnick MI, Palmer RM: Surgical decisions. In O'Donnell PD (ed): Geriatric Urology. Boston, Little, Brown, 1994.
2. O'Donnell PD: Biofeedback therapy. In Shlomo R (ed): Female Urology. Philadelphia, WB Saunders, 1996.
3. Burns PA: Biofeedback therapy. In O'Donnell PD. Urinary Incontinence. St. Louis, Mosby, 1997.
4. Fonda D, Benvenuti F, Cottenden A, et al: Urinary incontinence and bladder dysfunction in older persons. In Abrams P, Cardozo L, Khoury S, Wein A (eds): WHO Second International Consultation on Incontinence. Plymouth, UK, Health Publication, 2001, pp 627–695.
5. Bourcier A: Rééducation et urodynamique dans le postpartum. Dossiers de l'Obstétrique 85:19–33, 1982.
6. Laycock J: Clinical evaluation of the pelvic floor. In Schüssler B, Laycock J, Norton P, Stanton S (eds): Pelvic Floor Re-Education. New York, Springer-Verlag, 1994, p 42.
7. Kerschan-Schindl K, Uher E, Wiesinger G, et al: Reliability of pelvic floor muscle strength measurement in elderly incontinent women. Neurourol Urodyn 21:42–47, 2002.
8. O'Donnell PD: Goals of therapy and mechanisms of urethral incontinence. In Kursh ED, McGuire EJ (eds): Female Urology. Philadelphia, Lippincott-Raven, 1994.
9. O'Donnell PD: Geriatric issues in female incontinence. In Walters MD, Karram MM (eds): Clinical Urogynecology. St. Louis, Mosby, 1993.
10. Ouslander JG, Kane RL, Abass IB: Urinary incontinence in elderly nursing home patients. JAMA 248:1194–1198, 1992.
11. Ouslander JG: Geriatric considerations in the diagnosis and management of overactive bladder. Urology 60 (suppl 5A):50–55, 2002.
12. O'Donnell PD: Behavioral therapy for Incontinence. In O'Donnell PD (ed): Geriatric Urology. Boston, Little, Brown, 1994.
13. Fantl JA, Wyman JF, Mc Clich DK: Efficacy of bladder training in older women with urinary incontinence. JAMA 265:609–613, 1991.
14. Ouslander JG, Schnelle JF, Uman G: Does oxybutynin add to the effectiveness of prompted voiding for urinary incontinence among nursing home residents? A placebo-controlled trial. J Am Geriat Soc 43:610–617, 1995.
15. Burgio KL, Locher JL, Goode PS: Behavioral versus drug treatment for urge incontinence in older women: A randomized clinical trial. JAMA 280(23):1995–2000, 1998.
16. Cottenden AM: Aids and appliances for incontinence. In Roe BH (ed): Clinical Nursing Practice: The Promotion and Management of Continence. London, Prentice-Hall, 1992.
17. Gibb H, Wong G: How to choose: Nurses' judgement of the effectiveness of a range of currently marketed continence aids. J Clin Nurs 3:77–86, 1994.
18. Department of Health and Human Services: Practice Guidelines: Managing Acute and Chronic Urinary Incontinence. Washington DC, Agency for Health Care and Research, 1996.
19. O'Donnell PD: Incontinence in the elderly. In Appell RA, Bourcier A, La Torre F (eds): Pelvic Floor Dysfunction: Investigations and Conservative Treatment. Rome, Casa Editrice Scientifica Internazionale, 1999, pp 85–92.
20. Badlani GH: Surgical management decisions in geriatric incontinence. In O'Donnell PD: Urinary Incontinence. St. Louis, Mosby, 1997.

CHAPTER 37

Management of Male and Female Sexual Dysfunction

Jennifer R. Berman ■ Shalender Bhasin ■ Laura Berman ■
Cyrus A. Chowdhury ■ Wayne J. G. Hellstrom

MANAGEMENT OF MALE SEXUAL DYSFUNCTION

Erectile dysfunction (ED), previously referred to as impotence, is the inability of the male to attain or maintain an erection sufficient for satisfactory sexual intercourse. Sexual dysfunction is a more general term that also includes libidinal, orgasmic and ejaculatory dysfunction, in addition to the inability to attain or maintain penile erection.[1]

Evaluation of Patients with Erectile Dysfunction

History

The diagnostic workup of the patient with ED starts with an evaluation of general health.[2,3] The general medical history should be directed at identifying etiologic factors as well as factors that may affect the selection and response to therapy. The presence of diabetes mellitus, coronary artery disease, peripheral vascular disease, and hypertension may suggest a vascular cause. History of stroke, spinal cord or back injury, multiple sclerosis, or dementia may point to a neurologic disorder. Also relevant are a history of pelvic trauma, prostate surgery, or priapism. Social history must include ascertainment of recreational drug abuse, particularly tobacco, as well as use of cocaine, marijuana, and alcohol. Information about medications, particularly antihypertensives, antiandrogens, antidepressants, and antipsychotic drugs is important because nearly one fourth of all cases of impotence can be attributed to medications. Psychiatric illnesses such as depression, psychosis, and drugs used to treat these disorders might be associated with sexual dysfunction.

A detailed sexual history, including the nature of relationships, partner expectations, situational erectile failure, performance anxiety, and marital discord, must be elicited.[2,3] It is important to distinguish between inability to achieve erection, changes in sexual desire, failure to achieve orgasm and ejaculation, and dissatisfaction with the sexual relationship. The physician should ask about the onset, duration, quality, and duration of erections as well as the presence of nocturnal and early morning erections. Approximately 80% of cases of ED are primarily related to organic causes, whereas approximately 20% of cases stem from psychological factors. Most cases have both organic and psychologic components. During the history, any relationship between ED and chronic illness should be established based of the findings of the Massachusetts Male Aging Study. The main organic causes are diabetes, heart disease, and hypertension, and the main psychological causes are related to performance anxiety and poor communication with the partner.

The initial evaluation:

- Includes the patient's partner to facilitate education and communication
- Determines the nature and frequency of ED
- Evaluates the risk factors for ED (e.g., hypertension, diabetes, alcohol abuse, psychiatric illness)
- Identifies potential reversible causes of ED (e.g., depression, hyperprolactinemia)

Physical Examination

A directed physical examination should assess secondary sex characteristics, breast enlargement, and testicular volume. An evaluation of femoral and pedal pulses can provide clues to the presence of peripheral vascular disease. The neurologic examination focuses on motor weakness, perineal sensation, anal sphincter tone, and bulbocavernosus reflex. The penis is examined, and note is made of unusual curvature, palpable plaques, or superficial lesions.

The physical examination:

- Assesses secondary male sexual characteristics
- Measures femoral and lower extremity pulses

- Performs focused neurologic examination
- Performs genitourinary examination

Self-reporting Questionnaires

Over the last decade, there has been a general shift in most male sexual dysfunction clinics away from expensive, time-consuming, and invasive techniques (e.g., dynamic infusion cavernosometry, penile duplex Doppler ultrasonography, and RigiScan studies) and toward the use of simple, noninvasive, self-reporting questionnaires. The value of these questionnaires is that many men with ED do not voluntarily discuss their sexual symptoms with their physicians for a variety of reasons. Many men with ED are embarrassed, whereas others consider ED as an inevitable result of aging. Some physicians are uncomfortable discussing issues of such personal nature; this creates an atmosphere that is not conducive to effective communication. These self-reporting questionnaires can help to break the ice and facilitate communication. These instruments are widely available and easy to complete, and can complement or enhance the workup of sexual dysfunction.

The International Index of Erectile Function (IIEF) is a multidimensional scale consisting of 15 questions that address relevant domains of male sexual function.[4] This scale has been validated in several languages, used in many multinational clinical trials, and found to have adequate sensitivity and specificity for detecting treatment-related changes, including response to oral erectogenic agents in men with ED.

Considerable effort has been invested in the development of abbreviated questionnaires that take less time than the International Index of Erectile Dysfunction, but more concisely address similar aspects of male sexuality (e.g., Sexual Health Inventory for Men Questionnaire [SHIM]).[5]

Laboratory Tests

The diagnostic evaluation of a man with ED starts with a general health evaluation. This may include measurements of hemoglobin, white blood count, blood glucose, AST, ALT, bilirubin, alkaline phosphatase, BUN, and creatinine.

Measurement of serum total testosterone concentrations can help to detect androgen deficiency. Although there is no consensus on this issue, it is important to exclude androgen deficiency in men with ED because androgen deficiency may be a manifestation of serious underlying illness, such as a pituitary tumor or HIV infection. In addition, testosterone replacement is desirable in men with androgen deficiency to restore sexual function as well as to maintain bone mineral density, muscle mass and protein metabolism, and a sense of well-being.

Laboratory tests include:

- Morning serum testosterone
- Serum prolactin
- Glucose
- Complete blood count, tyroid function tests, and prostate-specific antigen test

If the history, physical examination, and ED questionnaire do not identify obvious medical concerns that need further workup, then a more cost-effective approach for a busy practitioner is to prescribe a trial of oral medication (e.g., sildenafil) if there are no contraindications (e.g., nitrate use).

Evaluation of Penile Vasculature and Blood Flow

Several tests are used to evaluate the integrity of penile vasculature and blood flow.[2,3] Of these, the penile brachial blood pressure index is a simple and specific, but not a very sensitive index of vascular insufficiency.[6-9] It is of historical interest and is rarely used today.

Intracavernosal injection of a vasoactive agent, such as prostaglandin E1, can be used as both a diagnostic tool and a potential therapeutic modality.[2,3] This procedure can show whether the patient will respond to this therapeutic modality and facilitate patient education about the procedure and its potential side effects. Failure to respond to intracavernosal injection can raise the suspicion of vascular insufficiency or a venous leak that might need further evaluation and treatment.

Most men with ED do not need duplex color sonography, cavernosography, or pelvic angiography.[2,3] These procedures should be reserved for patients where the results of these tests would alter the management or prognosis, and only by those with considerable experience with their use. For instance, angiography could be useful in a young man with arterial insufficiency associated with pelvic trauma. Similarly, suspicion of congenital or traumatic venous leak in a young man with ED would justify the use of cavernosography. In each instance, confirmation of the vascular lesion might lead to consideration of surgery. Duplex ultrasonography can provide a noninvasive evaluation of vascular function.[2]

Nocturnal Penile Tumescence

Although recording of formal nocturnal penile tumescence (NPT) in a sleep laboratory for successive nights can help to differentiate organic from psychogenic impotence, this test is expensive, labor-intensive and is not required in most men with ED. In most cases, formal NPT studies are reserved for medicolegal documentation.

The introduction of portable RigiScan devices in 1985 provided clinicians with a reliable means of continuously monitoring penile tumescence and rigidity at home. It is a multicomponent device that the patient wears at bedtime for 2 to 3 nights. It has two wire-gauge loops that are placed around the base and tip of the penis that record changes in penile circumference and rigidity. Data are stored and then downloaded via a software program that allows for sophisticated interpretation of the findings.

Nocturnal penile tumescence testing is not needed for most patients who are evaluated for ED, and is recommended only for patients with a high clinical suspicion of psychogenic ED, situational problems, or to document preoperatively poor penile rigidity. In most cases, a careful history eliciting nighttime or early morning erections provides a reasonable correlation with formal NPT and RigiScan studies.[10]

Diagnostic Tests to Exclude Androgen Deficiency and Hypothalamic–Pituitary Lesions

There is considerable debate about the usefulness and cost-effectiveness of hormonal evaluation and the extent to which androgen deficiency should be investigated in men with ED. Eight to ten percent of men with ED have low testosterone levels; the prevalence of androgen deficiency increases with advancing age.[11–17] The prevalence of low testosterone levels is not significantly different among men who have ED and in an age-matched population.[12,15] Urologic studies show that fewer than 6% of men with ED have an endocrine basis to their condition. These data are consistent with the proposal that ED and androgen deficiency are two common, but independently distributed disorders.[15]

However, it is important to exclude androgen deficiency in this patient population.[18] Androgen deficiency is a correctable cause of sexual dysfunction, and some men who have ED and low testosterone levels respond to testosterone replacement. Hypogonadism may have additional deleterious effects on health. For instance, hypogonadism might contribute to osteoporosis, loss of muscle mass and function, increased risk of disability, falls, and fracture, insulin resistance, and cardiovascular disease. Therefore, regardless of sexual dysfunction, androgen deficiency must be corrected by appropriate hormone replacement therapy. Furthermore, androgen deficiency may be a manifestation of a serious underlying disease, such as HIV infection or a hypothalamic–pituitary space-occupying lesion.

In large studies only a small fraction of men with ED and low testosterone levels had space-occupying lesions of the hypothalamic–pituitary region.[12,13,16] In one large survey, all of the hypothalamic–pituitary lesions were found in men with serum testosterone levels less than 150 ng/dL.[16] Therefore, the cost-effectiveness of the diagnostic workup to exclude an underlying lesion of the hypothalamic–pituitary region can be increased by limiting the workup to men with serum testosterone levels less than 150 ng/dL.

Treatment of Erectile Dysfunction

The selection of the therapeutic modality should be based on the underlying etiology, patient preference (goal-directed approach), the nature and strength of relationship with his sexual partner, underlying cardiovascular disease, and other comorbid conditions.[2] The ideal approach uses minimally invasive therapies that are easy to use and have fewer adverse effects and progresses to more invasive therapies that may require injections in some circumstances or surgical interventions after the first-line choices are exhausted.[2] The physician must discuss the risks, benefits, and alternatives of all the diagnostic procedures and therapies with the couple. In the execution of good medical practice, all associated medical disorders must be optimized. In men with diabetes mellitus, efforts to optimize glycemic control are instituted, although improving glycemic control may not improve sexual function. In men with hypertension, control of blood pressure is optimized and the therapeutic regimen may need to be modified to remove antihypertensive drugs that impair sexual function. This strategy is not always possible because almost all antihypertensive agents are associated with sexual dysfunction; the frequency of this adverse event is less with converting enzyme inhibitors than with other agents.

All patients with ED can benefit from psychosexual counseling.[2,3] Unfortunately, many couples are reluctant to pursue this avenue. When there is latent marital discord, the sensitive and astute clinician must direct affected couples appropriately.

First-line Therapies

Psychosexual Counseling

Counseling can be of benefit in both psychogenic and organic causes of sexual dysfunction. It can help decrease performance anxiety and increase the patient's ability to cope with the problem. Involving the partner in the counseling process can help to dispel misperceptions, decrease stress, enhance intimacy and the ability to talk about sex, and increase the chances of successful outcome. Counseling sessions are also helpful in uncovering conflicts in relationships, psychiatric problems, alcohol and drug abuse, and significant misperceptions about sex. Although psychobehavioral therapy is reported to relieve depression and anxiety, there is a striking paucity of outcome data on the effectiveness of this therapeutic modality.

Sildenafil

Sildenafil (Viagra, Pfizer, New York, NY) is the first effective oral agent for the treatment of ED. It was introduced to the US market in March 1998, and since that time, hundreds of millions of tablets have been dispensed. Sildenafil is a selective type 5 phosphodiesterase inhibitor that is a safe and effective first-line oral treatment for ED.[19–26]

Mechanism of Action. Sildenafil blocks the hydrolysis of cGMP induced by nitric oxide.[20–22] Therefore, sildenafil action requires an intact nitric oxide response as well as constitutive synthesis of cGMP by the smooth muscle cells of the corpora cavernosa. By selectively inhibiting cGMP catabolism in the cavernosal smooth muscle cells, sildenafil restores the natural erectile response to sexual stimulation, but importantly, does not produce an erection in the absence of sexual stimulation. Fidelity of the nitric oxide production pathway and sexual stimulation are necessary requirements for sildenafil to successfully induce an erection.

Efficacy. The efficacy of sildenafil was shown in a randomized dose-response study in which 532 men with organic, psychogenic, or mixed ED were randomized to receive placebo or 25, 50, or 100 mg sildenafil for 24 weeks. In this dose–response study, patients who received sildenafil performed better in increased rigidity, frequency of vaginal penetration, and maintenance of erection. Increasing doses of sildenafil were associated with higher mean scores for the questions assessing frequency of penetration and maintenance of erections after sexual penetration.[27] In a follow-up dose escalation study, 329 men were randomly assigned to receive placebo or 50 mg sildenafil for 12 weeks. At each follow-up, the dose of sildenafil was increased or decreased by 50%, depending on the therapeutic response or side effects. In men receiving sildenafil, 64% of attempts at intercourse were successful compared with 22% in men receiving placebo. The mean number of successful attempts per month was 5.9 for men receiving sildenafil and 1.5 for those receiving placebo. The mean scores for orgasms, intercourse satisfaction, and overall satisfaction domain were also significantly higher in the sildenafil group compared with placebo.[19]

In a separate randomized clinical trial, 268 men with diabetes mellitus and ED received either placebo or sildenafil for 12 weeks.[21] Fifty-six percent of men receiving sildenafil reported improved erections compared with 10% of those receiving placebo ($P < 0.001$). The percent of men who reported at least one successful attempt at intercourse was 61% for the sildenafil versus 22% for the placebo group. This study showed that sildenafil is an effective treatment for ED in patients with diabetes mellitus.[21]

Sildenafil is also effective in men with ED due to a variety of other causes, including spinal cord injury and post radical prostatectomy.[24,25] In general, baseline sexual function and the etiology of sexual dysfunction are good predictors of response to therapy.[25] However, no baseline characteristic predicts the likelihood of failure to respond to sildenafil therapy. Therefore, a therapeutic trial of sildenafil is warranted in all patients except in those in whom it is contraindicated.[25]

Adverse Effects Associated with Sildenafil Therapy. In clinical trials, the adverse effects reported with greater frequency in sildenafil-treated men than placebo-treated men include headaches, flushing, dyspepsia, respiratory tract disorders, and visual disturbances.[27] Sildenafil does not affect semen characteristics.[28] No cases of priapism were noted in the pivotal clinical trials.

Hemodynamic Effects of Sildenafil Citrate. In postmarketing surveillance, several cases of myocardial infarction and sudden death were reported in men using sildenafil. Forty-four of the 130 deaths reported by the U.S. Food and Drug Administration from March to November 1998 occurred in temporal relation to the ingestion of sildenafil; 16 of these deaths occurred in individuals who were taking nitrates.[29–33] Because most men with ED also have high prevalence of cardiovascular risk factors, it is unclear whether these events were causally related to the ingestion of sildenafil, underlying heart disease, or both.[32] In a rigorously controlled study, oral administration of 100 mg sildenafil to men with severe coronary artery disease produced only small decreases in systemic blood pressure and no significant changes in cardiac output, heart rate, coronary blood flow and coronary artery diameter.[34] This led the American Heart Association to conclude that the pre-existence of coronary artery disease by itself does not constitute a contraindication for the use of sildenafil.[32]

Guidelines for the Use of Sildenafil in Men with Coronary Artery Disease.[32] Before prescribing sildenafil, it is crucial to assess cardiovascular risk factors. If the patient has hypertension or symptomatic coronary artery disease, those clinical disorders must be treated first.[2,32] The physician must ask about the use of nitrates because sildenafil is absolutely contraindicated in individuals who take any form of nitrates and sildenafil should not be used within 24 hours of the use of nitrates.[32]

In men with pre-existing coronary artery disease, sexual activity can induce coronary ischemia[33]; these individuals should undergo assessment of their exercise tolerance. One practical way to assess exercise tolerance is to have the patient climb one or two flight of stairs. If he can safely climb one or two flights of stairs without angina or excessive shortness of breath, he can likely engage in sexual intercourse with a stable partner without similar symptoms. Exercise testing before prescribing sildenafil may be indicated in some men with significant heart disease to assess the risk of inducing cardiac ischemia during sexual activity.[32]

In men with congestive heart failure or those receiving vasodilator drugs or those who are on complex regimens of antihypertensive drugs, blood pressure must be monitored after initial administration of sildenafil.[32]

A number of reviews have been published on the safety of sildenafil therapy.[35–41]

Drug Interactions. Sildenafil is metabolized mostly by the P450 2C9 and the P450 3A4 pathways.[32] Cimetidine and erythromycin, inhibitors of P450 3A4, increase the plasma concentrations of sildenafil. Protease inhibitors may also alter the activity of the P450 3A4 pathway and affect the clearance of sildenafil.[32]

Conversely, sildenafil is an inhibitor of the P450 2C9 metabolic pathway, and its administration can affect the metabolism of drugs metabolized by this system, such as warfarin and tolbutamide.[32]

The most serious interactions of sildenafil are with nitrates. The vasodilator effects of nitrates are augmented by sildenafil; this also applies to inhaled forms of nitrates such as amyl nitrate and nitrites that are sold under the street name "poppers." Concomitant administration of the two drugs can cause a fatal decrease in blood pressure.[32]

Therapeutic Regimens. In most men with ED, sildenafil can be started at an initial dose of 50 mg. If this dose does not produce adverse effects, the dose can be titrated to 100 mg.[19,32] Further dose adjustment should be guided by the therapeutic response to therapy and occurrence of adverse effects. Typically, unit doses higher than 100 mg are not recommended. To minimize the risk of hypotension and adverse cardiovascular events in association with the use of sildenafil, the American Heart Association has prepared a list of recommendations, which should be followed rigorously.[32]

Sildenafil is taken at least 1 hour before sexual intercourse and not more than once in any 24-hour period.

Cost-effectiveness of Sildenafil Use for Erectile Dysfunction. A number of studies have evaluated the economic cost of treating ED in men in managed care organizations.[42-44] These analyses, using prevalence-based cost of illness approach, concluded that sildenafil and vacuum constriction devices are the most cost-effective of all the therapeutic options in managed care setting and should be considered first-line strategies.[42-44]

Vacuum Devices for Inducing Erection

Commercial vacuum devices consist of a plastic cylinder, a vacuum pump, and an elastic constriction band.[2,3] The plastic cylinder fits over the penis and is connected to a vacuum pump. The negative pressure created by the vacuum within the cylinder draws blood into the penis, producing an erection. An elastic band slipped around the base of the penis traps the blood in the penis, maintaining an erection as long as the rubber band is retained around the base. The constriction band should not be left in place for longer than 30 minutes.

These devices are safe, relatively inexpensive, and reasonably effective. However, they can impair ejaculation, resulting in entrapment of semen, and are difficult and awkward for some patients to use. Some couples dislike the lack of spontaneity engendered by the use of these devices. Partner cooperation is usually important for successful use of these devices.[45-49]

Testosterone Replacement in Androgen-deficient Men with Erectile Dysfunction

Testosterone replacement of healthy, young, androgen-deficient men restores sexual function.[50-59] In healthy young men, relatively low normal levels of serum testosterone can maintain sexual function.[52,57,59] In male rats, a decrease in serum testosterone concentrations to castrate levels is associated with marked impairment of all measures of mating behavior and testosterone replacement to levels that are at the lower end of the adult male range normalizes all measures of mating behavior.[58,59] In general, supraphysiologic doses of testosterone does not further improve sexual function. Increasing testosterone levels above the physiologic range may increase arousability; however, this has not been conclusively demonstrated.

As previously stated, androgen deficiency and ED are two common but independently distributed, clinical disorders in middle-aged and older men that often coexist. Eight to ten percent of men with ED have low testosterone levels.[11,12,15,16] The prevalence of low testosterone is not significantly different between middle-aged and older men with impotence and those without impotence.[12] The administration of testosterone is unlikely to improve sexual function in men with normal testosterone levels. Therefore, indiscriminate use of testosterone replacement in all older men with ED is not warranted. However, it is important to exclude testosterone deficiency in older men with ED. Androgen deficiency may be a manifestation of an underlying disease, such as a pituitary tumor. Additionally, therapies directed just at ED in men will not correct androgen deficiency which, if left uncorrected, will have deleterious effects on bone, muscle, energy level, and sense of well-being.

Many but not all impotent men with low testosterone levels experience improvements in their libido and overall sexual activity with androgen replacement therapy.[18,60] The response to testosterone supplementation, even in this group of men, is variable[12-16] because of the co-existence of other disorders, such as diabetes mellitus, hypertension, cardiovascular disease, and psychogenic factors. A meta-analysis of the usefulness of androgen replacement therapy concluded that testosterone administration is associated with greater improvements in sexual function than those associated with placebo in men with ED and low testosterone levels.[60]

Erectile dysfunction in middle-aged and older men is often a multifactorial disorder. Common causes of ED in men include diabetes mellitus, hypertension, medications, peripheral vascular disease, psychogenic factors, and end-stage renal disease. Many of these factors often coexist. Therefore, testosterone treatment alone may not improve sexual function in all men with androgen deficiency.

Testosterone treatment does not improve sexual function in impotent men who have normal testosterone levels.[11] It is not known whether testosterone replacement improves sexual function in impotent men with borderline serum testosterone levels.

Second-line Therapies

Intraurethral Therapies

An intraurethral system for delivery of alprostadil called MUSE (medicated urethral system for erection; VIVUS, Menlo Park, CA) was released in 1997. Alprostadil is a stable, synthetic form of prostaglandin E_1, which increases cAMP levels and thereby promotes cavernosal smooth muscle relaxation and penile erection. Alprostadil, when applied into the urethra, must be absorbed through the ventral side of the tunica albuginea and into the corpus cavernosum to cause an erection. High concentrations of PGE_1 must be used to maintain efficacy.

Typically, the initial MUSE dose of 500 µg is applied in the clinician's office to observe for changes in blood pressure or urethral bleeding secondary to misapplication of the MUSE device into the urethra. Depending on the erectile response, the clinician can increase the alprostadil dose to 1000 µg or decrease it to 250 µg.

Common side effects of transurethral alprostadil are penile pain and urethral burning in up to 30% of patients.[61-63] Initial randomized, placebo-controlled studies reported success rates of 40% to 60%, determined as having at least one successful sexual intercourse during a 3-month study period.[61-63] The use of a constriction device (Actis, VIVUS) at the time of application of transurethral alprostadil has been shown to increase efficacy. VIVUS is currently investigating a combination of alprostadil and prazosin (an alpha-blocking agent, Alibra) to further promote cavernosal smooth muscle relaxation and erectile response.

Intracavernosal Injection of Vasoactive Agents

The use of intracavernosal injections of vasoactive agents has been a cornerstone of the medical management of ED since the early 1980s. Patients are taught how to self-inject a vasoactive agent into their corpora cavernosa with a 27- or 30-gauge needle up to 3 times a week for sexual intercourse. Erections occur typically 15 minutes after intracorporal injection and ideally last 45 to 90 minutes. When appropriately titrated, the success rate of this therapy in producing a rigid erection is 80% to 90%. Early studies with intracavernosal injection therapy reported patient and partner satisfaction rates of 70% and 67%, respectively.

The main adverse effects include penile pain, hematoma, formation of corporal nodules, and the possibility of prolonged erections (priapism, if longer than 4 hours). Despite the effectiveness of this approach in producing rigid erections, many patients do not wish to inject a needle into their penis, and it is not surprising that long-term drop-out rates approach 60% to 70%.

Three different agents are commonly used alone or in combination by clinicians who prescribe injection therapy for the treatment of ED. Several formulations of alprostadil (PGE_1) are commercially available (Caverject, Pharmacia; Prostin VR, Pharmacia; Edex, Schwarz Pharma). PGE_1 is a powerful smooth muscle relaxant. The usual dose is 5 µg to 20 µg. Common side effects of intracavernosal PGE_1 injections include penile pain, fibrosis, and prolonged erections. Priapism occurs less commonly with PGE_1 than with other vasoactive agents.

Papaverine is a nonspecific phosphodiesterase inhibitor, which increases both intracellular cAMP and cGMP. Papaverine is derived from the poppy seed. As a single agent, it is efficacious and inexpensive, and it does not require refrigeration. It does not cause penile pain, but has a greater propensity to induce priapism and fibrosis with long-term use.

Phentolamine is a competitive alpha-1 and alpha-2 adrenergic antagonist that contributes to smooth muscle relaxation. As a single agent it is minimally efficacious, but it is commonly used in combination to potentiate papaverine or PGE_1.

To maximize efficacy and minimize side effects, many clinicians use a combination of PGE_1, papaverine, and phentolamine as a tri-mix, which allows the use of a lower dose of each agent. A common mixture is papaverine, 120 mg (4 mL of 30 mg/mL); phentolamine, 6 mg; and PGE_1, 120 µg (6 mL of 20 mg/mL) for a total volume of 10 mL. The reliable patient can titrate his intracavernosal dose from 0.2 mL to 0.5 mL to optimize erectile response.

The greatest concern with intracavernosal injection therapy is priapism. In the case of prolonged or painful erections with PGE_1, either brethane, 5 mg, or pseudoephedrine, 60 mg, self-administered orally may be of benefit. If priapism persists longer than 4 hours, patients are instructed to seek medical care in which aspiration alone or with the injection of an alpha-adrenergic agent is used to induce detumescence. Vital signs are always monitored. If this treatment fails, surgical therapy may be indicated to reverse a prolonged erection, otherwise anoxic damage to the cavernosal smooth muscle cells and permanent ED can occur.

Third-line Therapies

Penile Prosthesis

In the early part of the 20th century, the treatment of ED was virtually nonexistent. In the early 1970s, the introduction of semirigid and inflatable penile prostheses initiated the great strides that have been made in recent years in the treatment of ED. To some, penile prostheses are considered invasive and costly, but for many patients with advanced organic disease who are unresponsive to any contemporary form of therapy, have significant structural disorders of the penis (e.g., Peyronie's disease), or have suffered corporal loss from cancer or traumatic injury, prostheses remain a highly effective and predictable method for restoring erectile function.

Penile implants are paired supports that are placed one in each of the two erectile bodies. Two basic types are used: hydraulic or fluid-filled, referred to as inflatable prostheses; and semirigid, which are bendable and positionable, but always remain firm in the penis.

Inflatable prostheses include three-piece and two-piece models. The three-piece model uses a reservoir located in the pelvis behind the rectus muscle, a pump in the scrotum, and two inflatable cylinders. The two-piece device has the reservoir and pump combined, located in the scrotum, and two cylinders. Semirigid prostheses include malleable and mechanical versions.

Penile prostheses come in a variety of lengths and girths. The size selected for implantation is determined at the time of surgery, when each erectile body is measured. Implantation surgery usually takes less than an hour and in most cases can be done as an outpatient procedure under general or regional anesthesia.

With a number of recent modifications incorporating newer materials and designs, the likelihood of mechanical malfunction is only 5% to 10% in the first 10 years. Penile prostheses have a higher reliability than any other mechanical device implanted in the human body. The most feared complication by surgeons who implant prostheses is infection, which occurs in 1% to 3% of cases, but this can be higher in revision surgery, especially in diabetics.

The total cost of penile prosthesis implantation varies from $3,000 to $20,000, depending on the type of device and the community where the procedure is performed. If ED has an organic etiology, health or medical insurance in the United States often covers most of this cost.

Recent studies reported that greater than 80% of patients and 70% of partners are pleased with their prosthesis and the togetherness that it brings to their relationship.[64,65]

With an increasing aging population, a growing awareness of ED, and the availability of effective treatments, and more general practitioners prescribing oral ED agents, one can anticipate an increasing number of men with severe forms of ED who will need penile prosthesis procedures in the coming years.[64] This speculation is supported by a 1996 Dain Bosworth industry analysis report projecting an increase in the number of penile implant procedures performed through 2010. Ostensibly, there will always be a portion of the impotent population with advanced ED who will be candidates for penile prosthesis implantation.

Oral Therapeutic Agents under Development

In North America, the preferred route of administration for ED treatment is by mouth. The huge success of sildenafil (Viagra, Pfizer, NY) attests to the insatiable public demand for an effective oral erectogenic agent. Research and development in this field by other pharmaceutical enterprises has introduced a number of new phosphodiesterase (PDE) type 5 inhibitors with supposedly increased potency and fewer side effects.

Phosphodiesterases (PDE) have a ubiquitous presence in the human body. PDE type 5 inhibitors to enhance the effects of sexual stimulation through NO increases in cGMP in the penis. Besides acting in the corpus cavernosum of the penis, PDE type 5 inhibition is active in skeletal muscle, vascular smooth muscle, platelets, and visceral smooth muscle. PDE type 5 inhibition cross-reacting in other tissues causes most of the recognized side effects (e.g., headaches, gastroesophageal reflux, muscle cramps, and visual acuity changes).

The efficacy and side effects of PDE inhibitors are a function of pharmacologic specificity and bioavailability. Important parameters evaluated include t½, tmax, and IC50 (the concentration of a given agent to inhibit 50% of a given PDE). Vardenafil (Bayer) and Cialis (Lilly-ICOS) are two new PDE type 5 inhibitors that are currently available in the United States. Because of their reported increased selectivity, overall efficacy, and decreased number of adverse effects in phase II and III studies, they show clinical promise.

PDE type 5 inhibitors act as peripheral conditioners (i.e., enhance a local pathway to cause an erection). Another exciting area of research are drugs that initiate erections by actions directed within the central nervous system. Apomorphine SL (TAP Pharmaceuticals, Inc.) is an aporphine (not an opiate) that acts as a dopaminergic agonist. It is effective centrally at nanogram concentrations and has actions on the paraventricular and supraoptic nuclei of the midbrain. It was recently reformulated for sublingual absorption with an onset of action within 15 to 20 minutes. Adverse effects include nausea, vomiting, and rarely, syncope. Ongoing clinical research studies and experience from Europe since its approval in June 2001 may bring it to the US market in the near future.

Another central initiator of erection in early development is alpha-melanocyte–stimulating hormone (melonstan II). It has both dopaminergic agonist activity and beneficial effects on libido.

A double-blind, placebo-controlled, crossover study showed significant improvement in RigiScan events, penile rigidity, and sexual desire in 10 patients with documented ED risk factors receiving melanotan II compared with placebo. Nausea was the most common adverse event.[66]

Gene Therapy and Erectile Dysfunction

Gene therapy is the introduction of genetic material (RNA or DNA) into an appropriate cell type, thus altering gene expression of that cell to produce a therapeutic effect.[67] Gene therapy involves three steps: administration of a desired gene into the body, delivery of the gene to a targeted cell, and expression of the therapeutic product. Recently there has been an explosion in the amount of basic and clinical research in the field of gene therapy.[68] In the past, gene therapy approaches were used to treat disorders that had an underlying genetic component. However, gene therapy has evolved to the point where treatment of any disease process, genetic or acquired, can be theoretically accomplished as long as there exists a target gene that, when altered, can effectively restore or supplement defective functions. The goal of gene therapy for ED is to introduce novel genetic material into an appropriate cell in an attempt to restore normal cellular and physiologic function.

Gene therapy has been proposed as a viable treatment for diseases that have a vascular origin, such as arteriosclerosis, congestive heart failure, and pulmonary hypertension.[67,69,70] This, by biologic extension, suggests that gene therapy may also be used to treat vascular diseases of the penis. In most cases, ED is a manifestation of vascular disease. One advantage of treating ED with gene therapy is the easily accessible external location of the penis.[71,72] Hence, a tourniquet can be placed around the base of the penis and the desired gene can be administered directly into the corpora cavernosa without entering the systemic circulation. This is a distinct advantage over other gene therapy approaches in which a vector encoding a desired gene is introduced into the systemic circulation. This approach may cause numerous adverse systemic effects, including the gene being introduced into the incorrect organ or vascular bed. However, this potential adverse effect is minimized when gene therapy vectors are used to treat ED because the penis has its own external circulation, allowing a gene to be transferred and localized in one organ, thus lessening the risk of systemic spillover. Determination of the number of cells that must be transfected to produce a therapeutic effect is often difficult to determine. However, in the penis, only a small number of cells need to be transfected because the corpus cavernosum smooth muscle cells are interconnected by gap junctions that allow second messenger molecules and ions to be transferred to a number of interconnected smooth muscle cells, thus causing physiologically relevant changes in erectile function.[72] Moreover, the vascular smooth muscle cells of the penis have a relatively low turnover rate, thus allowing a desired gene to be expressed for long periods.

The concept of gene therapy for ED treatment focuses on preventing cavernosal tissue degradation and increasing cavernosal smooth muscle tone. Smooth muscle relaxation is the necessary step to achieve a normal erection. Therefore, molecules, enzymes, or growth factors that influence the signal transduction pathway of corporal smooth muscle relaxation represent possible targets for ED gene therapy. Nitric oxide is the principal mediator of penile erection.[73] However, other diverse mediators, such as the prostaglandins, vasoactive intestinal polypeptide (VIP), and calcitonin gene–related peptide (CGRP), play a role in erectile physiology. Only a few laboratories have used gene therapy to treat ED. Garban and associates first showed that gene therapy can be performed in the penis by using naked cDNA encoding the penile-inducible nitric oxide synthase gene, leading to physiologic benefit in the aging rat.[74] Christ and colleagues later showed that injection of hSlo cDNA, which encodes the human smooth muscle maxi-K+ channel, into the rat corpora cavernosa can increase gap junction formation and enhance erectile responses to nerve stimulation in the aged rat.[75] More recently, Bivalacqua and colleagues used an adenoviral gene transfer approach in which an adenoviral construct encoding the eNOS and CGRP genes reversed age-related ED in rats.[76-80] In these studies, cytomegalovirus and Rous sarcoma adenoviruses were used, and both eNOS and CGRP expression were sustained for at least 1 month in the corpora cavernosa of the rat penis. Five days after transfection with the AdCMVeNOS or AdRSVeNOS viruses, aged rats had significant increases in erectile function as determined by cavernosal nerve stimulation and pharmacologic injection with the endothelium-dependent vasodilator acetylcholine and the type 5 phosphodiesterase inhibitors zaprinast and sildenafil.[76-78]

Radical pelvic surgery is another common cause of ED due to injury to the cavernosal nerves. Lue and colleagues showed that intracavernous injection of adeno-associated virus-brain derived neurotrophic factor could improve erectile function after cavernosal nerve injury.[81] This neurotrophic factor purportedly restored neuronal NOS in the major pelvic ganglion, thus enhancing the recovery of erectile function after bilateral cavernous nerve injury. These early but innovative studies provide evidence that in vivo gene transfer can have beneficial physiologic effects on penile erection.

The use of gene therapy to treat ED represents an exciting new field that still requires significant basic research before in vivo gene therapy techniques can be applied to humans.

Other Male Sexual Disorders: Premature Ejaculation and Decreased Libido

The patient's history will help to establish if the condition is lifelong or acquired, as can happen with medication usage.[82] This is important in terms of treatment to determine whether the subject has primary or secondary ED. Men with ED may have secondary premature ejaculation when they can no longer maintain an erection for the completion of satisfactory intercourse. Premature ejaculation can also lead to secondary ED if it is not recognized and treated promptly.

Treatment of premature ejaculation has two primary approaches: behavioral and pharmacologic. Behavioral techniques include the "squeeze technique" that, once the desired outcome is achieved, progresses to the "stop/start technique." The pharmacologic approach is the use of antidepressants such as tricyclic clomipramine and the selective serotonin reuptake inhibitors (SSRIs), which is effective for treating premature ejaculation.[83]

Adverse effects associated with SSRI fluoxetine include drowsiness, insomnia, anxiety, and reduced sexual desire. Topical anesthetic such as lignocaine and prilocaine is moderately effective in retarding ejaculation.

Decreased libido is often associated with depression, sleep disturbance, loss of interest in normal activities, and alcohol abuse. Medications used to treat various disorders (antidepressants or antipsychotics) are also a common cause.

MANAGEMENT OF FEMALE SEXUAL DYSFUNCTION

Female sexual dysfunction is a multicausal and multidimensional medical problem that adversely affects physical health and emotional well-being.

Clinical Evaluation of the Female Sexual Response

Female sexual arousal causes a combination of vasocongestive and neuromuscular events that include increased clitoral, labial, and vaginal wall engorgement as well as increased vaginal luminal diameter and lubrication. Muscle tension, respiratory rate, heart rate, and blood pressure increase steadily during arousal, finally reaching their peak during orgasm. Historically, the evaluation of female patients with sexual dysfunction has been limited to psychological assessment. Physiologic evaluation of female sexual response in the clinical setting is complicated by the difficulty of objectively quantifying the changes that occur with arousal. Also, in contrast to the male erectile response, many genital changes that comprise the female sexual response are not only difficult to measure, but also may go unnoticed by the patient.

Previously described techniques for evaluating physiologic changes during female sexual arousal were preformed primarily by psychotherapists and physiologists and focused primarily on estimating vaginal engorgement.

Medical Evaluation

A comprehensive approach to the evaluation of physiologic changes during sexual arousal includes a full history and physical examination, including a pelvic examination, and when clinically indicated, a hormonal profile (FSH, LH, prolactin, free testosterone, SHBG and estradiol levels). Testosterone is bound to both albumin and serum hormone–binding globulin (SHBG) in the blood. Free testosterone levels correspond with the bioavailable active hormone. Medical conditions that disrupt the hypothalamic–pituitary axis or hormone deficiencies secondary to menopause, chemotherapy, or after bilateral salpingo-oophorectomy also affect female sexual dysfunction. The etiologies of these sexual symptoms are often not psychogenic and are amenable to medical therapy. Medications that adversely effect sexual function should also be addressed and changed if not contraindicated (Table 37-1).

TABLE 37-1 ■ Common Classes of Medications with Sexual Side Effects

Type of Agent	Drug Classes
Antihypertensive agents	Alpha-1 and alpha-2 blockers (clonidine, reserpine, prazosin)
	Beta blockers (metoprolol, propranolol)
	Calcium channel blockers (diltiazem, nifedipine)
	Diuretics (hydrochlorothiazide)
Chemotherapeutic agents	Alkylating agents (busulfan, chlorambucil, cyclophosphamide)
Central nervous system agents	Anticholinergics (diphenhydramine)
	Anticonvulsants (carbamazepine, phenobarbital, phenytoin)
	Antidepressants (MAOIs, TCAs, SSRIs)
	Antipsychotics (butyrophenones, phenothiazines)
	Narcotics (oxycodone)
	Sedatives and anxiolytics (benzodiazepines)
Medicines that affect hormones	Antiandrogens (cimetidine, spironolactone)
	Antiestrogens (raloxifene, tamoxifen)
	Oral contraceptives

MAOI, monoamine oxidase inhibitor; TCA, tricyclic antidepressant; SSRI, selective serotonin reuptake inhibitor.

Evaluating the female sexual response in the clinical setting both validates the patient's problem and potentially diagnoses organic disease such as vascular insufficiency, hormonal abnormalities, or neurologic disorders. Studies being undertaken at our institution seek to define ranges of normal for the following parameters:

- Genital blood flow. The clitoral, labial, urethral, and vaginal peak systolic velocities and end diastolic velocities can be measured with duplex Doppler ultrasound.
- Vaginal lubrication as reflected by pH.
- Vaginal compliance or elasticity (pressure–volume changes).
- Genital sensation and vibration perception thresholds.

These measurements are recorded before and after stimulation. Eventually, definition of the parameters before initiating medical therapy may become the standard of care.

Psychosocial and Psychosexual Assessment

In addition to the medical evaluations, all patients should be evaluated for emotional and relational issues. This includes the context in which the patient experiences her sexuality, her self-esteem and body image, and her ability to communicate her sexual needs to her partner. This is an integral component of the female sexual function evaluation. Emotional or relational issues should be addressed before treatment, and certainly before determining treatment efficacy. If ongoing therapy is desired or required, it should also be provided.

To assess subjective sexual function, in particular sexual arousal, several instruments are available. The Brief Index of Sexual Function Inventory (BISF-W), for example, is a validated 21-item, self-reported inventory of sexual interest, activity, satisfaction, and preference and discriminates among depressed, sexually dysfunctional, and healthy patients. Subjective sexual response data reflect the patient's experience, an important variable because the ultimate goal is to enhance the woman's sexual experience. Intervention is not considered successful unless the woman is able to subjectively experience sexual arousal, pleasure, and satisfaction. Thus, it is important to determine if physiologic changes or improvement in blood flow translate into an improved sexual experience. For instance, a physiologically documented increase in blood flow is irrelevant unless the patient experiences increased arousal, sensation, and satisfaction reflected by those physiologic processes.

Treatment

Treatment of female sexual dysfunction is gradually evolving as more clinical and basic science studies are dedicated to defining this problem. Thus, aside from hormone replacement therapy, medical management of female sexual dysfunction remains in the early experimental phases. Nonetheless, medical and health care professionals should realize that not all female sexual complaints are psychological and that there are potential therapeutic options. Aside from hormone replacement therapy, all medications discussed here used to treat male ED are still in the experimental phases for use in women.

Estrogen Therapy

This treatment is indicated in menopausal women (either spontaneous or surgical). Aside from relieving hot flashes, preventing osteoporosis, and lowering the risk of heart disease, estrogen replacement therapy improves clitoral sensitivity, increases libido, and decreases pain and burning during intercourse. Local or topical estrogen application relieves symptoms of vaginal dryness, burning, and urinary frequency and urgency. In menopausal or oophorectomized women, vaginal irritation, pain, or dryness is relieved with topical estrogen cream. A vaginal estradiol ring (Estring) is available that delivers low-dose estrogen locally and may benefit patients with breast cancer and other women who cannot take oral or transdermal estrogen.

Androgen Formulations

Methyltestosterone

17-Alpha-methyltestosterone is commonly used in combination with estrogen (Estrotest) in menopausal women for symptoms of inhibited desire, dyspareunia, or lack of vaginal lubrication, as well as for its vasoprotective effects. There are conflicting reports about the benefit of methyltestosterone for treatment of inhibited desire or vaginismus in premenopausal women. Topical vaginal testosterone is used to treat vaginal lichen planus. The suggested dose of methyltestosterone for premenopausal and postmenopausal women ranges from 0.25 to 1.25 mg/day. The dose should be adjusted according to symptoms, free testosterone levels, cholesterol levels, triglyceride HDL levels, and liver function tests. Topical testosterone (methyltestosterone or testosterone proprionate) preparations can be made in 1% to 2% formulations, and should be applied up to three times per week. Potential side effects include weight gain, clitoral enlargement, increased facial hair, and hypercholesterolemia. Increased clitoral sensitivity, decreased vaginal dryness, and increased libido are reported with the use of 2% testosterone cream. Side effects are similar to the oral preparation. The pharmacokinetics of these formulations have not been rigorously studied, and their clinical efficacy remains to be shown.

Two novel testosterone formulations are currently in early phases of clinical development. A transdermal matrix testosterone delivery system (patch) for women that is applied twice a week is being investigated.[81] Each patch provides a nominal delivery of 150 μg testosterone daily.[84,85] Thus, two patches applied simultaneously twice a week can achieve a daily delivery of 300 μg testosterone, approximating the daily production rates of testosterone in healthy women. The skin tolerability of the patch is excellent.[84] Initial pharmacokinetic studies showed that each 150 μg patch increases total serum testosterone concentrations by 25 to 30 ng/dL on average in healthy menstruating women and in surgically postmenopausal women.[84,86] For women who have undergone oophorectomy and hysterectomy, transdermal testosterone has been shown to improve both sexual function and psychological well-being.[87] A testosterone gel for women is in initial stages of development. Each milligram of testosterone applied to the nongenital skin can increase serum testosterone concentration by 7 to 8 ng/dL.

Sildenafil

Functioning as a selective type 5 (cGMP specific) phosphodiesterase inhibitor, sildenafil decreases the catabolism of cGMP, the second messenger in nitric oxide–mediated relaxation of clitoral and vaginal smooth muscle. Sildenafil may prove useful alone or possibly in combination with other vasoactive substances for the treatment of female sexual dysfunction. Studies assessing safety and efficacy of sildenafil have shown that the drug is safe and well tolerated in postmenopausal women with FSAD without concomitant HSDD or abuse issues.[88] Recent studies showed that sildenafil is successful in treating female sexual dysfunction associated with aging and menopause and secondary to the use of serotonin reuptake inhibitors (SSRI).[89]

l-Arginine

This amino acid functions as a precursor to the formation of nitric oxide, which mediates the relaxation of vascular and nonvascular smooth muscle. L-Arginine has not been tested in clinical trials in women; however, preliminary studies in men appear promising. A combination of L-arginine and yohimbine (an alpha-2 blocker) is under investigation in women.

Yohimbine

Yohimbine is an alkaloid agent that blocks presynaptic alpha-2-adrenergic receptors. It affects the peripheral autonomic nervous system, resulting in a relative decrease in adrenergic activity and an increase in parasympathetic tone. There have been mixed reports of its efficacy for inducing penile erections in men, and no formal clinical studies have been performed in women.

Prostaglandin E_1

An intraurethral application, absorbed via mucosa (MUSE), is now available for male patients. A similar application of prostaglandin E_1 delivered intravaginally is under investigation for use in women. Clinical studies are needed to determine the efficacy of this medication in the treatment of female sexual dysfunction.

Phentolamine

Currently available in an oral preparation, this drug functions as a nonspecific alpha-adrenergic blocker and causes vascular smooth muscle relaxation. This drug has been studied in men for the treatment of ED. A pilot study in menopausal women with sexual dysfunction showed enhanced vaginal blood flow and subjective arousal with medication.[90]

Apomorphine

This short-acting dopamine agonist facilitates erectile responses in both normal males and males with psychogenic ED, as well as males with organic impotence. Data suggest that dopamine is involved in the mediation of sexual desire and arousal. The physiologic effects of this drug are being tested in women with sexual dysfunction.

CONCLUSION

The ideal approach to female sexual dysfunction is a collaborative effort between therapists and physicians and should include a complete medical and psychosocial evaluation as well as inclusion of the partner or spouse in the evaluation and treatment.

Although there are significant anatomic and embryologic parallels between men and women, the multifaceted nature of female sexual dysfunction is clearly distinct from that of the male. Thus, we cannot approach female patients or their sexual function problems in the way that we do male patients. The context in which a woman experiences her sexuality is equally if not more important than the physiologic outcome she experiences, and these issues need to be determined before beginning medical therapy or attempting to determine treatment efficacies. Despite the presence of organic disease, psychosocial, emotional, or relational factors often contribute to female sexual dysfunction. For this reason, a comprehensive approach, addressing both psychological as well as physiologic factors is instrumental to the evaluation of female patients with sexual dysfunction. Whether sildenafil or other vasoactive agents are predictably effective in women with arousal disorder remains to be seen. There is a pressing need for more clinical and basic science research.

REFERENCES

1. Benet AE, Melman A: The epidemiology of erectile dysfunction. Urol Clin North Am 22:699–709, 1995.
2. Lue TF: Erectile dysfunction. N Engl J Med 342: 1802–1813, 2000.
3. NIH Consensus Conference. Impotence. NIH Consensus Development Panel on Impotence. JAMA 270(1):83–90, 1993.
4. Cappelleri JC, Rosen RC, Smith MD, et al: Diagnostic evaluation of the erectile function domain of the International Index of Erectile Function. Urology 54:346–351, 1999.
5. Rosen RC, Cappelleri JC, Smith MD, et al: Development and evaluation of an abridged, 5-item version of the International Index of Erectile Function (IIEF-5) as a diagnostic tool for erectile dysfunction. Int J Impot Res 11:319–326, 1999.
6. Ruutu ML, Virtanen JM, Lindstrom BL, Alfthan OS: The value of basic investigations in the diagnosis of impotence. Scand J Urol Nephrol 21:261–265, 1987.
7. Takasaki N, Kotani T, Miyazaki S, Saitou S: Measurement of penile brachial index (PBI) in patients with impotence. Hinyokika Kiyo 35:1365–1368, 1989.
8. Aitchison M, Aitchison J, Carter R: Is the penile brachial index a reproducible and useful measurement? Br J Urol 66:202–204, 1990.
9. Mueller SC, Wallenberg-Pachaly H, Voges GE, Schild HH: Comparison of selective internal iliac pharmaco-angiography, penile brachial index and duplex sonography with pulsed Doppler analysis for the evaluation of vasculogenic (arteriogenic) impotence. J Urol 143:928–932, 1990.
10. Brock G: Tumescence monitoring devices: Past and present. In Hellstrom W (ed): Handbook of Sexual Dysfunction. Lawrence, KS, Allen Press, 1999, pp 65–69.
11. Carani C, Zini D, Baldini A, et al: Effects of androgen treatment in impotent men with normal and low levels of free testosterone. Arch Sex Behav 19:223–234, 1990.
12. Korenman SG, Morley JE, Mooradian AD, et al: Secondary hypogonadism in older men: Its relation to impotence. J Clin Endocrinol Metab 71:963–969, 1990.
13. Buvat J, Lemaire A: Endocrine screening in 1,022 men with erectile dysfunction: Clinical significance and cost-effective strategy (see comments). J Urol 158:1764–1767, 1997.
14. Carani C, Bancroft J, Granata A, et al: Testosterone and erectile function, nocturnal penile tumescence and rigidity, and erectile response to visual erotic stimuli in hypogonadal and agonadal men. Psychoneuroendocrinology 17:647–654, 1992.
15. Kaiser FE, Viosca SP, Morley JE, et al: Impotence and aging: Clinical and hormonal factors. J Am Geriatr Soc 36:511–519, 1988.
16. Citron JT, Ettinger B, Rubinoff H, et al: Prevalence of hypothalamic-pituitary imaging abnormalities in impotent men with secondary hypogonadism. J Urol 155:529–533, 1996.
17. Morales A, Johnston B, Heaton JP, Lundie M: Testosterone supplementation for hypogonadal impotence: Assessment of biochemical measures and therapeutic outcomes. J Urol 157:849–854, 1997.
18. Hajjar RR, Kaiser FE, Morley JE: Outcomes of long-term testosterone replacement in older hypogonadal males: A retrospective analysis. J Clin Endocrinol Metab 82:3793–3796, 1997.
19. Goldstein I, Lue TF, Padma-Nathan H, et al: Oral sildenafil in the treatment of erectile dysfunction. Sildenafil Study Group. N Engl J Med 338(20):1397–1404, 1998.
20. Goldstein I: A 36-week, open label, non-comparative study to assess the long-term safety of sildenafil citrate (Viagra) in patients with erectile dysfunction. Int J Clin Pract Suppl 102:8–9, 1999.
21. Rendell MS, Rajfer J, Wicker PA, Smith MD: Sildenafil for treatment of erectile dysfunction in men with diabetes: A randomized controlled trial. Sildenafil Diabetes Study Group (see comments). JAMA 281:421–426, 1999.
22. Boolell M, Allen MJ, Ballard SA, et al: Sildenafil: An orally active type 5 cyclic GMP-specific phosphodiesterase inhibitor for the treatment of penile erectile dysfunction. Int J Impot Res 8:47–52, 1996.
23. Moreland RB, Goldstein I, Traish A: Sildenafil, a novel inhibitor of phosphodiesterase type 5 in human corpus cavernosum smooth muscle cells. Life Sci 62:PL309–PL318, 1998.
24. Giuliano F, Hultling C, El Masry WS, et al: Randomized trial of sildenafil for the treatment of erectile dysfunction in spinal cord injury: Sildenafil Study Group. Ann Neurol 46:15–21, 1999.
25. Jarow JP, Burnett AL, Geringer AM: Clinical efficacy of sildenafil citrate based on etiology and response to prior treatment (see comments). J Urol 162:722–725, 1999.
26. Dinsmore WW, Hodges M, Hargreaves C, et al: Sildenafil citrate (Viagra) in erectile dysfunction: Near normalization in men with broad-spectrum erectile dysfunction compared with age-matched healthy control subjects (erratum appears in Urology 53[5]:1072, 1999). Urology 53:800–805, 1999.
27. Morales A, Gingell C, Collins M, et al: Clinical safety of oral sildenafil citrate (Viagra) in the treatment of erectile dysfunction. Int J Impot Res 10:69–73, 1998.
28. Aversa A, Mazzilli F, Rossi T, et al: Effects of sildenafil (Viagra) administration on seminal parameters and post-ejaculatory refractory time in normal males. Hum Reprod 15:131–134, 2000.
29. Feenstra J, Drie-Pierik RJ, Lacle CF, Stricker BH: Acute myocardial infarction associated with sildenafil (letter) [see comments]. Lancet 352:957–958, 1998.
30. Zusman RM, Morales A, Glasser DB, Osterloh IH: Overall cardiovascular profile of sildenafil citrate. Am J Cardiol 83:35C–44C, 1999.
31. Arora RR, Timoney M, Melilli L: Acute myocardial infarction after the use of sildenafil (letter). N Engl J Med 341:700, 1999.
32. Cheitlin MD, Hutter AM Jr, Brindis RG, et al: Use of sildenafil (Viagra) in patients with cardiovascular disease: Technology and Practice Executive Committee (erratum appears in Circulation 100[23]:2389, 1999) [see comments]. Circulation 99:168–177, 1999.
33. Muller JE, Mittleman A, Maclure M, et al: Triggering myocardial infarction by sexual activity: Low absolute risk and prevention by regular physical exertion. Determinants of Myocardial Infarction Onset Study Investigators (see comments). JAMA 275:1405–1409, 1996.
34. Herrmann HC, Chang G, Klugherz BD, Mahoney PD: Hemodynamic effects of sildenafil in men with severe coronary artery disease. N Engl J Med 342:1622–1626, 2000.
35. Padma-Nathan H, Steers WD, Wicker PA: Efficacy and safety of oral sildenafil in the treatment of erectile dysfunction: A double-blind, placebo-controlled study of 329 patients. Sildenafil Study Group (see comments). Int J Clin Pract 52:375–379, 1998.
36. Goldenberg MM: Safety and efficacy of sildenafil citrate in the treatment of male erectile dysfunction. Clin Ther 20:1033–1048, 1998.

37. Conti CR, Pepine CJ, Sweeney M: Efficacy and safety of sildenafil citrate in the treatment of erectile dysfunction in patients with ischemic heart disease. Am J Cardiol 83:29C–34C, 1999.
38. Osterloh IH, Collins M, Wicker P, Wagner G: Sildenafil citrate (Viagra): Overall safety profile in 18 double-blind, placebo controlled, clinical trials. Int J Clin Pract Suppl 102:3–5, 1999.
39. Young J: Sildenafil citrate (Viagra) in the treatment of erectile dysfunction: A 12-week, flexible-dose study to assess efficacy and safety. Int J Clin Pract Suppl 102:6–7, 1999.
40. Kloner RA: Cardiovascular risk and sildenafil. Am J Cardiol 86:57F–61F, 2000.
41. McMahon CG, Samali R, Johnson H: Efficacy, safety and patient acceptance of sildenafil citrate as treatment for erectile dysfunction. J Urol 164:1192–1196, 2000.
42. McGarvey MR: Tough choices: The cost-effectiveness of sildenafil (editorial, comment). Ann Intern Med 132:994–995, 2000.
43. Smith KJ, Roberts MS: The cost-effectiveness of sildenafil (see comments). Ann Intern Med 132:933–937, 2000.
44. Tan HL: Economic cost of male erectile dysfunction using a decision analytic model for a hypothetical managed-care plan of 100,000 members. Pharmacoeconomics 17:77–107, 2000.
45. Witherington R: Vacuum devices for the impotent. J Sex Marital Ther 17:69–80, 1991.
46. Lewis JH, Sidi AA, Reddy PK: A way to help your patients who use vacuum devices. Contemp Urol 3:15–21, 1991.
47. Lewis RW, Witherington R: External vacuum therapy for erectile dysfunction: Use and results. World J Urol 15:78–82, 1997.
48. Ganem JP, Lucey DT, Janosko EO, Carson CC: Unusual complications of the vacuum erection device. Urology 51:627–631, 1998.
49. Morales A: Nonsurgical management options in impotence. Hosp Pract (Off Ed) 28:15–20, 23, 1993.
50. Davidson JM, Camargo CA, Smith ER: Effects of androgen on sexual behavior in hypogonadal men. J Clin Endocrinol Metab 48:955–958, 1979.
51. Kwan M, Greenleaf WJ, Mann J, et al: The nature of androgen action on male sexuality: A combined laboratory-self-report on hypogonadal men. J Clin Metab 57:557–562, 1983.
52. Bagatell CJ, Heiman JR, Rivier JE, Bremner WJ: Effects of endogenous testosterone and estradiol on sexual behavior in normal young men (erratum appears in J Clin Endocrinol Metab 78[6]:1520, 1994). J Clin Endocrinol Metab 78:711–716, 1994.
53. Skakkebaek NE, Bancroft J, Davidson DW, Warner P: Androgen replacement with oral testosterone undecenoate in hypogonadal men: A double blind controlled study. Clin Endocrinol (Oxf) 14:49–61, 1981.
54. McClure RD, Oses R, Ernest ML: Hypogonadal impotence treated by transdermal testosterone. Urology 37:224–228, 1991.
55. Nankin HR, Lin T, Osterman J: Chronic testosterone cypionate therapy in men with secondary impotence. Ferti Steril 46:300–307, 1986.
56. Arver S, Dobs AS, Meikle AW, et al: Improvement of sexual function in testosterone deficient men treated for 1 year with a permeation enhanced testosterone transdermal system. J Urol 155:1604–1608, 1996.
57. Buena F, Swerdloff RS, Steiner BS, et al: Sexual function does not change when serum testosterone levels are pharmacologically varied within the normal male range. Fertil Steril 59:1118–1123, 1993.
58. Bhasin S, Fielder T, Peacock N, et al: Dissociating antifertility effects of GnRH-antagonist from its adverse effects on mating behavior in male rats. Am J Physiol 254:E84–E91, 1988.
59. Fielder TJ, Peacock NR, McGivern RF, et al: Testosterone dose-dependency of sexual and nonsexual behaviors in the gonadotropin-releasing hormone antagonist-treated male rat. J Androl 10:167–173, 1989.
60. Jain P, Rademaker AW, McVary KT: Testosterone supplementation for erectile dysfunction: Results of a meta-analysis. J Urol 164:371–375, 2000.
61. Engelhardt PF, Plas E, Hubner WA, Pfluger H: Comparison of intraurethral liposomal and intracavernosal prostaglandin-E_1 in the management of erectile dysfunction. Br J Urol 81:441–444, 1998.
62. Kim ED, McVary KT: Topical prostaglandin-E_1 for the treatment of erectile dysfunction (see comments). J Urol 153:1828–1830, 1995.
63. Peterson CA, Bennett AH, Hellstrom WJ, et al: Erectile response to transurethral alprostadil, prazosin and alprostadil-prazosin combinations. J Urol 159:1523–1527, 1998.
64. Carson CC, Mulcahy JJ, Govier FE: Efficacy, safety and patient satisfaction outcomes of the AMS 700CX inflatable penile prosthesis: Results of a long-term multicenter study. AMS 700CX Study Group. J Urol 164:376–380, 2000.
65. Wilson SK, Cleves MA, Delk JR 2nd: Comparison of mechanical reliability of original and enhanced Mentor Alpha I penile prosthesis. J Urol 162:715–718, 1999.
66. Wessells H, Gralnek D, Dorr R, et al: Effect of an alpha-melanocyte stimulating hormone analog on penile erection and sexual desire in men with organic erectile dysfunction. Urology 56:641–646, 2000.
67. Nabel EG, Pompili VJ, Plautz GE, et al: Gene transfer and vascular disease. Cardiovasc Res 28(4):445–455, 1994.
68. Christ GJ: Gene therapy: Future strategies and therapies. Drugs Today (Barc) 36(2–3):175–184, 2000.
69. Heistad DD, Lentz SR, Rios CD: Atherosclerotic vascular disease: Will folate or gene therapy be useful? Trans Am Clin Climatol Assoc 108:69–76, 1996.
70. Champion HC, Bivalacqua TJ, D'Souza FM: Gene transfer of endothelial nitric oxide synthase to the lung of the mouse in vivo. Effect on agonist-induced and flow-mediated vascular responses. Circ Res 84(12)1422–1432, 1999.
71. Bivalacqua TJ, Hellstrom WJ: Potential application of gene therapy for the treatment of erectile dysfunction. J Androl 22:183–190, 2001.
72. Christ GJ, Melman A: The application of gene therapy to the treatment of erectile dysfunction. Int J Impot Res 10:111–112, 1998.
73. Burnett AL, Lowenstein CJ, Bredt DS, et al: Nitric oxide: A physiologic mediator of penile erection. Science 257:401–403, 1992.
74. Garban H, Marquez D, Magee T, et al: Cloning of rat and human inducible penile nitric oxide synthase: Application for gene therapy of erectile dysfunction. Biol Reprod 56:954–963, 1997.
75. Christ GJ, Rehman J, Day N, et al: Intracorporal injection of hSlo cDNA in rats produces physiologically relevant alterations in penile function. Am J Physiol 275:H600–H608, 1998.
76. Bivalacqua TJ, Champion HC, Mehta YS, et al: Adenoviral gene transfer of endothelial nitric oxide synthase (eNOS) to the penis improves age-related erectile dysfunction in the rat. Int J Impot Res 12 (suppl 3):S8–S17, 2000.
77. Champion HC, Bivalacqua TJ, Hyman AL, et al: Gene transfer of endothelial nitric oxide synthase to the penis augments erectile responses in the aged rat. Proc Natl Acad Sci U S A 96(20)11648–11652, 1999.

78. Champion HC, Bivalacqua TJ, D'Souza FM, et al: Gene transfer of endothelial nitric oxide synthase to the lung of the mouse in vivo: Effect on agonist-induced and flow-mediated vascular responses. Circ Res 84:1422–1432, 1999.
79. Champion HC, Bivalacqua TJ, Toyoda K, et al: In vivo gene transfer of prepro-calcitonin gene-related peptide to the lung attenuates chronic hypoxia-induced pulmonary hypertension in the mouse. Circulation 101:923–930, 2000.
80. Bivalacqua TJ, Rajasekaran M, Champion HC, et al: The influence of castration on pharmacologically induced penile erection in the cat. J Androl 19:551–557, 1998.
81. Bakircioglu ME, Lin CS, Fan P, et al: The effect of adeno-associated virus mediated brain derived neurotrophic factor in an animal model of neurogenic impotence. J Urol 165(6 Pt 1):2103–2109, 2001.
82. American Psychiatric Association: Diagnostic and Statistical Manual of Mental Disorders, ed 4. Washington DC, American Psychiatric Association, 1994, p 511.
83. McMahon CG, Samali R: Pharmacological treatment of premature ejaculation. Curr Opinion Urol 9:553–561, 1999.
84. Javanbakht M, Singh AB, Mazer NA: Pharmacokinetics of a novel testosterone matrix transdermal system in healthy, premenopausal women and women infected with the human immunodeficiency virus. J Clin Endocrinol Metab 85:2395–2401, 2000.
85. Simon JA, Mazer NA, Wekselman K: Safety profile: Transdermal testosterone treatment of women after oophorectomy. Obstet Gynecol 97:S10–S11, 2001.
86. Mazer NA: New applications of transdermal testosterone delivery in men and women. J Control Release 65:303–315, 2000.
87. Shifren JL, Braunstein GD, Simon JA, et al: Transdermal testosterone treatment in women with impaired sexual function after oophorectomy. N Engl J Med 343(10):682–688, 2000.
88. Berman JR, Berman LA, Toler SM, et al: Safety and efficacy of sildenafil citrate for the treatment of female sexual arousal disorder: A double-blind, placebo controlled study. J Urol 170(6 Pt1):2333–2338, 2003.
89. Berman JBL, Lin H, Cantey-Kiser J, et al: Effect of sildenafil on subjective and physiologic parameters of the female sexual response in women with sexual arousal disorder. J Sex Marital Ther 27(5):411–420, 2001.
90. Rosen RC, Phillips NA, Gendrano NC 3rd, et al: Oral phentolamine and female sexual arousal disorder: A pilot study. J Sex Marital Ther 25(2):137–144, 1999.

CHAPTER 38

Management of Vaginismus, Vulvodynia, and Childhood Sexual Abuse

DITZA KATZ ■ ROSS LYNN TABISEL

Optimal management of vaginismus, vulvodynia, and the outcomes of childhood sexual abuse necessitate a thorough understanding of these conditions because they represent a complex, intimate, and inseparable association between the body and the mind.

Physicians, therapists, and other health care practitioners who treat these conditions continually encounter that body–mind balance by virtue of their profession, yet diagnosis and treatment are often missed when the clinician is not acutely attuned to this delicate association. The patient, in turn, feels misunderstood, neglected, isolated, and hopeless, and is forced to either resign to living with the symptoms or embark on an endless quest for resolution.

The private and misunderstood nature of these conditions often brings about shame, feelings of inadequacy, "I am the only one who suffers from this," "even my doctor doesn't understand it," "I must be a freak," "weird," "deformed," "broken" . . . Thus, the patient's endless quest for answers is complicated by the emotional anguish of the condition and adds a traumatic aspect to the already distressing symptoms.

Living in secrecy is another common feature of these conditions. Although the patient is eager for explanation and resolution, there is often a reluctance to admit and disclose the presence and details of the problem. Unconsummated marriages are viewed as failure and inadequacy; pain and sexual dysfunction suggest abnormality; fear of touch means "danger," even in the hands of a well-meaning clinician. In dealing with these powerful emotions, the patient often presents only portions of the problem, and it is up to the treating clinician to be attuned and to ask questions while reassuring the patient of her safety and of the clinician's competency in understanding the condition.

VAGINISMUS

Definition

Vaginismus is the involuntary, instantaneous hypertonus of the pelvic floor musculature, occurring as a protective response to stress, apprehension, or fear associated with penetration, thus making it painful or impossible. This powerful reaction may be transient or ongoing, lasting from just a few seconds to most of the time. Vaginismus may be triggered from the body by a touch or an attempted penetration, or from the mind by thinking about penetration or by remembering an upsetting or traumatic experience.[1]

Regardless of the source of provocation, since vaginismus is a body–mind phenomenon, resolution requires treatment through both the body and the mind.

Etiology

The pelvic floor musculature is predominantly postural, containing an approximate 2:1 ratio of slow-twitch (type I) to fast-twitch (type II) fibers.[2] Neurologically, the efferent branch of the visceral (autonomic) nervous system supplies the urogenital system, sigmoid colon, rectum, and anal canal; its sympathetic nervous system (SNS) branch innervates the pelvic basin: the perineal musculature, sweat glands, and smooth muscles of blood vessels.[3] The pelvic floor musculature is known to have four functions: a mechanical support to the anus, perineal body, and the lower third of the vagina; a sphincter enhancement to the urinary system; a component of the micturition and defecating reflexes; and a vital component of the sexual response mechanism that produces orgasms. The fifth function is that of a defense mechanism, by virtue of its SNS innervation and the protective fight-or-flight reaction—a function in dire need of recognition.

In merging this information, one can clearly appreciate the intimate association between the pelvic floor and the instant activation of the SNS, especially when vaginal penetration is associated with apprehension, stress, fear, danger, or pain. Furthermore, repeated activation of this protective system lowers its threshold of response and establishes a conditioned pattern of reaction that is beyond any voluntary control or rational thinking.

Stated differently, vaginismus is the body's conditioned activation of the fight-or-flight response upon the slightest reminder, or presence, of impending stress or danger, be it real or imaginary, actual or remembered. Once established, this protective reaction is easily reactivated, sending the woman into a distressing body–mind experience with heart racing, trembling, excessive sweating, hip adduction, and a feeling of doom. Most important, being involuntary, vaginismus does not respond to suggestions such as "relax," "don't think about it," "it will go away," "have a drink," "just do it," and "take antianxiety medications"—common suggestions women are given by frustrated clinicians.

Vaginismus affects adolescent girls and women of all ages, all cultures, all religions, and all socioeconomic and educational levels. Family status is not a factor either: Vaginismus affects single people, married couples, and lesbian couples alike—there is no stereotype for the vaginismus sufferer. And, contrary to common belief, sexual abuse is not the major cause of vaginismus, although many women who were sexually abused present with vaginismus.

Dispelling another myth, vaginismus—the fear of penetration—is seldom caused by a pathology or organic lesions. Likewise, infections, allergic reactions, and other dermatologic concerns rarely cause vaginismus as they may be easily diagnosed and resolved with medical care, pharmacologic agents, proper hygiene, and lifestyle modifications. And while a rigid, imperforated hymen requires surgical intervention, vaginismus will not respond to a hymenectomy. Unfortunately, many clinicians operate under the assumption that a hymenectomy (often combined with an episiotomy and a labialectomy) will "open" the introitus, facilitate penetration, and bring about consummation of marriages/relationships. The truth, as patients will confess when encouraged to overcome their inadequacy and shame, is that while surgery eliminates genital tissue (body), it does not address the fear of the fight-or-flight response (mind) associated with penetration, leaving vaginismus intact yet with the added trauma of surgery, failed expectations, and body alterations.

The backdrop of vaginismus highlights a fundamental developmental difference between the sexes: Boys explore their genitals from an early age because they are external, easily palpable, and involved in the basic function of urination. Consequently, a man is usually quite clear on how his genitals look and react, which way he likes to be touched, and how he fares versus other males. Conversely, the female's genitals are internal, invisible, inexperienced, not usually involved in body exploration, and their function carries a notion of mystery, all of which may be too scary to some adolescents and women—a common feeling in vaginismus. Additionally, the individual's character and emotional makeup determine whether she will develop this condition or whether she is able to explore her body and emotions in a secure, healthy manner. Of course, traumatic life events adversely affect her development and emotional state and can bring about vaginismus as well.

Another feature of vaginismus is being the receiver of penetration, being "done to," a position that carries a tremendous emotional impact associated with a perceived lack of control and with being choiceless, even if the sexual encounter is consensual, loving, tender, and desired. Women who are shy or incapable of expressing their sexual preferences and women who perceive men as being overly powerful and sexually demanding will often send their bodies to speak up for them by developing vaginismus, assuming the ultimate control by rejecting penetration.

Finally, the pain associated with vaginismus warrants an explanation for a better understanding of the condition and in order to be able to ease the mind of the patient. At the same time, the pain should not be a deterrent to intervention because it is a symptom of the mechanism associated with the condition and not a warning sign of trouble.

Vaginismus pain is usually described as any combination of the following: vaginal or vulvar burning, pinching, or poking, "pain like hitting a brick wall," urinary urgency and frequency, and, although less often, pain radiating to the rectum or groin. All laboratory findings are negative, and there are usually no structural abnormalities.

The chief reason behind this symptomology, and the one that is always present, is the anterosuperior direction of pull of the pelvic floor musculature. When activated during a fight-or-flight response, this muscle contraction diminishes the lumen of the vagina and compresses the urethra into the pubic symphysis, resulting in urethral contusions and chafing that are manifested as this pain symptomology. This symptomology may be easily reproduced (once penetration is possible) by gliding a finger along the urethra, simulating the pressure exerted by the action of the pelvic floor musculature. In women who do not suffer from vaginismus, this digital experiment produces minimal urethral annoyance, but not the same pain as occurs with vaginismus. Treating clinicians should carefully differentiate between a true urinary tract infection (positive laboratory findings) and urethral contusions that do not require traditional pharmacologic intervention. Prolonged or unnecessary administration of antibiotics will negatively alter the eco system of the vaginal flora, predisposing it to breakdowns and to ongoing urethral contusions.

Other causes for the pain symptomology associated with vaginismus include the following:

- Inaccurate direction or angle of penetration resulting in pushing against the perineal body or the external urethral meatus
- Friction irritation due to forced or persistent penetration into a resistant vagina (diminished anterior-posterior diameter).

- Vaginal dryness, caused by reasons such as hormonal alterations, atrophic vaginitis, insufficient hydration, certain prescription drugs, chlorine in swimming pools, dry heat during winter months, insufficient lubrication during sexual arousal, etc.
- Associated muscle guarding in the pelvic girdle
- Body memories, or the psychophysical imprints of past traumatic experiences (for more, see the discussion under Sexual Abuse)

Remote pains that may also be present include the hypertonus of the other postural muscles in the body (temporomandibular joint, the cervical spine, and the lumbosacral region), and abdominal pains that are due to the neurophysiologic mechanisms associated with the fight-or-flight response.

Overall, one's ability to face, understand, manage, and cope with the sensation of pain is a determining fact in the development of vaginismus.

Considering the etiology of vaginismus, one should be attuned to any and all possible causes, as follows:

- Fear of the body or its functions
- Fear of pain
- Fear of the unknown (Where is my vagina? Will penetration hurt?)
- Past illness, surgery, other medical procedures with scary or painful memories
- Religious inhibitions and taboos regarding sex or a woman's body
- Cultural expectations of a woman's role (serve the man, sex is not for woman's pleasure, just do it for him, etc.)
- Parental or peer misrepresentation of sex and sexuality
- Inability to say no, thus feeling forced
- Sexual abuse or rape, whether witnessing it or being the victim
- Overprotective parents, limiting the child's ability to face challenges, to overcome fears, to face the unknown, and so on
- Traumatic sexual experiences (e.g., pain, infection)
- Failed attempts at inserting a tampon, which enhance the feeling of "I do not have an opening"
- Fear of pregnancy
- Fear of infection
- Social pressure to be sexually successful
- Fear of relationships or commitments
- Fear of loss of control
- Poor self-image, leading to body inhibitions and physical shutdown
- Pressure to have penetration despite discomfort, dyspareunia, reluctance, etc.
- Unresolved pathology or organic lesions

Manifestation

The following is a typical case presentation: "My wife and I have been married for almost 2 years and have had intimate relations for more than five, but in none of that time has she ever been able to have actual penetration with my finger, penis, a tampon, or a gynecologic exam. Upon initiation of sex, or any physical stimulation, my wife gets really nervous and tight, and there is no way I can get inside of her at all. She is very shy and doesn't want to go for help, but this issue is now causing strains in our marriage . . ."

Regardless of the cause, two common denominators unite all women who suffer from vaginismus: restricted or impossible vaginal penetration and the associated emotional stress. The level and severity of each component may vary from one woman to another, which is the explanation behind the differences in presentation among sufferers.

Penetration difficulties may occur during any or all of the following five activities that encompass the basic penetrations a woman should be able to handle if she chooses:

1. Using a tampon
2. Inserting a finger (own finger or someone else's)
3. Inserting an applicator with medication
4. Undergoing a pelvic examination
5. Having intercourse

The following are typical examples of varied presentations:

- Able to have a pelvic examination and use tampons but unable to have intercourse
- Able to have a pelvic examination despite a great deal of pain and anxiety yet unable to insert a tampon or have intercourse
- Able to have partial intercourse (head of penis only) with severe pain and distress
- Unable to have penetration of any kind; any attempt met with severe panic
- Resistant to any touch in the area, including pubic hair and inner thighs

Additional common difficulties may pertain to the following areas (in any combination):

- Looking at own genitals
- Touching own genitals (including daily hygiene and wiping after urination)
- Masturbation
- Accepting manual or oral sex from partner
- Reaching orgasm

The associated emotional stress may range from minimal apprehension and nervousness to severe anxiety or a panic attack, including flashbacks in cases of abuse. Because of the walls of silence that surround vaginismus and due to the limited resources for treatment, the prime belief of every sufferer is "I am the only one who has it," a devastating feeling that compounds the already complex makeup of the condition. Additional emotional manifestations may include the following in any combination:

- Self-blame, shame, and guilt
- Accepting pain as inseparable part of life, yet fearing and avoiding it
- Depression
- Living in secrecy
- Frustration, desperation
- Anger at the medical field for diminishing the magnitude of the problem or for placing the blame on the woman

- Avoidance (e.g., of intimacy, of relationships)
- Breakdown of intimacy, relationships, marriages
- Physical shutdown
- Sexual dysfunction
- Dissociation

For those in a relationship, there is quite an impact on the partner, who may feel at fault for causing the condition, or not being good enough sexually; he or she will be afraid to cause more pain, and may be frustrated, hopeless, angry, impatient, disappointed, and incapable of performing sexually. Cultural expectations may further complicate the situation, from ending a marriage to raping the wife—all underlining her lack of control.

Management

Vaginismus affects a woman's life on many levels, bringing with it physical pains, sexual dysfunctions, disruption of relationships. and the self-perception of being "abnormal." Fortunately, proper management of this condition will bring a complete resolution, making the woman feel "normal" and worthy. To reach this goal, however, intervention must adhere to the following guidelines:

- There is a dire need to recognize the body-mind presentation of vaginismus, to eliminate the fragmentation of rendered services, and to fill the voids in education and in practice by providing a comprehensive treatment approach to this condition.

  The ideal setup, touching the body and the mind at the same time for optimal resolution, is that of a team approach, consisting of a hands-on specialist and a psychotherapist or sex therapist, both highly trained by leading expert teams in the management of vaginismus.
- The clinician who wishes to treat vaginismus should be suitable emotionally and possess in-depth knowledge of the body and its function, with emphasis on body–mind interaction. Educational training should include in-depth study of the physiology of the pelvic floor and its reactions as well as human sexuality and sexual health. Training must also explore the psychological impact of trauma and, in turn, the impact of such traumatic events on the pelvic floor. Treatment techniques, modalities, and supplies are also very important, as is management of the patient's emotions. Most important, training must include the clinician's self-exploration regarding physical closeness, touch, intimacy, emotional balance, and compassion to secure a sense of comfort and confidence for treating vaginismus.
- It is imperative that the treating team be of the same sex as the patient to ensure an understanding "from within" of what it feels like to be a woman, to feel penetration, to be "done to," and so on. (Naturally, this would be true in the reverse—a female clinician will never be able to relate "from within" to the sensations of erection, penetrating a female, erectile dysfunction, and so on.) Furthermore, the emotional anguish that typifies vaginismus does not allow a male clinician to enter the private zone of a female patient, thus limiting the quality of the rendered care. However, annual or emergency medical exams may be rendered by any clinician, depending on the patient's comfort level.
- Office setup requires careful planning: Patient scheduling should be based on one patient per session (approximately 45 to 60 minutes) with direct contact for the duration of the treatment. Initial interview, meeting with patient and partner, and any structured counseling should take place in a comfortable family-room-like setting, which will radiate warmth and a personal atmosphere to ease the patient's feelings about exposing her upsetting condition. The hands-on treatment needs to be rendered in a separate room that will provide visual and auditory privacy. Also, there should be an adjacent bathroom for the patient's use during and after treatment. Additionally, it is highly recommended that the décor be pleasant and not alarming and void of anatomical posters, which may add to the patient's stressed state. An adjustable treatment bed, preferably without stirrups, and fresh linens add to the comfort. Of utmost importance is confidentiality—the receptionist and staff must be trained to be respectful and discreet.
- When none of the five basic penetrations noted above is possible, neuromuscular education must be integrated into the management of vaginismus as the vaginal canal is truly virgin, void of any kinematic input and frames of reference. Even if the woman is able to handle some of the basic penetrations, she will still need to experience and learn the body-mind sensations and reactions associated with the rest of the penetrations. Just as the developing infant establishes brain mapping of her body parts by way of repetitious touch and repetitious activities, so is the vaginal canal in need of establishing familiarity with various touches in and around it, including different textures, volumes, and pressures, similar to what a woman would experience vaginally in the course of a healthy life.
- The clinician must understand the body–mind involuntary nature of the protective reaction of the pelvic floor musculature, as described earlier, and resist the tendency to treat these muscles as if they were contracting in a voluntary, controllable fashion. In other words, vaginismus is not responsive to traditional treatment modalities such as heat, stretching, exercises, biofeedback, electrical stimulation, massage, tissue manipulation, and postural training; these do not address the cause of the problem and at best offer some physical relief but will never come close to curing the problem. Similarly, psychological counseling will offer only limited progress because it does not include touching the body where vaginismus occurs, and a hymenectomy will touch only the body but not the mind, where stress regarding penetration is centralized. Vaginal dilators have been a common treatment modality, often given or mailed to the patient, at best with verbal instructions for use. Unfortunately, except for marginal cases, the mere sight of the dilators is enough to send the woman into further distress, unable or fearful to try using them. If penetration exercises were so simple, vaginismus would not be such a common, complicated condition.

- The ideal, proven treatment for vaginismus may be defined as a guided tour of the woman's genitals in general, then the vagina in particular, including repeated practice of the five basic penetrations: finger, tampon, applicator, intercourse (with penis-size spacer if the woman does not have an intimate partner), and pelvic exam. The guides are the clinicians who offer explanations, demonstrations, hands-on practice, and the necessary emotional intervention. For the woman who suffers from vaginismus, the need for guidance and reassurance is what precludes self-treatment in the privacy of her own home.

The following is a sequential outline of the recommended intervention, highlighting the fact that because women can have vaginal penetrations in neutrality, without any sexual arousal, the treatment process is not about sex but rather about the woman assuming ownership of her genitals and their function.

1. Interview the patient regarding the nature of her problem, including input from the involved partner, if available. Assessment should explore all systems: eating habits, obstetric history, nutrition, exercise habits, hygiene, personal history, living arrangements, and sexual history. This step may take 1 hour or several weeks, depending on the severity of the condition and the patient's emotional state.
2. Have the patient draw a portrait of her genitals. This self-portrait is an excellent introduction to patient education, and it will bring to the surface her feelings about her body and her tools of stress management.
3. Educate the patient regarding the structure of the pelvic cavity using a three-dimensional model with removable internal organs for ease of visualization and clear understanding. This explanation should include physiology of the urogenital and digestive systems, specifically menstruation, ovulation, conception, birth control methods, the location and function of the pelvic floor musculature, and mechanisms of voiding and defecation. This educational session, which should take about 1 hour, is essential and may be optimized by inviting her partner to listen to it at the same time.
4. Introduce touch by exploring the external genitalia while looking at a mirror placed between the legs. The patient should be reclined, undressed from the waist down, on the treatment table. The entire genitalia are to be explored by vision and touch (never sexually!) by both patient and clinician: pubic hair, labia majora and minora, vulva, clitoris, perineal body, and anus. No vaginal penetration is introduced at this time so that the woman can focus on becoming familiar with her own body. This phase gives the clinician an excellent opportunity to assess the patient's external genitalia for structural defects, infections, dermatological concerns, evidence of self-mutilation, and so forth. Additionally, this is an ideal time to discuss the patient's genital hygiene and skin care, especially the common irritation due to shaving, and to allow her to get used to the clinician's hands on her body. The patient is encouraged to repeat this exploratory experience with her partner to eliminate misunderstandings about her body, typical of many relationships, especially when both partners are virgins. Unfortunately, some patients are reluctant to move on to this "being touched" phase because they need more time to establish trust in the clinicians or they have body fears due to abusive or traumatic encounters (see the section Childhood Sexual Abuse). Since lack of control is a major feature of vaginismus, the clinician should ensure the patient's comfort by inviting her to express her wishes while encouraging her to move on as soon as she is willing to try. Emotional counseling and further education about the body usually resolves this hesitation in a few sessions.
5. Proceed to a guided tour of the vagina, gradually moving from digital penetration (finger size) to the size of an erect penis, all while ensuring that the patient develops mental mapping of the tactile and emotional input of her vagina. The use of a lubricant for penetration activities is imperative in order to avoid vaginal and urethral chafing, a common painful sensation that amplifies the devastation of vaginismus.
6. Teach use of tampon, beginning with demonstrating how tampons are constructed to alleviate the common worry of them falling apart inside the vagina or getting lost in the vaginal canal, then proceed to practice insertion (lubricating the tip) and removal while introducing the patient to different brands and shapes for best fit and management. Finally, discuss menstrual hygiene and answer questions the patient may have about her body's reactions during menstruation, fears of using tampons, sexual activities while bleeding, and so on.
7. The final treatment detail is introducing the patient to the speculum, the bimanual palpation, and the rectal exam. Once proficient, the patient is confidently ready to undergo timely gynecologic examinations as part of her wellness program.

The goal of intervention is to guide the patient to a healthy, satisfying life, including an enjoyable sexual intimacy. This is achieved through continual body–mind guidance, education, and so forth. Sexually, the patient and her partner understand that her body will perform once her mind is free to allow it to happen.

Summary

Despite its prevalence, vaginismus—the reactive closure of the vaginal canal—remains a shameful, hopeless, and underdiagnosed condition. Clinicians must become familiar with and recognize its symptoms. If they cannot perform a pelvic examination or if a patient expresses undue anxiety with penetrations, as long as structural or infectious concerns have been ruled out, clinicians should make referrals to vaginismus specialists. The treatment of vaginismus consists of body–mind management of penetration simulations combined with necessary patient and partner education. The average duration of treatment is 12 to 18 hours. It is imperative that treatment not be viewed as physical "stretching" of a tight vaginal canal or a stiff pelvic floor musculature, but rather as internalizing the kinematic awareness of the five basic penetrations, and learning to view them as healthy, positive sensations that are anatomically safe and available.

VULVODYNIA

Definition

Vulvar symptoms can be puzzling and require differential diagnosis before the proper intervention can be offered. The following are the three generally recognized types of vulvodynia.[3]

1. Infectious vulvodynia includes Candida, cyclic vulvitis, chronic vaginitis, herpes simplex virus, herpes zoster, and so on. Intervention is by way of conventional medicine and pharmacology.
2. Vulvar dermatoses (formerly dystrophies) includes lichen sclerosus, lichen planus, lichen simplex chronicus, erosive vaginitis, and steroid rebound dermatitis. Intervention is well defined in the literature.
3. Dyesthetic (idiopathic) vulvodynia—the subject of this chapter—is a misunderstood disorder that benefits from body–mind intervention.

Symptoms

Dysethetic (idiopathic) vulvodynia presents a challenge to clinician and patient alike as each seeks definite explanations and clear resolutions. The patient commonly presents with any combination of the following complaints: burning, throbbing, itching, poking sensation as if a needle is stuck in her genitals, diffused vulvar pain, urinary urgency and frequency, dyspareunia, and vaginismus. Some claim that this area feels red and hot, yet visual inspection fails to identify such findings.

To complicate the situation, many patients present with psychophysical associations involving other systems that are responsive to stress, such as irritable bowel syndrome, headaches, interstitial cystitis, asthma, allergies, fibromyalgia, chronic fatigue syndrome, sleep disorders, eating disorders, and muscle pains.

Although the clinician shows interest in helping, the lack of answers often amplifies the patient's sense of helplessness and suffering, sending her into an emotional spin that includes depression, anger at the medical field, withdrawal from life's activities, and difficulties in sustaining intimate relationships. Her partner, family, and friends may soon exhaust their own emotional resources, becoming impatient, resentful, hopeless, angry, and withdrawn. Because of the condition's intimate mind–body aspect, such emotional upheaval can propel her vulvodynia into further complexity.

Etiology and Management

Idiopathic vulvodynia calls for a thorough investigation of the patient's daily habits and lifestyle to unearth the causes of her symptoms. Unfortunately, such a detailed assessment is beyond the scope of practitioners whose time with the patient is limited, in which case a referral should be made to clinicians who have the time and expertise to embark on this rather lengthy and challenging personal journey with the patient.

The following is a summary of the common causes of this vulvodynia and suggested management:

- Vulvar dryness, is caused by one or several factors, such as hormonal changes, insufficient hydration, certain prescription drugs, use of antibiotics, chemotherapy, chlorine from swimming pools, and excessive hygiene practice. Ongoing physical contact with the dry, brittle vulva causes friction and irritation, bringing about typical symptoms. When possible, hormonal and pharmacologic applications need to be modified to minimize dryness, and probiotics intake should be a standard to oppose the destructive effect of antibiotics on the ecosystem of the vulva and vagina. Patients are to be advised to drink enough fluids to support healthy skin and organ functions, and principles of healthy hygiene should be included in patient education. When vulvar dryness is inevitable, vaginal lubricants or moisturizers must be introduced in the hope of averting further damage.
- Alteration of the vulva's ecosystem away from the ideal balance among its organisms allows irritation and breakdowns. This is typically caused by frequent use of antibiotics, a diet rich in sugar and carbohydrates, vaginal estrogen preparations in excess of personal tolerance, prolonged exposure of the vulva to a moist warm environment such as wearing a wet bathing suit for many hours on a hot day, poor hydration, and infrequent change of bloody sanitary pads during menstruation. The focus of management is twofold: restoring the vulvar flora to its healthy balance and preventing future breakdowns. Probiotics and dietary modifications are the answer to the former, and patient education, behavior modifications, and life style changes to the latter.
- Excessive vulvar friction or irritation is a result of mechanical action such as rough hygiene (deep rubbing, etc.), use of abrasive agents, ill-fitting sanitary pads, very tight clothing, unwanted intercourse, manual sex despite lack of lubrication, unprotected cycling, and so on. Patient education, habit modification, sex education, and penetration practice are the recommended approaches, as is emotional counseling, which is aimed at unearthing and resolving any underlying psychologic conflicts.
- Poor vulvar hygiene, including reluctance to wipe after voiding, and limited or nonexisting bathing predisposes the vulva to irritation and breakdowns. The first step in managing this problem is getting to the root of it—not an easy task due to the private, secretive nature of the problem. The ideal clinician feels no inhibitions in exploring such an intimate subject while making the patient feel respected and protected.

- Hormonal influence, especially the glycogen-effect of topical vaginal estrogen, brings about irritation, stinging, and chafing in women who are more sensitive to it and in those with a compromised vaginal echo system. Hormonal adjustments and opposition with probiotics will usually remedy this situation.
- Substance sensitivity or allergies may be the hardest to explore because of the intricacy and the potential for masked interaction between substances. The clinician must patiently and methodically examine all facets of the patient's life, such as what she ingests, what she uses for hygiene, what substances she comes in contact with, including airborne particles; the offensive substance will cause systemic rejection commonly expressed in the urinary system and in its proximal environment, the vulva. This exploratory journey may take several weeks or even months to reach conclusions that may not be otherwise obvious, and may be helped by establishing a baseline, then gradually altering the presence of substances while watching for reactive interactions.
- Emotional stress regarding her own body and its functions, poor body image and low self-esteem, negative sexual experiences, fear of penetration, and negative body memories are all valid causes of vulvodynia. Furthermore, quite a few women use vulvodynia as a coping tool for attention, for avoiding intimacy, for expressing fears of illness, or for punishing the partner, often resulting in vaginismus with its psychophysical manifestations. Emotional counseling and hands-on treatments rendered as a team approach is the ideal management, touching the body and the mind at the same time for optimal effect.

Summary

Vulvar health is the key to the management of this multisystem condition, and clinician's proficiency is imperative. Although dysesthetic (idiopathic) vulvodynia may present as a puzzling condition, careful assessment by a knowledgeable clinician usually arrives at answers and resolutions, a superior approach to prescribing antidepressants that do not address the actual causes of the problem.

CHILDHOOD SEXUAL ABUSE

Childhood sexual abuse—invading a child's personal space or body for the sexual stimulation and gratification—is the most comprehensive of traumas yet the one so often missed by clinicians. It involves a youngster who is not yet aware of her bodily functions as they relate to sexuality, nor is she capable of perceiving the size of the abuser's genitals in realistic proportions. As a result, even as a grown woman, she is incapable of understanding sexual feelings beyond their concrete physical sensations because she has traveled only so far along the maturation process by the time the abuse began, halting her healthy development. Consequently, this trauma engenders a mix of persistent feelings, mainly negative, regarding sexual activity and feeling, such as secretiveness, shame, being bad, being punished, misinterpretation of love, and so forth.

The abused child is forced to embark on a lone struggle trying to understand her body's emotional reactions to the abuser, while endlessly drowning in unanswered questions about her responsibility for bringing about the abuse, the lack of protection, the existence of God, being "damaged," the motives of the abuser, her body's response, the intrusion on her private space, and being touched without permission.

Except when the perpetrator is violent, as is often the case when the abuse occurred once or twice only, the experienced pleasurable sexual stimulation creates a conflict in the child who is now drawn to this irresistible feeling and unable to stop her body from responding in favor of it. It is common for victims of long-term or repeated childhood abuse who were taken to orgasm by their abusers to want to feel that "nice" sensation again and again. Consequently, even the instilled fear imposed by the abuser does not keep the child from going back to the abuser, being trapped within her own confusing existence. Unfortunately, this sensation of "nice" is hidden so deeply by the child that traditional intervention cannot gain access to it, thus missing a fundamental component of the child's troubled being. However, a mind—body intervention allows access to this hidden component because it brings the true feelings and memories to the surface by virtue of touching the body and the mind at the same time, preventing the patient from escaping her physical sensations and emotional feelings.

Effect

Sexual abuse is an assault to the body and the mind whether it happens once or is an ongoing event in the child's life, and whether it is perpetrated by one or more people. Sexual abuse invades the skin, the largest organ in the body with its elaborate tactile network; it overwhelms the immature mind that must attempt to make sense of what is happening and of rights and wrongs; and it shatters the emotional being by imposing fear, intrusion, lack of safety, and helplessness. The perpetrator(s) in ongoing abuse relate to the child as a sexual partner, taking her through complete sexual acts (e.g., intercourse, manual sex, oral sex, anal sex), in various sexual positions, using sex toys, and so on. Consequently, to cope with her fear, guilt, shame, and confusion about her body's reactions, she will escape into the only component that she can manipulate—her mind. She blocks the bodily experiences, be they painful or pleasurable, turns her life into a journey of self-hurt, self-mutilation, body shutdown, and dissociation.

Symptoms

The devastating outcomes of childhood sexual abuse affect the child/woman on all levels of life, making it impossible for her either to escape or to hide from them. Clinicians must be attuned to the presentation of the patient and to modify their approach when sexual abuse is suspected or disclosed.

The following areas of great destruction can present in any combination and various levels of severity:

- Emotional outcomes include low self-esteem, immense sense of shame and guilt, feelings of helplessness and powerlessness, inability to trust, emotional shutdown and numbness, a sense of short life expectancy, and post traumatic stress disorder with its complicated symptomology including intense fear or horror, nightmares, flashbacks, inability to recall events, and increased arousal.
- Behavioral outcomes include living in a constant state of "racing" due to hyperexcitability of the sympathetic nervous system, getting involved in negative situations due to an inability to say no, inability to understand or to protect own space, self-defeating and self-destructive behaviors, dissociating, feeling victimized, making poor choices of mate/friends/jobs, holding on to negative situations or people in fear of rejection and pain, and operating in a fragmented disorganized fashion with poor focusing that worsens with increased stress.
- Spiritual outcomes usually manifest themselves as anger at God for abandoning her without protection and as an inert belief that life is bad and dangerous. Consequently, her life view becomes concrete and her feelings become fixed or stunted. She looks for a negative cause for any unfortunate occurrence, and there is no hope in sight. This may be the patient who radiates animosity or adversity and is rather combative and frightened.
- The physiologic outcomes range from the obvious to the hidden, from the simple to the complex, and highlight the need for a clinician who is not quick to draw conclusions or prescribe medications before exploring psychophysical causes for presenting symptomology such as:
  - Physical numbness and sensory detachment such as not responding to pinprick tests, alterations of body or skin temperature
  - Tactile hypersensitivity to the point of being unable to tolerate touch
  - Ongoing sympathetic nervous system activation; agitation, nervousness, anger, panic or anxiety attacks
  - Headaches
  - Gastrointestinal disorders
  - Eating disorders
  - Elimination disorders
  - Sleep disorders
  - Dermatologic concerns, including injuries by self-mutilation
  - Sudden, unexplained echymosis
  - Depression
  - Musculoskeletal dysfunctions
  - Pain anywhere or everywhere
  - Pelvic floor disorders: vaginismus, vulvodynia, sexual dysfunctions, dyspareunia, pelvic/perineal pain, vaginal dryness, chronic urinary tract infection–like symptoms, incontinence, levator ani syndrome, infertility
- Sexual outcomes illustrate the far-reaching impact of childhood sexual abuse, which robs the woman of the ability to experience herself as a healthy sexual being. Sexuality is a life-long process of maturation, experience, and established preferences; it develops as an integral part of intimacy, of body and mind, not just sex. Sexual intimacy is the ultimate of self-expression and self-assurance; it combines vulnerability with confidence, trust with trying the unknown, feeling and sharing feelings, and experiencing the utmost of body awareness while giving up control. These experiences are not available to the woman who was sexually abused in childhood because her body and mind have been fighting to make sense of what happened while sorting out the confusing sexual feelings associated with the abuse. For her, what happened was not sexual but rather "body games," playing with bodies in different ways, just like with toys. This is the only way children may understand sex abuse because they lack the emotional understanding of an adult regarding sexuality, feeling sexy, giving pleasure, and so forth. For her, sexual activities are dangerous and confusing, and she'll cope with them by bringing about psychophysical ailments, pelvic floor dysfunctions, and promiscuity. Confusion involves questions such as, is sexuality a tool for showing love or being loved? At what price? Should I allow myself to feel the nice? Am I bad for wanting it?

Clinical Manifestation

A clinician attuned to the presentation of sexual abuse and to the patient's body language can identify classic signs of sexual abuse, although not all patients present with all of them, or at least not overtly:

- Vocabulary, or description of the problem, that includes child's lexicon such as "fix me" and "I'm broken," referring to the genitals as "that part" or "down there," alluding to men as "bad, mean, dangerous," and voice intonation resembling a young child speaking
- Presentation and behavior that appear unfocused, a disorganized description of medical and personal history, and poor time perception (late for appointments, forgetting appointments, unsure of time sequences, etc.). Observing her personal belongings, one may notice (if allowed to look) excessive luggage, which may contain all sorts of medications or remedies, extra clothing, objects she may use for self-mutilation, and more. Overall behavior reveals either agitation or resignation, commonly accompanied by body picking and frequent trips to the bathroom to stimulate or hurt herself or because of her conditioned incontinence.
- Body memories, the psychophysical imprints of trauma, are another paramount feature of any traumatic event, and childhood sexual abuse in particular. Each

traumatic episode establishes neurologic pathways for recording it, while lowering the threshold for activation of the fight-or-flight reaction. Left to her immature understanding of the abuse, the child tries to run away from the confusing bodily sensations; unfortunately, the body remembers without alterations and she cannot truly escape her body memories. The only solution she sees is to ask her mind to edit, filter, and choose what to consciously remember, enlisting dissociation as the cover-up and the escape mechanism, never really erasing the memories but leaving them accessible through the basic senses of touch, smell, vision, taste, and hearing.

- Flashbacks, or reliving experiences, are powerful, frightening, and uncontrolled phenomena caused by an environmental reminder of the abuse or by an inner provocation (e.g., a thought, a fear, or a body memory). Although flashbacks are time-limited events, they are devastating to the woman who experiences them and to the clinician who may have brought them on by virtue of a touch, a conversation, office décor, body scent, and so on. The unpredictability of flashbacks and the physical changes they bring about are often the reason that clinicians are reluctant to treat abused women, which can make the women feel even more "dirty, bad, crazy."

Treatment Considerations

Familiarity with child development is essential for management because sexual abuse arrests the process, leaving the child "stuck" at the maturation level that corresponds to her age when the abuse began. Healing calls for revisiting the earliest affected developmental milestone and offering age-appropriate trust and explanations before moving onto the next milestone, then the next.

Management is based on a body–mind intervention with both the hands-on clinician and the psychotherapist present during all treatments to avoid fragmentation of services in this complex process and to allow the patient to benefit from their combined resources.

Keeping in mind the maturation process of the child who may now be in the body of an adult, the following steps are recommended, in the order most suitable for each patient:

- Patient interview: Watch and listen carefully without offering ideas as to what happened; tune in to body language, physical expressions, tempo of speech, emotional display, and eye contact; skillfully stir the conversation by exploring topics the patient seems to avoid; explore all body systems for breakdowns; explore eating habits, obstetric history, nutrition, exercise habits, and hygiene; discuss personal history; identify living arrangements; explore sexual history; and perform emotional assessment. Remember the concept of layers: what you hear at first will not be the same once layers of protection begin to peel off. Last, during any step of the process, offer comfort and reassurance and ask for permission to touch.
- Dissociation, if present, does not allow the patient and clinician to "connect" and must therefore be addressed as early as possible. Once the clinician identifies the mode of dissociation that is unique to that patient, the clinician should explain it to her while reassuring her of its protective nature instead of making her feel "crazy" because of it. As soon as the patient is able to realize when she dissociates and loses time, measures should be taken to practice focusing while resolving the need to "run away" into dissociation.
- Intervention must also close the gaps and resolve perceptual fallacies that developed due to the abrupt cessation of the maturation process. One method is to teach anatomy, physiology, and sexology as it pertains to the body while distinguishing true facts (reality) from her traumatic perceptions and visualizations that are the result of her lone struggle to understand what was done to her. This teaching needs to be theoretical and physical, taking her through exploring her own body and letting her feel it in a safe, guided way. Her psychophysical complaints should be addressed through this process as well, differentiating true pathologies from emotion-based reactions in the body.
- Neuromuscular desensitization and touch reeducation, important components of repairing the alterations caused by the abuse, is done by introducing the patient to her body through tactile exercises with emphasis on eventually feeling the touch without dissociating or being fearful. Just as the developing infant experiences each new touch thousands of time before it is integrated, so will the sexually abused need to practice to acclimate herself to healthy touch. But her process is more complex because she also needs to undo body memories before she can embark on reclaiming the safety of the many kinds of touch by her own hand and by others.
- Teaching self-care and toileting may be difficult because she will often reject help to her body that betrayed her by wanting the "nice," or because she may be afraid of the stimulation and body memories that the clinician's touch may stir up in her charged, confused body. Before proceeding, the clinician needs to gain her trust and acknowledge her fears and worries about being touched and reassure her that it is safe to feel and to express her feelings and her thoughts.
- Pelvic floor rehabilitation is necessary to normalize its sensations and functions. This usually includes all the components mentioned earlier about vaginismus management, yet with adjustments appropriate to the patient's sexual experience, which is associated with fear and body memories. This aspect of the treatment process is the one most likely to bring about flashbacks and crises, which emphasizes the need for the presence of a specialized team trained to treat the body and the mind, regardless of how devastating the presentation may be. When treating flashbacks, the clinician must realize that the patient is removed from reality, not aware of her present surroundings or the people around her; she is re-experiencing a trau-

matic event to its fullest including feeling and acting the age she was at the time of the actual event. Clinically, this is an opportunity for the skilled clinician to "join" the patient in her flashback in order to get a closer view of the events that took place and to guide her through them by offering explanations of what she feels and sees but without altering the facts of the abusive event. Doing this would be the ultimate journey to resolution, merging the past and the present through bodily experiences and emotional guidance.

- Wound care is imperative when self-mutilation is present. The clinician needs to keep an observing eye on the patient's body and attempt a visual screening in full every so often. Self-mutilation is a secretive coping tool that may cause tremendous disfiguration and medical symptomology, especially when it involves the genitals. Ideal intervention identifies and confronts the pattern and methods of self-mutilation and assists the patient in ridding herself of this negative tool as she learns to cope with life in a constructive, healthy way.
- Restoring spiritually refers to the process of internalizing trust and safety, outgrowing destructive coping tools, being able to reach to the abstract instead of being stuck in the concrete life similar to that of a child, and finding the good even in bad situations. This is the culmination of closing all the gaps in her maturation process while diffusing the victimization and the "betrayal by God," thus allowing her to develop a healthy spiritual self.
- Develop the patient's sexuality by freeing her of body memories, of confusions, and of inhibitions that stem from the abuse. Provide her with sex education, teach her principles of sexual health and guide her, body and mind, as she experiences relationships and her own emerging sexuality, all the way to feeling confident and secure.

Summary

The management of childhood sexual abuse is a long and intricate process that may take years to complete. Adult women who were victims may present with various pelvic floor disorders; however, the effects of sexual abuse are never only physical. Clinicians must be aware of the emotional contributors to such conditions. Optimal treatment addresses the woman as a physical and emotional whole, and is best rendered by a specialized team that addresses the inseparable body–mind complexity of this unfortunate trauma.

CONCLUSION

Vaginismus, vulvodynia, and childhood sexual abuse are powerful forces with destructive impact on a woman's quality of life. Inasmuch as they are different, they are unified by their body–mind manifestations. Since women have been known to suffer in silence, especially when faced with such shameful, devastating problems, it is up to the treating clinician to guide them toward disclosure, treatment, and a cure in a reassuring, trustworthy manner. Being instrumental in helping the woman reclaim her body and her life should be the most rewarding aspect of patient care.

REFERENCES

1. Katz D, Tabisel RL: Private Pain. New York, Women's Therapy Center, 2002, p 57.
2. Dixon J, Goling J: Histomorphology of pelvic floor muscle. In Schussler B, Laycock J, Norton P, Stanton S (eds): Pelvic Floor Re-education. London, Springer-Verlag, 1994, pp 30–31.
3. Roger RM Jr: Basic pelvic neuroanatomy. In Steege JF, Metzger DA, Levy BS (eds): Chronic Pelvic Pain. Philadelphia, WB Saunders, 1998, pp 31–68.

PART V

Pharmacology and Surgical Techniques

CHAPTER 39

Pharmacologic Treatment of Urinary Incontinence

KARL-ERIK ANDERSSON ■ CHRISTOPHER R. CHAPPLE ■ ALAN J. WEIN

Theoretically, disturbed filling or storage function can be improved by agents that decrease detrusor activity, increase bladder capacity, or increase outlet resistance.[1]

Many drugs have been tried, but the results are often disappointing, partly because of poor treatment efficacy or side effects. The development of pharmacologic treatments for the different forms of urinary incontinence has been slow, and the use of some currently prescribed agents is based more on tradition than on evidence from controlled clinical trials.[1]

This chapter describes the pharmacotherapeutic options for the management of disorders of bladder filling or storage based on the deliberations of the International Consensus meeting. Agents that are specifically used to treat urinary tract infections and interstitial cystitis have not been included. Drugs have been evaluated using different types of evidence based on evaluations made with a modification of the Oxford system, which emphasizes the quality of the trials assessed. (Tables 39-1 and 39-2). Evidence of pharmacologic or physiologic efficacy means that a drug had the desired effects in relevant preclinical experiments, in healthy volunteers, or in experimental situations in patients.

CENTRAL NERVOUS CONTROL

The normal micturition reflex in adults is mediated by the spinobulbospinal pathway that passes through relay centers in the brain. Studies in humans and animals show areas in the brain stem and diencephalon that are specifically implicated in micturition control, namely, Barrington's nucleus and the pontine micturition center in the dorsomedial pontine tegmentum, which directly excites bladder motor neurons and indirectly inhibits urethral sphincter motor neurons through inhibitory interneurons in the medial sacral cord; the periaqueductal gray, which receives bladder filling information; and the preoptic area of the hypothalamus, which is probably involved in the initiation of micturition. Positron emission tomography scans in humans show that these supraspinal regions are active during micturition.[2]

PERIPHERAL NERVOUS CONTROL

Bladder emptying and urine storage involve a complex pattern of efferent and afferent signaling in the parasympathetic, sympathetic, and somatic nerves (Figs. 39-1 and 39-2). These nerves are part of the reflex pathways that either maintain the bladder in a relaxed state, enabling urine storage at low intravesical pressure, or initiate micturition by relaxing the outflow region and contracting the bladder smooth muscle. Contraction of the detrusor smooth muscle and relaxation of the outflow region are caused by activation of parasympathetic neurons located in the sacral parasympathetic nucleus in the spinal cord at the level of S2–S4.[3] Postganglionic neurons in the pelvic nerve mediate excitatory input to human detrusor smooth muscle by releasing acetylcholine, which acts on muscarinic receptors. However, an atropine-resistant component has been shown, particularly in functionally and morphologically altered human bladder tissue. The pelvic nerve also conveys parasympathetic fibers to the outflow region and urethra. These fibers exert an inhibitory effect and thereby relax the outflow region. This effect is mediated partly by the release of nitric oxide,[4] although other transmitters may be involved.[5]

Most sympathetic innervation of the bladder and urethra originates from the intermediolateral nuclei in the thoracolumbar region (T10–L2) of the spinal cord. The axons either travel through the inferior mesenteric ganglia and the hypogastric nerve or pass through the paravertebral chain and enter the pelvic nerve. Thus, sympathetic signals are conveyed in both the hypogastric and pelvic nerves.[6] The predominant effects of sympathetic innervation of the lower urinary tract in humans are inhibition of the parasympathetic pathways at the spinal and ganglion levels and mediation of contraction of the bladder base and

TABLE 39-1 ■ Types of Evidence

Pharmacodynamic
    In vitro
    In vivo
Pharmacokinetic
    Absorption
    Distribution
    Metabolism
    Excretion
Physiologic
    Animal models
    Clinical phase I trials
Clinical
    Oxford guidelines

urethra. However, in several animals, adrenergic innervation of the bladder body is believed to inactivate the contractile mechanisms in the detrusor directly.[4] Noradrenaline is released in response to electrical stimulation of detrusor tissues in vitro, and relaxation is the normal response of detrusor tissues to released noradrenaline.[4]

Most sensory innervation of the bladder and urethra reaches the spinal cord through the pelvic nerve and dorsal root ganglia. In addition, some afferents travel in the hypogastric nerve. The sensory nerves of the striated muscle in the rhabdosphincter travel in the pudendal nerve to the sacral region of the spinal cord.[6] The most important afferents for the micturition process are myelinated A delta fibers and unmyelinated C-fibers that travel in the pelvic nerve to the sacral spinal cord, conveying information from receptors in the bladder wall to the spinal cord. The A delta fibers respond to passive distension and active contraction, conveying information about bladder filling.[7] C-fibers have a high mechanical threshold and respond primarily to either chemical irritation of the bladder mucosa[8] or cold.[9] After chemical irritation, the C-fiber afferents exhibit spontaneous firing when the bladder is empty and exhibit increased firing during bladder distension.[8] Because these fibers are normally inactive, they are known as silent fibers.

TABLE 39-2 ■ International Consultation on Incontinence Assessments: Oxford Guidelines (modified)

Level of evidence
1   Randomized, controlled clinical trials
2   Good-quality prospective studies
3   Retrospective case–control studies
4   Case series
5   Expert opinion

Grade of recommendation
A   Based on level 1 evidence (highly recommended)
B   Consistent level 2 or 3 evidence (recommended)
C   Level 4 studies or "majority evidence" (recommended with reservation)
D   Evidence inconsistent or inconclusive (not recommended)

From Anderson KE, Appell R, Awad S, et al: Pharmacological treatment of urinary incontinence. In Abrams P, Khoury S, Wein A (eds): Incontinence, First Consultation on Incontinence. Plymouth, UK, Plymouth Distributors LTD, 2000, pp 479–512.

FIGURE 39-1 During filling, there is continuous and increasing afferent activity from the bladder. There is no spinal parasympathetic outflow that can contract the bladder. Sympathetic outflow to urethral smooth muscle and somatic outflow to urethral and pelvic floor striated muscles keep the outflow region closed. Whether sympathetic innervation to the bladder (not indicated) contributes to bladder relaxation during filling in humans has not been established. PAG, periaqueductal gray.

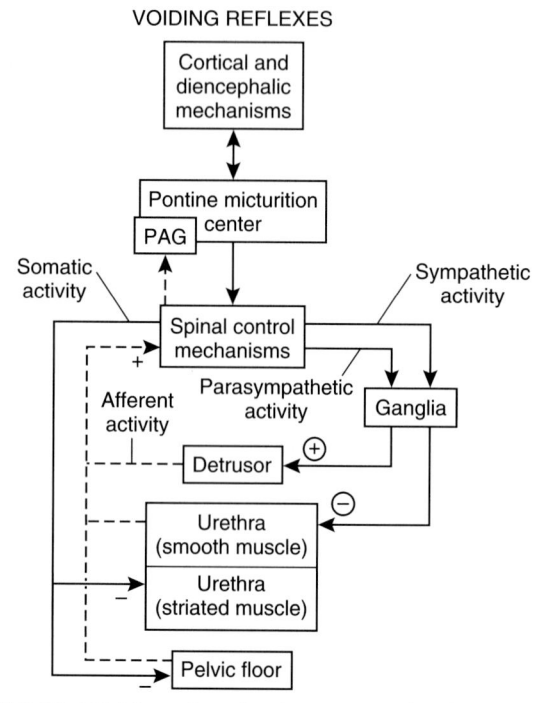

FIGURE 39-2 Voiding reflexes involve supraspinal pathways, and are under voluntary control. During bladder emptying, spinal parasympathetic outflow is activated, leading to bladder contraction. Simultaneously, sympathetic outflow to urethral smooth muscle and somatic outflow to urethral and pelvic floor striated muscles are turned off, and the outflow region relaxes. PAG, periaqueductal gray.

PATHOGENESIS OF BLADDER CONTROL DISORDERS

Bladder control disorders can be divided into two general categories: disorders of filling or storage and disorders of voiding.[1] Storage problems can occur as a result of weakness or anatomic defects in the urethral outlet, causing stress urinary incontinence, which may account for one third of cases. Failure to store also occurs if the bladder is unstable or overactive, and this may affect more than 50% of incontinent men and 10% to 15% of incontinent young women. Overactive bladder can occur as a result of sensitization of afferent nerve terminals in the bladder or outlet region, changes of the bladder smooth muscle as a result of denervation, or damage to central nervous system (CNS) inhibitory pathways, as seen in various neurologic disorders, such as multiple sclerosis, cerebrovascular disease, Parkinson's disease, brain tumors, and spinal cord injury. Overactive bladder may also occur in elderly patients as a result of aging-related changes in the brain or bladder. Urinary retention and overflow incontinence may occur in patients with urethral outlet obstruction (e.g., prostate enlargement), neural injury, or diseases that damage nerves (e.g., diabetes mellitus) as well as in those who take drugs that depress neural control of the bladder.[1]

BLADDER CONTRACTION

Normal bladder contraction in humans is mediated mainly through stimulation of muscarinic receptors in the detrusor muscle. Atropine resistance (i.e., contraction of the isolated bladder muscle in response to electrical nerve stimulation after pretreatment with atropine) is seen in most animal species, but seems to be of little importance in normal human bladder muscle.[4] However, atropine-resistant (nonadrenergic, noncholinergic) contractions have been reported in normal human detrusor muscle, and may be caused by adenosine triphosphate (ATP).[10] $P2X_3$ receptors, which have been identified in small-diameter afferent neurons in dorsal root ganglia, have also been detected immunohistochemically in the wall of the bladder and ureter in a suburothelial plexus of afferent nerves. In $P2X_3$ knockout mice, afferent activity induced by bladder distension was significantly reduced.[11] These data show that purinergic receptors are involved in mechanosensory signaling in the bladder in these animals.

A significant degree of atropine resistance may exist in the morphologically or functionally changed bladder, the hypertrophic bladder,[12] interstitial cystitis,[13] the neurogenic bladder,[14] and the aging bladder.[15] The importance of the nonadrenergic, noncholinergic component to detrusor contraction, in vivo, normally, and in different micturition disorders, remains to be established.

Muscarinic Receptors

Molecular cloning studies show five distinct genes for muscarinic receptors in rats and humans, and it is now generally accepted that five receptor subtypes correspond to these gene products.[16] Muscarinic receptors are coupled to G-proteins (Fig. 39-3). The signal transduction systems involved vary, but M_1, M_3, and M_5 preferentially couple to phosphoinositide hydrolysis, leading to mobilization of intracellular calcium. In contrast, activation of muscarinic M_2 and M_4 receptors inhibits adenylyl cyclase activity. Muscarinic receptor stimulation may also inhibit K_{ATP} channels in smooth muscle cells from the urinary bladder through activation of protein kinase C.[17]

Bladder Muscarinic Receptors

Detrusor smooth muscle from various species contains muscarinic receptors of the M_2 and M_3 subtypes.[18] In the human bladder, the occurrence of messenger ribonucleic acid (mRNA) encoding M_2 and M_3 subtypes has been shown, whereas no mRNA encoding M_1 receptors was found.[19] The M_3 receptors in the human bladder are believed to cause direct smooth muscle contraction through phosphoinositide hydrolysis,[20] whereas the role of M_2 receptors is not clear. However, through beta-adrenoceptors, M_2 receptors may oppose sympathetically mediated smooth muscle relaxation, because in rats, activation of M_2 receptors inhibits adenylyl cyclase.[21]

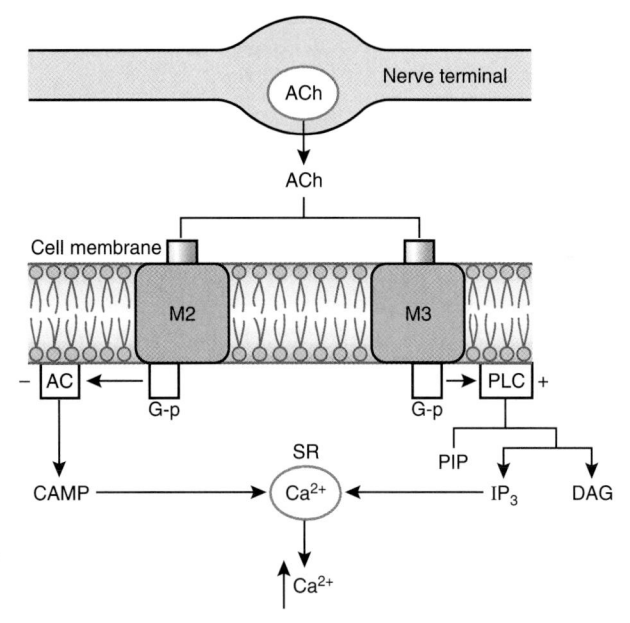

FIGURE 39-3 Acetylcholine (ACh) is released from cholinergic nerve terminals, and acts on muscarinic receptors (M_2 and M_3) in the detrusor. Both M_2 and M_3 receptors are coupled to G-proteins (G-p) and may contribute to bladder contraction, but different signal transduction pathways are involved. M_2 receptors inhibit adenylyl cyclase (AC), decreasing the intracellular level of cyclic adenosine monophosphate (cAMP), which mediates bladder relaxation. Stimulation of M_3 receptors activates phospholipase C (PLC) to generate inositol triphosphate (IP_3). IP_3 can release calcium ions (Ca^{2+}) from the sarcoplasmic reticulum (SR), activating the contractile machinery within the cell and causing bladder contraction. The voiding contraction is believed to be mediated mainly through M_3 receptors. DAG, diacylglycerol; PIP, phosphatidyl inositol phosphate.

Contractile mechanisms involving M_2 muscarinic receptors, such as activation of a nonspecific cationic channel and inactivation of potassium channels, may operate in the bladder.[18] However, there is general agreement that M_3 receptors are mainly responsible for the normal contraction that occurs with micturition.[18] Even in the obstructed rat bladder, M_3 receptors play a predominant role in mediating detrusor contraction.[22] On the other hand, in certain disease states, M_2 receptors may contribute to contraction of the bladder. Thus, in the denervated rat bladder, M_2 receptors, or a combination of M_2 and M_3 receptors, mediate contractile responses.[23] Also, in patients with neurogenic bladder dysfunction, detrusor contraction can be mediated by M_2 receptors.[24] Muscarinic receptors may also be located on the presynaptic nerve terminals and participate in the regulation of transmitter release. Inhibitory prejunctional muscarinic receptors have been classified as the muscarinic M_2 subtype in the rabbit[25] and rat[26] and as the M_4 subtype in the guinea pig urinary bladder.[27] Prejunctional facilitatory muscarinic receptors appear to be of the M_1 subtype in the rat and rabbit urinary bladder.[25,26] Prejunctional muscarinic facilitation has also been detected in the human bladder.[28] The muscarinic facilitatory mechanism seems to be upregulated in hyperactive bladders in rats with chronic spinal cord transection. The facilitation in these preparations is primarily mediated by M_3 muscarinic receptors.[28]

Muscarinic receptor function may be altered in different urologic disorders (e.g., outflow obstruction, neurogenic bladder, bladder overactivity without an overt neurogenic cause, diabetes). However, it is not always clear how these changes affect detrusor function.

DRUGS USED TO TREAT BLADDER OVERACTIVITY

It has been estimated that more than 50 million people in the developed world are affected by urinary incontinence. Even though it affects 30% to 60% of patients older than 65 years of age, it is not a disease exclusive to aging. Detrusor overactivity may be caused by several mechanisms, both myogenic[29] and neurologic.[30] Both factors probably contribute to the development of the disease.

Many drugs have been used to treat detrusor hyperactivity (Table 39-3). However, for many, clinical use is based on the results of preliminary, open studies rather than randomized, controlled clinical trials. In many trials on both detrusor instability and detrusor hyperreflexia, there has been such a high placebo response that meaningful differences between placebo and active drug cannot be shown. However, drug effects in individual patients may be both distinct and useful. Drugs may be efficacious in some patients, but they have side effects, and often are not continued indefinitely. Hence, it would be worth considering drugs as an adjunct to conservative therapy. The role of pharmacotherapy is even more contentious in older patients, particularly frail older people.

TABLE 39-3 ■ Drugs Used to Treat Detrusor Overactivity*

Drug	Level of Evidence	Grade of Recommendation
Antimuscarinic drugs		
Tolterodine	1	A
Trospium	1	A
Propantheline	2	B
Atropine, hyoscyamine	2	D
Darifenacin, solifenacin	Under investigation	
Drugs that act on membrane channels		
Calcium antagonists	Under investigation	
Potassium channel openers	Under investigation	
Drugs with mixed actions		
Oxybutynin	1	A
Propiverine	1	A
Dicyclomine	4	C
Flavoxate	4	D
Alpha-adrenoceptor antagonists		
Alfuzosin	4	D
Doxazosin	4	D
Prazosin	4	D
Terazosin	4	D
Tamsulosin	4	D
Beta-adrenoceptor agonists		
Terbutaline	4	D
Clenbuterol	4	D
Salbutamol	4	D
Antidepressants		
Imipramine	2	C†
Prostaglandin synthesis inhibitors		
Indomethacin	4	C
Flurbiprofen	4	C
Vasopressin analogues		
Desmopressin	1	A
Other drugs		
Baclofen	2‡	C‡
Capsaicin	3	C
Resiniferatoxin	Under investigation	

*Assessments according to the Oxford system (modified).
†Use with caution.
‡For intrathecal use.

Antimuscarinic (Anticholinergic) Drugs

Voluntary and involuntary bladder contractions are mediated mainly by acetylcholine-induced stimulation of muscarinic receptors on bladder smooth muscle. Antimuscarinic drugs depress both types of contraction, regardless of how the efferent part of the micturition reflex is activated. In patients with involuntary bladder contractions, the volume needed to induce the first contraction is increased, the amplitude of the contraction is decreased, and total bladder capacity is increased.

Several studies support the idea that antimuscarinics can depress involuntary bladder contractions.[32] On the other hand, several reports show insufficient efficacy of oral antimuscarinics in patients with unstable detrusor contractions.[33,34] It is unclear to what extent this finding can be attributed to low bioavailability of the drugs used, dose-limiting side effects, or atropine resistance.

Atropine and related antimuscarinics are tertiary amines that are well absorbed from the gastrointestinal tract and pass into the CNS. Therefore, CNS side effects may limit their use. Quaternary ammonium compounds are not well absorbed, pass into the CNS to a limited extent, and have a lower incidence of CNS side effects.[35] They still cause well-known peripheral antimuscarinic side effects, such as accommodation paralysis, constipation, tachycardia, and dry mouth. All antimuscarinic drugs are contraindicated in patients with narrow-angle glaucoma.

Antimuscarinics are still the most widely used treatment for urge and urge incontinence.[36] However, currently used drugs lack selectivity for the bladder, and effects on other organ systems may result in side effects that limit their usefulness. Theoretically, drugs with selectivity for the bladder could be obtained, if the subtypes that mediate bladder contraction and those that produce the main side effects of antimuscarinic drugs were different. One way to avoid many antimuscarinic side effects is to administer the drugs intravesically. However, this is practical only in a limited number of patients.

Several antimuscarinic drugs are used to treat bladder overactivity. For many of them, documentation of effects is not based on randomized, controlled trials that satisfy currently required criteria, and some drugs can be considered obsolete (e.g., emepronium). Information on these drugs has not been included in this chapter, but can be found elsewhere.[36,37]

Atropine

Atropine (D, L-hyoscyamine) is rarely used to treat detrusor overactivity because its systemic side effects preclude its use. However, in patients with detrusor hyper-reflexia, intravesical atropine may be effective for increasing bladder capacity without causing systemic adverse effects, as shown in open pilot trials.[38,39]

The pharmacologically active antimuscarinic half of atropine is L-hyoscyamine. Although it is still used, few clinical studies are available to evaluate the antimuscarinic activity of L-hyoscyamine sulfate.

Propantheline

Propantheline bromide is a quaternary ammonium compound that is nonselective for muscarinic receptor subtypes and has low (5%–10%), individually varying biologic availability.[40] It is usually given in a dose of 15 to 30 mg four times daily. However, to obtain an optimal effect, individual titration of the dose is necessary, and higher dosages are often needed. Using this approach in an open study of 26 patients with uninhibited detrusor contractions, Blaivas and colleagues[41] obtained complete clinical response in all patients but one, who did not tolerate propantheline at a dose of higher than 15 mg four times daily. Dosages varied from 7.5 to 60 mg four times daily. In contrast, in a randomized, double-blind, multicenter study of the treatment of frequency, urgency, and incontinence as a result of detrusor overactivity (154 patients with idiopathic detrusor instability or detrusor hyper-reflexia), Thüroff and associates[42] compared the effects of oxybutynin 5 mg three times daily, propantheline 15 mg three times daily, and placebo. They found no differences between the placebo and propantheline groups. In another randomized comparative trial with a crossover design (23 women with idiopathic detrusor instability) and dose titration, Holmes and associates[43] found no differences in efficacy between oxybutynin and propantheline. The Agency of Health Care Policy and Research Clinical Practice Guidelines (Urinary Incontinence Guideline Panel) list five randomized, controlled trials of propantheline that showed a reduction of urge (percent drug effect minus percent placebo effect) of 0% to 53%. Although the effect of propantheline on detrusor overactivity has not been well documented in controlled trials that meet current standards, this drug can be considered effective, and in individually titrated doses, may be clinically useful.

Trospium

Trospium chloride is a quaternary ammonium compound that has antimuscarinic actions on detrusor smooth muscle as well as effects on ganglia. However, the clinical importance of the ganglionic effects has not been established. In isolated detrusor muscle, it was more potent than oxybutynin and tolterodine in inhibiting carbachol-induced contractions.[44] Trospium has no selectivity for muscarinic receptor subtypes. Its biologic availability is low, approximately 5%,[45] and it does not cross the blood–brain barrier. It seems to have no negative cognitive effects.[45,46] Several open studies show that the drug may be useful in the treatment of detrusor overactivity.[47,48] In a placebo-controlled, double-blind study of patients with detrusor hyper-reflexia,[48] the drug was given twice daily at a dose of 20 mg over a 3-week period. It increased maximum cystometric capacity, decreased maximum detrusor pressure, and increased compliance in the treatment group, whereas no effects were seen in the placebo group. Side effects were few, and were comparable in both groups. In a randomized, double-blind multicenter trial in patients with spinal cord injuries and detrusor hyper-reflexia, trospium and oxybutynin were equally effective; however, trospium seemed to have fewer side effects.[49]

The effect of trospium in urge incontinence has been documented in placebo-controlled, randomized studies. Allousi and colleagues[50] compared the effects of the drug with those of placebo in 309 patients in a urodynamic study lasting 3 weeks. Trospium 20 mg was given twice daily. Significant increases were noted in volume at first unstable contraction and in maximum bladder capacity. Cardozo and associates[51] studied 208 patients with bladder instability who were treated with trospium 20 mg twice daily for 2 weeks. Significant increases were found in volume at first unstable contraction and in maximum bladder capacity in the trospium-treated group. Trospium was well tolerated, and the frequency of adverse effects was similar to that in the placebo group. Höfner and associates[52] compared the effects of oxybutynin 5 mg twice daily with those of trospium 20 mg twice daily in a double-blind, randomized study performed over 12 months in 358 patients with urge symptoms or urge incontinence. Urodynamic improvements were comparable, but oxybutynin produced a significantly higher rate of side effects, and the drop-out rate was higher in the oxybutynin group. Jünemann and Al-Shukri[53] compared trospium 20 mg twice daily with tolterodine 2 mg twice daily in a placebo-controlled, double-blind study in 232 patients with urodynamically proven bladder overactivity, sensory urge incontinence, or mixed incontinence. Trospium reduced the frequency of micturition, which was the primary end point, more than tolterodine or placebo, and also reduced the number of episodes of incontinence more than the other drugs. The incidence of dry mouth was comparable in the trospium and tolterodine groups (7% and 9%, respectively). Trospium chloride has a documented effect on detrusor overactivity, and seems to be well tolerated.

Tolterodine

Tolterodine is a potent and competitive muscarinic receptor antagonist that was developed for the treatment of urinary urgency and urge incontinence.[54] The drug has no selectivity for muscarinic receptor subtypes, but shows some selectivity for the bladder over the salivary glands in an animal model[55] and possibly in humans.[56] Tolterodine has a major active metabolite with a pharmacologic profile similar to that of the mother compound.[57] This metabolite significantly contributes to the therapeutic effect of tolterodine.[58] Tolterodine is rapidly absorbed and has a half-life of 2 to 3 hours, but the effects on the bladder seem to be more long-lasting than could be expected based on the pharmacokinetic data. The main metabolite also has a half-life of 2 to 3 hours.[58] In healthy volunteers, orally administered tolterodine in a high dose (6.4 mg) had a powerful inhibitory effect on micturition and also reduced stimulated salivation 1 hour after administration.[56] However, 5 hours after administration, the effects on the urinary bladder were maintained, whereas no significant effects on salivation were seen.

The relatively low affinity for lipids exhibited by tolterodine implies a limited propensity to penetrate the CNS, which may explain the low incidence of cognitive side effects.[54,59]

Several randomized, double-blind, placebo-controlled studies of patients with idiopathic detrusor instability and detrusor hyper-reflexia show a significant reduction in micturition frequency and number of episodes of incontinence.[54] Tolterodine seems to be well tolerated when used at 1 to 4 mg daily. Chancellor and colleagues[60] reported the results of a double-blind, randomized study of 1022 patients that compared tolterodine 2 mg twice daily with placebo. Active drug reduced the number of episodes of urge incontinence by 46% versus baseline, and the effect compared with placebo was also significant. Withdrawals were essentially the same in the two treatment groups.

A once-daily formulation of tolterodine was recently developed, and the first large-scale (1529 patients) clinical trial compared the effects of this agent with placebo and the twice-daily formulation.[61] Extended-release tolterodine 4 mg once daily and immediate-release tolterodine 2 mg twice daily both significantly reduced the mean number of episodes of urge incontinence per week compared with placebo. The median reduction in these episodes, as a percentage of baseline value, was 71% for extended-release tolterodine, 60% for immediate-release tolterodine, and 33% for placebo. Treatment with both formulations of tolterodine was also associated with statistically significant improvements in all other micturition diary variables compared with placebo. The rate of dry mouth (of any severity) was 23% for extended-release tolterodine, 30% for immediate-release tolterodine, and 8% for placebo. The rates of withdrawal were comparable for the two active drug groups and the placebo group. No safety concerns were noted.

In a placebo-controlled study comparing tolterodine 2 mg twice daily and oxybutynin 5 mg three times daily in 293 patients with detrusor instability, both drugs were equally effective in reducing the frequency of micturition and the number of episodes of incontinence. However, tolterodine appeared to have a better efficacy and tolerability profile.[62] These findings were largely confirmed by other investigators.[63] Malone-Lee and associates[63] compared oxybutynin and tolterodine in 378 patients who were 50 years of age or older and had symptoms of overactive bladder. These patients received 10 weeks of treatment with tolterodine 2 mg twice daily or oxybutynin 5 mg twice daily (final doses). Patients treated with tolterodine had significantly fewer adverse events (69% vs. 81%), notably, dry mouth (37% vs. 61%), than those in the oxybutynin group. The drugs had comparable efficacy for improving urinary symptoms. The authors concluded that tolterodine was as effective as oxybutynin for improving the symptoms of overactive bladder, but had superior tolerability. These data contrast with those of Appell and colleagues,[64] who compared extended-release oxybutynin chloride and immediate-release tolterodine in a 12-week randomized, double-blind, parallel-group study in 378 patients with overactive bladder. Participants who had 7 to 50 episodes of urge incontinence per week and 10 or more voids in 24 hours received extended-release oxybutynin 10 mg once daily or tolterodine 2 mg twice daily. Outcome measures included the number of episodes of urge incontinence, total incontinence, and micturition frequency at 12 weeks, adjusted for baseline. At the end of the study, extended-release oxybutynin was significantly more effective than tolterodine in each of the main outcome measures, adjusted for baseline. Dry mouth, the most common adverse event, was reported in 28.1% and 33.2% of participants who took extended-release oxybutynin and tolterodine, respectively. Rates of CNS and other adverse events were low, and were similar in both groups. The authors concluded that extended-release oxybutynin was more effective than tolterodine and that rates of dry mouth and other adverse events were similar in both treatment groups.

No comparative trials have evaluated extended-release tolterodine and the extended-release form of oxybutynin. However, comparison of the immediate-release forms indicates that efficacy is no different, whereas the side effect profile of tolterodine is more favorable.[59,65] Head-to-head comparisons between the two extended-release preparations are required to compare efficacy and tolerability adequately between the two agents. Tolterodine, in both the immediate- and extended-release forms, has a well-documented effect on detrusor overactivity, and the side effect profile seems acceptable.

Darifenacin

Darifenacin is a selective muscarinic M_3 receptor antagonist that was developed for the treatment of bladder overactivity.[66] In vitro, it is selective for human cloned muscarinic M_3 receptors relative to M_1, M_2, M_4, or M_5. Theoretically, M_3 versus M_1 selectivity may provide an advantage over nonselective agents, because both M_3 and M_1 receptors have been implicated in salivary secretion of mucus,[67] and an anesthetized dog model showed selectivity for the urinary bladder over the salivary gland.[68] M_3 versus M_1 selectivity may be associated with a low rate of cognitive impairment (M_1[69]). M_3 versus M_2 selectivity can provide little effect on heart rate (M_2), and M_3 versus M_5 selectivity may reduce impairment of visual accommodation (M_5).[70] However, the clinical importance of these potential advantages has not been established.

Published clinical information on the effect of darifenacin is scarce. In a pilot study of patients with detrusor instability, the drug reduced the total number, maximum amplitude, and duration of unstable bladder contractions.[71] A randomized, double-blind study of 25 patients with detrusor instability compared the effects of darifenacin 15 mg and 30 mg daily with those of oxybutynin 5 mg three times daily on ambulatory urodynamic findings and salivary flow.[72] Both drugs had similar urodynamic efficacy, but oxybutynin reduced salivary flow significantly more than darifenacin. Another controlled study of 27 healthy men investigated the effects of darifenacin 7.5 and 15 mg daily, dicyclomine 20 mg four times daily, and placebo on cognitive and cardiac function.[73] Unlike dicyclomine, darifenacin had no detectable effects on cognitive or cardiovascular function.

Darifenacin is currently being evaluated in a phase III global clinical evaluation program for the treatment of bladder overactivity to identify the optimal dose regimen and assess its potential clinical benefits.

Solifenacin (YM-905)

Solifenacin is a long-acting muscarinic receptor antagonist for the treatment of overactive bladder that is currently in development. In guinea pig urinary bladder smooth muscle preparations, solifenacin inhibited cholinergic responses with nanomolar potency. When tested in anesthetized mice, both solifenacin and oxybutynin potently inhibited carbachol-induced increases in urinary bladder pressure. However, only oxybutynin was associated with potent inhibition of carbachol-stimulated salivary secretion.[74] In cellular systems, solifenacin appears to be more potent as a muscarinic receptor antagonist for bladder smooth muscle than for salivary gland when compared with reference molecules, such as oxybutynin or tolterodine. This finding indicates a potentially beneficial efficacy and tolerability profile. The clinical relevance of these findings is being investigated in phase III clinical studies.

Drugs that Act on Membrane Channels

Calcium Antagonists

Activation of detrusor muscle, through both muscarinic receptor and nonadrenergic, noncholinergic pathways, seems to require influx of extracellular Ca^{2+} through Ca^{2+} channels as well as through mobilization of intracellular Ca^{2+}. The influx of extracellular calcium can be blocked by calcium antagonists that block L-type Ca^{2+} channels. Theoretically, this would be an attractive way to inhibit detrusor overactivity.[75] However, there have been few clinical studies of the effects of calcium antagonists in patients with detrusor overactivity.[36] Intravesical instillation of verapamil increased bladder capacity and decreased the degree of leakage during cystometry in patients with detrusor hyper-reflexia.[76] The effect was less pronounced in patients with non-neurogenic overactivity.[77]

Available information does not suggest that systemic therapy with calcium antagonists is an effective way to treat detrusor overactivity, but controlled clinical trials are lacking. However, intravesical therapy with these drugs could be useful, and calcium antagonists may enhance the effects of anticholinergic agents.[78] Oral nifedipine has been used effectively as prophylaxis for autonomic hyper-reflexia during urologic instrumentation in patients with spinal cord injury.[1]

Potassium Channel Openers

Opening of K^+ channels and subsequent efflux of K^+ causes hyperpolarization of various smooth muscles, including the detrusor.[79] This leads to a decrease in Ca^{2+} influx by reducing the probability that Ca^{2+} channels will open, with subsequent relaxation or inhibition of contraction. Theoretically, these drugs may be active during the filling phase of the bladder, abolishing bladder overactivity, with no effect on normal bladder contraction. K^+ channel openers, such as pinacidil and cromakalim, have been effective in animal models,[79] but clinically, the effects have not been encouraging.

The first generation of drugs that open ATP-sensitive K^+ channels, such as cromakalim and pinacidil, were more potent as inhibitors of vascular smooth muscle preparations than of detrusor muscle, and clinical trials showed no bladder effects at doses that already lowered blood pressure.[80] However, new drugs with K_{ATP} channel-opening properties have been described, and may be useful for the treatment of bladder overactivity.[81]

Opening of K^+ channels is an attractive way to treat bladder overactivity, because it would make it possible to eliminate undesired bladder contractions without affecting normal micturition. However, no evidence from controlled clinical trials suggests that K^+ channel openers are a treatment alternative.

Drugs with Mixed Actions

Some drugs that are used to block bladder overactivity have more than one mechanism of action. They all have a more or less pronounced antimuscarinic effect, and in addition, an often poorly defined direct action on bladder muscle. For several of these drugs, the antimuscarinic effects can be seen at much lower drug concentrations than the direct action, which may involve blockade of voltage-operated Ca^{2+} channels. The clinical effects of these drugs can be explained mainly by their antimuscarinic action. Among the drugs with mixed actions was terodiline, which was withdrawn from the market because it was suspected to cause polymorphic ventricular tachycardia (torsade de pointes) in some patients.[82]

Oxybutynin

Oxybutynin has several pharmacologic effects, some of which seem difficult to relate to its effectiveness in the treatment of detrusor overactivity. It has both an antimuscarinic effect and a direct muscle relaxant effect, in addition to local anesthetic actions. The latter effect may be important when the drug is administered intravesically, but probably plays no role when it is given orally. In vitro, oxybutynin was 500 times weaker as a smooth muscle relaxant than as an antimuscarinic agent. When given systemically, oxybutynin acts mainly as an antimuscarinic drug. Oxybutynin has a high affinity for muscarinic receptors in human bladder tissue, and effectively blocks carbachol-induced contractions.[83] The drug has higher affinity for muscarinic M_1 and M_3 receptors than for M_2 receptors,[84] but the clinical significance of this finding is unclear.

Oxybutynin is a tertiary amine that is well absorbed, but undergoes extensive first-pass metabolism (biologic availability 6% in healthy volunteers). Its plasma half-life is approximately 2 hours, but with wide individual variation.[85] Oxybutynin has an active metabolite, N-desethyl oxybutynin, which has pharmacologic properties similar to those of the parent compound, but occurs in much higher concentrations.[85] Therefore, it seems reasonable to assume that, to a large extent, the effect of oral oxybutynin is exerted by the metabolite. The occurrence of an active metabolite may also explain the lack of correlation between plasma concentrations of oxybutynin and the side effects in elderly patients reported by Ouslander and colleagues.[86]

Several controlled studies show that oxybutynin is effective in controlling detrusor overactivity, including hyper-reflexia.[1,31,43,87] The recommended oral dose of the immediate-release form is 5 mg three or four times daily, even if lower doses have been used. Thüroff and colleagues[31] summarized 15 randomized, controlled studies in a total of 476 patients treated with oxybutynin. The mean decrease in incontinence was 52%, and the mean reduction in frequency over 24 hours was 33%. The overall rate of subjective improvement was 74% (range, 61%–100%). A mean of 70% of patients reported side effects (range, 17%–93%). Oxybutynin 7.5 to 15 mg daily significantly improved the quality of life in patients with overactive bladder in a large, open, multicenter trial. In this study, patient compliance was 97%, and side effects, mainly dry mouth, were reported in only 8% of patients.[88] In nursing home residents ($n = 75$), Ouslander and associates[89] found that oxybutynin did not add to the clinical effectiveness of prompted voiding in a placebo-controlled, double-blind, crossover trial. On the other hand, in another controlled trial in elderly subjects ($n = 57$), oxybutynin with bladder training was superior to bladder training alone.[90]

Several open studies in patients with spinal cord injury suggest that oxybutynin, given orally or intravesically, can be of therapeutic benefit.[91] The therapeutic effect of immediate-release oxybutynin on detrusor overactivity is associated with a high incidence of side effects ($\leq 80\%$ with oral administration). These are typically antimuscarinic (dry mouth, constipation, drowsiness, blurred vision), and are often dose-limiting.[92] Oxybutynin crosses the blood–brain barrier and may have effects on the CNS.[46] The drug can cause cognitive impairment,[93] which may be particularly troublesome in the geriatric population.[94] The electrocardiographic effects of oxybutynin were studied in elderly patients with urinary incontinence, and no changes were found.[95] The commonly recommended dose of 5 mg three times daily may be unnecessarily high in some patients, and a starting dose of 2.5 mg twice daily, followed by dose titration, may reduce the number of adverse effects.[88]

Once-daily formulations of oxybutynin have been developed. Extended-release oxybutynin (Ditropan XL) uses an innovative osmotic drug delivery system to release the drug at a controlled rate over 24 hours. This formulation overcomes the marked peak-to-trough fluctuations in plasma levels of both drug and the major metabolite that occur with immediate-release oxybutynin.[96] A trend toward a lower incidence of dry mouth with extended-release oxybutynin was attributed to reduced first-pass metabolism and to the maintenance of lower and less fluctuating plasma levels of drug. Clinical trials of extended-release oxybutynin have concentrated primarily on comparing this drug with immediate-release oxybutynin. Anderson and associates[97] reported a multicenter, randomized, double-blind study of 105 patients with urge incontinence or mixed incontinence with a clinically significant urge component. The number of episodes of urge urinary incontinence was the primary efficacy parameter. The number of weekly episodes of urge incontinence decreased from 27.4 to 4.8 after extended-release oxybutynin, and from 23.4 to 3.1 after immediate-release oxybutynin. The total number of episodes of incontinence decreased from 29.3 to 6 and from 26.3 to 3.8, respectively. Weekly episodes of urge incontinence from baseline to the end of the study also decreased by 84% after controlled-release oxybutynin and by 88% after immediate-release oxybutynin. Because only patients who had previously responded to treatment with oxybutynin were selected for treatment, these figures do not represent normal clinical practice. Dry mouth of any severity was reported by 68% and 87% of the controlled-release and immediate-release groups, respectively, and moderate or severe dry mouth occurred in 25% and 46%, respectively.

Another controlled study comparing the efficacy and safety of controlled-release oxybutynin with conventional, immediate-release oxybutynin included 226 patients with urge incontinence.[98] These patients responded to anticholinergic therapy and had seven or more episodes of urge incontinence per week. Reductions in the number of episodes of urge urinary incontinence from baseline to the end of treatment were 18.6 to 2.9 per week (mean decrease, 83%) and 19.8 to 4.4 per week (mean decrease, 76%) in the controlled-release and immediate-release oxybutynin groups (difference nonsignificant), respectively. The incidence of dry mouth increased with dose in both groups, but there was no difference in the rates of dry mouth between the groups (47.7% and 59.1% for the controlled-release and immediate-release groups, respectively). However, a significantly lower proportion of patients taking controlled-release oxybutynin had moderate to severe dry mouth or dry mouth of any severity compared with those taking immediate-release oxybutynin.

As discussed earlier, Appell and colleagues[64] compared extended-release oxybutynin chloride 10 mg daily and tolterodine 2 mg twice daily in a 12-week randomized, double-blind, parallel-group study in 378 patients with overactive bladder. Extended-release oxybutynin was significantly more effective than tolterodine in each of the main outcome measures (number of episodes of urge incontinence, total incontinence, and micturition frequency at 12 weeks), adjusted for baseline, and the rates of dry mouth and other adverse events were similar in both treatment groups.

A different extended-release form of oxybutynin was used by Birns and colleagues,[99] who reported comparable efficacy of a 10-mg preparation with immediate-release oxybutynin 5 mg twice daily. Efficacy was similar, but the extended-release formulation was better tolerated, with patients reporting approximately half the total number of adverse effects than with the immediate-release preparation.

Other forms of oxybutynin have also been introduced. Rectal administration[100] led to fewer adverse effects than the conventional tablet form. A transdermal preparation is in clinical trials.

Administered intravesically, in several studies, oxybutynin increased bladder capacity and produced clinical improvement with few side effects, in both hyperreflexia and other types of bladder overactivity, and in both children and adults,[101–104] although adverse effects may occur. Cognitive impairment can also occur in children treated with intravesical oxybutynin. Because these effects may differ from those seen with oral administration,[105] these patients should be monitored closely. Oxybutynin has well-documented efficacy in the treatment of detrusor overactivity, and is, together with tolterodine, the drug of first choice in patients with this disorder.

Dicyclomine

Dicyclomine has both a direct relaxant effect on smooth muscle and an antimuscarinic action.[106] Favorable results in detrusor overactivity were shown in several studies[107] performed more than a decade ago that do not satisfy the current criteria for good-quality randomized controlled trials (RCTs). Even if published experiences of the effect of dicyclomine on detrusor overactivity are favorable, the drug is not widely used, and few RCTs document its efficacy and side effects.

Propiverine

Propiverine has combined anticholinergic and calcium antagonistic actions.[108] The drug is rapidly absorbed, but has a high first-pass metabolism. Several active metabolites are formed,[109] and their pharmacologic characteristics remain to be established. These metabolites probably contribute to the clinical effects of the drug.

In several studies, propiverine showed beneficial effects in patients with detrusor overactivity. Thüroff and colleagues[31] collected nine randomized studies on a total of 230 patients, and found reductions in frequency (30%) and number of micturitions per 24 hours (17%), a 64-mL increase in bladder capacity, and a subjective improvement rate of 77% (range, 33%–80%). Side effects occurred in 14% of patients (range, 8%–42%). In patients with hyperreflexia, controlled clinical trials show the superiority of propiverine over placebo, with symptomatic improvement occurring in approximately 50% and 25% of cases, respectively.[110] Propiverine also increased bladder capacity and decreased maximum detrusor contractions. Controlled trials comparing propiverine, flavoxate, and placebo,[111] and propiverine, oxybutynin, and placebo,[112] confirm the efficacy of propiverine, and suggest that it may have the same efficacy as oxybutynin, with fewer side effects.

Stohrer and associates[113] reported a double-blind, randomized, prospective, multicenter trial comparing propiverine 15 mg three times daily with placebo in 113 patients with spinal cord injury and detrusor hyperreflexia. Maximal cystometric capacity increased significantly in the propiverine group, by an average of 104 mL. Changes in bladder capacity at first contraction and in maximum bladder contraction were likewise statistically significant. Bladder compliance showed a more pronounced increase with propiverine compared with placebo. Sixty-three percent of patients in the propiverine group reported subjective improvement, compared with 23% of the placebo group. Dry mouth (37% in the propiverine group and 8% in the placebo group) and accommodation disorders (28% and 2%, respectively) were reported side effects.

Madersbacher and associates[112] compared the tolerability and efficacy of propiverine (15 mg three times daily), oxybutynin (5 mg twice daily), and placebo in 366 patients with urgency and urge incontinence in a randomized, double-blind, placebo-controlled clinical trial. The urodynamic efficacy of propiverine was similar to that of oxybutynin, but the incidence and severity of dry mouth were less with propiverine than with oxybutynin.

Dorschner and associates[114] performed a double-blind, multicenter, placebo-controlled, randomized study of the efficacy and cardiac safety of propiverine in 98 elderly patients (mean age, 68 years) with urgency, urge incontinence, or mixed urge and stress incontinence. After a 2-week placebo run-in period, the patients received propiverine 15 mg three times daily or placebo three times daily for 4 weeks. Propiverine significantly reduced micturition frequency (from 8.7 to 6.5) and significantly decreased the number of episodes of incontinence (from 0.9 to 0.3 daily). Resting and ambulatory electrocardiograms indicated no significant changes. The incidence of adverse events was very low, with 2 of 49 patients (2%) who received propiverine reporting dry mouth.

Propiverine has a documented beneficial effect in the treatment of detrusor overactivity, and seems to have an acceptable side effect profile. Its complex pharmacokinetic profile, with several active, poorly characterized metabolites, requires further study.

Flavoxate

The main mechanism of the effect of flavoxate on smooth muscle has not been established. The drug has moderate calcium antagonistic activity, inhibits phosphodiesterase, and has local anesthetic properties. No anticholinergic effect has been found. Pertussis-toxin-sensitive G-proteins in the brain may be involved in the flavoxate-induced suppression of the micturition reflex in rats.[115] Its main metabolite (3-methylflavone-8-carboxylic acid) has low pharmacologic activity.[116]

The clinical effects of flavoxate in patients with detrusor instability and frequency, urge, and incontinence have been studied in both open and controlled investigations, with varying rates of success.[117] Stanton[118] compared emepronium bromide and flavoxate in a double-blind, crossover study of patients with detrusor instability, and reported improvement rates of 83% and 66% with flavoxate and emepronium bromide, respectively, both administered as 200 mg three times daily. No difference in efficacy was found between the two groups, but flavoxate had fewer and milder side effects. However, the lack of a placebo arm in these studies reduces the value of conclusions about efficacy.

Other investigators compared the effects of flavoxate with those of placebo. They found no beneficial effect of flavoxate at dosages of up to 400 mg three times daily.[119] Few side effects have been reported with flavoxate, but its efficacy compared with other therapeutic alternatives is not well documented.

Alpha-adrenoceptor Antagonists

The normal human detrusor responds to noradrenaline by relaxing,[120] probably because of the effect on both alpha- and beta-adrenoceptors. Stimulation of alpha-2-adrenoceptors on cholinergic neurons may lead to a decreased release of acetylcholine, and stimulation of postjunctional beta-adrenoceptors may lead to direct relaxation of the detrusor muscle.[4,121]

Drugs that stimulate alpha-adrenoceptors have little contractile effect on isolated normal human detrusor muscle. However, this may change in bladder overactivity associated with, for example, hypertrophic bladder and outflow obstruction[120] or a neurogenic bladder.[4] Significant subtype-selective alpha-1D-adrenoceptor mRNA upregulation was found in rats with outflow obstruction,[122] but functional correlates were not reported. Factors such as the degree and duration of obstruction may have an important effect on the alpha-adrenoceptors in the detrusor, but the functional consequences have not been established.

Even if alpha-adrenoceptor antagonists can ameliorate lower urinary tract symptoms in men with benign prostatic hypertrophy[121] and occasionally can abolish detrusor overactivity in these patients,[120] no controlled clinical trials show that they are an effective alternative in the treatment of bladder overactivity in these patients. In an open-label study, Arnold[123] evaluated the clinical and pressure-flow effects of tamsulosin 0.4 mg once daily in patients with lower urinary tract symptoms caused by benign prostatic obstruction. He found that tamsulosin can produce a significant decrease in detrusor pressure, an increase in flow rate, and symptomatic improvement in patients with lower urinary tract symptoms and confirmed obstruction. Alpha-adrenoceptor antagonists have been used to treat patients with neurogenic bladder and bladder overactivity[124]; however, success has been moderate. Abrams and the European Tamsulosin NLUTD Study Group[124] reported results from a 4-week, placebo-controlled study of the effects of tamsulosin in 263 patients with suprasacral spinal cord lesions and neurogenic lower urinary tract dysfunction. A trend was noted, but there was no statistically significant reduction in maximum urethral pressure with tamsulosin after 4 weeks. In 134 patients who completed a 1-year, open-label study, significant positive urodynamic and symptomatic effects were found. No definitive conclusions can be drawn about the efficacy of alpha-1-adrenoceptor antagonists in the treatment of neurogenic bladder until further information is available.

Lower urinary tract symptoms in women respond favorably to treatment with alpha-adrenoceptor antagonists. In an open, prospective study of 34 women with urgency and frequency who were evaluated by an expanded American Urological Association symptom score, a combination of doxazosin and hyoscyamine was more effective than either drug given alone.[125] The value of such a combination should be evaluated in a controlled clinical trial.

Although alpha-adrenoceptor antagonists may be effective in some cases of bladder overactivity, convincing effects documented in randomized clinical trials are lacking. In women, these drugs may cause stress incontinence.[126]

Beta-adrenoceptor Agonists

In isolated human bladder, non-subtype-selective beta-adrenoceptor agonists, such as isoprenaline, have a pronounced inhibitory effect, and administration of these drugs can increase bladder capacity in humans. However, the beta-adrenoceptors of the human bladder have functional characteristics that are typical of neither beta-1-adrenoceptors nor beta-2-adrenoceptors, because they can be blocked by propranolol, but not by practolol or metoprolol (beta-1) or butoxamine (beta-2).[127] On the other hand, receptor-binding studies with subtype-selective ligands suggested that the beta-adrenoceptors of the human detrusor are primarily of the beta-2 subtype,[128] and favorable effects on bladder overactivity were reported in open studies with selective beta-2-adrenoceptor agonists, such as terbutaline.[129] In a double-blind study, clenbuterol 0.01 mg three times daily had a good therapeutic effect in 15 of 20 women with motor urge incontinence.[130] However, other investigators have not shown that beta-adrenoceptor agonists are effective in elderly patients with unstable bladder[131] or in young patients with myelodysplasia and detrusor overactivity.

Atypical beta-adrenoceptor-mediated responses, reported in early studies of beta-adrenoceptor antagonists, are mediated by a beta-3-adrenoceptor that was cloned, sequenced, expressed in a model system, and extensively characterized functionally.[132] Both normal and neurogenic human detrusors express beta-1-, beta-2-, and beta-3-adrenoceptor mRNAs, and selective beta-3-adrenoceptor agonists effectively relax both types of detrusor muscle.[133] Thus, the atypical beta-adrenoceptor of the human bladder may be the beta-3-adrenoceptor. Whether this is of importance in humans, and whether beta-3-adrenoceptor stimulation is an effective way to treat the overactive bladder, has yet to be shown in controlled clinical trials.

Antidepressants

Several antidepressants have beneficial effects in patients with detrusor overactivity.[134] However, imipramine is the only drug that has been widely used clinically to treat this disorder.

Imipramine has complex pharmacologic effects, including marked systemic anticholinergic actions and blockade of the reuptake of serotonin and noradrenaline, but its mode of action in detrusor overactivity has not been established.[135] Good results were reported in elderly patients with detrusor instability who received oral imipramine in doses of up to 150 mg daily. Even if imipramine is generally considered a useful drug in the treatment of detrusor overactivity, no high-quality randomized clinical trials have shown its usefulness. Imipramine has favorable effects in the treatment of nocturnal enuresis in children, with a success rate of 10% to 70% in controlled trials.[135]

Therapeutic doses of tricyclic antidepressants, including imipramine, may cause serious toxic effects on the cardiovascular system (orthostatic hypotension, ventricular arrhythmias). Imipramine prolongs QTc intervals and has an antiarrhythmic and proarrhythmic effect similar to that of quinidine.[136] Children seem particularly sensitive to the cardiotoxic effects of tricyclic antidepressants.[137]

The risks and benefits of imipramine in the treatment of voiding disorders have not been assessed. Few studies were performed during the last decade,[135] and no high-quality randomized clinical trials show that the drug is effective in the treatment of detrusor overactivity. However, a beneficial effect has been shown in the treatment of nocturnal enuresis.

Prostaglandin Synthesis Inhibitors

Human bladder mucosa can synthesize eicosanoids, and these agents can be liberated from bladder muscle and mucosa in response to different types of trauma.[138,139] Even if prostaglandins cause contraction of human bladder muscle, it is unclear whether prostaglandins contribute to the pathogenesis of unstable detrusor contractions.

Because few controlled clinical trials have been done to evaluate the effects of prostaglandin synthesis inhibitors in the treatment of detrusor overactivity, and few drugs have been tested, it is difficult to evaluate their therapeutic value. No new information has been published during the last decade.

Vasopressin Analogues

Desmopressin

Desmopressin (1-desamino-8-D-arginine vasopressin) is a synthetic vasopressin analogue with a pronounced antidiuretic effect, but few vasopressor actions.[140] It is now widely used to treat primary nocturnal enuresis.[141] Studies show that one factor that can contribute to nocturnal enuresis in children, and probably in adults, is lack of a normal nocturnal increase in plasma vasopressin, which leads to high nocturnal urine production.[142] Decreasing nocturnal production of urine may improve enuresis and nocturia. Several controlled, double-blind studies show that intranasal administration of desmopressin is effective in the treatment of nocturnal enuresis in children.[143] The dose that is used in most studies is 20 µg intranasally at bedtime. However, the drug is orally active, even if bioavailability is low (<1% compared with 2%–10% after intranasal administration), and its oral efficacy in primary nocturnal enuresis in children and adolescents has been documented in randomized, double-blind, placebo-controlled studies.[144]

Positive effects of desmopressin on nocturia in adults have been documented. Nocturnal frequency and enuresis as a result of bladder instability responded favorably to intranasal desmopressin therapy, even when previous treatment with antispasmodics was unsuccessful. In controlled studies in patients with multiple sclerosis, desmopressin reduced nocturia and micturition frequency.[145,146] Furthermore, desmopressin was successful in treating nocturnal enuresis in patients with spina bifida and diurnal incontinence.[147] Oral desmopressin is effective in the treatment of nocturia of polyuric origin. In addition to prolonging the sleep duration to first void, desmopressin reduced the number and frequency of nocturnal voids as well as nocturnal urine volume in both men and women.[148,149]

Desmopressin is a well-documented therapeutic alternative in pediatric nocturnal enuresis, and also seems to be effective in adults with nocturia of polyuric origin. Although side effects are uncommon, water retention and hyponatremia may occur,[150] and consideration should be given to these potential side effects, particularly in elderly patients.

Other Drugs

Baclofen

Baclofen depresses monosynaptic and polysynaptic motor neurons and interneurons in the spinal cord by acting as a gamma-aminobutyric acid agonist, and has been used in voiding disorders, including detrusor hyper-reflexia caused by spinal cord lesions.[40] The drug may also be used to treat idiopathic detrusor overactivity, although published experience is limited. Intrathecal baclofen may be useful in patients with spasticity and bladder dysfunction, and may increase bladder capacity.[151]

Capsaicin and Resiniferatoxin

Capsaicin, the pungent ingredient of red peppers, has identified a pharmacologic classification of subpopulations of primary afferent neurons innervating the bladder and urethra, the capsaicin-sensitive nerves. Capsaicin exerts a biphasic effect on sensory nerves. Initial excitation is followed by a long-lasting blockade that renders sensitive primary afferents (C-fibers) resistant to activation by natural stimuli.[152] Capsaicin is believed to exert these effects by acting on specific receptors known as vanilloid receptors.[153] At high concentrations (mM), capsaicin may have additional nonspecific effects.[154]

Cystometric evidence that capsaicin-sensitive nerves may modulate the afferent branch of the micturition reflex in humans was originally presented by Maggi and colleagues,[155] who instilled capsaicin (0.1–10 μM) intravesically in five patients with hypersensitivity disorders, with attenuation of their symptoms a few days after the administration of capsaicin. Intravesical capsaicin, given at considerably higher concentrations (1–2 mM) than those administered by Maggi and colleagues,[155] has been used with success in neurologic disorders, such as multiple sclerosis and traumatic chronic spinal lesions.[156] The effect of treatment may last for 2 to 7 months.[157] DeRidder and associates[158] recommended that the drug should not be given to severely disabled, bedridden patients.

Side effects of intravesical capsaicin administration include discomfort and a burning sensation at the pubic or urethral level during instillation, an effect that can be overcome by previous instillation of lidocaine, which does not interfere with the beneficial effects of capsaicin.

Resiniferatoxin is a phorbol-related diterpene that is isolated from some species of *Euphorbia*, a cactus-like plant with effects similar to those of capsaicin. Given intravesically, resiniferatoxin is approximately 1000 times more potent than capsaicin in stimulating bladder activity. Moreover, resiniferatoxin seems to be able to desensitize bladder sensory fibers with less C-*fos* expression in the rat spinal cord.[159] Currently, it is not in clinical development because of formulation problems.

Botulinum Toxin

Botulinum toxin is considered to act by inhibiting acetylcholine release from cholinergic nerve terminals. However, botulinum toxin also inhibits release of several other transmitters. This results in decreased muscle contractility and muscle atrophy at the injection site. The produced chemical denervation is a reversible process, and axons are regenerated in about 3 to 6 months. The botulinum toxin molecule cannot cross the blood-brain barrier and therefore has no CNS effects.

Botulinum toxin injected into the external urethral sphincter was initially used to treat patients with spinal cord injuries who had detrusor-external sphincter dyssynergia, but the use of the toxin has increased rapidly. Successful treatment of neurogenic detrusor overactivity by intravesical botulinum toxin injections has now been reported by several groups, and toxin injections may also be effective in refractory idiopathic detrusor overactivity.[160]

DRUGS USED TO TREAT STRESS INCONTINENCE

Many factors seem to be involved in the pathogenesis of stress urinary incontinence, including urethral support, vesical neck function, and urethral muscle function. These anatomic factors cannot be treated pharmacologically. However, women with stress incontinence have lower resting urethral pressures than age-matched continent women. Because most women with stress incontinence likely have reduced urethral closure pressure, it seems logical to increase urethral pressure to improve the condition. Factors that may contribute to urethral closure include urethral smooth muscle tone and the passive properties of the urethral lamina propria, in particular, the vascular submucosal layer. The relative contribution of these factors to intraurethral pressure is subject to debate. However, pharmacologic evidence shows that a substantial part of urethral tone is mediated through stimulation of alpha-adrenoceptors in the urethral smooth muscle by released noradrenaline. Lack of mucosal function may contribute to stress incontinence, mainly in elderly women who have low levels of estrogen. The role of striated urethral and pelvic floor muscles has not been established.

The goal of pharmacologic treatment of stress incontinence (Table 39-4) is to increase intraurethral pressure by increasing tone in urethral smooth muscle or by affecting tone of the striated muscles in the urethra and pelvic floor. Although several drugs may contribute to an increase in intraurethral pressure, including beta-adrenoceptor antagonists and imipramine,[40] only alpha-adrenoceptor agonists and estrogens, alone or together, are more widely used.

Alpha-adrenoceptor Agonists

Although several drugs that have agonistic effects on alpha-adrenoceptors have been used to treat stress incontinence (e.g., midodrine,[161] norfenefrine[162]), ephedrine and norephedrine seem to be the most widely used.[40] Ephedrine, pseudoephedrine (a stereoisomer of ephedrine), and norephedrine (phenylpropanolamine) directly stimulate alpha- and beta-adrenoceptors, but can

TABLE 39-4 ■ Drugs Used in the Treatment of Stress Incontinence*

Drug	Level of Evidence	Grade of Recommendation
Alpha-adrenoceptor agonists		
Ephedrine	3	C
Norephedrine (phenylpropanolamine)	2	NR
Other drugs		
Imipramine	4	C†
Clenbuterol	4	C
Duloxetine	Under investigation	
Hormones		
Estrogens	2	D

*Assessments according to the Oxford system (modified).
†Use with caution.
NR, not recommended.

also release noradrenaline from adrenergic nerve terminals. They are effective in stress incontinence, as reported in open and controlled clinical trials[163,164] of ephedrine, at a dose of 25 to 50 mg three to four times daily, and phenylpropanolamine, at a dose of 50 to 100 mg two to three times daily. These drugs lack selectivity for urethral alpha-adrenoceptors, and may increase blood pressure. They also can cause sleep disturbances, headache, tremor, and palpitations. No drug with appropriate subtype selectivity is currently available, and the role of alpha-adrenoceptor agonists in the treatment of stress incontinence has yet to be established.

Alpha-adrenoceptor agonists have been used in combination with estrogens[165] and with other nonsurgical treatments of stress incontinence, such as pelvic floor exercises and electrical stimulation. Hilton and colleagues[166] used vaginal or oral estrogen, alone or in combination with phenylpropanolamine, to treat 60 postmenopausal women with genuine stress incontinence in a double-blind, placebo-controlled study. Subjectively, stress incontinence improved in all groups, but objectively, it improved only in the women given combination therapy. In selected patients, selective alpha-1-adrenoceptor antagonists may be used on an on-demand basis in situations that provoke leakage.

Imipramine

Among other pharmacologic effects, imipramine inhibits the reuptake of noradrenaline and serotonin in adrenergic nerve endings. In the urethra, this effect can be expected to enhance the contractile effects of noradrenaline on urethral smooth muscle. Theoretically, this action may also affect the striated muscles in the urethra and pelvic floor by acting at the spinal cord level (Onuf's nucleus). No randomized clinical trials on the effects of imipramine are available.

Clenbuterol

Because beta-adrenoceptor antagonists have been used to treat stress incontinence, it seems paradoxical that the selective beta-2-adrenoceptor agonist clenbuterol caused significant clinical improvement and increased Maximal Urethral Closure Pressure (MUCP) in 165 women with stress incontinence.[167] Additional well-designed RCTs documenting the effects of clenbuterol are needed to assess its potential as a treatment for stress incontinence because this agent may have a novel, undefined mechanism of action.

Duloxetine

In animal experiments, duloxetine, a combined noradrenaline and serotonin reuptake inhibitor, increased neural activity to the external urethral sphincter and increased bladder capacity through effects on the CNS.[168] In a double-blind, placebo-controlled study in women with stress ($n = 140$) or mixed ($n = 146$) incontinence, duloxetine (20–40 mg daily) caused significant improvements in several efficacy measures (International Continence Society [ICS] 1-hour stress pad test, 24-hour pad weight, number of incontinence episodes, quality-of-life assessment).[169] The drug was well tolerated, and there were few discontinuations as a result of side effects (8% for duloxetine and 3% for placebo). The drug is undergoing clinical trials.

DRUGS USED TO TREAT OVERFLOW INCONTINENCE

According to the definition of the ICS, overflow incontinence is "leakage of urine at greater than normal bladder capacity. It is associated with incomplete bladder emptying due to either impaired detrusor contractility or bladder outlet obstruction." Two types of overflow incontinence are recognized. One is caused by mechanical obstruction, and the other is caused by functional disorders. Occasionally, both types coexist.

The clinical presentation of overflow incontinence may vary depending on the age of the patient and the cause of incontinence. In children, overflow incontinence may be caused by congenital obstructive disorders (e.g., urethral valve disorders) or neurogenic vesical dysfunction (e.g., myelomeningocele, Hinman syndrome). In adults, overflow incontinence may be associated with outflow obstruction caused by benign prostatic hypertrophy or can be caused by diabetes mellitus. Mixed forms are seen in disorders associated with motor spasticity (e.g., Parkinson's disease).

Pharmacologic treatment (Table 39-5) is based on previous urodynamic evaluation. The aim of treatment is to prevent damage to the upper urinary tract by normalizing voiding and urethral pressures. Drugs used to increase intravesical pressure include parasympathomimetics (acetylcholine analogues, such as bethanechol, or acetylcholine esterase inhibitors) and beta-adrenoceptor antagonists. These agents have no documented benefit.[170] Stimulation of detrusor activity by intravesical instillation of prostaglandins has been successful; however, the effect is controversial, and no randomized clinical trials have been done.[1,40]

TABLE 39-5 ■ Drugs Used to Treat Overflow Incontinence*

Drug	Level of Evidence	Grade of Recommendation
Alpha-adrenoceptor antagonists		
Alfuzosin	4	C
Doxazosin	4	C
Prazosin	4	C
Terazosin	4	C
Tamsulosin	4	C
Phenoxybenzamine	4	NR
Muscarinic receptor agonists		
Bethanechol	4	D
Carbachol	4	D
Anticholinesterase inhibitors		
Distigmine	4	D
Other drugs		
Baclofen	4	C
Benzodiazepines	4	C
Dantrolene	4	C

*Assessments according to the Oxford system (modified).
NR, Not recommended.

HORMONAL TREATMENT OF URINARY INCONTINENCE

Estrogens and the Continence Mechanism

The estrogen-sensitive tissues of the bladder, urethra, and pelvic floor play an important role in continence. For a woman to remain continent, urethral pressure must exceed intravesical pressure at all times, except during micturition.[171] The urethra has four estrogen-sensitive functional layers that play a part in the maintenance of positive urethral pressure: (1) epithelium, (2) vasculature, (3) connective tissue, and (4) muscle.

Estrogens in the Treatment of Urinary Incontinence

Estrogens may be useful in the treatment of women with urinary incontinence. In addition to improving the "maturation index" of urethral squamous epithelium,[172] estrogens increase urethral closure pressure and improve the transmission of abdominal pressure to the proximal urethra.[173] The sensory threshold of the bladder may also be increased. Salmon and colleagues[174] were the first to report the successful use of estrogens to treat urinary incontinence more than 50 years ago. Intramuscular estrogen therapy was administered to 16 women with dysuria, frequency, urgency, and incontinence for 4 weeks. Symptoms improved in 12 women until treatment was discontinued, at which time, symptoms recurred.

Lower urinary tract disorders in postmenopausal women have many causes. There is poor correlation between symptoms and the subsequent diagnosis after appropriate investigation. Unfortunately, initial trials were conducted before the widespread introduction of urodynamic studies. Therefore, these early studies almost certainly included a heterogeneous group of patients with a variety of pathologies. The lack of objective outcome measures also limits their interpretation.

Estrogens in the Treatment of Stress Incontinence

The role of estrogen in the treatment of stress incontinence is controversial, although there are a number of reported studies.[175] Some show promising results, but this may be because they were observational, not randomized, blinded, or controlled. The situation is further complicated because many types of estrogen have been used, with varying doses, routes of administration, and durations of treatment.

Two meta-analyses have helped to clarify the situation. In the first, a report by the Hormones and Urogenital Therapy Committee, examined the use of estrogens to treat all types of incontinence in postmenopausal women.[176] Of 166 articles identified that were published in English between 1969 and 1992, only 6 were controlled trials and 17 were uncontrolled series. The results showed significant subjective improvement in all patients and in those with genuine stress incontinence. However, assessment of the objective parameters showed no change in the volume of urine lost. Maximum urethral closure pressure increased significantly, but only one study showed a large effect. In the second meta-analysis, Sultana and Walters[177] reviewed 8 controlled and 14 uncontrolled prospective trials and included all types of estrogen treatment. They also found that estrogen therapy was not effective in the treatment of stress incontinence, but may be useful for the often associated symptoms of urgency and frequency.

Therefore, when given alone, estrogen does not appear to be an effective treatment for stress incontinence. However, several studies show that it may have a role in combination with other therapies (e.g., alpha-adrenoceptor agonists; discussed earlier). In a randomized trial, Ishiko and associates[178] compared the effects of the combination of pelvic floor exercise and estriol 1 mg daily in 66 patients with postmenopausal stress incontinence, and concluded that combination therapy was effective and capable of serving as first-line treatment for mild stress incontinence.

Estrogens in the Treatment of Urge Incontinence

Estrogen has been used to treat postmenopausal urgency and urge incontinence for many years, but few controlled trials confirm its benefit.[175] Estrogen has an important physiologic effect on the female lower urinary tract, and estrogen deficiency is an etiologic factor in the pathogenesis of many conditions. However, the use of estrogens alone to treat urinary incontinence has led to disappointing results.

CONCLUSION

In the last decade, the search for new therapies to treat voiding disorders has been intensive. Despite this, few drugs with modes of action other than antimuscarinic have passed the proof of concept stadium. A major problem has been to find drugs exhibiting "clinical uroselectivity," meaning a good clinical effect relative to side effects. Most drugs do not affect only the smooth or striated muscles of the bladder and bladder outlet or the reflexes/pathways controlling their activities, but have additional effects on other organ systems. This lack of selectivity is responsible for a given agent's side effects, and limits its ability to be used in dosages above a certain level. Useful drugs should not interfere with the ability to empty the bladder in a normal manner.

For control of micturition, many potential drug targets have been defined, both in the central nervous system and peripherally. However, micturition control is complex, and most probably several classes of drugs will eventually be used to treat voiding problems. Since drug development is a time-consuming process, and since the potential of the treatment targets defined so far is promising, there are reasons to believe that new drugs effective for treatment of voiding disorders will be introduced in the coming decade.

REFERENCES

1. Wein AJ: Pathophysiology and categorization of voiding dysfunction. In Walsh PC, Retik AB, Vaughan ED, Wein AJ: Campbell's Urology, 8th ed. Philadelphia, WB Saunders, 2002, pp 887–899.
2. Nour S, Svarer C, Kristensen JK, et al: Cerebral activation during micturition in normal men. Brain 123:781, 2000.
3. de Groat WC, Booth AM, Yoshimura N: Neurophysiology of micturition and its modification in animal models of human disease. In Maggi CA (ed): The Autonomic Nervous System, vol. 6: Nervous Control of the Urogenital System. Chur, Switzerland, Harwood, 1993, pp 227–289.
4. Andersson KE, Persson K: The L-arginine/nitric oxide pathway and non-adrenergic, non-cholinergic relaxation of the lower urinary tract. Gen Pharmacol 24:833, 1993.
5. Werkstrom V, Persson K, Ny L, et al: Factors involved in the relaxation of female pig urethra evoked by electrical field stimulation. Br J Pharmacol 116:1599, 1995.
6. Lincoln J, Burnstock G: Autonomic innervation of the urinary bladder and urethra. In Maggi CA (ed): The Autonomic Nervous System, vol. 6: Nervous Control of the Urogenital System, Chur, Switzerland, Harwood, 1993, pp 33–68.
7. Janig W, Morrison JF: Functional properties of spinal visceral afferents supplying abdominal and pelvic organs, with special emphasis on visceral nociception. Prog Brain Res 67:87, 1986.
8. Habler HJ, Janig W, Koltzenburg M: Activation of unmyelinated afferent fibres by mechanical stimuli and inflammation of the urinary bladder in the cat. J Physiol 425:545, 1990.
9. Fall M, Lindstrom S, Mazieres L: A bladder-to-bladder cooling reflex in the cat. J Physiol 427:281, 1990.
10. Hoyle CHV, Chapple C, Burnstock G: Isolated human bladder: Evidence for an adenine dinucleotide acting on P_{2x}-purinoceptors and for purinergic transmission. Eur J Pharmacol 174:115, 1989.
11. Cockayne DA, Hamilton SG, Zhu QM, et al: Urinary bladder hyporeflexia and reduced pain-related behaviour in P2X3-deficient mice. Nature 407:1011, 2000.
12. Smith DJ, Chapple CR: In vitro response of human bladder smooth muscle in unstable obstructed male bladders: A study of pathophysiological causes? Neurourol Urodynam 134:14, 1994.
13. Palea S, Artibani W, Ostardo E, et al: Evidence for purinergic neurotransmission in human urinary bladder affected by interstitial cystitis. J Urol 150:2007, 1993.
14. Wammack R, Weihe E, Dienes H-P, et al: Die Neurogene Blase in vitro. Aktuel Urol 26:16, 1995.
15. Yoshida M, Homma Y, Inadome A, et al: Age-related changes in cholinergic and purinergic neurotransmission in human isolated bladder smooth muscles. Exp Gerontol 36:99, 2001.
16. Caulfield MP, Birdsall NJ: International Union of Pharmacology: XVII. Classification of muscarinic acetylcholine receptors. Pharmacol Rev 50:279, 1998.
17. Bonev AD, Nelson MT: Muscarinic inhibition of ATP-sensitive K+ channels by protein kinase C in urinary bladder smooth muscle. Am J Physiol 265:C1723, 1993.
18. Hegde SS, Eglen RM: Muscarinic receptor subtypes modulating smooth muscle contractility in the urinary bladder. Life Sci 64:419, 1999.
19. Yamaguchi O, Shisda K, Tamura K, et al: Evaluation of mRNAs encoding muscarinic receptor subtypes in human detrusor muscle. J Urol 156:1208, 1996.
20. Harriss DR, Marsh KA, Birmingham AT, et al. Expression of muscarinic M3-receptors coupled to inositol phospholipid hydrolysis in human detrusor cultured smooth muscle cells. J Urol 154:1241, 1995.
21. Hegde SS, Choppin A, Bonhaus D, et al: Functional role of M2 and M3 muscarinic receptors in the urinary bladder of rats in vitro and in vivo. Br J Pharmacol 120:1409, 1997.
22. Krichevsky VP, Pagala MK, Vaydovsky I, et al. Function of M3 muscarinic receptors in the rat urinary bladder following partial outlet obstruction. J Urol 161:644, 1999.
23. Braverman A, Legos J, Young W, et al: M2 receptors in genito-urinary smooth muscle pathology. Life Sci 64:429, 1999.
24. Braverman, AS, Ruggieri MR, Pontari MA: The M2 muscarinic receptor subtype mediates cholinergic bladder contractions in patients with neurogenic bladder dysfunction (abstract 147). J Urol 165 (suppl):36, 2001.
25. Tobin G, Sjögren C: In vivo and in vitro effects of muscarinic receptor antagonists on contractions and release of [3H]acetylcholine in the rabbit urinary bladder. Eur J Pharmacol 28:1, 1995.
26. Somogyi GT, de Groat WC: Evidence for inhibitory nicotinic and facilitatory muscarinic receptors in cholinergic nerve terminals of the rat urinary bladder. J Auton Nerv Syst 37:89, 1992.
27. Alberts P: Classification of the presynaptic muscarinic receptor that regulates ^{3}H-acetylcholine secretion in the guinea pig urinary bladder in vitro. J Pharmacol Exp Ther 274:458, 1995.
28. Somogyi GT, de Groat WC: Function, signal transduction mechanisms and plasticity of presynaptic muscarinic receptors in the urinary bladder. Life Sci 64:411, 1999.
29. Brading AF: A myogenic basis for the overactive bladder. Urology 50 (suppl 6A):57, 1997.
30. de Groat WC: A neurological basis for the overactive bladder. Urology 50 (suppl 6A):36, 1997.
31. Thüroff JW, Chartier-Kastler E, Corcus J, et al: Medical treatment and medical side effects in urinary incontinence in the elderly. World J Urol 16 (suppl 1):S48, 1998.
32. Cardozo LD, Stanton SL: An objective comparison of the effects of parenterally administered drug in patients suffering from detrusor instability. J Urol 122:58, 1979.

33. Bonnesen T, Tikjøb G, Kamper AL, et al: Effect of emepronium bromide (Cetiprin) on symptoms and urinary bladder function after transurethral resection of the prostate: A double-blind randomized trial. Urol Int 39:318, 1984.
34. Zorzitto ML, Jewett MAS, Fernie GR, et al: Effectiveness of propantheline bromide in the treatment of geriatric patients with detrusor instability. Neurourol Urodynam 5:133, 1986.
35. Pietzko A, Dimpfel W, Schwantes U, et al: Influence of trospium chloride and oxybutynin on quantitative EEG in healthy volunteers. Eur J Clin Pharmacol 47:337, 1994.
36. Andersson KE, Appell R, Cardozo LD, et al: Pharmacological treatment of urinary incontinence. In Abrams P, Khoury S, Wein A (eds): Incontinence: 1st International Consultation on Incontinence. Plymouth, UK, Plymbridge, 1999, pp 447–486.
37. Andersson KE, Appell R, Cardozo LD, et al: The pharmacological treatment of urinary incontinence. BJU Int 84:923, 1999.
38. Ekström B, Andersson K-E, Mattiasson A: Urodynamic effects of intravesical instillation of atropine and phentolamine in patients with detrusor hyperactivity. J Urol 149:155, 1992.
39. Enskat R, Deaney CN, Glickman S: Systemic effects of intravesical atropine sulphate. BJU Int 87:613, 2001.
40. Andersson K-E: Current concepts in the treatment of disorders of micturition. Drugs 35:477, 1988.
41. Blaivas JG, Labib KB, Michalik J, et al: Cystometric response to propantheline in detrusor hyperreflexia: Therapeutic implications. J Urol 124:259, 1980.
42. Thüroff JW, Bunke B, Ebner A, et al: Randomized, double-blind, multicenter trial on treatment of frequency, urgency and incontinence related to detrusor hyperactivity: Oxybutynin versus propantheline versus placebo. J Urol 145:813, 1991.
43. Holmes DM, Montz FJ, Stanton SL: Oxybutinin versus propantheline in the management of detrusor instability: A patient-regulated variable dose trial. Br J Obstet Gynaecol 96:607, 1989.
44. Ückert S, Stief CG, Odenthal KP, et al: Responses of isolated normal human detrusor muscle to various spasmolytic drugs commonly used in the treatment of the overactive bladder. Arzneimittelforschung 50:456, 2000.
45. Fusgen I, Hauri D: Trospium chloride: An effective option for medical treatment of bladder overactivity. Int J Clin Pharmacol Ther 38:223, 2000.
46. Todorova A, Vonderheid-Guth B, Dimpfel W: Effects of tolterodine, trospium chloride, and oxybutynin on the central nervous system. J Clin Pharmacol 41:636, 2001.
47. Lux B, Wiedey KD: Trospium chloride (Spasmex®) in the treatment of urine incontinence. Therapiewoche 42:302, 1992.
48. Stöhrer M, Bauer P, Giannetti BM, et al: Effect of trospium chloride on urodynamic parameters in patients with detrusor hyperreflexia due to spinal cord injuries: A multicentre placebo controlled double-blind trial. Urol Int 47:138, 1991.
49. Madersbacher H, Stöhrer M, Richter R, et al: Trospium chloride versus oxybutynin: A randomized, double-blind, multicentre trial in the treatment of detrusor hyperreflexia. Br J Urol 75:452, 1995.
50. Allousi S, Laval K-U, Eckert R: Trospium chloride (Spasmo-lyt) in patients with motor urge syndrome (detrusor instability): A double-blind, randomised, multicentre, placebo-controlled study. J Clin Res 1:439, 1998.
51. Cardozo L, Chapple CR, Toozs-Hobson P: Efficacy of trospium chloride in patients with detrusor instability: A placebo-controlled, randomized, double-blind, multicentre clinical trial. BJU Int 85:659, 2000.
52. Höfner K, Halaska M, Primus G, et al: Tolerability and efficacy of trospium chloride in a long-term treatment (52 weeks) in patients with urge-syndrome: A double-blind, controlled, multicentre clinical trial. Neurourol Urodynam 19:487, 2000.
53. Jünemann KP, Al-Shukri S: Efficacy and tolerability of trospium chloride and tolterodine in 234 patients with urge-syndrome: A double-blind, placebo-controlled multicentre clinical trial. Neurourol Urodynam 19:488, 2000.
54. Clemett D, Jarvis B: Tolterodine a review of its use in the treatment of overactive bladder. Drugs Aging 18:277, 2001.
55. Nilvebrant L, Andersson K-E, Gillberg P-G, et al: Tolterodine: A new bladder selective antimuscarinic agent. Eur J Pharmacol 327:195, 1997.
56. Stahl MMS, Ekström B, Sparf B, et al: Urodynamic and other effects of tolterodine: A novel antimuscarinic drug for the treatment of detrusor overactivity. Neurourol Urodynam 14:647, 1995.
57. Nilvebrant L, Gillberg PG, Sparf B: Antimuscarinic potency and bladder selectivity of PNU-200577, a major metabolite of tolterodine. Pharmacol Toxicol 81:169, 1997.
58. Brynne N, Dalen P, Alvan G: Influence of CYP2D6 polymorphism on the pharmacokinetics and pharmacodynamics of tolterodine. Clin Pharmacol Ther 63:529, 1998.
59. Chapple CR: Muscarinic receptor antagonists in the treatment of overactive bladder. Urology (suppl 5A):33, 2000.
60. Chancellor M, Freedman S, Mitcheson HD, et al: Tolterodine, an effective and well tolerated treatment for urge incontinence and the overactive bladder symptoms. Drug Invest 19:83, 2000.
61. Van Kerrebroeck P, Kreder K, Jonas U, et al: Tolterodine once-daily: Superior efficacy and tolerability in the treatment of the overactive bladder. Urology 57:414, 2001.
62. Abrams P, Freeman R, Anderstrom C, et al: Tolterodine, a new antimuscarinic agent: As effective but better tolerated than oxybutynin in patients with an overactive bladder. Br J Urol 81:801, 1998.
63. Malone-Lee J, Shaffu B, Anand C, et al: Tolterodine: Superior tolerability than and comparable efficacy to oxybutynin in individuals 50 years old or older with overactive bladder. A randomized controlled trial. J Urol 165:1452, 2001.
64. Appell RA, Sand P, Dmochowski R, et al: Prospective randomized controlled trial of extended-release oxybutynin chloride and tolterodine tartrate in the treatment of overactive bladder: Results of the OBJECT Study. Mayo Clin Proc 76:358, 2001.
65. Wein AJ: Pharmacological agents for the treatment of urinary incontinence due to overactive bladder. Exp Opin Invest Drugs 10:65, 2001.
66. Alabaster VA: Discovery and development of selective M_3 antagonists for clinical use. Life Sci 60:1053, 1997.
67. Culp DJ, Luo W, Richardson LA, et al: Both M1 and M3 receptors regulate exocrine secretion by mucous acini. Am J Physiol 271:C1963, 1996.
68. Newgreen DT, Anderson CWP, Carter AJ, et al: Darifenacin: A novel bladder-selective agent for the treatment of urge incontinence. Neurourol Urodynam 14:95, 1995.
69. Pavia J, de Ceballos ML, Sanchez de la Cuesta F: Alzheimer's disease: Relationship between muscarinic cholinergic receptors, beta-amyloid and tau proteins. Fundam Clin Pharmacol 12:473, 1998.

70. Choppin A, Eglen RM: Pharmacological characterisation of muscarinic receptors in feline and human isolated ciliary muscle. Br J Pharmacol 129:206P, 2000.
71. Rosario DJ, Leaker BR, Smith DJ, et al: A pilot study of the effects of multiple doses of the M3 muscarinic receptor antagonist darifenacin on ambulatory parameters of detrusor activity in patients with detrusor instability. Neurourol Urodynam 14:464, 1995.
72. Mundy AR, Abrams P, Chapple CR, et al: Darifenacin, the first selective M_3 antagonist for overactive bladder: Comparison with oxybutynin on ambulatory urodynamic monitoring and salivary flow. In Proceedings of the 31st International Continence Society, International Continence Society, September 18–21, 2001.
73. Nichols D, Colli E, Goka J, et al: Darifenacin demonstrates no effect on cognitive and cardiac function: Results from a double-blind, randomised, placebo controlled study. In Proceedings of the 31st International Continence Society, International Continence Society, September 18–21, 2001.
74. Ikeda K, Kobayashi S, Suzuki M, et al: Effect of YM905, a novel muscarinic receptor antagonist, on salivary gland and bladder. Jpn J Pharmacol 76 (suppl 1):243, 1998.
75. Andersson K-E, Forman A: Effects of calcium channel blockers on urinary tract smooth muscle. Acta Pharmacol Toxicol 43 (suppl II):90, 1978.
76. Mattiasson A, Ekström B, Andersson K-E: Effects of intravesical instillation of verapamil in patients with detrusor hyperactivity. J Urol 141:174, 1989.
77. Babu R, Vaidyanathan S, Sankaranarayan A, et al: Effect of intravesical instillation of varying doses of verapamil (20 mg, 40 mg, 80 mg) upon urinary bladder function in chronic traumatic paraplegics with overactive detrusor function. Int J Clin Pharmacol 28:350, 1990.
78. Andersson K-E, Fovaeus M, Morgan E, et al: Comparative effects of five different calcium channel blockers on the atropine resistant contraction in electrically stimulated rabbit urinary bladder. Neurourol Urodynam 5:579, 1986.
79. Andersson K-E: Clinical pharmacology of potassium channel openers. Pharmacol Toxicol 70:244, 1992.
80. Komersova K, Rogerson JW, Conway EL, et al: The effect of levcromakalim (BRL 38227) on bladder function in patients with high spinal cord lesions. Br J Pharmacol 39:207, 1995.
81. Gilbert AM, Antane MM, Argentieri TM, et al: Design and SAR of novel potassium channel openers targeted for urge urinary incontinence: 2. Selective and potent benzylaminocyclobutenediones. J Med Chem 43:1203, 2000.
82. Stewart DA, Taylor J, Ghosh S, et al: Terodiline causes polymorphic ventricular tachycardia due to reduced heart rate and prolongation of QT interval. Eur J Clin Pharmacol 42:577, 1992.
83. Waldeck K, Larsson B, Andersson K-E: Comparison of oxybutynin and its active metabolite, N-desethyloxybutynin, in the human detrusor and parotid gland. J Urol 157:1093, 1997.
84. Norhona-Blob L, Kachur, JF: Enantiomers of oxybutynin: In vitro pharmacological characterization at M1, M2 and M3 muscarinic receptors and in vivo effects on urinary bladder contraction, mydriasis and salivary secretion in guinea pigs. J Pharmacol Exp Ther 256:562, 1991.
85. Hughes KM, Lang JCT, Lazare R, et al: Measurement of oxybutynin and its N-desethyl metabolite in plasma, and its application to pharmacokinetic studies in young, elderly and frail elderly volunteers. Xenobiotica 22:859, 1992.
86. Ouslander JG, Blaustein J, Connor A, et al: Pharmacokinetics and clinical effects of oxybutynin in geriatric patients. J Urol 140:47, 1988.
87. Tapp AJS, Cardozo LD, Versi E, et al: The treatment of detrusor instability in post menopausal women with oxybutynin chloride: A double blind placebo controlled study. Br J Obstet Gynaecol 97:521, 1990.
88. Amarenco G, Marquis P, McCarthy C, et al: Qualité de vie des femmes souffrant d'mpériosité mictionelle avec ou sans fuites: Étude prospective aprés traitement par oxybutinine (1701 cas). Presse Med 27:5, 1998.
89. Ouslander JG, Schnelle JF, Uman G, et al: Does oxybutynin add to the effectiveness of prompted voiding for urinary incontinence among nursing home residents? A placebo-controlled trial. J Am Geriatr Soc 43:610, 1995.
90. Szonyi G, Collas DM, Ding YY, et al: Oxybutynin with bladder retraining for detrusor instability in elderly people: A randomized controlled trial. Age Aging 24:287, 1995.
91. Kim YH, Bird ET, Priebe M, et al: The role of oxybutynin in spinal cord injured patients with indwelling catheters. J Urol 158:2083, 1996.
92. Baigrie RJ, Kelleher JP, Fawcett DP, et al: Oxybutynin: Is it safe? Br J Urol 62:319, 1988.
93. Katz IR, Sands LP, Bilker W, et al: Identification of medications that cause cognitive impairment in older people: The case of oxybutynin chloride. J Am Geriatr Soc 46:8, 1998.
94. Ouslander JG, Shih YT, Malone-Lee J, et al: Overactive bladder: Special considerations in the geriatric population. Am J Manag Care 6 (suppl 11):S599, 2000.
95. Hussain RM, Hartigan-Go K, Thomas SHL, et al: Effect of oxybutynin on the QTc interval in elderly patients with urinary incontinence. Br J Clin Pharmacol 37:485P, 1994.
96. Gupta SK, Sathyan G: Pharmacokinetics of an oral once-a-day controlled-release oxybutynin formulation compared with immediate-release oxybutynin. J Clin Pharmacol 39:289, 1999.
97. Anderson RU, Mobley D, Blank B, et al: Once daily controlled versus immediate release oxybutynin chloride for urge urinary incontinence: OROS Oxybutynin Study Group. J Urol 161:1809, 1999.
98. Versi E, Appell R, Mobley D, et al: Dry mouth with conventional and controlled-release oxybutynin in urinary incontinence. The Ditropan XL Study Group. Obstet Gynecol 95:718, 2000.
99. Birns J, Lukkari E, Malone-Lee JG: A randomized controlled trial comparing the efficacy of controlled-release oxybutynin tablets (10 mg once daily) with conventional oxybutynin tablets (5 mg twice daily) in patients whose symptoms were stabilized on 5 mg twice daily of oxybutynin. BJU Int 85:793, 2000.
100. Winkler HA, Sand PK: Treatment of detrusor instability with oxybutynin rectal suppositories. Int Urogynecol J Pelvic Floor Dysfunct 9:100, 1998.
101. Weese DL, Roskamp DA, Leach GE, et al: Intravesical oxybutynin chloride: Experience with 42 patients. Urology 41:527, 1993.
102. Buyse G, Verpoorten C, Vereecken R, et al: Treatment of neurogenic bladder dysfunction in infants and children with neurospinal dysraphism with clean intermittent (self) catheterisation and optimized intraversical oxybutynin hydrochloride therapy. Eur J Pediatr Surg 5 (suppl 1):31, 1995.
103. Madersbacher H, Knoll M: Intravesical application of oxybutynin: Mode of action in controlling detrusor hyperreflexia. Eur Urol 28:340, 1995.

104. Palmer LS, Zebold K, Firlit CF, et al: Complications of intravesical oxybutynin chloride therapy in the pediatric myelomeningocele population. J Urol 157:638, 1997.
105. Ferrara P, D'Aleo CM, Tarquini E, et al: Side-effects of oral or intravesical oxybutynin chloride in children with spina bifida. BJU Int 87:674, 2001.
106. Downie JW, Twiddy DAS, Awad SA: Antimuscarinic and noncompetitive antagonist properties of dicyclomine hydrochloride in isolated human and rabbit bladder muscle. J Pharmacol Exp Ther 201:662, 1977.
107. Castleden CM, Duffin HM, Millar AW: Dicyclomine hydrochloride in detrusor instability: A controlled clinical pilot study. J Clin Exper Gerontol 9:265, 1987.
108. Tokuno H, Chowdhury JU, Tomita T: Inhibitory effects of propiverine on rat and guinea-pig urinary bladder muscle. Naunyn Schmiedebergs Arch Pharmacol 348:659, 1993.
109. Muller C, Siegmund W, Huupponen R, et al: Kinetics of propiverine as assessed by radioreceptor assay in poor and extensive metabolizers of debrisoquine. Eur J Drug Metab Pharmacokinet 18:265, 1993.
110. Richter R, Madersbacher H, Stohrer M, et al: Double-blind, placebo-controlled clinical study of propiverine in patients suffering from detrusor hyperreflexia. International Medical Society of Paraplegia, 36th Annual Scientific Meeting, May 14–16, 1997, Innsbruck.
111. Wehnert J, Sage S: Comparative investigations to the action of Mictonorm (propiverin hydrochloride) and Spasuret (flavoxat hydrochloride) on detrusor vesicae. Z Urol Nephrol 82:259, 1989.
112. Madersbacher H, Halaska M, Voigt R, et al: A placebo-controlled, multicentre study comparing the tolerability and efficacy of propiverine and oxybutynin in patients with urgency and urge incontinence. BJU Int 84:646, 1999.
113. Stohrer M, Madersbacher H, Richter R, et al: Efficacy and safety of propiverine in SCI-patients suffering from detrusor hyperreflexia. A double-blind, placebo-controlled clinical trial. Spinal Cord 37:196, 1999.
114. Dorschner W, Stolzenburg JU, Griebenow R, et al: Efficacy and cardiac safety of propiverine in elderly patients: A double-blind, placebo-controlled clinical study. Eur Urol 37:702, 2000.
115. Oka M, Kimura Y, Itoh Y, et al: Brain pertussis toxin-sensitive G proteins are involved in the flavoxate hydrochloride-induced suppression of the micturition reflex in rats. Brain Res 727:91, 1996.
116. Caine M, Gin S, Pietra C, et al: Antispasmodic effects of flavoxate, MFCA, and Rec 15/2053 on smooth muscle of human prostate and urinary bladder. Urology 37:390, 1991.
117. Ruffmann R: A review of flavoxate hydrochloride in the treatment of urge incontinence. J Int Med Res 16:317, 1988.
118. Stanton SL: A comparison of emepronium bromide and flavoxate hydrochloride in the treatment of urinary incontinence. J Urol 110:529, 1973.
119. Chapple CR, Parkhouse H, Gardener C, et al: Double-blind, placebo controlled, cross-over study of flavoxate in the treatment of idiopathic detrusor instability. Br J Urol 66:491, 1990.
120. Perlberg S, Caine M: Adrenergic response of bladder muscle in prostatic obstruction. Urology 20:524, 1982.
121. Andersson K-E, Lepor H, Wyllie M: Prostatic α-adrenoceptors and uroselectivity. Prostate 30:202, 1997.
122. Schwinn DA, Michelotti GA: Alpha1-adrenergic receptors in the lower urinary tract and vascular bed: Potential role for the alpha1d subtype in filling symptoms and effects of ageing on vascular expression. BJU Int 85 (suppl 2):6, 2000.
123. Arnold EP: Tamsulosin in men with confirmed bladder outlet obstruction: A clinical and urodynamic analysis from a single centre in New Zealand. BJU Int 87:24, 2001.
124. Abrams P, European Tamsulosin NLUTD Study Group: Tamsulosin efficacy and safety in neurogenic lower urinary tract dysfunction (NLUTD) [abstract 1137]. J Urol 165 (suppl):276, 2001.
125. Serels S, Stein M: Prospective study comparing hyoscyamine, doxazosin, and combination therapy for the treatment of urgency and frequency in women. Neurourol Urodynam 17:31, 1998.
126. Marshall HJ, Beevers DG: Alpha-adrenoceptor blocking drugs and female urinary incontinence: Prevalence and reversibility. Br J Clin Pharmacol 42:507, 1996.
127. Larsen JJ: α-and β-adrenoceptors in the detrusor muscle and bladder base of the pig and β-adrenoceptors in the detrusor of man. Br J Urol 65:215, 1979.
128. Levin RM, Ruggieri MR, Wein AJ: Identification of receptor subtypes in the rabbit and human urinary bladder by selective radio-ligand binding. J Urol 139:844, 1988.
129. Lindholm P, Lose G: Terbutaline (Bricanyl®) in the treatment of female urge incontinence. Urol Int 41:158, 1986.
130. Grüneberger A: Treatment of motor urge incontinence with clenbuterol and flavoxate hydrochloride. Br J Obstet Gynaecol 91:275, 1984.
131. Castleden CM, Morgan B: The effect of β-adrenoceptor agonists on urinary incontinence in the elderly. Br J Clin Pharmacol 10:619, 1980.
132. Strosberg D, Pietri-Rouxel F: Function and regulation of the β3-adrenoceptor. Trends Pharmacol Sci 17:273, 1997.
133. Igawa Y, Yamazaki Y, Takeda H, et al: Relaxant effects of isoproterenol and selective beta3-adrenoceptor agonists on normal, low compliant and hyperreflexic human bladders. J Urol 165:240, 2001.
134. Lose G, Jorgensen L, Thunedborg P: Doxepin in the treatment of female detrusor overactivity: A randomized double-blind crossover study. J Urol 142:1024, 1989.
135. Hunsballe JM, Djurhuus JC: Clinical options for imipramine in the management of urinary incontinence. Urol Res 29:118, 2001.
136. Giardina EG, Bigger JT Jr, Glassman AH, et al: The electrocardiographic and antiarrhythmic effects of imipramine hydrochloride at therapeutic plasma concentrations. Circulation 60:1045, 1979.
137. Baldessarini KJ: Drugs in the treatment of psychiatric disorders. In Gilman A, Goodman LS, Rall TW, Murad F et al (eds): The Pharmacological Basis of Therapeutics, 7th ed. New York, McMillan, 1985, pp 387–445.
138. Leslie CA, Pavlakis AJ, Wheeler JS, et al: Release of arachidonate cascade products by the rabbit bladder: Neurophysiological significance? J Urol 132:376, 1984.
139. Downie JW, Karmazyn M: Mechanical trauma to bladder epithelium liberates prostnoids which modulate neurotransmission in rabbit detrusor muscle. J Pharmacol Exp Ther 230:445, 1994.
140. Andersson K-E, Bengtsson B, Paulsen O: Desamino-8-D-arginine vasopressin (DDAVP): Pharmacology and clinical use. Drugs Today 24:509, 1988.
141. Neveus T, Lackgren G, Tuvemo T, et al: Enuresis: Background and treatment. Scand J Urol Nephrol Suppl 206:1, 2000.
142. Hjalmas K: Desmopressin treatment: Current status. Scand J Urol Nephrol Suppl 202:70, 1999.

143. Moffat ME, Harlos S, Kirshen AJ, et al: Desmopressin acetate and nocturnal enuresis: How much do we know? Pediatrics 92:420, 1993.
144. Skoog SJ, Stokes A, Turner KL: Oral desmopressin: A randomized double-blind placebo controlled study of effectiveness in children with primary nocturnal enuresis. J Urol 158:1035, 1997.
145. Hilton P, Hertogs K, Stanton SL: The use of desmopressin (DDAVP) for nocturia in women with multiple sclerosis. J Neurol Neurosurg Psychiatry 46:854, 1983.
146. Kinn A-C, Larsson PO: Desmopressin: A new principle for symptomatic treatment of urgency and incontinence in patients with multiple sclerosis. Scand J Urol Nephrol 24:109, 1990.
147. Horowitz M, Combs AJ, Gerdes D: Desmopressin for nocturnal incontinence in the spina bifida population. J Urol 158:2267, 1997.
148. Weiss J, Blaivas JG, Abrams P, et al: Oral desmopressin (Miririn, DDAVP) in the treatment of nocturia in men (abstract 1030). J Urol 165 (suppl):250, 2001.
149. Van Kerrebroeck P, Bäckström T, Blaivas JG, et al: Oral desmopressin (Miririn, DDAVP) in the treatment of nocturia in women (abstract 1031). J Urol 165 (suppl):250, 2001.
150. Schwab M, Ruder H: Hyponatraemia and cerebral convulsion due to DDAVP administration in patients with enuresis nocturna or urine concentration testing. Eur J Pediatr 156:668, 1997.
151. Steers WD, Meythaler JM, Haworth C, et al: Effects of acute bolus and chronic continuous intrathecal baclofen on genitourinary dysfunction due to spinal cord pathology. J Urol 148:1849, 1992.
152. Maggi CA: The dual, sensory and "efferent" function of the capsaicin-sensitive primary sensory neurons in the urinary bladder and urethra. In Maggi CA (ed): The Autonomic Nervous System, vol. 3: Nervous Control of the Urogenital System. Chur, Switzerland, Harwood, 1993, pp 383–422.
153. Szallasi A: The vanilloid (capsaicin) receptor: Receptor types and species differences. Gen Pharmacol 25:223, 1994.
154. Kuo H-C: Inhibitory effect of capsaicin on detrusor contractility: Further study in the presence of ganglionic blocker and neurokinin receptor antagonist in the rat urinary bladder. Urol Int 59:95, 1997.
155. Maggi CA, Barbanti G, Santicioli P, et al: Cystometric evidence that capsaicin-sensitive nerves modulate the afferent branch of micturition reflex in humans. J Urol 142:150, 1989.
156. Igawa Y, Komiyama I, Nishizawa S, et al: Intravesical capsaicin inhibits autonomic dysreflexia in patients with spinal cord injury. Neurourol Urodynam 15:374, 1996.
157. Fowler CJ, Jewkes D, McDonald WI, et al: Intravesical capsaicin for neurogenic bladder dysfunction. Lancet 339:1239, 1992.
158. DeRidder D, Chandiramani V, Dasgupta P, et al: Intravesical capsaicin as a treatment for refractory detrusor hyperreflexia: A dual center study with long-term followup. J Urol 158:2087, 1997.
159. Cruz F: Desensitization of bladder sensory fibers by intravesical capsaicin or capsaicin analogs: A new strategy for treatment of urge incontinence in patients with spinal detrusor hyperreflexia or bladder hypersensitivity disorders. Int Urogynecol J Pelvic Floor Dysfunct 9:214, 1998.
160. Smith CP, Somogyi GT, Chancellor MB: Emerging role of botulinum toxin in the treatment of neurogenic and non-neurogenic voiding dysfunction. Curr Urol Rep 3(5):382, 2002.
161. Gnad H, Burmucic R, Petritsch P, et al: Conservative therapy of female stress incontinence: Double-blind study with the alpha-sympathomimetic midodrin. Fortschr Med 102:578, 1984 (in German).
162. Lose G, Lindholm D: Clinical and urodynamic effects of norfenefrine in women with stress incontinence. Urol Int 39:298, 1984.
163. Collste L, Lindskog M: Phenylpropanolamine in treatment of female stress urinary incontinence: Double-blind placebo controlled study in 24 patients. Urology 40:398, 1987.
164. Siltberg H, Larsson G, Hallen B, et al: Validation of cough-induced leak point pressure measurement in the evaluation of pharmacological treatment of stress incontinence. Neurourol Urodynam 18:591, 1999.
165. Ahlström K, Sandahl B, Sjöberg B, et al: Effect of combined treatment with phenylpropanolamine and estriol, compared with estriol treatment alone, in postmenopausal women with stress urinary incontinence. Gynecol Obstet Invest 30:37, 1990.
166. Hilton P, Tweddel AL, Mayne C: Oral and intravaginal estrogens alone and in combination with alpha adrenergic stimulation in genuine stress incontinence. Int Urogynecol J 12:80, 1990.
167. Yasuda K, Kawabe K, Takimoto, et al, and the Clenbutrol Clinical Research Group: A double-blind clinical trial of a β-adrenergic agonist in stress incontinence. Int Urogynecol J 4:146, 1993.
168. Thor KB, Katofiasc MA: Effects of duloxetine, a combined serotonin and norepinephrine reuptake inhibitor, on central neural control of lower urinary tract function in the chloralose-anesthetized femal cat. J Pharmacol Exp Ther 274:1014, 1995.
169. Zinner N, Sarshik S, Yalcin I, et al: Efficacy and safety of duloxetine in stress urinary incontinent patients: Double-blind, placebo-controlled multiple dose study. ICS 28th Annual Meeting, Jerusalem, Israel, September 14–17, 1998.
170. Wein AJ, Longhurst PA, Levin RM: Pharmacologic treatment of voiding dysfunction. In Mundy AR, Stephenson TP, Wein AJ (eds): Urodynamics: Principles, Practice, and Application, 2nd ed, 1994, pp 43–70.
171. Abrams P, Blaivas JG, Stanton SL, et al: The standardisation of terminology of lower urinary tract function. Br J Obstet Gynecol 97:1, 1990.
172. Bergman A, Karram MM, Bhatia NN: Changes in urethral cytology following estrogen administration. Gynecol Obstet Invest 29:211, 1990.
173. Karram MM, Yeko TR, Sauer MV, et al: Urodynamic changes following hormone replacement therapy in women with premature ovarian failure. Obstet Gynecol 74:208, 1989.
174. Salmon UL, Walter RI, Gast SH: The use of estrogens in the treatment of dysuria and incontinence in postmenopausal women. Am J Obstet Gynecol 14:23, 1941.
175. Hextall A: Oestrogens and lower urinary tract function. Maturitas 36:83, 2000.
176. Fantl JA, Cardozo LD, McClish DK, et al: Estrogen therapy in the management of urinary incontinence in postmenopausal women: A meta-analysis. First report of the Hormones and Urogenital Therapy Committee. Obstet Gynecol 83:12, 1994.
177. Sultana CJ, Walters MD: Estrogen and urinary incontinence in women. Maturitas 20:129, 1990.
178. Ishiko O, Hirai K, Sumi T, et al: Hormone replacement therapy plus pelvic floor muscle exercise for postmenopausal stress incontinence: A randomized, controlled trial. J Reprod Med 46:213, 2001.

Surgical Treatment of Stress Urinary Incontinence in Women

CHRISTOPHER E. KELLY ■ PHILLIPE E. ZIMMERN

SURGICAL MANAGEMENT OF STRESS URINARY INCONTINENCE

Surgical Management of Urethral Hypermobility

Retropubic Suspensions

Indications and Techniques

The goal of surgery for stress urinary incontinence (SUI) caused by urethral hypermobility is to stabilize the bladder neck and proximal urethra to prevent sudden descent when intra-abdominal pressure increases. A more controversial indication is to offer prophylaxis against urethral hypermobility during procedures to repair anterior compartment or vault prolapse.[1]

Urethral hypermobility can be corrected with a retropubic approach. Indications for this approach are concomitant abdominal surgery and vaginal pathology (e.g., stenosis) precluding a direct vaginal approach. Patient preference and the surgeon's level of familiarity with retropubic or vaginal procedures can also affect the final decision.

The Marshall-Marchetti-Krantz (MMK) and Burch colposuspension procedures are the two most common retropubic procedures. In the original MMK procedure, double-bite sutures that incorporate paravaginal tissues and the vaginal wall are taken on either side of the urethra, bladder neck, and anterior bladder wall.[2] These sutures are anchored into the cartilage of the symphysis pubis or periosteum on the posterior aspect of the pubis. Inserting fingers into the vagina to elevate the anterior vaginal wall helps to bring the bladder neck in contact with the pubis while the sutures are tied down.

The Burch procedure[3] and its modifications[4-6] involve placing two to four sets of absorbable sutures into the anterior vaginal wall, on either side of the proximal urethra and at the bladder neck. These suspension sutures are secured to Cooper's ligament and tied while the anterior vaginal wall is elevated to avoid excessive tension. In a successful procedure, the anterior vaginal wall acts as a broad sling that supports the bladder neck and proximal urethra.[7]

Results

Table 40-1 summarizes studies with the longest follow-up data on the MMK and Burch retropubic suspensions. Both procedures have success rates of 70% to 90%. Factors that appear to limit their success include previous incontinence surgery and preoperative detrusor instability.[8]

Transvaginal Needle Suspensions

Introduction and Techniques

In 1959, Pereyra described the first transvaginal needle suspension to correct SUI caused by urethral hypermobility.[9] Table 40-2 lists variations of the original suspension procedure and outlines their unique features. All of the procedures that have been introduced since the Pereyra technique have incorporated cystoscopic assessment to verify suture placement and exclude penetration or injury of the bladder wall.

Results

The initial results with transvaginal needle suspension were excellent. However, this enthusiasm did not last. Long-term results have been disappointing, with "dry" rates ranging from 53% to 79%. Thus, fewer needle suspension procedures are being performed.[10] However, the Raz four-corner suspension and its variants (e.g., in situ vaginal wall sling,[11] anterior vaginal wall suspension[12]), all of which incorporate the vaginal wall as an anchor, continue to have their proponents.

Complications of Retropubic and Transvaginal Suspension Procedures

Complications associated with retropubic and transvaginal needle suspensions can be categorized according to whether they occur intraoperatively, early, or late.

TABLE 40-1 ■ Long-term Results of Marshall-Marchetti-Krantz (MMK) and Burch Retropubic Suspensions

Procedure	Study	No. of Patients	Mean Follow-up (mo)	Results
MMK	Milani et al[83] (1985)	42	39 (22–73)	Cured (71%)
	Mainprize and Drutz[18] (1988)	2712	Unclear	Cured and improved (89%)
	Colombo et al[84] (1994)	40	42 (24–84)	Subjective cure (85%)
				Objective cure (65%)
Burch colposuspension				
	Eriksen et al[85] (1990)	86	60	Cured and improved (63%)
				De novo instability (26%)
	Herbertsson and Iosif[86] (1993)	72	67 (96–144)	Cured and improved (90%)
	Alcalay et al[21] (1995)	109	165 (120–240)	Cured and improved (69%)
	Kinn[87] (1995)	141	60 (38–102)	Cured and improved (89%)
	Drouin et al[88] (1999)	79	91 (63–130)	Cured and improved (69%)

Intraoperative injuries to the bladder and urethra can occur with either approach, although they are more common in patients with previous retropubic surgery. Ureteric injury is rare, and has been mainly associated with MMK and Burch procedures.[13,14] Cystoscopy to confirm efflux of intravenously administered methylene blue can help to exclude ureteral injury. Although blood loss is seldom reported, the incidence of significant blood loss requiring transfusion is rare.

Nerve injury can be categorized as secondary to nerve entrapment or secondary to nerve compression (from either insufficient padding or nonphysiologic positioning). Entrapment of the sensory branches of the ilioinguinal nerve or the genital branch of the genitofemoral nerve can occur when suspension sutures are passed too far laterally and tied tightly over the anterior rectus sheath, or when bone anchors are drilled too closely to the nerve.[5,15]

Outflow obstruction, a complication of retropubic suspension, is caused by urethral overcorrection or by placement of sutures too close to the urethral wall, which results in distortion.[16] De novo detrusor instability ranges from 7% to 27%, and may be related to obstruction or disruption of the autonomic nerves around the urethrovesical junction.[17] Osteitis pubis occurs in up to 2.5% of MMK procedures.[18] Burch[19] and others[20–22] report a significant incidence of secondary enterocele. In some studies, the rate is as high as 26%.

Surgical Management of Intrinsic Urethral Deficiency

Pubovaginal Sling

Introduction

Von Giordano[23] first described the use of the pubovaginal sling procedure to treat urinary incontinence in 1907. Not surprisingly, since that time, the technique and choice of materials have evolved. Among autologous materials, only the fascia lata, rectus fascia, and vaginal wall are currently used. Other sling materials include cadaveric fascia and newer synthetics.[24,25] These materials are discussed later in this chapter.

The traditional indication for a pubovaginal sling procedure is SUI as a result of intrinsic sphincteric deficiency (ISD). Recently, however, indications have broadened to include SUI as a result of urethral hypermobility (type II), with or without ISD.[26–30]

Technique

Although individual techniques vary, all pubovaginal sling techniques share some fundamental features:

- Adequate proximal urethral and bladder neck exposure is crucial, regardless of the method of anterior vaginal wall dissection (i.e., inverted U-shaped flap,[31] midline incision,[32] parallel bladder neck incision,[33] sandwich technique[34]).

Table 40-2 ■ Technical Differences among Various Transvaginal Needle Suspensions

Procedure (Year)	Support	Retropubic Dissection	Needle Passage	Suture Exposed on Vaginal Side	Foreign Material
Pereyra (1959)	PUT	No	Blind	Yes	Steel wire
Modified Pereyra (1967)	EPF	Yes	Finger control	No	NAS
Stamey (1973)	PCF	No	Blind	No	Pledgets and NAS
Raz (1981)	EPF/AVW	Yes	Finger control	No	None
Gittes (1987)	AVW (FT)	No	Blind	Yes	NAS
Four-corner suspension (1994)	EPF/PUT	Yes	Finger control	No	None
Bone Fixation (1994)	AVW (FT)	No	Blind	Yes	Bone anchor or NAS
AVWS (1997)	AVW	Yes	Finger control	No	None

AVW, anterior vaginal wall; AVWS, anterior vaginal wall suspension; EPF, endopelvic fascia; FT, full thickness; NAS, nonabsorbable suture; PCF, pubocervical fascia; PUT, periurethral tissue.

- Fixation of the sling with suture material is crucial to prevent sling migration, rolling, or bunching, all of which could cause obstruction, persistent incontinence, or erosion (Figs. 40-1 and 40-2).
- The choice of sling material is important (Table 40-3).
- The significance of sling length has not been established. Sling length varies from a long fascial strip attached to itself over an abdominal fascial bridge[35] to a small patch of sling material secured beneath the proximal urethra. However, the use of smaller strips of autologous fascia decreases skin incision length, operative harvesting time, and the overall morbidity of the procedure.
- Whether to anchor the sling to a fixed point (i.e., the pubis) or to a more compliant surface (i.e., the anterior rectus fascia[36]) is debated. Neither technique shows a significant increase in cure rate. Advantages of anchoring the sling to the pubis include the stability of the pubis and the minimal need for retropubic dissection. Disadvantages include the potential risk of infection (osteitis pubis and osteomyelitis) and the limited data on durability. Conversely, securing the sling to the anterior rectus sheath has proven durability. Moreover, the compliant nature of the sheath may decrease the likelihood of suture pull-through. Disadvantages of using the rectus fascia include the need for greater retropubic dissection and the risk of nerve entrapment.
- The need for retropubic dissection during a pubovaginal sling procedure is also debated. To some clinicians, this type of dissection is attractive because it allows finger guidance during retropubic suture transfer with a ligature carrier. Moreover, it promotes the formation of retropubic scarring, which may enhance the strong support from the sling. Opponents of retropubic dissection argue that avoiding dissection can minimize the risks of blood loss and bladder injury while preserving existing urethropelvic support and innervation.[37]
- No standardized adjustment exists to create sling tension. Cough or Crede maneuvers,[38] intraoperative urodynamic measurements,[39] adjustment until hypermobility ceases,[28] suture knot spacing techniques,[30] and endoscopic "tricks"[33,40,41] are used to achieve the correct sling tension. However, the rate of postoperative chronic retention is 6% to 11% and the rate of persistent stress incontinence is 5%, indicating that a reliable and reproducible method for placing proper tension has yet to be identified.[42]

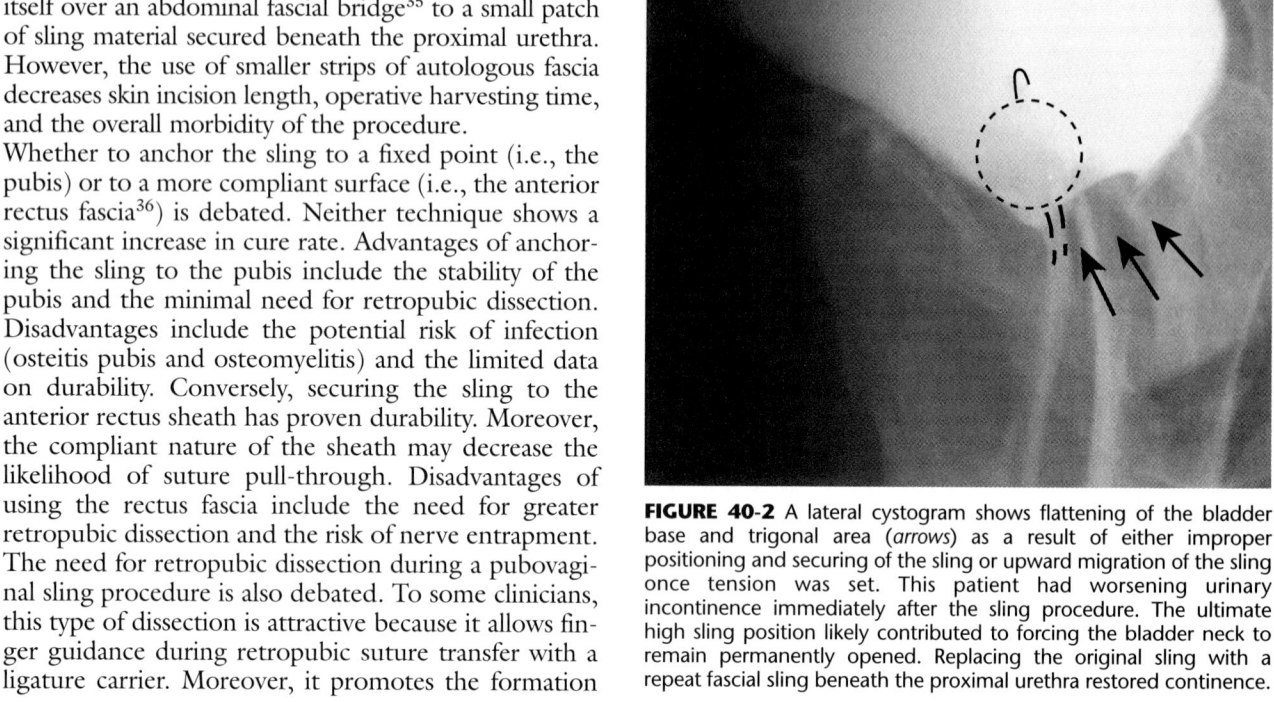

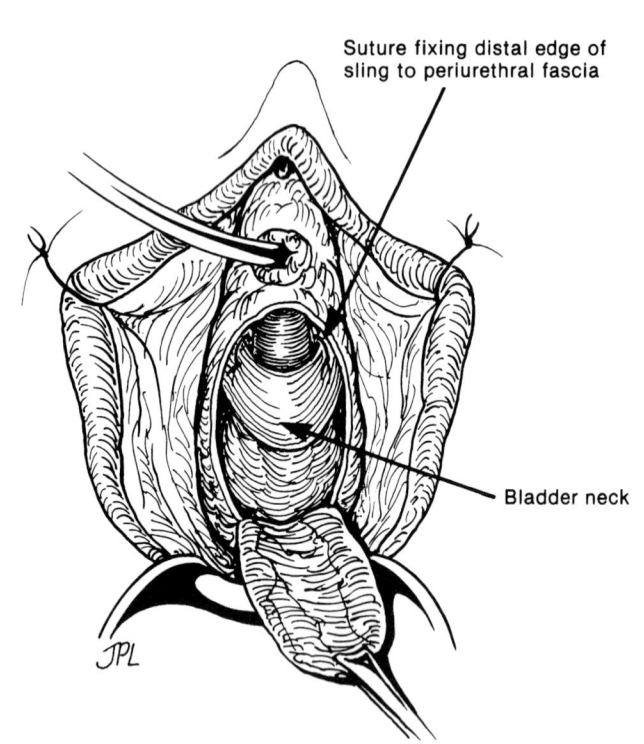

FIGURE 40-2 A lateral cystogram shows flattening of the bladder base and trigonal area (*arrows*) as a result of either improper positioning and securing of the sling or upward migration of the sling once tension was set. This patient had worsening urinary incontinence immediately after the sling procedure. The ultimate high sling position likely contributed to forcing the bladder neck to remain permanently opened. Replacing the original sling with a repeat fascial sling beneath the proximal urethra restored continence.

FIGURE 40-1 Successful outcome depends greatly on proper positioning and suturing of the fascial sling beneath the proximal urethra. However, sling tension is also crucial, and unfortunately, there is no reproducible technique for adjusting sling tension. (From Leach GE, Sirls L: Pubovaginal sling procedures. Atlas Urol Clin North Am 2(1):61–71, 1994.)

Results

Based on an extensive meta-analysis of 282 articles, the Female Stress Urinary Incontinence Clinical Guidelines Panel reported an overall cure or dry rate of 83% and an overall cure, dry, or improvement rate of 85% to 91% for pubovaginal slings.[42]

Complications

The complication rate for pubovaginal sling procedure is 2% to 29%. The incidence of transient urinary retention (lasting >4 weeks) is approximately 8% (range, 6%–11%), whereas permanent urinary retention occurs in fewer than 5% of patients.[41] Other significant

TABLE 40-3 ■ Pros and Cons of Various Pubovaginal Sling Materials

Type of Material	Pros	Cons
Autologous (fascial slings, in situ vaginal wall)	Easily available Biocompatible Cost-effective	Harvesting morbidity (wound complications, pain) except for in situ sling Longer operative time
Cadaveric	Easily available Length and side adjustment Orthopedic outcome data available No harvesting Shorter procedure	Tensile strength unknown Potential risk of infection (HIV, prions) Cost Durability and efficacy unknown Cost
Synthetic	Easily available Length and size adjustment No harvesting Shorter procedure	Durability and efficacy unknown Risk of urethral, bladder neck, or vaginal erosion and infection

HIV, human immunodeficiency virus.

complications are de novo urge or urge incontinence (range, 3%–45%) and worsening urge (range, 13%–68%).[42] Such urgency is related to detrusor overactivity and could herald bladder outlet obstruction. Rarer complications include wound dehiscence, common peroneal nerve injury (fascia lata harvesting) or nerve entrapment, bleeding, and urethral or vaginal erosion.

Prosthetic slings have been particularly associated with infection, erosion,[43] and fistula formation. The incidence of these complications appears to vary with the type and size of the material used. Polymeric silicon, polytetrafluoroethylene (Gore-Tex, Gore, Newark, DE), and polyester slings (ProteGen) have the highest incidence of infection or erosion, with rates ranging from 11% to 18%.[44-47] Efforts to reduce the rate of infection or erosion of synthetic slings by reducing the amount of material used, decreasing vaginal exposure time, and using antimicrobial mesh have been described.[29,48]

Artificial Urinary Sphincter

Introduction

The artificial urinary sphincter (AUS) is infrequently recommended for the treatment of ISD in women. Candidates for the AUS should have the mental capacity, motivation, and manual dexterity needed to manipulate the device. The AUS is most suitable for patients with pure ISD, a stable bladder with normal capacity and compliance, and no vesicoureteral reflux. The AUS may be ideal for patients with ISD and detrusor hypocontractility, in whom the risk of permanent retention after the pubovaginal sling procedure is high. Contraindications to the AUS include previous irradiation to the sphincter area, steroid dependency,[49] chronic and frequent need for instrumentation or manipulation of the urinary tract (e.g. active stone disease),[50] uncontrolled detrusor hyper-reflexia, and high-grade vesicoureteral reflux.

The current model, the AMS Sphincter 800, is composed of an inflatable, polyester (Dacron, DuPont, Wilmington, DE)-reinforced cuff; a pressure-regulating balloon; and a manual pump. Recent modifications to the AUS include a deactivation button; a surface-treated silicone urethral cuff designed to reduce urethral erosion; color-coded, kink-resistant tubing; and various connectors.[51]

Technique

The most common approach used for the AUS procedure is abdominal, although other approaches, such as the transvaginal approach[52,53] and the combined suprapubic transvaginal approach,[54] have been described. Critical intraoperative steps include meticulous urethral dissection, cuff sizing, pump placement, perfusion sphincterometry (optional), and deactivation.

In the abdominal approach, dissection around the bladder neck is begun with two parallel incisions of the endopelvic fascia on either side of the bladder neck. Methods to achieve the circumferential dissection include using a Cutter[50] or right-angle clamp, making an anterior cystotomy,[51] dissecting above the urethral meatus,[51] and proceeding anterograde from the vaginal apex.[55,56] The cuff is then sized (range, 4–11 cm long). A 61- to 70-cm H_2O balloon reservoir is often used for bladder neck cuffs. The pump is usually placed into a subcutaneous labia majoral pocket on the side of the patient's preference supersedes this general rule.

The device is tested intraoperatively with perfusion sphincterometry to identify unrecognized urethral injury and document appropriate function of the AUS.[57] The pump is deactivated for 4 to 6 weeks to allow for primary healing at the cuff site before intermittent compression begins.

Results

The few available studies report dry rates of 59% to 100% and patient satisfaction rates of 78% to 100%. Table 40-4 shows the long-term results of the AUS.

Complications

The most significant intraoperative complication during AUS placement is injury to the urethra, bladder, and vagina during dissection. During dissection, palpation of the area between the urethral catheter and the pre-placed vaginal pack can assist in localizing the proper plane for cuff placement (Fig. 40-3). Some authors report that repair of vaginal or urethral injuries can be followed by immediate dissection of another suburethral plane without compromising the final result.[58]

Late complications associated with the AUS in women are similar to those in men, and can be classified under the general headings of infection, erosion, and mechanical malfunction. Reported rates of infection and mechanical failure in women are similar to those in men.[59,60] Placing the cuff transvaginally does not appear to increase the infection rate.[50,54] The cuff erosion rate in women is approximately 2.3%,[60] and is commonly attributed to vascular compromise, infection, or unrecognized intraoperative injury. Erosion may be more common in women because, unlike men, the bladder neck or proximal urethral tissues have undergone multiple previous

TABLE 40-4 ■ Artificial Urinary Sphincter: Long-term Results

Study	No. of Patients	Mean Follow-up (mo)	Dry (%)	Satisfied (%)	Reoperations(%)
Diokno et al[89] (1987)	32	30	91	NA	21
Appell[54] (1988)	34	>36 (56% of patients)	100	100	3
Webster et al[90] (1992)	24	31	92	100	17
Stone et al[91] (1995)	54	67	59	78	18
Heitz et al[92] (1997)	144	Unclear	86	86	3
Costa et al[93] (1998)	141*	37	79	NA	9
Venn et al[59] (2000)	30	120	73	NA	80

*Non-neurogenic patients.
NA, not applicable.

anti-incontinence procedures and, therefore, may be at risk for poor wound healing.[61]

SURGICAL MANAGEMENT OF VAGINAL PROLAPSE

Surgery for Anterior Vaginal Wall Prolapse

Introduction

Cystocele, which is commonly associated with urethral hypermobility, occurs because of lateral or central defects in the pubocervical fascia. Various classification systems have been described (Table 40-5). For this chapter, we have adopted the halfway system of Baden and Walker, which is practical and widely used. Other systems, such as the International Continence Society System (POPQ[62]), which was recently challenged by Scotti and associates[63] are useful for research purposes, but cumbersome in clinical practice.

Indications for cystocele repair are symptomatic prolapse, associated stress incontinence, hydronephrosis, and outflow obstruction with incomplete emptying. The natural history and risk of progression of cystocele are unknown.[64] For this reason, debate exists as to whether a grade 1 cystocele should be observed or repaired[65] with a bladder neck suspension procedure. Grade 2 and 4 cystoceles can be repaired transabdominally or transvaginally with various procedures (Table 40-6).

Cystocele Repair: Abdominal Approach

The abdominal approach to cystocele repair is sometimes preferable in patients who need concurrent abdominal surgery or hernia repair, those with ovarian or uterine pathology, and those with recurrent anterior compartment or vault prolapse requiring mesh interposition. Although the Burch procedure is designed to resuspend the relaxed anterior vaginal wall, not to repair the actual fascial defect, it shows good long-term results in most series.[21] This technique produces better results in patients with mild to moderate cystocele than in those with severe cystocele.[66]

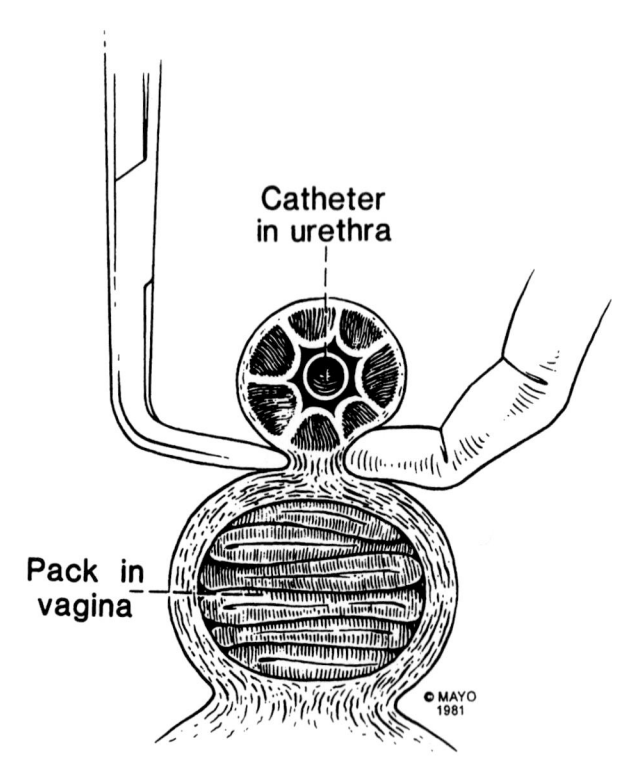

FIGURE 40-3 Performing circumferential dissection of the female urethra before placement of an artificial urinary sphincter can be challenging if the patient has scar tissue from previous anti-incontinence procedures. The use of a preplaced vaginal pack can help to identify the plane between the undersurface of the urethra and the anterior vaginal wall. (From Petrou SP, Elliott DS, Barrett DM: Artificial urethral sphincter for incontinence. Urology 56:353–359, 2000.)

TABLE 40-5 ■ Classification Systems for Pelvic Organ Prolapse

Study	Classification	Grading	Method
Baden and Walker[94] (1972)	Halfway system	0-4	Physical examination
Raz and Erickson[95] (1992)	SEAPI incontinence score	0-3	Physical examination and lateral cystogram
Bump et al[62] (1996)	Pelvic organ prolapse quantitation (POPQ)	0-4 and grid	Physical examination with precise measurements
Scotti et al[63] (2000)	Scotti	0-4 and grid	Physical examination with precise measurements

SEAPI, Stress, Emptying, Anatomic, Protection, and Instability

TABLE 40-6 ■ Technical Differences among Various Cystocele Repair Approaches

Approach	Procedure	Cystocele Grade (Baden System)	Defect Fixed	Support	Anchor	Retropubic Dissection	Foreign Material
Abdominal	Burch colposuspension	I-II	No	Vaginal wall	ARF	Yes	No
	Paravaginal repair	I-II	Lateral	Lateral vaginal sulcus	ATFP	Yes	No
	Sacrocolpopexy	II-IV	Central	Vaginal cuff or AVW	Sacrum	No	Mesh, or occasionally bone anchors
Vaginal	Four-corner suspension	II-III	No	Bladder neck and PCF or CL	ARF	Yes	No
	AVWS	II-III	No	Bladder neck and PCF or CL	ARF	Yes	No
Anterior colporrhaphy		II-IV	Central	PCF	PCF	No	No
	Polypropylene mesh (Nicita, 1998)[74]	II-IV	Central	Mesh	ATFP	Limited	Mesh
	Cadaveric fascia lata (Kobashi et al, 2000)[65]	II-IV	Central or lateral	Mesh	ATFP or pubis	Limited	Cadaveric tissue and bone anchors

ARF, anterior rectus fascia; ATFP, arcus tendinous fascia pelvis; AVW, anterior vaginal wall; AVWS, anterior vaginal wall suspension; CL, cardinal ligament; PCF, pubocervical fascia.

Paravaginal repair, a technique popularized by Richardson and colleagues,[67] corrects the lateral fascial defect by using a series of interrupted nonabsorbable sutures to reapproximate the anterolateral vaginal sulcus to the pelvic side wall at the level of the arcus tendineus fasciae pelvis. When SUI as a result of urethral hypermobility coexists with a large cystocele, a Burch colposuspension can be added to the paravaginal repair to stabilize the urethra. Paravaginal repair, although traditionally a retropubic procedure, has been described using a transvaginal approach.[68,69]

Sacral colpopexy, which was designed to correct vault prolapse, can include an anterior mesh extension between the bladder base and vaginal wall.[70] Various mesh materials have been advocated (autologous, allogenic, or synthetic).

Cystocele Repair: Vaginal Approach

The four-corner suspension procedure,[71] which is an extension of the modified Pereyra bladder neck suspension, resuspends the anterior vaginal wall without repairing the fascial defect. One set of suspension sutures is placed on either side of the proximal urethra and bladder neck, and another set is placed on either side of the cystocele bulge at the apex, incorporating the vaginal wall, pubocervical fascia, and cardinal ligaments.[72] The four sets of sutures are transferred suprapubically with a ligature carrier and secured to the anterior rectus fascia. Anterior vaginal wall suspension, a modification of four-corner suspension, incorporates more of the anterior vaginal wall, with continuous helical bites from the vaginal apex to the bladder neck. With this technique, sutures are not placed near the urethra, avoiding the risk of obstruction[12] (Fig. 40-4).

Traditional anterior colporrhaphy can correct moderate to severe cystocele by reapproximating the pubocervical fascia beneath the reduced herniated bladder. However,

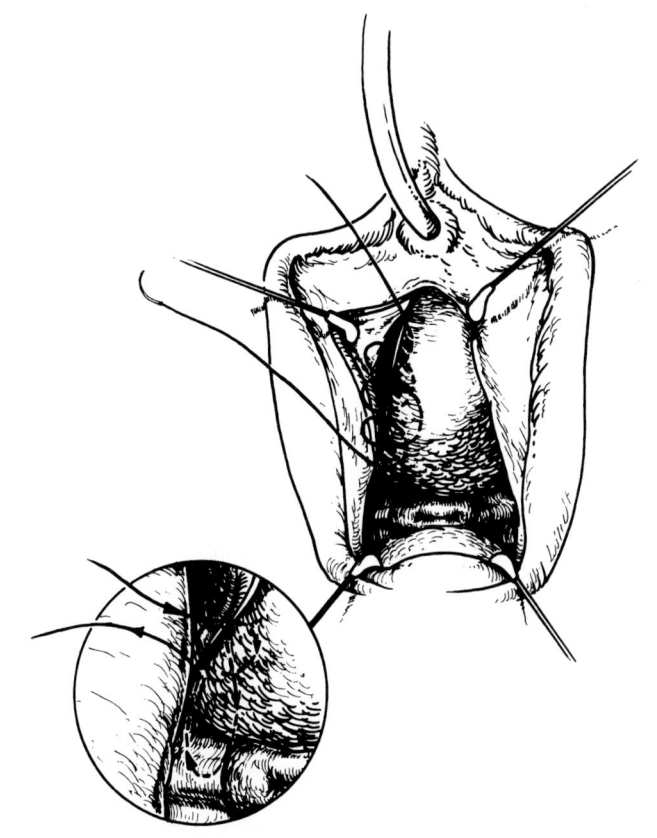

FIGURE 40-4 The goals of anterior vaginal wall suspension are to correct laxity of the anterior vaginal wall and to stabilize the proximal urethra and bladder neck while supporting the bladder base (to reduce the cystocele). Bladder neck suspension sutures incorporate the anterior vaginal wall (excluding the epithelium) lateral to, and on each side of, the bladder neck, with several passes of nonabsorbable suture. More proximal sutures, placed closer to the vaginal apex, are placed in the anterior vaginal wall and the cardinal ligaments (or the cuff, in patients who have undergone hysterectomy).

this procedure may be challenging when the fascia is weak or poorly defined. Because anterior colporrhaphy does not adequately support the urethra or bladder neck, it is often used in conjunction with anti-incontinence procedures (e.g., transvaginal bladder neck suspension or sling) when cystocele and SUI coexist.

Newer procedures involve adding a support beneath the formal cystocele repair before vaginal closure is performed. This support can be absorbable,[71,73] or made of polypropylene[74] or cadaveric fascia.[65] Nicita[74] and Migliari and colleagues[75] recently described a method to repair moderate to severe cystoceles with a polypropylene mesh hammock anchored laterally between the two arcus tendineus of the endopelvic fascia and anteroposteriorly between the bladder neck and cervix. Kobashi and Leach[65] recently used a broad piece of cadaveric fascia lata as a urethral sling to correct the cystocele.

Results

Table 40-7 shows the long-term surgical results of the various techniques described.

Complications

Intraoperative complications of cystocele repair include bleeding and injuries, mostly to the bladder or ureter. Cystoscopy with intravenous indigo carmine is critical for the assessment of bladder integrity and ureteral patency. Ureteral injury, a major concern during anterior colporrhaphy and mesh procedures, is rarely seen with four-corner or anterior vaginal wall suspension because there is no formal bladder base dissection. Short- and long-term complications are similar to those for surgery for urethral hypermobility (discussed earlier). Other complications include sacral osteomyelitis after sacrocolpopexy,[76] dyspareunia, obstruction of the small bowel, decreased vaginal length, and erosion of mesh into the vagina,[77] bladder, or sigmoid colon.[78]

Surgical Management of Rectocele

Introduction

A rectocele is a herniation of the rectum through the posterior vaginal wall. This defect is often seen in multiparous women, possibly as a result of stretching of the posterior wall during vaginal childbirth.[79] Patients are often asymptomatic, and are typically diagnosed during evaluation for another symptom (i.e., SUI or prolapse). However, some have vaginal protrusion, difficulty defecating, constipation, dyspareunia, or the need for manually assisted stool evacuation.[80] Constipation rarely causes rectocele, although they may coexist.

During vaginal examination, a single speculum blade is used to retract the anterior vaginal wall upward while the patient bears down. Rectal examination may detect

TABLE 40-7 ■ Comparison of Surgical Outcomes among Cystocele Repair Approaches in Large Series

Approach	Procedure	Study	No. of Patients	Mean Follow-up (mo)	Results at Follow-up	Outcome Measure
Abdominal						
	Burch colposuspension	Wiskind et al[96] (1992)	131	61 (36-168)	Mild cystocele or less (72%)	PE
		Alcalay et al[21] (1995)	109	66 (120-240)	Grade II cystocele or less (96%)	PE
		Colombo et al[66] (2000)	35	60	Grade I cystocele or less (66%)	PE
	Paravaginal repair	Richardson et al[67] (1976)	60	20 (3-48)	Cured (92%)	PE
		Shull and Baden[97] (1989)	149	(6-48)	Cured (95%)	PE
		Bruce et al[98] (1999)	52	17	Prolapse cured or improved (85%)	PE
	Sacrocolpopexy	Creighton and Stanton[99] (1991)	23	17.1	Vault prolapse cured (91%)	PE
		Valaitis and Stanton[100] (1994)	43	21 (3-91)	Vault prolapse cured (100%)	PE
		Winters et al[78] (2000)	20	11.3 (6-27)	Grade I cystocele or less (85%)	PE
Vaginal						
	Four-corner bladder neck suspension	Raz et al[71] (1989)	120	24 (6-60)	Cystocele cured (98%)	PE
	Anterior vaginal wall suspension	Dmochowski et al[12] (1997)	47	37 (15-80)	Grade I or II cystocele (57%)	PE and VCUG
	Anterior colporrhaphy	Walter et al[101] (1982)	86	14 (12-30)	No recurrence (100%)	PE
		Porges and Smilen[102] (1994)	299	31 (12-240)	Cystocele cured (97%)	PE
		Colombo et al[66] (2000)	33	60	Grade 1 cystocele or less (97%)	PE
	Polypropylene mesh	Nicita[74] (1998)	44	13.9 (9-23)	Cystocele cured (100%)	PE
		Migliari et al[75] (2000)	12	20.5 (15-32)	Cystocele cured (75%)	PE
	Cadaveric fascia lata	Kobashi and Leach[65] (2000)	50	<18	Cystocele cured (100%)	PE

PE, physical examination; VCUG, voiding cystourethrogram.

site-specific herniation. The configuration of the perineal body[81] and the strength of the levator muscles are noted.

Surgical repair is considered if the rectocele is symptomatic, although several authors have long debated the prophylactic merit of surgical correction during repair of other vaginal wall prolapses. The risks of dyspareunia and rectal injury should be discussed with the patient preoperatively.

Techniques

There are two general approaches to rectocele correction: traditional posterior colporrhaphy[81] and site-specific defect repair.[79] During posterior colporrhaphy, a midline mucosal incision is made, and the vaginal wall is dissected off the rectum. The levator ani muscles are approximated in the midline with absorbable sutures. The rectal wall is pushed downward as the sutures are tied across the midline. Excess vaginal wall is excised, and the vaginal edges are reapproximated with absorbable sutures.

With the site-specific method, the rectocele is repaired at one of five potential break sites in the rectovaginal fascia[79] (Fig. 40-5). Using a midline incision, the vaginal wall is dissected off the rectovaginal fascia and the edges of the fascial defect are identified and sewn together with a series of interrupted sutures. The edges of the vaginal wall are then reapproximated over the repair site.[82]

When perineorrhaphy is indicated, it is performed as the last step of posterior vaginal wall reconstruction. Two Allis clamps are applied to the mucocutaneous junction on each side of the midline and pulled together medially to allow for an adequately sized introitus. Then, a transverse incision is made at the mucocutaneous junction between the clamps, and a thin strip of epithelial tissue is removed. An inverted-V-shaped incision is made to join the edges of the incision to the apex of the rectocele. The perineal body is reconstructed by reapproximating the superficial and deep perineal muscles over the midline with U-shaped absorbable sutures. The mucocutaneous junction is carefully reapproximated to avoid misalignment, which could cause introital dyspareunia.[81]

Results

No study has directly compared posterior colporrhaphy with site-specific fascial defect repair. Table 40-8 lists the surgical outcomes with these two approaches.

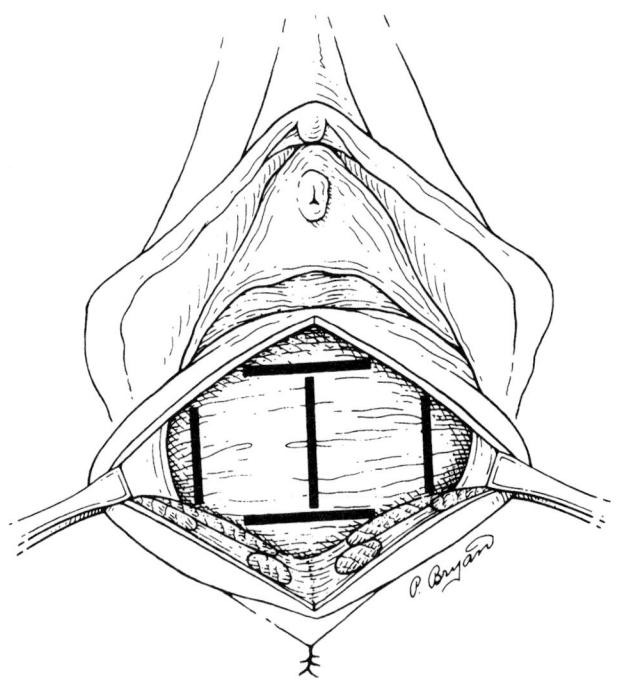

FIGURE 40-5 The recognition of site-specific tears in the rectovaginal fascia (*bold straight lines*) has led to selective repair of defects. Not reapproximating the levator muscles over the midline, as classically performed during posterior repair, may prevent dyspareunia. However, the reliability and durability of this site-specific technique cannot be determined until more long-term follow-up data are reported. (From Cundiff GW, Weidner AC, Visco AG, et al: An anatomic and functional assessment of the discrete defect rectocele repair. Am J Obstet Gynecol 179(6):1451–1457, 1998.)

Complications

The main intraoperative complication of rectocele repair is rectal injury. When unrecognized, a rectovaginal fistula may occur. Hydrodissection of the posterior vaginal wall and localization of the yellow prerectal fat can help to avoid rectotomy. Dyspareunia may occur as a result of excessive tightening of the introitus, when a shelf-like ridge is created along the posterior wall because the levator ani edges are approximated too tightly, or when the posterior horizontal angle of the upper vagina is not respected.[65]

TABLE 40-8 ■ Outcomes of traditional posterior colporrhaphy versus site-specific rectocele repair

Procedure	Study	No. of Patients	Follow-up (mo)	Herniation Repaired	Symptom Improvement
Posterior colporrhaphy	Arnold et al[103] (1990)	22	Not stated	Not stated	Overall (77%)
	Mellgren et al[104] (1994)	25	12 (4-32.4)	96%	Constipation (88%)
Rectovaginal fascia defect repair	Cundiff et al[82] (1998)	69	36	82%	Difficulty defecating (49%) Constipation (75%) Dyspareunia (33%)
	Kenton et al[105] (1999)	46	12	85%	Protrusion (90%) Difficulty defecating (54%) Constipation (43%) Dyspareunia (92%)

REFERENCES

1. Mostwin JL, Genadray R, Sanders R, Yang A: Anatomic goals in the correction of female stress urinary incontinence. J Endourol 10(3):207–212, 1996.
2. Marshall VF, Marchetti AA, Krantz KF: The correction of stress incontinence by simple vesicourethral suspension. Surg Obstet Gynecol 88:509–518, 1949.
3. Burch JC: Urethrovaginal fixation to Cooper's ligament for correction of stress incontinence, cystocele, and prolapse. Am J Obstet Gynecol 81:281–290, 1961.
4. Tanagho EA: Colpocystourethropexy: The way we do it. J Urol 116:751–753, 1976.
5. Stanton SL, Williams JE, Ritchie D: The colposuspension operation for urinary incontinence. Br J Obstet Gyneaecol 83:890–895, 1976.
6. Bhatia NN, Bergman A: Modified Burch versus Pereyra retropubic urethropexy for stress urinary incontinence. Obstet Gynecol 66:255–261, 1985.
7. Dainer M, Hall CD, Choe J, Bhatia NN: The Burch procedure: A comprehensive review. Obstet Gynecol Surg 54(1):49–60, 1998.
8. Stanton SL, Cardozo L, Williams JE, et al: Clinical and urodynamic features of failed incontinence surgery in the female. Obstet Gynecol 51:515–520, 1978.
9. Pereyra AJ: A simplified surgical procedure for the correction of stress incontinence in women. West J Surg 67:223–226,1959.
10. Kim HL, Gerber GS, Patel RV, et al: Practice patterns in the treatment of urinary incontinence: A postal and internet survey. Urology 57(1):45–48, 2001.
11. Raz S, Siegel AL, Short JL, Synder JA: Vaginal wall sling. J Urol 141:43–46, 1989.
12. Dmochowski RR, Zimmern PE, Ganabathi K, et al: Role of the four-corner bladder neck suspension to correct stress incontinence with a mild to moderate cystocele. Urology 49:35–40, 1997.
13. Erikson BC, Hagen B, Eik-Nes SH, et al: Long-term effectiveness of coloposuspension in stress incontinence. Acta Obstet Gynecol Scand 69:45–50, 1990.
14. Persky L, Guerriere K: Complications of Marshall-Marchetti-Krantz urethropexy. Urology 8:469, 1976.
15. Bernier PA, Zimmern PE: Bone anchor removal after bladder neck suspension. Br J Urol; 82(2):303–303, 1998.
16. Zimmern PE, Hadley HR, Leach GE, Raz S: Female urethral obstruction after Marshall-Marchetti-Krantz operation. J Urol 138:517–520, 1987.
17. Vierhout ME, AFP Mulder: De novo detrusor instability after Burch colposuspension. Acta Obstet Gynecol Scand 71:414–416, 1992.
18. Mainprize TC, Drutz HP: The Marshall-Marchetti-Krantz procedure: A critical review.; 43(12):724–729, 1988.
19. Burch JC: Cooper's ligament urethrovesical suspension for stress incontinence. Am J Obstet Gynecol 100:764–773, 1968.
20. Langer R, Ron-El R, Newman M, et al: Detrusor instability following colposuspension for urinary stress incontinence. Br J Obstet Gynaecol 95:607–610, 1988.
21. Alcalay M, Monga A, Stanton SL: Burch colposuspension: A 10-20 year follow up. Br J Obstet Gynaecol 102:740–745, 1995.
22. Wiskind AK, Creighton SM, Stanton SL: The incidence of genital prolapse after the Burch colposuspension. Am J Obstet Gynecol 167(2):399–404, 1992.
23. Ridley JH: The Goebll-Stoeckel Sling Operation. In Mattingly RF, Thompson JD (eds): TeLinde's Operative Gynecology. Philadelphia, Lippincott, 1985.
24. Hilton P, Stanton SL: Clinical and urodynamic evaluation of the polypropylene (Marlex) sling for genuine stress incontinence. Neurourol Urodynam 2:145, 1983.
25. Norris JP, Breslin DS, Staskin DR: Use of synthetic material in sling surgery: A minimally invasive approach. J Endourol 10(3):227–230, 1996.
26. Kreder KJ, Austin JC: Treatment of stress urinary incontinence in women with urethral hypermobility and intrinsic sphincter deficiency. J Urol 156:1995–1998, 1996.
27. Appell RA: Argument for sling surgery to replace bladder suspension for stress urinary incontinence. Urology 56:360–363, 2000.
28. Zaragoza MR: Expanded indications for the pubovaginal sling: Treatment of type 2 or 3 stress incontinence. J Urol 156(5):1620–1622, 1996.
29. Choe JM, Staskin DR: Gore-Tex patch sling: 7 years later. Urology 54(4):641–646, 1999.
30. Morgan TO, Westney OL, McGuire EJ: Pubovaginal sling: Four year outcome analysis and quality of life assessment. J Urol 163:1845–1848, 2000.
31. Raz S: Modified bladder neck suspension for female stress incontinence. Urology 17(1):82–85, 1981.
32. Cespedes RD, McGuire EJ: Pubovaginal fascial slings. In Graham SD (ed): Glenn's Urologic Surgery, 5th ed. Philadelphia, Lippincott-Raven, 1998, pp 337–341.
33. Carr LK, Walsh PJ, Abraham VE, Webster GD: Favorable outcome of pubovaginal slings for geriatric women with stress incontinence. J Urol 157:125–128, 1997.
34. Sousa-Escandron A: 'Sandwich technique' for the suburethral placement of Mersilene mesh sling during pubovaginal suspension surgery: preliminary results. Urology 57(1):49–54, 2001.
35. Payne CK: A transvaginal sling procedure with bone anchor fixation. Urol Clin North Am 26(2):423–430, 1999.
36. Blaivas JG, Jacobs BZ: Pubovaginal fascial sling for the treatment of complicated stress urinary incontinence. J Urol 145:1214–1217, 1991.
37. Winters JC, Scarpero HC, Appell RA: Use of bone anchors in female urology. Urology 56 (suppl 6A):15–22, 2000.
38. Schonauer S: Correction of stress incontinence in women by simple sling operation. Urology 32(3):189–191, 1988.
39. Mcguire EJ, Lytton B: Pubovaginal sling procedure for stress incontinence. J Urol 119:82–84, 1978.
40. Rovner ES, Ginsberg DA, Raz S: A method for intraoperative adjustment of sling tension: Prevention of outlet obstruction during vaginal wall sling. Urology 50:273–276, 1996.
41. Leach GE, Sirls L: Pubovaginal sling procedures. Atlas Urol Clin North Am 2(1):61–71, 1994.
42. Leach GE, Dmochowski RR, Appell RA, et al: Female stress urinary incontinence clinical guidelines panel: Summary report on surgical management of female stress urinary incontinence. J Urol 158:875–880, 1997.
43. Melnick I, Lee RE: Delayed transection of urethra by Mersilene tape. Urology 8(6):580–581, 1976.
44. Chin YK, Stanton SL: A follow up of silicone sling for genuine stress incontinence. Br J Obstet Gynaecol 102:143–147, 1995.
45. Bent AE, Ostergard DR, Zwick-Zaffuto M: Tissue reaction to expanded polytetrafluoroethylene suburethral sling for urinary incontinence: Clinical and histologic study. Am J Obstet Gynecol 169:1198–1204, 1993.
46. Morgan JE, Farrow GA, Stewart FE, et al: The Marlex sling operation for the treatment of recurrent stress urinary incontinence: A 16 year review. Am J Obstet Gynecol 151:224–226, 1985.

47. Kobashi KC, Dmochowski R, Mee SL, et al: Erosion of woven polyester pubovaginal sling. J Urol 162(6): 2070–2072, 1999.
48. Choe JM, Ogan K, Battino BS: Antimicrobial mesh versus vaginal wall sling: A comparative outcomes analysis. J Urol 163:1829–1834, 2000.
49. Long RL, Barrett DM: Artificial sphincter: Abdominal approach. In Raz S (ed): Female Urology. Philadelphia, Saunders, 1996, pp 428–434.
50. Elliott DS, Barrett DM: The artificial urinary sphincter in the female: Indications for use, surgical approach and results. Int Urogynecol J 9:409–415, 1998.
51. Petrou SP, Elliott DS, Barrett DM: Artificial urethral sphincter for incontinence. Urology 56:353–359, 2000.
52. Abbassian A: A new operation for insertion of the artificial urinary sphincter. J Urol 140:512–513, 1988.
53. Wang Y, Hadley HR: Artificial sphincter: Transvaginal approach. In Raz S (ed): Female Urology. Philadelphia, Saunders, 1996, pp 428–434.
54. Appell RA: Techniques and results in the implantation of the artificial urinary sphincter in women with type III stress urinary incontinence by vaginal approach. Neurourol Urodynam 7:613–619, 1988.
55. Fishman IJ: Female incontinence and the artificial urinary sphincter. In Seidmon EJ, Hanno PM (eds): Current Urologic Therapy, 3rd ed. Philadelphia, Saunders, 1994, pp 312–315.
56. Light JK, Scott FB: Management of urinary incontinence in women with the artificial urinary sphincter. J Urol 134:476–478, 1985.
57. Leach GE: Incontinence after artificial urinary sphincter placement: The role of perfusion sphincterometry. J Urol 138:529–532, 1987.
58. Diokno AC, Hollander JB, Alderson TP: Artificial urinary sphincter for recurrent female urinary incontinence: Indications and results. J Urol 138:778–780, 1987.
59. Venn SN, Greenwell TJ, Mundy AR: The long-term outcome of artificial urinary sphincters. J Urol 164:702–707, 2000.
60. Petrou SP, Elliott DS, Barrett DM: Artificial urethral sphincter for incontinence. Urology 56:353–359, 2000.
61. Nurse DE, Mundy AR: One hundred artificial sphincters. Br J Urol 61:318–325, 1988.
62. Bump RC, Bo K, Brubaker L, et al: The standardization of terminology of female pelvic organ prolapse and pelvic floor dysfunction. Am J Obstet Gynecol 175:10–17, 1996.
63. Scotti RJ, Flora R, Greston WM, et al: Characterizing and reporting pelvic floor defects: The revised New York classification system. Int Urogynecol J Pelvic Floor Dysfunct 11(1):48–60, 2000.
64. Zimmern PE, Leach GE, Ganabathi K: The urological aspects of vaginal wall prolapse: Part 1. Diagnosis and surgical indications. AUA Update Series XII(25):193, 1993.
65. Kobashi, KC, Leach GE: Pelvic prolapse. J Urol 164:1879–1890, 2000.
66. Colombo M, Vitobello D, Proietti F, Milani R: Randomised comparison of Burch colposuspension versus anterior colporrhaphy in women with stress urinary incontinence and anterior vaginal wall prolapse. Br J Obstet Gynaecol 107(4):544–551, 2000.
67. Richardson AC, Lyon JB, Williams NL: A new look at pelvic relaxation. Am J Obstet Gynecol 126(5):568–573, 1976.
68. White GR: Cystocele: A radical cure by suturing lateral sulci of vagina to the white line of pelvic fascia. JAMA 21:1707–1710, 1909.
69. Shull BL, Benn SJ, Kuehl TJ: Surgical management of prolapse of the anterior vaginal segment: An analysis of support defects, operative morbidity, and anatomic outcome. Am J Obstet Gynecol 171:1429–1439, 1994.
70. Richardson AC: Pelvic support defects in women (urethrocele, cystocele, uterine prolapse, enterocele and rectocele). In Skandalakis J, Gray S, Mansberger A Jr, et al (eds): Hernia: Surgical Anatomy and Technique. New York, McGraw-Hill, 1989, pp 238–263.
71. Raz S, Klutke C, Golumb J: Four-corner bladder and urethral suspension for moderate cystocele. J Urol 142:712–715, 1989.
72. Leach GE, Zimmern PE: Vaginal suspension procedures. AUA Update Series IX(40):313–320, 1990.
73. Benizri EJ, Volpe P, et al: A new vaginal procedure for cystocele repair and treatment of stress urinary incontinence. J Urol 156:1623–1625, 1996.
74. Nicita G: A new operation for genitourinary prolapse. J Urol 160:741–745, 1998.
75. Migliari R, DeAngelis M, Madeddu G, Verdacchi T: Tension-free vaginal mesh repair for anterior vaginal wall prolapse. Eur Urol 38:151–155, 2000.
76. Timmons MC: Transabdominal sacral colpopexy. Oper Tech Gynecol Surg 1:92–96, 1996.
77. Kohli N, Walsh PM, Roat TW, et al: Mesh erosion after abdominal sacrocolpopexy. Obstet Gynecol 92(6):999–1004, 1998.
78. Winters JC, Cespedes RD, Vanlangendonck R: Abdominal sacral colpopexy and abdominal enterocele repair in the management of vaginal vault prolapse. Urology 56 (6 suppl 1):55–63, 2000.
79. Richardson AC: The rectovaginal septum revisited: Its relationship to rectocele and its importance in rectocele repair. Clin Obstet Gynecol 36:976–983, 1993.
80. Kenton K, Shott S, Brubaker L: Outcome after rectovaginal fascia reattachment for rectocele repair. Am J Obstet Gynecol 181(6):1360–1364, 1999.
81. Zimmern PE, Leach GE: Repair of enterocele and rectocele, perineal repair, and vault suspension. Atlas Urol Clin North Am 2(1):47–60, 1994.
82. Cundiff GW, Weidner AC, Visco AG, et al: An anatomic and functional assessment of the discrete defect rectocele repair. Am J Obstet Gynecol 179(6):1451–1457, 1998.
83. Milani R, Scalambrino S, Quadri G, Algeri M: Marshall-Marchetti-Krantz procedure and Burch colposuspension in the surgical treatment of female urinary incontinence. Br J Obstet Gynecol 92:1050–1053, 1985.
84. Colombo M, Scalambrino S, Maggioni A, et al: Burch colposuspension versus modified Marshall-Marchetti-Krantz urethropexy for primary genuine stress urinary incontinence: A prospective, randomized clinical trial. Am J Obstet Gynecol 171(6):1573–1579, 1994.
85. Eriksen BC, Hagen B, Eik-Nes SH, et al: Long-term effectiveness of the Burch colposuspension in female urinary stress incontinence. Acta Obstet Gynecol Scand 69:45–50, 1990.
86. Herbertsson G, Iosif CS: Surgical results and urodynamic studies 10 years after retropubic colposystourethropexy. Acta Obstet Gynecol Scand 72:298–301, 1993.
87. Kinn AC: Burch colposuspension for stress urinary incontinence: 5 year results in 153 women. Scand J Urol Nephrol 29:449–455, 1995.
88. Drouin J, Tessier J, Bertrand PE, et al: Burch colposuspension: Long-term results and review of published reports. Urology 54(5):808–814, 1999.
89. Diokno AC, Hollander JB, Alderson TP: Artificial urinary sphincter for recurrent female urinary incontinence. J Urol 138(4):778–780, 1987.

90. Webster GD, Perez LM, Khoury JM, et al: Management of type III stress urinary incontinence using an artificial urinary sphincter. Urology 39:499–503, 1992.
91. Stone KT, Diokno AC, Mitchell BA: J Urol 153 (suppl):433A, 1995.
92. Heitz M, Olianas R, Schreiter F: Therapie der weiblichen Harninkontinenz mit dem artifiziellen Sphinter AMS 800: Indikationen, ergebnesse, komplikationen und risikofaktoren. Urologe A 36(5):426–431, 1997.
93. Costa P, Naoum KB, Mottet N, et al: Efficacy and safety of artificial urinary sphincter AMS 800 in females: Medium and long term follow-up (abstract). J Urol 159 (suppl 5):37, 1998.
94. Baden WF, Walker TA: Genesis of the vaginal profile: A correlated classification of vaginal relaxation. Clin Obstet Gynecol 15(4):1048–1054, 1972.
95. Raz S, Erickson DR: SEAPI QMM incontinence classification system. Neurourol Urodynam 11:187–199, 1992.
96. Wiskind AK, Creighton SM, Stanton SL: The incidence of genital prolapse after the Burch colposuspension. Am J Obstet Gynecol 167(2):399–405, 1992.
97. Shull BL, Baden WF: A six-year experience with paravaginal defect repair for stress urinary incontinence. Am J Obstet Gynecol 160:1432–1435, 1989.
98. Bruce RG, El-Galley RES, Galloway NTM: Paravaginal defect repair in the treatment of female stress urinary incontinence and cystocele. Urology 54(4):647–651, 1999.
99. Creighton SM, Stanton SL: The surgical management of vaginal vault prolapse. Br J Obstet Gynaecol 98:1150–1154, 1991.
100. Valaitis SR, Stanton SL: Sacrocolpopexy: A retrospective study of a clinician's experience. Br J Obstet Gynaecol 101:518–522, 1994.
101. Walter S, Olesen KP, Hald T, et al: Urodynamic evaluation after vaginal repair and colposuspension. Br J Urol 54:377–380, 1982.
102. Porges RF, Smilen SW: Long-term analysis of the surgical management of pelvic support defects. Am J Obstet Gynecol 171:1518–1528, 1994.
103. Arnold MW, Stewart WR, Aguilar PS: Rectocele repair: Four years' experience. Dis Colon Rectum 33:684–687, 1990.
104. Mellgren A, Anzen B, Nilsson B-Y, et al: Results of rectocele repair. Dis Colon Rectum 38:7–13, 1995.
105. Kenton K, Shott S, Brubaker L: Outcome after rectovaginal fascia reattachment for rectocele repair. Am J Obstet Gynecol 181(6):1360–1364, 1999.

CHAPTER 41

The Tension-Free Vaginal Tape Technique

FRANÇOIS HAAB ■ OLIVIER TRAXER ■ CALIN CIOFU

The treatment of female stress urinary incontinence is still a controversial issue in the medical literature. According to many authors, hypermobility of the urethra would be the main cause of urinary leakage when abdominal pressure increases.[1] Therefore, most surgical procedures aim to restore urethral support to prevent leakage. A technique that has been remarkably rapidly adopted by many surgeons is the tension-free vaginal tape (TVT) procedure described by Ulmsten and colleagues in 1996.[2] This technique is based on a series of experimental investigations of the urethral closure mechanisms in the female.

ANATOMICAL BASIS

Until the early 1980s, the pathophysiology of stress incontinence was based mainly on Enhorning's theory.[3] Enhorning suggested that pressure transmission from the bladder to the urethra occurs because the urethra lies with the bladder in the abdomen. According to this theory, stress incontinence was due to descent of the bladder neck and proximal urethra, therefore escaping from the influence of increases in abdominal pressure, causing urine leakage. Thus, most surgical procedures aimed not only to support but to elevate the bladder neck and urethra so that they would respond once again to changes in abdominal pressure.

The 1980s saw a change in approach inspired by De Lancey's hammock theory.[4] In De Lancey's view, stress continence was due to tension arising within a subcervical hammock composed of a muscle (the anterior pubourethral bundle of the levator ani) held by two ligaments (pubourethral and conjunctive) connected to the endopelvic fasciae. In the normal continent female, increases in urethral closure pressure during a cough arise because the urethra is compressed rather than being truly intra-abdominal as previously stated by Enhorning. The tissue that supports the urethra constitutes a sling under the urethra in its upper and mid portions. This sling is composed with a segment of the anterior vaginal wall that is attached to the muscles of the pelvic floor (levator ani muscles principally) and to the arcus tendineus fascia pelvis. The levator ani muscles not only help to support the visceral structures at rest because of a constant tone, but they act as a backup to the endopelvic fasciae and probably serve as the principal support during sudden increases in intra-abdominal pressure. The connection of the urethra to the arcus tendineus assists the levator support and limits the descent of vesical neck when the levator muscles are relaxed or overcome.

Since the support of the bladder neck and proximal urethra is both muscular and ligamentous, proper intrapelvic support relies on an active component of muscular contraction during stress along with the firm strength of the ligaments and vaginal wall. When both active or passive supports are altered, the urethra and bladder base are no longer well supported, resulting in a defect in transmission of the intra-abdominal pressure to the urethra. This type of incontinence is described as type II SUI in Blaivas and Olsson classification.[1] Based on the hammock theory, to ensure continence the bladder neck and proximal urethra did not have to be elevated but should be provided with underlying support. This view explained the renewed appeal of placing slings beneath the bladder neck.

The TVT procedure stems from a careful analysis of the physiology of female urinary continence and of the mechanisms possibly causing stress incontinence.[5] It is based on the idea that the opening and closure of the inner urethra and bladder neck are controlled mainly by three anatomical mechanisms: the tension in the pubourethral ligaments, the activity of the pubococcygeus and levator ani muscles, and the condition of the suburethral vaginal hammock. All these three structures are connected by connective tissues. According to this theory, the tension in the pubourethral ligaments ensures that the muscular component of the support and the vaginal hammock interact correctly. If tension is adequate, forward contraction of the pubococcygeus muscles and backward contraction via the levator ani muscles kink the inner urethra and the bladder neck, leading to closure. Urethral pressure profile measurements and lateral urethrocystography have established the presence of the kink in the urethra, called the urethral "knee," indicating the position of insertion of the pubourethral ligaments.

According to the hammock theory, the TVT procedure was described to correct the lack of tension in the pubourethral ligaments, and then to restore the support of the urethra to the pubic bone and also to restore the connections of the urogenital structures.

THE TVT TECHNIQUE

The TVT technique is easy to learn; but to ensure its maximal efficacy, the surgeon has to follow the original principle.

The TVT device is made of a polypropylene tape attached to two needles that measure 4 mm in diameter (Fig. 41-1). The tape is protected by a plastic sheath, which facilitates placement of the tape through the tissues and theoretically decreases the risk of infection.

The technique is performed under local anesthesia plus intravenous sedation. Diluted lidocaine is injected in the vaginal skin toward the endopelvic fascia but also in the retropubic space. Wang recently reported more favorable results when the surgery was performed under local anesthesia than with epidural anesthesia.[6] The mode of anesthesia remains controversial; some authors argue that the procedure could be done with local, epidural, or even general anesthesia with the same efficacy.

The patient is put in lithotomy position, and the bladder is drained. The vaginal skin is incised beneath the mid urethra. The incision is usually 1.5 cm to 2 cm long (Fig. 41-2). A minimal dissection is performed to create a small tunnel under the vaginal skin toward the endopelvic fascia. The endopelvic fascia should not be opened at this stage of the procedure. The tape is therefore placed, using the special needles, at the level of the mid urethra. When passing the needles from the vagina toward the retropubic space, care should be taken to follow the posterior surface of the pubic bone and to stay as medial as possible (Fig. 41-3). This is critical to prevent major complications such as vascular or bowel injuries. An intra-operative cystoscopy should be performed to verify no bladder injury. A 70° lens or a flexible scope is recommended. The tape is left beneath the urethra without tension (Fig. 41-4). When the procedure is performed under local or epidural anesthesia, an intra-operative stress test could be performed to adjust the tension of the tape for each patient. When the procedure is performed under general anesthesia or when the patient is not able to cough hard enough to have a leakage, the tape should be left without tension, and a space of 0.5 cm to 1 cm is left between the urethra and the tape. The vaginal skin should be closed carefully with long-lasting absorbable sutures to prevent tape exposure in the vagina.

The TVT technique is considered minimally invasive surgery. The duration of the operation is usually less than 30 minutes and the duration of hospitalization varies between 1 and 3 days. Complication rates

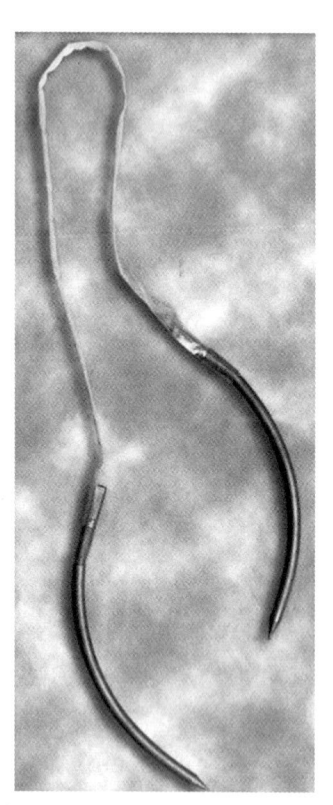

FIGURE 41-1 The tension-free vaginal tape (TVT) device.

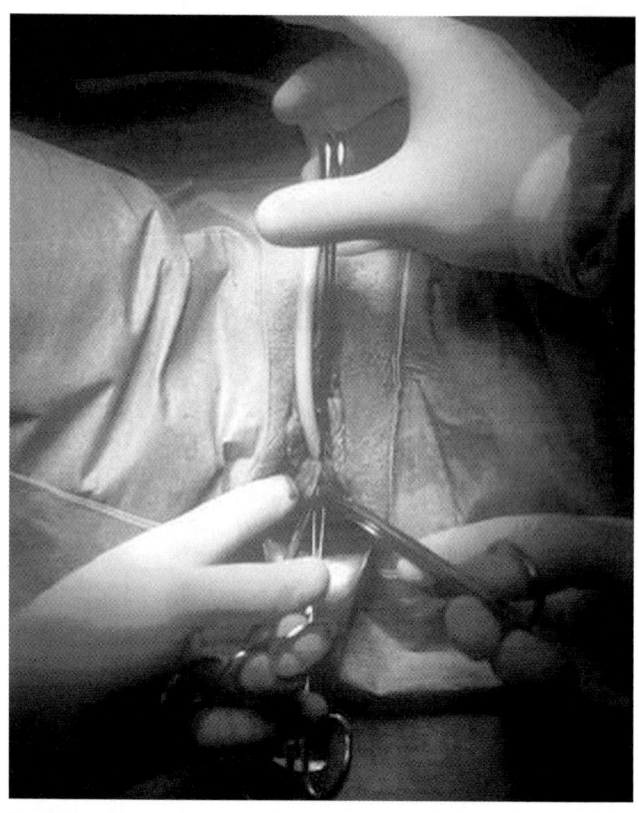

FIGURE 41-2 Incision in the vaginal skin beneath the mid urethra to perform the tension-free vaginal tape procedure.

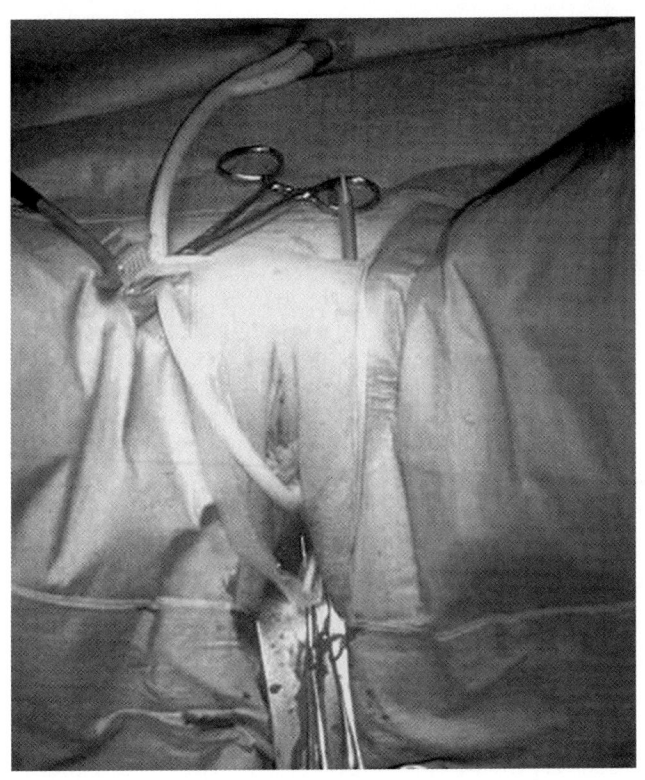

FIGURE 41-3 Passing the needle from the vagina toward the retropubic space during the tension-free vaginal tape procedure.

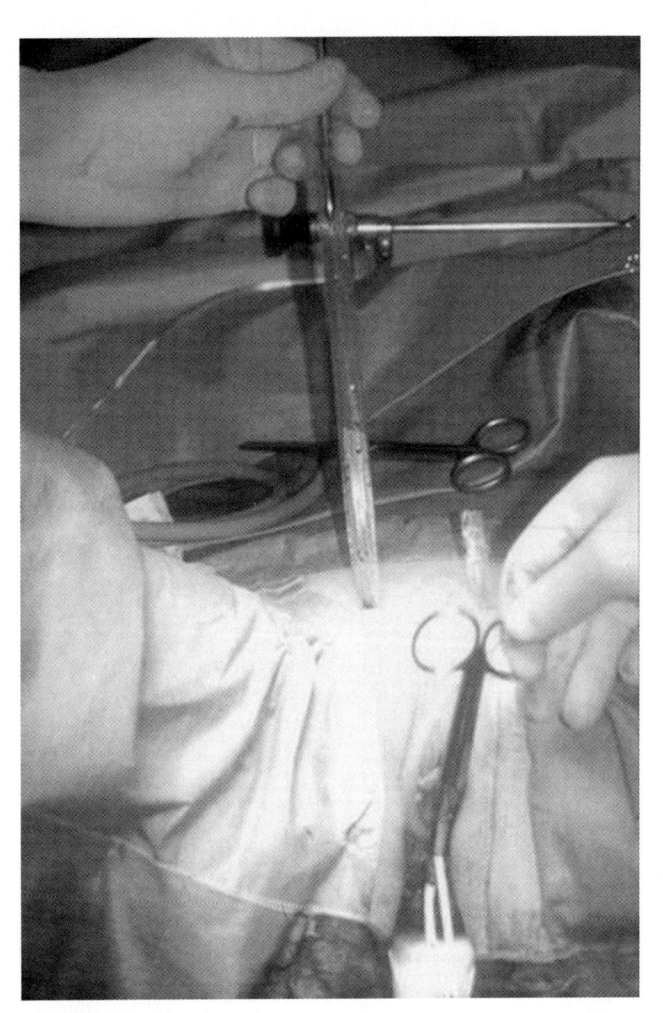

FIGURE 41-4 During the tension-free vaginal tape procedure, leaving the tape without tension beneath the urethra.

reported on large series of patients are low (see Box 41-1). Bladder perforation is the most common complication, according to a study presented by Kuuva and Nilsson at the International Continence Society meeting.[7] The prevalence of intra-operative bladder perforation was estimated at 6%, but it is not serious if noted during surgery. Previous surgery seems to increase that risk.[8] Haab and colleagues reported up to 30% bladder perforation in patients with history of anti-incontinence procedures versus 2.1% in patients who had had no surgery before this ($P < 0.05$).[8] Notwithstanding, severe complications such as injury to the intestines, large vessels, or nerves have been reported in the literature. Moran and colleagues reported on few unusual complications: one right obturator nerve damage recognized by postoperative electromyography and one left groin pain due to periostitis.[9] More recently Peyrat and colleagues described one bowel injury during the needle placement, which was recognized after the procedure and necessitated another operation.[10] These severe complications nearly always occurred in patients who had already undergone surgery, at least once, for incontinence or who had undergone pelvic surgery. Extreme caution should be exercised, however, when dealing with patients who have had multiple operations.

A Synthetic Mesh: Pros and Cons

A suburethral hammock (colposuspension or suburethral sling) should be a solid and durable foundation. Initial

> **BOX 41-1** **COMPLICATIONS OF THE TVT: A Prospective Assessment in a Series of 100 Consecutive Patients: A Multicenter Study**
>
> Urinary infection: 10%
> Bladder injury: 6%
> Prolonged pain: 3%
> Complete retention >1 month: 1%
> Retropubic hematoma: 1%
> Major labia hematoma: 1%
> Healing problems: 1%
> Bleeding >200 cc: 1%

simple procedures like the Gites procedure, the modified Peyreyra procedure as developed by Raz, and the Burch procedure relied on the support of the vaginal wall, but patients with stress incontinence may have damaged connective structures. Sling procedures have been successful partly because they provide undamaged, often autologous tissue (mainly rectus fascia or fascia lata) beneath the urethra. Clearly, however, an interesting option was to employ synthetic material to reduce the morbidity related to autologous tissue use. Initial attempts with semisynthetic biological tissue or with purely artificial material were not very promising. The risk of endovaginal, even endourethral, rejection was significantly increased. Explantation rates up to 20% were noted during the year following surgery.[11] Most rejections of the synthetic slings happened within the first year after the procedures. With the woven polyester pubovaginal sling, Kobashi and colleagues reported on 34 women that required removal of the sling secondary to erosion, infection, or pain.[11] The most common presenting complaints were delayed vaginal discharge in 21 patients (62%), vaginal pain in 21 (62%), suprapubic pain in 11 (32%), and recurrent urinary tract infections in 5 (15%). In this large series, complications happened at a mean of 8 months after the sling placement with extremes of 1 to 22 months. Clemens and colleagues reported the same experience using mainly polyester slings but also Goretex or cadaveric fasciae.[12] The erosions happened at a median follow-up of 9 months after the initial operation. Intravaginal slingplasty, the precursor procedure to TVT, which uses either Dacron or Goretex, also gave poor results. There were two cases of rejection and explantation of the Goretex tapes. In fact, the current TVT procedure differs from intravaginal slingplasty in only one respect. It uses a wide-mesh polypropylene tape instead of Dacron or Goretex.[2] So far no cases of rejection have been reported in the literature. The reasons for the biocompatibility of polypropylene are not known but may reside in the very loose mesh that allows fibroblasts to colonize. When laterourethral biopsies taken during surgery and 2 years later were compared, a significant increase in collagen synthesis (from 41.2% to 66.3%, $P < 0.001$) was noted.[13]

The use of synthetic material for sling procedures also carries the risk of bladder outlet obstruction and urine retention, and the TVT procedure is no exception in this respect. In a recent study by Haab and colleagues,[8] the rate of clinical voiding dysfunction fringed on 25%, but urine flow rate was less than 15 mL/sec in only 5% of patients.[8] Longer-term studies are required to address this issue. The relationship between pressure and flow also needs to be analyzed to evaluate the prevalence of post-TVT subvesical obstruction and its possible consequences. Although the rates of severe outlet obstruction and retention seem to be lower with the TVT procedure than with other sling procedures,[14] it is important to note that no comparative study has been published yet. Other controversial points relate to the mode of anesthesia and the possibility of performing an intra-operative cough stress test. Although surgery under local anesthesia tends to be the rule, preliminary data suggest that bladder outlet obstruction and retention rates are not influenced by the mode of anesthesia provided that the tape is positioned loosely.[8] Spinal and local anesthesia have yielded comparable results but no prospective randomized controlled trials comparing these two options have been published. Moreover, no data are available on the risk of obstruction when the TVT procedure is performed under general anesthesia.

RESULTS OF THE TVT PROCEDURE

Most published results on the TVT procedure relate to stress incontinence due to a hypermobile urethra recognized as type II stress urinary incontinence in Blaivas and Olsson classification. The cure rate in these patients is above 80% (see Table 41-1). The failure rate usually ranges from 5% to 10% mainly due to persistent or de novo urgency symptoms.[8] However, it is notable that overall results are remarkably consistent throughout the literature (see Table 41-1). This suggests that the procedure is highly reproducible and well standardized and no doubt accounts for its rapid and widespread diffusion. Moreover, unlike laparoscopic Burch colposuspension or suburethral slings that are not easy to position, the TVT procedure does not appear to be operator dependent.

Few studies have evaluated long-term follow-up. In a study published by Ulmsten and colleagues,[15] none of 50 patients cured by the TVT procedure had relapsed at 3 years. A recent update[16] found no deterioration at 5 years. The use of a synthetic tape, which allows fibroblasts to colonizes, probably accounts for the stability of the results over time.

Only one study has compared the results of the Burch colposuspension and the TVT procedure. The preliminary results were presented at the International Continence Society meeting by Ward and colleagues in 2002.[17] The trial was conducted in 14 centers in the United Kingdom and Ireland with a total of 344 randomly selected patients. Finally, 170 patients underwent a TVT procedure and 146 a Burch colposuspension. At 6 months follow-up, the continence rates based on objective and subjective criteria were not statistically different in the two groups. Bladder injury was more common during the vaginal tape procedure. The TVT procedure appeared significantly better than the Burch on the following items: postoperative opiate analgesia (21% versus 91%), mean duration of hospital stay (2.2 days versus 6.5 days), and number of rehospitalizations (9 versus 18 patients). However, longer follow-up will be necessary to address the continence issues precisely.

Few prognostic factors have been identified. In a recently published series, Rezapour and colleagues reported the results of the TVT procedure in stress incontinent women with intrinsic sphincteric deficiency. Forty-nine women were enrolled in the study. Sphincteric deficiency was defined by a low urethral closure pressure. At 4 years follow-up, the cure rate was

TABLE 41-1 ■ **Results of the TVT procedure**

	Patients	Follow-up (months)	Cure (%)	Improved (%)	Failed (%)	De novo DI* (%)
Olsson[18]	51	36	90	6	4	–
Ulmsten[19]	131	12	91	7	2	–
Haab[20]	62	16	87	10	3	6
Klutke[21]	20	12	85	10	5	–
Ulmsten[19]	50	36	86	12	2	–
Moran[9]	40	12	80	17	3	12

*DI, detrusor instability.

74%. The authors concluded that patients older than 70 years with a low resting urethral closure pressure and an immobile urethra seem to constitute a risk group where TVT surgery is less successful.[22] Another study was conducted on 39 patients with genuine stress urinary incontinence and 32 patients with mixed incontinence. A total of 21 patients had a low urethral closure pressure below 20 cm of water.[23] The cure rate among patients with low closure pressure was 86% while cure rate for patients with a closure pressure higher than 20 cm was 94%. The difference between the two groups was statistically significant.[23] However, the number of previous surgeries did not seem to alter significantly the results as long as there was a hypermobile urethra. As previously discussed, however, the risk of intra-operative complication is significantly increased.[24]

CONCLUSION

The surgical treatment of female stress urinary incontinence has changed dramatically in the 5 years after Ulmsten introduced the tension-free vaginal tape procedure. The procedure is easy to learn, can be performed on an outpatient basis, and is minimally invasive. Despite these advantages, the most probable reason for the present success is the reproducibility of the results in the various series published in the literature. The success rate is estimated between 85% and 95% for correction of genuine stress urinary incontinence. Longer follow-up is necessary to confirm these preliminary, very exciting results, and probably to determine the most valuable prognostic factors.

REFERENCES

1. Haab F, Zimmern PE, Leach GE: Female stress urinary incontinence due to intrinsic sphincteric deficiency: Recognition and management. J Urol 156(1):3–17, 1996.
2. Ulmsten U, Henriksson L, Johnson P, et al: An ambulatory surgical procedure under local anesthesia for treatment of female urinary incontinence. Int Urogynecol J 7:81–86, 1996.
3. Enhorning G: Simultaneous recording of the intravesical and intraurethral pressure. Acta Obstet Gynecol Scand 276(suppl):1–69, 1961.
4. De Lancey JOL: Structural support of the urethra as it relates to stress urinary incontinence: The hammock hypothesis. Am J Obstet Gynecol 170:1713–1723, 1994.
5. Petros P, Ulmsten U: An integral theory and its method for the diagnosis and management of female urinary incontinence. Scand J Urol Nephrol 153:1–93, 1993.
6. Wang AC, Chen MC: Randomized comparison of local versus epidural anesthesia for tension-free vaginal tape operation. J Urol 165:1177–1180, 2001.
7. Kuuva N, Nilsson CG: A nationwide analysis of complications associated with the tension-free vaginal tape procedure. Neurourol Urodyn 19:394–395, 2000.
8. Haab F, Sananes S, Amarenco G, et al: Results of the tension-free vaginal tape procedure for the treatment of type II stress urinary incontinence at a minimum follow-up of 1 year. J Urol 165:159–162, 2001.
9. Moran PA, Ward KL, Johnson D, et al: Tension-free vaginal tape procedure for primary genuine stress incontinence: A two center follow-up study. BJU Int 86:39–42, 2000.
10. Peyrat L, Boutin JM, Bruyere F, et al: Intestinal perforation on a complication of tension free vaginal tape procedure for urinary incontinence. Eur Urol 39:603–605, 2001.
11. Kobashi KC, Dmochowski R, Mee SL, et al: Erosion of woven polyester pubovaginal sling. J Urol 162:2070–2072, 1999.
12. Clemens JQ, De Lancey JOL, Faerber GJ, et al: Urinary tract erosions after synthetic pubovaginal slings: Diagnosis and management strategy. Urology 56:589–595, 2000.
13. Falconer C, Ekman-Ordeberg G, Malmstrom A, et al: Clinical outcome and changes in connective tissue metabolism after intravaginal slingplasty in stress incontinent women. Int Urogynecol J 7:133–137, 1996.
14. Nilsson CG. The tension-free vaginal tape procedure (TVT) for treatment of female urinary incontinence. A minimal invasive surgical procedure. Acta Obstet Gynecol Scand Suppl 168:34–47, 1998.
15. Ulmsten U, Johnson P, Rezapour M: A three-year follow-up of tension-free vaginal tape for surgical treatment of female stress urinary incontinence. Brit J Obstet Gynecol 106:345–350, 1999.
16. Nilsson CG, Kuuva N, Falconer C, et al: Long-term results of the tension-free vaginal tape procedure for surgical treatment of female stress urinary incontinence. Int Urogynecol J Suppl 2:S5–S8, 2001.
17. Ward KL, Hilton P, Browning J: A randomised trial of colposuspension and tension-free vaginal tape for primary genuine stress incontinence. Neurourol Urodyn 19:386–388, 2000.
18. Olsson I, Kroon U: A three-year postoperative evaluation of tension-free vaginal tape. Gynecol Obstet Invest 48:267–269, 1999.
19. Ulmsten U, Falconer C, Johnson P, et al: A multicenter study of tension-free vaginal tape for surgical treatment of stress urinary incontinence. Int Urogynecol J 9:210–213, 1998.
20. Haab F, Blanchet P, Cortesse A, et al: Morbidité péri-opératoire du TVT: Étude prospective multicentrique. Prog Urol 10:47A, 2000.
21. Klutke JJ, Carlin BI, Klutke CG: The tension-free vaginal tape procedure: Correction of stress incontinence with minimal alteration in proximal urethral mobility. Urology 55:512–514, 2000.
22. Rezapour M, Falconer C, Ulmsten U: Tension-free vaginal tape in stress incontinent women with intrinsic sphincteric deficiency: A long-term follow-up. Int Urogynecol J Suppl 2:S12–S14, 2001.
23. Kulseng-Hanssen S, Kristoffersen M, Larsen E: Tension-free vaginal tape operation: Results and possible problems. Neurourol Urodyn 19:300–301, 2000.
24. Rezapour M, Ulmsten U: Tension-free vaginal tape in women with recurrent stress urinary incontinence. A long-term follow-up. Urogynecol J Suppl 2:S9–S11, 2001.

CHAPTER 42

Artificial Sphincter: Transvaginal Approach

H. ROGER HADLEY

The artificial urinary sphincter (AUS) is an effective alternative to the urethral sling or periurethral injection therapy for the treatment of urinary incontinence in women with primary urethral sphincter insufficiency (type III stress urinary incontinence).[1,2] In patients with anatomic (type II) urinary incontinence that results from poor bladder neck support, the AUS is rarely inserted in deference to the more common urethral sling or standard bladder neck suspension.

Primary urethral sphincter dysfunction in women may be associated with scarring following multiple anti-incontinence operations, neurologic causes (myelomeningocele, sacral cord tumor, or peripheral neuropathy), radical pelvic operations (abdominoperineal resection or radical hysterectomy), pelvic radiation therapy, and possibly estrogen deficiency or senile changes. Because primary urethral sphincter dysfunction results in inadequate urethral closure, a standard bladder neck suspension will not alleviate the patient's stress urinary incontinence. Operative management, therefore, is directed toward improving direct urethral closure with a urethral sling, periurethral bulking agents, or insertion of the AUS.

The artificial urinary sphincter is a synthetic device that includes a cuff designed to provide a uniform circumferential compression on the urethra and bladder neck. The patient manipulates a labially placed pump to open the cuff prior to voiding. The American Medical System AS-800 is the only currently used model and can be implanted using either a transvaginal or transabdominal approach.

This chapter describes the technique of transvaginal implantation of the artificial urinary sphincter in the treatment of type III stress urinary incontinence.

EVALUATION OF THE PATIENT

Preoperative evaluation of the patient should include a history, physical examination, radiographic evaluation, and urodynamic studies. The patient with genuine stress urinary incontinence due to primary urethral insufficiency will report loss of urine with abdominal straining that may or may not be associated with urgency. Previous anti-incontinence procedures, radical pelvic operations, orthopedic or neurologic disorders, and currently used medications (including replacement hormones), are important historical information.

The physical examination includes measurement of postvoid residual urine and an assessment of vaginal wall integrity and pelvic floor support. With the bladder full, the patient is assessed for stress urinary incontinence in the supine or upright position. The Q-tip deflection test is used to measure urethral mobility. Neurologic examination of the lower extremities and perineum is performed to evaluate the lower lumbar and sacral cord segments. Cystourethroscopy is done to assess urethral coaptation, bladder trabeculation, and the unlikely presence of a fistula.

Radiographic evaluations may include a standing voiding cystourethrogram with resting and straining views. A well-supported urethra with an open bladder neck not associated with a bladder contraction is consistent with primary urethral insufficiency.

Urodynamic studies include a filling cystometrogram and measurement of urethral leak-point pressure. Leakage of urine associated with a leak-point pressure of less than 80 cm to 100 cm H_2O in the absence of a detrusor contraction supports the diagnosis of intrinsic sphincter insufficiency. Video urodynamics, if available, combines fluoroscopic radiography and urodynamics to allow a simultaneous and perhaps a more accurate assessment of the cause and type of urinary incontinence.

The patient best suited for implantation of an artificial urinary sphincter is one who has genuine stress urinary incontinence despite a well-supported bladder neck and no significant bladder instability. If the incontinent patient has concomitant vesical instability, simultaneous pharmacologic or operative management may be required to achieve urinary continence.

For urinary incontinence caused by primary urethral insufficiency, conservative measures should be tried before operative intervention. These nonoperative measures include timed voiding, fluid restriction, pelvic floor exercises, systemic or topical estrogens, alpha-receptor agonists, and anticholinergic medications. If the patient continues to be incontinent despite conservative treatment, placement of the artificial urinary sphincter may be considered.

TECHNIQUE

The artificial urinary sphincter is composed of three parts: the inflatable cuff, the pressure-regulating balloon, and the pump (Fig. 42-1). The cuff is placed circumferentially around the bladder neck, the pressure-regulating balloon is positioned in the prevesical space, and the pump is put in the labia majora. When the pump is squeezed, fluid moves from the cuff to the balloon reservoir. This decompression of the cuff opens the bladder neck and allows the patient to void. After 1 to 2 minutes the pressure-regulating balloon automatically reinflates the cuff, which then reestablishes urethral coaptation and continence.

Three techniques have been described for the transvaginal placement of the artificial urinary sphincter.[1,3,4] The inherent advantage of the transvaginal approach is the possibility of dissection of the urethrovaginal plane, which is often obliterated after previous anti-incontinence procedures. The transvaginal technique allows dissection of the urethrovaginal plane under direct vision.

A vertical incision is made in the anterior vaginal wall (Fig. 42-2). The incision extends from a point midway between the bladder neck and the external meatus to the proximal bladder neck. A plane under the vaginal wall is created on each side of the incision with sharp dissection. The dissecting scissors are first pointed laterally to the pubis ramus and then upward toward the ipsilateral shoulder of the patient (Fig. 42-3). Sufficiently thick vaginal flaps are created in anticipation of closure of the vagina over the soon-to-be-placed cuff of the artificial urinary sphincter. If the patient has not had a bladder neck operation, blunt finger dissection may be performed to separate the endopelvic fascia from its lateral attachments to the pubic rim. The finger should sweep from lateral to medial, creating a window into the retropubic space. If the patient has dense scar tissue, sharp dissection will be required to enter the retropubic space. The urethra and bladder neck can then be

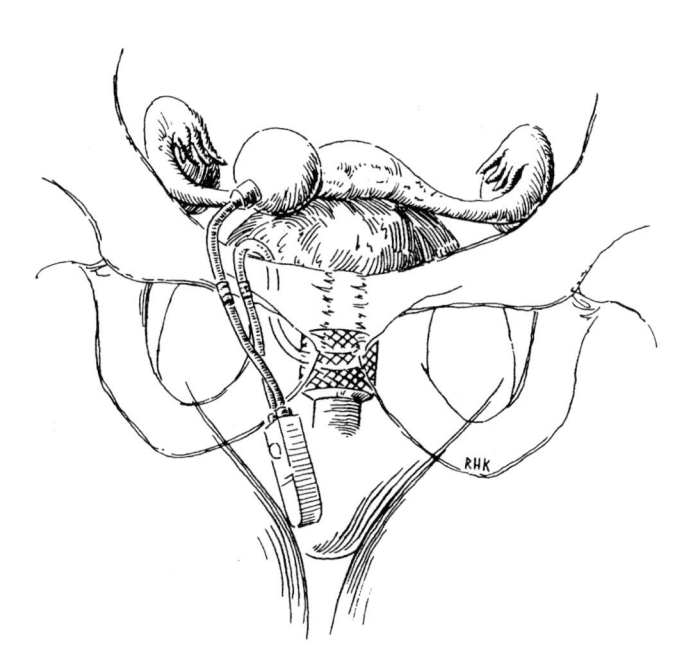

FIGURE 42-1 The AS-800 artificial urinary sphincter in a woman. The cuff is placed around the bladder neck, the pressure-regulating balloon in the prevesical space, and the pump in the labia majora. (From Wang Y, Hadley HR: Artificial sphincter: Transvaginal approach. In Raz S [ed]: Female Urology, 2nd ed. Philadelphia, WB Saunders, 1996.)

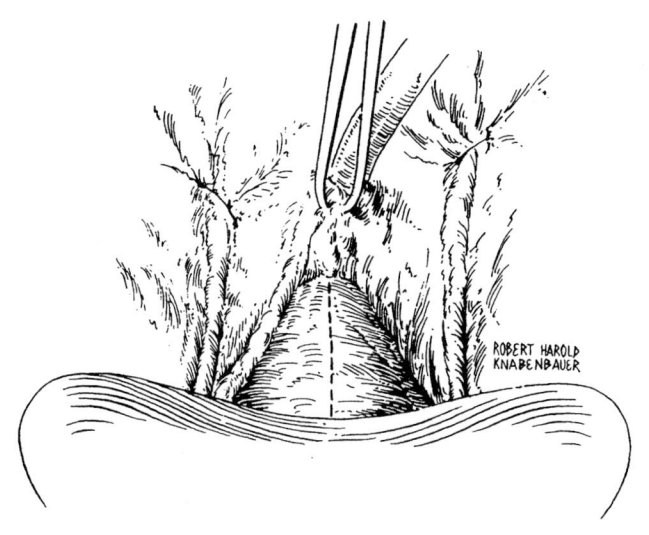

FIGURE 42-2 With the patient in the modified dorsolithotomy position, a vertical incision is made in the anterior vaginal wall. (From Wang Y, Hadley HR: Artificial sphincter: Transvaginal approach. In Raz S [ed]: Female Urology, 2nd ed. Philadelphia, WB Saunders, 1996.)

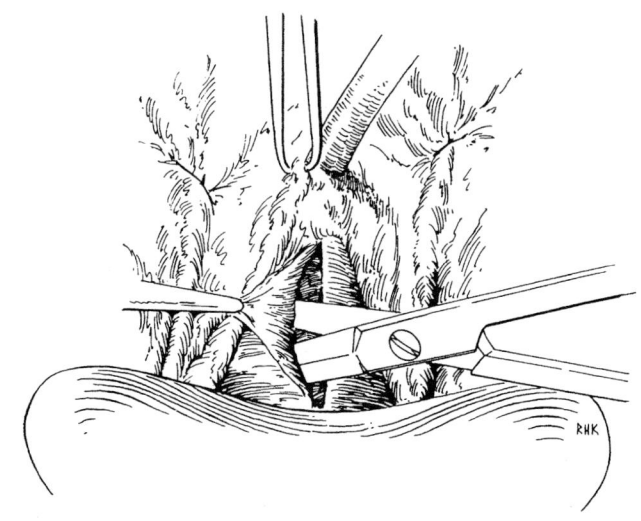

FIGURE 42-3 Using a combination of sharp and blunt dissection, the retropubic space is entered lateral to the bladder neck. (From Wang Y, Hadley HR: Artificial sphincter: Transvaginal approach. In Raz S [ed]: Female Urology, 2nd ed. Philadelphia, WB Saunders, 1996.)

separated posteriorly and laterally from the vagina and the pelvic side wall with sharp and blunt dissection. A similar procedure is followed on the opposite side.

The posterior aspect of the bladder neck is dissected free from the underlying anterior vaginal wall. It is important to mobilize the bladder from the vaginal wall without extending the vaginal incision toward the apex of the vagina. Leaving an intact thick vaginal wall underneath the bladder neck will lessen the likelihood of cuff erosion into the vagina.

Attention is next directed to the anterior aspect of the proximal urethra or bladder neck to free its attachments from the overlying symphysis pubis. If possible, blunt finger dissection should be used to perform this part of the procedure. However, if the patient has had a retropubic operation, dense scarring may be encountered in the anterior portion of the urethra. Overly aggressive dissection may lead to unintentional bladder opening or urethral tear. The dissection on the anterior side of the urethra may be particularly difficult because of its relative inaccessibility through the transvaginal approach. To facilitate exposure of the top side of the urethra, a separate suprameatal incision may be used. The Foley catheter is retracted downward, and a small (1 cm to 2 cm) crescent-shaped incision is made above the external meatus (Fig. 42-4A). Sharp dissection is then done in the midline below the symphysis pubis (Fig. 42-4B). After the bladder is allowed to drop away from its attachments to the symphysis, lateral blunt dissection can easily be performed to complete the dissection to the retropubic space previously opened through the vaginal incision. Thus, a circumferential dissection is completed around the bladder neck. This suprameatal dissection is not necessary, however, if one is readily able to free the urethra from its anterior attachments through the vaginal incision alone.

After the proximal urethra has been freed circumferentially, a broken-back small vascular clamp (Dale femoral-popliteal anastomosis clamp, Pilling 35-3543) is passed around the urethra from the left to right. The cuff-measuring tape is grasped and passed around the urethra (Fig. 42-5), and the circumference of the urethra is measured. If the circumference is equivocal, it is best to err in favor of a slightly larger cuff size. Using a curved clamp, the appropriate size cuff of the artificial urinary sphincter is placed around the proximal urethra (Fig. 42-6). If the pump of the artificial urinary sphincter is to be inserted into the right labium majorus, the cuff is withdrawn from right to left. If, however, the pump is to be placed in the left labia majora, the cuff should be withdrawn from left to right. The cuff is then locked in place (see Fig. 42-6) and rotated 180 degrees so that the hard-locking button lies on the anterior aspect of the urethra, away from the anterior vaginal wall (Fig. 42-7).

A 4-cm transverse suprapubic incision is made on the side that the pressure-regulating balloon and pump mechanism will be implanted. The tubing passer is passed antegrade under fingertip guidance from the suprapubic incision lateral to the midline and down to the vaginal incision on the ipsilateral side of the bladder neck. (This operative step is similar to passing a needle

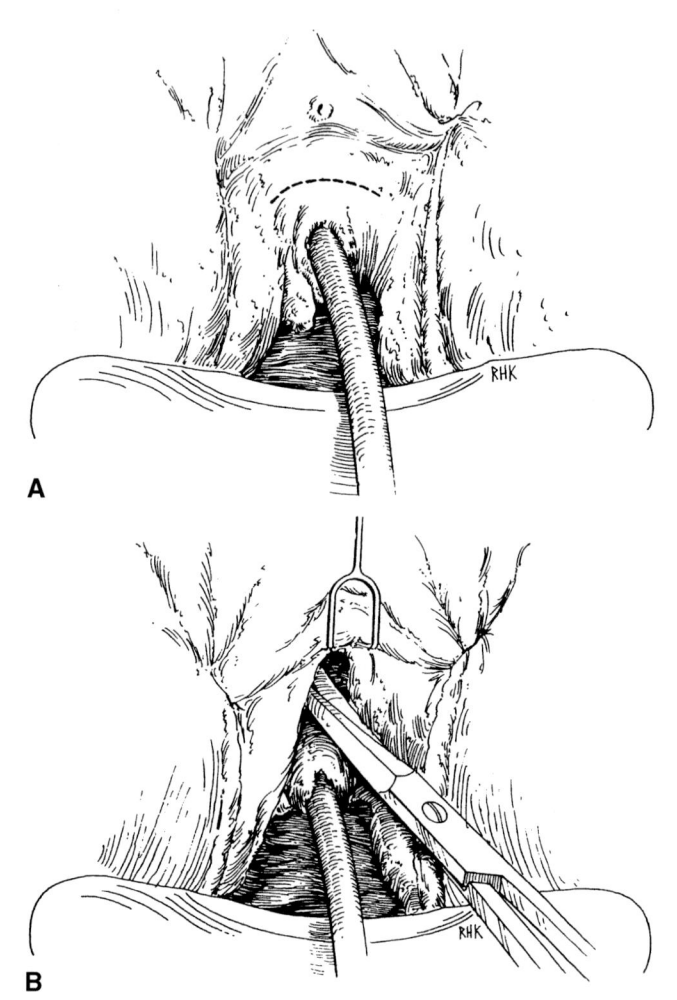

FIGURE 42-4 **A**, If dense scarring is encountered anterior to the urethra, a separate incision is made above the urethral meatus. **B**, The suprameatal dissection is done in the midline just below the symphysis pubis. (From Wang Y, Hadley HR: Artificial sphincter: Transvaginal approach. In Raz S (ed): Female Urology, 2nd ed. Philadelphia, WB Saunders, 1996.)

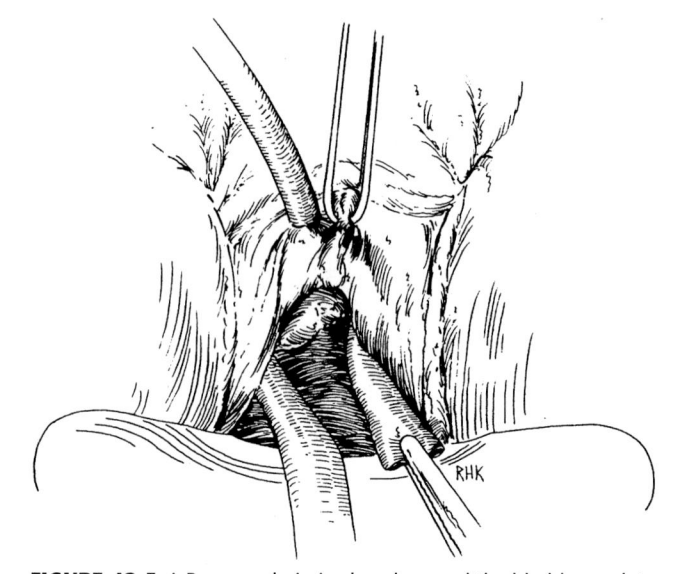

FIGURE 42-5 A Penrose drain is placed around the bladder neck to demonstrate the completed circumferential dissection. (From Wang Y, Hadley HR: Artificial sphincter: Transvaginal approach. In Raz S (ed): Female Urology, 2nd ed. Philadelphia, WB Saunders, 1996.)

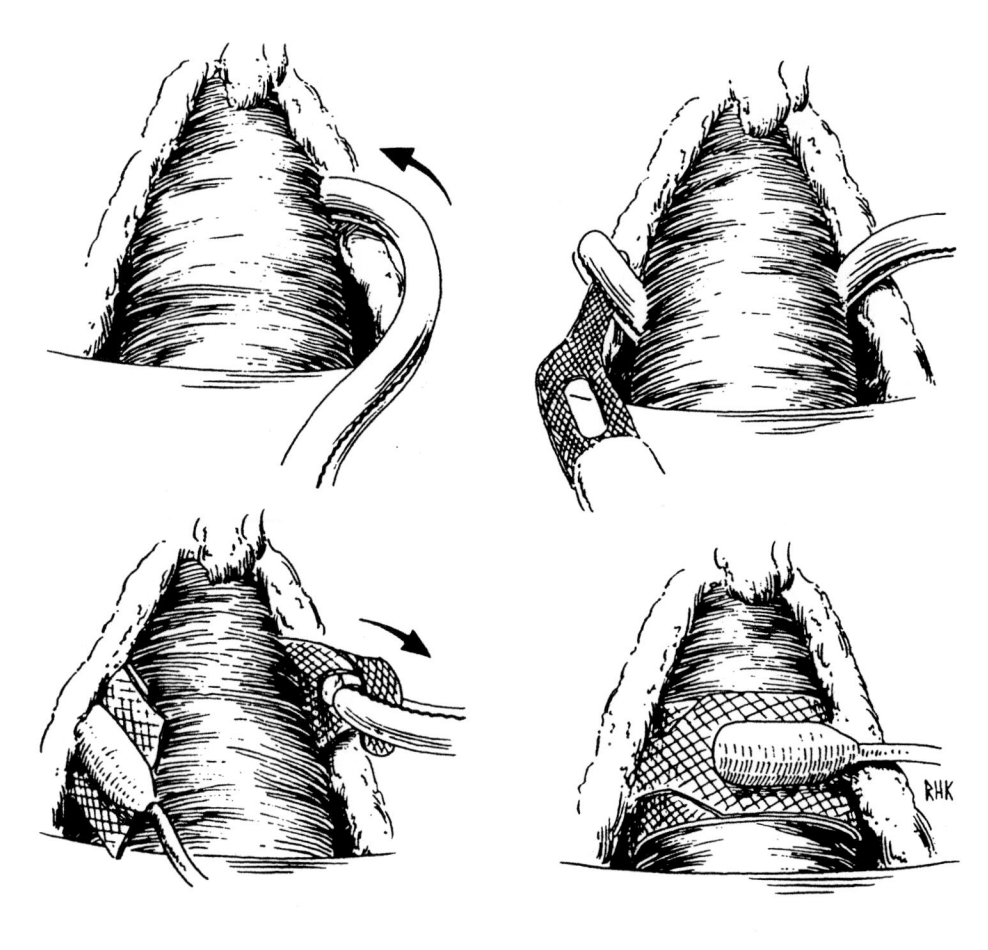

FIGURE 42-6 The cuff of the artificial urinary sphincter is passed around the bladder neck and then locked in place. (From Wang Y, Hadley HR: Artificial sphincter: Transvaginal approach. In Raz S (ed): Female Urology, 2nd ed. Philadelphia, WB Saunders, 1996.)

carrier under fingertip guidance during a Pereyra-type bladder neck suspension.) The cuff tubing is attached to the tubing passer and then withdrawn up to the suprapubic incision. The anterior rectus sheath is incised transversely, and the prevesical space is developed adjacent to the bladder. The pressure-regulating balloon is then inserted in the prevesical space. In women, the 51 cm to 60 cm H_2O pressure balloon reservoir is routinely used.

From the suprapubic incision a subcutaneous tunnel is created through which the pump will be inserted into the labia majora. The pump is passed into the labia majora to the level of the meatus with the deactivation button facing anteriorly.

Filling of the cuff and reservoir are performed according to the instructions specified by the manufacturer. The tubings are trimmed to the appropriate lengths and then irrigated to remove any air or debris from the system.

The suprapubic and vaginal wounds are irrigated with copious amount of antibiotic solution. The wounds are then closed in multiple layers with absorbable sutures to ensure good coverage of the prosthesis with healthy overlying tissue. If the integrity of the vaginal wall appears to be compromised, an interposition of a vascularized flap (e.g., Martius flap) should be considered. The pump is left in the deactivated mode for 6 weeks.

A vaginal gauze pack is placed and removed on the first postoperative day. The Foley catheter is removed on the third postoperative day. The principles and technical steps of the transvaginal placement of the artificial urinary sphincter are outlined in Box 42-1.

FIGURE 42-7 The cuff is rotated 180 degrees clockwise so that the hard-locking button lies anterior to the urethra, away from the anterior vaginal wall. (From Wang Y, Hadley HR: Artificial sphincter: Transvaginal approach. In Raz S (ed): Female Urology, 2nd ed. Philadelphia, WB Saunders, 1996.)

DISCUSSION

The few published reports of the artificial urinary sphincter implanted through the transvaginal approach report

> **BOX 42-1** **Technical Steps for Placement of Artificial Urinary Sphincter**
>
> 1. Vertical incision in the anterior vaginal wall.
> 2. Entrance into the retropubic space lateral to the bladder neck.
> 3. If dense scar tissue is encountered, the circumferential bladder neck dissection is completed with a suprameatal incision to facilitate direct vision of the anterior surface of the urethra and bladder neck.
> 4. Placement of the cuff around the bladder neck with rotation of the hard-locking button of the cuff 180 degrees away from the vaginal wall incision.
> 5. Placement of the low-pressure balloon reservoir (51 cm to 60 cm water pressure) and the labial pump through a small suprapubic incision.
> 6. Interposition of Martius flap if necessary.
> 7. Delayed cuff activation for 6 weeks.
>
> Patients with prior pelvic radiotherapy are excluded.

favorable outcomes. Appell reported a series of 34 patients in whom the AUS was placed through simultaneous vaginal and abdominal incisions.[1] Nineteen patients underwent follow-up of 3 years. The overall continence rate was 100%. Three patients, however, required revisionary operations for inadequate cuff compression and connector leak. Abbassian used the vaginal incision alone to implant the artificial urinary sphincter in four patients.[4] At mean follow-up of 14 months all patients were dry.

The potential advantage of the artificial urinary sphincter over the urethral sling is the capability to place a known circumferential compressive force around the entire urethra rather than a single force on the posterior surface of the urethra. Also a probable decreased likelihood of urinary retention and bladder instability is associated with the artificial urinary sphincter. The incidence of prolonged postoperative urinary retention after the urethral sling operation has been reported to be up to 10%, especially in patients with a preoperative hypotonic bladder.[5] Persistent postoperative urinary frequency and urgency due to bladder instability has been demonstrated in 6% to 18% of patients after placement of the pubovaginal sling in the treatment of type III stress urinary incontinence.[6,7] In our experience of 25 patients who underwent transvaginal placement of the AS-800 artificial urinary sphincter for primary urethral insufficiency, 7 patients had preoperative hypotonic bladder documented on urodynamic studies. Follow-up lasted from 3 to 16 months (mean, 7.3 months). None of the patients developed clinically significant postoperative frequency or urgency. All 7 patients were dry and able to void spontaneously with or without abdominal straining. Prolonged (i.e., more than 1 month) urinary retention requiring intermittent catheterization was not demonstrated by any of the patients who had hypocontractile bladders preoperatively.[8]

The continence rate of the AUS successfully implanted either by the transvaginal or transabdominal approach in women who have not had an erosion in either the bladder or vagina has been very good. A recent series of more than 200 women undergoing a transabdominal placement of the AUS reported a continence rate greater than 90% with a mean follow-up of 3.9 years. In this same series the explantation rate was 6%.[9]

Long-term reliability of the artificial sphincter, regardless of the technique of implantation, is reported sparingly in the urological literature. Our experience with the artificial sphincter in both men and women indicates that the revision rate from all causes is approximately 50% at 5 years and over 90% at 10 years. Similar 10-year revision rates have been reported by Fulford and colleagues.[10]

One major disadvantage of the artificial urinary sphincter is the risk of erosion of the device. This complication can occur if the pump erodes through the skin of the labium or the cuff erodes into the urethra or the vagina. Device erosion has been attributed to poor circulation, low-grade infection, technical difficulties, and shifting of the cuff.[4] Cuff erosion commonly occurs in patients who have undergone prior pelvic irradiation.[11] Our earlier experience included two patients who had been previously irradiated for cervical carcinoma. Both patients developed repeated cuff erosion into the vagina despite multiple revisionary operations. With the use of a low-pressure-regulating balloon (51 cm to 60 cm H_2O pressure), delayed primary activation of the cuff, and exclusion of the patient with prior pelvic radiotherapy, the incidence of device erosion may be much reduced.[1,10] In the past, mechanical malfunction of the artificial urinary sphincter has been common, revision occurring in 31% to 43% of women with the device.[12,13] However, since the introduction of the newly improved cuff design and the in situ activation-deactivation control assembly of the AS-800 model in 1983, the incidence of mechanical malfunction has dramatically decreased.[2]

CONCLUSION

The management of female stress urinary incontinence associated with a nonmobile well-supported urethra and bladder neck is certainly a challenge to the surgeon. Many of these patients have undergone previous unsuccessful anti-incontinence operations. For these difficult situations, the artificial urinary sphincter is a viable alternative treatment modality to the urethral sling or periurethral injection therapy.

The advantage of the transvaginal approach in the placement of the artificial urinary sphincter is that it offers the surgeon the ability to dissect through the difficult urethrovaginal plane under direct vision. If the patient has abundant scar tissue, the addition of a suprameatal incision reduces the likelihood of an inadvertent cystotomy or urethral injury during the anterior dissection of the urethra. With familiarization of implantation technique, the use of a low-pressure-regulating balloon reservoir (51 cm to 60 cm H_2O pressure), delayed primary activation of the cuff, and selective patient criteria (e.g., exclusion of patients with prior pelvic irradiation), the artificial urinary sphincter can result in reasonable long-term social continence in patients with urinary incontinence due to intrinsic urethral insufficiency. In the subgroup of patients with a combination of hypotonic bladder and intrinsic sphincteric incompetence, the artificial urinary sphincter may be the initial treatment of choice over the urethral sling because of its lower incidence of prolonged postoperative urinary retention and vesical instability.

REFERENCES

1. Appell RA: Techniques and results in the implantation of the artificial urinary sphincter in women with type III stress urinary incontinence by a vaginal approach. Neurourol Urodyn 7:613, 1988.
2. Webster GD, Perez LM, Khoury JM, et al: Management of type III stress urinary incontinence using artificial urinary sphincter. Urology 39(6):499, 1992.
3. Hadley R: Transvaginal placement of the artificial urinary sphincter in women. Neurourol Urodyn 7:292, 1988.
4. Abbassian A: A new operation for insertion of the artificial urinary sphincter. J Urol 140:512, 1988.
5. Blaivas JG, Jacobs BZ: Pubovaginal fascial sling for the treatment of complicated stress urinary incontinence. J Urol 145:1214, 1991.
6. Blaivas JG, Olsson CA: Stress incontinence: Classification and surgical approach. J Urol 139:727, 1988.
7. McGuire EJ, Bennett CJ, Konnak JA, et al: Experience with pubovaginal slings for urinary incontinence at the University of Michigan. J Urol 138:525, 1987.
8. Wang Y, Hadley HR: Artificial urinary sphincter in the female: Is it procedure of choice for the patient with type III urinary incontinence associated with an acontractile bladder? J Urol 147(4):377A, 1992.
9. Costa P, et al: The use of an artificial urinary sphincter in women with type III incontinence and a negative Marshall test. J Urol 165(3):1172–1176, 2001.
10. Fulford SC, et al: The fate of the "modern" artificial urinary sphincter with a follow-up of more than 10 years. Br J Urol 79(5):713–716, 1997.
11. Duncan HJ, Nurse DE, Mundy AR: Role of the artificial urinary sphincter in the treatment of stress incontinence in women. Br J Urol 69:141, 1992.
12. Donovan MG, Barrett DM, Furlow WL: Use of the artificial urinary sphincter in the management of severe incontinence in females. Surg Gynecol Obstet 161:17, 1985.
13. Light JK, Scott FB: Management of urinary incontinence in women with the artificial urinary sphincter. J Urol 134:476, 1985.

CHAPTER 43

Conventional and Minimized Pubovaginal Sling in Patients with Severe Stress Urinary Incontinence

DMITRY PUSHKAR ■ OLEG LORAN

Much information has been published on the management of complex stress urinary incontinence (SUI). Usually, this problem is associated with type III stress incontinence.[1-7] Pubovaginal sling (PVS) procedures are the optimum treatment choice for patients with type III SUI.

Various organic and synthetic materials have been used for sling formation during the development of this procedure.[8-12] Some of them are shown in Table 43-1.

In Russia, most patients are treated for type IIB or type III SUI. Since 1977, in our department, we have used conventional sling procedures for patients with type III SUI. In 1989, we started to use minimized sling procedures for patients with type IIB and type III SUI. Minimized procedures lead to shorter hospital stays and are associated with less morbidity. We have used various materials, and in 1985, we started to use autologous skin taken from the anterior abdominal wall of the patient.

This chapter describes our experience with this conventional and minimized PVS procedure, and describes the technique for the minimized PVS procedure that we developed.[13]

RATIONALE FOR USING PUBOVAGINAL SLING PROCEDURES IN PATIENTS WITH TYPE IIB STRESS URINARY INCONTINENCE

Measurement of abdominal leak-point pressure in patients with primary forms of SUI and severe anatomic abnormalities showed a decrease of leak-point pressure to a mean value of 75.6 cm H_2O.[14] This finding allowed us to consider this group of patients with intrinsic sphincter dysfunctions. Periurethral tissue biopsy specimens showed fibrotic changes in the periurethral area. Since the majority of the patients had prior anti-stress incontinence surgery and periurethral fibrosis was demonstrated on biopsy, standard pubovaginal suspension procedures were deemed unacceptable because of the potential for a high rate of failure. Therefore, these patients were offered minimized pubovaginal sling procedures.

THE TECHNIQUE OF MINIMIZED PUBOVAGINAL SKIN SLING PROCEDURE (FIGS. 43-1 TO 43-7)

The first step in this procedure is the formation of 2-cm-wide and 4-cm-long skin flap from the lower anterior abdominal wall. Subcutaneous fat is removed from the

Text continued on page 418

TABLE 43-1 ■ Materials Used for Sling Procedures

Type of Material	Material	Study
Organic		
	Pyramidalis muscle	Goebell (1910)
		Steckel (1917)
	Rectus fascia	Thompson (1923)
		Aldridge (1942)
		Shaw (1949)
		McGuire (1978)
	Round ligaments	Barns (1950)
		Hodgkinson (1957)
	Autologous skin	Loran (1993)
Synthetic		
	Nylon	Bracht (1951)
	Mersilene mesh	Moir (1968)
	Marlex mesh	Morgan (1970)
	Silastic	Stanton (1985)

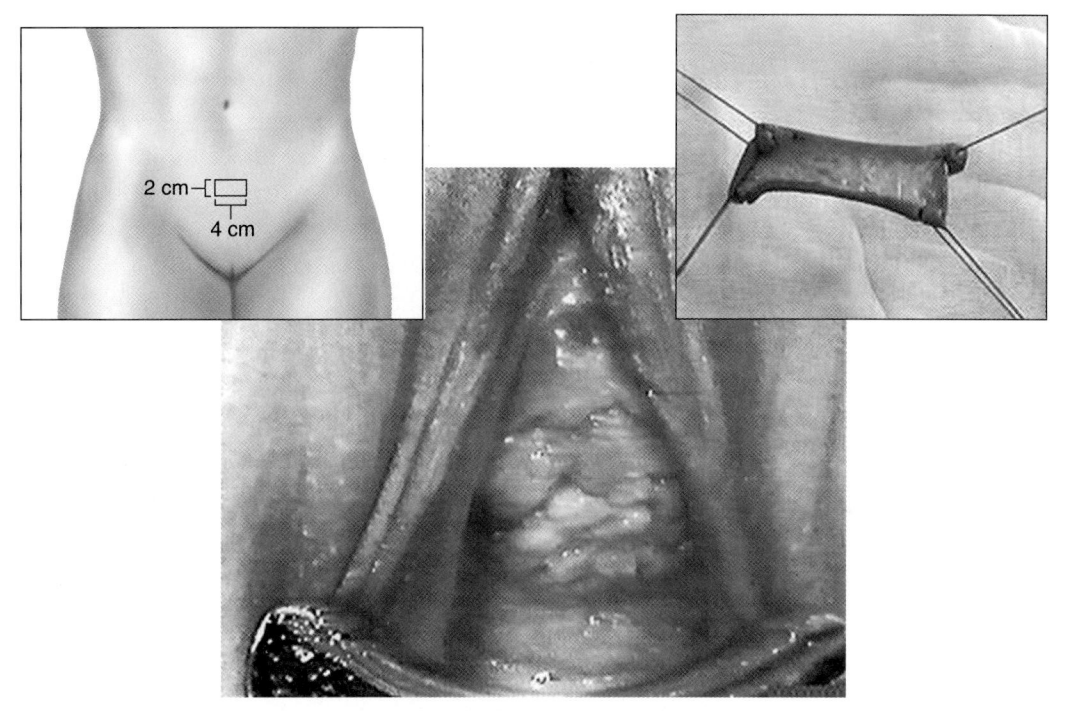

FIGURE 43-1 A rectangular skin flap is created in the lower abdominal area. The average flap size is 1.5 to 2 cm × 4 cm. Four Prolene 0 sutures are attached to each corner of the flap.

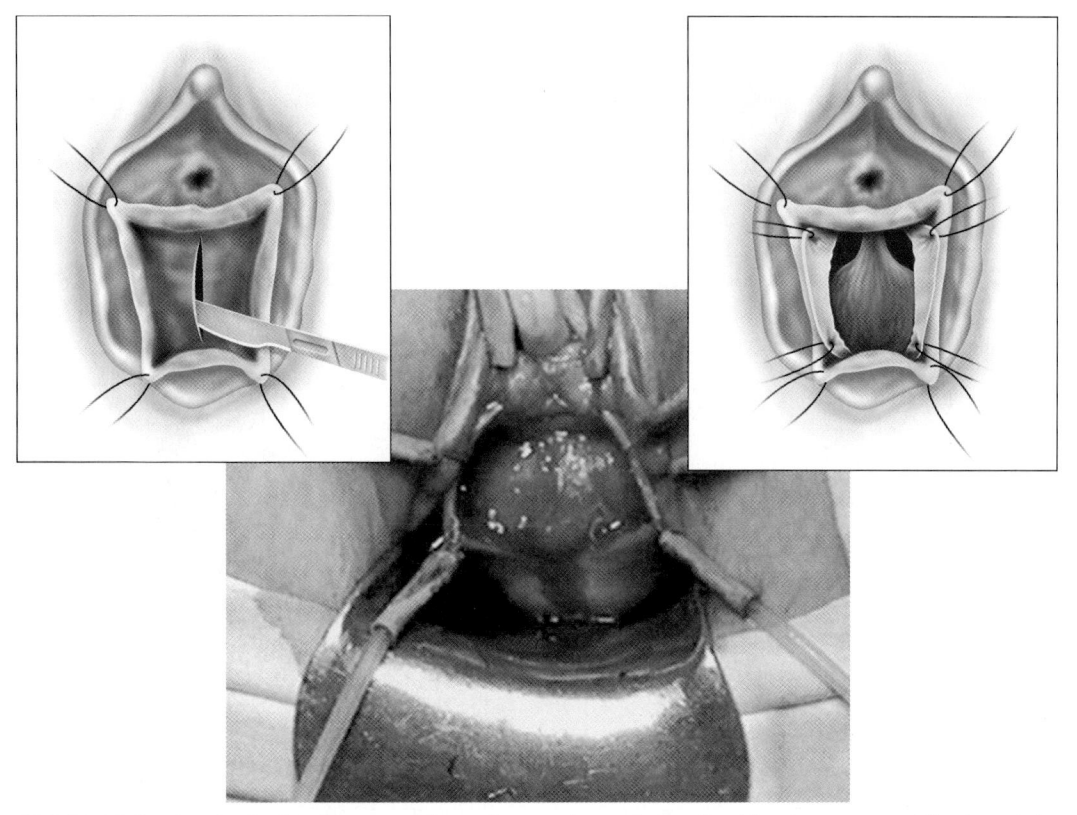

FIGURE 43-2 A longitudinal incision is made on the anterior vaginal wall, with subsequent mobilization of the periurerhral and bladder neck areas.

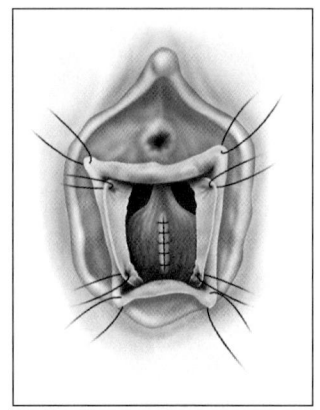

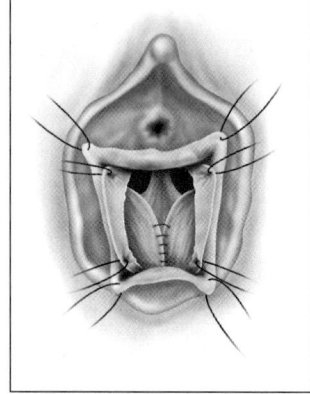

FIGURE 43-3 A standard cystocele repair, which can be performed at the time of the procedure, if necessary.

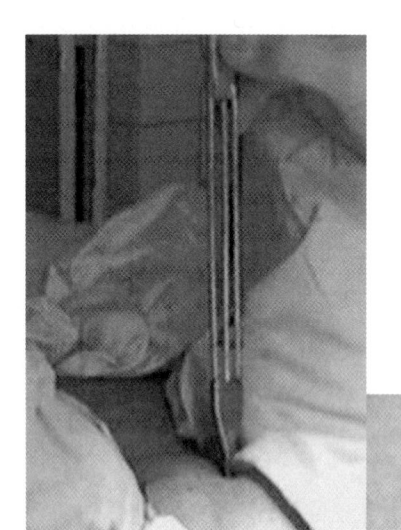

FIGURE 43-4 Two Pereyra ligature carriers are passed from the suprapubic area to the vaginal wound.

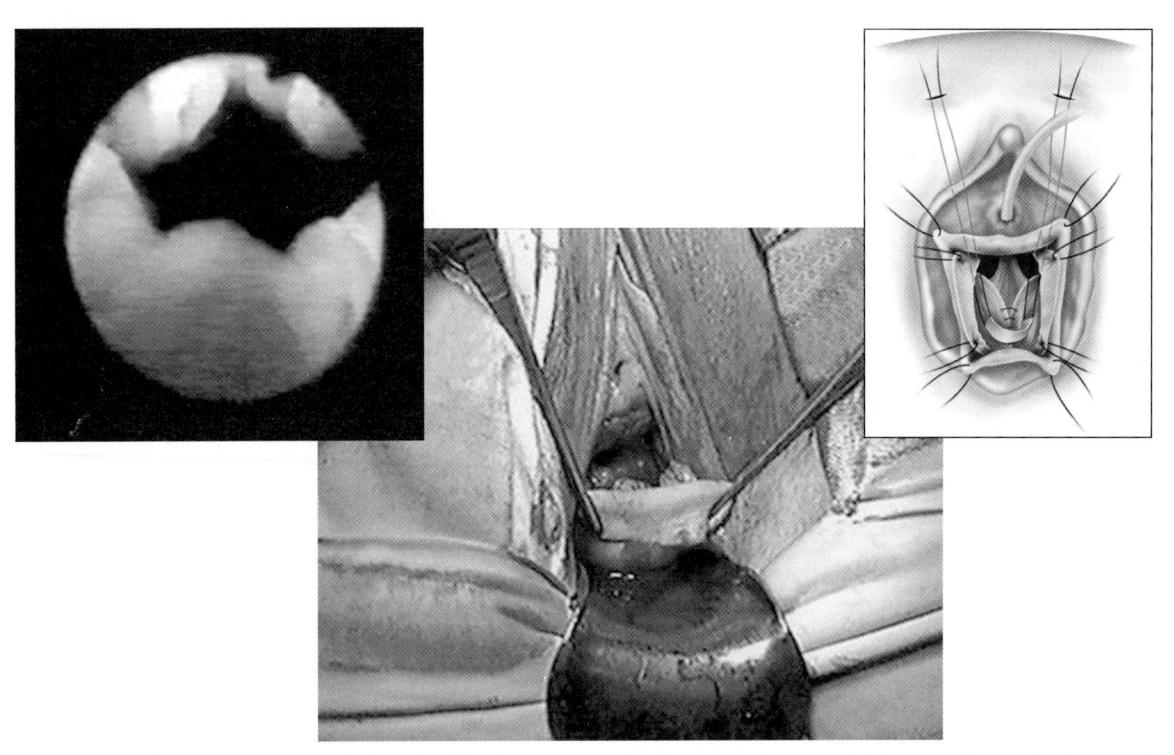

FIGURE 43-5 Prolene sutures attached to the skin flap are passed to the suprapubic area. Cystoscopy shows the absence of bladder perforation and a wide open bladder neck.

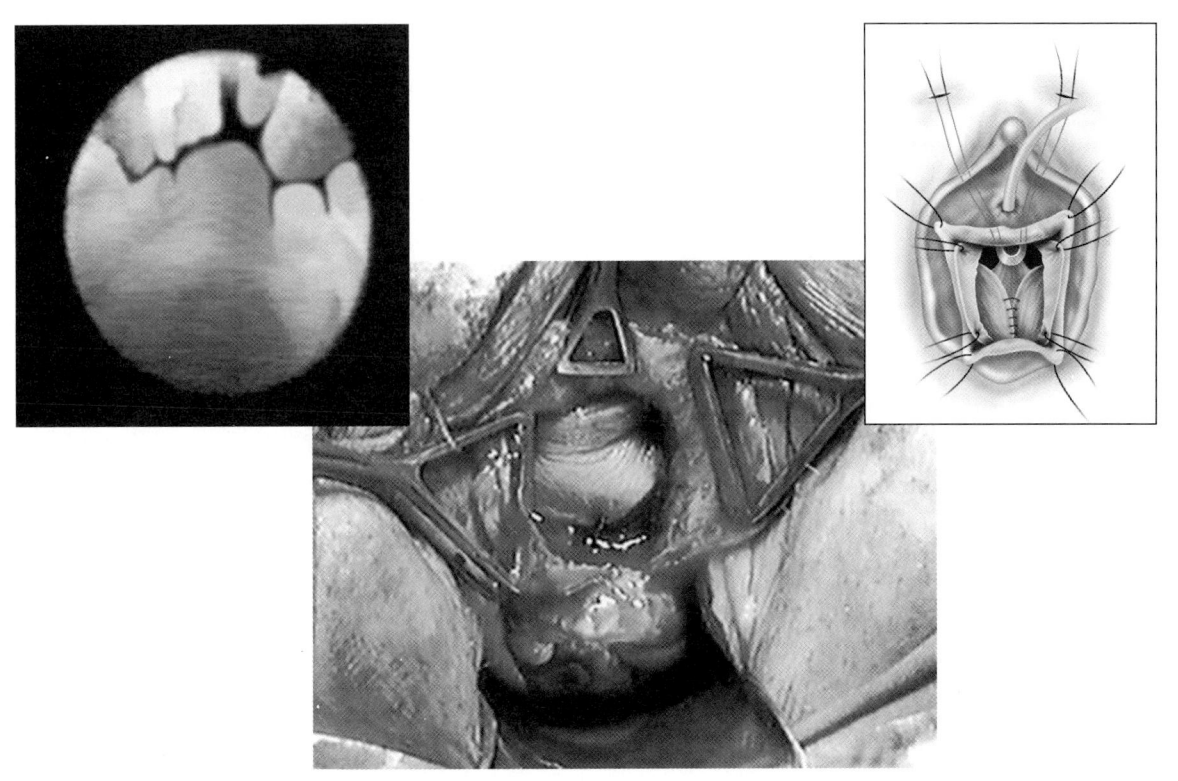

FIGURE 43-6 The flap is located in the bladder neck and part of the proximal urethra area, and fixed by two absorbable sutures to the periurethral tissues.

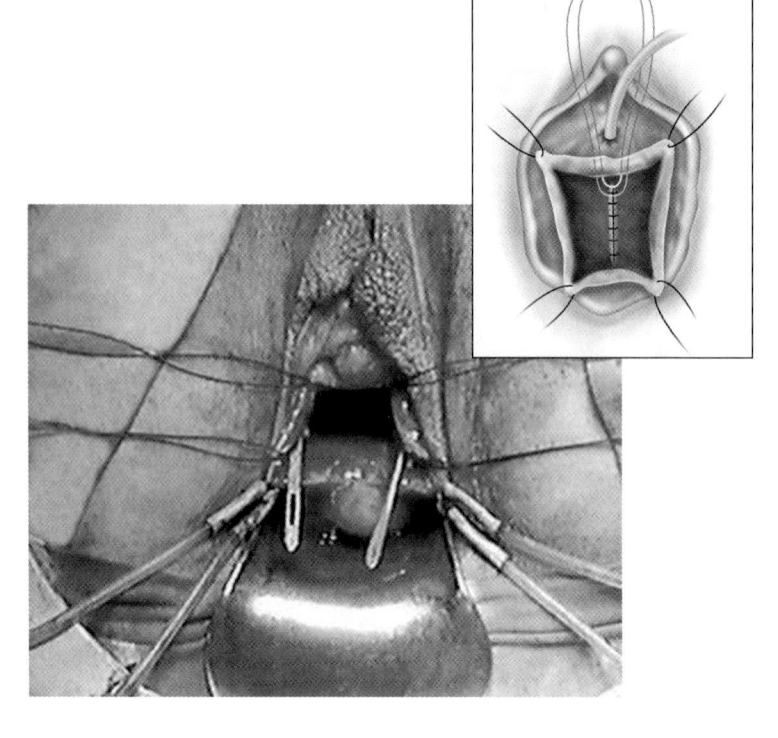

FIGURE 43-7 The final steps of the procedure are closure of the vaginal wall, followed by tying of the Prolene sutures under the skin with no tension.

Text continued from page 414

flaps, and they are left in an antiseptic solution for 10 to 15 minutes. Four polypropylene ligatures are placed on the tips of the skin flap so that they can be guided from the vagina to the suprapubic area by Pereyra ligature carrier.

The vaginal part of the procedure provides both mobilization of the bladder neck area and standard cystocele repair. If necessary, a hysterectomy or hysterosuspension may be performed at this stage. Further on, the mobilization of the perivesical and periurethral tissue continues to create tunnels to guide the Pereyra ligature carrier.

The Prolene sutures fixed on the tips of the flap are guided from the vaginal wound to the suprapubic area, and the skin flap is fixed in the bladder neck area. Cystoscopy shows an open bladder neck before and a closed bladder neck after the Prolene ligature is stretched subcutaneously in the suprapubic area with no tension. The final step is closure of the vaginal wall and insertion of a Foley catheter for 24 hours.

PATIENT CHARACTERISTICS AND FOLLOW-UP

In total, 531 patients with type IIB and type III SUI underwent PVS procedures. Of these, 392 patients with a mean age of 52.9 years underwent conventional PVS and 139 patients with a mean age of 49 years underwent minimized PVS.

Long-term follow-up data were analyzed for 176 patients who underwent conventional PVS (group 1) and 105 patients who underwent minimized PVS (group 2).

The mean follow-up period for both groups of patients was 5.7 years (range, 5–7 years). Long-term outcome was evaluated according to the responses on an annual standard subjective questionnaire and the findings on physical examination. On average, all patients completed the questionnaire 5.1 times, and no less than 3 times, during the follow-up period. Figure 43-8 shows the questionnaire that was used for annual patient evaluations. Table 43-2 shows additional data for patients studied. Table 43-3 shows intraoperative and postoperative complications in both groups of patients.

Two patients suffered distal ureteral obstruction requiring percutaneous nephrostomy and subsequent ureteroneocystostomy. One patient developed a pelvic hematoma, which was successfully drained percutaneously. Bladder instability was corrected by secondary medical treatment with oxybutynin (Ditropan).

Mean hospital stay was 6.7 days for patients in group 1 and 3.5 days for those in group 2. Follow-up evaluation included physical examination, cystometry, and urethral pressure profiles. For both groups, maximal urethral pressure and functional urethral length were not statistically different before surgery and 1 year later.

RESULTS

In total, 85% of patients had good results during the first year of follow-up. Long-term follow-up data were available for both groups of patients. In postoperative years 1 and 2, positive results (defined as no sign of SUI) were reported in 87% of patients in both groups. In postoperative years 3 and 4, positive results were reported in 77% of patients in

1. Do you have SUI symptoms now?

☐ yes   ☐ no   ☐ one-two times a month   ☐ more than two times a month

___

2. Do you use pads?

☐ no   ☐ sometimes (specify)   ☐ yes (how many, how often)

___

3. Did you develop new micturition disorders after operation?

☐ no   ☐ yes (specify)

___

4. Are you satisfied with operative results?

☐ yes   ☐ no

___

5. Would you recommend this procedure to other patients with similar symptoms?

☐ yes   ☐ no

___

FIGURE 43-8 A standard simplified postoperative questionnaire. SUI, stress urinary incontinence.

group 1 and 71% of patients in group 2. In postoperative years 5 to 7, positive results were reported in 61% of patients in group 1 and 62% of patients in group 2.

Positive results indicate total patients satisfaction and complete restoration of continence. The latest annual survey showed that approximately 10% of patients in group 2 were satisfied with the operative results, despite mild SUI symptoms and pad use. All of the patients said that they would recommend this procedure to other patients with similar symptoms.

Axial magnetic resonance imaging performed 6 months after the minimized procedure in 27 patients showed a well-supported urethra and normal anatomic position of the bladder neck. In most cases, imaging also showed a skin flap that was localized around the urethrovesical junction (Fig. 43-9).

TABLE 43-2 ■ Patients Studied

Prior and Simultaneous Procedures	Group 1	Group 2
Previous antistress procedures (1–5)	154 (87.5%)	51 (48.6%)
Previous successful urethral restoration	6 (3.4%)	39 (37.1%)
Previous hysterectomy	37 (21.0%)	16 (15.2%)
Previous vaginal gynecologic procedures	12 (6.8%)	42 (40%)
Previous cystocele repair	89 (50.6%)	41 (39.05%)
Previous prolapse repair	19 (10.8%)	8 (7.6%)
Simultaneous vaginal hysterectomy	21 (11.9%)	7 (6.7%)
Simultaneous hysterocolpo-suspension (Kozminski procedure)	7 (4.0%)	2 (1.9%)
Simultaneous cystocele repair	89 (50.6%)	41 (39.05%)

TABLE 43-3 ■ Intraoperative and Postoperative Complications in Both Groups of Patients

Complication	Group 1	Group 2
Wound infection	6 (3.4%)	3 (2.9%)
Distal ureteral obstruction	2 (1.1%)	
Vesicovaginal fistula	1 (0.6%)	
Skin flap necrosis	1 (0.6%)	
Pelvic hematoma	1 (0.6%)	1 (1.0%)
Prolonged postoperative urinary retention (>1 mo)	14 (8.0%)	5 (4.8%)
De novo bladder instability	11 (6.3%)	7 (6.7%)

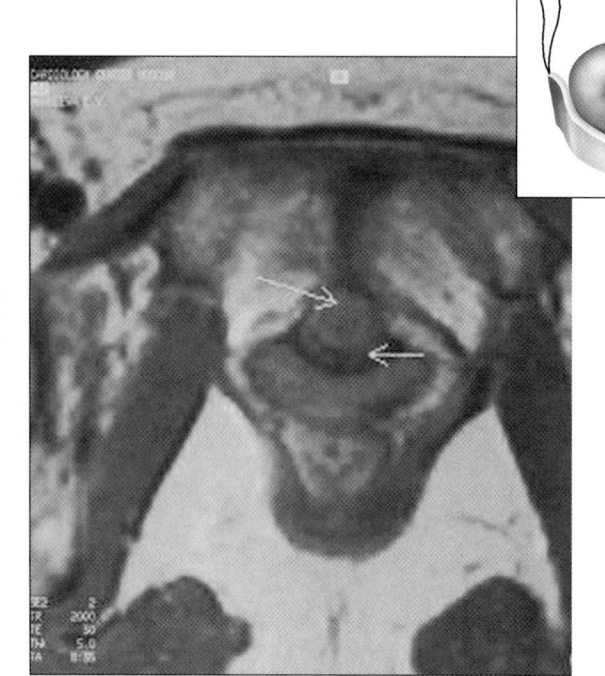

FIGURE 43-9 Pelvic magnetic resonance imaging scan performed 6 months after the procedure and line drawing, showing satisfactory flap position at the bladder neck. *Arrows* show the urethra and the well-placed skin flap.

CONCLUSION

We prefer to use the PVS procedure to correct complex SUI. Patient preference and technical limitations are the defining factors that determine the appropriateness of minimized procedures, which offer decreased morbidity and a shorter hospital stay. The minimized PVS procedure produced good results in 62% of patients, which is comparable to the finding of good results in 61% of patients who underwent conventional PVS.

We do not currently practice conventional PVS in our department because minimized PVS is simpler and offers lower morbidity rates, a lower complication rate, and equal efficacy. We believe that minimized procedures will replace conventional PVS and could become the treatment of choice for patients with type III SUI. In our department, widespread use of synthetic materials for both the treatment of stress urinary incontinence and cystocele repair began in 1996. Today, minimized skin sling procedure is reserved for those patients who prefer autologous tissue for their surgery.

REFERENCES

1. Blaivas JC, Olsson CA: Stress incontinence: Classification and surgical approach. J Urol 139(4):727–731, 1988.
2. Hodgkinson CP: Recurrent stress urinary incontinence. Am J Obstet Gynecol 132(8):844–860, 1978.
3. Horbach NS, Blanco JS, Ostergard DR, et al: A suburethral sling procedure with polytetrafluoroethylene for the treatment of genuine stress incontinence in patients with low urethral closure pressure. Obstet Gynecol 71(4):648–652, 1988.
4. Iosif CS: Sling operation for urinary incontinence. Acta Obstet Gynecol Scand 64(2):187–190, 1985.
5. Juma S, Little NA, Raz S: Vaginal wall sling: Four years later. Urology 39(5):424–428, 1992.
6. McGuire EJ, Bennett CJ, Konnak JA, et al: Experience with pubovaginal slings for urinary incontinence at the University of Michigan. J Urol 138(3):525–526, 1987.
7. Raz S, Siegel AL, Short JL, Snyder JA: Vaginal wall sling. J Urol (141):43–46, 1989.
8. Aldridge AH: Transplantation of fascia for relief of urinary stress incontinence. Am J Obstet Gynecol (44):398–411, 1942.
9. Blaivas JG, Jacobs BZ: Pubovaginal fascial sling for the treatment of complicated stress urinary incontinence. J Urol (145):1214–1218, 1991.
10. Farrow GA, Morgan JE, Heritz D: Marlex sling for recurrence stress urinary incontinence: Late results. AUA abstracts. J Urol 149(4):291, 1993.
11. Morgan JE, Farrow GA, Stewart FE: The Marlex sling operation for the treatment of recurrent stress urinary incontinence: A 16 year review. Am J Obstet Gynecol 151(2):224–226, 1985.
12. Stanton SL, Brindley GS, Holmes DM: Silastic sling for urethral sphincter incompetence in women. Br J Obstet Gynaecol 92(7):747–750, 1985.
13. Loran OB, Pushkar DU: Pubovaginal skin sling in patients with artificial urethra. AUA abstracts. J Urol 149(4):403, 1993.
14. Nitti VW, Combs AJ: Correlation of Valsalva leak point pressure with subjective degree of stress urinary incontinence in women. J Urol 155(1):281–285, 1996.

CHAPTER 44

Surgical Treatment in Men

JOANNA K. CHON ■ GARY E. LEACH

Pelvic floor disorders in men are usually a complication of surgery, most commonly occurring after prostatectomy for benign or malignant prostate disease or other pelvic surgery, such as abdominoperineal resection or pelvic exenteration for colorectal cancer. Neurogenic dysfunction, including myelodysplasia, spinal cord injury, and suprapontine disorders, can also result in retention or incontinence. Earlier chapters discussed the anatomy, physiology, evaluation, and conservative management of pelvic floor disorders. This chapter briefly summarizes the etiology of pelvic floor disorders and details their surgical treatment.

In choosing the appropriate therapy, it is necessary to establish several goals. Maintenance of low storage pressure to reduce the risk of upper-tract damage is essential. Other therapeutic goals include decreasing the incidence of urinary tract infections, achieving adequate emptying at low intravesical pressure, achieving adequate urinary control, and avoiding a catheter or stoma when possible.

A logical classification of voiding dysfunction is to categorize it functionally as a failure to facilitate storage or a failure to empty. These categories can be further classified according to whether the defect is at the level of the bladder or at the bladder outlet (the sphincter). Some diseases are the result of both storage and emptying problems and are treated with a combination of treatment modalities.

FAILURE TO EMPTY

Failure to Empty because of the Bladder

Any injury to the sacral spinal cord (S2–S4) or the pelvic nerves can cause sacral arc denervation and result in a poorly compliant bladder or an acontractile bladder. Bladder emptying is impeded by acontractility of the detrusor. The smooth sphincter is the smooth muscle of the bladder neck and proximal urethra, and is under involuntary control. The striated sphincter is the muscle that surrounds the urethra at the level of the membranous urethra, which is under voluntary control. In patients with sacral arc denervation, the smooth sphincter is nonrelaxing and the striated sphincter retains some fixed tone, but is not under voluntary control. Chronic overdistension of the bladder in patients who have bladder outlet obstruction causes a "myogenic bladder" as a result of overstretching. This overstretching may leave the bladder temporarily or permanently acontractile.

After abdominoperineal resection, injury to the pelvic plexus can occur and cause voiding dysfunction. Urinary and sexual dysfunction are common problems after surgery for rectal cancer and are caused by damage to the pelvic autonomic nerves during surgery.[1] Lower urinary dysfunction is reported in 10% to 60% of patients after abdominoperineal resection and radical hysterectomy, and approximately 15% to 20% of these patients have permanent voiding dysfunction.[2,3] The most common type of voiding dysfunction is impaired bladder contractility.

Usually, patients with myelodysplastic diseases have an acontractile bladder with an open bladder neck.[4] However, approximately 10% to 15% of patients with myelodysplasia have detrusor–external sphincter dyssynergia (DESD), which causes a functional obstruction because the external sphincter does not open with bladder contraction, whereas 62% have detrusor hyperreflexia and 39% have detrusor areflexia.[5]

Treatment for Failure to Empty at the Bladder Level

Nonsurgical therapy is the most appropriate treatment for patients with acontractile bladders. A program of clean intermittent catheterization (CIC) should be instituted. When patients cannot catheterize themselves because of impaired dexterity or insufficient nursing assistance, chronic catheter drainage may be indicated as a last resort. In the patient who has complications from a chronic indwelling catheter, urinary diversion may be beneficial. A variety of continent and incontinent diversions using different intestinal segments can be tailored to suit the needs of the individual patient. Other therapy, such as sacral nerve stimulation with the Interstim implant (Medtronic, Minneapolis, MN), may be considered. The details of this therapeutic modality are discussed in Chapters 46 and 47.

Failure to Empty because of the Outlet

Anatomic obstruction at the outlet may result in poor emptying, and is the most common cause of failure to empty. Benign prostatic hyperplasia affects approximately 85% of men older than 50 years of age, and by the ninth decade of life, 50% of American men become symptomatic.[6] Patients with urethral stricture disease may have retention as a result of outlet obstruction. For patients with outlet obstruction, the surgical treatment is transurethral resection of the prostate or simple prostatectomy for patients with benign prostatic hyperplasia, or internal urethrotomy for patients with urethral stricture disease.

Complete suprasacral spinal cord injury results in a characteristic pattern in which DESD and detrusor hyper-reflexia are present. In patients with DESD, the goal is to paralyze the bladder with anticholinergic agents to decrease bladder pressure and increase storage volume. CIC is performed to empty the bladder. In patients who have severe DESD and can perform CIC, eliminating the dysfunctional sphincter surgically (i.e., sphincterotomy) is an alternative that, in theory, converts a combined problem with emptying and storage to one of storage alone.

Treatment for Failure to Empty at the Outlet Level

Sphincterotomy

Approximately 8% to 60% of patients with spinal cord injuries undergo sphincterotomy.[7] Sphincterotomy may be indicated in a select group of patients with detrusor hyper-reflexia who cannot perform CIC or lack the necessary assistance to perform CIC. Before the advent of CIC combined with anticholinergic therapy, transurethral sphincterotomy was one of the most popular therapeutic modalities used for patients with spinal cord injury and DESD. The goal of the operation is to transform high-pressure incontinence to low-pressure incontinence, thereby protecting the upper urinary tracts.

Preoperative Considerations. Sphincterotomy is an irreversible therapeutic procedure, and the decision to perform it must be made carefully, after all possibilities to restore continence are exhausted. Patients with spinal cord lesions above T6, the level of the sympathetic outlet, can have problems with autonomic dysreflexia. A spinal anesthetic should be used to prevent autonomic dysreflexia from occurring during sphincterotomy. The patient must understand that a sphincterotomy may achieve low bladder pressure, but at the expense of continence. In addition to decreased bladder contractility, persistently high postvoid residuals are reported after sphincterotomy,[8–10] and a suprapubic tube may be a simpler alternative, if continence is desired.

Procedure. External sphincterotomy is performed with a Collins knife. A single incision is made at the 12 o'clock position rather than the bilateral posterolateral position, which had been reported.[11,12] Making the incision at the 12 o'clock position results in decreased complications of hemorrhage and erectile dysfunction. The sphincterotomy incision must be 2 cm long and 6 mm deep to transect the striated muscle fibers of the external sphincter completely.[13] This incision is basically made from the bladder neck to the bulbar urethra. A catheter is left in place and removed when the urine is clear.

Results. Vapnek and colleagues[14] examined the results of sphincterotomy in patients with spinal cord injuries. Long-term follow-up showed a significant reoperation rate of 15% to 50%. Most sphincterotomy "failures" are caused by detrusor areflexia. Consequently, at least 10% of patients do not empty the bladder sufficiently, even after the decrease in outlet resistance after sphincterotomy.[8–10] Incomplete emptying after sphincterotomy may be caused by decreased detrusor contractility. Detrusor contractility may be dependent on a sensory feedback mechanism that is dependent on filling of the bladder. Therefore, sphincterotomy may prevent the bladder from reaching a critical volume that triggers a detrusor contraction and, over time, leads to decreased contractility and emptying.[8]

After sphincterotomy, patients are incontinent and require long-term condom catheter use. Patients with a small or retracted phallus may have difficulty keeping the catheter in place. For patients who do not use external collection devices, a chronically wet diaper can lead to skin breakdown and dissatisfaction with the outcome. We do not routinely perform sphincterotomy for patients with DESD because of the high failure and reoperation rates. We prefer to paralyze the bladder with anticholinergic agents and use CIC, which may be performed by the patient or a caregiver. If the patient cannot perform CIC, we prefer to treat patients with DESD with a suprapubic tube. Urinary diversion is an option for patients who have major complications with indwelling catheters.

Intraurethral stent

The use of an intraurethral sphincter stent prosthesis as an alternative treatment for DESD has been available since 1990. The UroLume (AMS, Minnetonka, MN) device is a superalloy mesh tube that produces a radial force to keep the urethral sphincter in an open position. The stent expands to a luminal diameter of 42 Fr.

Procedure. The patient is placed in the dorsal lithotomy position. A 3-cm UroLume stent is inserted with a 22 Fr cystoscopic insertion tool. The deployment tool is prepackaged and loaded with the prosthesis and placed in the urethra, at the level of the verumontanum, under direct vision. The proximal margin of the stent is used to cover the distal half of the verumontanum. The distal end of the stent is usually placed in the bulbar urethra to bridge the length of the external sphincter (Fig. 44-1). Postoperatively, a condom catheter is used for urinary collection.

Results. Chancellor and associates[15] evaluated the results with the sphincteric stent and reported findings that were comparable to those with sphincterotomy. In this study, 25 patients were treated with sphincterotomy and 31 patients were treated with the sphincteric stent. The preoperative maximum detrusor pressure was

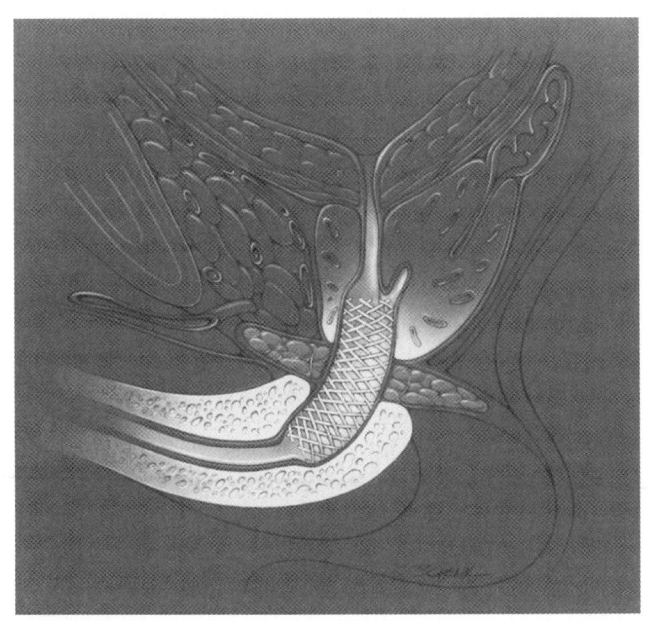

FIGURE 44-1 UroLume endoprosthesis. (Courtesy of American Medical Systems, Inc., Minnetonka, MN. Artist: Michael Schenk.)

98.3 cm H$_2$O for patients who underwent sphincterotomy and 95.7 cm H$_2$O for those who had sphincteric stents. At 24 months of follow-up, the maximum detrusor pressure decreased to 41.6 and 71.6 cm H$_2$O for the sphincterotomy and stent groups, respectively. Mean residual volumes at 24 months were 112 and 132 mL for the sphincterotomy and stent groups, respectively. Although improved from preoperative pressures, detrusor pressures were still elevated and patients still had increased postvoid residual volumes.

Device retrieval was required in 13% of patients because of misplacement or migration during the initial insertion of the stent, but was performed with minimal complications. Of 158 men who had the device placed, 31 (19.6%) eventually required removal.[16] The UroLume is removed cystoscopically by grasping the distal end of the stent with alligator forceps and gently pulling the stent. Even with complete epithelialization of the stent, the investigators reported no significant difficulty with removal of the stent. The epithelialized tissue was resected at a low generator setting. To prevent the stent wires from melting, the loop did not remain in the same area for more than 1 to 2 seconds. Once the stent was exposed, it was grasped and removed.

An advantage of the UroLume procedure is its reversibility. However, problems similar to those associated with sphincterotomy (persistent detrusor hyper-reflexia and high postvoid residuals) make this option less attractive than anticholinergic therapy with CIC for patients who desire continence.

Other options

CIC in addition to anticholinergic therapy is preferred to sphincterotomy for patients with DESD, but when CIC is not an option, suprapubic drainage may be considered. In most cases, consideration of a suprapubic tube in lieu of sphincterotomy can be justified on the basis of the complications of sphincterotomy. These complications include recurrent infections, inadequate emptying, autonomic dysreflexia, and penile skin problems that result from chronic condom catheter wear. Suprapubic catheterization has been criticized as a form of bladder management because it was previously associated with a high complication rate.[17,18] However, MacDiarmid and colleagues[19] found that suprapubic catheterization is a safe and effective alternative form of bladder management, and patients did well, with no renal deterioration, vesicoureteral reflux, or bladder carcinoma. These authors evaluated 44 patients with spinal cord injury who had suprapubic catheters in place for 12 to 150 months (mean, 58 months). Uncomplicated symptomatic urinary tract infection was the most common complication, occurring in 43% of patients. Complicated urinary tract infection occurred in only 9% of patients. Suprapubic catheterization is safer and more effective for bladder drainage than urethral catheterization. However, clean intermittent catheterization is a significantly better method of bladder management and should be initiated for patients who are able to perform self-catheterization.[20]

FAILURE TO STORE

Failure to Store because of the Bladder

The presence of involuntary detrusor contractions as a result of neurologic disease is known as detrusor hyper-reflexia. If no neurologic disease is present, it is known as detrusor instability. Suprasacral cord injuries, cortical injuries as a result of cerebral ischemic attacks, and other neurologic disorders can cause detrusor hyper-reflexia and incontinence. Among patients treated for benign prostate disease, bladder outlet obstruction is the most likely cause of bladder dysfunction. Approximately 52% to 80% of patients with bladder outlet obstruction as a result of benign prostatic hyperplasia have detrusor instability. After prostatectomy, 25% of patients have persistent detrusor instability.[21] A significant de novo decrease in bladder wall compliance occurs after radical prostatectomy.[22] Hellstrom and colleagues[23] postulated that partial bladder decentralization or denervation might play a role in this decrease in bladder wall compliance. Kirby and associates[24] found a 60% reduction in the density of detrusor innervation after major pelvic surgery. Aging is also associated with bladder instability, and Jones and Schoenberg[25] estimated that aging may account for 11% of cases. Regardless of the presence of outflow obstruction, Abrams[21] reported an increasing incidence of detrusor instability with age. The incidence of detrusor instability in elderly people may also be explained by the fact that concomitant neurologic disorders, such as Parkinson's disease, stroke, and herniated intervertebral disk, are more common in the elderly population.[26]

Treatment

Patients who primarily have failure to store as a result of bladder dysfunction are treated with conservative therapy, such as biofeedback and anticholinergic agents. Surgical management is an option only in severe cases that do not respond to conservative treatment, and bladder augmentation can be considered in patients with low bladder volume and detrusor instability.[27] Diversion should be reserved for patients in whom all other types of therapy have failed.

Patients with severe detrusor overactivity and decreased bladder capacity, as seen with congenital diseases such as myelomenigocoele, are treated with bladder augmentation. Bladder augmentation is an attempt to decrease intravesical pressure by increasing storage volume, thereby preserving the upper tracts. However, because bladder augmentation may interfere with spontaneous voiding, patients must be willing to perform self-catheterization permanently.

Failure to Store because of the Outlet

Postprostatectomy incontinence is the diagnosis in most patients who are seen for surgical treatment of incontinence, and its management is discussed in detail. After prostatectomy, some patients have obstruction as a result of residual adenoma, urethral or anastomotic stricture, or bladder neck contracture. These patients may be cured by appropriate endoscopic procedures, such as transurethral resection of the prostate, incision, or dilation. Bladder augmentation should be considered for patients who have detrusor instability after failure of conservative measures, such as fluid restriction, anticholinergic drugs and CIC, and sacral nerve root stimulation.

Postprostatectomy Incontinence

Incidence

Prostate cancer is the most common solid tumor in US men. Approximately 220,900 men will be diagnosed as having the disease in 2003.[28] The Prostate Cancer Outcomes Study completed a longitudinal assessment of functional status in a large community-based cohort of patients with prostate cancer who were treated with radical prostatectomy for clinically localized disease.[29] At 24 months, 8.7% of patients had incontinence that was rated as moderate to significant. Overall, 40.2% of patients reported occasional urinary leakage, 6.8% had frequent urinary leakage, and 1.6% had no urinary control at 24 months. Many other studies assessed urinary incontinence and reported rates of 4% to 40%.[30-35] In patients with benign disease, the incidence of total incontinence after transurethral prostatectomy is approximately 1%.[36] Rates of urinary incontinence are highly variable because most reports vary in the definition of incontinence. The level of continence as reported by physicians may differ from that reported with the use of patient questionnaires.

All forms of prostatectomy, whether simple, radical, or endoscopic, ablate all parts of the proximal urethral sphincter. The proximal urethral sphincter includes the bladder neck, prostate gland, and prostatic urethra to the verumontanum. The distal, or external, sphincter, which extends from the distal aspect of the verumontanum to the bulbar urethra, is primarily responsible for continence after prostatectomy. The maintenance of urinary continence depends on the ability of urethral resistance to exceed intravesical pressure.[36] Incontinence occurs when intravesical pressure is greater than the urethral resistance exerted by the distal sphincter.

Preoperative Considerations

Urodynamic studies are used to differentiate between sphincter and bladder dysfunction. Different rates of bladder dysfunction with postprostatectomy incontinence are reported in different studies. Some studies show a high rate of bladder dysfunction, ranging from 40% to 90%,[26,37] whereas others report a lower incidence of 3%.[38-40] Bladder dysfunction is important to identify because treatment for incontinence caused by an incompetent sphincter mechanism, such as an artificial urinary sphincter (AUS), may be perceived as a failure without appropriate treatment of bladder dysfunction. Detrusor instability can override the resistance provided by the sphincter, and incontinence may persist. Therefore, anticholinergic agents should be used initially to control detrusor instability. If detrusor instability persists despite anticholinergic therapy, bladder augmentation should be considered.

Treatment of Postprostatectomy Incontinence

The treatment of significant sphincteric incompetence is mainly surgical, with the goal of augmentation of outlet resistance. Figure 44-2 shows a suggested algorithm for the treatment of postprostatectomy incontinence.

Urethral Bulking Agents. In patients with sphincteric dysfunction, injectable materials can improve the ability of the urethra to resist abdominal pressure as an expulsive force without changing voiding pressure or detrusor pressure at the time of leakage.[41] Initially, polytetrafluoroethylene (PTFE) was used. However, migration of PTFE particles[42] and granuloma formation in the lung[43] led to concern about the use of this material. PTFE is now rarely used in the United States for urethral injections. Bovine collagen has been used for many years, with minimal morbidity. Migration of particles or granuloma formation has not been demonstrated with Bovine collagen. At 12 weeks, collagen begins to degrade, and it is completely degraded in 19 months.[44] Degradation of collagen probably accounts for the need for multiple injections to achieve continence.

A new product, Durasphere (Advanced UroScience, St. Paul, MN), has been used for periurethral injection. This material, which consists of pyrolytic carbon-coated microbeads, is not absorbed over time. Furthermore, it is biocompatible, nonmigratory, and permanent. The radio-opaque quality of Durasphere allows visualization of the beads, and retention of the particles in tissue can be assessed radiographically (Fig. 44-3).

We rarely use periurethral injections in men because of the low rate of success associated with this technique. The need for multiple injections can increase the cost substantially, to equal or exceed the cost of an AUS, thereby diminishing the utility of periurethral injections in men. In comparison, the AUS is highly successful.[45]

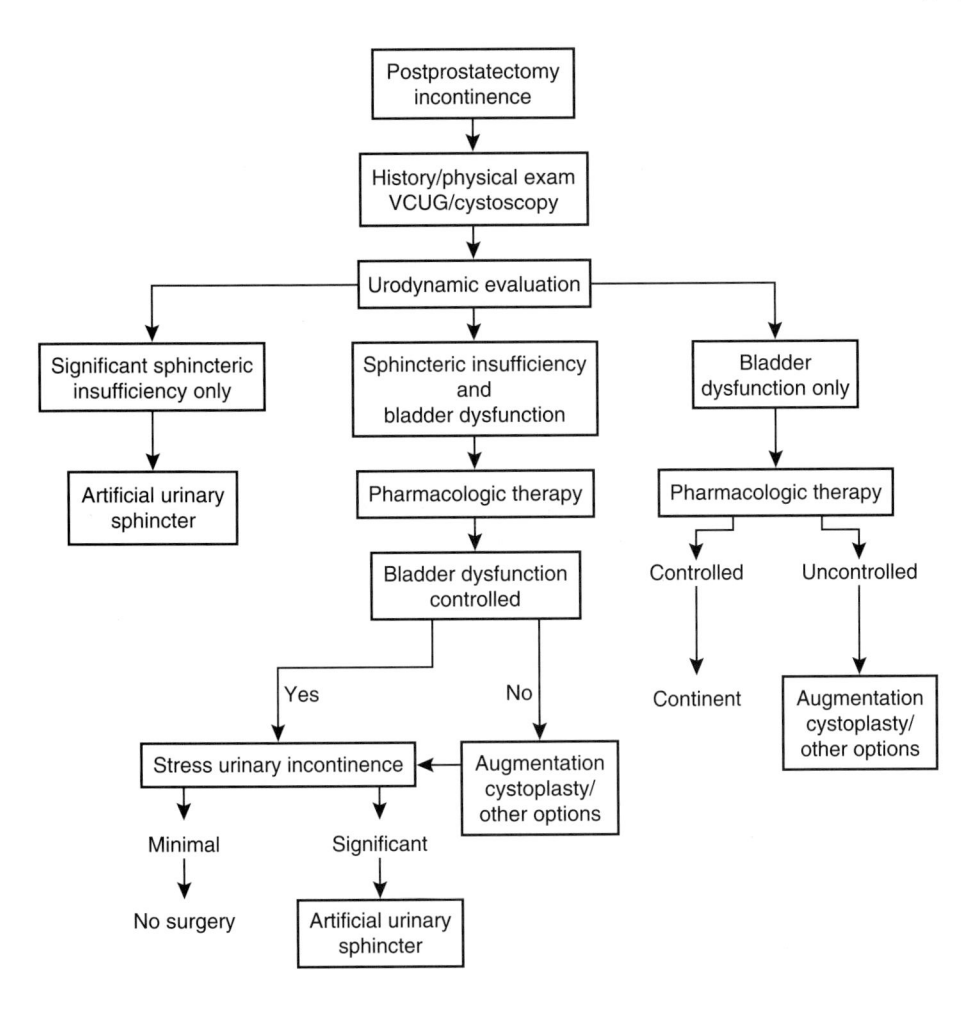

FIGURE 44-2 Suggested algorithm for the management of postprostatectomy incontinence. VCUG, voiding cystourethrogram.

PREOPERATIVE CONSIDERATIONS. The ideal candidate for periurethral injection therapy is a patient with mild stress urinary incontinence and normal detrusor function. To be effective, an injectable material must be placed in the urethra, proximal to the external sphincter. The depth of injection is important, because the material must bulk the urethral mucosa so that there is coaptation of the urethral lumen. An injection that is placed too deep does not sufficiently bulk up the lumen, and is ineffective.

PROCEDURE. Patients are placed in the dorsal lithotomy position and prepared in standard surgical fashion. A standard cystoscope sheath or resectoscope sheath is

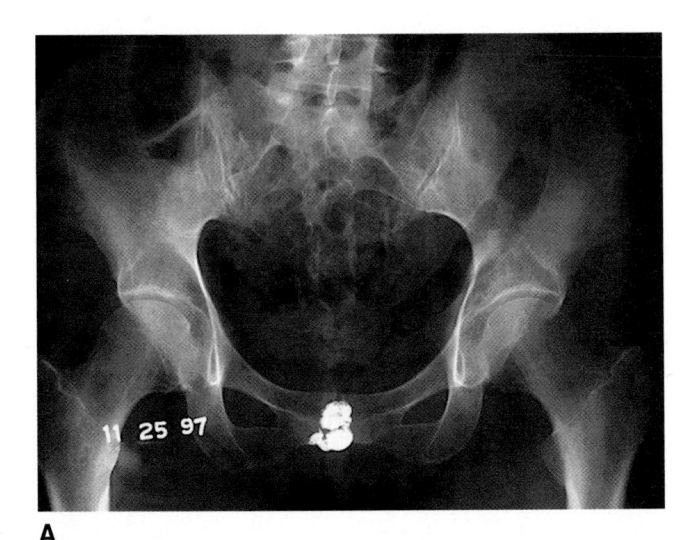

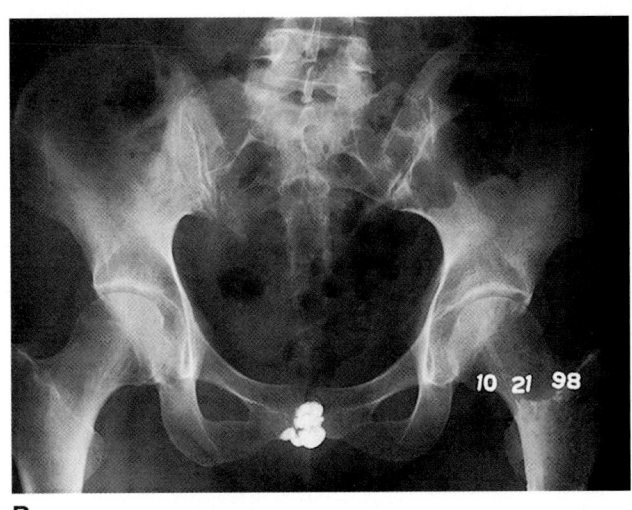

FIGURE 44-3 One-year (**A**) and 2-year (**B**) plain frontal supine views after the injection of Durasphere. (Courtesy of Advanced UroScience, St. Paul, MN.)

FIGURE 44-4 Coaptation of the urethral lumen before and after the injection of Durasphere. (Courtesy of Advanced UroScience, St. Paul, MN.)

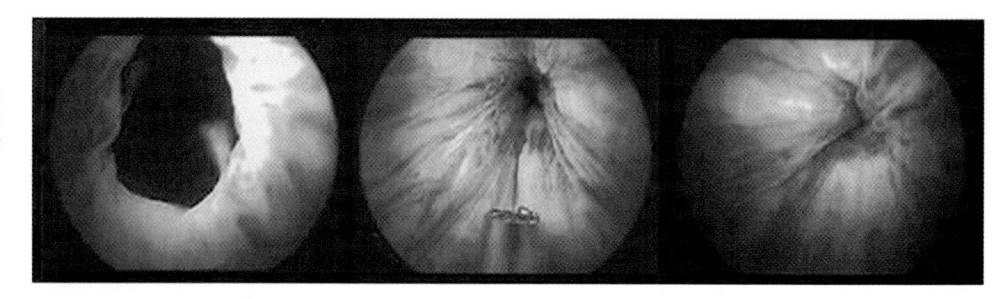

used, and collagen or Durasphere is injected proximal to the external sphincter. The needle is advanced under the urethral mucosa, with the beveled portion of the needle facing the lumen of the urethra to bulk the suburethral tissue (Fig. 44-4). Multiple injections placed circumferentially may be used to coapt the urethral tissue. Minimizing the number of puncture sites is important to prevent leakage of the injectable material.

Antegrade injection in the area of the bladder neck is another injection technique that was initially described in 1996 by Appell and colleagues.[46] Antegrade injection is performed by placing a flexible cystoscope through a suprapubic cystostomy and injecting the material into the more supple, less scarred bladder neck.

After periurethral injection, indwelling catheters should be avoided because they can "mold" the injectable agent and impair coaptation of the urethral tissue. When urinary retention occurs, CIC with a small (10 Fr) catheter should be performed.

RESULTS. The success rate for transurethral retrograde collagen injection ranges from 8% to 63%.[47,48] Sanchez-Ortiz and colleagues[49] evaluated the role of Valsalva leak-point pressure (VLPP) as a predictor of success of collagen injection. They evaluated 31 men with incontinence after radical prostatectomy, with a mean follow-up of 15 months. In their study, 35% of patients were successfully treated. Of these patients, 6% were completely dry and 29% were improved after a mean of 2.6 collagen sessions (number of different procedures) and a mean cumulative volume of 27.9 mL collagen. Of the patients with pretreatment VLLP of 60 cm or greater, 70% responded favorably to collagen injection, whereas those with VLLP less than 60 cm H_2O had a 19% cure rate. Because VLLP is highly predictive of beneficial outcome, it can be used to select men who would benefit most from injection therapy. Often, patients need at least four collagen sessions to notice improvement.

Cespedes and associates[50] reviewed the data for 257 postprostatectomy patients who were treated with collagen. Mean follow-up was 28 months. The patients had an average of 4.4 collagen sessions, with a mean cumulative volume of 36.6 mL. The overall rate of improvement was 39%. Approximately 20% of men were completely dry, and 39% showed significant improvement.

Durasphere appears to be an efficacious injectable agent. In a study of 355 women and 22 men, multiple treatments resulted in an improvement rate of 80.3% at 12 months.[51] Long-term results with Durasphere were not stratified by sex; therefore, the outcome in men is not available. Urethral injections in women are usually more successful. Efficacy may be decreased in men because men lack the periurethral fascia that is present in women and may prevent diffusion of the injectable material to surrounding tissue.

Artificial urinary sphincter. In 1973, the Scott AUS was a major breakthrough in the treatment of urinary incontinence.[52] Since that time, improvements to the AUS have been made, and the AMS800 urinary sphincter (American Medical Systems, Minnetonka, MN) is now the gold standard for neurogenic and postprostatectomy incontinence caused by sphincteric weakness. (Fig. 44-5). The pump is used to deflate the cuff by transferring fluid from the cuff to the balloon pressure reservoir. The cuff is automatically refilled by the passage of fluid through a delay-fill resistor to the cuff. The pump mechanism has a deactivation button.

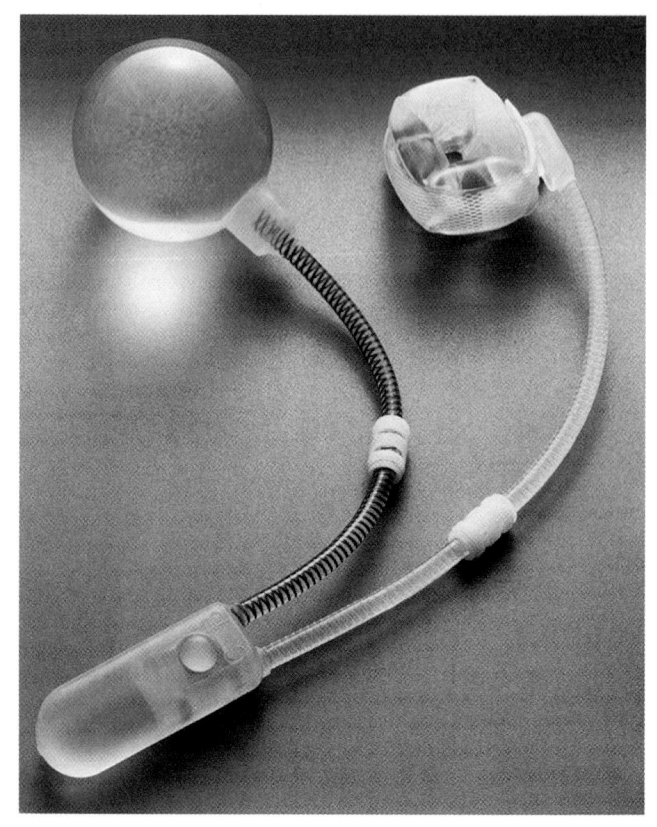

FIGURE 44-5 AMS Sphincter 800 urinary prosthesis. (Courtesy of American Medical Systems, Inc., Minnetonka, MN.)

PREOPERATIVE CONSIDERATIONS. A formal urodynamic study must be performed before placement of the AUS to identify patients who will benefit from the sphincter. The ideal candidate has stress urinary incontinence, no evidence of detrusor instability, adequate bladder capacity, and the ability to empty the bladder completely. Detrusor instability must be controlled with pharmacologic agents to ensure success of the operation because detrusor instability may overcome the resistance provided by the sphincter. If a sphincter is placed in a patient with high bladder pressure, the pressure may be transmitted to the kidney and result in upper-tract damage.

Patients with decreased bladder compliance and small functional capacity are poor candidates for AUS alone. They should receive anticholinergic agents or undergo augmentation cystoplasty, either before or at the time of AUS placement. Patients with uncontrolled, recurrent urethral stricture disease are also poor candidates. Evaluation of patient compliance and mental capability to operate the device is essential, and the patient must have both the manual dexterity and mental faculty to operate the pump after implantation.

PROCEDURE. Strict aseptic technique must be followed, because infection of an artificial prosthesis can be devastating. The urine must be sterile before the prosthesis is placed. To prevent infections, antibiotic prophylaxis is essential. The patient is instructed to shower preoperatively at home with an iodine soap solution. Intraoperatively, a full 10-minute iodine skin scrub is performed, and an intravenous antibiotic to cover *Staphylococcus epidermidis* is used. Traffic of personnel in the operating room is limited to decrease the risk of contamination.

BULBAR URETHRAL PLACEMENT OF CUFF. The cuff is most commonly placed at the bulbar urethra. This site is ideal for use in postprostatectomy, postsurgical, and trauma patients (Fig. 44-6). The patient is placed in the lithotomy position, and a midline perineal incision is made to the bulbocavernosus muscle. The bulbocavernosus muscle is dissected to expose the urethra. A length of urethra (≈ 2 cm) is sharply dissected and mobilized to accommodate the cuff. Care must be taken at the 12 o'clock position because this is the area that is most susceptible to iatrogenic injury. A Babcock clamp is used to retract the urethra to allow circumferential dissection of the spongiosum. Once the urethra is mobilized, the urethral measuring tape is passed, and the circumference of the urethra is measured. The appropriate cuff (typically 4.0–4.5 cm) is then placed around the urethra and snapped into place. All parts of the prosthetic device must be handled with care, and only silicone rubber–shod clamps should be used on the tubing.

A suprainguinal incision is made on the side of the dominant hand and carried down to the fascia. The anterior rectus fascia is opened in a transverse fashion, and the preperitoneal space is bluntly dissected to create a space for the reservoir. We use the lowest pressure balloon, 51 to 60 cm H_2O, to minimize the risk of cuff erosion and urethral atrophy from excessive pressure. The subdartos layer of the scrotum is bluntly dissected, and the pump is placed in a dependent position. The reservoir is filled with 23 mL isotonic contrast fluid, and all connections are made in the inguinal incision. The use of contrast material in the reservoir is helpful in postoperative follow-up and facilitates troubleshooting that may be needed after the procedure. The bulbocavernosus muscle and

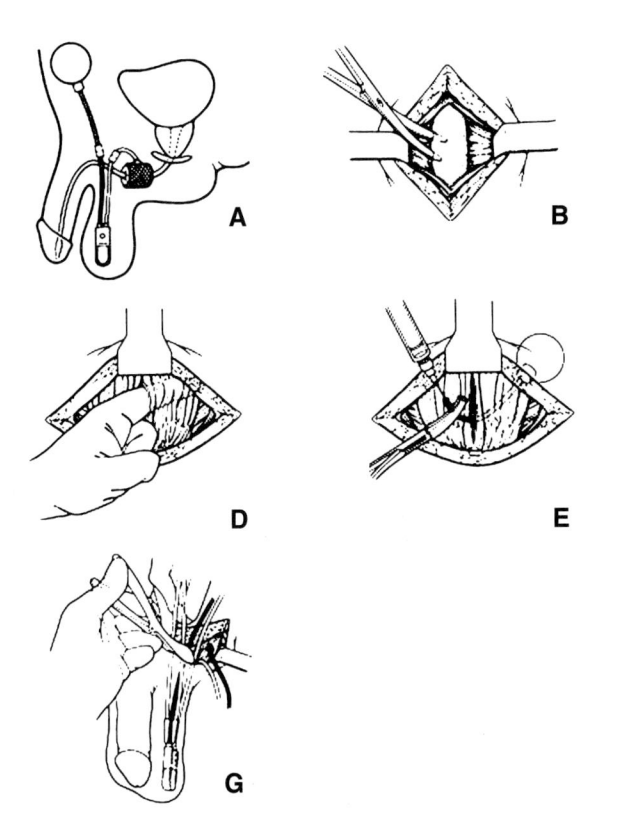

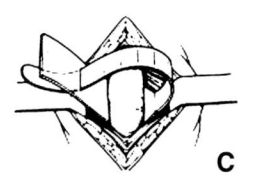

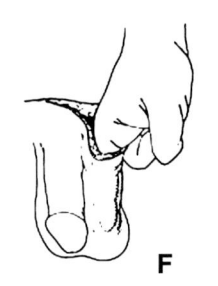

FIGURE 44-6 Placement of an artificial urinary sphincter. **A,** The bulbar urethral cuff is placed. **B,** The bulbar urethra is dissected. **C,** A urethral measuring tape is used to determine the cuff size. **D,** The rectus fascia is divided to reach the preperitoneal space through a suprainguinal incision. **E,** The balloon is filled with 23 mL isotonic contrast solution. **F,** Blunt dissection is performed to create a dependent subdartos pouch. **G,** The pump is placed in a dependent position. (Courtesy of American Medical Systems. Inc., Minnetonka, MN.)

subcutaneous tissue are approximated, and the skin is closed with a subcuticular stitch. A generous amount of antibiotic irrigation is used throughout the procedure.

The device is tested by compressing the pump three times to transfer the cuff fluid to the reservoir. Retrograde perfusion sphincterometry is then performed to document the closure pressure of the cuff around the urethra.[53] The closure pressure should be within the range generated by the pressure-regulating balloon. An 8 Fr Foley catheter is placed in the distal urethra and attached to irrigation fluid. The level of irrigation fluid is adjusted to the level at which the fluid just starts to drip into the drip chamber. The difference between the level of the cuff and the level of the fluid is the closure pressure. Within 30 seconds, the pump refills, and when only a small dimple is felt in the pump, the deactivation button is pressed to deactivate the device.

In 1993, Brito and associates[54] described a novel method in which a double cuff was used to treat persistent severe incontinence after sphincter placement. To increase the surface area of compression and provide greater outlet resistance, the additional cuff was joined by a three-way connector to the original cuff and a single pressure-regulating balloon (Fig. 44-7).

BLADDER NECK PLACEMENT. Patients with neuropathic disease and stress urinary incontinence who are candidates for bladder augmentation and patients who are wheelchair-bound and have increased perineal pressure may be considered for bladder neck placement. Men who wish to maintain fertility should have the AUS placed at the bladder neck to preserve antegrade ejaculation.

A Pfannenstiel incision is made to expose the retropubic space. The bladder neck is dissected sharply until it is circumferentially isolated. In patients who have had previous surgery or trauma, it may be necessary to open the bladder to aid in dissection. An umbilical tape is passed around the bladder neck, and hemostasis is achieved. The catheter is removed, and a right-angle clamp is passed under the bladder neck. The urethral measuring tape is passed around the urethra with the right angle clamp. The circumference of the bladder neck is measured, and the sizer is removed. In men, an 8- to 14-cm cuff is used for the bladder neck, and the higher-pressure balloon (61–70 cm H_2O) is typically used. The pump is placed and connected to the urethral cuff and reservoir as described earlier. The rectus fascia and skin are closed.

POSTOPERATIVE CARE. A pelvic x-ray is obtained postoperatively to confirm the radiographic appearance of the AUS and to ensure that the device is deactivated and the cuff is open. A condom catheter or small Foley catheter is placed for 24 hours. Oral antibiotics should be continued for 1 week, and the patient is seen at follow-up 1 week and 1 month after the surgery. The patient is instructed to pull the pump to a dependent scrotal position several times daily to prevent upward migration of the pump. Approximately 4 to 6 weeks after the operation, when scrotal pain has resolved, the AUS is activated with a firm compression of the pump.

RESULTS AND COMPLICATIONS. This procedure has a success rate of 60% to 80% in postprostatectomy patients.[55,56] Haab and associates[57] evaluated 68 men who underwent AUS placement. They found that 80% were continent, and 52 patients (76%) showed significant improvement on a quality-of-life index. In an overview of the long-term outcome of AUS placement, Venn and associates[58] reported that the overall success rate 10 years after implantation was 84%. In males, the success rate was 92% for bulbar urethral implantation and 84% for bladder neck placement. In patients with neuropathic bladder dysfunction, the 10-year continence rate was 86%. Excellent outcome was seen in the postprostatectomy group, with an overall success rate of 91%. Device survival was 66% at 10 years. Overall, 36% of the prostheses were removed because of infection or erosion during the 10-year period. In an analysis of all published results, Hajivassiliou[59] corroborated these findings and noted continence in 73% of men, with an overall improvement rate of 88%.

Although success rates are excellent after proper placement of an AUS, approximately 15% of patients do not achieve satisfactory continence. Incontinence may be a result of poor outflow resistance because of late tissue atrophy at the cuff site, which can lead to poor coaptation of the urethra.

The addition of a second sphincter cuff around the bulbar urethra in patients with persistent urinary incontinence resulted in symptom improvement, with 80% of patients becoming satisfactorily dry.[60] The erosion rate of the double-cuff AMS800 was evaluated to determine whether the additional cuff increased the risk of erosion.

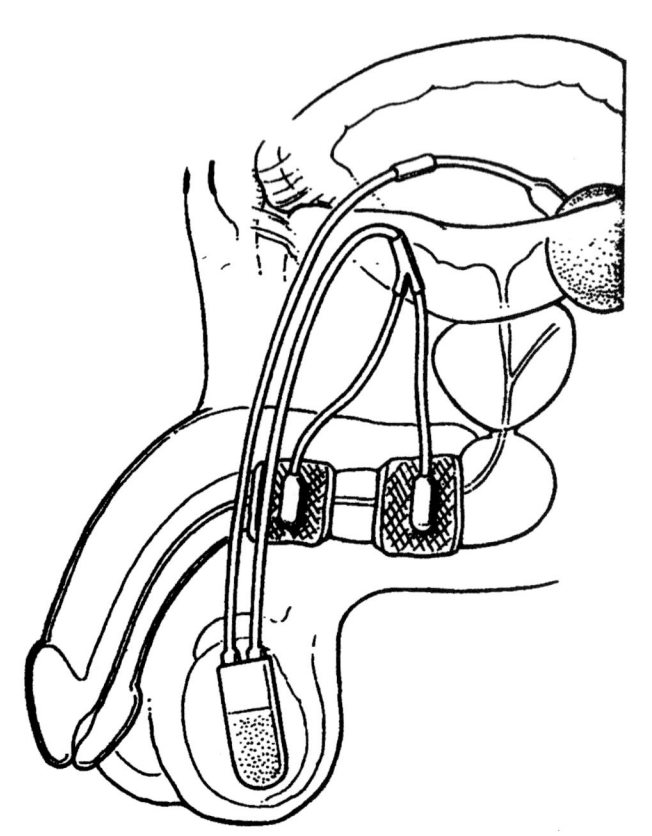

FIGURE 44-7 A urinary sphincter with two cuffs in tandem.

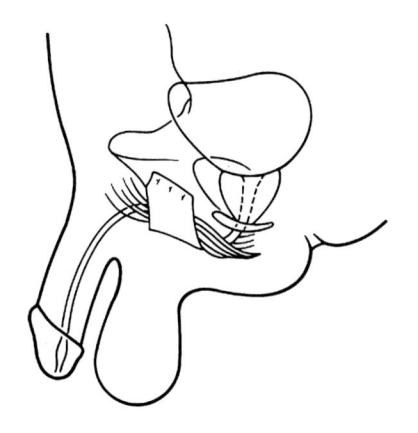

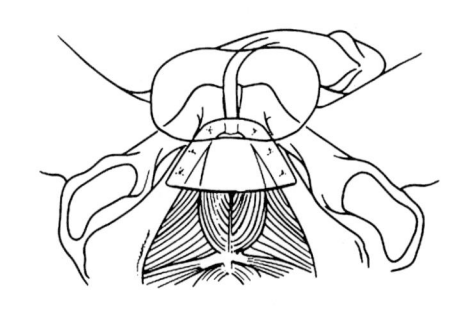

FIGURE 44-8 The male sling procedure with bone fixation using titanium bone anchors. (Courtesy of American Medical Systems, Minnetonka, MN.)

Of the 95 patients who were followed for 1 to 119 months (mean, 28.5 months), only 10.5% had cuff erosion.[61] This low rate of erosion is well within the range of rates reported with a single cuff (3.9%–14.3%).[57,62,63]

With increasing device improvements and the advent of delayed activation, erosion rates have declined. Persistent burning perineal pain, swelling, or erythema suggests erosion of the cuff, and the patient should be evaluated with cystoscopy and a retrograde urethrogram. When erosion occurs, the entire prosthesis should be removed because it may become infected. An indwelling catheter is placed to promote healing, and after a period of 3 to 6 months, another AUS may be placed.

Male sling. The male sling is a potential alternative in men who are averse to having artificial devices placed and in patients who cannot operate the AUS. Multiple sling operations for male stress urinary incontinence have been described.[60,64] The goal is to provide urethral compression to maintain continence.

DESCRIPTION. The patient is placed in the dorsal lithotomy position, and a 16 Fr Foley catheter is placed. A midline perineal incision is made (Fig. 44-8). The bulbocavernosus muscle is dissected off of the underlying bulbar urethra. Dissection is continued laterally to expose the inner portion of the descending ramus of the pubic bone. With the use of the Straight-In Bone Screw Inserter and the In-Fast Bone Screw System (American Medical Systems), three bone screws are placed on both the right and the left sides of the descending ramus. Once the screw is seated, the sling material, which may be cadaveric fascia lata or dermis, is prepared. Usually, a graft of 4 × 7 cm is sufficient. Each end of the three Prolene sutures from the bone screws is threaded through the sling material by passing the suture through an 18-gauge needle. The three sutures on one side are tied down tightly to the pubic bone.

The sutures on the contralateral side are used to adjust the tension of the sling. Retrograde perfusion sphincterometry is used to assess adequate closing pressure and sling tension. A Foley catheter is placed in the fossa navicularis, and the balloon is inflated with 1 to 3 mL water to form a seal to hold the catheter in position. The fluid level of the infusion fluid bag is raised 60 cm above the level of the bladder. The sling tension is adjusted by tying the second set of Prolene sutures on the contralateral side just tight enough so that the fluid is no longer seen dripping in the drip chamber. After the sling is placed, the perineum is closed. A catheter is left indwelling for 1 day, and postvoid residuals are evaluated postoperatively.

RESULTS. The male sling is a relatively new procedure, and preliminary results appear promising. Jacoby and colleagues[65] evaluated 23 men who underwent the male sling procedure, with a mean follow-up of 3.65 months (range, 1–11 months). In this study, 87% of men showed moderate to significant improvement or resolution of stress urinary incontinence, with 48% of patients achieving complete dryness and 13% showing no improvement. Preliminary results are encouraging, but long-term follow-up is needed to determine the durability of the procedure.

CONCLUSION

A number of surgical procedures are highly successful in patients with pelvic floor disorders, particularly men with postprostatectomy incontinence. To determine the most effective therapy, it is important to evaluate both the bladder and sphincteric function urodynamically. With the wide array of methods available to improve continence, patients no longer need to accept incontinence as a fixture in their lives, but can improve their quality of life by seeking treatment.

REFERENCES

1. Havenga K, Mass CP, DeRuiter MC, et al: Avoiding long-term disturbance to bladder and sexual function in pelvic surgery, particularly with rectal cancer. Semin Surg Oncol 18:235, 2000.
2. Mundey AR: Pelvic plexus injuries. In Mundy AR, Stephenson TP, Wein AJ (eds): Urodynamics: Principles, Practice, and Application. London, Churchill Livingstone, 1984, p 273.
3. McGuire EJ: Clinical evaluation and treatment of neurogenic vesical dysfunction. In Libertino J (ed): International Perspectives in Urology. Baltimore, Williams & Wilkins, 1984, p 11.
4. McGuire EJ, Denil J: Adult myelodyplasia. AUA Update Series 10:298, 1991.

5. Webster GD, El-Mahrovky A, Stone AR, Zakrzewski C: The urological evaluation and management of patients with myelodysplasia. Br J Urol 58:261, 1986.
6. Oesterling JE: Benign prostate hyperplasia: A review of its histogenesis and natural history. Prostate (suppl) 6:67, 1996.
7. Catz A, Luttwak ZP, Agranov E, et al: The role of external sphincterotomy for patients with a spinal cord lesion. Spinal Cord 35:48, 1997.
8. Light JK, Beric A, Wise PG: Predictive criteria for failed sphincterotomy in spinal cord injury patients. J Urol 138:1201, 1987.
9. Lockhart JL, Vorstman B, Weinstein D, Politano VA: Sphincterotomy failure in neurogenic bladder disease. J Urol 135:86, 1986.
10. Nanninga JB, O'Conor VJ Jr, Rosen JS: An explanation for the persistence of residual urine after external sphincterotomy. J Urol 118:821, 1977.
11. Kiviat MC: Transurethral sphincterotomy: relationship of site of incision to postoperative potency and delayed hemorrhage. J Urol 49:721, 1978.
12. Yalla SV, Fam BA, Gabilondo FB, et al: Anteromedian external urethral sphincterotomy: Technique, rationale, and complications. J Urol 117:489, 1977.
13. Linker DG, Tangho EA: Complete external sphincterotomy: Correlation between endoscopic observation and the anatomic sphincter. J Urol 113:348, 1975.
14. Vapnek JM, Couillard DR, Stone AR: Is sphincterotomy the best management of the spinal cord injured bladder? J Urol 151:961, 1994.
15. Chancellor MB, Bennett C, Simoneau AR, et al: Sphincteric stent versus external sphincterotomy in spinal cord injured men: Prospective randomized multicenter trial. J Urol 161:1893, 1999.
16. Gajewski JB, Chancellor MB, Ackman CF, et al: Removal of UroLume endoprosthesis: Experience of the North American Study Group for detrusor-sphincter dyssynergia application. J Urol 163:773, 2000.
17. Hackler RH: Long-term suprapubic cystostomy drainage in spinal cord injury patients. Br J Urol 48:120, 1982.
18. Dewire DM, Owens RS, Anderson GA, et al: A comparison of the urological complications associated with long-term management of quadriplegics with and without chronic indwelling urinary catheters. J Urol 147:1069, 1992.
19. MacDiarmid SA, Arnold EP, Palmer NB, Anthony A: Management of spinal cord injured patients by indwelling suprapubic catheterization. J Urol 154:492, 1995.
20. Weld KJ, Dmochowski RR: Effect of bladder management on urological complications in spinal cord injured patients. J Urol 163:768, 2000.
21. Abrams P: Detrusor instability and bladder outlet obstruction. Neurourol Urodynam 4:317, 1985.
22. Leach GE, Yip CM, Donovan BJ: Post-prostatectomy incontinence: The influence of bladder dysfunction. J Urol 138:574, 1987.
23. Hellstrom P, Lukkarinen O, Kontturi M: Urodynamics in radical retropubic prostatectomy. Scand J Urol 23:21, 1989.
24. Kirby RS, Fowler CJ, Gilpin SA, et al: Bladder muscle biopsy and urethral sphincter EMG in patients with bladder dysfunction after pelvic surgery. J R Soc Med 79:270, 1986.
25. Jones KW, Schoenberg HW: Comparison of the incidence of bladder hyperreflexia in patients with benign prostatic hypertrophy and age matched female controls. J Urol 133:125, 1985.
26. Goluboff ET, Chang DT, Olsson CA, Kaplan SA: Urodynamics and the etiology of post-prostatectomy urinary incontinence: The initial Columbia experience (see comments). J Urol 153:1034, 1995.
27. Linder A, Leach GE, Raz S: Augmentation cystoplasty in the treatment of neurogenic bladder dysfunction. J Urol 129:491, 1983.
28. Jemal A, Murray T, Samuels A, et al: Cancer Statistics, 2003. Ca Cancer J Clin 53:5–26, 2003.
29. Stanford JL, Feng Z, Hamilton AS, et al: Urinary and sexual function after radical prostatectomy for clinically localized prostate cancer: The Prostate Cancer Outcomes Study. JAMA 283:354, 2000.
30. Wahle GR: Urinary incontinence after radical prostatectomy. Semin Urol Oncol 18:66, 2000.
31. Walsh PC: Patient-reported urinary continence and sexual function after anatomic radical prostatectomy. J Urol 164:242, 2000.
32. Catalona WJ, Carvalhal GF, Mager DE, Smith DS: Potency, continence and complication rates in 1,870 consecutive radical retropubic prostatectomies. J Urol 162:433, 1999.
33. Goluboff ET, Saidi JA, Mazer S, et al: Urinary continence after radical prostatectomy: The Columbia experience. J Urol 159:1276, 1998.
34. Benoit RM, Naslund MJ, Cohen JK: Complications after radical retropubic prostatectomy in the medicare population. Urology 56:116, 2000.
35. Fowler FJ, Barry MJ, Lu-Yao G, et al: Patient-reported complications and follow-up treatment after radical prostatectomy. Urology 42:622, 1993.
36. Foote J, Yun S, Leach GE: Postprostatectomy incontinence: Pathophysiology, evaluation, and management. Urol Clin North Am 18:229, 1991.
37. Leach GE, Trockman B, Wong A, et al: Post-prostatectomy incontinence: Urodynamic findings and treatment outcomes. J Urol 155:1256, 1996.
38. Ficazzola MA, Nitti VW: The etiology of post-radical prostatectomy incontinence and correlation of symptoms with urodynamic findings. J Urol 160:1317, 1998.
39. Gudziak MR, McGuire EJ, Gormley EA: Urodynamic assessment of urethral sphincter function in post-prostatectomy incontinence. J Urol 156:1131, 1996.
40. Desautel MG, Kapoor R, Badlani GH: Sphincteric incontinence: The primary cause of post-prostatectomy incontinence in patients with prostate cancer. Neurourol Urodynam 16:153, 1997.
41. McGuire EJ, Appell RA: Transurethral collagen injection for urinary incontinence. Urology 413, 1994.
42. Malizia AAJ, Riman JM, Myers RP, et al: Migration and granulomatous reaction after periurethral injection of polytef (Teflon). JAMA 251:3277, 1984.
43. Mittleman RE, Marraccini JV: Pulmonary Teflon granulomas following periurethral Teflon injection for urinary incontinence. Arch Pathol Lab Med 107:611, 1983.
44. Remacle M, Marbaix E: Collagen implants in the human larynx. Arch Otorhinolaryngol 245:203, 1988.
45. Brown JA, Elliot DS, Barrett DM: Postprostatectomy urinary incontinence: A comparison of the cost of conservative versus surgical management. Urology 51:715, 1998.
46. Appell RA, Vasavada SP, Rackely RR, Winters JC: Percutaneous antegrade collagen injection therapy for urinary incontinence following radical prostatectomy. Urology 48:769, 1996.
47. Aboseif SR, O'Connell HE, Usui A, McGuire EJ: Collagen injection for intrinsic sphincteric deficiency in men. J Urol 155:10, 1996.
48. Cummings JM, Boullier JA, Parra RO: Transurethral collagen injections in the therapy of post-radical prostatectomy stress incontinence. J Urol 155:1011, 1996.

49. Sanchez-Ortiz RF, Broderick GA, Chaikin DC, et al: Collagen injection therapy for post-radical retropubic prostatectomy incontinence: Role of Valsalva leak point pressure. J Urol 158:2132, 1997.
50. Cespedes RD, Leng WW, McGuire EJ: Collagen injection therapy for postprostatectomy incontinence. Urology 54(4):597–602, 1999.
51. Lightner D, Diokno A, Snyder J, et al: Study of Durasphere in the treatment of stress urinary incontinence: A multi-center, double-blind, randomized, comparative study (abstract). AUA Meeting, Atlanta, GA, 2000.
52. Scott FB, Bradley WE, Timm GW: Treatment of urinary incontinence by an implantable prosthetic sphincter. Urology 1:252, 1973.
53. Leach GE: Incontinence after artificial urinary sphincter placement: The role of perfusion sphincterometry. J Urol 138:529, 1987.
54. Brito CG, Mulcahy JJ, Mitchell ME, Adams MC: Use of a double cuff AMS800 urinary sphincter for severe stress incontinence. J Urol 149:283, 1993.
55. Marks JL, Light JK: Management of urinary incontinence after prostatectomy with the artificial urinary sphincter. J Urol 142:302, 1989.
56. Montague DK: The artificial urinary sphincter (AMS800): Experience in 166 consecutive patients. J Urol 147:380, 1992.
57. Haab F, Trockman BA, Zimmern PE, Leach GE: Quality of life and continence assessment of the artificial urinary sphincter in men with minimum 3.5 years of followup. J Urol 158:435, 1997.
58. Venn SN, Greenwell TJ, Mundy AR: The long-term outcome of artificial urinary sphincters. J Urol 164:702, 2000.
59. Hajivassiliou CA: A review of the complications and results of implantation of the AMS artificial urinary sphincter. Eur Urol 35:36, 1999.
60. Schaeffer AJ, Clemens JQ, Ferrari M, Stamey TA: The male bulbourethral sling procedure for post-radical prostatectomy incontinence (erratum appears in J Urol 160[1]:136, 1998). J Urol 159:1510, 1998.
61. Kowalczyk JJ, Spicer DL, Mulcahy JJ: Erosion rate of the double cuff AMS800 artificial urinary sphincter: Long-term followup. J Urol 156:1300, 1996.
62. Fishman IJ, Shabsigh R, Scott FB: Experience with the artificial urinary sphincter model AS800 in 158 patients. J Urol 141:307, 1989.
63. Diokno AC, Sonda LP, MacGregor RJ: Long-term followup of the artificial urinary sphincter. J Urol 131:283, 1984.
64. Mizuo T, Ando M, Tanizawa A, et al: Sling operation for male stress incontinence by utilizing modified Stamey technique. Urology 39:211, 1992.
65. Jacoby K, Franco N, Westney L: Male sling: A new perineal approach (abstract). Society of Urodynamics, Female Urology Meeting, Atlanta, 2000.

CHAPTER 45

Surgical Management of Children with Urinary and Fecal Incontinence

STUART B. BAUER ■ HIEP T. NGUYEN

Functional or anatomic abnormalities of the detrusor muscle, bladder neck, or external sphincter may result in disabling incontinence. In children, abnormal development of the spinal column, with associated impairment of spinal cord function, is the most common cause of urinary incontinence. Other functional etiologies include sacral agenesis, tumors of the spinal cord, iatrogenic injury, and trauma to the spinal cord. These children may have incontinence as a result of poor detrusor compliance, detrusor hyper-reflexia, or low or excessive urethral resistance. Anatomic abnormalities that cause incontinence include bladder exstrophy–epispadias complex, cloacal malformation, urogenital sinus anomalies, bilateral ureteral ectopia, cecoureterocele, and traumatic or iatrogenic injury to the sphincter. Although clean intermittent catheterization combined with pharmacotherapy provides satisfactory urinary control in many children with neurogenic or anatomic urinary incontinence, some require surgical intervention to achieve socially acceptable continence. Moreover, many children with urinary incontinence have concomitant fecal incontinence that does not respond to routine medical management. This chapter discusses options for the surgical treatment of urinary and fecal incontinence in children.

PREOPERATIVE ASSESSMENT

To achieve urinary continence, it is important to determine whether the child has a compliant large-capacity reservoir, a competent bladder neck or sphincteric mechanism, and a reliable mechanism for effectively emptying the bladder. Careful preoperative assessment is necessary to determine which surgical intervention is needed. Options include increasing bladder capacity, thus, improving compliance; improving bladder outlet resistance; creating a continent catheterizable urinary stoma; or any combination thereof.

Simple physical examination is often inadequate to assess the etiology of urinary incontinence, and properative urodynamic studies must be performed before surgery is undertaken. In children with spinal dysraphism, the resultant neurologic lesion is dependent on which neural elements have everted into the meningocele sac. However, the assessment of bladder function cannot be reliably based on just the level of the bony abnormality, because the neurologic deficit can extend higher or lower than the observed vertebral abnormality and spinal cord function may be preserved for up to three vertebral levels below the bony abnormality.[1] Sacral function remains intact in as many as 75% of children with thoracic or cervical vertebral defects, despite the lack of brain stem or cortical control.[2] Consequently, careful urodynamic assessment is necessary to determine the etiology of urinary incontinence in children with spinal dysraphism.

A thorough urodynamic evaluation includes water cystometry, static and dynamic urethral pressure profilometry, and sphincter electromyography. Water cystometry is performed with a 7 Fr trilumen urodynamic catheter with a filling rate of 10% of expected capacity $[(\{1/2\} \times \text{age in years} + 6) \times 30 \text{ mL}]$ for children older than 2 years of age and $[(2 \times \text{age in years} + 2) \times 30 \text{ mL}]$ per minute for children younger than 2 years of age.[3] Static urethral pressure profile testing is performed with the same urodynamic catheter withdrawn at 0.5 mm/sec while saline is infused at 2 mL/sec to determine the maximal urethral resistance and functional urethral length. Dynamic urethral pressure profiles are measured with the side port of the urodynamic catheter positioned at the point of maximal resistance in the urethra while the pressure is monitored continuously throughout bladder filling and emptying. Sphincter electromyography is assessed with a 24-gauge concentric needle electrode placed at the level of the external urethral sphincter. Provocative maneuvers, such as coughing, straining, and standing, are used to assess the adequacy of outlet resistance. Fluoroscopic images of the bladder, obtained during filling, voiding, and straining, are helpful in evaluating the competency of the bladder neck and external urethral sphincter.

In an attempt to achieve urinary continence, two additional goals should be sought concurrently: preserving renal function and establishing a reliable mechanism for effectively emptying the bladder. Achieving urinary continence should not be accomplished at the expense of compromising renal function. Increasing bladder outlet resistance can drastically alter bladder dynamics, resulting in elevated detrusor filling pressure that can impede ureteral drainage and lead to obstruction and, consequently, renal impairment. In a poorly compliant bladder, augmentation cystoplasty may be required at the time of bladder outlet surgery. Because low-pressure storage of urine is dependent on the compliant properties of the bladder wall as well as appropriate modulation by neural pathways, bladder compliance and tonicity must be assessed before continence surgery is undertaken. However, accurate assessment of bladder compliance or capacity with urodynamic studies is often difficult in the presence of low bladder outlet resistance. In children with poor outlet resistance, leakage of urine from the urethra often occurs before the bladder is filled to its full capacity. As a result, bladder pressure at functional capacity cannot be assessed. In these cases, occlusion of the bladder outlet with a Foley balloon catheter allows the bladder to be filled to its full capacity and bladder compliance to be accurately assessed. Furthermore, appropriate bladder capacity depends not only on the age of the patient but also on the amount of urine that the patient produces. Urine production in patients with vesicoureteral reflux or hydronephrosis may be higher than expected as a result of the associated nephrogenic diabetes inspidus. Therefore, the appropriate bladder capacity in these patients is sometimes larger than normal to accommodate their excessive urine production.

Before continence surgery is undertaken, it should be determined whether the patient has a reliable channel for effective and efficient evacuation of urine. Most children with a neurogenic bladder and those who undergo augmentation cystoplasty require intermittent catheterization to empty their bladder because they cannot spontaneously void to completion. In most cases, catheterization via the native urethra can be performed readily; however, when it cannot, an alternative method of catheterization is required to empty the bladder. Bladder emptying may be achieved with the creation of a continent catheterizable stoma fashioned from the appendix, small bowel, colon, or ureter at the time of continence surgery. The importance of systematic catheterization cannot be overstated. Failure to empty the bladder regularly may lead to bladder perforation, peritonitis, and even death. Therefore, continence surgery is often delayed until the child reaches an age at which social continence is normally achieved and understands the importance of adhering to scheduled bladder emptyings by intermittent catheterization.

SURGICAL CORRECTION OF ABNORMALITIES OF BLADDER CAPACITY AND COMPLIANCE

Urinary continence cannot be achieved without a low-pressure, appropriate-capacity bladder. Initial attempts to improve bladder capacity should include anticholinergic drugs. When a poorly compliant bladder is unresponsive to medical treatment, augmentation cystoplasty must be considered. Tissue sources for bladder augmentation include the ileum, stomach, colon, and ureter. In selecting which donor tissue to use, it is important to consider which segment can be removed from the gastrointestinal tract with the least effect on bowel function and which segment, once placed into the urinary tract, would cause the least metabolic disturbance. In children with neurogenic bladder dysfunction, derangements in bowel function are common. Removal of the ileocecal valve in these patients may precipitate intractable diarrhea and severe fecal incontinence.[4] Thus, in these children, the use of the ileocecal segment should be avoided because of its profound effect on bowel function. In children with cloacal anomalies, use of the colon should be avoided because it may be needed for reconstruction of the lower gastrointestinal tract. In these cases, augmentation cystoplasty with ileum may be preferable.

Placement of gastrointestinal segments into the urinary tract can have drastic long-term metabolic effects. When small bowel or colon is placed in contact with urine for an extended period, chloride absorption increases and can overwhelm the ability of the kidney to maintain acid–base equilibrium, leading to a state of metabolic acidosis. In contrast, when stomach is interposed into the urinary tract, a net increase in acid excretion into the urine occurs, leading to metabolic alkalosis. Thus, in children with concomitant renal failure and metabolic acidosis, the use of stomach may be advantageous. The acid urine also limits the incidence of urinary infection and reduces the risk of stone formation. However, gastric augmentation should not be performed in children who have full sensation in the perineum, because the urine produced is acidic and can lead to significant dysuria (hematuria–dysuria syndrome). Gastric augmentation should be avoided in children who have low urine output as a result of either renal failure or surgical removal of the native kidneys. In these patients, minimal urine is available to dilute the secreted acid load, putting the residual bladder tissue at risk for ulceration, inflammation leading to hematuria, and possibly perforation.

Another consideration is the physical properties of the bowel segment selected. The sigmoid colon and stomach are thick-walled, allowing for reimplantation of the ureters or a continent catheterizable stoma into these segments. However, the thick-walled colon may have intractable contractions, despite being detubularized.[5] Moreover, ileal and colonic segments produce mucus, which can predispose the patient to recurrent urinary tract infection and stone formation. In contrast, gastric segments do not secrete much mucus; this feature, combined with acid secretion, limits infection and stone formation.

To minimize the potential complications associated with the use of a specific bowel segment, bladder augmentation can be performed with a combination of bowel segments, such as ileum or colon, in combination with stomach. The opposing metabolic effects of the bowel segments tend to neutralize each other.[6] Other alternatives include removal of the mucosal lining of the bowel segment or stomach and using the seromuscular portion of the segment for bladder augmentation.[7,8] Removing the mucosal lining limits the absorptive and secretion properties of the bowel or stomach; however, long-term results with this procedure have not been reported. A promising new technology for bladder augmentation involves the use of tissue-engineered biomaterials.[9,10] Before augmentation cystoplasty, bladder smooth muscle cells and urothelial cells are harvested from the patient and expanded in cell culture. The expanded smooth muscle and urothelial cells are then seeded onto an acellular matrix, such as donor bladder submucosa. After the cells are established, the engineered tissue is augmented to the patient's bladder. Preliminary results with tissue-engineered bladder augmentation are promising; however, long-term results have not been reported.

The final decision about which type of bowel segment to use is often made at the time of laparotomy, and is based on the underlying condition of the patient and the availability and accessibility of a particular bowel segment. Consequently, all patients should receive a standard mechanical and antibiotic bowel preparation to avoid limiting surgical options. Adequate exposure of the entire gastrointestinal tract is achieved through a low midline incision that exposes the retropubic space first to expedite bladder or ureteral surgery that is needed before the peritoneum is entered. In addition, the delay in opening the abdomen will reduce heat and fluid loss through exposed peritoneal surfaces, which is particularly important in small children. It also maintains excellent surgical exposure of the true pelvis and its contents. After bladder or ureteral surgery is completed, the midline incision is extended cephalad and the abdomen is entered. If the patient has a ventriculoperitoneal shunt, the tubing is wrapped with an antibiotic-soaked sponge and packed away in the upper abdominal quadrant to avoid infection. Usually, it is not necessary to extraperitonealize the shunt, unless areas of infection are uncovered.

A segment of bowel is then selected. If ileum is to be used, a segment approximately 15 to 20 cm long is isolated on its blood supply, approximately 15 cm from the ileocecal valve (Fig. 45-1). Avoiding removal of the terminal portion of the ileum preserves the ileocolic artery and several important absorptive functions in the distal ileum. If colon is selected, a 10-cm segment is isolated from the sigmoid colon because of its proximity to the bladder (Fig. 45-2). The isolated ileal or colonic segment is then opened along its antimesenteric border and reconfigured into a U-shaped cap.[11] Detubularization prevents the bowel segment from generating high-pressure intraluminal contractions.[12] If stomach is used, an 8-cm, diamond-shaped patch is isolated from the greater curvature of the body of the stomach, and its blood supply is based

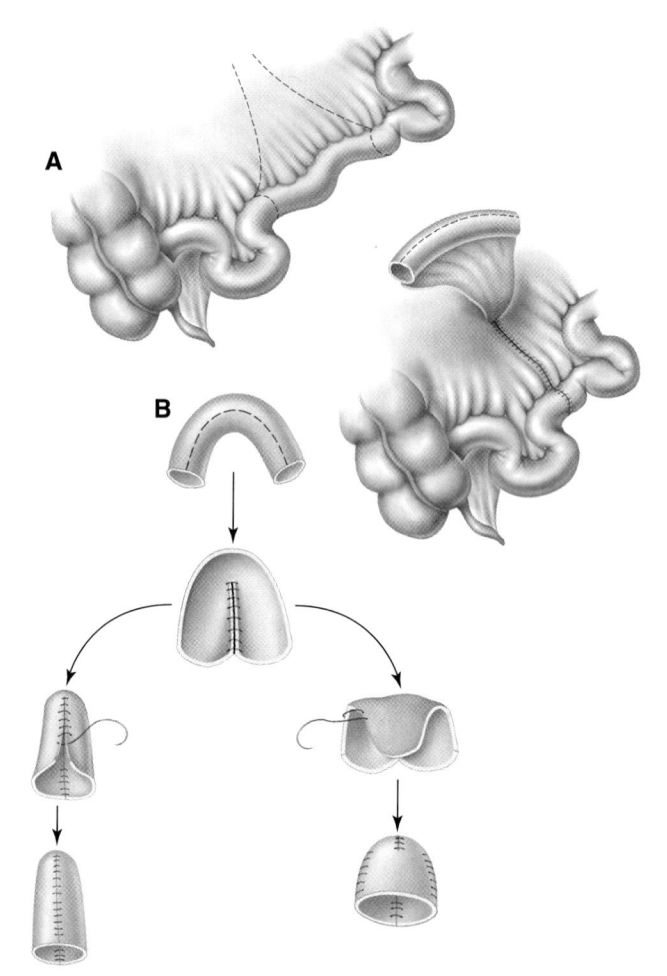

FIGURE 45-1 Ileocystoplasty. **A**, A 15- to 20-cm segment is isolated on its blood supply, approximately 15 cm from the ileocecal valve. **B**, The segment is opened along the antimesenteric border and reconfigured into a U-shaped cap, before being anastomosed to the bivalved bladder. (From Kaefer M, Bauer SB: The surgical correction of incontinence in myelodysplastic children. In King LR [ed]: Urologic Surgery in Infants and Children. Philadelphia, Saunders, p 122, 1998.)

on either the right or the left gastroepiploic vessel (Fig. 45-3). To minimize acid secretion in the isolated patch, it is best to avoid removing the antral portion of the stomach. The gastric segment should extend to approximately 2 to 3 cm below the lesser curvature of the stomach. Short gastric vessels that extend into the greater curvature of the stomach are ligated proximal to the harvested segment to allow the gastroepiploic vessel to be mobilized. The isolated segment is then brought down through the transverse mesocolon and small bowel mesentery, with the gastroepiploic vessels placed retroperitoneally. This maneuver prevents acute angulation of the vessels and entrapment of small bowel. The continuity of the gastrointestinal tract is re-established, and the isolated ileal, colonic, or gastric segment is anastomosed to the bivalved bladder. Efforts should be made to obtain a spherical storage reservoir. This configuration allows the greatest volume with the least surface area, resulting in a low-pressure, large-capacity bladder.[13] To ensure optimal

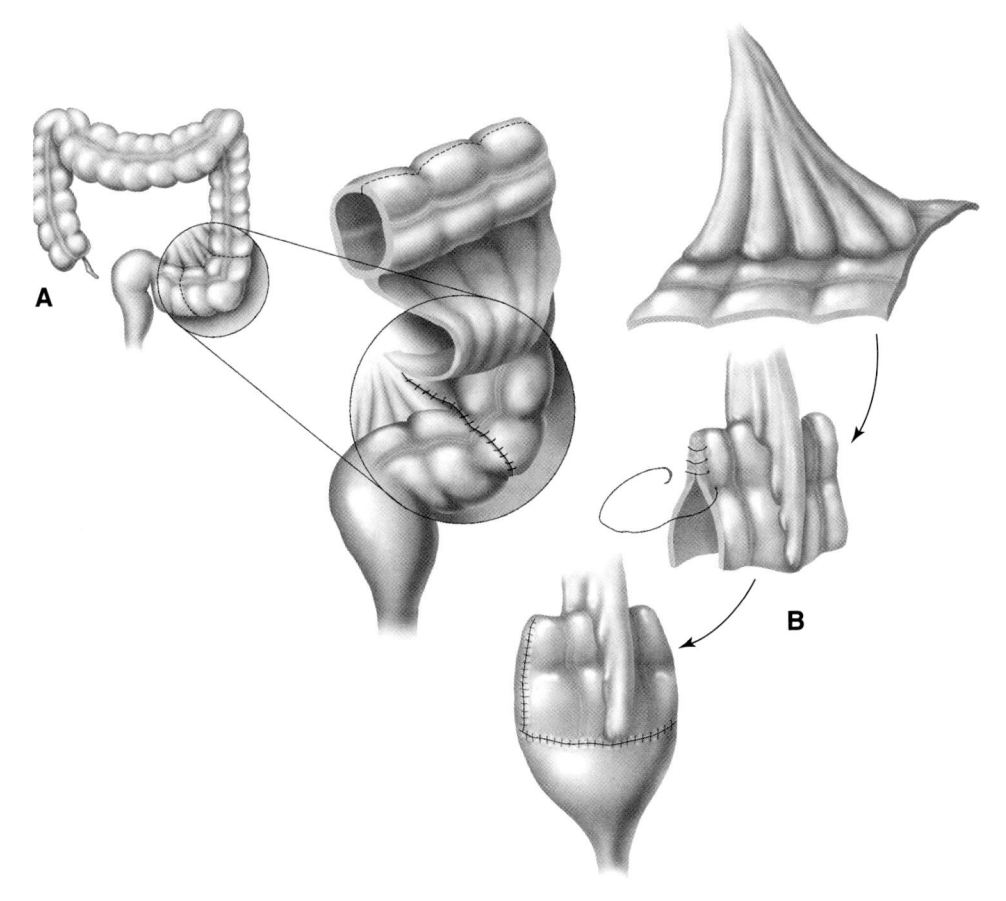

FIGURE 45-2 Colocystoplasty. **A**, A 10-cm segment is isolated on its blood supply and opened along the antimesenteric border. **B**, The colonic segment is then reconfigured into a U-shaped cap, before being anastomosed to the bivalved bladder. (From Kaefer M, Bauer SB: The surgical correction of incontinence in myelodysplastic children. In King LR [ed]: Urologic Surgery in Infants and Children. Philadelphia, Saunders, p 123, 1998.)

postoperative drainage, a suprapubic catheter is usually brought out through the native bladder.

An alternative to using portions of the gastrointestinal tract is to augment the bladder with ureteral tissue. This approach has significant advantages. Using ureteral tissue for bladder augmentation does not require disruption of bowel function and thus allows for more rapid recovery. Furthermore, ureteral augments have minimal metabolic complications.[14] Because they are lined with urothelium, these augments do not absorb electrolytes, secrete acid, or produce mucus. Thus, they avoid many complications associated with bowel augments. However, only an occasional patient is a candidate for this procedure, one who has an abnormally dilated ureter associated with a nonfunctioning renal unit. Ureteral augmentation can be performed with the distal dilated ureter of a functional renal unit in conjunction with a transureteroureterostomy or with a dilated lower or upper pole ureter in a duplex system. During this procedure, the ureter is mobilized, with care taken to preserve its medially positioned blood supply (Fig. 45-4). The ureter is detubularized longitudinally, along its anterior wall, from the renal pelvis or the upper third to the intramural segment. The ureter is then reconfigured as a U-shaped patch and anastomosed to the bladder. As with bowel augmentation, a suprapubic catheter is brought out through the native bladder.

Whether ileum, stomach, colon, or ureter is used for bladder augmentation, the suprapubic catheter is left in place for 3 to 4 weeks after surgery, after which time, a cystogram is performed to check for anastomotic leaks. The suprapubic catheter should not be removed until the bladder can be emptied reliably with either catheterization or voiding. Routine bladder irrigation should be performed beginning 5 to 7 days after surgery to remove mucus from the bladder, particularly when colon or ileum has been used for augmentation. Bladder irrigation should be maintained after removal of the suprapubic tube to remove mucus and reduce the risk of infection and stone formation. In patients with gastric augments, H2 blockers are administered for up to 6 months postoperatively.

SURGICAL CORRECTION OF BLADDER OUTLET ABNORMALITIES

The surgical management of urinary incontinence caused by inadequate bladder outlet resistance remains a technical challenge. Multiple surgical options are available, indicating the lack of universal success with any one procedure. The choice of technique depends on the patient's diagnosis and neurourologic findings and the familiarity of the surgeon with specific operative approaches. Bladder outlet resistance can be increased by the transurethral submucosal injection of artificial materials to narrow the urethral lumen; tubularization of the bladder neck; creation of a flap-valve mechanism; elevation or compression of the urethra and bladder neck with a

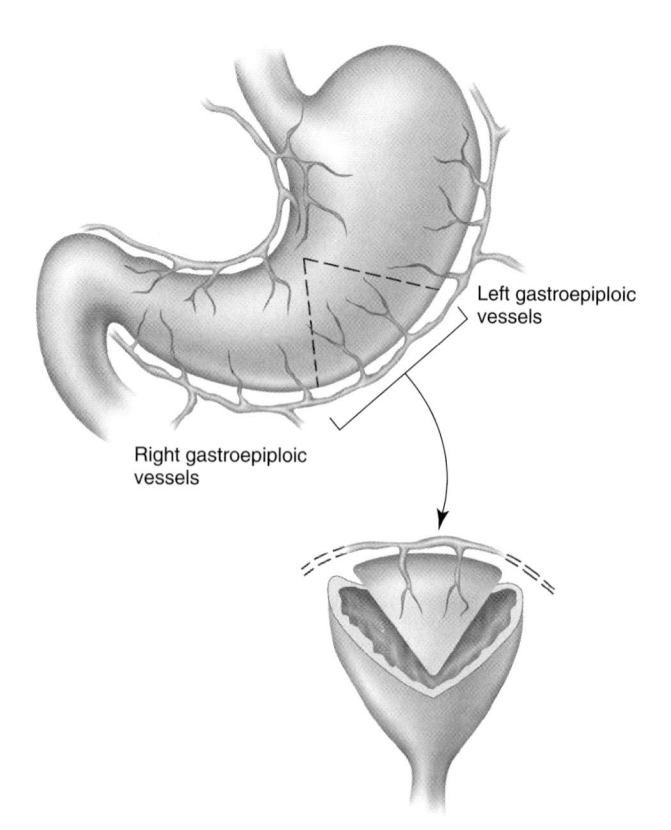

FIGURE 45-3 Gastrocystoplasty. A 8-cm, diamond-shaped segment is isolated from the greater curvature of the stomach, with the blood supply from either the right or the left gastroepiploic vessel. The segment is then anastomosed to the bivalved bladder. (From Kaefer M, Bauer SB: The surgical correction of incontinence in myelodysplastic children. In King LR [ed]: Urologic Surgery in Infants and Children. Philadelphia, Saunders, p 123, 1998.)

fascial sling; or the use of an artificial urinary sphincter. However, when all reasonable efforts to achieve acceptable continence have failed, closure of the bladder neck with the creation of a continent catheterizable stoma may be the only reliable alternative. Table 45-1 lists general indications for the selection of specific bladder neck surgery to improve incontinence.

Injection of Bulking Agents

Endoscopic placement of artificial materials periurethrally was first introduced in the 1960s, and its use in children was first reported in 1985.[15] Improvement in continence was achieved with this minimally invasive procedure in both adults and children. Injection of bulking agents into the urethra or bladder neck area facilitates coaptation of the mucosa of the bladder neck and proximal urethra, thereby increasing bladder outlet resistance and competency.[16] Initially, polytetrafluoroethylene (Teflon, Dupont, Wilmington, DE) was injected periurethrally as a bulking agent. However, the use of this material was largely abandoned when animal and human studies showed evidence of regional and distant migration (i.e., liver, lung, spleen, kidney, and brain) of polytetrafluoroethylene particles.[17,18] Alternative materials were evaluated, with gluteraldehyde cross-linked bovine collagen being the most used and studied. The modification of collagen with gluteraldehyde cross-linking helps to prevent breakdown by endogenous collagenase, and the collagen provides a matrix for host collagen deposition and neovascularization.[19]

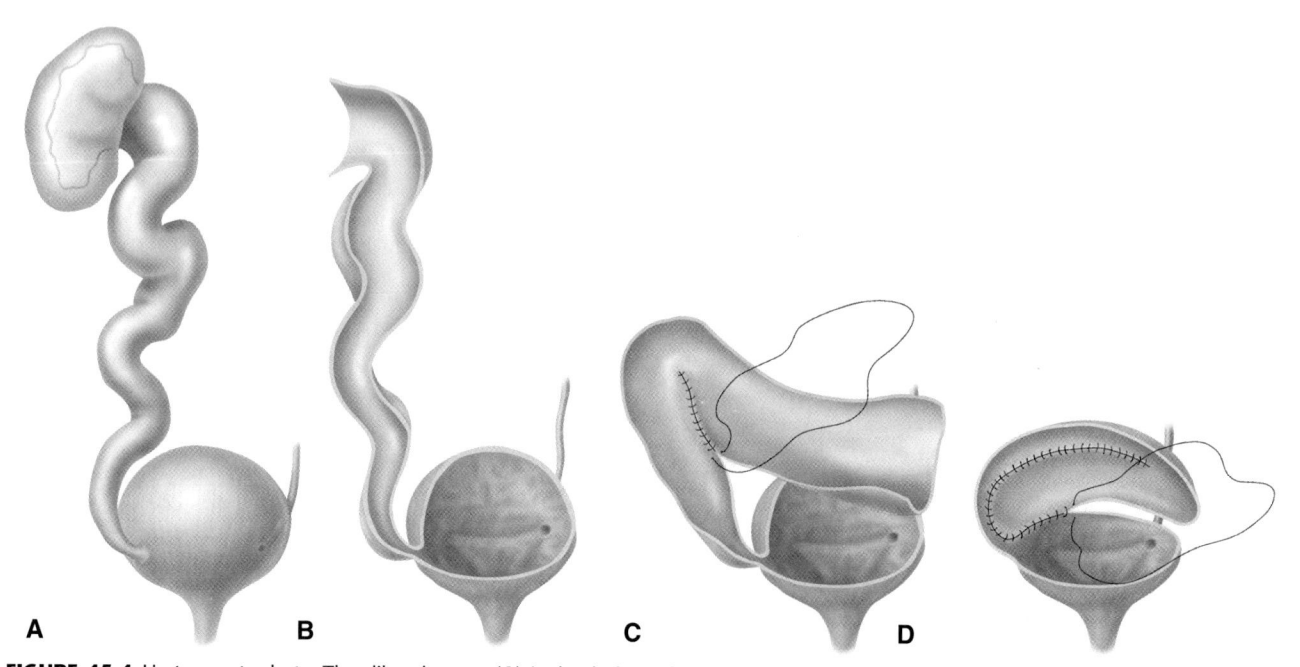

FIGURE 45-4 Ureterocystoplasty. The dilated ureter (**A**) is detubularized longitudinally (**B**), in conjunction with an ipsilateral nephrectomy or a transureteroureterostomy. The segment is then reconfigured into a U-shaped patch (**C**) and anastomosed to the bladder (**D**). (From Kaefer M, Bauer SB: The surgical correction of incontinence in myelodysplastic children. In King LR [ed]: Urologic Surgery in Infants and Children. Philadelphia, Saunders, p 124, 1998.)

TABLE 45-1 ■ Indications for Bladder Neck Surgery to Improve Continence

Type of Bladder Neck Procedure	Salient Indications
Fascial sling	No reflux
	Open bladder neck
	Stress incontinence
	Marginal capacity
	Compliant bladder
	Urethral resistance > 20 cm H_2O
Young-Dees-Leadbetter bladder neck reconstruction	Reflux
	Open bladder neck
	Reactive external sphincter (no denervation)
	Good capacity
	Compliant bladder
	Urethral resistance > 40 cm H_2O
Kropp/Pippi Salle procedure	Reflux
	Small capacity requiring augmentation
	Low urethral resistance (<20 cm H_2O) as a result of denervation
Artificial urinary sphincter	No reflux
	Areflexic, good capacity
	Highly compliant bladder
	Empties by straining
	Prefers no Clean Intermittent Catheterization (CIC)
	Urethral resistance ≤ 30 cm H_2O
Endoscopic injection	Good capacity
	Compliant bladder
	Mild or moderate stress incontinence
	Urethral resistance > 40 cm H_2O

Potential candidates for this procedure first undergo a skin test (0.1 mL injected intradermally) to exclude hypersensitivity to bovine collagen, and their urine is cultured. Approximately 3% of children have a positive skin reaction to the collagen. Children with a negative result on skin testing and infection-free urine undergo the procedure under general anesthesia. Prophylactic antibiotics are given, and a suprapubic tube is placed to avoid deforming the periurethral injections of collagen by postoperative placement of a urethral catheter. In boys, the collagen is placed transurethrally. Through one channel of a cystoscope, a 5-gauge needle is positioned beneath the urothelium, just distal to the bladder neck, at the 3 and 9 o'clock positions. Care is taken not to perforate the urothelium, which would allow an exit point for the collagen. The collagen is then delivered until visual occlusion of the urethral lumen is achieved. In girls, a periurethral approach is preferred because of the short urethra. A cystoscope is positioned just distal to the bladder neck, and a 22-gauge needle is inserted transvaginally into the periurethral tissue. Once movement of the needle tip is visualized endoscopically, the collagen is delivered until visual occlusion of the urethral lumen is achieved. Once the collagen is injected, the cystoscope is not advanced into the bladder to avoid displacement of the injected collagen.

Studies show that continence (defined as dryness for 4 hours between episodes of voiding or catheterization) is achieved in 5% to 63% of patients, using periurethral collagen injection.[20] Most of these studies were done in children with neurogenically impaired sphincters who had a relatively short follow-up (<5 years). The wide range in success rates suggests that many children showed an improvement in the severity of their incontinence, but did not fully achieve dryness. Moreover, the durability of collagen injections is unknown. As with adults, collagen injections appear to be more successful in girls than in boys. The efficacy of the treatment depends largely on the urodynamic findings of the patients selected. Children with detrusor areflexia and good compliance had a higher success rate than those with detrusor hyper-reflexia or poor compliance.[21] Many children in these studies required multiple treatments to achieve or maintain continence. An average of 1.6 to 2.1 injection treatments was needed per patient, with some children requiring up 5 treatments each. Reported complications have been rare, and include infection and migration of the collagen.

The advantages of periurethral collagen injection include its relative ease of administration, the ability to perform the procedure on an outpatient basis, and its low complication rate. However, these advantages are offset by its limited success in selected patients, the need for multiple treatments, and the cost of the procedure (average cost per treatment, $3000–$5000[16]). Because of these factors, we prefer not to use this method as first-line therapy in most patients. We reserve the use of periurethral collagen injections for improvement of residual incontinence in patients who have undergone a partially successful open procedure and who have minimal residual leakage. However, as with its use in the primary treatment of incontinence, the success of collagen injections in a previously operated bladder neck is variable.[22] Alternative artificial agents, such as chondrocytes and self-detachable balloons,[23] are being studied in hopes of identifying a more successful material for use in the endoscopic treatment of urinary incontinence.

Bladder Neck Tubularization and Urethral Lengthening: Young-Dees-Leadbetter Procedure

In 1907, Young[24] proposed the concept of improving bladder outlet resistance by increasing the functional length of the urethra. Subsequent modifications by Dees[25] and Leadbetter[26] resulted in the current technique that is used for bladder neck reconstruction. The patient is placed in the supine position, and the perivesical space is exposed. The vesical neck and urethra are dissected free from the surrounding tissue. Posterior mobilization is limited to prevent inadvertent injury to the rectum, vagina, or penile neurovascular bundles. The bladder is opened vertically. The ureters are then reimplanted more cephalad in a cross-trigonal manner to allow for further tubularization of the bladder neck (Fig. 45-5). A posterior strip of bladder (1.4 cm wide × 4 cm long) is outlined, and the triangular segments of mucosa are denuded on both sides of this strip. The resultant

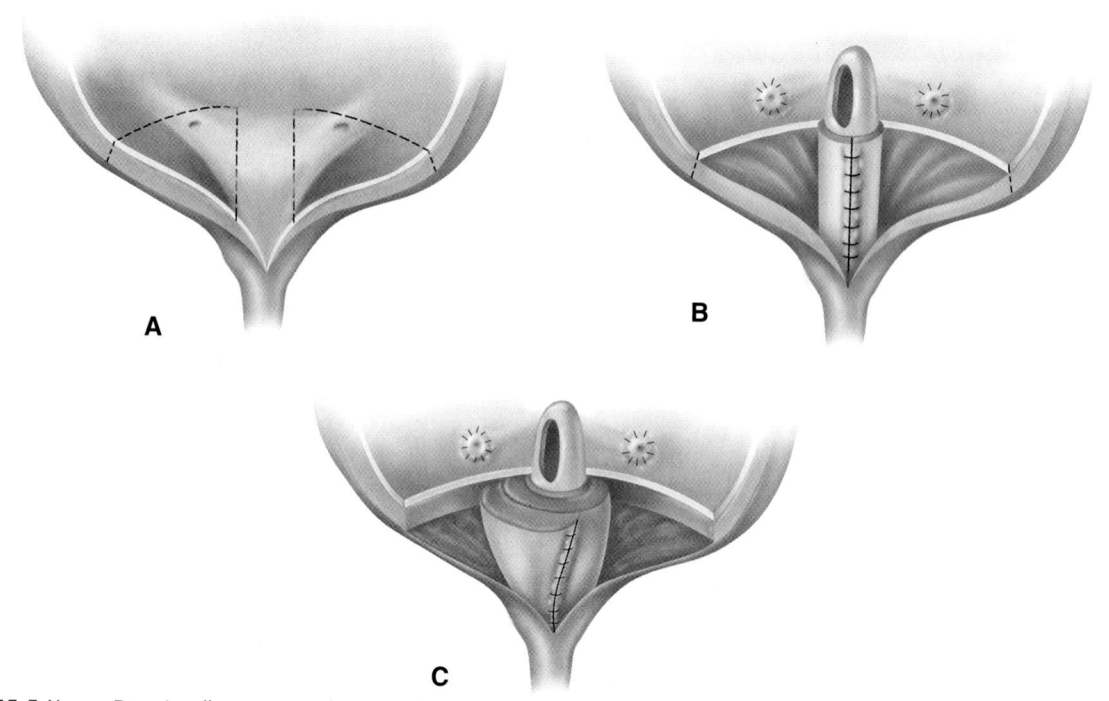

FIGURE 45-5 Young-Dees-Leadbetter procedure. **A,** The ureters are reimplanted more cephalad in a cross-trigonal manner. **B,** A posterior strip of bladder is outlined, and the triangular segments of mucosa are denuded on both sides of this strip. The posterior strip is then tubularized over an 8 Fr catheter. **C,** The triangular segments of muscle are then closed over the neourethra in a pants-over-vest fashion. (From Kaefer M, Bauer SB: The surgical correction of incontinence in myelodysplastic children. In King LR [ed]: Urologic Surgery in Infants and Children. Philadelphia, Saunders, p 127, 1998.)

triangular segments of muscle are then incised transversely along their cephalad border. The posterior strip of bladder mucosa is then tubularized over an 8 Fr feeding tube with a running 4–0 chromic suture. The triangular muscular segments are then closed over the neourethra, in a pants-over-vest fashion, with interrupted 3–0 polyglactin 910 (Vicryl) suture, reinforcing the muscular layer of the neourethra. If augmentation cystoplasty is not needed, the bladder is closed. A suprapubic catheter provides postoperative drainage while the urethral stent acts as a mold for the neourethra. Both catheters remain in place for 3 weeks. The stent is removed first, and the suprapubic tube is removed once reliable catheterization or voiding to completion is achieved.

This procedure has been used primarily in children with bladder exstrophy–epispadias and those with traumatic or iatrogenic injury to the bladder neck. In these children, continence rates vary from 40% to 75%.[27-30] Few studies report the use of this procedure in children with neurogenic sphincteric dysfunction.[31] Initial studies suggested that bladder neck reconstruction is much less likely to be successful when performed in a patient with a neurogenic bladder[32,33] because bladder neck reconstruction is dependent on good bladder neck and trigone muscular tone, which when properly reconfigured, provides some component of sphincteric control. However, subsequent studies[34] showed that 64% of children with neurogenic sphincteric deficiency who underwent this procedure remain dry for more than 4 hours or have only minor stress incontinence or night dampness.

A very poor success rate is reported with this technique in children with incontinence as a result of bilateral ureteral ectopia.[35] The complication rate for Young-Dees-Leadbetter procedure is high (≤45%[34]). The main complication appears to be difficulty with catheterization, requiring additional surgery.

This procedure uses native tissue to reconstruct the bladder neck, avoiding the complications inherent in the use of artificial materials. Advantages of this procedure include the use of healthy muscle around the bladder neck and the achievable outcome of 2- to 4-hour continence intervals. The success of the procedure depends on the availability of normally innervated tissue at the bladder neck. Disadvantages include the need for ureteral reimplantation, reduced bladder capacity, and a high complication rate, mainly as a result of difficulty with catheterization. The failure to achieve very high success rates has led to innovative surgical procedures that provide more reliable outcomes.

Kropp Procedure

In an attempt to improve the surgical continence rate for bladder neck reconstruction, the Kropp procedure, first described in 1986,[36] combines urethral lengthening and flap-valve dynamics. This procedure involves the creation of an anterior bladder wall tube, which is in continuity with the bladder neck and is reimplanted into a posterior submucosal tunnel that extends above the trigone. This anatomic arrangement provides an excellent continence mechanism that allows for the efficient transmission of dynamic bladder pressure changes to the neourethral tube located in the submucosal space. As intravesical pressure increases, the neourethral tube is effectively compressed, allowing for increased outlet resistance and eliminating both stress incontinence and leakage.

When this procedure is performed, a catheter is placed in the bladder and the bladder is filled to capacity. The anterior surface of the bladder is then exposed down to the bladder neck. The bladder neck is identified with the assistance of an inflated Foley balloon catheter. The aerolar tissue overlying this area is then removed. A rectangular strip of bladder (2 cm wide × 6 cm long) is developed along the anterior bladder wall, leaving the bladder mucosa and its distal attachments to the posterior urethra intact (Fig. 45-6). The incised bladder musculature retracts and separates, leaving the mucosa exposed. The mucosa is then incised on the outer edge of the separation. This maneuver allows sufficient bladder mucosa to be rolled into a tube around the catheter. Once the bladder is opened, the ureteral orifices are identified and the ureters are cannulated with feeding tubes. The ureters may need to be reimplanted laterally to accommodate the neourethral tube. The Foley balloon catheter is then grasped and pulled over the pubis. The bladder mucosa is incised around the bladder neck posteriorly and upward to meet the two lateral incisions. The developed rectangular anterior bladder wall strip is then tubularized around the catheter, using a running 4–0 Vicryl suture proximally and interrupted sutures distally. The cystotomy is opened further in the midline, extending to the dome of the bladder. A transverse incision is made in the mucosa of the original bladder neck. A submucosal tunnel is developed on the posterior wall of the bladder, between the ureteral orifices, and an opening is created in the mucosa, near the cephalad end of the tunnel. The neourethral tube opening is then brought through the submucosal tunnel. Excess tissue is excised, and the muscle of the neourethral tube is sutured to the bladder musculature posteriorly. The mucosa of the new bladder tube is reapproximated to the mucosa of the bladder, maturing the new bladder neck opening. Augmentation cystoplasty is performed as needed. We prefer not to create the two lateral wings of musculature in the bladder neck, as initially described by Kropp and Angwafo.[36] Leaving the posterior bladder musculature intact causes less difficulty with postoperative catheterization. Two ureteral feeding tubes, the suprapubic catheter, and the Foley balloon catheter, are left in place for postoperative drainage. The ureteral catheters are removed postoperatively once the edema subsides and adequate quantities of urine begin to drain into the bladder. The Foley catheter is removed 3 weeks after surgery. The suprapubic tube is removed once reliable catheterization is achieved.

Studies show that the continence rate for this procedure ranges from 78% to 81%.[37,38] The efficacy of this procedure is durable, with a continence rate of 72% to 77% in patients with more than 5 years of follow-up.[39,40] Concomitant bladder augmentation cystoplasty is needed in 88% to 100% of patients. Several studies show that without augmentation, these bladders become noncompliant postoperatively, with low capacity and high pressure.[39] Furthermore, intermittent catheterization is required in all patients. The most common complications reported include difficulty with catheterization (28%–45%); new onset of vesicoureteral reflux (22%–45%) despite concomitant ureteral reimplantation initially; peritonitis (38%); febrile urinary tract infection (38%); and struvite calculi (33%).[20] Seventy-six percent of patients required a second operation for one of these complications. Although the Kropp procedure is effective in achieving urinary continence, its use is limited because of the difficulty associated with catheterization and its complexity in construction.

Pippi Salle Procedure

To decrease the difficulty associated with catheterization while maintaining the flap-valve mechanism, in 1994, Pippi Salle and associates[41] proposed a "flip-flap" technique to lengthen the urethra. With the bladder partially filled, a 7-cm-long flap is isolated from the anterior bladder wall, beginning at the bladder neck and extending superiorly (Fig. 45-7). The flap is 2.5 cm wide at its base and tapers to 1.5 cm at the tip. In patients with previous bladder neck surgery, a lateralized anterior bladder wall flap is developed to obtain a more vascularized flap. A posterior midline bladder mucosal strip is isolated, and mucosal flaps on both sides of the strip are elevated to facilitate their approximation in the midline, without tension, over the newly created urethral tube. The mucosa of the anterior bladder wall flap is sutured to the posterior mucosal strip with a running 4–0 Vicryl suture. The muscle layer of the anterior bladder wall flap is then sutured to the exposed posterior trigonal muscle on either side of the posterior mucosal strip with interrupted 4–0 Vicryl sutures. The elevated mucosal flaps on each side of the neourethra are reapproximated over the tube to create a submucosal tunnel, and the opening of the new bladder tube is matured onto the mucosal surface of the bladder. The bladder is closed in two layers, and a pocket of bladder neck is allowed to extend down to the base of the new bladder tube. As with the Kropp procedure, two ureteral stents and suprapubic and urethral catheters are left in place to provide postoperative drainage. The urethral catheter is removed 5 weeks postoperatively, and intermittent catheterization is initiated.

Studies of children who underwent this procedure reported a continence rate of 50% to 69%.[42-44] However, many of these studies had a relatively short follow-up time and involved a small number of patients. Problems of incontinence are not uncommon, and have been associated with the formation of a urethrovesical fistula or with partial necrosis of the intravesical bladder tube. As with the Kropp procedure, 75% to 83% of patients require concomitant bladder augmentation, and all patients need intermittent catheterization to empty the bladder completely. Commonly reported complications include urethrovesical fistulas (12%–17%), new-onset vesicoureteral reflux (12%–17%), and bladder calculi (12%).[20]

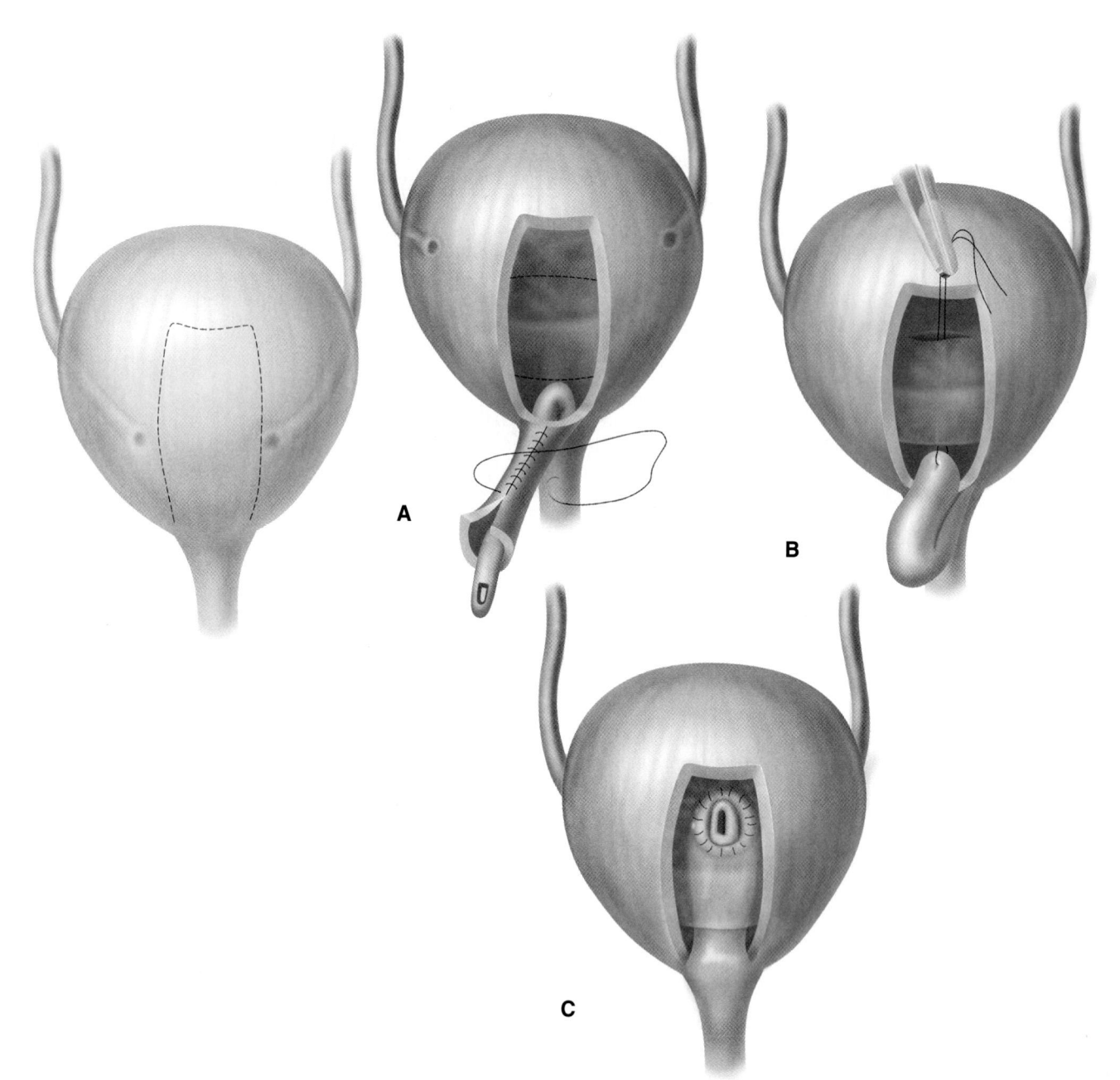

FIGURE 45-6 Kropp procedure. **A**, A rectangular strip of bladder developed from the anterior bladder wall is tubularized. **B**, After the ureters are reimplanted more cephalad, a submucosal tunnel is developed in the trigonal area. **C**, The neourethra is pulled through this tunnel. The mucosa of the new bladder tube is reapproximated to the mucosa of the bladder, maturing the new bladder neck opening. (From Kaefer M, Bauer SB: The surgical correction of incontinence in myelodysplastic children. In King LR [ed]: Urologic Surgery in Infants and Children. Philadelphia, Saunders, p 128, 1998.)

The revision rate is 12% to 17%, probably due to urethrovesical fistulas. Compared with the Kropp procedure, less difficulty with catheterization is reported after the Pippi Salle procedure; however, its continence rate is worse in children with neurogenic sphincter incompetence.

Bladder Neck Sling Suspension

Another method to improve bladder outlet resistance is to elevate and maintain the bladder neck in an intraabdominal position with a fascial sling. This maneuver provides static compression of the urethral lumen, increases dynamic urethral compression during abdominal straining, and improves the transmission of sudden increases in abdominal pressure to the bladder outlet.[45] This method was first popularized in women with stress urinary incontinence,[46] and the procedure soon gained popularity in children. In 1982, Woodside and Borden[47] first reported its use in children with neurogenic sphincter deficiency.

The procedure involves suspending the bladder neck with a small rectangular strip of fascia, usually obtained from the rectus fascia. In boys and prepubertal girls,

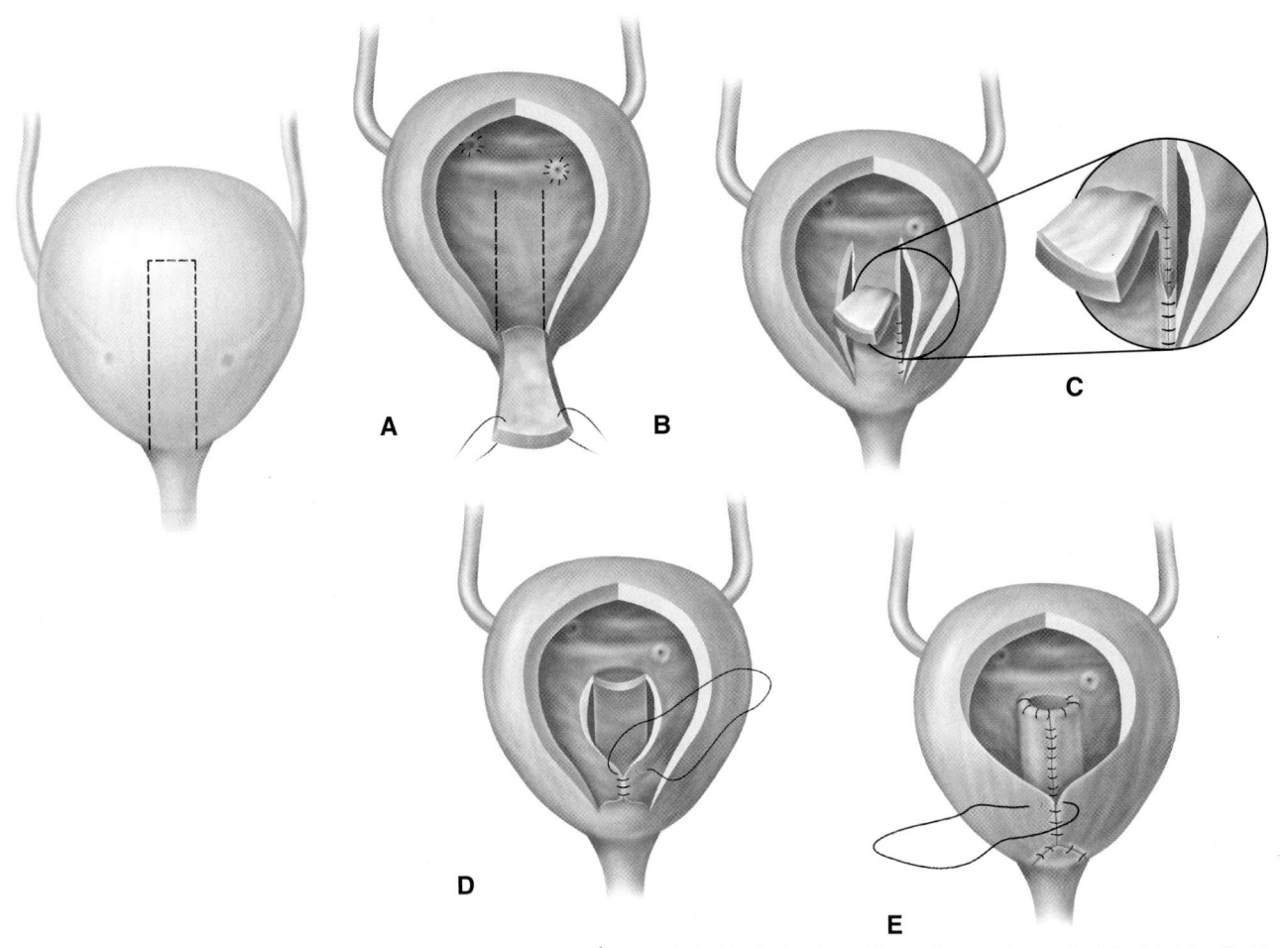

FIGURE 45-7 Pippi Salle procedure. **A**, A 7-cm-long rectangular strip of bladder is developed from the anterior wall of the bladder. **B**, After the ureters are reimplanted more cephalad, a submucosal tunnel is developed in the trigonal area. **C**, The mucosa of the anterior bladder strip is sutured to the posteriorly outlined strip. The muscle of the anterior bladder strip is sutured to the posterior musculature of the bladder wall. **D**, The mobilized lateral mucosal flaps are reapproximated over the neourethra. **E**, The mucosa of the new bladder tube is reapproximated to the mucosa of the bladder, maturing the new bladder neck opening. (From Kaefer M, Bauer SB: The surgical correction of incontinence in myelodysplastic children. In King LR [ed]: Urologic Surgery in Infants and Children. Philadelphia, Saunders, p 129, 1998.)

a strip of rectus fascia (15 cm long × 1.5 cm wide) is completely isolated 5 cm above the pubis. The strip may be transverse or vertical, depending on the skin incision. The sling is placed via a suprapubic approach by first incising the endopelvic fascia and developing the plane between the posterior urethra (just below the bladder neck) and rectum (Fig. 45-8). The sling is then positioned around the bladder neck and passed through the rectus fascia, near the pubic bone. The ends of the sling are tied over the rectus fascia in a crisscross fashion so that the sling fits snugly under the urethrovesical junction. In postpubertal girls, especially those who are sexually active, a vaginal approach is preferred (Fig. 45-9). When the bladder neck is exposed in this manner, a smaller strip of rectus fascia (3 × 4 cm) is needed. Access to the bladder neck is obtained by making an inverted U-shaped incision in the vaginal mucosa, with the apex at the level of the midurethra. A vaginal flap is raised, and the periurethral fascia is identified. The anterior vagina is dissected laterally and superiorly to the level of the bladder neck. The endopelvic fascia is then opened, mobilizing the urethra and vagina away from the pubic bone. After a small transverse suprapubic incision is made and the anterior rectus fascia is exposed adequately, a ligature carrier is passed through the rectus fascia from the suprapubic space and out of the vaginal incision. Sutures on the fascial sling are transferred suprapubically by withdrawing the ligature carrier after engaging the sutures in it. Cystoscopy is performed to exclude inadvertent bladder perforation and to assess how tightly to suspend the bladder neck. The sutures are then tied snugly over the rectus fascia. In the suprapubic and vaginal approaches, a urethral catheter and suprapubic tube are left indwelling after the procedure. The urethral catheter is removed 4 to 7 days later, and intermittent catheterization is either begun or resumed. The suprapubic catheter is removed when the patient resumes regular emptying of the bladder. Additional modifications to the fascial sling procedure include the use of prefabricated materials, such as intestinal submucosa; combining the sling procedure with tapering of the bladder neck[48]; wrapping the bladder neck circumferentially with the sling[49]; and wrapping a pedicle strip of anterior bladder wall around the bladder neck and suspending it to the pubis symphysis.[50]

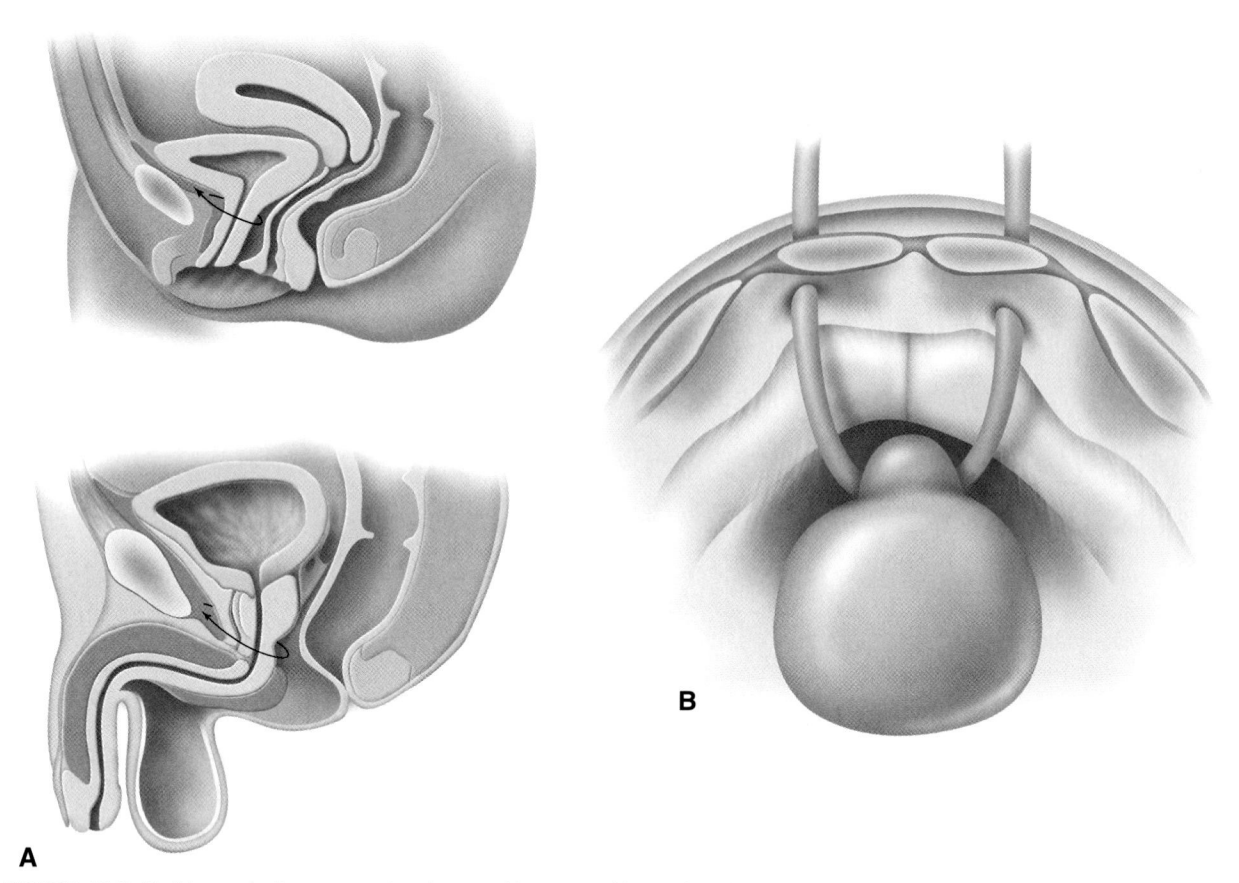

FIGURE 45-8 Bladder neck sling suspension (suprapubic approach). **A,** The plane between the urethra and vagina in girls or between the urethra and rectum in boys is developed. **B,** The harvested strip of fascia is positioned around the bladder neck (*arrows*) and passed through the rectus fascia, near the pubic bone. The ends of the strip are secured to the rectus sheath at each lateral edge before being tied over the rectus fascia in a crisscross fashion. (From Kaefer M, Bauer SB: The surgical correction of incontinence in myelodysplastic children. In King LR [ed]: Urologic Surgery in Infants and Children. Philadelphia, Saunders, p 130, 1998.)

Studies show that continence rates for a fascial sling procedure are 40% to 100%, depending on patient selection.[20] The sling procedure has been mainly limited to children with neurogenic urinary incontinence. In children with bladder exstrophy–epispadias, the sling procedure is not advised because of the lack of lower abdominal wall and anterior pubic symphysis support. Although it was initially thought that the sling was best suited for girls, several studies show that it is also effective in boys.[51-53] Previously, it was thought that dissection around the bladder neck would be difficult and that the risk of bladder neck, urethral, or rectal injury would be high in males, especially postpubertal boys. However, we and others[54] have found the dissection to be straightforward; furthermore, it was not made more difficult by the size and fixation of the prostate. Of children who underwent the sling procedure, 55% to 93% had concomitant bladder augmentation, and 78% to 100% required intermittent catheterization. These findings likely reflect the underlying pathology of neurogenic bladder dysfunction rather than the effects of the sling procedure on bladder dynamics. However, the long-term effects of a fascial sling procedure on bladder dynamics are not clear. Some studies[55] report significant decreases in bladder compliance after a sling procedure, whereas others do not.[56]

The complication rate for a fascial sling procedure is relatively low. Anecdotal reports of intraoperative complications include bladder neck, urethral, or rectal injury; wound infection; and difficulty with catheterization.[52,53,55-57] Placement of a fascial sling creates an acute angulation in the proximal urethra, increasing the chances of creating a false passage when passing a catheter. This problem may be avoided by placing the sling at the level of the bladder neck, avoiding pulling the sling too tightly against the abdominal wall, and using a soft coudé catheter for intermittent postoperative catheterization. Several studies[54,57] reported that the fascial sling may interfere with urethral access for endoscopic procedures involving the bladder in these patients, noting that it is difficult to visualize the trigone without a 70-degree lens or a flexible cystoscope. A potential complication associated with the use of a fascial sling in males is injury to the periprostatic neurovascular bundle, with resultant impotence. Dik and colleagues[53] reported that in 14 boys with spinal dysraphism who underwent bladder neck sling suspension, erectile function was preserved in all who had normal erections preoperatively. The neurovascular bundle is preserved by leaving Denonvilliers' fascia on the prostate and passing the fascial sling lateral to the prostate.

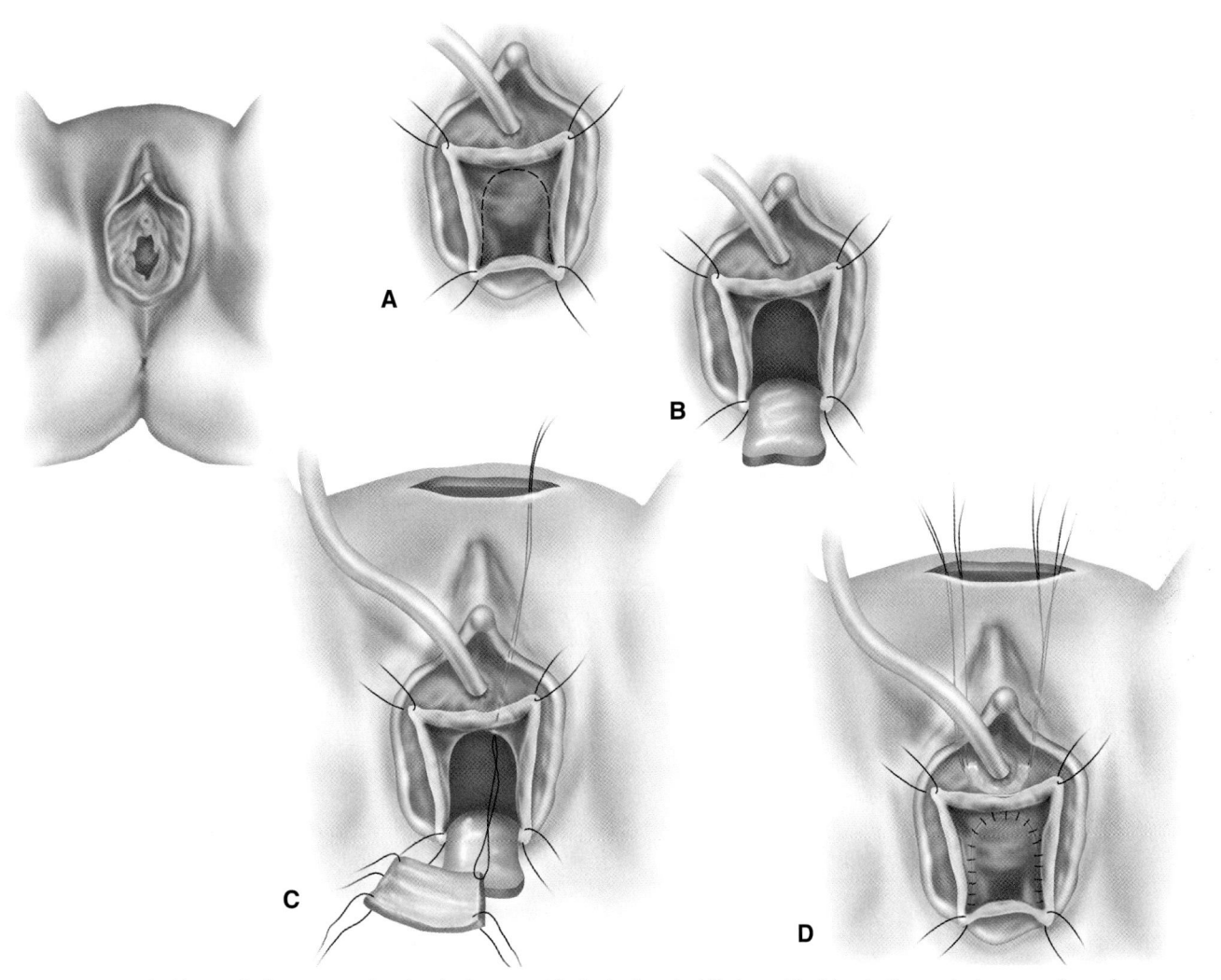

FIGURE 45-9 Bladder neck sling suspension (vaginal approach). **A**, An inverted U-shaped incision in the vaginal mucosa is made to expose the urethra. **B**, The endopelvic fascia is opened, mobilizing the urethra and vagina away from the pubic bone. **C**, Sutures on the fascial sling are transferred suprapubically. **D**, The sutures are then tied snugly over the rectus fascia. (From Kaefer M, Bauer SB: The surgical correction of incontinence in myelodysplastic children. In King LR [ed]: Urologic Surgery in Infants and Children. Philadelphia, Saunders, p 131, 1998.)

This procedure has several advantages: it is not technically complicated, it is reliable and durable, it does not markedly reduce bladder capacity nor require ureteral reimplantation, and it avoids the use of artificial materials in the reconstruction of the bladder neck. The sling procedure has a low complication rate, with an overall revision rate of 15%.[20]

Placement of an Artificial Urinary Sphincter

In 1973, Scott and colleagues[58] described the first use of a reliable, pressure-controlled artificial urinary sphincter (AUS). Since that time, many modifications in biomaterials and product design have been made to reduce treatment failures and decrease the need for periodic revision. With this technique, continence is achieved by static compression of the bladder neck or proximal urethra, thereby increasing urethral resistance.

When an artificial device is implanted, meticulous technique to maintain sterility is paramount; otherwise, infection rates can be high. The bladder is exposed through a Pfannenstiel or midline incision. The bladder neck is cleared of loose aerolar tissue, and the endopelvic fascia is incised. A plane is then developed between the proximal urethra and the rectum in boys or the vagina in girls. After the circumference of the bladder neck is measured with a sphincter cuff sizer, a sphincter cuff of appropriate length is selected and placed snugly around the proximal urethra (Fig. 45-10). In postpubertal boys, the cuff can be placed around the bulbous urethra, because it is well developed and easier to access. The AUS pump and the tubing that connects it to the cuff are placed into the hemiscrotum or labia opposite the child's dominant hand. The pressure reservoir balloon is placed into a retroperitoneal pouch on the same side as the pump. The tubing from the reservoir is brought through the rectus fascia and connected to the pump. The pressure-regulating balloon reservoir is chosen to be below the patient's diastolic blood pressure to maintain

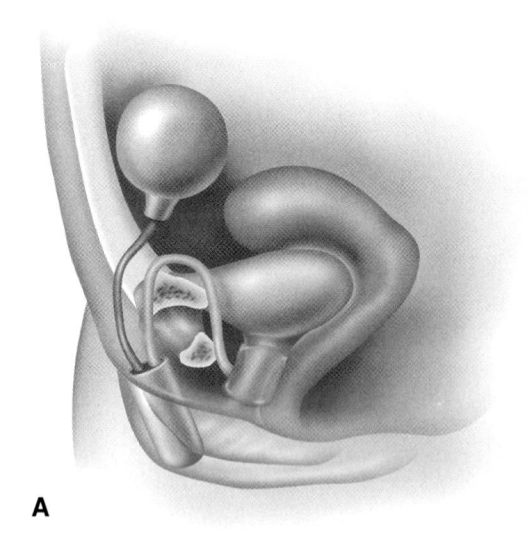

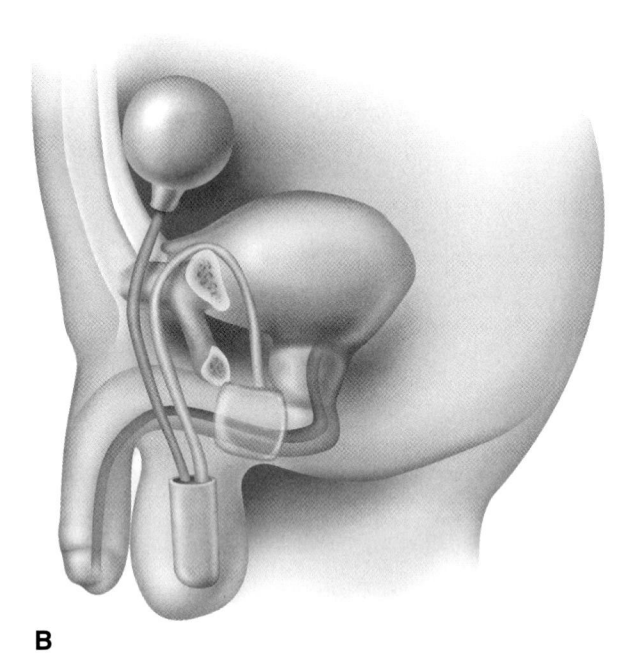

FIGURE 45-10 Artificial urinary sphincter placement. A sphincter cuff of appropriate length is placed snugly around the proximal urethra. In postpubertal boys, the cuff may be placed around the bulbous urethra. The pump can be placed (**A**) in the labia for girls or (**B**) in the scrotum in boys. (From Kaefer M, Bauer SB: The surgical correction of incontinence in myelodysplastic children. In King LR [ed]: Urologic Surgery in Infants and Children. Philadelphia, Saunders, p 132, 1998.)

adequate perfusion of the tissues beneath the cuff once it is inflated. The AUS is left deactivated for 10 to 12 weeks to allow for healing of tissues beneath the cuff and in the scrotum. The AUS is activated easily, by squeezing the pump to release the deactivation button.

Studies show that the continence rate for the AUS procedure is 76% to 95%.[20] This continence rate is maintained in patients with more than 10 years of follow-up.[59,60] After placement of an AUS, 63% to 74% of patients perform intermittent catheterization; 26% to 37% can void spontaneously. Placement of an AUS can markedly alter bladder compliance, especially in patients who had detrusor hyper-reflexia or decreased compliance preoperatively.[61-63] However, standard preoperative urodynamic studies cannot predict which patients will require bladder augmentation after placement of an AUS.[64] Thus, all patients who undergo sphincter placement should be followed routinely with radiologic imaging to detect upper urinary tract deterioration and should undergo urodynamic evaluation to detect changes in bladder function. Approximately 35% of patients require bladder augmentation after AUS placement,[59,60] and 2% to 15% have hydronephrosis or renal failure.[59,60,62,65]

Commonly reported complications include erosion of the AUS into the urethra (5%–15% incidence in contemporary studies), infection (5%), fluid loss, and mechanical failure. Risk factors for erosion include infection, previous bladder neck surgery, high balloon pressure, previous radiation therapy, and placement of the sphincter around the bulbous urethra in prepubertal boys.[20] Because of these complications, the revision rate for AUS procedures is 19% to 28% in contemporary series, which is much lower than that reported previously (79%). This decreased revision rate is the result of a number of product modifications, such as a dip-coated silicone cuff, a seamless reservoir, nonkink tubing, and a narrow back design for the cuff.[66,67] Like the sling procedure, placement of an AUS does not alter sexual function or development,[68] even in boys who underwent the procedure before puberty.

The advantage of the AUS compared with other bladder neck reconstruction techniques is that it provides adequate outlet resistance that can be lowered periodically to allow catheterization or voiding. In addition, the AUS can be readily deactivated indefinitely using the deactivation button on the pump; this feature is especially helpful in patients who require an indwelling urethral catheter for a prolonged time. Placement of the AUS is highly effective in achieving urinary continence. However, the associated risks of infection, erosion, product failure, and alteration of bladder dynamics limit the usefulness of this procedure.

Closure of the Bladder Neck and Creation of a Catheterizable Stoma

When surgery of the bladder neck does not provide adequate outlet resistance, it may be necessary to completely close off the bladder outlet to achieve urinary continence. This procedure is used only after all other options are exhausted, because closure of the bladder neck mandates dependence on an alternative access into the bladder.

Reliable bladder neck closure requires complete disruption of the epithelial and muscular continuity between the urethra and bladder and a meticulous multiple-layer closure with interposition of vascularized tissue (omentum, if possible) to avoid fistula formation. In most children who undergo this procedure, the bladder neck is approached retropubically, through a Pfannenstiel or midline incision. The endopelvic fascia is incised, and the proximal urethra is mobilized off of the rectum or vagina and the surrounding supporting ligaments. Mobilization of a longer segment of urethra allows for easier subsequent closure. The urethra is then divided and the posterior wall of the bladder mobilized. The cut edges of the bladder neck then spring apart, helping to create a separation between the urethral stump and bladder. The urethra is closed with 4–0 Vicryl sutures, in several imbricating layers. The bladder neck is also closed in several layers. Omentum or other vascularized tissue is then brought down and interposed between the urethral stump and bladder neck.

Occasionally, the proximal urethra cannot be approached retropubically because of extensive fibrosis from previous bladder neck surgery. In these cases, bladder neck closure should be approached transvesically or, in girls, transvaginally. In the transvesical approach, the bladder neck is visualized once the bladder is opened. The bladder neck is incised circumferentially and the mucosa around the bladder neck excised. The urethra is then inverted into the lumen of the bladder. The urethra and its mucosa are trimmed as much as possible. The urethral stump is then closed in multiple layers. The bladder neck muscle is closed over the urethral stump, obliterating the mucosal layer. In girls, bladder neck closure can be performed transvaginally. An inverted U-shaped incision is made in the anterior vaginal wall. A second incision is made circumferentially around the urethra, and the anterior vaginal wall flap is mobilized. The urethra is dissected to the bladder neck and transected. The bladder is then closed in several layers, and the vaginal flap is reapproximated. Transurethral cautery obliteration of the bladder neck mucosa is an ineffective way to close off the bladder neck. To achieve continence, extensive dissection and interposition of vascularized tissue between the bladder and urethral stump must be performed.

Once the bladder neck is closed, alternative access into the bladder must be established by constructing a continent catheterizable stoma. This stoma can be constructed using the flap-valve, or Mitrofanoff principle. With this procedure, a vascularized, catheterizable conduit is positioned in the bladder submucosa, providing access from the abdominal wall surface into the bladder. Continence is achieved when increasing pressure in the bladder during filling is transmitted to the submucosal portion of the conduit, compressing its lumen. A minimum of 2 cm for the intramural tunnel is needed to create a continent stoma.[69] Structures that can be used as a vascularized, catheterizable conduit include appendix, ureter, tapered ileum, stomach, colon, and fallopian tube. In patients with a large-capacity, highly compliant bladder, a detrusor tube can also be fashioned.[70]

The appendix is most commonly used to create a continent catheterizable conduit (appendicovesicostomy, Fig. 45-11). A midline laparotomy is made, and the appendix is identified and isolated from the cecum, on its blood supply. If the appendix is not long enough, a segment of cecum may be taken with the appendix and tubularized to extend the proximal end of the conduit. After the cecum is closed and the distal end of the appendix is opened, a catheter is placed into the appendix tube to ensure patency and ease of catheterization. The distal

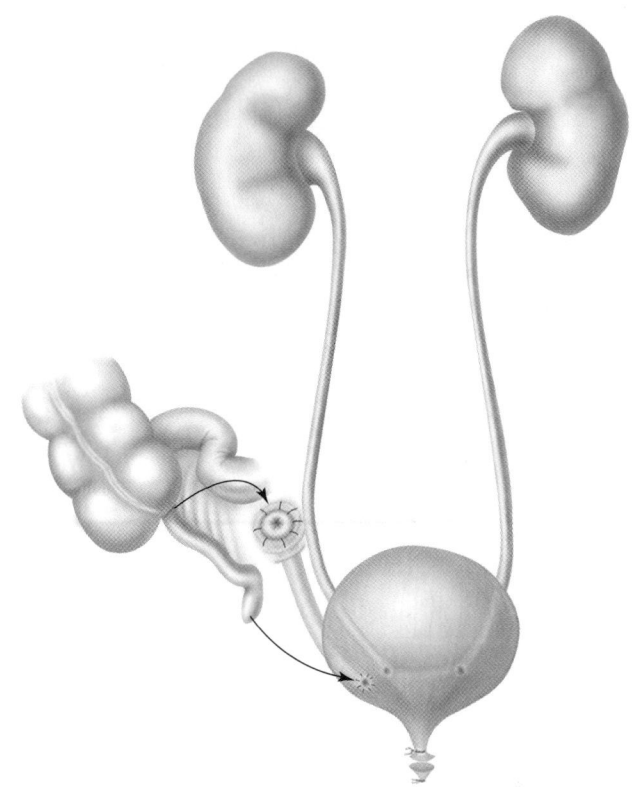

FIGURE 45-11 Appendicovesicostomy. The appendix (*arrows*) is isolated from the cecum, on its blood supply. The proximal end is brought through the abdominal wall, and the distal end is implanted into the bladder submucosa. (From Kaefer M, Bauer SB: The surgical correction of incontinence in myelodysplastic children. In King LR [ed]: Urologic Surgery in Infants and Children. Philadelphia, Saunders, p 134, 1998.)

end of the appendix is implanted into the bladder submucosa. The proximal end of the appendix is brought through the abdominal wall to a previously identified stoma site in the right lower quadrant or to the umbilicus, and sutured at both the level of fascia and the skin. This reverse direction for the appendix is used to minimize stomal stenosis. A U-shaped skin flap is advanced into the spatulated end of the appendix to prevent stomal stenosis. To facilitate catheterization, the bladder is fixed to the anterior abdominal wall at the site where the appendix traverses the rectus fascia.

When the appendix is not available or is not long enough, a vascularized, catheterizable conduit can be fashioned out of ileum (Monti procedure[71,72]). With this procedure, a 2-cm ileal segment is isolated with a good vascular pedicle (Fig. 45-12). The segment is detubularized through a longitudinal incision halfway up the anterior side of the ileal segment. The flap is tubularized transversally over a 12 Fr catheter, with a running 4–0 chromic suture used proximally and interrupted sutures used distally. Closure of the second layer is performed with a 4–0 Vicryl suture. The resultant tube is implanted into the bladder and brought out onto the skin, as described earlier for the appendicovesicostomy procedure.

Several studies reported a 98% continence rate for the catheterizable stoma.[73–75] Using this procedure, continence is durable with long-term follow-up.[73] Commonly

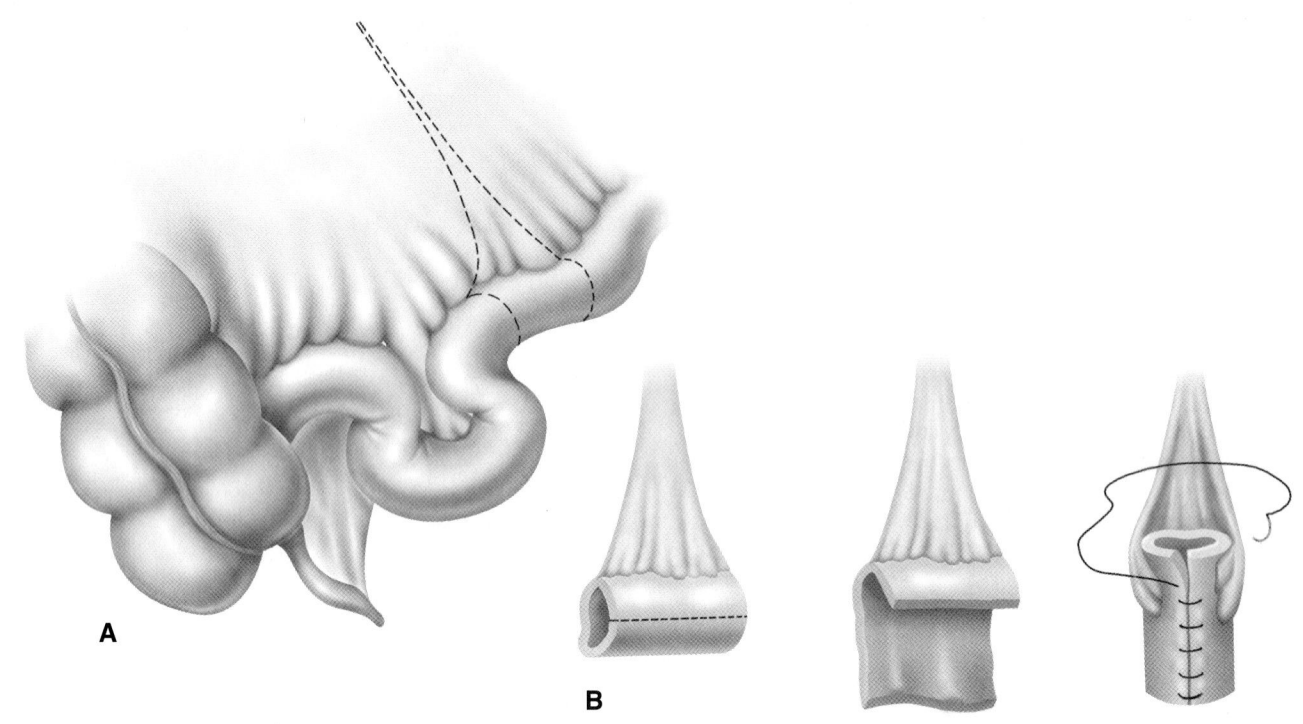

FIGURE 45-12 Monti procedure. **A**, A 2-cm segment of ileum is isolated with its blood supply. **B**, The segment is detubularized through a longitudinal incision halfway up the anterior side of the ileal segment. The flap is tubularized transversely over a 12 Fr catheter and then implanted into the bladder submucosa.

reported complications include stomal stenosis (10%–25%), stricture formation, and perforation. The revision rate for the continent catheterizable conduit procedure is 16% to 28%. Overall, this procedure is reliable and has an acceptable complication rate. We prefer to use the appendix as the first option, but also have had good results with the tapered or reconfigured ileum.

Surgical Correction of Fecal Incontinence

Many children with urinary incontinence have concomitant fecal incontinence, especially those with spinal dysraphism. Medical management is based on controlled constipation with regular periodic evacuation. Diet and therapy with drugs, such as fiber additives, are used to control stool consistency, and laxatives and enemas are used to empty the colon. Many children with neurogenic bowel dysfunction are treated successfully with this regimen, although some remain incontinent. In 1990, Malone and associates[76] described a technique in which a continent catheterizable channel is created between the skin and the cecum to allow for antegrade administration of an enema (Malone Antegrade Continence Enema or MACE). The MACE procedure allows reliable and complete evacuation of stool from the colon, resulting in fecal continence. This procedure is appropriate for children who have an adequate length of colon to act as a reservoir between flushes and who do not have distal obstruction that would impair complete rectal emptying, prolong flushes, or promote ongoing leakage. This procedure should be considered only after dietary and medical management does not result in reliable and predictable bowel movements. When surgery is considered to correct urinary incontinence, bowel function should be assessed and MACE should be considered. It would be distressing for the child to achieve urinary incontinence only to remain in diapers because of fecal soiling.

With this procedure, the appendix is identified and isolated on its blood supply (Fig. 45-13). The appendix is opened distally, and its patency is evaluated with a 10 Fr catheter. Next, the appendix is tunneled into the tinea of the cecum or adjacent serosal flaps that are created to place it in a submucosal tunnel. Alternatively, the appendix is detached proximally and reimplanted into the cecum. Our preference is to leave the appendix in situ. The distal end of the appendix is brought through the anterior abdominal wall to a preselected stoma site or to the umbilicus. A U-shaped skin flap is advanced into the spatulated end of the appendix to prevent stomal stenosis. In children who require both appendicovesicostomy and MACE, we divide the appendix, using the distal portion for the former procedure and the proximal portion for the latter. A small portion of the cecum may be tubularized to elongate the MACE conduit.

The MACE procedure has been performed laparoscopically, with good success.[77] With the laparoscopic technique, the appendix is brought out of the skin without the need for reimplantation into the tinea of the colon. A catheter is left in the conduit for 3 weeks, after which, daily catheterizations are performed. In the postoperative period, while the catheter is still in place, daily flushes are initiated once bowel sounds return. After the catheter is removed, antegrade flushes are conducted

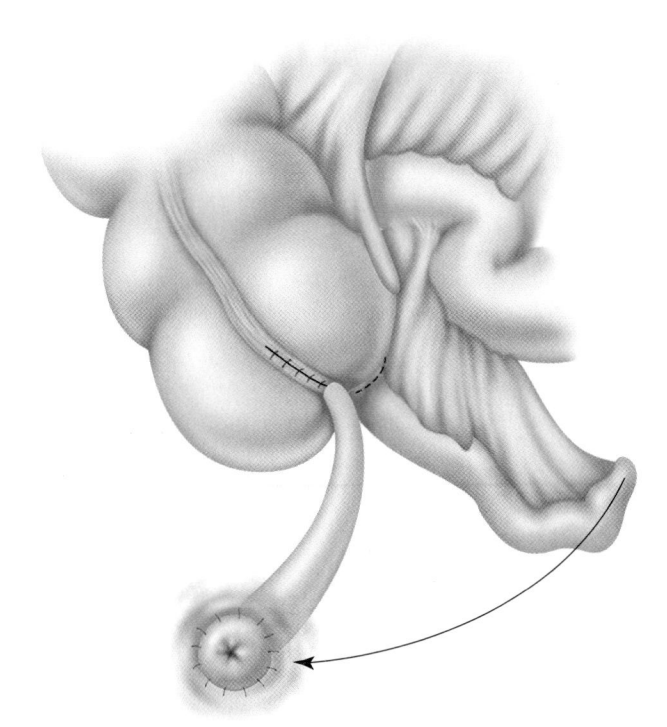

FIGURE 45-13 Antegrade continent enema procedure. The appendix (*arrows*) can be tunneled into the tinea of the cecum or adjacent serosal flaps. Alternatively, the appendix can be detached proximally and then implanted into the cecum. (From Kaefer M, Bauer SB: The surgical correction of incontinence in myelodysplastic children. In King LR [ed]: Urologic Surgery in Infants and Children. Philadelphia, Saunders, p 136, 1998.)

daily. Some patients remain continent and free of constipation with flushes performed every other day. Less commonly, some children, usually those with decreased anal sphincter tone (e.g., imperforate anus), need to perform the procedure twice daily to prevent fecal soiling.

Several studies report a fecal continence rate of 61% to 80% with this technique.[78-81] After undergoing the MACE procedure, more than 90% of children report improvements in bowel habits and a better quality of life.[79] Most become independent of daily diaper use. Major complications associated with this procedure include stomal stenosis (10%–33%) and leakage from the stoma (6%–15%). Iatrogenic metabolic complications of enema administration (e.g., fatal hypernatremia) may occur[82]; however, most are mild and are not clinically significant. When the MACE procedure is performed laparoscopically, the results are comparable with the results of the open technique.[77,83] Children with motility disorders, such as Hirschsprung's disease, severe chronic idiopathic constipation, or neuronal intestinal dysplasia, may have poor results with the MACE procedure.[84]

CONCLUSION

Many options are available to treat children with urinary and fecal incontinence. A treatment plan, progressing from the least invasive to the most invasive procedure, should be designed for each child. Some treatment options are more appropriate for some children than for others, based on individual anatomy, physiology, level of function, home environment, and motivation. An understanding of the surgical options, techniques, and associated complications will allow the physician to select the most appropriate treatment with the highest rate of success. If surgical treatment is undertaken, close follow-up is needed to ensure optimal results for children with urinary and fecal incontinence.

REFERENCES

1. Bauer SB, Labib KB, Dieppa RA, Retik AB: Urodynamic evaluation of a boy with myelodysplasia and incontinence. Urology 10:354, 1977.
2. Pontari MA, Keating M, Kelly M, et al: Retained sacral function in children with high level myelodysplasia. J Urol 154:775, 1995.
3. Kaefer M, Zurakowski D, Bauer SB, et al: Estimating normal bladder capacity in children. J Urol 158:2261, 1997.
4. Roth S, Semjonow A, Waldner M, Hertle L: Risk of bowel dysfunction with diarrhea after continent urinary diversion with ileal and ileocecal segments. J Urol 154:1696, 1995.
5. Roth JA, Borer JG, Hendren WH, et al: Is gastric augmentation a good long-term urodynamic solution to the poorly functioning bladder? 2000 Annual Meeting of the American Academy of Pediatrics, Section in Urology, Oct 28, 2000, Chicago, IL.
6. Austin PF, Lockhart JL, Bissada NK, et al: Multi-institutional experience with the gastro-intestinal composite reservoir. J Urol 165:2018–2021, 2001.
7. Duel BP, Gonzalez R, Barthold JS: Alternative techniques for augmentation cystoplasty. J Urol 159:998, 1998.
8. Dayanc M, Kilciler M, Tan O, et al: A new approach to bladder augmentation in children: Seromuscular enterocystoplasty. BJU Int 84:103, 1999.
9. Atala A: Creation of bladder tissue in vitro and in vivo: A system for organ replacement. Adv Exp Med Biol 462:31, 1999.
10. Yoo JJ, Meng J, Oberpenning F, Atala A: Bladder augmentation using allogenic bladder submucosa seeded with cells. Urology 51:221, 1998.
11. Decter RM, Bauer SB, Mandell J, et al: Small bowel augmentation in children with neurogenic bladder: An initial report of urodynamic findings. J Urol 138:1014, 1987.
12. Goldwasser B, Barrett DM, Webster GD, Kramer SA: Cystometric properties of ileum and right colon after bladder augmentation, substitution or replacement. J Urol 138:1007, 1987.
13. Hinman F Jr: Selection of intestinal segments for bladder substitution: Physical and physiological characteristics. J Urol 139:519, 1988.
14. Churchill BM, Aliabadi H, Landau EH, et al: Ureteral bladder augmentation. J Urol 150:716, 1993.
15. Vorstman B, Lockhart J, Kaufman MR, Politano V: Polytetrafluoroethylene injection for urinary incontinence in children. J Urol 133:248, 1985.
16. Bomalaski MD, Bloom DA, McGuire EJ, Panzl A: Glutaraldehyde cross-linked collagen in the treatment of urinary incontinence in children. J Urol 155:699, 1996.
17. Malizia AA Jr, Reiman HM, Myers RP, et al: Migration and granulomatous reaction after periurethral injection of polytef (Teflon). JAMA 251:3277, 1984.

18. Claes H, Stroobants D, Van Meerbeek J, et al: Pulmonary migration following periurethral polytetrafluoroethylene injection for urinary incontinence (see comments). J Urol 142:821, 1989.
19. Leonard MP, Canning DA, Epstein JI, et al: Local tissue reaction to the subureteral injection of glutaraldehyde cross-linked bovine collagen in humans. J Urol 143:1209, 1990.
20. Kryger JV, Gonzalez R, Barthold JS: Surgical management of urinary incontinence in children with neurogenic sphincteric incompetence. J Urol 163:256, 2000.
21. Silveri M, Capitanucci ML, Mosiello G, et al: Endoscopic treatment for urinary incontinence in children with a congenital neuropathic bladder. Br J Urol 82:694, 1998.
22. Duffy PG, Ransley PG: Endoscopic treatment of urinary incontinence in children with primary epispadias. Br J Urol 81:309, 1998.
23. Diamond DA, Bauer SB, Retik AB, Atala: Initial experience with the transurethral self-detachable balloon system for urinary incontinence in pediatric patients. J Urol 164:942, 2000.
24. Young H: Suture of the urethral and vesical sphincters for the cure of incontinence of urine, with a report of a case. Trans South Surg Gynecol Assoc 20:210, 1907.
25. Dees JE: Congenital epispadias with incontinence. J Urol 62:513, 1949.
26. Leadbetter GWJ: Surgical correction of total urinary incontinence. J Urol 91:261, 1964.
27. Donnahoo KK, Rink RC, Cain MP, Casale AJ: The Young-Dees-Leadbetter bladder neck repair for neurogenic incontinence. J Urol 161:1946, 1999.
28. Husmann DA, Vandersteen DR, McLorie GA, Churchill BM: Urinary continence after staged bladder reconstruction for cloacal exstrophy: The effect of coexisting neurological abnormalities on urinary continence. J Urol 161:1598, 1999.
29. Ahmed S, Fouda-Neel K, Borghol M: Continence after bladder-neck reconstruction in patients with bladder exstrophy and pubic diastasis. Br J Urol 77:896, 1996.
30. Mathews R, Sponseller PD, Jeffs D, Gearhart JP: Bladder neck reconstruction in classic bladder exstrophy: The role of osteotomy in the development of continence. BJU Int 85:498, 2000.
31. Rink RC, Mitchell ME: Surgical correction of urinary incontinence. J Pediatr Surg 19:637, 1984.
32. Tanagho EA, Smith DR: Clinical evaluation of a surgical technique for the correction of complete urinary incontinence. J Urol 107:402, 1972.
33. Leadbetter GW Jr: Surgical reconstruction for complete urinary incontinence: A 10 to 22-year followup. J Urol 133:205, 1985.
34. Sidi AA, Reinberg Y, Gonzalez R: Comparison of artificial sphincter implantation and bladder neck reconstruction in patients with neurogenic urinary incontinence. J Urol 138:1120, 1987.
35. Jayanthi VR, Churchill BM, Khoury AE, McLorie GA: Bilateral single ureteral ectopia: Difficulty attaining continence using standard bladder neck repair. J Urol 158:1933, 1997.
36. Kropp KA, Angwafo FF: Urethral lengthening and reimplantation for neurogenic incontinence in children. J Urol 135:533, 1986.
37. Mollard P, Mouriquand P, Joubert P: Urethral lengthening for neurogenic urinary incontinence (Kropp's procedure): Results of 16 cases. J Urol 143:95, 1990.
38. Belman AB, Kaplan GW: Experience with the Kropp anti-incontinence procedure. J Urol 141:1160, 1989.
39. Nill TG, Peller PA, Kropp KA: Management of urinary incontinence by bladder tube urethral lengthening and submucosal reimplantation. J Urol 144:559, 1990.
40. Kropp KA: Bladder neck reconstruction in children. Urol Clin North Am 26:661, 1999.
41. Salle JL, de Fraga JC, Amarante A, et al: Urethral lengthening with anterior bladder wall flap for urinary incontinence: A new approach. J Urol 152:803, 1994.
42. Salle JL, McLorie GA, Bagli DJ, Khoury AE: Urethral lengthening with anterior bladder wall flap (Pippi Salle procedure): Modifications and extended indications of the technique. J Urol 158:585, 1997.
43. Rink RC, Adams MC, Keating MA: The flip-flap technique to lengthen the urethra (Salle procedure) for treatment of neurogenic urinary incontinence. J Urol 152:799, 1994.
44. Mouriquand PD, Boddy S: Salvage procedures for failed Benchekroun hydraulic valves: Experience in four patients. Br J Urol 77:740, 1996.
45. McGuire EJ, Wang CC, Usitalo H, Savastano J: Modified pubovaginal sling in girls with myelodysplasia. J Urol 135:94, 1986.
46. McGuire EJ, Lytton B: Pubovaginal sling procedure for stress incontinence. J Urol 119:82, 1978.
47. Woodside JR, Borden TA: Pubovaginal sling procedure for the management of urinary incontinence in a myelodysplastic girl. J Urol 127:744, 1982.
48. Herschorn S, Radomski SB: Fascial slings and bladder neck tapering in the treatment of male neurogenic incontinence. J Urol 147:1073, 1992.
49. Walker RD III, Flack CE, Hawkins-Lee B, et al: Rectus fascial wrap: Early results of a modification of the rectus fascial sling. J Urol 154:771, 1995.
50. Kurzrock EA, Lowe P, Hardy BE: Bladder wall pedicle wraparound sling for neurogenic urinary incontinence in children. J Urol 155:305, 1996.
51. Nguyen HT, Bauer SB, Diamond DA, Retik AB: Rectus fascial sling for the treatment of neurogenic sphincteric incontinence in boys: Is it effective? J Urol 166:658–661, 2000.
52. Perez LM, Smith EA, Broecker BH, et al: Outcome of sling cystourethropexy in the pediatric population: A critical review. J Urol 156:642, 1996.
53. Dik P, Van Gool JD, De Jong TP: Urinary continence and erectile function after bladder neck sling suspension in male patients with spinal dysraphism. BJU Int 83:971, 1999.
54. Elder JS: Periurethral and puboprostatic sling repair for incontinence in patients with myelodysplasia. J Urol 144:434, 1990.
55. Decter RM: Use of the fascial sling for neurogenic incontinence: Lessons learned. J Urol 150:683, 1993.
56. Kakizaki H, Shibata T, Shinno Y, et al: Fascial sling for the management of urinary incontinence due to sphincter incompetence (see comments). J Urol 153:644, 1995.
57. Gosalbez R, Castellan M: Defining the role of the bladder-neck sling in the surgical treatment of urinary incontinence in children with neurogenic incontinence. World J Urol 16:285, 1998.
58. Scott FB, Bradley WE, Timm GW: Treatment of urinary incontinence by implantable prosthetic sphincter. Urology 1:252, 1973.
59. Kryger JV, Spencer Barthold J, Fleming P, Gonzalez R: The outcome of artificial urinary sphincter placement after a mean 15-year follow-up in a paediatric population. BJU Int 83:1026, 1999.
60. Levesque PE, Bauer SB, Atala A, et al: Ten-year experience with the artificial urinary sphincter in children. J Urol 156:625, 1996.

61. Bauer SB, Reda EF, Colodny AH, Retik AB: Detrusor instability: A delayed complication in association with the artificial sphincter. J Urol 135:1212, 1986.
62. Light JK, Pietro T: Alteration in detrusor behavior and the effect on renal function following insertion of the artificial urinary sphincter. J Urol 136:632, 1986.
63. Roth DR, Vyas PR, Kroovand RL, Perlmutter A: Urinary tract deterioration associated with the artificial urinary sphincter. J Urol 135:528, 1986.
64. Kronner KM, Rink RC, Simmons G, et al: Artificial urinary sphincter in the treatment of urinary incontinence: Preoperative urodynamics do not predict the need for future bladder augmentation. J Urol 160:1093, 1998.
65. Churchill BM, Gilmour RF, Khoury AE, McLorie GA: Biological response of bladders rendered continent by insertion of artificial sphincter. J Urol 138:1116, 1987.
66. Singh G, Thomas DG: Artificial urinary sphincter in patients with neurogenic bladder dysfunction (see comments). Br J Urol 77:252, 1996.
67. Simeoni J, Guys JM, Mollard P, et al: Artificial urinary sphincter implantation for neurogenic bladder: A multi-institutional study in 107 children. Br J Urol 78:287, 1996.
68. Jumper BM, McLorie GA, Churchill BM, et al: Effects of the artificial urinary sphincter on prostatic development and sexual function in pubertal boys with meningomyelocele. J Urol 144:438, 1990.
69. Watson HS, Bauer SB, Peters CA, et al: Comparative urodynamics of appendiceal and ureteral Mitrofanoff conduits in children. J Urol 154:878, 1995.
70. Casale A: Continent vesicostomy: A new method utilizing only bladder tissue (abstract 72). 60th Annual Meeting of the American Academy of Pediatrics, New Orleans, 1991.
71. Yang WH: Yang needle tunneling technique in creating antireflux and continent mechanisms. J Urol 150:830, 1993.
72. Monti PR, Lara RC, Dutra MA, de Carvalho JR: New techniques for construction of efferent conduits based on the Mitrofanoff principle. Urology 49:112, 1997.
73. Harris CF, Cooper CS, Hutcheson JC, Snyder HM III: Appendicovesicostomy: The Mitrofanoff procedure: A 15-year perspective. J Urol 163:1922, 2000.
74. Cain MP, Casale AJ, King SJ, Rink RC: Appendicovesicostomy and newer alternatives for the Mitrofanoff procedure: Results in the last 100 patients at Riley Children's Hospital. J Urol 162:1749, 1999.
75. Suzer O, Vates TS, Freedman AL, et al: Results of the Mitrofanoff procedure in urinary tract reconstruction in children. Br J Urol 79:279, 1997.
76. Malone PS, Ransley PG, Kiely EM: Preliminary report: The antegrade continence enema. Lancet 336:1217, 1990.
77. Van Savage JG, Yohannes P: Laparoscopic antegrade continence enema in situ appendix procedure for refractory constipation and overflow fecal incontinence in children with spina bifida. J Urol 164:1084, 2000.
78. Curry JI, Osborne A, Malone PS: The MACE procedure: Experience in the United Kingdom. J Pediatr Surg 34:338, 1999.
79. Shankar KR, Losty PD, Kenny SE, et al: Functional results following the antegrade continence enema procedure (see comments). Br J Surg 85:980, 1998.
80. Hensle T, Reiley EA, Chang DT: The Malone antegrade continence enema procedure in the management of patients with spina bifida. J Am Coll Surg 186:669, 1998.
81. Malone PS, Curry JI, Osborne A: The antegrade continence enema procedure: Why, when and how? World J Urol 16:274, 1998.
82. Schreiber CK, Stone AR: Fatal hypernatremia associated with the antegrade continence enema procedure. J Urol 162:1433; discussion 1433, 1999.
83. Lynch AC, Beasley SW, Robertson RW, Morreau PN: Comparison of results of laparoscopic and open antegrade continence enema procedures. Pediatr Surg Int 15:343, 1999.
84. Curry JI, Osborne A, Malone PS: How to achieve a successful Malone antegrade continence enema. J Pediatr Surg 33:138, 1998.

CHAPTER 46

Neuromodulation

PHILIP EDWARD VICTOR VAN KERREBROECK ■ EMMANUEL CHARTIER-KASTLER

Many neurologic disorders can affect bladder and pelvic floor function. Although the incidence of lower urinary tract dysfunction is different among the various neurologic entities, an important percentage of patients have voiding dysfunction.[1] Incontinence and poor evacuation of urine, with residual urine and recurrent urinary tract infections, are important sources of morbidity. One of the most prominent features in patients with spinal cord injury is the inability to control the storage and evacuation function of the bladder. Besides these bladder problems that have a proven neurologic basis, many patients have lower urinary tract dysfunction without an evident neurologic cause. These are patients with different forms of idiopathic dysfunctional voiding.

Therapy includes pharmacologic treatment, eventually in combination with clean intermittent catheterization. However, lifelong continuation of this therapy is a problem, mainly because of side effects. Furthermore, in most patients, especially women, incontinence remains a problem, even with maximal pharmacologic treatment. The failure of pharmacologic treatment has led to the development of surgical approaches, such as augmentation cystoplasty, sphincteric incisions, and artificial sphincter implantation. However, many patients with neurogenic bladder dysfunction continue to have significant urologic problems, despite the use of maximal classic therapy.

The use of electrical stimulation to control the storage and evacuation of urine has become an important tool in the urologic treatment of voiding dysfunction. The aim of electrical stimulation for voiding dysfunction is to treat incontinence caused by lack of activity of the striated muscles of the urethral closure mechanism by improving contraction of the sphincter mechanism or to overcome incontinence as a result of detrusor hyperactivity by reducing detrusor contractions. Furthermore, electrical stimulation can be used to permit evacuation of a paraplegic bladder by provocation of detrusor contractions or to control micturition in the hyper-reflexic bladder by a combination of dampening of spontaneous reflex excitability and controlled activation of the detrusor.

These aims can be fulfilled by stimulation of the efferent nerves to the lower urinary tract or by modulation of reflex activity as a result of stimulating afferent nerves.

Different modalities to apply electrical current to the lower urinary tract are available. Surface electrodes can be used as nonimplantable devices,[2] and insertable plugs in the anal canal or vagina can be used to treat incontinence.[3-5] Intravesical electrostimulation is performed in children with meningomyelocele.[6-8] Implantable prostheses are available to induce bladder contraction to evacuate urine in paraplegic bladders or to control detrusor contraction in hyper-reflexic bladders.[9-11] Another type of prosthesis permits the modulation of symptomatic voiding dysfunction, such as urge incontinence, urgency, frequency, and retention.[12,13]

ELECTRICAL STIMULATION IN SPINAL CORD INJURY

The development of systems for electrical stimulation of the bladder in spinal cord injury coincided with better knowledge about the pathophysiology of neurogenic bladder dysfunction. In patients with complete spinal cord injury and bladder hyper-reflexia, the complete micturition cycle must be controlled. In other words, in addition to electrostimulation for evacuation, bladder capacity and compliance must be increased.

Two approaches for stimulation of the bladder in patients with spinal cord injury are available, one of which is intradural and the other extradural. Brindley,[14] from London, started with animal experiments to try to develop a system for intradural sacral anterior root stimulation in 1969. The first successful sacral anterior root stimulator for a patient with traumatic paraplegia was implanted in 1978.[15] The clinical results have improved since the 1986 introduction of complete intradural sacral posterior root rhizotomy to control the reservoir function of the bladder in combination with implantation of the sacral posterior root stimulator.[16]

Because of the anatomic features of the sacral roots, separation of their anterior (motoric) and posterior (sensory) parts only is possible in their intradural part. Therefore, the actual technique of intradural sacral anterior root stimulation consists of the combination of complete posterior rhizotomy with implantation of the Finetech-Brindley electrodes in the remaining anterior roots.[17] After a development period of 14 years in the Neurological Prostheses Unit in London, an anterior root stimulator has been commercially available since 1986. The Finetech-Brindley bladder controller (Finetech, Hertfordshire, Great Britain; Neuro-Control, Brussels, Belgium) consists of an implanted system of electrodes for sacral anterior root stimulation. This system contains no implanted power supply, but is driven by an external radio transmitter.

The internal equipment, or implant, consists of three parts. The electrode mounts are called books because of their shape, in which the anterior sacral roots are trapped intradurally. The electrode book is designed to be implanted intradurally at about L5–S1. The radio receiver block, which contains three radio receivers, is implanted subcutaneously in a pouch in the lower thoracic or abdominal wall. Three silicone-coated cables form the connection between the electrode book and the radio receiver block. Together with the implant, a sleeve is delivered to pass the cables through the dura mater and prevent leakage of cerebrospinal fluid.

The external equipment consists of a transmitter block with three coils connected through an isolated cable with the control box. The control box contains the electronic components and rechargeable batteries, and generates electrical impulses that are transmitted to the transmitter block. The transmitter block transforms these high-frequency signals back into electrical impulses that are transmitted to the motor spinal nerve roots.

The control box permits the installation of three different programs. Normally, the first program aids in micturition, the second program aids in defecation, and the third program can be used for erection in men and lubrication of the vagina in women. After the programs are installed by the physician, the patient uses a command to select a program.

A laminectomy from L3–L4 to S2 is necessary to implant the material intradurally. The interlaminar joints are spared on both sides because they are essential for the stability of the spine.

The results of this technique in approximately 700 patients who have undergone this operation worldwide have been published.[18] In a personal series of 52 patients and also in the review of 184 patients from different centers, more than 80% of patients achieved sufficient intravesical pressure and efficient voiding.[19] In nearly all patients with a functioning implant, the incidence of infection was decreased. In patients who had a posterior rhizotomy, the occurrence of reflex-uninhibited detrusor contractions is abolished because the reflex arc is no longer intact. As a result, patients had increased functional capacity without involuntary detrusor contractions. Therefore, continence can be achieved in most patients without previous surgery to reduce urethral closure function. Most patients become appliance-free, which enhances dignity and self-image.[20,21]

Long-term follow-up of the original 50 patients described by Brindley[14] shows that persistent results of bladder stimulation can be achieved with a limited number of technical problems.[22]

Another type of sacral root stimulation for the evacuation of urine in spinal cord injury was developed by the San Francisco group of researchers.[13] As a result of their research, electrodes were placed extradurally in combination with selective posterior rhizotomy of sacral root S3, S4, or both. The extradural approach is an easier surgical technique with less risk of cerebrospinal fluid leak. However, exact separation of the anterior and posterior parts of the sacral roots is more difficult in the extradural segment of S3 and nearly impossible at the S4 level. In a group of 22 patients, complete success (i.e., normal reservoir function, continence, and evacuation of urine with electrical stimulation) was achieved in 8 (42%).[11] Voiding with this type of stimulation is claimed to be synchronous, and would occur with low voiding pressure. This extradural stimulation system is not available commercially. Further experimental and clinical work is ongoing.

ELECTRICAL STIMULATION FOR CHRONIC LOWER URINARY TRACT DYSFUNCTION

Chronic lower urinary tract dysfunction, such as urge incontinence, urgency, frequency, and problems with bladder evacuation, present a challenge. Initially, most patients are treated conservatively with bladder retraining, pelvic floor exercises, and biofeedback. In most patients, this regimen is supplemented with drugs. However, approximately 40% of patients with these forms of lower urinary tract dysfunction do not achieve acceptable improvement with these forms of treatment, and remain a therapeutic challenge. Alternative procedures with variable success rates, such as bladder transection, transvesical phenol injection of the pelvic plexus, augmentation cystoplasty, and even urinary diversion, are being advocated.

During the last few decades, functional electrical stimulation has gained interest in the treatment of this type of lower urinary tract dysfunction. Different stimulation sites, such as the vagina or anus, have been reported to be successful. Since the 1960s, transcutaneous neurostimulation applied to the foramen S3 or S4 has been attempted in an effort to control functional lower urinary tract disorders.[23] Unilateral sacral segmental stimulation with a permanent electrode at the level of sacral foramen S3 or S4 (sacral neuromodulation) offers an alternative nondestructive mode of treatment for patients with voiding dysfunction and chronic pelvic pain that is resistant to conservative measures. Since 1981, a clinical trial has been underway to evaluate the effectiveness of this method. Since that time, experience has been gained in the evaluation, surgical treatment, and follow-up of patients with voiding dysfunction and pelvic pain who have been treated with sacral foramen electrode implants.[24] The goal of this treatment is to relieve the symptoms by rebalancing micturition control.

The mode of action of this "sacral neuromodulation" is unclear, but it has been hypothesized that the electrical current modulates reflex pathways involved in the filling and evacuation phases of the micturition cycle.[25]

Stimulation of A-delta myelinated fibers of sacral roots S3 and S4 decreases the spastic behavior of the pelvic floor and enhances the tone of the urethral sphincter. The threshold for the somatic component of the spinal nerve that innervates the pelvic floor is lower than that for the automatic component of the bladder. Therefore, simultaneous bladder contraction is avoided during stimulation. In many subjects, the primary voiding dysfunction appears to begin with unstable urethral activity, which activates the voiding reflexes and leads to detrusor instability and the associated urgency, frequency, and incontinence. The inhibitory effect of the enhanced urethral sphincter tone suppresses detrusor instability and stabilizes detrusor activity.

Ideal candidates for neuromodulation are patients with urge incontinence, urinary urgency, frequency, and problems with evacuation. Patients who underwent numerous other unsuccessful therapies should not be excluded from neuromodulation because they often have an excellent response to this technique.

Sacral neuromodulation is planned as a long-term treatment, but patients are first tested with a temporary trial stimulation for 3 to 7 days. This trial stimulation has two steps: acute testing, followed by the subchronic phase. During an outpatient procedure and under local anesthesia, one of the sacral foramina, preferably S3, is punctured with a 20-gauge hollow needle. The proximal and distal tip of the needle is not isolated, and allows electrical stimulation.

Typical responses to stimulation of each nerve level are seen at both the local (perineum) and distant (foot and toe) sites. S3 stimulation produces a bellows-like contraction of the levator muscles as well as contraction of the detrusor and urethral sphincter. Signs of S3 stimulation in the lower extremities include plantar flexion of the great toe. Subjectively, patients report a pulling sensation in the rectum during S3 stimulation, with variable sensations being perceived in the scrotum and the tip of the penis by men or the labia and vagina in women. S4 stimulation causes a bellows-like contraction of the levator ani muscle, with no activity noted in the foot or leg. The sacral root at the site with the best clinical (subjective) or urodynamic response is selected, and the intensity of the current is adapted to the sensation of stimulation.

A temporary electrode is placed through the needle, and the needle is removed. This electrode remains in the vicinity of the sacral root that is selected, and passes through the sacral foramen, subcutaneous tissue, and skin. When the acute motoric responses with stimulation are confirmed, the electrode is connected to an external stimulator. Then the subchronic phase of the trial stimulation starts. Patients check the effect over a period of 3 to 7 days, based on voiding diaries. Urodynamic examination is possible as an extra control of the effect.

Patients with a good clinical and preferably urodynamic result are candidates for a permanent implant, which consists of a surgically implanted electrode with four contact points (Pisces quad lead Model 3886, Medtronic, Minneapolis, MO) connected to a pace-maker (Interstim stimulator, Medtronic Interstim, Maastricht, The Netherlands).

Implantation is performed under general anesthesia. After a midline incision is made over the sacrum, the fascia overlying the foramina at one side of the sacrum is opened, giving access to the foramen selected. Acute stimulation with a needle is repeated to confirm the motoric responses. The permanent electrode is positioned in the foramen with the four contact points near the sacral bone (or sacrum). The electrode is fixed to the posterior wall of the sacral bone (or sacrum) with nonresorbable sutures, and passed subcutaneously to an incision in one of the flanks. After wound closure, the patient is placed in a lateral position. A subcutaneous pocket is created lateral to the umbilicus. The flank wound is opened, and the electrode is connected to the pulse generator with a connection cable that is passed subcutaneously to an abdominal pocket. The pacemaker is fixed to the rectus fascia. Recently, an alternative technique was presented in which a gluteal pocket is created to receive the pulse generator. The advantage of this method is that the surgery can be performed in one position. Furthermore, morbidity, especially pain at the side, seems to be reduced.

Usually, low amplitudes (1.5–5.5 V; 210-µsec pulse duration at 10–15 cycles/sec) are sufficient for stimulation of the somatic nerve fibers. With these parameters, no dyssynergia of the bladder and striated urethral musculature is induced, even when voiding is initiated with the stimulator on.

Previous reports showed an overall success rate of 60% to 75% at initial trial stimulation.[24] Of the patients selected after subchronic trial stimulation who underwent permanent implantation, as many as 83% derived major benefit from the definitive procedure.[26] This effect appears to be durable, as evidenced by the late results. However, approximately 20% of patients who respond well to trial stimulation do not have the same result after chronic stimulation. Based on clinical parameters, it appears that patients with detrusor overactivity and urethral instability have the best result.[27]

Recently, the results of a multinational, multicenter clinical trial of this method were presented.[28] In a group of 155 patients with treatment-resistant urge incontinence, 98 (63%) had good results on the temporary trial stimulation. Of these, 38 were followed up for 1 year, with a successful outcome in 30 (79%).

Similar multicenter, multinational studies in patients with urgency, frequency, and chronic voiding problems reported similar results.[29,30] Also, with long-term follow-up, results seem to be persistent over time.[31] However, after permanent implantation, approximately 20% of patients with initially favorable percutaneous nerve evaluation test results do not respond for unknown reasons. Further research is needed to identify additional parameters that can be used as reliable predictors of success.

Neuromodulation seems to be an effective treatment modality in patients with various forms of lower urinary tract dysfunction. This technology is a valuable addition to the current treatment options when conservative measures fail.

REFERENCES

1. Wein AJ, Raezer DM, Benson GS: Management of neurogenic bladder dysfunction in the adult. Urology 8:432, 1976.

2. Bradley WE, Timm GW, Chou SN: A decade of experience with electronic stimulation of the micturition reflex. Urol Int 26:283, 1971.
3. Godec C, Cass AS, Ayala GF: Electrical stimulation for incontinence: Technique, selection and results. Urology 7:388, 1976.
4. Merrill DC: The treatment of detrusor incontinence by electrical stimulation. J Urol 122:515, 1979.
5. Fall M: Does electrical stimulation control incontinence? J Urol 131:664, 1984.
6. Katona F: Stages of vegetative afferentation in reorganization of bladder control during intravesical electrotherapy. Urol Int 30:192, 1975.
7. Seiferth J, Heising J, Larkamp H: Experiences and critical comments on the temporary intravesical electrostimulation of neurogenic bladder in spina bifida children. Urol Int 33:27, 1978.
8. Madersbacher H, Pauer W, Reiner E: Rehabilitation of micturition by transurethral electrostimulation of the bladder in patients with incomplete spinal cord lesions. Paraplegia 20:191, 1982.
9. Caldwell KPS: Urinary incontinence following spinal injury treated by electronic implant. Lancet 1:846, 1985.
10. Brindley GS, Polkey CE, Rushton DN, Cardozo L: Sacral anterior root stimulators for bladder control in paraplegia: The first 50 cases. J Neurol Neurosurg Psychiatry 49:1104, 1986.
11. Tanagho EA, Schmidt RA, Orvis BR: Neural stimulation for control of voiding dysfunction: A preliminary report in 22 patients with serious neuropathic voiding disorders. J Urol 142:340, 1989.
12. Markland C, Merrill D, Chou S, Bradley W: Sacral nerve root stimulation: A clinical test of detrusor innervation. J Urol 107:772, 1972.
13. Schmidt RA: Advances in genitourinary neurostimulation. Neurosurgery 18:1041, 1986.
14. Brindley GS: Experiments directed towards a prosthesis which controls the bladder and the external sphincter from a single site of stimulation. Proceedings of the Biological Engineering Society 46th Meeting, Liverpool, 1972.
15. Brindley GS, Polkey CE, Rushton DN: Sacral anterior root stimulation for bladder control in paraplegia. Paraplegia 20:365, 1982.
16. Sauerwein D: Die operative Behandlung der spastischen Blasenlahmung bei Querschnittlahmung. Urologe A 29:196, 1990.
17. Van Kerrebroeck PEV, Koldewijn EL, Wijkstra H, Debruyne FMJ: Intradural sacral rhizotomies and implantation of an anterior sacral root stimulator in the treatment of neurogenic bladder dysfunction after spinal cord injury. World J Urol 9:126, 1991.
18. Van Kerrebroeck PEV, Debruyne FMJ: World-wide experience with the Finetech-Brindley bladder stimulator. Neurourol Urodynam 12:497–503, 1993.
19. Van Kerrebroeck PhEV, Koldewijn EL, Rosier P, et al: Results of the treatment of neurogenic bladder dysfunction in spinal cord injury by sacral posterior root rhizotomy and anterior sacral root stimulation. J Urol 155:1378–1381, 1996.
20. Van Kerrebroeck PhEV, van der Aa HE, Bosch JLHR, et al: Sacral rhizotomies and electrical bladder stimulation in spinal cord injury: Part I. Clinical and urodynamic analysis. Eur Urol 31:263–271, 1997.
21. Wielink G, Essink-Bot ML, Van Kerrebroeck PhEV, et al: Sacral rhizotomies and electrical bladder stimulation in spinal cord injury: Part II. Cost-effectiveness and quality of life analysis. Eur Urol 31:441–446, 1997.
22. Brindley GS, Rushton DN: Long-term follow-up of patients with sacral anterior root stimulator implants. Paraplegia 28:469, 1990.
23. Habib HN: Experiences and recent contributions in sacral nerve stimulation for both human and animal. Br J Urol 39:73, 1967.
24. Schmidt RA: Applications of neurostimulation in urology. Neurourol Urodynam 7:585, 1988.
25. Thon WF, Baskin LS, Jonas U, et al: Neuromodulation of voiding dysfunction and pelvic pain. World J Urol 9:38, 1991.
26. Bosch JLHR, Groen J: Sacral (S_3) segmental nerve stimulation as a treatment for urge incontinence in patients with detrusor instability: Results of chronic electrical stimulation using an implantable neural prosthesis. J Urol 154:504, 1995.
27. Koldewijn EL, Rosier PFWM, Meuleman EJH, et al: Predictors of success with neuromodulation in lower urinary tract dysfunction: Results of trial stimulation in 100 patients. J Urol 152:2071, 1994.
28. Janknegt RA, Van Kerrebroeck PhEV, Lyckama à Nijeholt AA, et al: Sacral nerve modulation for urge incontinence: A multinational, multicenter randomized study. J Urol 157(4):1237, 1997.
29. Hassouna MM, Siegel SW, Lyckama à Nijeholt AA, et al: Sacral neuromodulation in the treatment of urgency-frequency symptoms: A multicenter study on efficacy and safety. J Urol 163(6):1849–1854, 2000.
30. Jonas U, Fowler CJ, Chancellor MB, et al: Efficacy of sacral nerve stimulation for urinary retention: Results 18 months after implantation. J Urol 165:15–19, 2001.
31. Bosch JL, Groen J: Sacral nerve neuromodulation in the treatment of patients with refractory motor urge incontinence: Long-term results of a prospective longitudinal study. J Urol 163(4):1219–1222, 2000.

CHAPTER 47

Management of Neurogenic Voiding Dysfunction

KEVIN V. CARLSON ■ VICTOR W. NITTI

DETRUSOR OVERACTIVITY

Detrusor hyper-reflexia and impaired compliance presents clinically in several ways, depending on the resistance of the bladder outlet and the presence of detrusor–external sphincter–dyssynergia (DESD). Depending on the degree of neurological impairment, patients may present with urinary frequency and urgency as well as various degrees of incontinence. When outlet resistance is high, such as in DESD, there may also be impaired emptying. The goals of management of detrusor overactivity are to protect the upper tracts and relieve or reduce symptoms. This is accomplished by lowering storage pressures either by improving compliance, reducing or abolishing involuntary contraction, or increasing the volume at which they occur. This may be achieved by a variety of methods including oral pharmacotherapy, intravesical agents, augmentation cystoplasty, sacral rhizotomy, and perhaps neuromodulation.

Oral Pharmacotherapy

Anticholinergic (antimuscarinic) agents have been the mainstay of treatment for neurogenic detrusor overactivity for years. In 1996 the Agency for Health Care Policy and Research (AHCPR) recommended that anticholinergics be the first-line treatment for detrusor overactivity.[1] Anticholinergic agents act primarily by blocking postganglionic muscarinic receptors in bladder smooth muscle. They have been shown to suppress both normal and involuntary bladder contractions and to increase bladder capacity.[2] Several subpopulations of muscarinic receptors have been identified (M_1 M_5). It appears, at least from animal studies, that M_3 and M_2 receptors predominate in the bladder[3]; however, currently pharmacotherapy is not subtype specific, leading to the variety of unwanted side effects related to blockade of muscarinic receptors in the salivary glands and ciliary muscle, as well as the gastrointestinal, cardiovascular and central nervous systems. These include dry mouth, impaired visual accommodation, constipation, tachycardia, and drowsiness. Treatment with oral anticholinergics is therefore unfortunately often limited by these dose-related side effects, particularly dry mouth, which often leads to discontinuation or suboptimal dosing of medication.

Oxybutynin chloride has been the most widely used anticholinergic agent for the treatment of detrusor overactivity. In addition to its antimuscarinic effect, it causes direct smooth muscle relaxation and has a local anesthetic effect.[4] It has been reported to produce good or excellent results in 61% to 86% of patients with detrusor instability or hyper-reflexia.[5] Propantheline bromide is another anticholinergic agent with variable efficacy reported in the literature, but it is no longer widely used. Both of these agents are limited by side effects, particularly dry mouth. A once-daily formulation of oxybutynin chloride (Ditropan XL) has been shown in two large trials to have similar efficacy to conventional oxybutynin for the treatment of urinary urge incontinence, with a lower rate of anticholinergic side effects[6,7]: This is thought to be due to more consistent serum levels, avoiding peaks thought to be responsible for side effects. Tolterodine (Detrol) is a potent muscarinic antagonist that has no muscarinic subtype selectivity, but has been shown to have some selectivity for bladder over salivary glands in an animal model.[8] Clinical studies have shown its efficacy to equal oxybutynin's with reduced dry mouth at a dose of 2 mg BID in patients with non-neurogenic bladder overactivity.[9,10] A study using tolterodine in patients with neurogenic detrusor overactivity showed a dose-dependent benefit on two critical urodynamic parameters, volume at first detrusor contraction and maximum cystometric capacity, using doses from 0.5 mg BID to 4 mg BID.[11] Tolterodine is now available in a time-release once daily formulation (Detrol LA), which, in the non-neurogenic population, is comparable in efficacy to once daily oxybutynin.[12] The latest developments in antimuscarinic drugs have focused on M_3 subtype-specific blockade. Several compounds have been developed and are under investigation, with darifenacin[13,14] and solifenacin[15] appearing the most promising. It remains to be seen if these subtype-specific agents will offer improved efficacy or reduced side effects.

Alpha-adrenergic receptor antagonists have also been used to treat patients with neurogenic voiding dysfunction. Theoretically, these agents offer three potentially beneficial effects in the management of the neurogenic lower urinary tract: (1) facilitation of storage by reducing hyper-reflexic contractions and improving compliance and capacity, (2) facilitation of emptying by reducing detrusor–internal (and perhaps external) sphincter–dyssynergia, and (3) amelioration of symptoms of autonomic dysreflexia.[16] In vitro and animal studies have suggested that in the decentralized bladder, there may be a change in receptor distribution such that alpha-1 receptors play a more prominent role and may facilitate loss of compliance and hyperreflexia.[17] It has subsequently been shown in human clinical trials that the alpha blockers phentolamine, prazosin, and phenoxybenzamine can reduce autonomous detrusor contractions, lower filling pressure, and improve capacity.[16,18] Alpha blockers have not gained widespread use in the treatment of neurogenic detrusor overactivity to date, but they may have a future therapeutic role, perhaps in combination with anticholinergic agents.

Intravesical Therapy

In the past, treatment options for patients failing oral pharmacotherapy were limited to bladder augmentation or urinary diversion. Recently, however, several new approaches to this challenging problem have been described. Intravesical pharmacotherapy, particularly for patients already performing self-catheterization, has gained popularity as a second-line treatment for patients refractory to or unable to tolerate side effects of oral agents. Oxybutynin chloride was the first agent to be widely used. Intravesical instillation of oxybutynin chloride has been used extensively in children, who have difficulty tolerating oral agents. Recent studies with long-term follow-up have shown reduction of storage pressures and improved continence,[19] with few systemic side effects (due to reduced first-pass metabolism to metabolites that are active in the salivary glands).[20] Studies in adults with detrusor hyper-reflexia refractory to oral anticholinergics have shown that intravesical oxybutynin is effective in reducing involuntary contractions, lowering storage pressures, improving capacity, and reducing or eliminating incontinence.[21,22] The use of electromotive drug administration may improve the durability of response, but this requires further investigation.[23] A recent small, uncontrolled study using modified intravesical oxybutynin (with hydropropylcellulose) suggests that this preparation may reduce absorption of oxybutynin from the bladder mucosa (and retain it longer in the bladder), thus reducing systemic side effects and increasing efficacy.[24] By eliminating the need for oral drugs and external collection devices, this therapy has improved quality of life and enhanced sexuality in these patients.[25]

An exciting new approach to the patient with refractory detrusor hyper-reflexia is the intravesical instillation of vanilloid compounds, such as capsaicin or resiniferatoxin (RTX). Capsaicin is the active ingredient in red-hot chili peppers, while RTX is isolated from the cactuslike plant Euphorbia Resinifera, and is 1000 times more potent than capsaicin. Intravesically, these compounds bind the vanilloid receptor subtype 1 on the bladder mucosa, which excites unmyelinated C afferent fibers. The C fibers are responsible for the detection of noxious signals and trigger painful sensations and normally have no role in triggering the micturition reflex, which is mediated by myelinated A delta fibers. However, following spinal cord injury, there is reorganization of micturition neural pathways, and C fibers assume the role of afferent signaling.[26] Ablation of this afferent stimulation therefore holds potential for suppressing hyper-reflexic contractions. Besides these afferent effects, vanilloids have an efferent action by causing release of neuropeptides locally, which induces inflammation.[27] Furthermore, they have neuromodulatory activity through inhibition of nuclear factor kappa B–mediated responses.[28] Much of the early work on vanilloids involved capsaicin, which is diluted in ethanol and saline and instilled into the bladder. There is an initial excitatory phase, whereby vanilloid receptors signal a painful stimulus.[29] This excitation is short-lived, however, and soon the neurons become insensitive to further drug application. This secondary neurotoxic effect is reversible, but it may last for several months.[30] Capsaicin does cause a painful burning sensation and may cause hemorrhagic cystitis immediately after instillation. Most patients are treated under local anesthesia with a dose of 50 mL to 100 mL of 1 to 2 mM capsaicin dissolved in 30% ethanol in saline.[29] A dwell time of 30 minutes is generally used, and the bladder neck is occluded with a catheter balloon to avoid skin irritation. Patients typically experience short-lived pain and irritative symptoms, followed by improvement in continence and capacity. Chancellor and de Groat have summarized the clinical experience with capsaicin in treating neurogenic bladder.[29] A double-blind, placebo-controlled trial in 20 patients with neurogenic bladder confirmed the efficacy and safety of capsaicin.[31] Besides being more potent than capsaicin, RTX has fewer initial side effects. It seems to desensitize nerve endings without the initial excitation, which accounts for its lack of initial side effects.[29] The initial clinical trials on RTX have shown it to be effective in treating hyper-reflexia, including that of patients who were initially refractory to capsaicin instillations.[32] Rivas and colleagues reported a multicenter, double-blind, placebo-controlled study using multiple single doses of RTX (0.005 μmolar − 1 μmolar) in 36 patients with refractory detrusor hyper-reflexia.[33] They noted significant improvements in mean cystometric capacity and incontinence episodes, which appears to be dose-dependent. The ideal dosing of RTX, however, has not yet been established. Recently, the first randomized, double-blind, controlled study comparing capsaicin and RTX was published.[34] These authors believe that the poor tolerability of capsaicin is at least partly due to the solvent effect of the 30% alcohol solution required to dilute the drug. They dissolved synthetic capsaicin in a glucidic solution and compared its effect to that of RTX in 10% ethanol. Thirty-nine spinal cord injury patients with hyper-reflexia were evaluated. At 30 days, clinical and urodynamic improvement was observed in 78% and 83% respectively of the capsaicin group versus 80% and 60% of the RTX group. These improvements persisted in two-thirds of patients at 3 months. While suprapubic pain was more common and prolonged following capsaicin administration, it was never severe enough to require symptomatic management. It is our opinion that these agents have a promising future in the treatment of refractory detrusor hyper-reflexia when issues of drug stability, dosing, and administration can be refined.

Miscellaneous Conservative Therapy

Botulinum A toxin directly blocks postsynaptic acetylcholine receptors and is used to treat a variety of spastic conditions and movement disorders. Having had success in using botulinum injections for the treatment of detrusor–external sphincter dyssynergia, Schurch and colleagues have now injected it directly into the bladders of patients with hyper-reflexia.[35] These authors improved urodynamic parameters of the entire group and cured neurogenic incontinence in 19 of 21 patients, durable up to 36 weeks. Intrathecal clonidine[36] and acupuncture[37] have also been evaluated for use in detrusor hyper-reflexia, and further trials are awaited.

Surgery for Overactive Detrusor

When pharmacologic or minimally invasive therapies fail to correct detrusor hyper-reflexia or impaired compliance, surgical approaches should be considered in order to establish a low-pressure storage vesical of adequate capacity and complete evacuation of urine. There are four basic surgical options for this difficult problem, each of which will be considered separately:

1. Augmentation cystoplasty with or without self-catheterization via the urethra, or continent catheterizable stoma
2. Autoaugmentation (detrusor myectomy)
3. Urinary diversion (continent or incontinent)
4. Sacral rhizotomy with implantation of anterior sacral root stimulator or neural reconstruction

Mickulicz first performed augmentation cystoplasty on humans in 1898.[38] It remains the most successful means of creating a low-pressure, high-capacity reservoir. Augmentation can be performed using a variety of intestinal segments including stomach, ileum, cecum, and sigmoid colon.[39] Regardless of the segment selected, it must be detubularized and reconfigured into a spherical shape to maximize volume, minimize bowel contractions, and achieve optimal compliance. The bladder is either resected, sparing the trigone, or more commonly, widely opened. Continence can be expected in 78% to 95% of patients,[40–42] and overall 75% of patients can expect an excellent result, with another 20% being improved.[43] Complications of bladder augmentation include failure to adequately lower storage pressures, incontinence secondary to bowel contractions, metabolic abnormalities (depending on the bowel segment used), wound infection or pyelonephritis, spontaneous perforation, mucus production, calculi, tumor formation, and bowel obstruction or dysfunction.[42,44]

Alternatives to enterocystoplasy include ureterocystoplasy, autoaugmentation, and seromuscular enterocystoplasty.[42] Ureterocystoplasty provides a highly compliant and locally available augment when associated vesicoureteral reflux has resulted in massive hydronephrosis and a nonfunctioning kidney. Autoaugmentation (detrusor myectomy) involves extraperitoneal excision of a segment of detrusor muscle, leaving the underlying mucosa intact. This procedure avoids the complications associated with enterocystoplasty and is an alternative for the select few patients with impaired compliance but adequate capacity. From the recent literature, it appears that autoaugmentation is more successful in patients with idiopathic overactivity than those with neuropathic hyper-reflexia, although success rates as high as 80% have been reported for this latter group.[45] Seromuscular enterocystoplasty combines autoaugmentation with enterocystoplasty by laying a demucosalized detubularized segment of bowel over the exposed bladder mucosa following detrusor myectomy.[46] This theoretically prevents the complications associated with exposure of urine to gastrointestinal mucosa, and may prevent the loss in capacity seen over time with simple autoaugmentation. Although recent literature cites encouraging results,[40] this technique remains limited to a few centers, and long-term follow-up on significant numbers of patients is still pending.

Careful consideration of the bladder outlet and functional status of the patient must be undertaken in planning an augmentation cystoplasty.[47] Patients who are able to empty their bladder preoperatively must be instructed that they may require intermittent catheterization postoperatively because the augmented bladder may not contract with as much force as the native bladder. Patients with DESD, regardless of preoperative emptying status, should be advised to expect bladder emptying via catheterization after bladder augmentation. Patients who are unwilling or mentally or physically unable to perform self-catheterization should not be considered good candidates for augmentation cystoplasty. If patients are unable to catheterize the urethra, but are able to catheterize via an abdominal stoma (e.g., female paraplegics), then consideration should be given to creation of a continent catheterizable abdominal stoma. We prefer to tunnel the appendix into the bladder (Mitrofanoff procedure) whenever it is available. In cases where the appendix is unavailable or too short, one or two transverse tubularized ileal segments can be used (Monti procedure).[48] This technique is gaining acceptance, and early results are encouraging.[49,50] Other authors have had success with continent ileocecal augmentation cystoplasty.[51] When the outlet is incompetent, a simultaneous bladder neck sling procedure may be performed at the time of augmentation. For patients with neurologic disability, this will most likely require permanent intermittent catheterization postoperatively. When there is complete urethral destruction (e.g., following chronic indwelling catheterization in women), the bladder neck may be closed and a continent or incontinent limb brought up to the skin from the augmented bladder. Bladder neck closure can be achieved transvaginally in women, transperineally in men, or retropubically in either sex.

An alternative to bladder augmentation, especially in cases where the native bladder is thought to not be feasible for enlargement or when an incompetent bladder outlet cannot be closed, continent urinary diversion with or without cystectomy may be performed.[52]

In select cases of neurogenic voiding dysfunction, where catheterization is not possible, incontinent urinary diversion may offer the best solution. Stein and colleagues recently confirmed the long-term success of colonic conduit diversion in children and young adults with neurogenic bladder, with 91% of the renal units remaining stable or improving over 11.8 years follow-up.[47] Ileal and colonic conduits are disadvantaged because they require uretero-intestinal anastamoses, which can portend to complications including pyelonephritis, renal scarring, stone formation, fistula, abscess, urinoma, and uretero-intestinal stricture.[53] To avoid these problems, the ileocystoplasty (ileal "chimney") was developed and has become popular for patients who require incontinent diversion. Along with reduced morbidity, ileocystoplasty has the advantages of preserving native bladder and being reversible in the case of neural recovery; alternatively, it can be converted easily to a conventional ileal conduit if necessary. Several small studies indicate that this operation provides low-pressure urinary drainage with acceptable complication rates.[54–56]

An entirely different surgical approach to the patient with neurogenic voiding dysfunction is to manipulate the nervous system so as to suppress the micturition reflex, and then activate it "voluntarily." This may be accomplished by severing the peripheral afferent nerves (posterior rhizotomy) from the bladder as they enter the spinal cord, then providing some means of voluntary stimulation of the motor efferents. This technique of deafferentiation and neurostimulation was developed by Brindley, beginning in 1969.[57] Typically, an L4–L5 laminectomy is performed, the dura is opened, and the anterior and posterior sacral roots are identified and isolated using in situ stimulation.[58] The posterior roots of S2, S3, and S4 are then transsected, and a segment of the roots is removed. The anterior roots are then placed in an electrode "book," and the electrodes are connected to a Brindley stimulator. The stimulator is driven by electromagnetic induction and delivers intermittent bursts of stimulation to the anterior roots, timed in such a way as to offset the peaks of detrusor contraction and sphincter contraction, allowing the patient to void. The device can also facilitate defecation and erection. Egon and colleagues reported a large series of patients with neurogenic bladder treated with posterior sacral rhizotomy and implantation of Brindley-Finetech sacral anterior root stimulators.[59] Of 90 evaluable patients, 83 voided using their implants, and 82 were continent. Bladder capacity was significantly increased, and vesicoureteral reflux disappeared. Reoperation was required in 3 patients with cerebrospinal fluid (CSF) leaks, and another two devices were explanted due to infection.

Neuromodulation

Neuromodulation is an accepted treatment for symptoms of frequency, urgency, and urge incontinence secondary to detrusor instability, idiopathic urinary retention, and pelvic pain.[60–63] There is less clinical experience with neurogenic voiding dysfunction and detrusor hyper-reflexia. Neuromodulation involves chronic stimulation of the sacral nerve roots, which supply the bladder and pelvic floor. Simply put, it entails the placement of a wire electrode into the sacral foramen (usually S3), through which a current is either continuously or intermittently applied.[60] Patients are first evaluated for suitability of the procedure with an external wire placed as an outpatient (peripheral nerve evaluation), and those who respond favorably have a permanent electrode and subcutaneous stimulator implanted. The stimulator can be activated and adjusted via an external magnet placed over the device. The exact mechanism of action of neuromodulation is not fully understood. Neuromodulation likely restores the balance between inhibitory and excitatory impulses to and from the pelvis through a combination of mechanisms. These include stimulation of inhibitory pudendal somatic afferent interneurons in the sacral spinal cord, stimulation of inhibitory hypogastric sympathetic nerves in the pelvic ganglia, induction of muscular hypertrophy of the pelvic floor, and reflex recruitment of central inhibitory pathways.[60]

To date neuromodulation has been used primarily to treat non-neurogenic bladder overactivity and voiding dysfunction with favorable results. Its role in select cases of neurogenic voiding dysfunction has not yet been clearly defined. In an experimental model, Zvara and colleagues recently demonstrated that chronic electrostimulation of the S3 nerve root in spinal transsected rats reduced bladder hyper-reflexia.[64] In humans, Spinelli and colleagues showed significant improvement in incontinence episodes in 50% of patients with hyper-reflexia at 12 months follow-up.[65] Hohenfellner and colleagues, while observing 50% improvement in symptoms in 8 of 12 patients with chronic implants, noted that these results did not persist with longer follow-up.[66]

DETRUSOR–EXTERNAL SPHINCTER–DYSSYNERGIA

Detrusor–external sphincter–dyssynergia (DESD) causes a functional obstruction of the bladder outlet, and therefore has the potential to cause incomplete emptying, recurrent urinary tract infections, bladder calculi, and incontinence. It occurs in conjunction with detrusor hyper-reflexia and often results in high-pressure detrusor contractions and incomplete bladder emptying. Furthermore, storage pressures may be elevated, as bladder compliance worsens over time secondary to the obstruction. The combination of high storage and voiding pressures puts the upper tracts at risk of decompensation. It is critical, therefore, to relieve this functional obstruction when detrusor pressures are elevated to the point of putting the upper tracts at risk or when incomplete emptying leads to bothersome sequela. There are six basic approaches to managing DESD:

- Intermittent catheterization usually combined with medical or surgical therapy to control detrusor overactivity
- Indwelling catheterization
- Medical therapy
- Sphincterotomy
- Stent placement across the sphincter
- Urinary diversion

Before World War II, patients who sustained spinal cord injuries (SCI) faced an 80% early mortality rate. Most of these deaths were secondary to urological complications, particularly urosepsis.[67] The introduction of indwelling catheter drainage improved survival in this group and shifted the major cause of death to renal failure. Lapides then showed that clean intermittent catheterization (CIC) could safely manage the lower urinary tract in these patients and dramatically reduce the urologic complications following SCI.[68] Unfortunately, many patients with neurologic disease lack the manual dexterity or support required to perform CIC. In such cases, indwelling catheterization is an option; however, this subjects patients to the risks of urethral erosion (avoided with suprapubic catheters), calculus formation, infection, and malignancy.[69] In a heterogeneous group of patients with neurogenic voiding dysfunction, Weld and Dmochowski showed intermittent catheterization to be the safest bladder management method in spinal cord injury patients in terms of urologic complications.[70]

Although no definitive medical treatment is available for DESD, variable success has been observed with the use of alpha-adrenergic antagonists.[16] Not only can these agents improve DESD, but they may also improve emptying by relaxing the bladder neck and by improving contractility. Yasuda and colleagues evaluated the alpha-blocker urapidil on 136 patients with neurogenic voiding dysfunction.[18] Eight of 28 patients in the treatment group with DESD were improved, compared to 1 of 16 in the placebo arm. Flow rates and residual volumes for the entire treatment group were also modestly improved versus the placebo group. In another study, Al-Ali and colleagues treated 46 SCI patients with phenoxybenzamine, noting improvement in bladder emptying in 41%, with urethral closure pressures dropping by a mean of 22 cm H_2O (10–32 cm H_2O).[71] Most failures were limited to those with areflexic bladders. Abrams and colleagues completed a large, randomized, placebo-controlled trial of the selective alpha blocker tamsulosin for SCI in Europe.[72] They enrolled 263 patients, of which 244 were evaluated at 4 weeks. Another 186 continued on in an open label study, of which 134 were evaluated at 1 year. In the 4-week RCT, there was a greater drop in the maximum urethral pressure (MUP) in the tamsulosin groups (−12.2 cm H_2O with 0.4 mg and −9.6 cm H_2O with 0.8 mg) than in the placebo groups (−6.5 cm H_2O), albeit not statistically significant. In the 1-year open label study, the MUP was reduced by 18.0 cm H_2O from baseline (p < 0.001). Furthermore, other urodynamic parameters of bladder storage and emptying, as well as quality of life scores and symptoms of autonomic dysreflexia were all improved. This study supports the use of alpha blocker therapy in this population of patients.

Other oral agents used to treat DESD in the past include muscle relaxants such as diazepam, dantrolene, and baclofen.[73] These drugs not only proved ineffective, but also are associated with significant side effects. Continuous infusion intrathecal baclofen has been used successfully to treat spasticity in a variety of neurologic disorders, and it has yielded some success (40% in one study) in managing DESD.[74] Several studies have highlighted the use of transperineal[75] and transurethral[76] botulinum toxin injections to treat sphincter–dyssynergia. Although injections have to be repeated every 2 to 3 months, this treatment appears to offer an effective alternative for refractory cases of DESD in patients unwilling to accept more invasive measures.

Surgical sphincterotomy, using electocautery at the 12 o'clock position, remains the gold standard for treating male patients with DESD who cannot perform CIC (e.g., some quadraplegics). Sphincterotomy is not a good option for women because of the lack of an effective external collection device. It may be performed by standard electrosurgical technique or with a laser to minimize bleeding.[77] Following sphincterotomy, patients typically require an external collection device for continence. Complications of sphincterotomy include hemorrhage (5% to 20%), erectile dysfunction (5%), and urinary extravasation. Early failures may result from inadequate incision or unrecognized bladder neck obstruction or impaired detrusor contractility. Late failures may result from fibrosis, prostatic obstruction, or a change in detrusor or sphincter function. Thus long-term urodynamic follow-up is necessary.[78] These patients may also be subjected to the complications of condom catheter drainage itself, ranging from skin excoriation to urethrocutaneous fistula and penile gangrene.

To circumvent these problems, a variety of minimally invasive procedures for the treatment of DESD have been reported, the most popular being intraluminal stenting with the UroLume endoprosthesis (American Medical Systems, Minneapolis, MN). One to three wire mesh stents are placed endoscopically across the external sphincter with a special insertion device. In 1999, long-term follow-up of the North American Multicenter UroLume Trial, which began in 1990, was reported.[79] This study enrolled 160 spinal cord injured men and followed them prospectively, with follow-up to 5 years in 41 patients. The UroLume was effective in reducing voiding pressures and residual volumes while maintaining cystometric capacity, and these results were maintained over 5 years. Eighty-five percent of patients previously requiring indwelling catheter drainage were rendered catheter-free. Overall, an 84% subjective improvement rate was noted. Surgical complications were minimal, and no adverse effects on sexual function were reported; however, 19.6% of patients required stent explantation over the study period for a variety of reasons, mainly migration.[80] Stent removal is easily performed endoscopically and does not preclude reimplantation. The first study comparing the UroLume stent with conventional sphincterotomy was also reported in 1999.[81] Both subjective and objective outcome measures were equal among the two treatment groups at 2 years follow-up. Length of hospital stay was longer overall in the sphincterotomy group; however, 22% of patients in the stent group required more than one insertion procedure, and another 19% required explantation. The UroLume stent thus appears to offer an effective and minimally invasive alternative to formal sphincterotomy, and it has the added advantage of reversibility. Patients must be aware, however, that multiple procedures, including explantation, may be required.

DETRUSOR AREFLEXIA

The areflexic lower motor neuron bladder remains a significant challenge to the urologist, and few advances have been made in treating this condition over the past decade or more. These patients typically present with symptoms of incomplete emptying or sequela of residual urine, including recurrent urinary tract infections (UTIs), bladder calculi, and overflow incontinence. The goal of management is to improve evacuation of urine, and this is best accomplished by intermittent catheterization; when this fails, indwelling catheterization or urinary diversion is required. Like others, we have had no success in using cholinomimetic agents, such as bethanacol, to improve bladder contractility.

A remote-controlled intraurethral valve pump (American Medical Systems, Minneapolis, MN) was developed for use in women to assist in bladder emptying, and this device has now been tested in clinical practice.[82] Two series reported the early results using this device on a total of 110 patients, 40 of whom had neurogenic hyporeflexia.[83,84] Of the 110 patients, only 53 (47%) continued to use the implant at less than 2 years follow-up. Many devices required removal secondary to local irritation or significant incontinence around the catheter. Bacteriuria developed in 34 (31%), and 20 (18%) had symptomatic UTIs. The long-term consequences to the urethra of leaving such an implant in place is unknown, but presumably urethral erosion would be a risk, as it is with indwelling catheters. Plans for development of this device are not known.

Neuromodulation has been used in a limited number of cases of neurogenic detrusor areflexia. In the studies by Spinelli and colleagues[65] and Hohenfeller and colleagues,[66] promising results were achieved in the subset of patients with areflexia; however, as noted above, the latter study indicates poor durability of results. This application of neuromodulation requires further review.

Bladder myoplasty represents another novel approach to the treatment of detrusor areflexia and is being investigated at several centers. Based on successes with animal models, Stenzl and colleagues wrapped a free flap of latissimus dorsi muscle around the bladders of three patients and were able to restore voiding.[85] This technique obviously remains investigational, and further research is necessary to determine its role in the management of detrusor areflexia.

REFERENCES

1. Urinary Incontinence in Adults Guideline Update Panel: Urinary Incontinence in Adults: Acute and Chronic Management. Clinical Practice Guideline, #2, 1996 Update. Rockville, MD, Agency for Health Care Policy and Research, Public Health Service, U.S. Department of Health and Human Services, 1996. AHCPR Publication No. 96-0682.
2. Andersson KE: Current concepts in the treatment of disorders of micturition. Drugs 35:477–494, 1988.
3. Eglen RM, Hedge SS, Watson N: Muscarinic receptor subtypes and smooth muscle function. Pharmacol Rev 48:531–565, 1996.
4. Wein AJ: Pharmacologic options for the overactive bladder. Urology 51 (2A suppl):43–47, 1998.
5. Thuroff JW, Bunke B, Ebner A, et al: Randomized, double-blind, multicenter trial on treatment of frequency, urgency and incontinence related to detrusor hyperactivity: Oxybutynin versus propantheline versus placebo. J Urol 145:813–816, 1991.
6. Anderson RU, Mobley D, Blank B, et al: Once-daily controlled versus immediate-release oxybutynin chloride for urge urinary incontinence. OROS Oxybutynin Study Group. J Urol 161:1809–1812, 1999.
7. Gleason DM, Susset J, White C, et al: Evaluation of a new once-daily formulation of oxybutynin for the treatment of urinary urge incontinence. Ditropan XL Study Group. Urology 54:420–423, 1999.
8. Nilverbrant L, Hallen B, Larsson G: Tolterodine: A new bladder selective, muscarinic receptor antagonist: Preclinical pharmacological and clinical data. Life Sci 60:1129–1136, 1997.
9. Appell RA: Clinical efficacy and safety of tolterodine in the treatment of overactive bladder: A pooled analysis. Urology 50 (suppl 6A):90–96, 1997.
10. Ruscin JM, Morgenstern NE: Tolterodine use for symptoms of overactive bladder. Ann Pharmacother 33:1073–1082, 1999.
11. Van Kerrebroeck PEVA, Amarenco G, Thuroff JW, et al: Dose-ranging study of tolterodine in patients with detrusor hyperreflexia. Neurourol Urodynam 17:499–512, 1998.
12. Diokno AC, Appell RA, Sand PK, et al: Prospective, randomized, double-blind study of the efficacy and tolerability of the extended-release formulations of oxybutynin and tolterodine for overactive bladder: Results of the OPERA trial. Mayo Clin Proc 78(6):687–695, 2003.
13. Alabaster VA: Discovery and development of selective M_3 antagonists for clinical use. Life Sci 60:1053–1060, 1997.
14. Newgreen DT, Anderson CWP, Cartet AJ, et al: Darifenicin—a novel bladder-selective agent for the treatment of urge incontinence. Neurourol Urodyn 14:95–96, 1995.
15. Chapple CR, Arano P, Bosch JL, et al: Solifenacin appears effective and well tolerated in patients with symptomatic idiopathic detrusor overactivity in a placebo- and tolterodine-controlled phase 2 dose-finding study. BJU Int 93(1):71–77, 2004.

16. Sullivan J, Abrams P: Alpha-adrenoceptor antagonists in neurogenic lower urinary tract dysfunction. Urology 53 (suppl 3A):21–28, 1999.
17. Skehan AM, Downie JW, Awad SA: Control of detrusor stiffness in the chronic decentralized feline bladder. J Urol 149:1165–1173, 1993.
18. Yasuda K, Yamanishi T, Kawabe K, et al: The effect of urapidil on neurogenic bladder: A placebo-controlled double-blind study. J Urol 156:1125–1130, 1996.
19. Amark P, Bussman G, Eksborg S: Follow-up of long-time treatment with intravesical oxybutynin for neurogenic bladder in children. Eur Urol 34:148–153, 1998.
20. Buyse G, Waldeck K, Verpoorten C, et al: Intravesical oxybutynin for neurogenic bladder dysfunction: Less systemic side effects due to reduced first-pass metabolism. J Urol 160:892–896, 1998.
21. Pannek J, Sommerfeld HJ, Botel U, et al: Combined intravesical and oral oxybutynin chloride in adult patients with spinal cord injury. J Urol 55:358–362, 2000.
22. Szollar SM, Lee SM: Intravesical oxybutynin for spinal cord injury patients. Spinal Cord 34:284–287, 1996.
23. Riedl CR, Knoll M, Plas E, et al: Intravesical electromotive drug administration technique: Preliminary results and side effects. J Urol 159:1851–1856, 1998.
24. Saito M, Tabuchi F, Otsubo K, Miyagawa I: Treatment of overactive bladder with modified intravesical oxybutynin. Neurourol Urodynam 19:683–688, 2000.
25. Vaidyananthan S, Soni BM, Brown E, et al: Effect of intermittent urethral catheterization and oxybutynin bladder instillation on urinary continence status and quality of life in a selected group of spinal cord injury patients with neuropathic bladder dysfunction. Spinal Cord 36:409–414, 1998.
26. de Groat WC, Kawatani M, Hisamitsu T, et al: Mechanisms underlying the recovery of urinary bladder function following spinal cord injury. J Auto Nerv Syst 30 (suppl):S71–S77, 1990.
27. Buck SH, Burks TF: The neuropharmacology of capsaicin: Review of some recent observations. Pharmacol Rev 38:179–226, 1986.
28. Singh A, Nataraja K, Aggarwal BB: Capsaicin (8-methyl-N-vanillyl-6-nonenamide) is a potent inhibitor of nuclear transcription factor-kappa B activation by diverse agents. J Immunol 157:4412–4420, 1996.
29. Chancellor MB, de Groat WC: Intravesical capsaicin and resiniferatoxin therapy: Spicing up the ways to treat the overactive bladder. J Urol 162:3–11, 1999.
30. Craft RM, Cohen SM, Porreca F: Long-lasting desensitization of bladder afferents following intravesical resiniferatoxin and capsaicin in the rat. Pain 61:317–323, 1995.
31. de Seze M, Wiart L, Joseph PA, et al: Capsaicin and neurogenic detrusor hyperreflexia: A double-blind placebo-controlled study in 20 patients with spinal cord lesions. Neurourol Urodynam 17:513–523, 1998.
32. Lazzeri M, Spinelli M, Beneforti P, et al: Intravesical resiniferatoxin for the treatment of detrusor hyperreflexia refractory to capsaicin in patients with chronic spinal cord diseases. Scand J Urol Nephrol 32:331–334, 1998.
33. Rivas DA, Shenot PJ, Vasavada SP, et al: Intravesical resiniferatoxin (RTX) improves bladder capacity and decreases incontinence in patients with refractory detrusor hyperreflexia (DH): A multicenter, blinded, randomized, placebo-controlled trial. J Urol 163 (4 suppl):244, 2000.
34. de Seze M, Wiart L, de Seze MP, et al: Intravesical capsaicin versus resiniferatoxin for the treatment of detrusor hyperreflexia in spinal cord injured patients: A double-blind, randomized, controlled study. J Urol 171(1):251–255, 2004.
35. Schurch B, Schmid DM, Stohrer M: Treatment of neurogenic incontinence with botulinum toxin A. N Engl J Med 342:556, 2000.
36. Denys P, Chartier-Kastler C, Azouvi P, et al: Intrathecal clonidine for refractory detrusor hyperreflexia in spinal cord injured patients: A preliminary report. J Urol 160:2137–2138, 1998.
37. Cheng PT, Wong MK, Chang PL: A therapeutic trial of acupuncture in neurogenic bladder of spinal cord injured patients—a preliminary report. Spinal Cord 36:476–480, 1998.
38. Orr LM, Thomley MW, Campbell MF: Ileocystoplasty for bladder enlargement. J Urol 79:250, 1958.
39. Rink RC, Adams MC: Augmentation cystoplasty. In Walsh PC, Retik AB, Vaughan ED, et al (eds): Campbell's Urology, 7th ed. Philadelphia, WB Saunders, 1998, pp 3167–3189.
40. Shekarriz B, Upadhyay J, Demirbilek S, et al: Surgical complications of bladder augmentation: Comparison between various enterocystoplasties in 133 patients. Urology 55:123–128, 2000.
41. Venn SN, Mundy AR: Long-term results of augmentation cystoplasty. Eur Urol 34 (suppl 1):40–42, 1998.
42. Rink RC: Bladder augmentation: Options, outcomes, future. Urol Clin North Am 26:111–123, 1999.
43. Flood HD, Malhotra SJ, O'Connell HE, et al: Long-term results and complications using augmentation cystoplasty in reconstructive urology. Neurourol Urodynam 14:297–309, 1995.
44. N'Dow J, Leung HY, Marshall C, et al: Bowel dysfunction after bladder reconstruction. J Urol 159:1470, 1998.
45. Swami KS, Feneley RCL, Hammonds JC, et al: Detrusor myectomy for detrusor overactivity: A minimum 1 year follow-up. Brit J Urol 81:68–72, 1998.
46. Buson H, Manivel JC, Dayanc M, et al: Seromuscular colocystoplasty lined with urothelium: Experimental study. Urology 44:743–748, 1994.
47. Stein R, Fisch M, Ermert A, et al: Urinary diversion and orthotopic bladder substitution in children and young adults with neurogenic bladder: A safe option for treatment? J Urol 163:568–573, 2000.
48. Gerharz EW, Woodhouse CR: The transverse ileal tube as second-line modification of the Mitrofanoff principle. World J Urol 16:231–234, 1998.
49. Sugarman ID, Malone PS, Terry TR, et al: Transversely tubularized ileal segments for the Mitrofanoff or Malone antegrade colonic enema procedures: The Monti principle. Brit J Urol 81:253–256, 1998.
50. Monti PR, DeCarvalho JR, Arap S: The Monti procedure: Applications and complications. Urology 55:616–621, 2000.
51. Sutton MA, Hinson JL, Nickell KG, et al: Continent ileocecal augmentation cystoplasty. Spinal Cord 36:246–251, 1998.
52. Plancke HR, Delaere KP, Pons C: Indiana pouch in female patients with spinal cord injury. Spinal Cord 37:208–210, 1999.
53. McDougall WS: Use of intestinal segments and urinary diversion. In Walsh PC, Retik AB, Vaughan ED, et al (eds): Campbell's Urology, 7th ed. Philadelphia, WB Saunders, 1998, pp 3121–3161.
54. Atan A, Konety BR, Nangia A, et al: Advantages and risks of ileovesicostomy for the management of neuropathic bladder. Urology 54:636–640, 1999.
55. Gudziak MR, Tiguert R, Puri K, et al: Management of neurogenic bladder dysfunction with incontinent ileovesicostomy. Urology 54:1008–1011, 1999.
56. Gauthier AR Jr., Winters JC: Incontinent ileovesicostomy in the management of neurogenic bladder dysfunction. Neurourol Urodyn 22(2):142–146, 2003.

57. Brindley GS, Polkey CE, Rushton DN: Sacral anterior root stimulators for bladder control in paraplegia. Paraplegia 20:365–381, 1982.
58. Van der Aa HE, Alleman E, Nene A, et al: Sacral anterior root stimulation for bladder control: Clinical results. Arch Physiol Biochem 107:248–256, 1999.
59. Egon G, Barat M, Colombel P, et al: Implantation of anterior sacral root stimulators combined with posterior sacral rhizotomy in spinal injury patients. World J Urol 16:342–349, 1998.
60. Bemelmans BLH, Mundy AR, Craggs MD: Neuromodulation by implant for treating lower urinary tract symptoms and dysfunction. Eur Urol 36:81–91, 1999.
61. Schmidt RA, Jonas U, Oleson KA, et al: Sacral nerve stimulation for treatment of refractory urinary urge incontinence. J Urol 162:352–357, 1999.
62. Weil EHJ, Ruiz-Cerda JL, Eerdmans PHA, et al: Sacral root neuromodulation in the treatment of refractory urinary urge incontinence: A prospective randomized clinical trial. Eur Urol 37:161–171, 2000.
63. Bosch JLHR, Groen J: Sacral nerve neuromodulation in the treatment of patients with refractory motor urge incontinence: Long-term results of a prospective longitudinal study. J Urol 163:1219–1222, 2000.
64. Zvara P, Sahi S, and Hassouna MM: An animal model for the neuromodulation of neurogenic bladder dysfunction. Br J Urol 82(2):267–271, 1998.
65. Spinelli M, Bertapelle P, Cappellano F, et al: Chronic sacral neuromodulation in patients with lower urinary tract symptoms: Results from a national register. J Urol 166(2):541–545, 2001.
66. Hohenfellner M, Humke J, Hampel C, et al: Chronic sacral neuromodulation for treatment of neurogenic bladder dysfunction: Long-term results with unilateral implants. Urology 58(6):887–892, 2001.
67. McGuire EJ, Savastano JA: Urodynamic findings and long-term outcome management of patients with multiple sclerosis-induced lower urinary tract dysfunction. J Urol 132:713–715, 1984.
68. Lapides J, Diokno AC, Silber SJ, et al: Clean, intermittent self-catheterization in the treatment of urinary tract disease. Trans Am Assoc Genitourin Surg 63:92–96, 1971.
69. Perkash I: Long-term urologic management of the patient with spinal cord injury. Urol Clin North Am 20:423–424, 1993.
70. Weld KJ, Dmochowski RR: Effect of bladder management on urological complications in spinal cord injured patients. J Urol 163:768–772, 2000.
71. Al-Ali M, Salman G, Rasheed A, et al: Phenoxybenzamine in the management of neuropathic bladder following spinal cord injury. Aust N Z J Surg 69:660–663, 1999.
72. Abrams P, Amarenco G, Bakke A, et al: Tamsulosin: Efficacy and safety in patients with neurogenic lower urinary tract dysfunction due to suprasacral spinal cord injury. J Urol 170 (4 Pt 1):1242–1251, 2003.
73. Wein AJ: Neuromuscular dysfunction of the lower urinary tract and its treatment. In Walsh PC, Retik AB, Vaughan ED, et al (eds): Campbell's Urology, 5th ed. Philadelphia, WB Saunders, 1998, pp 953–1006.
74. Steers WD, Meythaler JM, Haworth C, et al: Effects of acute bolus and chronic continuous intrathecal baclofen on genitourinary dysfunction due to spinal cord pathology. J Urol 148:1849–1855, 1992.
75. Gallien P, Robineau S, Verin M, et al: Treatment of detrusor sphincter dyssynergia by transperineal injection of botulinum toxin. Arch Phys Med Rehabil 79:715–717, 1998.
76. Petit H, Wiart L, Gaujard E, et al: Botulinum A toxin treatment for detrusor-sphincter dyssynergia in spinal cord disease. Spinal Cord 36:91–94, 1998.
77. Rivas DA, Chancellor MB, Staas WE, et al: Contact neodynium:yttrium-aluminum-garnet laser ablation of the external sphincter in spinal cord injured men with detrusor-sphincter dyssynergia. Urology 45:1028–1031, 1995.
78. Kim YH, Kattan MW, Boone TB: Bladder leak-point pressure: The measure for sphincterotomy success in spinal cord injured patients with external detrusor-sphincter dyssynergia. J Urol 159:493–497, 1998.
79. Chancellor MB, Gajewski J, Ackman CFD, et al: Long-term followup of the North American Multicenter UroLume Trial for the treatment of external detrusor-sphincter dyssynergia. J Urol 161:1545–1550, 1999.
80. Gajewski JB, Chancellor MB, Ackman CF, et al: Removal of UroLume endoprosthesis: Experience of the North American Study Group for detrusor-sphincter dyssynergia application. J Urol 163:773–776, 2000.
81. Chancellor MB, Bennett C, Simoneau AR, et al: Sphincteric stent versus external sphincterotomy in spinal cord injured men: Prospective randomized multicenter trial. J Urol 161:1893–1898, 1999.
82. Nativ O, Moskowitz B, Issaq E, et al: New intraurethral sphincter prosthesis with a self-contained urinary pump. ASAIO J 43:197–203, 1997.
83. Madjar S, Sabo E, Halachmi S, et al: A remote-controlled intraurethral insert for artificial voiding: A new concept for treating women with voiding dysfunction. J Urol 161:895–898, 1999.
84. Schurch B, Suter S, Dubs M: Intraurethral sphincter prosthesis to treat hyporeflexic bladders in women: Does it work? BJU Int 84:789–794, 1999.
85. Stenzl A, Ninkovic M, Kolle D, et al: Restoration of voluntary emptying of the bladder by transplantation of innervated free skeletal muscle. Lancet 351:1483–1485, 1998.

INDEX

Note: Page numbers followed by f refer to figures; page numbers followed by t refer to tables; page numbers followed by b refer to boxes.

A

Absorbent products, in urinary incontinence, 58, 315–318, 315f–317f, 337, 345
Acetylcholine, in penile erection, 95
Acidosis, erectile dysfunction and, 104
Adrenocorticotropin, in penile erection, 97
Alcohol
　erectile dysfunction and, 127, 252–253, 253t
　urinary incontinence and, 272–273
Alfuzosin, in urinary incontinence, 376t
Alpha-adrenoceptor agonists, in stress urinary incontinence, 384–385, 385t
Alpha-adrenoceptor antagonists, in urinary incontinence, 376t, 382
Alprostadil
　in erectile dysfunction, 351, 352
　in female sexual dysfunction, 110
Anal canal, 14–16
　hypotonia of, 325–326
　pressure in, 15–16, 16f, 17, 17f. See also Anorectal manometry.
Anal fistula, 237
Anal incontinence. See Fecal incontinence.
Anal re-education, 323–324, 323f, 325–326
Anal reflex, 139, 239, 240f
Anal sphincter(s), 14–16
　electromyography of, 219, 220, 220f, 221f
　external, 15, 15f
　　in fecal incontinence, 75–76
　　manometric testing of, 238–239, 239f
　　re-education of, 324
　　transanal ultrasonography of, 235–237, 236f, 237f
　in patient evaluation, 139–140
　internal, 14, 15f
　　in fecal incontinence, 75–76
　　manometric testing of, 238–239, 239f
　　transanal ultrasonography of, 235–237, 236f
　trauma to, 78
　　during childbirth, 35–37, 36f
Androgens
　female sexual function and, 23–24, 99, 109
　male sexual function and, 97
Anejaculation, 89
Anesthesia, for childbirth, 38
Angiography, in erectile dysfunction, 262–263
Angiotensin II
　in female sexual function, 98
　in male sexual function, 95–96

Anismus, 79, 238, 240f
Anorectal manometry, 237–241
　in constipation, 240–241
　in fecal incontinence, 241
　indications for, 240–241
　instruments for, 237–238
　pressure units in, 238
　recordings of, 238–239, 239f, 241f
　rectal compliance on, 239–240, 241f
　rectoanal reflexes on, 239, 240f
Anorexia nervosa, rectal prolapse and, 86
Anorgasmia, 89, 109
Anoxia, erectile dysfunction and, 103–104
Anticonvulsants, erectile dysfunction and, 252–253, 253t
Antidepressants
　erectile dysfunction and, 127, 252–253, 253t
　female sexual dysfunction and, 109, 124
　in urinary incontinence, 376t, 383
Antihypertensive agents, erectile dysfunction and, 127, 252–253, 253t
Anti-incontinence devices, 337
Antimuscarinic (anticholinergic) drugs, in urinary incontinence, 376–379, 376t
Antipsychotic agents, erectile dysfunction and, 105, 127, 252–253, 253t
Anus. See also Anal canal; Anal sphincter(s).
　anatomy of, 235–236, 236f
　sensation in, fecal incontinence and, 75
　surgery on, anal sphincter defects with, 236–237
　trauma to, 78
　ultrasonography of, 235–236, 236f
Apomorphine
　in erectile dysfunction, 353
　in female sexual dysfunction, 356
Appendicovesicostomy, in pediatric urinary incontinence, 445, 445f
Arcus tendineus fascia pelvis, 5
L-Arginine, in female sexual dysfunction, 356
Arterial insufficiency, erectile dysfunction and, 100–102
Artificial urinary sphincter, 395–396, 396f, 396t, 408–413
　continence rate with, 412b
　erosion of, 412b
　in children, 443–444, 444f
　in male, 426–429, 426f–428f
　outcomes for, 411–412
　patient evaluation for, 408–409
　physical examination for, 408

463

results of, 411–412, 428–429
technique of, 409–411, 409f–411f, 412b
urodynamic studies for, 408
Atherosclerosis
erectile dysfunction and, 100–102
female sexual dysfunction and, 110, 123
Athletes, urinary incontinence in, 274–275
Atropine, in urinary incontinence, 376t, 377
Augmentation cystoplasty
in neurogenic voiding dysfunction, 456–457
in pediatric urinary incontinence, 433–435, 434f–436f
in severe detrusor overactivity, 424

B

Baclofen
in neurogenic voiding dysfunction, 458
in urinary incontinence, 376t, 384
Barbiturates, erectile dysfunction and, 252–253, 253t
Bartholin's glands, 92
Behavioral therapy. *See* Biofeedback; Bladder retraining; Pelvic floor exercises.
Benign prostatic hyperplasia, 49–53
alpha-1 receptor blockade in, 10
AUA Symptoms Index in, 51
clinical manifestations of, 50–51
diagnosis of, 51–53, 52f, 53f
differential diagnosis of, 51–52
mechanical obstruction in, 50, 205–206, 205f
neurogenic bladder and, 52–53
pathophysiology of, 49–50
physical findings in, 51
smooth muscle obstruction in, 50
urinary retention in, 51
urinary tract infection in, 51
urodynamic evaluation in, 52–53, 52f, 53f
Beta-adrenoceptor agonists, in urinary incontinence, 376t, 382–383
Biofeedback therapy
bladder control by, 297–308
clinical results of, 306–308
cystometric methods of, 298, 298f, 299f
equipment for, 300–301, 300f, 301f
methods of, 297–300, 298f, 299f
pelvic floor methods of, 298–300, 299f, 300f
position variation and, 305–306, 305f
stage 1 (awareness) of, 302
stage 2 (muscle strengthening) of, 302–304, 303f
stage 3 (reflex contraction) of, 304–305, 304f
stage 4 (skill performance), 305–306, 305f
technique of, 301–306, 303f–305f
video-assisted methods in, 305
in age-related urinary incontinence, 344
in anal canal re-education, 325–326
in pelvic floor re-education, 321–322, 321f, 332, 335f
Biothesiometry, in erectile dysfunction, 253, 257
Bladder. *See also* Detrusor.
acontractile, 421
adrenergic activity in, 9–10
afferent activity in, 8–9, 8f, 67
atropine resistance in, 375
C fibers of, 9
cancer of, 195
cholinergic activity in, 9
contraction of, 375–376, 375f
diverticulum of, 209, 210f
efferent activity in, 8f, 9–11, 67
electrical stimulation of, 281–288. *See also* Electrical stimulation.
emptying of, in patient evaluation, 135
endometriosis of, 195–196
endoscopy of, 192, 192f. *See also* Endoscopy.
extracorporeal electromagnetic stimulation therapy effects on, 295
extrinsic compression of, 193
hernia of. *See* Cystocele.
incomplete emptying of, in patient evaluation, 135
innervation of, 373–374, 374f
muscarinic receptors of, 375–376, 375f
neurogenic. *See* Neurogenic voiding dysfunction.
neuropeptides in, 10
overactive, 45, 45t, 46b, 47. *See also* Urinary incontinence.
pressure in, 9. *See also* Cystometry, filling.
sensory disorders of, 46b–47b, 47
underactive, 45, 45t, 46b, 47
urodynamic evaluation of, 209–210, 209f–211f. *See also* Urodynamic studies.
Bladder leak point pressure, 213–214, 213f, 214f
bladder volume in, 214
in neurogenic voiding dysfunction, 68, 69f
Bladder neck. *See also* Bladder outlet obstruction.
funneling of
cystography for, 153, 154f
ultrasonography for, 158, 159f
incompetence of
cystocele and, 156, 156f
radiologic evaluation for, 152–153, 153f, 154f
ultrasonography for, 158–159, 159f, 159t, 161
Bladder neck closure, in pediatric urinary incontinence, 444–446
Bladder neck sling suspension, in pediatric urinary incontinence, 440–443, 442f, 443f
Bladder neck tubularization, in pediatric urinary incontinence, 437–438, 437t, 438f
Bladder outlet obstruction, 49–55
benign prostatic hyperplasia and, 49–53, 205–206. *See also* Benign prostatic hyperplasia.
neurologic lesions and, 53, 62
overflow urinary incontinence and, 56
pressure-flow study in, 205–206, 205f
primary, 54
treatment of, 422–423
uroflowmetry in, 199, 199f
Bladder retraining, 311–312, 333, 344
results of, 336
Body mass index, urinary incontinence and, 270–271
Botulinum A toxin, in neurogenic voiding dysfunction, 456
Bradykinin, in penile erection, 96
Brain, in male sexual function, 26–27
Brief Male Sexual Function Inventory, 254
Brindley stimulator, in neurogenic voiding dysfunction, 457
Broad ligaments, 165

Bulbocavernosus reflex, 225–226
    in cauda equina lesions, 229–230
    in conus medullaris lesions, 229–230
    in erectile dysfunction, 231, 257
    in patient evaluation, 140
Bulbourethral glands, 92
Bulimia nervosa, rectal prolapse and, 86
Burch colposuspension, 392–393, 393t, 396–397, 397t, 398t

C

C fibers, of bladder, 9
Caffeine, in urinary incontinence, 272
Calcium antagonists, in urinary incontinence, 376t, 379
Cancer, bladder, 195
Capsaicin
    in neurogenic voiding dysfunction, 455–456
    in urinary incontinence, 376t, 384
Carbonated beverages, urinary incontinence and, 272
Cardinal ligaments, 4, 165
Cardiovascular disease, erectile dysfunction and, 127
Catheterization
    in age-related urinary incontinence, 345
    in pediatric urinary incontinence, 433
    in spinal cord injury, 423
Cauda equina
    lesions of
        bulbocavernosus reflex in, 229–230
        electromyography in, 229
        erectile dysfunction and, 106
        neurogenic voiding dysfunction and, 71–72
    transcutaneous stimulation of, 227
Cavernosal artery, 90–91
    insufficiency of, 100–102
Cavernosal ischemia, erectile dysfunction and, 103
Cavernosal nerves, 91
Cavernosometry, 261, 262, 262f
Central nervous system, 217–218
Cerebral cortex, in male sexual function, 26–27
Cerebral somatosensory evoked potentials, 228
Cerebrovascular accidents, micturition disorders with, 52–53
Cervicocystoptosis, 155, 155f
Cervix, 21
Childbirth, 33–39, 34f
    anal sphincter defects with, 35–37, 36f, 236
    anesthesia for, 38
    episiotomy for, 37–38, 39f
    fecal incontinence and, 36–37, 76–77
    forceps for, 38
    maternal position for, 38
    pelvic floor distension with, 33, 34f
    pelvic floor re-education after, 337, 338
    pelvic magnetic resonance imaging after, 177
    pudendal nerve damage during, 34
    rectocele and, 82, 85, 398
    urethral sphincter and, 34–35
    urinary stress incontinence after, 35
    vacuum extraction for, 38
Children
    sexual abuse of, 366–369. *See also* Sexual abuse, childhood.
    urinary incontinence in, 432–446. *See also* Urinary incontinence, pediatric.
Cigarette smoking
    cessation of, 269–270
    erectile dysfunction and, 126, 252–253, 253t
Clenbuterol, in urinary incontinence, 376t, 382–383
Clitoris, 20–21, 92–93
    blood supply to, 21, 93, 97
    histochemistry of, 93
    innervation of, 93
    tone of, 98
Clotting factors, in diabetes mellitus, 101
Cocaine, erectile dysfunction and, 252–253, 253t
Coffee, in urinary incontinence, 272, 273
Collagen, in pelvic floor dysfunction, 6
Collagen injection
    in pediatric urinary incontinence, 436–437
    periurethral, 196, 424–426
Colonic motility
    constipation and, 78
    rectal prolapse and, 84
Colpocystodefecography, 156–157, 156f, 157f, 161
    analysis of, 150–151, 151b
    technique of, 149–150
Colporectocystourethrography, 145–146, 164–174
    after incontinence surgery, 172, 172f, 173f
    in cystocele, 170, 170f
    in enterocele, 171–172, 172f
    in postsurgical stricture, 173
    in puborectalis muscle dysfunction, 172
    in rectocele, 171, 171f
    in urethral diverticula, 173, 173f
    in uterine prolapse, 170–172, 171f
    in vaginal vault prolapse, 170–172, 171f
    in vesicovaginal fistula, 173, 174f
    indications for, 174
    normal findings on, 168–170, 169f, 170f
    technique of, 167–168, 168f
Condyloma acuminatum, 193
Connective tissue disease, rectal prolapse and, 85
Constipation, 78–79
    colonic dysmotility and, 78
    definition of, 78
    dietary therapy for, 328
    disease associations of, 79
    drug-related, 328
    electromyography in, 231
    in rectal prolapse, 87
    pathogenesis of, 78–79
    pelvic floor abnormalities and, 79
    pelvic floor re-education in, 324–326
    rectal inertia and, 78–79
    rectal prolapse and, 86
    re-reduction for, 324–326, 326f
    slow-transit, 78–79
    urinary incontinence and, 62, 270b, 273–274
Conus medullaris, lesions of
    bulbocavernosus reflex in, 229–230
    electromyography in, 229
Corpora cavernosa, 90
    veno-occlusive dysfunction of, 102–104
Corpus spongiosum, 90
Cowper's glands, 92
Crohn's disease, rectal compliance and, 75

Cystectomy, erectile dysfunction and, 101–102
Cystitis, interstitial, endoscopy in, 195, 195f
Cystocele
  colporectocystourethrography of, 170, 170f
  grade of, 155, 155t, 159–160, 160f, 165, 165f
  incontinence with, 156
  magnetic resonance imaging in, 185–186, 186f, 187f
  paravaginal repair of, 397, 398t
  pathophysiology of, 165, 165f
  radiologic evaluation of, 154–155, 155f, 155t, 156f
  sacral colpopexy in, 397, 398t
  surgical treatment of, 396–398, 397f, 397t
    abdominal approach to, 396–397, 397t, 398t
    provocative stress testing after, 141, 141f
    uterine prolapse after, 172, 173f
    vaginal approach to, 397–398, 397f, 397t, 398t
  types of, 155
  urodynamic evaluation of, 209–210, 209f, 211f
  with rectocele, 141, 141f
Cystography
  descending, 149
  retrograde dynamic and voiding, 149, 150, 150t, 151f, 161
Cystometry, filling, 200–204
  ambulatory, 203–204
  artifacts on, 203
  bladder capacity with, 203
  bladder compliance with, 203, 203f
  bladder sensation with, 202
  cough spikes for, 203
  detrusor activity with, 202–203, 202f
  for biofeedback, 298, 298f, 299f
  quality control during, 203, 204f
  technique of, 201–203
  urethral function with, 203
Cystoplasty, augmentation
  in neurogenic voiding dysfunction, 456–457
  in pediatric urinary incontinence, 433–435, 434f–436f
  in severe detrusor overactivity, 424
Cystoprostatectomy, erectile dysfunction and, 101–102, 107
Cystoscopy. *See* Endoscopy.

D
Darifenacin, in urinary incontinence, 376t, 379
Deep tendon reflexes, in patient evaluation, 140, 140f
Defecation, 16–17, 17f
  disorders of. *See* Constipation; Fecal incontinence.
  frequency of, 78
  in urinary incontinence treatment, 270b, 273–274
  normal, 74
  radiography of, 242, 243f. *See also* Pelvic viscerography.
  re-education for, 324–326
Defectography. *See* Pelvic viscerography.
Dementia, urge incontinence in, 62
Depression
  female sexual dysfunction and, 109, 124
  male sexual dysfunction and, 127
Descending perineum syndrome
  defecography in, 242, 244
  fecal incontinence in, 77–78, 241
Desmopressin, in urinary incontinence, 376t, 383–384

Detrusor
  cystometric evaluation of, 202–203, 202f
  electrical stimulation of, 281–288. *See also* Electrical stimulation.
  electromyography of, 208, 219
  electron microscopy of, in urge incontinence, 63
  extracorporeal electromagnetic stimulation of, 293–294, 295
  instability of, 46b, 154, 423–424
  overactivity of, 45, 45t, 46b, 47, 423–424. *See also* Urinary incontinence.
    drug treatment of, 376–384, 376t
    extracorporeal electromagnetic stimulation therapy in, 293
    on filling cystometry, 202–203, 202f
    surgical treatment of, 457–458
    with impaired contractility, 63
  underactivity of, overflow incontinence and, 64
  uninhibited contraction of, in urge incontinence, 60, 62
Detrusor areflexia, 293–294, 459
Detrusor hyper-reflexia, 423–424. *See also* Detrusor, overactivity of.
Detrusor–external sphincter dyssynergia, 54, 55f, 421–423, 423f
  biofeedback therapy in, 308
  complications of, 54
  electromyography in, 219
  suprasacral spinal cord lesions and, 70–71, 71t
  treatment of, 54, 422–423, 423f, 457–459
  urodynamic study in, 54, 55f, 69, 70f
Diabetes mellitus
  constipation and, 79
  erectile dysfunction and, 101, 103, 106–107, 108, 126–127
  female sexual dysfunction and, 109–110
Dicyclomine, in urinary incontinence, 376t, 381
Diet
  in constipation, 328
  in urinary incontinence, 270b, 271–274
Digoxin, erectile dysfunction with, 252–253, 253t
Dihydrotestosterone, in benign prostatic hyperplasia, 50
Disposable incontinence pads, 315–318, 315f–317f
Diuretics, erectile dysfunction and, 127, 252–253, 253t
Diverticula
  bladder
    urge incontinence and, 62
    urodynamic evaluation of, 209, 210f
  urethral, 139
    colporectocystourethrography in, 173, 173f
    endoscopy of, 193
    magnetic resonance imaging in, 189, 189f
Dopamine
  in female sexual function, 98
  in penile erection, 96
Dorsal penile nerve, 107–108
  electroneurography of, 227–228
Dorsal penile vein, 91
Doxazosin, in urinary incontinence, 376t
Dribble, postmicturition, 135
Drugs. *See also specific drugs*.
  constipation and, 79, 328
  erectile dysfunction and, 127, 252–253, 253t
  female sexual dysfunction with, 354, 355t
  in patient evaluation, 136
  urinary incontinence and, 59

Duloxetine, in stress urinary incontinence, 385, 385t
Dyspareunia, 122
    after rectocele repair, 399
Dysuria, in patient evaluation, 135

E

Ejaculation
    premature, 354
    retrograde, 89
Electrical stimulation, 281–288
    clinical applications of, 284–288, 285f, 286f
    contraindications to, 286
    duty cycle in, 283
    electrodes for, 282, 283–284
    faradism in, 283
    frequencies for, 282–283, 285
    home-based, 285, 286f
    in age-related urinary incontinence, 344–345
    in chronic lower urinary tract dysfunction, 450–451
    in detrusor areflexia, 459
    in neurogenic voiding dysfunction, 457
    in pelvic floor re-education, 332–333, 335–336
    in spinal cord injury, 450–451
    in urinary incontinence, 450–451
    interferential, 283
    mechanism of, 281–284, 282f, 284f
    nonacceptance of, 286
    office-based, 284, 285f
    on-to-off time in, 283
    patient selection for, 286
    probes for, 284–285, 285f
    results of, 286–288
    transcutaneous, 283–284, 284f, 344
    variant technology for, 283
    voltage setting in, 283
Electrodiagnostic testing, 146, 216–232, 217t. *See also* Electromyography.
    anterior sacral root stimulation for, 227
    bulbocavernosus reflex for, 225–226
    cerebral somatosensory evoked potentials for, 228
    classification of, 218, 219f
    clinical assessment before, 216–217
    corpus cavernosum electromyography for, 228–229
    dorsal penile nerve electroneurography for, 227–228
    electroneurography for, 227–228
    in cauda equina lesions, 229–230
    in central nervous system disease, 231
    in constipation, 231
    in conus medullaris lesions, 229–230
    in erectile dysfunction, 231
    in fecal incontinence, 231
    in myopathy, 230
    in Parkinson's disease, 229
    in urinary incontinence, 230–231
    in urinary retention, 230
    limitations of, 217t
    magnetic stimulation for, 227
    motor cortex stimulation for, 227
    motor nerve conduction studies for, 226–227
    of anterior sacral root, 227
    of autonomic nervous system, 228–229
    of dorsal penile nerve, 227–228
    of dorsal sacral roots, 228
    of pudendal nerve, 226–227
    of sacral motor system, 226–227
    of sacral reflexes, 225–226
    of sacral sensory system, 227–228
    physiology of, 218
    pudendal nerve terminal motor latency for, 226–227
    pudendal somatosensory evoked potentials for, 226
    sacral root electroneurography for, 228
    sympathetic skin response for, 228
Electromyography, 145, 146, 208–209, 218–225
    clinical assessment before, 216–217
    concentric needle, 219–224, 220f, 221f
    in constipation, 231
    in erectile dysfunction, 231
    in fecal incontinence, 231
    in Parkinson's disease, 229
    in urinary incontinence, 230–231
    in urinary retention, 230
    interference pattern (IP) analysis in, 223–224, 224f
    kinesiologic, 218–219
    motor unit potential (MUP) analysis in, 222–223, 222f
    motor unit potential in, 221–222, 221f
    of corpus cavernosum, 228–229
    single-fiber, 224–225
Electrotherapy, in pelvic floor re-education, 322
Emissary veins, of corpora cavernosa, 91
Endometriosis, 195–196
Endopelvic fascia, 4–5, 4f, 6f
Endoscopy, 191–196
    equipment for, 191–192
    in benign prostatic hyperplasia, 53
    in bladder cancer, 195
    in bladder compression, 193
    in ectopic ureter, 192–193
    in endometriosis, 195–196
    in interstitial cystitis, 195, 195f
    in intrinsic sphincter deficiency, 194, 194f
    in periurethral bulking, 196
    in stress urinary incontinence, 194
    in ureterocele, 193, 194f
    in urethral diverticula, 193
    in urethral tumors, 193
    in urethritis, 193
    in urethrovesical fistula, 194
    in vesicovaginal fistula, 194
    in vesioenteric fistula, 194, 195f
    indications for, 191
    intraoperative, 196
    normal findings on, 192, 192f, 193f
Endothelial cell dysfunction, erectile dysfunction and, 100
Endothelin
    in diabetes mellitus, 101
    in penile erection, 95
Enterocele
    colporectocystourethrography in, 171–172, 172f
    magnetic resonance imaging in, 184–185, 185f
    pathophysiology of, 165–166, 166f
    radiography of, 244–245, 245f
Enterocystoplasty, in neurogenic voiding dysfunction, 456
Enuresis. *See* Urinary incontinence.
Ephedrine, in stress urinary incontinence, 384–385, 385t

Epilepsy, erectile dysfunction and, 105
Episiotomy, 37–38, 39f, 137–138
Erectile dysfunction, 89, 99–108, 125–128
   acidosis and, 104
   aging and, 103, 106, 107
   anoxia and, 103–104
   antipsychotic agents and, 105
   bulbocavernosus reflex in, 231
   cardiovascular disease and, 127
   cauda equina syndrome and, 106
   cavernosal ischemia and, 103
   cigarette smoking and, 126, 252–253, 253t
   classification of, 250, 250b
   corporal veno-occlusive dysfunction and, 102–104
   diabetes mellitus and, 101, 103, 106–107, 108, 126–127
   diagnostic evaluation of, 251–263, 251f, 347–349
      angiography in, 262–263
      biothesiometry in, 253, 257
      blood flow testing in, 259–263, 260f, 262f
      bulbocavernosus reflex in, 231, 257
      cavernosometry in, 261, 262, 262f
      color duplex Doppler testing in, 260
      cystometrography in, 257
      electromyography in, 231
      endocrine testing in, 255–257, 256b
      neurologic testing in, 257–258
      neurotransmitter study in, 258
      nocturnal penile tumescence in, 255, 348–349
      papaverine testing in, 258
      patient history in, 251–253, 252t, 347
      peak systolic velocity in, 260
      penile artery pressure in, 259
      penile brachial index in, 259
      pharmacotesting in, 258, 261, 348
      physical examination in, 253–255, 347–348
      plethysmography in, 253, 259
      prostaglandin E testing in, 258
      psychometry in, 254–255, 254b
      RigiScan in, 261
      self-administered questionnaires for, 250, 254–255, 254b, 348
      serum testosterone in, 348, 349
      somatosensory evoked potential testing in, 231, 258
      structured interview in, 254–255, 254b
      venous testing in, 260–262, 260f
   drug-related, 127, 252–253, 253t
   endocrinopathy in, 255–257, 256b
   epilepsy and, 105
   fistulae and, 104
   hormonal factors in, 126
   hyperprolactinemia and, 257
   hypoxia and, 103–104
   incidence of, 125–126
   lifestyle factors in, 126
   multiple sclerosis and, 106
   nerve root compression and, 106
   nerve trauma and, 107
   neurogenic, 104–108, 104t, 127
   organic, 250, 252, 252t
   Parkinson's disease and, 105
   pathophysiology of, 250
   penile fracture and, 102
   Peyronie's disease and, 102–103
   polyneuropathy and, 106
   prevalence of, 125–126
   priapism and, 104
   psychogenic, 99, 99t, 100t, 250, 252, 252t
      pharmacotesting in, 258
   renal failure and, 101, 128
   risk factors for, 126–128, 127b
   sensory nerve deficits and, 107–108
   social status and, 126
   spinal cord trauma and, 105–106
   spinal dysraphism and, 105
   testosterone, 126
   trauma and, 101, 105–106, 107
   treatment of, 349–354
      adeno-associated virus-brain derived neurotrophic factor in, 354
      alprostadil in, 351
      apomorphine SL in, 353
      Cialis in, 353
      counseling in, 349
      gene therapy in, 353–354
      intracavernosal injections in, 352
      melanotan II in, 353
      MUSE device in, 351
      penile prosthesis in, 352–353
      priapism with, 352
      sildenafil in, 349–351. *See also* Sildenafil.
      testosterone replacement in, 351
      vacuum devices in, 351
      vardenafil in, 353
      vasoactive agents in, 352
   vasculogenic, 100–104
      arterial insufficiency and, 100–102
      cystoprostatectomy and, 101–102, 107
      diabetes mellitus and, 101
      endothelial cell dysfunction and, 100
      evaluation of, 260–263, 260f, 262f
      hypercholesterolemia and, 100–101
      hypertension and, 101
      radiation therapy and, 102
      trauma and, 101
      uremia and, 101
Estradiol, in epilepsy, 105
Estrogen
   deficiency of, female sexual dysfunction and, 108–109, 123
   in age-related urinary incontinence, 345
   in female sexual function, 23, 98–99
   in urinary incontinence, 385t, 386
Exercise
   incontinence and, 274–275
   pelvic floor, 277–280, 331–332. *See also* Pelvic floor exercises.
Extracorporeal electromagnetic stimulation therapy, 291–295
   bladder capacity effects of, 295
   historical perspective on, 291–292
   in areflexic bladder, 293–294
   in overactive bladder, 293
   in pelvic floor re-education, 333–334, 334f, 336–337
   in pelvic pain syndrome, 292

Extracorporeal electromagnetic stimulation therapy (*cont.*)
   in spinal cord injury, 294
   in urinary incontinence, 292, 294, 295
   mechanism of action of, 293
   safety of, 295
   technique of, 292–293
   tissue density and, 292
   tissue effects of, 292
   urethral pressure effects of, 294–295

F
Fecal continence, 14–16. *See also* Defecation; Fecal incontinence.
   anal sphincters in, 14–16, 15f
   rectosphincteric reflexes in, 16
   rectum in, 14
Fecal incontinence, 73–78
   anal re-education for, 323–324, 323f
   anal sensation and, 75
   anal sphincter injury and, 78
   anorectal manometry in, 241
   childbirth and, 36–37, 76–77
   classification of, 74–75
   definition of, 73
   disease associations of, 74
   electromyography in, 231
   etiology of, 76–78, 76b, 77b
   excessive straining and, 77–78
   external anal sphincter in, 76
   idiopathic, 73
   in descending perineum syndrome, 241
   in rectal prolapse, 86–87
   incidence of, 73–74
   infection-related, 75
   internal anal sphincter in, 75–76
   major, 75
   minor, 75
   neurogenic, 73
   pathophysiology of, 74–78
   pediatric, 446–447, 447f
   pelvic floor muscle exercises in, 278
   pelvic floor re-education for, 337–338
   prevalence of, 73–74
   psychological effect of, 74
   puborectalis muscle in, 76
   rectal compliance and, 75
   rectal sensation and, 75
   rectoanal inhibitory reflex and, 75
   stool consistency and, 75
   surgical associations of, 74
   transanal ultrasonography in, 236, 236f, 237f
   trauma and, 78
Fiber, dietary, in constipation, 328
Fibroid, uterine, bladder compression by, 193
Filling cystometry. *See* Cystometry, filling.
Finasteride, erectile dysfunction and, 252–253, 253t
Fistula
   anal, 237
   erectile dysfunction and, 104
   urethrovesical, 194
   vesicovaginal, 173, 174f, 194
   vesicoenteric, 194, 195f
Flavoxate, in urinary incontinence, 376t, 382
Fluid intake, urinary incontinence and, 270b, 271–272, 272b
Flurbiprofen, in urinary incontinence, 376t
Forceps, during childbirth, 38
Four-corner suspension, in cystocele repair, 397–398, 397f, 397t
Fracture, penile, 102
Functional stop test, of pelvic floor, 144

G
Gene therapy, in erectile dysfunction, 353–354
Genitalia. *See also specific structures.*
   female, 92–93
   male, 89–92
G-spot, 22
Gynecologic history, in patient evaluation, 136

H
Halban's fascia, 22
Helicine arteries, 91
Hematuria, in patient evaluation, 135
Hemodialysis, erectile dysfunction and, 101
Hesitancy, in patient evaluation, 135
Hirschsprung's disease, 16
Histamine-2 receptor antagonists, erectile dysfunction and, 127
Hormone replacement therapy, female sexual function and, 23
Hunner's ulcer, 195, 195f
Hymenectomy, in vaginismus, 361
Hyoscyamine, in urinary incontinence, 376t, 377
Hypercalcemia, constipation and, 79
Hypercholesterolemia, erectile dysfunction and, 100–101
Hyperparathyroidism, constipation and, 79
Hypertension, erectile dysfunction and, 101
Hypoactive sexual desire disorder, 122
Hypogastric nerve, 91
   section of, penile erection and, 107
Hypoxia, erectile dysfunction and, 103–104
Hysterectomy
   sexual function after, 21
   vaginal support after, 4, 4f

I
Imipramine, in urinary incontinence, 376t, 383, 385, 385t
Immobility, urinary incontinence and, 59, 64
Impotence, 89. *See also* Erectile dysfunction.
Indomethacin, in urinary incontinence, 376t
Infection, after pubovaginal sling, 395
Inflammation, in urge incontinence, 61–62
International Index of Erectile Function, 254
Intestinal transit
   constipation and, 78–79
   rectal prolapse and, 84
Intra-abdominal pressure
   in patient evaluation, 135
   rectal prolapse and, 85
Intraurethral stent, 422–423, 423f
Intraurethral valve pump, in detrusor areflexia, 459
Intravaginal resistance devices, in pelvic floor re-education, 332, 335
Introitus, laxity of, 137, 138f
Intussusception, rectal prolapse and, 82–83, 84f
Irritable bowel syndrome, 328–329

K

Kegel exercises, 277–280. *See also* Pelvic floor exercises.
Kegel perineometry, 144
Kinesitherapy
    in anal canal re-education, 325
    in pelvic floor re-education, 320–321
Kropp procedure, in pediatric urinary incontinence, 438–439, 440f

L

Labia majora, 92
Labia minora, 92
Labor. *See* Childbirth.
Lamotrigine, in epilepsy, 105
Leak-point pressure, 68, 69f, 213–214, 213f, 214f
Leiomyoma, urethral, 193
Levator ani, 3–4, 81. *See also at* Pelvic floor.
    electrical stimulation of, 281–288. *See also* Electrical stimulation.
    evaluation of, 142–146, 143b, 143f. *See also* Electrodiagnostic testing; Electromyography.
    exercises for, 277–280. *See also* Pelvic floor exercises.
    female sexual function and, 22, 123
    fibers of, 142
    in constipation, 79
    innervation of, 4
Libido, 89, 354
Limbic system, in sexual function, 27
Littre's glands (periurethral glands), 92
Luteinizing hormone, in benign prostatic hyperplasia, 50

M

MACE procedure, 446–447, 447f
Magnetic resonance imaging, 146, 176–181, 178f, 180f
    after minimized pubovaginal sling procedure, 419, 420f
    anatomy for, 176–177
    dynamic, 177–181, 178f, 183–189
    in cystocele, 185–186, 186f, 187f
    in enterocele, 184–185, 185f
    in pelvic mass, 188–189
    in pelvic organ prolapse, 164, 184–188, 185f–188f
    in postpartum patient, 177
    in rectocele, 186–187, 188f
    in urethral diverticula, 189, 189f
    in uterine prolapse, 187–188, 188f
    normal findings on, 184, 184f
    technique of, 179–181, 180f, 183–184
    urethral diverticula on, 189, 189f
Male sling procedure, 429, 429f
Manometry
    anorectal. *See* Anorectal manometry.
    in biofeedback therapy, 298–300, 299f, 300f
Marshall-Marchetti-Krantz colposuspension, 392–393, 393t
Massage, in anal canal re-education, 325
Maximum urethral closure pressure, 206
Meatus, postoperative stricture of, 173
Melanocortin, in penile erection, 97
Melanotan II, in erectile dysfunction, 353
Mental status, evaluation of, 139
Metoclopramide, erectile dysfunction with, 252–253, 253t

Micturition cycle, 7–12, 373–374, 374f
    adrenergic activity in, 8f, 9–10
    afferent activity in, 8–9, 8f, 67, 373–374, 374f
    cholinergic activity in, 8f, 9
    efferent activity in, 8f, 9–11
    inhibition in, 8, 11
    interruption of, 10, 12
    neurophysiology of, 66–67
    nonadrenergic noncholinergic activity in, 8f, 10
    pontine center in, 11–12, 66–67
    radiography of, 242, 243f
    somatic nerve activity in, 8f, 10–11
Military training, urinary incontinence and, 275
Monti procedure, in pediatric urinary incontinence, 445, 446f
Motor cortex stimulation, for electrodiagnostic testing, 227
Motor examination, in patient evaluation, 140
Motor nerve conduction studies, 226–227
Motor neurons, 217–218
Motor unit, 218
Motor unit potential, 221–222, 221f
    analysis of, 222–223, 222f
    duration of, 223
    phases of, 221f, 223
    size of, 223
Mucilage, in irritable bowel syndrome, 328–329
Multiple sclerosis, erectile dysfunction in, 106, 127
Muscarinic receptors, of bladder, 9, 375–376, 375f
Muscular dystrophy, electromyography in, 230
MUSE device, in erectile dysfunction, 351
Myelodysplasia, leak-point pressure in, 213, 214f
Myoplasty, bladder, in detrusor areflexia, 459

N

Nerve root compression, erectile dysfunction and, 106
Nerve trauma, erectile dysfunction and, 107
Neurogenic voiding dysfunction, 66–72, 67b
    cauda equina lesions and, 71–72
    clinical assessment of, 67–69
    cystometrography in, 68, 69f
    laboratory tests in, 68
    management of, 454–457
        botulinum A toxin in, 456
        intravesical therapy in, 455–456
        neuromodulation in, 457
        pharmacotherapy in, 454–455
        surgical therapy in, 456–457
    patient history in, 67–68
    pelvic plexus lesions and, 71–72
    sacral spinal cord lesions and, 71, 71t
    suprapontine lesions and, 70
    suprasacral spinal cord lesions and, 70–71, 71t
    urodynamic study in, 68–69, 69f–71f
    videourodynamic study in, 69, 71f
    vs. benign prostatic hyperplasia, 52–53
Neurologic examination, 139–140
Neurologic history, in patient evaluation, 135–136
Neuromodulation, 450–452. *See also* Electrical stimulation.
Neuropathy
    erectile dysfunction and, 106–107
    female sexual dysfunction and, 110

Neuropeptides
　in bladder, 10
　in penile erection, 95
Neurotransmitters, in penile erection, 96–97
Nitrates, sildenafil interactions with, 350
Nitric oxide
　in female sexual function, 22
　in male sexual function, 28, 95, 96
　in urethral relaxation, 10
Nocturia
　fluid intake and, 272
　in patient evaluation, 134
Nocturnal penile tumescence, 255, 348–349
Nonsteroidal anti-inflammatory agents, erectile dysfunction with, 252–253, 253t
Norephedrine, in stress urinary incontinence, 384–385, 385t
Norepinephrine, in penile erection, 95, 96

O
Obesity, urinary incontinence and, 270–271
Occupational stress, urinary incontinence and, 275
Onuf's nucleus, 218
Oophorectomy, female sexual function and, 98–99
Opioids
　in penile erection, 97
　micturition effects of, 11
Orgasm, male, 27
Orgasmic disorder, 122
Oxybutynin
　in neurogenic voiding dysfunction, 454, 455
　in urinary incontinence, 345, 376t, 380–381
Oxytocin
　in female sexual function, 98
　in penile erection, 96

P
Pads, incontinence, 58, 315–318, 315f–317f, 345
Pain
　sexual, 122–123
　suprapubic, 47, 135
Pants, incontinence, 315–318, 315f, 316f
Papaverine, in erectile dysfunction, 258, 352
Paracolpium, 4
Parkinson's disease
　electrodiagnostic testing in, 229
　erectile dysfunction in, 105, 127
　urge incontinence in, 62
　voiding symptoms in, 53
Patient evaluation, 133–146
　bladder emptying in, 135
　bladder pain in, 135
　coital incontinence in, 134
　colporectocystourethrography in, 145–146. See also Colporectocystourethrography.
　deep tendon reflexes in, 140
　dribble in, 135
　drug history in, 136
　dysuria in, 135
　electrodiagnosis in, 146, 216–232. See also Electrodiagnostic testing.
　electromyography in, 145, 146, 208–209, 218–224. See also Electromyography.
　endoscopy in, 191–196, 192f–195f. See also Endoscopy.
　functional stop test in, 144
　general physical examination in, 137
　giggle incontinence in, 134–135
　gynecologic symptoms in, 136
　hematuria in, 135
　history in, 133–136, 134b
　magnetic resonance imaging in, 146, 176–181. See also Magnetic resonance imaging.
　manual muscle testing in, 142, 143, 143f
　mental status in, 139
　mixed incontinence in, 134
　motor function in, 140
　neurologic examination in, 139–140, 140f
　neurologic history in, 135–136
　nocturia in, 134
　nocturnal enuresis in, 135
　pelvic examination in, 137–139, 138f
　pelvic floor muscle assessment in, 142–146, 143b, 143f
　pelvic organ prolapse in, 139
　pelvic relaxation in, 139
　perineometry in, 144, 145
　physical examination in, 136–142
　poor urinary stream in, 135
　postvoid residual measurement in, 142
　provocative stress testing in, 140–141, 141f
　Q-tip test in, 141–142, 145
　questionnaire in, 133
　radiologic studies in, 149–157, 150t, 151f–157f
　risk factor assessment in, 136
　sensory function in, 139–140
　stress incontinence in, 134
　surgical history in, 136
　ultrasonography in, 145, 157–161, 158f–160f, 162f
　urethral pressures in, 145, 206, 206f, 211–213, 213f
　urge incontinence in, 134
　urinary frequency in, 133
　urinary hesitancy in, 135
　urinary incontinence in, 134–135
　urinary symptoms in, 133–135
　urodynamic studies in, 198–206, 208–214. See also Urodynamic studies.
　vaginal cones in, 144
　voiding difficulties in, 135
Pelvic examination, 137–139, 138f
Pelvic floor
　anatomy of, 3–6, 4f–6f, 81, 82f, 142
　connective tissue of, 5–6
　evaluation of, 142–146, 143b, 143f. See also Patient evaluation.
　exercises for. See Pelvic floor exercises.
　function of, 277–278
　functional anatomy of, 4–6, 4f, 5f, 6f
　gross anatomy of, 3–4
　histology of, 5–6
　manual evaluation of, 142, 143, 143f
　re-education of. See Pelvic floor re-education.
Pelvic floor exercises, 277–280, 331–332, 334–335
　abdominal muscle activity during, 279
　adverse effects of, 280
　effectiveness of, 280
　frequency of, 279

in age-related urinary incontinence, 344
in fecal incontinence, 278
in urinary stress incontinence, 278
in urinary urge incontinence, 278
instruction methods for, 279
principles of, 278–279
results of, 334–335
training period for, 280
work-rest phase for, 279–280
Pelvic floor re-education, 320–329, 331–338
after vaginal delivery, 337
biofeedback in, 321–322, 321f, 332, 335
bladder retraining in, 333, 336
contraindications to, 320
electrical stimulation in, 322, 332–333, 335–336
extracorporeal electromagnetic stimulation in, 333–334, 334f, 336–337
in constipation, 324–326
in fecal incontinence, 337–338
in sexual dysfunction, 338
indications for, 320
intravaginal resistance devices in, 332, 335
kinesitherapy in, 320–321
manual techniques in, 321
pelvic floor muscle training in, 331–332, 334–335
results of, 334–337
vaginal cones in, 332, 335, 336
vs. anti-incontinence devices, 337
Pelvic mass, magnetic resonance imaging of, 188–189
Pelvic organ prolapse. *See also* Cystocele; Enterocele; Rectocele; Uterine prolapse.
colpocystodefecography in, 156–157, 156f, 157f
colporectocystourethrography in, 167–174. *See also* Colporectocystourethrography.
evaluation of, 136–137, 164–165
ICS system for, 136–137
in lithotomy position, 137
magnetic resonance imaging in, 184–188, 185f–188f
pathophysiology of, 165–167, 165f–167f
radiologic evaluation of, 154–157, 155f, 155t, 156f, 157f
stages of, 136–137
Pelvic plexus lesions, neurogenic voiding dysfunction and, 71–72
Pelvic relaxation syndrome, 139
Pelvic viscerography, 241–246
enterocele on, 244–245, 245f
functional abnormalities on, 242
in descending perineum syndrome, 242, 244
normal results on, 242, 243f
positional abnormalities on, 242, 244
rectocele on, 244, 244f, 245–246, 245f, 246f
technique of, 241–242
Penile artery, 90
Penile artery pressure, 259
Penile brachial index, 259
Penile nerve, electroneurography of, 227–228
Penile sheath, for incontinence, 317–318, 317f, 318f
Penile shell, for incontinence, 317, 317f
Penis
anatomy of, 26, 89–92
angiography of, 262–263
blood supply to, 28, 90–91
corpora cavernosa of, 90
corpus spongiosum of, 90
detumescence of, 28, 94
erection of, 26, 27, 28–29, 93–97, 258–259. *See also* Erectile dysfunction.
acetylcholine in, 95
adrenergic activity in, 95
adrenocorticotropin in, 97
androgens in, 97
angiotensin II in, 95–96
arterial phase of, 94
bradykinin in, 96
castration effects on, 97
cavernosal phase of, 94
cholinergic activity in, 94–95
detumescence phase of, 94
dopamine in, 96
endothelin in, 95
hemodynamics of, 93–94, 94f
in spinal cord trauma, 105–106
melanocortin in, 97
neuropeptides in, 95
neurophysiology of, 94–97
neurotransmitters in, 96–97
nitric oxide in, 95, 96
norepinephrine in, 95, 96
opioids in, 97
oxytocin in, 96
paracrine factors in, 95–96
peptidergic activity in, 95
prostaglandins in, 96
resting phase of, 94
serotonin in, 96
spinal mechanisms in, 96
supraspinal mechanisms in, 96
testosterone in, 97
fracture of, 102
histochemistry of, 92
innervation of, 26, 27, 91–92
motor nerves of, 92
parasympathetic nerves of, 91
prosthetic, 352–353
sensory nerves of, 91–92
sensory thresholds of, 107–108
sympathetic nerves of, 91
veins of, 91
Perineal body, support for, 5, 5f
Perineal membrane, 5, 5f, 6f
Perineometry, 144, 145
Perineum
abnormal descent of, 77–78
examination of, 137, 138f
trauma to, 78
during childbirth, 35–37
erectile dysfunction and, 101
Peripheral nerves, in micturition, 8–11, 8f
Peripheral neuropathy, erectile dysfunction in, 127
Peritoneocele, 156–157, 156f
Peyronie's disease, 102–103
Phenoxybenzamine, in neurogenic voiding dysfunction, 455, 458

Phentolamine
  in erectile dysfunction, 352
  in female sexual dysfunction, 356
  in neurogenic voiding dysfunction, 455
Physical examination, 136–142
  vs. imaging, 160–161
Pippi Salle procedure, in pediatric urinary incontinence, 439–440, 441f
Plethysmography, in erectile dysfunction, 253, 259
Polyneuropathy, erectile dysfunction and, 106
Pontine micturition center, 11
Postvoid residual measurement, 142
Potassium channel openers, in urinary incontinence, 376t, 379–380
Prazosin, in neurogenic voiding dysfunction, 455
Prazosin, in urinary incontinence, 376t
Pregnancy. See also Childbirth.
  fecal incontinence and, 77
  rectal prolapse and, 85
Premature ejaculation, 354
Pressure
  anorectal. See Anorectal manometry.
  bladder. See Cystometry, filling.
  urethral. See Urethral pressures.
Pressure-flow study, 204–206, 205f
  artifacts during, 206
  in detrusor–external sphincter dyssynergia, 205
  in dysfunctional voiding, 205
  in mechanical urethral obstruction, 205–206
  in nonrelaxing sphincter obstruction, 205
  pressure curves on, 204, 205f
Priapism, 104
Primary degenerative internal sphincter syndrome, 237
Prolapse. See Cystocele; Enterocele; Rectocele; Uterine prolapse.
Prompted voiding, in age-related urinary incontinence, 344
Propantheline
  in neurogenic voiding dysfunction, 454
  in urinary incontinence, 376t, 377
Propiverine, in urinary incontinence, 376t, 381–382
Prostaglandin, in penile erection, 96
Prostaglandin E
  in erectile dysfunction, 258
  in female sexual dysfunction, 356
Prostaglandin synthesis inhibitors, in urinary incontinence, 376t, 383
Prostate gland, 92
  benign hyperplasia of, 49–53. See also Benign prostatic hyperplasia.
Prostatectomy
  erectile dysfunction and, 101–102, 107
  incontinence and, 64, 346, 424–429
    artificial urinary sphincter in, 426–429, 426f–428f
    incidence of, 424
    male sling in, 429, 429f
    urethral bulking agents in, 424–426, 425f, 426f
Prostatitis, 54
Provocative stress testing
  after cystocele repair, 141, 141f
  in patient evaluation, 140–141, 141f
Psychiatric drugs
  in female sexual dysfunction, 109
  in male sexual dysfunction, 105

Psychometry, in erectile dysfunction, 254–255, 254b
Psychotherapy, anorectal re-education and, 329
Pubocervical fascia, 4, 5
Puborectalis. See also at Pelvic floor.
  anatomy of, 81, 82f
  colporectocystourethrography of, 172
  in constipation, 79
  in fecal incontinence, 76
  in female sexual function, 22
Pubovaginal sling, 393–395, 394f, 394t, 414–420
  colporectocystourethrography of, 172, 172f, 173f
  in type IIB stress incontinence, 414
  materials for, 414, 414t
  minimized, 414–419, 415f–418f, 418t
    follow-up of, 418–419, 419f
    results of, 419, 420f
Pudendal artery, 90
Pudendal nerve
  childbirth-related injury to, 34
  electrical stimulation of, 281–288. See also Electrical stimulation.
  in male sexual function, 27–28
Pudendal nerve terminal motor latency, 226–227
  childbirth and, 34, 76–77
Pudendal somatosensory evoked potentials, 226
  in erectile dysfunction, 231

Q
Q-tip test, 141–142, 145

R
Radiation therapy, erectile dysfunction and, 102
Receptors, muscarinic, 375–376, 375f
Rectal compliance, 239–240, 241f
Rectal re-education, 322–324
  contraindications to, 322–323
  principles of, 322
Rectal ulcer syndrome, 86
Rectoanal angle, during straining, 17, 17f
Rectoanal excitatory reflex, 16, 239, 240f
  fecal incontinence and, 241
Rectoanal inhibitory reflex, 16, 239, 240f
  fecal incontinence and, 75, 241
  re-education of, 325
Rectocele, 81–87
  age and, 81
  childbirth and, 82, 85, 398
  colonic motility and, 84
  colporectocystourethrography in, 171, 171f
  connective tissue disorders and, 85
  constipation and, 86, 87
  electrophysiology of, 83, 84
  epidemiology of, 81–82
  etiology of, 82–86, 83f–85f
  fecal incontinence and, 78, 86–87
  female-to-male ratio in, 81–82
  intra-abdominal pressure in, 85
  intussusception theory of, 82–83, 84f
  labor and, 82, 85, 398
  levator hiatus in, 83, 85f
  magnetic resonance imaging in, 186–187, 188f

neurologic disorders and, 85–86
parity and, 82
pathophysiology of, 166, 167f
pelvic anatomy and, 86
pelvic floor disorders and, 83, 85, 85f, 87
predisposing factors for, 85
pregnancy and, 85
psychiatric illness and, 86
radiography of, 244, 244f, 245–246, 245f, 246f
re-education for, 326–327
sliding hernia theory of, 82, 83f
surgical treatment of, 398–399, 399f, 399t
Rectorectal reflex, 16, 239, 240f, 241
Rectovaginal fascia, 4, 5
Rectum, 14. *See also* Defecation; Fecal continence; Fecal incontinence.
balloon dilation re-education of, 323–324, 323f
complicance of
fecal incontinence and, 75
testing of, 240, 241f
digital examination of, in female, 138–139
distension of, 14, 16
prolapse of. *See* Rectocele.
sensation in
fecal incontinence and, 75
testing of, 239–240, 241f
support for, 5
Reflexes
in patient evaluation, 139–140, 140f
rectoanal, 16, 239, 240f, 241
sacral, 225–226
Renal failure, erectile dysfunction and, 101, 128
Resiniferatoxin
in neurogenic voiding dysfunction, 455–456
in urinary incontinence, 376t, 384
Retrograde dynamic and voiding cystography
advantages of, 161
analysis of, 150, 150t, 151f
disadvantages of, 161
method of, 149
Retropubic suspensions, in stress urinary incontinence, 392–393, 393t
Rhizotomy, posterior, in neurogenic voiding dysfunction, 457
RigiScan, in erectile dysfunction, 261

S
Sacral colpopexy, 397, 398t
Sacral nerve roots
electroneurography of, 228
stimulation of, 227
in neurogenic voiding dysfunction, 457
Sacral reflex, 225–226
Salbutamol, in urinary incontinence, 376t
Samples perineometry, 144
Sampling reflex, in anal continence, 16
Seminal vesicle, 92
Sensory examination, in patient evaluation, 139–140
Sensory neurons, 218
Serotonin
in micturition cycle, 11
in penile erection, 96

Sexual abuse
childhood, 366–369
clinical manifestations of, 367–368
dissociation in, 368
effect of, 366
patient interview for, 368
pelvic floor rehabilitation in, 368–369
physiologic symptoms of, 367
self-mutilation in, 369
sexual effects of, 367
spiritual restoration in, 369
symptoms of, 366–367
touch re-education in, 368
treatment of, 368–369
wound care in, 369
fecal incontinence with, 237
Sexual arousal disorder, 122
Sexual aversion disorder, 122
Sexual dysfunction
fecal incontinence and, 74
female, 108–110, 121–124, 354–356
androgen level and, 109
apomorphine in, 356
classification of, 108, 121–123
diabetes mellitus and, 109–110
drug-induced, 109
estrogen therapy in, 355
estrogen withdrawal and, 108–109
etiology of, 123–124
evaluation of, 354–355, 355t
incidence of, 121
L-arginine in, 356
methyltestosterone in, 355–356
neurologic factors in, 109–110
pathophysiology of, 108–109
pelvic floor re-education in, 338
phentolamine in, 356
prevalence of, 121
prostaglandin E_1 in, 356
psychological factors in, 109
sildenafil in, 110, 356
spinal cord injury and, 109
treatment of, 354–356
vasculogenic, 110
yohimbine in, 356
male, 99–108, 347–354. *See also* Erectile dysfunction.
Sexual function. *See also* Sexual dysfunction.
female, 19–24, 97–99, 98f
adrenergic responses in, 23
anatomy of, 19–22
androgen in, 99
angiotensin II in, 98
arterial phase of, 97
clitoris in, 21, 98
dopamine in, 98
estrogen in, 23, 98–99
evaluation of, 354–355, 355t
hemodynamics of, 97
labial changes during, 21
levator ani muscle in, 22
neurogenic mediators of, 22–23
neurophysiology of, 98

Sexual function (cont.)
   female (cont.)
      oophorectomy effects on, 98–99
      oxytocin in, 98
      plateau phase of, 97
      resolution phase of, 97
      response cycle of, 19
      resting phase of, 97
      testosterone in, 23–24
      uterine changes during, 21
      vaginal changes during, 20, 97, 98
   male, 26–29, 93–97, 94f. See also Penis, erection of.
      cerebrocortical function and, 26–27
      hemodynamics of, 28–29, 93–94, 94f
      hormonal factors in, 97
      limbic system and, 27
      neurophysiology of, 94–97
      somatic nerves and, 27–28
      spinal cord and, 27
Shy-Drager syndrome, erectile dysfunction in, 127
Sildenafil, 349–351
   adverse effects of, 350
   cost-effectiveness of, 351
   dosage of, 350
   drug interactions with, 350
   efficacy of, 349–350
   hemodynamic effects of, 350
   in coronary artery disease patient, 350
   in female sexual dysfunction, 110, 356
   in spinal cord trauma patient, 106
   mechanism of action of, 349
   nitrate interactions with, 350
Sims speculum, 138, 138f
Skene's glands (paraurethral glands), 92
Skin, sympathetic response of, 228
Solifenacin, in urinary incontinence, 376t, 379
Somatosensory evoked potentials
   cerebral, 228
   pudendal, 226, 231, 258
Sphincter. See Anal sphincter(s); Artificial urinary sphincter; Urethral sphincter.
Sphincterotomy, 422, 458
Spinal cord, in male sexual function, 27
Spinal cord injury
   acontractile bladder in, 421
   electrical stimulation in, 450–451
   erectile dysfunction and, 105–106, 127
   extracorporeal electromagnetic stimulation therapy in, 294
   female sexual dysfunction and, 109, 123
   intraurethral stent in, 422–423, 423f
   rectal prolapse and, 85–86
   sphincterotomy in, 422
   suprapubic catheterization in, 423
Spinal dysraphism, erectile dysfunction and, 105
Spinal roots, sacral
   electroneurography of, 228
   stimulation of, 227
      in neurogenic voiding dysfunction, 457
Spinal stenosis, urge incontinence and, 62
Squamous metaplasia, cake-icing appearance of, 192, 193f
Stent, intraurethral, 422–423, 423f
Stoma, in pediatric urinary incontinence, 444–446, 445f, 446f

Stool. See Constipation; Defecation; Fecal incontinence.
Stop test, of pelvic floor, 144
Stroke, incontinence after, 59, 62
Subtunical veins, 91
Suprapubic pain, in patient evaluation, 47, 135
Surgical history, in patient evaluation, 136
Suspensory ligament of clitoris, 92–93
Sympathectomy, penile erection and, 107
Sympathetic skin response, 228

T
Tamsulosin, in urinary incontinence, 376t, 382
Temporal lobe epilepsy, erectile dysfunction and, 105
Tension-free vaginal tape, 161, 162f, 403–407, 404f, 405f, 406t
   anatomical basis for, 403–404
   complications of, 405, 405b
   evaluation of, 405–406
   results of, 406–407, 406t
   technique for, 404–406, 404f, 405f
Terazosin, in urinary incontinence, 376t
Terbutaline, in urinary incontinence, 376t
Testosterone
   erectile dysfunction and, 126, 257, 348, 349, 351
   female sexual dysfunction and, 123, 355–356
   in female sexual function, 23–24
   in penile erection, 97
   penile sensory thresholds and, 108
Tolterodine
   in age-related urinary incontinence, 345
   in neurogenic voiding dysfunction, 454
   in urinary incontinence, 376t, 378–379
Transanal ultrasonography, 235–237, 236f, 237f
Transcutaneous electrical stimulation, 283–284, 284f. See also Electrical stimulation.
Transurethral prostatectomy
   erectile dysfunction and, 107
   stress incontinence and, 64
Transvaginal needle suspensions, in stress unitary incontinence, 392–393, 393t
Trauma
   at childbirth, 35–38, 36f, 39f
   erectile dysfunction and, 101, 105–106, 107
   with anal penetration, 78
Tricyclic antidepressants, in urinary incontinence, 383
Trigone
   colporectocystourethrography of, 172, 173f
   squamous metaplasia of, 192, 193f
Trospium, in urinary incontinence, 376t, 377–378

U
Ultrasonography, 145, 157–160
   in urinary incontinence, 157–159, 158f–160f, 161
   transanal, 235–237, 236f, 237f
Urapidil, in neurogenic voiding dysfunction, 458
Uremia, erectile dysfunction and, 101
Ureter, ectopic, 192–193
Ureterocele, 193, 194f
Ureterocystoplasty, in neurogenic voiding dysfunction, 456
Urethra. See also Urethral sphincter.
   afferent activity in, 8–9, 8f
   bulking agent injection for, 424–426, 425f, 426f

condyloma acuminata of, 193
diverticula of, 139
  colporectocystourethrography in, 173, 173f
  endoscopy of, 193
  magnetic resonance imaging in, 189, 189f
efferent activity in, 8f, 9–11
endoscopy of, 192, 192f, 193. *See also* Endoscopy.
female, 5, 21–22, 93
involuntary relaxation of, in urge incontinence, 62
leiomyoma of, 193
neuropeptides in, 10
pressure in, 9
sling-related distortion of, 172, 173f
urodynamic evaluation of, 210–213, 212f, 213f
Urethral hypermobility
  retropubic suspensions for, 392–393, 393t
  transvaginal needle suspensions for, 392–393, 393t
Urethral notch, in cystocele, 155, 155f
Urethral pressures, 145, 206, 206f, 211–213, 213f
  extracorporeal electromagnetic stimulation therapy effects on, 294–295
Urethral sphincter
  after childbirth, 34
  distal, 44–45
  electrical stimulation of, 281–288. *See also* Electrical stimulation.
  electromyography of, 219, 221
  in detrusor-sphincter dyssynergia, 54, 55f
  intrinsic deficiency of, 63, 153, 194
  proximal, 44–45
  ultrasonography of, 159, 160f
Urethrectomy, erectile dysfunction and, 101–102
Urethritis, 62, 193
Urethrovesical fistula, 194
Urethrovesical junction, mobility of
  evaluation of, 139, 141–142
  radiology for, 152, 152f
  ultrasonography for, 157–158, 158f
Urinary diversion, in neurogenic voiding dysfunction, 457
Urinary incontinence
  age-related, 57–64
    absorbent products for, 58, 345
    behavioral therapy in, 343–344
    biofeedback therapy in, 344
    bladder emptying and, 62–63
    bladder retraining in, 344
    catheterization in, 345
    clinical evaluation of, 342–343
    detrusor hyperactivity and, 59
    disease associations of, 343
    drug treatment of, 345
    drug use and, 59
    electrical stimulation in, 344–345
    female, 57–58
      estrogen deficiency and, 62
      incidence of, 57
      pelvic organ prolapse and, 62
      prevalence of, 57
      risk factors for, 59
      types of, 57–58
    functional status and, 342
    immobility and, 59, 64
    intrinsic sphincter deficiency and, 63
    male, 58, 346
      incidence of, 58
      prevalence of, 58
      prostatectomy and, 64
      risk factors for, 59
      types of, 58
    mental status and, 62, 342
    MESA incontinence questionnaire in, 60, 61f
    neurologic factors in, 62, 343
    nonmedical strategies for, 58–59
    overflow, 64
    pathophysiology of, 59–64, 375
    pelvic muscle exercise in, 344
    physical examination in, 342–343
    physical status and, 342
    prevalence of, 57, 58, 59
    prompted voiding in, 344
    prostate surgery and, 59, 64
    risk factors for, 59
    spinal stenosis and, 62
    stress, 63–64
    stroke and, 59, 62
    surgical treatment of, 345–346
    treatment of, 341–346. *See also* Urinary incontinence, treatment of.
      in chronic-care patient, 341–342
      in community-dwelling patient, 341
    types of, 57–58, 60–64
    urge, 60–63
  alcohol and, 272–273
  caffeine and, 272, 273
  cigarette smoking and, 269–270
  classification of, 43, 44b, 44t, 45t, 46b–47b
  coital, 134
  diary record of, 273, 274f
  electromyography in, 230–231
  evaluation of, 134–135. *See also* Patient evaluation.
  functional, 44b
  giggle, 134–135
  in athletes, 274–275
  magnetic resonance imaging in, 179–181, 180f
  mixed, 134, 154, 154t
  neurogenic. *See* Neurogenic voiding dysfunction.
  nocturnal
    evaluation of, 134, 135
    prevention of, 272, 272b
  obesity and, 270–271
  occupational stress and, 275
  overflow, 44b, 385
    drug treatment of, 385, 386t
    etiology of, 45–47, 46b
  pediatric, 432–446
    appendicovesicostomy in, 445, 445f
    artificial urinary sphincter in, 443–444, 444f
    augmentation cystoplasty in, 433–435, 434f, 435f
    bladder neck closure in, 444–446
    bladder neck sling suspension in, 440–443, 442f, 443f
    bladder neck tubularization in, 437–438, 437t, 438f
    catheterization in, 433
    collagen injections in, 436–437

Urinary incontinence (cont.)
  pediatric (cont.)
    Kropp procedure in, 438–439, 440f
    Monti procedure in, 445, 446f
    Pippi Salle procedure in, 439–440, 441f
    preoperative assessment of, 432–433
    renal function and, 433
    stoma creation in, 444–446, 445f, 446f
    Young-Dees-Leadbetter procedure in, 437–438, 437t, 438f
  pharmacologic treatment of, 373–387
  stress. See also Urinary incontinence, age-related.
    artificial urinary sphincter in, 395–396, 396f, 396t, 408–413, 409f–411f, 412b
    bladder neck incompetence and, 152–153
    childbirth and, 35, 77
    classification of, 44b, 46b
    cystocele and, 156, 156f, 396–398, 396t, 397t
    electrical stimulation in, 281–288. See also Electrical stimulation.
    endoscopy in, 194
    etiology of, 44–45, 46b
    evaluation of, 134
    fecal incontinence and, 76–77
    magnetic resonance imaging in, 179–181, 180f
    neural factors in, 181
    pathophysiology of, 45, 45t, 46b, 63–64, 166–167, 167f
    pelvic floor muscle exercises in, 278
    postpartum, 35
    pubovaginal sling in, 393–395, 394f, 394t, 414–420, 414t, 415f–420f
    radiologic evaluation of, 152–153, 152f, 153f
    retropubic suspensions in, 392–393, 393t
    surgical treatment of, 392–396, 393t, 394f, 394t, 396t
    tension-free vaginal tape for, 161, 162f, 403–407, 404f, 405f, 406t
    transvaginal needle suspensions in, 392–393, 393t
    urethral support in, 5
    urethrovesical junction hypermobility and, 139, 152, 157–158
  treatment of
    biofeedback therapy in, 297–308. See also Biofeedback therapy.
    bladder retraining in, 311–312
    bowel regularity in, 270b, 273–274
    diary for, 273, 274f
    diet in, 270b, 271–274
    electrical stimulation in, 281–288, 450–451. See also Electrical stimulation.
    extracorporeal electromagnetic stimulation in, 292, 294, 295
    fluid intake in, 270b, 271–272
    in athletes, 274–275
    irritant avoidance in, 272–273
    lifestyle interventions in, 269–275, 274f
    pads and appliances for, 314–318, 315f–318f, 345
    pelvic floor exercises in, 277–280. See also Pelvic floor exercises.
    pharmacologic, 376–387, 376t, 385t
    smoking cessation in, 269–270
    surgical, 392–396, 393t, 394f, 394t, 396t, 429, 429f
    weight loss in, 270–271
    ultrasonography in, 157–159, 158f–160f
  urge, 44b. See also Urinary incontinence, age-related.
    electrical stimulation in, 281–288. See also Electrical stimulation.
    etiology of, 45–47, 46b
    evaluation of, 134
    pathophysiology of, 60–63
    pelvic floor muscle exercises in, 278
    pharmacologic treatment of, 376–384, 376t
    urodynamic evaluation of, 210–211, 210f, 212f, 213f
Urinary retention
  female, 230, 395
  male, 51, 421–423, 423f. See also Detrusor–external sphincter dyssynergia.
Urinary stream, in patient evaluation, 135
Urinary tract
  infection of
    fluid intake and, 271–272
    in benign prostatic hyperplasia, 51
  lower
    dysfunction of. See also Urinary incontinence.
      in female, 43–47, 44b, 46b–47b
      in male, 49–55, 50t, 52f, 53f, 55f
    innervation of, 7–12. See also Micturition cycle.
Urination
  disorders of. See Neurogenic voiding dysfunction; Urinary incontinence.
  frequency of, 133
    after age 60, 58
    in patient evaluation, 133
  functional stop test of, 144
  pressure-flow studies of, 204–206, 205f
  residual measurement after, 142
Urine, pad and device collection of, 58, 314–318, 315f–318f, 345
Urodynamic studies, 198–206, 208–214. See also Electromyography.
  filling cystometry for, 200–204, 202f–204f
  in benign prostatic hyperplasia, 52–53, 52f, 53f
  in bladder diverticulum, 209, 210f
  in cystocele, 209–210, 211f
  in detrusor–external sphincter dyssynergia, 54, 55f, 69, 70f
  in neurogenic voiding dysfunction, 68–69, 69f
  in vesicoureteral reflux, 209, 210f
  of bladder volume, 214
  of detrusor leak-point pressure, 213–214, 214f
  of urethral function, 210–211
  of urethral pressures, 211–213
  pressure-flow study for, 204–206, 205f
  urethral pressure profilometry for, 206, 206f
  uroflowmetry for, 198–200, 199f, 200f
  video in, 209, 209f
Uroflowmetry, 198–200, 199f
  artifacts on, 200, 200f
  equipment for, 199
  in bladder outlet obstruction, 199–200, 199f
  in detrusor instability, 199
  in detrusor underactivity, 200
  in straining, 200

in urethral overactivity, 200
indications for, 198–199
interpretation of, 199–200, 199f, 200f
UroLume endoprosthesis, in neurogenic voiding dysfunction, 458–459
Uterine prolapse
   after cystocele repair, 172, 173f
   colporectocystourethrography of, 170–172, 171f
   magnetic resonance imaging in, 187–188, 188f
   pathophysiology of, 166, 166f
Uterosacral ligaments, 4
Uterus, during sexual arousal, 21

V

Vacuum extraction, during childbirth, 38
Vagina
   anatomy of, 19–20, 93, 165
   blood supply to, 20, 93
   examination of, 137–139, 138f
   histochemistry of, 93
   innervation of, 20, 93
   pelvic wall attachment of, 4–5
   tone of, 98
   vestibule of, 92
Vaginal cones
   in pelvic floor evaluation, 144
   in pelvic floor re-education, 332, 335, 336
Vaginal delivery. *See* Childbirth.
Vaginal tape, in stress urinary incontinence, 161, 162f, 403–407, 404f, 405f, 406t
Vaginal vault prolapse
   colporectocystourethrography of, 170–172, 171f
   pathophysiology of, 166
Vaginal wall, 5
   anterior descent of. *See also* Cystocele.
      evaluation of, 139, 170, 170f
      pathophysiology of, 165, 165f
   apical descent of. *See also* Enterocele; Uterine prolapse; Vaginal vault prolapse.
      evaluation of, 139, 141, 141f, 171–172, 172f
      pathophysiology of, 165–166, 166f
   posterior descent of. *See also* Rectocele.
      evaluation of, 139, 171, 171f
      pathophysiology of, 165–166, 166f, 167f
Vaginismus, 122, 360–365
   clinical manifestations of, 362–363
   definition of, 360
   etiology of, 360–362
   hymenectomy in, 361
   management of, 363–364
   pain of, 361–362
   psychological aspects of, 361
   sympathetic nervous system in, 360–361
Vas deferens, 92
Vasoactive intestinal polypeptide, in female sexual function, 22
Vesicoureteral reflux, 209, 210f, 212f
Vesicovaginal fistula, 173, 174f, 194
Vesioenteric fistula, 194, 195f
Vestibular bulbs, 21, 93
Viscerography. *See* Pelvic viscerography.
Voiding. *See also* Micturition cycle.
   dysfunctional. *See also* Urinary incontinence.
      evaluation of, 135. *See also* Patient evaluation.
      in male, 421–429
      neurogenic. *See* Neurogenic voiding dysfunction.
   pressure-flow studies of, 204–206, 205f
   residual measurement after, 142
Vulva, 92
Vulvodynia, 365–366

Y

Yohimbine, in female sexual dysfunction, 356
Young-Dees-Leadbetter procedure, in pediatric urinary incontinence, 437–438, 437t, 438f